PRAISE FOR *THE POLITICS OF CANCER Revisited*

From leading voices in the medical, labor, and women's health fields —

Some twenty years later, we have a most worthy sequel to the ground-breaking *The Politics of Cancer.* This work is muscular, relentless, and compelling. Its thesis: billions of public dollars are being misspent in an ill-conceived "war on cancer" — a war we are losing because we are not addressing the increasingly carcinogenic environment that man has created. We have introduced these creations into our water and air, our food chain, our habitation, our workplace, and into the products produced there.

In failing to allocate these resources for prevention, we are fighting the wrong war.

The author documents that opposition from powerful corporate interests, and their allies in government and the academy, has sustained this strategy.

We have here a must-read for the scientist and the citizen concerned with the public's health.

> – Quentin D. Young, M.D.
> President, American Public Health Association

Cancer continues to be the scourge of many workplaces; this book is an extraordinary weapon to mount an attack on this deadly disease. It minces no words in indicting the cancer establishment whose misdirected efforts have contributed to the ongoing cancer epidemic.

Dr. Epstein's work is a strong rebuttal to the self-interested Pollyannas in the cancer establishment and provides worker advocates with essential knowledge that will serve to protect the lives of those we represent.

> – Robert Wages
> President, Oil, Chemical, and Atomic
> Workers Union International Union, AFL-CIO

A unique and superbly documented indictment of the National Cancer Institute and the American Cancer Society for their reckless indifference to cancer prevention, for their incestuous relationship with the cancer drug industry, and for their false claims for miracle cancer drugs and for winning the war against cancer. This is essential reading for every concerned woman and man on how to reverse the cancer epidemic by personal and political initiatives.

– Barbara Seaman
Co-founder, National Women's Health Network
and author, *The Doctors' Case Against the Pill*

Every journalist reporting on cancer (as it should be covered) has within easy reach, a shop-worn, dog-eared, heavily underlined 1978 edition of Sam Epstein's *Politics of Cancer*. For twenty years we have waited impatiently for the day when we would no longer have to update old findings. Our wait is over. Not only has Dr. Epstein provided new data, charts, epidemiology, and science, but he has refortified his contention that the war on cancer is unfinished, and far from triumphant.

– Mark Dowie
Former publisher and editor, *Mother Jones* and
author, *Losing Ground: American
Environmentalism at the Close of the
Twentieth Century*

Samuel Epstein's book *The Politics of Cancer* blew the lid off the "cancer establishment" when it was published in 1978. Twenty years later, the new *POLITICS OF CANCER Revisited* is a blockbuster. It exposes the rampant industrial pollution that causes many preventable cases of cancer. It also shows the frightening power of industry in keeping us from winning the war against cancer. We all owe Professor Epstein a debt of gratitude for almost single-handedly keeping this issue alive and before the public for all these years.

– Ralph W. Moss, Ph.D.
Director, *The Moss Reports*

In *THE POLITICS OF CANCER Revisited*, Professor Samuel Epstein delivers a devastating attack on the cancer establishment. He provides damning evidence, in extraordinary detail, of the rising tide of cancer incidence and death. With scholarly precision, he delivers a ringing indictment of the National Cancer Institute and the American Cancer Society. Epstein details their fixation on diagnosis and treatment, and their complete failure to focus on prevention by research and education on eliminating the poisons from our food, air, water, and environment.

While the original *Politics of Cancer* was a tremendously important work, as influential as Rachel Carson's *Silent Spring, THE POLITICS OF CANCER Revisited* is even more chilling — in the face of rising cancer incidence and death, Epstein documents that the cancer establishment resists all efforts toward reform and continues its failed policies of the past.

In 1998, nearly 1,500,000 Americans will be diagnosed with cancer and 750,000 will die. As a nation, we can not afford to overlook Epstein's recommendations.

To the health of our nation this is a book of tremendous importance.

– Frank D. Wiewel
Founder, People Against Cancer

A remarkable scientifically documented analysis of the failing war against cancer and the reasons for the failure. This book also provides a practical road map for personal and political opportunities for turning the tide of the modern cancer epidemic.

– Devra Lee Davis, Ph.D., M.P.H.
World Resources Institute
Washington, D.C.

THE POLITICS
OF CANCER *Revisited*

THE POLITICS
OF CANCER *Revisited*

Samuel S. Epstein, M.D.

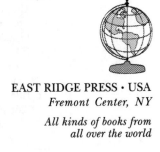

EAST RIDGE PRESS · USA
Fremont Center, NY

*All kinds of books from
all over the world*

The author gratefully acknowledges the financial support
of the Sauve and JMG Foundations.

East Ridge Press • USA
1998

Library of Congress Cataloging-in-Publication Data

Epstein, Samuel S.
   The politics of cancer revisited / Samuel S. Epstein.
     p.   cm.
   Includes bibliographical references and index.
   ISBN 0-914896-46-6   0-914896-47-4 (pbk)
    1. Cancer — Prevention — Political aspects — United States.
  2. American Cancer Society.   3. National Cancer Institute (U.S.)
  I. Title.
  RC268.E673   1998
  362. 1 ' 96994 ' 00973 — dc21   98-41094
                                            CIP

To my wondrous wife Catherine,
who has made all things possible,
and our splendid children Mark, Julian, and Emily

Contents

Appendices

Acknowledgments

I would like to thank my friend, the late Dr. Irving Selikoff, pioneer in occupational cancer, who was not only most helpful in critically reviewing the 1978 edition of *The Politics of Cancer* but also for repeatedly urging me to update it with a new book, advice on which I have belatedly acted.

As importantly, I would like to acknowledge the group of sixty-five distinguished public health experts on the causes and prevention of cancer for endorsing my statement on "Losing the War Against Cancer; A Need for Public Policy Reforms," released at a February 4, 1992 press conference at the National Press Club in Washington, D.C. These scientists include: past directors of three Federal agencies — Dr. Eula Bingham, former Assistant Secretary of Labor, Occupational Safety and Health Administration; Dr. David Rall, former Director of the National Institutes of Environmental Health Sciences and former Assistant Surgeon General USPHS; and Dr. Anthony Robbins, past Director of the National Institute for Occupational Safety and Health; — Dr. Irwin Bross, former Director of Biostatistics, Roswell Park Memorial Institute, Buffalo, NY; Dr. Nicholas Ashford, MIT, Cambridge, MA; Dr. Marvin Legator, University of Texas, Galveston; Dr. Vicente Navarro, John Hopkins University, Baltimore, MD; Dr. Thomas Mancuso, University of Pittsburgh; and the late Nobel Laureate, Dr. George Wald, Harvard University, Cambridge, MA. Warm acknowledgment is also due to the late Dr. Wally Burnstein for his enthusiastic support and assistance with the logistics of the experts' press conference.

I would also like to thank many members of the experts' group for supporting the creation of the Cancer Prevention Coalition in 1993 to implement the recommended reforms. Notably, these include: Dr. Legator; Dr. William Lijinsky, former Director Chemical Carcinogenesis, Frederick Cancer Research Center, Frederick, MD; and Dr. Thomas Mancuso. In this connection, I also express strong appreciation to the late Sir James Goldsmith, and the Goldsmith and Gillian and Ellis Goodman Foundations for very generous financial support of the Coalition, and also support from the Tides, Gaia, Oestreicher, and Cashman Foundations, and from Tom Mower, besides other generous donors.

Others I also thank include: Ralph Nader, for co-sponsoring the September, 1995 Cancer Prevention Coalition, Washington, D.C. press conference on the "Dirty Dozen" consumer products; Anthony Mazzocchi, Presidential Assistant to the Oil Chemical Atomic Workers Union, for long-standing support and activities in prevention of occupational cancer; Thomas J. Moore, George Washington University Medical Center, for invaluable comments on prescription drugs in Chapters 17 and 18; Martin Walker, distinguished British author of *Dirty Medicine* for permission to include his article on Sir Richard Doll in Chapter 14, and for the listing of British activist and resource groups; and the indomitable Studs Terkel, for frequent invitations to discuss cancer politics and avoidable causes of cancer on his highly celebrated radio program series.

Gratitude is also due to: Cong. David Obey (D-WI) for his insight and tireless scrutiny of NCI policies and priorities; Cong. Henry Waxman (D-CA) for long-standing concerns on consumer product safety and escalating cancer rates, and for his 1987 request for a report to Congress on the status of the cancer war and for its publication — "Losing the Winnable War against Cancer: Who is Responsible and What to do About It" — in the Congressional Record; Cong. John Conyers, for his 1979 invitation to draft legislation on "White Collar Crime" in relation to industry malpractice in knowingly exposing millions of citizens and workers to avoidable risks of cancer from industrial chemicals, for long-standing interest in *The Politics of Cancer,* and for warm friendship; and Dr. Ralph Moss for his scholarly research and publications on the cancer industry, the questionable efficacy of most cancer drugs, and on the largely un-explored utility of a wide range of non-patented alternative and complementary treatments. I would also like to acknowledge the important contributions of Drs. John Bailar and Devra Davis to the urgent national and international need for developing higher priorities for cancer prevention.

I find difficulty in adequately expressing my deep gratitude to Edward Goldsmith, a leading international ecologist, erudite environmental scholar, and editor and publisher of *The Ecologist,* for decades-long deep friendship and enthusiastic encouragement.

Thanks are also due to the University of Illinois, Chicago for staunch support of my academic freedom, and to the School of Public Health and its scholarly and activist Dean Susan Scrimshaw, for providing me with a hospitable academic base for scientific research and public policy initiatives; Natalie Chapman, former publisher and editor of Macmillan Books for her editorial skills and warm support of citizens' right-to-know embodied in two recent books I coauthored — the 1995 *Safe Shopper's Bible,* and the 1998 *Breast Cancer Prevention Program.*

Finally, it is with great pleasure that I pay tribute to Tom Powers, publisher, and Meredith Powers, editor, of East Ridge Press, who inspired this new book and worked indefatigably with an extraordinary sense of dedication, for valuable editorial guidance.

Author's Note

In 1978, the Sierra Club Books landmark *The Politics of Cancer* documented the relation between increasing cancer rates and avoidable exposures to environmental and occupational carcinogens, and exposed the reckless culpability of the petrochemical industry and the unresponsiveness of the cancer establishment — the National Cancer Institute (NCI) and the American Cancer Society (ACS).

THE POLITICS OF CANCER Revisited proceeds from that point with an analysis of subsequent scientific and public policy developments over the last two decades, on the basis of which it incriminates the cancer establishment with major responsibility for losing the winnable war against cancer.

The incidence of cancer, including a wide range of nonsmoking cancers, has escalated to epidemic proportions with lifetime cancer risks now approaching 50%. Meanwhile, there has been little, if any, improvement in the treatment and survival of most common cancers in spite of an increase in NCI's budget from $870 million in 1978 to $2.6 billion in 1998; NCI is now insisting that it must have $5 billion by 2003. Furthermore, NCI and ACS policies have remained myopically fixated on damage control — diagnosis and treatment — and on basic genetic research with, not always benign, indifference to cancer prevention, coupled with pervasive conflicts of interest, particularly with the cancer drug industry.

The cancer establishment has misled the public and Congress with long-standing claims for winning the war against cancer based on intermittent extravagant claims of success with a series of "miracle cancer drugs," unsupported by evidence of prolonged survival rates. At the same time, the establishment has blocked funding of research and clinical trials on promising alternative or complementary treatments, contrary to the strong 1991-1992 recommendations of the Congressional Office of Technology Assessment and the National Institutes of Health Office of Alternative Medicine; very recently, bowing to strong protests from patient advocacy groups and their Congressional supporters, NCI announced a newfound interest in research on alternative therapies.

The NCI has made widely divergent claims for its 1998 prevention budget, ranging from $480 million to $1 billion, while more realistic estimates are well under $100 million and while its admitted budget for occupational cancer — the most avoidable of all cancers — is a mere $20 million. These inflated budgetary claims are in striking contrast to NCI's minimalistic research on cancer prevention. Furthermore, NCI and ACS have failed to research and systematize information on risk factors for those many cancers whose rates have escalated over recent decades, and to undertake systematic epidemiological research on populations exposed to environmental and occupational carcinogens identified in National Toxicology Program and other valid bioassay tests. The establishment has even gone so far as to denigrate the human relevance of experimental carcinogenicity data.

Most critical of all, the cancer establishment has failed to provide Congress and regulatory agencies with well-documented scientific information on a wide range of unwitting exposures to avoidable carcinogens in air, water, the workplace, and consumer products — food, cosmetics and toiletries, and household products—with the result that corrective legislative and regulatory action has not been taken. The cancer establishment has also failed to provide the public, particularly African American and other underprivileged ethnic groups with their disproportionately higher incidence and mortality rates, with such information on avoidable causes of cancer, thus denying their right-to-know and to take necessary action to protect themselves — a flagrant rejection of environmental justice.

These basic criticisms of cancer establishment policies have been unanimously endorsed by a group of 65 leading national experts in public health and cancer prevention, including past directors of Federal agencies.

Such concerns are not just restricted to the U.S., as illustrated by the book's analysis of parallel developments in Great Britain. Moreover, in view of the powerful influence of the U.S. cancer establishment on policies of most other major industrialized nations, the book's message is truly global rather than national.

In addition to a blueprint for drastic reforms of the cancer establishment, the book proposes practical strategies for winning the losing cancer war, based on right-to-know personal and political initiatives.

The factual basis of the book is documented in detail. In addition to extensive previously unpublished material, the book also presents information from a wide range of relatively inaccessible sources including Congressional testimony, reports to the World Trade Organization, citizen petitions and press releases. The book also reflects the author's longstanding scientific and public policy research and outreach activities on the causes and prevention of cancer.

For historical perspective and background and for thematic continuity, and in response to continuing requests for its availability, the long out-of-print 1978 *The Politics of Cancer* is incorporated in this book.

Introduction

In 1970, when the Environmental Protection Agency was first created, I was among a small group of active members of Congress who understood we were at the precipice of a new era in public health. The disasters of Love Canal and Times Beach Missouri — in which the environmental sins of chemical manufacturing plants left entire communities homeless and stricken with fatal diseases — hit the nation like a tidal wave. For the first time, we were beginning to comprehend the sheer vastness and complexity of environmental dangers of the modern industrial era and the perils — many of them invisible to the naked eye — that were lurking in our air, waterways, consumer products, and workplaces.

During that pivotal decade in which the modern environmental movement came to the forefront of the nation's political agenda, Dr. Epstein wrote the epochal *Politics of Cancer.* It was a bombshell both inside and outside of Washington officialdom, and its vast media coverage sent warning bells throughout the nation.

What made *The Politics of Cancer* so unique was its fusion of science with politics. For the first time, the intimidatingly complex scientific data and facts of asbestos, vinyl chloride, benzene, and hundreds of other toxic threats were demystified and explained in the context of a political, social, and cultural evolution. Any layperson who knew nothing about which chemicals were dangerous and how Washington was reacting to the grave dangers could come away after having read the *Politics* with an expertise in both. The book was an education for the public and a handbook for decision-makers. It also carefully documented startling evidence of decisions made by U.S. corporations to deliberately withhold from Congress and the public information about public health dangers.

When this disclosure was made, public outrage spawned new legislation to criminalize the withholding of vital health and safety data. Thus Congress was able to protect and inform the public of this vast array of industrial, occupational, and manufacturing health hazards.

This milestone work was not just a wake-up call to the nation, it was also a call to arms for those of us both inside and outside the beltway, Republican and Democrat, young and old, to reclaim our fundamental rights to a safe environment for ourselves and our families. The work served as a treatise for us in the Congress as we fought in the 1980s for the enactment of a half dozen landmark environmental laws, including the Clean Air and Clean Water Acts, the Toxic Substances Control Act, the Resource Conservation and Recovery Act, and much else.

During the intervening two decades since Dr. Epstein first wrote the book, there has been a major shift in the political and cultural landscape. As we enter the year 2000, cancer is well on its way to becoming the nation's number one killer, taking 500,000 lives and bilking our purses of well over $110 billion every year. A sense of crisis — sometimes even panic — grips the public when the word "cancer" is spoken, but a sense of paralysis seems to characterize our institutional ability to confront this aggressor.

Inevitably, any public crisis will spawn institutions. During the past two decades, we have seen the birth and maturation of what Dr. Epstein calls the "Cancer Establishment" — the National Cancer Institute, the American Cancer Society, and the myriad of research centers — all of whom have been trusted explicitly by the government and implicitly by the American people as the high generals in the war against cancer. What Dr. Epstein charges is that these generals are losing the war, and losing it badly. As we did in 1978 when *The Politics of Cancer* was first published, we should today hear this clarion call.

Most disturbingly, Dr. Epstein chronicles how the Cancer Establishment has nearly totally ignored cancer prevention, ignored the most common sense proposition that we should simply keep poison out of our communities and immediate surroundings. Every parent tells their child the common-lore adage that a "stitch in time saves nine," but according to Dr. Epstein, this simple truth seems to have eluded those entrusted with waging one of the most important public policy objectives of the latter part of the century.

Simply put, the evidence seems to adduce that our ability to cure and treat cancer has not materially changed in recent decades, while the incidence of fatal cancers spins out of control as our communities become increasingly drenched with carcinogens. Given this evidence, which fundamentally questions our ability to "cure" our way out of the cancer problem, it appears clear that no solution will work without a comprehensive national program to prevent our people from being exposed to poisons in the first place.

With all the data available clearly demonstrating environmental causes of cancer, one might reasonably ask why there has been less focus on cancer prevention both in and out of the Cancer Establishment. *THE POLITICS OF CANCER Revisited* attempts to answer that question, and in so doing, attempts to show us the way out of our current fix.

In short, this new book argues that the Cancer Establishment has become beset with a range of myopic institutional pressures which prevent it from devoting more research and capital to prevention: the common quest to amass more resources and build bigger empires by the research institutions which promise what may be a mythical pot of gold at the end of the research rainbow; the apparently growing and somewhat disturbing interlocking corporate interests of pharmaceutical industries who benefit from public optimism that an elixir is near; and chemical industries that want as little prevention through environmental regulation as possible. While political scientists commonly theorize that all institutions may be subject to these pressures, no one has attempted to systematically document these problems in the context of the war against cancer until now.

None of this is to say that research into the mechanisms, treatment, and potential cures of cancer is not critical or that it should not continue. It should. None of this is to say that there are not noble people struggling to find cures. There are. But *THE POLITICS OF CANCER Revisited* argues that, as important as the research is, it cannot eclipse prevention. We should not in our emotionally understandable hope for a cure become transfixed with a Nero-like neglect for the simple truth that preventing cancer appears to be well within our grasp. This is the thesis of *THE POLITICS OF CANCER Revisited*, and Americans in all quarters would be well advised to heed it very carefully.

Congressman John Conyers, Jr.
August 1998

PART I

THE POLITICS OF CANCER: 1978

"Many difficult decisions will have to be made in the years ahead about how we live with the new chemical hazards in our environment. There is a point where questions like these become political and ethical, as well as scientific. Those questions should not be resolved without broad-based public understanding and participation. This discussion has not yet taken place, and it will not until the scientific questions have been more thoroughly understood. . . . I hope that by reading this book more citizens will understand and become involved in the complex and difficult decisions that lie ahead."

Congressman David Obey

Preface
(*The Politics of Cancer, 1978*)

If one thousand people died every day of cholera, swine flu, or food poisoning, an epidemic of major proportions would be at hand and the entire country would mobilize against it. Yet cancer claims that many lives daily, often in prolonged and agonizing pain, and most people believe they can do nothing about it. Cancer, they think, strikes where it will, with no apparent cause. Some take out a cancer insurance policy, all hope not to be one of its victims.

But cancer has distinct, identifiable causes. It is not just another degenerative disease associated with aging. It can largely be prevented, but this requires more than just scientific effort or individual action. The control and prevention of cancer will require a concerted national effort. This book is offered as a contribution to that essentially political process.

There are four basic axioms of cancer causation which will be continually referred to:

1. *Cancer is caused mainly by exposure to chemical or physical agents in the environment.* To be sure, there are genetic aspects to cancer, and some cancers are suspected to be caused by viruses, but these factors account for only a small fraction of all cases.* Just as germs cause infections, so do certain chemical and physical agents, *carcinogens,* cause cancer.† While some carcinogens, such as arsenic, asbestos, afla-toxins, and ionizing radiation, occur naturally, there is increasing recognition of the dangers of synthetic petrochemical carcinogens, such as vinyl chloride and bischloromethylether, which have been introduced into the workplace and environment in growing numbers over the last few decades.

2. *The more of a carcinogen present in the human environment, hence the greater the exposure to it, the greater is the chance of developing cancer from it.*

3. *Although environmental carcinogens are the predominant causes of human cancer, the incidence of cancer in any population of animals or humans exposed to a carcinogen may be influenced by a variety of factors.* The development of cancer is of course profoundly influenced by genetic, endocrine, immunological, viral, biochemical, and possibly even psychological factors. Additionally, there are a wide range of other external factors which can increase individual sensitivity to a given carcinogen or carcinogens. Among these are excesses or deficiencies in certain dietary components, exposure to other carcinogens which enhance the effects of a particular carcinogen, and exposure to *promoting* (or *co-carcinogenic*) agents which, while not carcinogenic in themselves, may enhance the effect of an already present carcinogen.‡ These factors do

---

* There is little or no evidence that chemical carcinogens cause cancer by activating latent viruses in human cells.

† The relation of carcinogens to cancer is pragmatic and has been established by observation of human and animal populations, and not by prior understanding of the biological mechanisms involved. To be sure, a great deal is known about the biochemical, immunological, and other effects of many carcinogens at the cellular level. It now seems that the carcinogenic action of certain chemicals is due to their direct interaction with cellular genes. Large research programs and institutions have been built upon studies yielding such information. However, the promise of improved treatment and prevention of cancer based upon this knowledge of the mechanism of carcinogenesis has not yet been fulfilled.

‡ For example, alcohol, which does not itself appear to cause cancer, other than possibly in the

not themselves cause cancer, but they can and do affect when a certain carcinogen will trigger cancer in an individual and how rapidly or slowly the course of the clinical symptoms and the disease will progress.

4. *There is no known method for measuring or predicting a "safe" level of exposure to any carcinogen below which cancer will not result in any individual or population group.* That is, there is no, basis for the threshold hypothesis which claims that exposure to relatively low levels of carcinogens is safe and therefore justifiable.

This book has been shaped by the author's long-standing scientific involvement in toxicology and carcinogenesis, including several of the case studies discussed in this book. (It does not deal with nuclear radioactivity, a potent source of carcinogens, which would require a book in itself. Certainly, issues raised in this book apply directly to the dangers of radiation, but the solutions to the problems posed by nuclear materials are different than those that apply to chemicals.) *The Politics of Cancer* is also based on the author's support of attempts to control human exposure to carcinogenic and other toxic chemicals, including many of those discussed in the following pages. In these efforts, he has worked with Congressional committees and regulatory agencies, and also with public interest groups and organized labor.

---

liver, increases the risk of cancer of the mouth, larynx, and esophagus, particularly in tobacco smokers. The "fertile ground" concept expresses the possible influence of such factors on the response of the host to any specific carcinogen.

Foreword

No word in the English language is more chilling than cancer. It's hard to imagine anyone not wanting "war" waged against this disease. Yet those closely associated with the National Cancer Program and our regulatory efforts to control cancer-causing chemicals have found it increasingly difficult to agree on how that war should be fought.

The chemical causation of cancer was hardly mentioned eight years ago when Congress was debating the National Cancer Attack Act. Most Americans and members of Congress were impressed with the optimism voiced by physicians and clinical research spokesmen. There was widespread belief that there could be major breakthroughs in the treatment of cancer victims in a matter of years, possibly in the form of a Salk-type vaccine. Such an approach made some sense in the '60s, when it was commonly believed that much cancer was caused by a virus.

But at least since 1970, it has been generally accepted that the majority of all cancer is caused by chemicals and environmental factors — what we touch, breathe, eat, drink, work with, or otherwise absorb. Some of these factors occur naturally in the environment; most do not. They are put there by man.

Those same factors also cause other damage. For example, recent research relating to birth defects suggests that many cancer-causing chemicals also cause heritable mutations. In 1974, vinyl chloride, which had already been linked to liver cancer, was also tied to lung and brain cancer and birth defects. Most scientists believe that reversing such extensive damage is far beyond the scope of current technology.

For that reason, those involved in formulating the government's cancer research policy have become adamant about the need to better understand the risks of cancer-causing chemicals and to prevent exposure to them.

But such efforts have faced serious obstacles. One problem has been the orientation of many individuals who have played a dominant role in shaping our national cancer policy. For the most part, they are surgeons, radiologists, chemotherapists, and well-intentioned survivors of cancer. However, these people usually fail to have a basic understanding of the concept of cancer as an environmentally induced disease. In some instances, they fear that a major new emphasis in the National Cancer Program toward the environment will reduce visibility and funding for other research efforts. Thus, for one reason or another, there has been considerable resistance against moving the study of environmental causes of cancer from the back burner of the National Cancer Program.

Another obstacle has been the large expenditures required to eliminate these environmental hazards. Most Americans probably would favor the elimination of a clearly established cancer hazard, regardless of the cost. But some people in both government and industry, including some top economists in the current (Carter) administration, feel that "economic considerations" should be given greater weight, despite clear evidence that additional cancer deaths will result.

The trump card of a few opponents of tighter governmental regulation of cancer-causing chemicals is that evidence of carcinogenicity is rarely 100 percent conclusive. There is usually some element of doubt as to whether a particular chemical causes cancer. Thus, while initial tests with animals will strongly suggest a cancer link in humans, conclusive proof of that link often is years or even decades away. Regulatory action to protect workers and the general public from further exposure to a potential hazard may add millions of dollars to the cost of producing needed products, and the possibility would remain that further research might conceivably show that the chemical does not cause cancer. In either case, the stakes are enormous.

To err on the side of "economic considerations" could mean millions of lives. An extreme example of these costs can be seen in the case of asbestos. Prior to World War II, there was already considerable scientific evidence that asbestos posed serious health problems. In fact, Henry Johns, one of the co-founders of the Johns-Manville Corp., the major asbestos supplier in the United States, died apparently of asbestosis.

During the 1930s, the German government agreed to pay compensation claims to workers who had been exposed to asbestos and were suffering from respiratory diseases. American and other scientific literature at that time contained numerous descriptions of asbestos-induced diseases, yet during and after World War II we continued to use asbestos in shipbuilding and other industries with virtually no controls. A study recently released by the Department of Health, Education and Welfare shows that approximately 2 million asbestos-related cancer deaths will occur during the next thirty to thirty-five years as a result of exposures that have already occurred. That means about 60,000 deaths per year from now until the year 2013 — more than the combined death rate from all automobile, airplane, ship, and railroad accidents.

Failure to heed the early warning signs about asbestos has cost us continuing suffering and deaths. And the economic consequences of our failure have also been monstrous: increased medical bills, lost income and productivity, higher Medicaid and Medicare costs, and additional Social Security and SSI payments. Together, these cost Americans billions of dollars each year, and will continue to do so in the coming few decades.

So the cost of erring on the side of "economic considerations" is high, but erring on the side of stopping possibly harmful exposures can also be expensive. Redesigning our factories and manufacturing processes, developing safe chemical substitutes, and monitoring chemical concentrations is not cheap. Cost estimates of controlling worker exposure to cancer-causing coke emissions, for example, range from $150 million to $1 billion. The cost of controlling worker exposure to arsenic is estimated at $100 million to $225 million. Private industry has also recently claimed that it will cost more than $88 billion to control exposure to all workplace carcinogens.

In at least two instances, those of benzidine dyes and drywoven asbestos textiles, carcinogens have been virtually eliminated in the United States because of health problems which apparently could not be resolved cheaply enough to permit American factories to continue competing with the international market. So with these cases, the profits — together with the health problems — have been, in one sense, exported. Imports of these two products from Taiwan, Mexico, India, Rumania, and other countries have steadily increased.

Our errors, however, have seldom if ever been on the side of worker health. We have now identified, for instance, dozens of chemicals that probably are carcinogenic, but there is no regulation of their use, and hundreds of thousands of workers are being exposed to them daily.

Take trichloroethylene, for example. Congressmen don't even have to leave their offices to see workers using this chemical to clean carpets. It is also widely used in dry cleaning, and as an industrial solvent. We know it is similar to vinyl chloride in its chemical structure, and that when fed to rats or mice, they develop liver cancer. Most scientists would conclude from these data that the odds are good that this chemical also causes cancer in humans. Yet our response to finding out more about trichloroethylene has been to wait for more "conclusive evidence" that human beings would die from this exposure. Regulations have not been issued, and workers have not even been warned about the danger. The majority of those working with trichloroethylene are as ignorant today of the potential danger from this chemical as the shipyard workers were decades ago of the potential hazards they faced from asbestos.

Many difficult decisions will have to be made in the years ahead about how we live with the new chemical hazards in our environment. There is a point where questions like these become political and ethical, as well as scientific. Those questions should not be resolved without broad-based public understanding and participation. This discussion

has not yet taken place, and it will not until the scientific questions have been more thoroughly understood.

Dr. Epstein's book clearly explains the scientific problems involved in environmentally induced cancer and carcinogenesis. Equally important, it analyzes the wide range of political and social considerations involved in our failure to regulate carcinogens and stem the growing tide of cancer. I hope that by reading this book more citizens will understand and become involved in the complex and difficult decisions that lie ahead.

Congressman David Obey
September 1979

Chapter One

The Impact of Cancer

A Bittersweet Example

On March 9, 1977, an agency of the federal government, the U.S. Food and Drug Administration (FDA), proposed a ban on the use of saccharin, an artificial sweetener in foods. The public responded loudly. In outrage, citizens demanded that the government withdraw the proposal. Congress and the agency were barraged with thousands of letters, cables, and phone calls. The diet-soda generation had risen in arms.

Hearings were held. The news media were flooded with reports. The soft-drink industry paid for full-page advertisements in leading national newspapers to protest the FDA decision. Industry lobbies, responding to and organizing public opinion, gathered in strength.

Much of the controversy surrounding the saccharin ban arose from the public's sudden awareness and astonishment that this regulatory decision was based solely on the results of animal feeding tests. Further, the public was surprised that these tests were carried out using what seemed to be excessively high quantities of saccharin. In the case of the most recent study, rats had been fed concentrations of saccharin equivalent to a daily dose of 800 cans of diet soda. Predictably, comedians and editorial cartoonists had a field day. Johnny Carson joked that Canadian researchers who fed rats large quantities of saccharin in their coffee went broke paying for the coffee. The nation simultaneously laughed and stormed over the FDA decision.

Some people, though, weren't laughing. Public health activists were concerned that the standard scientific practices which had been used in the study of saccharin, in particular the use of rodents to test for cancer, were under attack. In turn, they were concerned that public misconception about the nature of this scientific research might cause legislative backlash and weaken the government's power to limit exposure to other chemicals suspected of causing cancer. This was not an idle concern. The scientific community lined up on opposite sides and issued conflicting statements about the saccharin question with the same vigor as the public. Statisticians, toxicologists, cancer researchers, environmental scientists, physicians, and chemists all joined in the fray.

Two quotations illustrate how far apart apparently informed scientific opinions could be. In March, 1977, Guy Newell, Jr., then acting director and now deputy director of the National Cancer Institute (NCI), testified: "Based on human data, we do not believe saccharin is a potent carcinogen for humans, if it is one at all."[1] David Rall, director of the National Institute of Environmental Health Sciences, a sister institute of the NCI, clearly disagreed with Newell:

It may be that drinking just a couple of bottles [of a diet cola] a day may be risky for some people. FDA certainly should get saccharin out of diet pop. . . . When one looks at the data that have been accumulated from animal experiments over the years, there is plenty of reason to doubt that saccharin is safe. . . . In practically all of the studies that have been done, including those in which animals were fed saccharin at much lower doses than in the Canadian study, you find tumors in more of the saccharin-fed animals than in the controls.

Such diversity of opinion among scientists fed the public's concern and confusion. After all, how could the lay press and the nation be expected to make a decision on an issue about which the nation's leading scientists couldn't agree? What's more, why couldn't they agree? Isn't science by nature exact?*

The fact is, much cancer research at its present stage of development must focus on statistical trends and tendencies in animal and human populations to link, in a causal chain, a particular agent or agents with a particular type of cancer. As was so clearly seen with saccharin, the ultimate judgment whether a substance causes cancer in humans is not always easy. The public has found, and scientists have had to admit, that there are many subjective and judgmental decisions being made about cancer — its causes, prevention, and control. Many of these judgments, particularly when regulation comes under discussion, have little to do with pure science. The economic impact of banning a substance or requiring its strict control, the technological feasibility of substituting new processes, the desirability of low-calorie foods in the nation's diet — all these topics are implicit in the saccharin issue. In short, the science of the saccharin decision is clearly mixed up with nonscientific considerations. Even the very basis of the research into saccharin's carcinogenicity is mixed up with economics and politics.

It is vital that the public learn where the science of cancer ends and social policy considerations begin. Further, it is important to realize that the basis of many so-called "scientific" decisions are in fact economic considerations, and not science. When regulatory judgments are made and laws are passed (or not passed) which touch on our lives and welfare, we must understand the real basis of the decision-making process.

Cancer is a problem which touches each of us in some way. We and our families are daily exposed to agents that cause cancer (called carcinogens), often unknowingly, while we breathe, eat, drink, work, and sleep. Moreover, we usually have no knowledge of what we are being exposed to. In order for us to respond to the cancer threat, we must all be equipped with the basic information needed to demand preventive policies and actions. If action is to be effective, it must be based on information and directed within the realistic limits of the political system.

The Impact of Cancer

The Human Costs

Cancer is now a killing and disabling disease of epidemic proportions.† More than

---

* The popular notion that science is strictly a logical process has largely been abandoned by philosophers of science, yet the idea still retains an iron grip on the public mind.

† The impact of cancer is often expressed in terms of mortality or of incidence rates. (Cancer incidence data comes from the NCI; mortality data from the National Center for Health Statistics.) The mortality rate is the number of people in a particular population who die of cancer in a given time period, usually specified as a number per 100,000 population. The incidence rate is the number of new cases per year in the population, again usually per 100,000 population. Incidence rates are a more meaningful measure of the impact of cancer than are mortality rates, which also reflect curability. The longer the survival or the greater the cure rate for a given cancer, the more the incidence rate will exceed the mortality rate. Skin cancer, for example, has the highest incidence rate of all cancers, but because the chances of catching and curing the disease at an early stage are good, its mortality rate is small. Lung cancer, on the other hand, occurs less often than skin cancer, but once detected its prognosis is poor; hence its mortality rate approaches its incidence rate.

53 million people in the United States (over a quarter of the population) will develop some form of cancer, from which approximately 20 percent of the U.S. population will die.[2] It is estimated that 765,000 new cancer cases will be diagnosed in 1979,‡ and there will be 395,000 cancer deaths. Cancer deaths this year alone were about five times higher than the total U.S. military deaths in all the Vietnam and Korean war years combined.

Cancer strikes not only the elderly, but also other age groups, including infants. Among males, cancer is the second leading cause of death for all age groups except 15-34 years, where it is exceeded by violent deaths, accidents, homicide, and suicide (Table 1.1). Among females, cancer is the leading cause of death for ages 35-54 years and the second leading cause for all other ages up to 75.

Black males, as a group, experience the highest incidence of cancer in the United States, while black females experience the lowest; whites are intermediate between these two, with males higher than females.[3] Strong racial variations exist for cancer at almost every body site. For instance, blacks have three to four times as much cancer of the esophagus as whites, twice as much cancer of the cervix, and prostate, and higher rates of cancer of the stomach, pancreas, and lung.[4]

The most common sites of fatal cancer are the lung and large bowel in men, and the breast and large bowel in women (see Tables 1.2 and 1.3 and Figure 1.1). Virtually every other organ in the body is also a potential site for cancer's attack. Leukaemia is the leading cause of fatal cancer in children.

A high and unmeasurable cost is the fear of contracting cancer oneself. Such fears are particularly well founded in individuals or groups at "high risk" of developing cancer from past exposures to carcinogens: hundreds of thousands of workers currently or previously exposed to occupational carcinogens; women treated with estrogens for "menopausal symptoms"; and premenopausal women who have received repeated breast x-rays (mammography).

The Financial Costs

Obviously, cancer also places an enormous economic and social burden on the cancer victim, on the victim's family, and on society. It is a disease which can begin unobtrusively and linger on for years. Specialized treatment is often necessary. The total direct cost of treatment for an individual case continues to increase, with current estimates averaging $20,000 and ranging between $5,000 and $30,000.[5] Indirect costs to the family are often much greater still, including loss of earnings from premature disability and death and the depletion of family financial resources. Dollar costs aside, the agony of watching a loved one die is an incalculable emotional burden.

Total national costs from cancer, both direct and indirect, were estimated by HEW in 1971 to be about $15 billion annually. Projections for 1978 are in the region of $30 billion.*[6]

The Static Cure Rate of Cancer

Many cancers are lethal, even when di-

---

‡ This figure excludes about 300,000 new cases of non-melanoma skin cancer and carcinoma in situ.
* These figures underestimate the true costs, which are still largely unrecognized. For example, a recent National Occupational Hazards Survey by the National Institute for Occupational Safety and Health estimated that the costs of surveillance of workers exposed to just those few carcinogens currently regulated by the Department of Labor are as high as $8.5 billion. (The results of this survey are summarized in an NIOSH document, "The Right to Know," July, 1977.)

Table 1.1 Top Three Causes of Death in 1971

Age in Years	Sex	First	Percent of All Deaths*	Most Frequent Causes of Death		Third	Percent of All Deaths*
				Second	Percent of All Deaths*		
1-14	M	Accidents	49	Cancer	12	Congenital malformation	7
	F	Accidents	38	Cancer	12	Congenital malformation	8
15-34	M	Accidents	48	Homicide	13	Suicide	9
	F	Accidents	30	Cancer	13	Suicide	8
35-54	M	Heart disease	34	Cancer	18	Accidents	11
	F	Cancer	33	Heart disease	18	Stroke	7
55-74	M	Heart disease	43	Cancer	22	Stroke	8
	F	Heart disease	38	Cancer	26	Stroke	11
75+	M	Heart disease	46	Cancer	14	Stroke	14
	F	Heart disease	50	Stroke	18	Cancer	11

Source: *Vital Statistics of the United States, 1971.* Vol. II, Mortality, Pt. A, U.S. DHEW, Public Health Service, 1975.

* Percent of all deaths for the given age group and sex.

Table 1.2 U.S. Mortality for the Three Leading Cancer Sites in Major Age Groups by Sex in 1975

Rank	Under 15 Male	Under 15 Female	15-34 Male	15-34 Female	35-54 Male	35-54 Female	55-74 Male	55-74 Female	75+ Male	75+ Female
1	Leukaemia	Leukaemia	Leukaemia	Breast	Lung	Breast	Lung	Breast	Lung	Colon and rectum
2	Brain and nervous system	Brain and nervous system	Brain and nervous system	Leukaemia	Colon and rectum	Lung	Colon and rectum	Colon and rectum	Prostate	Breast
3	Lympho- and recticulo-sarcoma	Bone	Testis	Brain and nervous system	Pancreas	Colon and rectum	Prostate	Lung	Colon and rectum	Lung

Source: American Cancer Society, "1978 Cancer Facts and Figures," New York, 1977.

Table 1.3 Estimates of New Cancer Cases and Cancer Deaths in 1979

Site	No. of Cases*	Deaths*
Lung	112,000	98,000
Colon-rectum	112,000	52,000
Breast	107,000	35,000
Uterus	53,000†	11,000
Mouth	24,000	9,000
Skin	14,000‡	6,000
Leukaemia	22,000	15,000

Source: American Cancer Society, "1979 Cancer Facts and Figures," New York, 1978.
* Figures rounded to the nearest 1,000.
† If carcinoma in situ is included, cases total over 98,000.
‡ Estimated new cases of non-melanoma over 300,000. Incidence estimates are based on rates from NCI SEER Programs, 1973-76.

prostate, and some relatively uncommon cancers such as Hodgkin's disease, acute lymphocytic leukaemia in children, (and also choriocarcinoma and Wilm's tumor), where in some instances prolonged regressions, if not cures have been achieved, no substantial overall progress has been made in treating cancer.[7]

Particularly for the major cancer killers, such as lung, breast, and colon, the odds of a cure have not improved much over the last two decades. The prognosis for lung cancer, the most common fatal type among men, remains poor; only about one of ten victims survives for five years after diagnosis. Victims of Hodgkin's disease now agnosed early and treated with the best modern techniques. Our ability to treat cancer effectively has not markedly increased on an overall basis over the last four or so decades. Even the improvements in cancer cure rates which were achieved from the mid-1930s to the mid-1950s, from an approximate overall 20 percent to a 33 percent five-year survival rate, seem to have been due not so much to the early detection or specialized treatment of cancer with drugs or radiation therapy as largely to advances in general surgical and postoperative procedures, particularly blood transfusion and antibiotics.

Modern figures on cancer survival rates are not encouraging, in spite of common claims to the contrary. When the percentage of people who have survived for five years after cancer diagnosis and treatment in the period 1970-73 are compared to similar figures for 1960-63, it can be seen (Table 1.4) that with the exception of cancer of the

Table 1.4 Five-Year Survival Rates for Cancer* (Whites)

Type of Cancer	Sex	5-Year Survival Rates %	
		1950-59	1965-69
Lung	M	7	8
	F	11	12
Breast	F	60	64
Cervix	F	59	56
Uterus (Body)	F	71	74
Prostate	M	47	56
Colon	M	42	43
	F	46	46
Stomach	M	12	12
	F	13	14
Hodgkin's disease	M	31	52
	F	38	56
Childhood leukaemia*	M	1	4
	F	2	8

Source: M. H. Myers, NCI, May 1979.

* These data are composite of results from three participants in the SEER program: Connecticut Tumor Registry; Registry of the University of Iowa; and Registry of the Charity Hospital of New Orleans. Results reflect rates with a standard error of less than 5 percent.

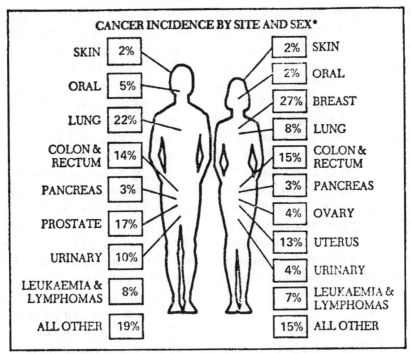

CANCER INCIDENCE BY SITE AND SEX*

	Male		Female	
SKIN	2%	2%	SKIN	
ORAL	5%	2%	ORAL	
LUNG	22%	27%	BREAST	
COLON & RECTUM	14%	8%	LUNG	
PANCREAS	3%	15%	COLON & RECTUM	
PROSTATE	17%	3%	PANCREAS	
URINARY	10%	4%	OVARY	
LEUKAEMIA & LYMPHOMAS	8%	13%	UTERUS	
ALL OTHER	19%	4%	URINARY	
		7%	LEUKAEMIA & LYMPHOMAS	
		15%	ALL OTHER	

*Excluding non-melanoma skin cancer and carcinoma in situ of uterine cervix.

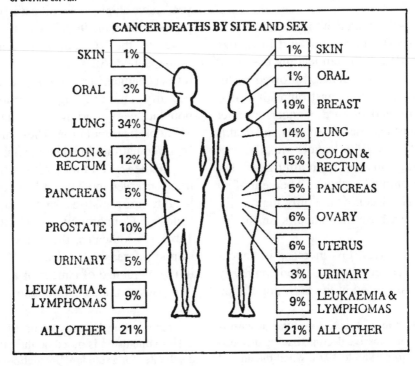

CANCER DEATHS BY SITE AND SEX

	Male		Female	
SKIN	1%	1%	SKIN	
ORAL	3%	1%	ORAL	
LUNG	34%	19%	BREAST	
COLON & RECTUM	12%	14%	LUNG	
PANCREAS	5%	15%	COLON & RECTUM	
PROSTATE	10%	5%	PANCREAS	
URINARY	5%	6%	OVARY	
LEUKAEMIA & LYMPHOMAS	9%	6%	UTERUS	
ALL OTHER	21%	3%	URINARY	
		9%	LEUKAEMIA & LYMPHOMAS	
		21%	ALL OTHER	

Figure 1.1 Estimates of Cancer Incidence and Deaths by Site and Sex in 1979

Source: American Cancer Society, "1979 Cancer Facts and Figures," New York, 1978.

have about a 60 percent five-year survival rate, but Hodgkin's disease represents only about 1 percent of all cancers. Table 1.4 reflects the best available data on historical trends in cancer patient survival from the NCI Cancer Surveillance Epidemiology and End Results (SEER) program.[8] (Results are much less encouraging than those claimed by the American Cancer Society on the basis of the same NCI Data.) This is the case despite the vast sums of money spent over the last 30 years, despite the high priorities for cancer research set by Congress, despite devotion of an entire federal agency (the National Cancer Institute) to the cancer problem, and in the face of continuing misleading and optimistic reassurances by the American Cancer Society.

The Increasing Incidence of Cancer

The Facts

Cancer is the plague of the twentieth century. In 1900, pneumonia and influenza headed the list of the ten leading causes of death in the United States, followed by tuberculosis, infectious gastrointestinal diseases, and heart disease. Cancer, number eight, caused less than 4 percent of all deaths (Table 1.5). By 1976, cancer was the second leading cause of death after heart disease, accounting for about 20 percent of all deaths. Cancer is now the only major killing disease whose incidence is on the increase.†

To some extent, this increase in cancer mortality reflects the increased longevity which has occurred in the U.S. population during this century. Living longer increases the chances of developing cancer. However, there is also a greater cancer risk in each specific age group.[9] Thus a fifty-year-old man today is more likely to die of cancer than was a fifty-year-old man in 1950. It has been recently calculated, by Marvin Schneiderman, Assistant Director for Field Studies and Statistics of the NCI, that between 9.5 percent and 27 percent of the increase in the death rate from cancer over the past few decades is due to the increased cancer risk of specific age groups. The increased cancer death rate, therefore holds true despite the factor of age.‡ Standardized cancer death rate data, adjusted for age and based on the total U.S. population, also show an overall and progressive increase of about 11 percent over the last four decades.

Table 1.6 shows how the standardized cancer incidence rates (the number of newly detected cases per 100,000 population each year) have changed over the thirty-two-year period ending in 1969. These data were collected by the NCI during its periodic National Cancer Surveys and are adjusted to reflect changes in regions surveyed and, especially, changing age structures of the populations, i.e., to discount the effects of aging of the population. These are the most accurate nationwide data available on cancer incidence, and they reflect the general trend observed more recently in regional and local tumor registries, such as those of the states of Connecticut and California. As Table 1.6 indicates, there have been substantial increases between 1937 and 1969 in the incidence of cancer of a wide range of organs in males and females, both black

---

† The death rate from cardiovascular disease is now on the progressive decline, having dropped 20 percent from 1968 to 1975, when the annual toll (994,513) fell below one million for the first time in more than a decade. The death rate from cirrhosis of the liver and crimes of violence, including suicide, are also on the increase, but these

are minor killing diseases compared with cancer.
‡ This conclusion is based on the calculation of death rates for a standard population with a fixed percentage of people in each age category. Statisticians can then adjust the data to reflect a hypothetical constant age distribution and thus compensate for differences in aging.

Table 1.5 The Ten Leading Causes of Death in the U.S. in 1900 and in 1976

1900

Rank	Cause of Death	Crude Death Rate per 100,000 Population	Percent of Total Deaths
	All causes	1,719.1	100.0
1	Influenza and pneumonia	202.2	11.8
2	Tuberculosis	194.4	11.3
3	Gastroenteritis	142.7	8.3
4	Diseases of heart	137.4	8.0
5	Cerebral hemorrhage	106.9	6.2
6	Chronic nephritis	81.0	4.7
7	Accidents	72.3	4.2
8	Cancer	64.0	3.7
9	Certain diseases of infancy	62.6	3.6
10	Diphtheria	40.3	2.3

Source: "Facts of Life and Death," National Center for Health Statistics, Public Health Service Publication no. 600, 1970, Table 12.

1976

Rank	Cause of Death	Crude Death Rate per 100,000 Population	Percent of Total Deaths
	All causes	889.5	100.0
1	Diseases of heart	337.1	37.9
2	Cancer	175.8	19.8
3	Stroke	87.9	9.9
4	Accidents	46.9	5.3
5	Influenza and pneumonia	28.7	3.2
6	Diabetes mellitus	16.1	1.8
7	Cirrhosis of liver	14.7	1.6
8	Arteriosclerosis	13.9	1.5
9	Suicide	12.5	1.4
10	Diseases of infancy	11.6	1.3

Source: American Cancer Society, "1979 Cancer Facts and Figures," New York, 1978.

Table 1.6 Changes in Age-Standardized Cancer Incidence from 1937 to 1969

Cancer Site	Group*	Percent Changes 1937-1947	Percent Changes 1947-1969	Net Change 1937-1969
Esophagus	WM	6	-28	Down
	WF	19	-18	Up
	BM	62	101	Up†
	BF	57	89	Up†
Stomach	WM	-23	-59	Down
	WF	-30	-67	Down
	BM	3	-48	Down
	BF	3	-56	Down
Colon	WM	17	26	Up
	WF	16	-1	Up
	BM	5	90	Up†
	BF	37	129	Up†
Rectum	WM	16	-22	Down
	WF	25	-29	Down
	BM	59	3	Up
	BF	62	-27	Up
Pancreas	WM	33	22	Up
	WF	12	21	Up
	BM	132	30	Up†
	BF	88	127	Up†
Lung	WM	115	133	Up†
	WF	63	108	Up†
	BM	202	234	Up†
	BF	71	213	Up†
Breast	WF	10	4	Up
	BF	9	25	Up
Ovary	WF	16	-10	Up
	BF	80	16	Up
Prostate	WM	17	23	Up
	BM	63	55	Up†
Bladder	WM	22	21	Up
	WF	8	-26	Down
	BM	25	118	Up†
	BF	44	-43	Up

Source: S. J. Cutler and S. S. Devesa, "Trends in Cancer Incidence and Mortality in the USA," in R. Doll and I. Voldopija, eds., *Host Environment Interactions in the Etiology of Cancer in Man,* International Agency for Research on Cancer, Lyon, France, 1973, pp. 15-34.

* WM=white male; WF=white female; BM=black male; BF=black female.

† Total increase exceeds 75 percent.

and white. Of the 34 categories of cancer type by sex and race listed in the left-hand columns of Table 1.6, the incidence of cancer has increased in about two-thirds of them (twenty-four categories). In half of these (twelve categories) the incidence rate has increased by more than 75 percent. Similar substantial increases have occurred for malignant melanoma and thyroid cancer in white males and for lymphoma in black males and females.

These major increases in cancer incidence up to 1969 have been maintained progressively and more recently have become even more marked for certain sites.

As can be seen from Table 1.7, the increase in cancer incidence from 1970 to 1975 involves not only the lung but a wide range of organs in both sexes and racial groups and therefore cannot be largely due to smoking. In fact, the overall increase in total cancer incidence for all sites is comparable to that when cancer of the lung is excluded (see Table 1.8).

The differences between the increased incidence rates for cancer of all sites and all sites excluding the lung reflect the relative increase in the incidence of lung cancer compared to all other cancers. For white males, lung cancer and all other cancers are increasing at about the same rate, whereas in black males, lung cancer is now increasing less rapidly. For white and black females, lung cancer is increasing more rapidly than all other cancers, reflecting the increase in smoking by females.

The rate of increase in the incidence and mortality of cancer seems to be sharper in blacks, particularly males, than in whites. Esophageal and bladder cancers are on the increase in blacks, although they are declining among whites. Cancer of the breast is also increasing among blacks at a time when it has leveled off among whites. Cancers of other sites including prostate, pancreas, lung,

and ovary are also on the increase in blacks.

The actual probability, at today's death rates, of a person born today getting cancer by the age of eighty-five is 27 percent for both men and women. This is up from 19 percent for men and 22 percent for women in 1950.[10]

It is clear that there has been a real and absolute increase in cancer incidence and mortality during this century which cannot be explained away by increased life span or by smoking. A significant acceleration in the long-term upward trend of cancer mortality is now underway. The increase offers additional support for the conclusion by most independent experts that cancer is environmental in origin and that the recent increase in the incidence of cancer is due to industrial pollutants.

Attempts to Deny the Facts

Many industry groups have tried to argue away this increase in cancer. Their arguments were summarized in an anonymous January, 1978, report by the American Industrial Health Council, an organization recently created by the chemical industry to fight effective regulation of carcinogens in the workplace:

> If we use the turn of the century as a time against which to compare today's cancer problem, there has indeed been an increase in the incidence of cancer . . . but the increase is predominantly attributable to (1) greater longevity (the incidence of cancer increases with age), and (2) pandemic cigarette smoking.[11]

The American Industrial Health Council attempts to support its arguments with graphs that show a decrease in cancer death rates when lung cancer (which in the general population is largely due to smoking) is excluded. The council argues that cancer

Table 1.7 Changes in Standardized Cancer Incidence (for Some Major Sites) from 1970 to 1975

Cancer Site	Annual Percent Changes in Incidence Rates, 1970-1975*			
	WM†	BM	WF	BF
Lung	1.0	0.7	8.5	11.6
Bladder	2.4	8.2	3.2	10.0
Rectum	0.3	4.5	2.3	9.9
Colon	0.8	4.9	1.0	4.9
Melanoma (skin)	6.0	36.6‡		
Cervix			-6.5	-6.1
Uterus			9.0	12.0
Breast			2.3	8.9
All sites	0.9	2.3	2.2	6.1

Source: NCL Third National Cancer Survey, 1969-1971, and Cancer Surveillance Epidemiology and End Results (SEER) Program.
* The 1975 standardized overall cancer incidence rate (per 100,000) is 359.8 for white males; 413.2 for black males; 299.8 for white females; and 329.1 for black females.
† WM=white male; BM=black male; WF=white female; BF=black female
‡ Estimate unreliable as based on small number of cases.

Table 1.8 Changes in Cancer Incidence Rates from 1970 to 1975

Group	Average Percent Increase in Incidence Rates, 1970-1975			
	Cancers of All Sites		Cancers of All Sites except Lung	
	Annual	5-Year	Annual	5-Year
White male	0.9	4.7	0.9	4.6
Black male	2.3	11.9	2.7	14.3
White female	2.2	11.6	1.8	10.2
Black female	6.1	34.6	5.7	32.2

Source: As for Table 1.7. NCI, Third National Cancer Survey, 1969-1971; SEER Program; and statement of M. A. Schneiderman before the U.S. Department of Labor, Occupational Safety and Health Administration, OSHA Docket 090, April 4, 1978.

is on the decline, that its present incidence can largely be attributed to smoking and diet, and that industrial chemicals are responsible for no more than 5 percent of all cancers in the United States. However, it is easy to see from industry data that two sites have accounted for most of the decrease, stomach and cervix, and that this decrease has been more than matched by increases at other sites. The lower rate of cervix cancer is due in part to widespread Pap screening programs which detect and treat precancerous conditions, not to the disappearance of its possible environmental causes.* The decline in stomach cancer is still unexplained. As is obvious from Tables 1.7 and 1.8, smoking is not a significant cause of the increased incidence of cancer in the past decade.

The industry position is based on oversimplification of a complex statistical problem. Cancer is probably not one disease but a spectrum of diseases with common features but different — though proximate — causes. Cancer strikes different parts of the population with different force. Any attempt to represent the effect of cancer with a single summary statistic for many cancer sites lumped together necessarily masks the real situation. As Table 1.6 shows, the incidence of many different types of cancer has risen dramatically in recent decades. There is also growing evidence incriminating the role of industrial chemicals as major causes of cancer. Further confirmation of this was provided by a September 15, 1978, blue-ribbon HEW report, "Estimates of the Fraction of Cancer in the United States Related to Occupational Factors," prepared by ten leading experts in the NCI, the National Institute of Environmental Health Sciences, and the National Institute for Occupational Safety and Health. The report conservatively

estimates (with detailed epidemiological and statistical evidence) that up to about 38 percent of total cancer mortality over the next three decades will be associated with asbestos and five other "high exposure" carcinogens (arsenic, benzene, chromium, nickel oxides, and petroleum fractions). These estimates, however, exclude the effects of radiation and a wide range of other known occupational carcinogens. Furthermore, these estimates fail to consider the effect of occupational carcinogens on the general community (community cancer), due to their discharge or escape from industrial plants and hazardous waste disposal sites.

Environmental Causes of Cancer

An informed consensus has gradually developed that most cancer is environmental in origin and is therefore preventable. The striking increase in cancer death rates in this century cannot be accounted for by aging alone and cannot be due to genetic changes in the population, which would take generations to propagate throughout the population. Furthermore, a series of epidemiological studies have concluded that environmental factors cause from 70 percent to 90 percent of all cancers. Such estimates are derived from a comparison of cancer incidence and mortality in different countries all over the world.[12] Countries at low risk for a given type of cancer are assumed to establish the background rate for that cancer type. A higher cancer rate in other countries is then attributed to environmental factors peculiar to them. Genetic differences between countries or regions are largely discounted in view of evidence that groups which migrate from one country to another tend to develop cancers at the sites and rates

---

* The decrease in cervix cancer rates is less real than apparent, as a large portion of older women (perhaps as many as 30-50 percent in some areas of the country) have had hysterectomies.

prevalent in their adopted countries.[13]

Striking geographical variations in the incidence and mortality of a wide range of specific organ cancers (sometimes as much as 2,000 percent) are now well recognized, and in some instances the environmental causes for its excess rates in certain regions have been discovered.[14] The high incidence of cancer of the mouth in Asia, representing some 35 percent of all Asiatic cancers (in contrast to less than 1 percent of European and North American cancers), is clearly due to the common habit of chewing betel nuts and tobacco leaves. The high incidence of liver cancers in the Bantu and in Guam is well recognized and is likely to be due to dietary contamination with aflatoxin, a potent fungal carcinogenic toxin, and to eating cycad plants containing naturally occurring (azoxyglucoside) carcinogens, respectively. The high incidence of cancer of the esophagus in Zambians drinking a homemade alcoholic brew (kachasu) and in residents of the Calvados area of France incriminates strong alcoholic spirits, possibly contaminated with carcinogens such as nitrosamines.

Environmental factors incriminated as causes of human cancer encompass a wide range of influences including background and man-made radiation, smoking, naturally occurring plant, fungal, bacterial, and chemical carcinogens, and industrial chemical carcinogens contaminating air, water, food, consumer products, and the workplace. While it is known that smoking is associated with up to 80,000 lung cancer deaths each year, there is no reliable method for calculating the numbers of deaths caused by other classes of carcinogens. For instance, it has been claimed, particularly by the chemical industry, that industrial chemicals are a relatively trivial cause of cancer, accounting for only about 5 percent of all cancers in adult males.[15] This figure is based on estimates of the effects of those workplace chemicals *known* to cause cancer. But in view of the very limited number of epidemiological studies that have been carried out in the workplace there is every reason to suspect that many other industrial chemicals are carcinogenic, but not yet so identified. Also, there is no way of currently determining how many workers are unknowingly exposed to industrial carcinogens, so figures based on known workplace carcinogens will seriously underestimate the carcinogenic hazards of industrial chemicals.† Two or more carcinogens, furthermore, can interact synergistically and thus greatly increase the carcinogenic effects over those induced by either carcinogen alone. For example, the incidence of lung cancer among asbestos workers who smoke cigarettes is many times greater than either that of nonsmoking asbestos workers or of smokers among the general population.[16] The additional lung cancers due to synergistic effects would not have occurred in the absence of the occupational exposure to asbestos.

The Cancer Maps

Cancers caused by industrial chemicals are not restricted to the workers immediately exposed to them. These chemicals are discharged or escape from plants handling

---

† The majority of industries has not been evaluated for cancer and other chronic effects. This alone makes it impossible to estimate the number of cancers that are industrially related. Furthermore, it seems premature to assume that the effects of more recently introduced industrial chemicals can be gauged through current cancer rates. It must also be stressed that the majority of epidemiological studies so far undertaken in the workplace have been in larger industries which are likely to be less hazardous than the innumerable small plants manufacturing, handling, or processing carcinogenic chemicals under even more poorly controlled conditions.

them into the air, water, and soil of the surrounding communities, and also to hazardous waste disposal sites of distant communities. (Workers also carry them home on contaminated clothes to their families.) Examination of overall cancer death rates on a state and county basis, using the recently published maps of the National Cancer Institute showing the geographical distribution of overall cancer mortality rates and rates for most major sites in men and women between 1950 and 1969, clearly shows excess rates for people living in industrialized areas, particularly in the vicinity of petrochemical plants.‡[17] While some of the excess cancers in males are due to exposures within the plant, the excess female cancers are most likely due to contamination of the community air or water by carcinogens originating from the plant. In a growing number of instances, chemical monitoring has demonstrated the presence of occupational carcinogens such as asbestos, vinyl chloride, benzene, arsenic, benzidine, Kepone and nitrosamines in the air outside plants.

An additional major source of community exposure to carcinogens that is becoming belatedly recognized are hazardous waste disposal sites and the innumerable sites where hazardous wastes have been improperly dumped, such as municipal landfills, industrial dumps, and abandoned mines. Recent EPA estimates indicate that as much as 90 percent of hazardous wastes continue to be improperly discarded, in some cases in the immediate vicinity of populated areas.

More recent NCI cancer-mortality data for 1969 to 1971 generally confirms previous findings in the NCI maps of markedly higher overall cancer-mortality rates in urbanized and industrialized states than in rural and agricultural states. The most striking recent change is the marked increase in rates in many southern and southwestern states, presumably corresponding to their rapid industrialization during the previous two decades. Additionally, rates in New York have edged up, and now rank with those of New Jersey.

The extent and importance of proximity of residence to industry, and possibility of exposure to industrial chemical carcinogens, as a substantial factor in causes of cancer in the general public is becoming increasingly recognized. Table 1.9 lists the five states with the highest overall cancer death rates for both men and women during the period 1950-69 and contrasts these with the five states with the lowest rates. As can be seen, the five highest rates, both for men and women, are all found in the northeast in some of the country's most heavily industrialized states. In contrast, the states with the lowest cancer death rates are in predominantly rural western and southern states, where there is relatively little industry. The combined cancer death rate for the five highest states is 45 percent greater than that for the five lowest among males, and 38 percent greater among females. These large differences between urban industrial and rural environments, taken in the aggregate, point strongly to an important role of industrial pollution, possibly together with pollution from nonindustrial sources, such as automobiles. One would be hard pressed to explain away differences of this large magnitude on the basis of possible differences in smoking, medical care, lifestyle patterns, or other such factors. New Jersey and Wyoming, for instance, have almost identical per capita tobacco sales (New Jersey's sales are 2 percent higher), but New Jersey's female cancer death rate is 36 percent higher than that

---

‡ The pattern of distribution for each cancer site and sex and ethnic group tends to be distinctive.

of Wyoming.*

Differences in cancer mortality rates among states and counties are even more striking when specific types of cancer rates are compared. As Table 1.10 shows, the excess rates for lung, bladder, and colon-rectal cancers are much greater for females living in New Jersey than in Wyoming or North Carolina. Similar but less marked excesses are also seen for breast cancer, a cancer not generally considered to result from exposure to industrial chemicals. When comparisons are extended to the United States as a whole, the strongest association in any county between cancer death rates and the location of petrochemical plants are found for bladder cancer.

Use of only the state-by-state data masks much of the association between industrialization and excess cancer mortality rates. All states contain some areas that are urbanized and industrialized, and other areas that are predominantly rural. The cancer maps show that, within any given state, there are much higher cancer mortality rates in industrialized than in rural counties. For example, the state of Maryland has the highest male lung cancer mortality rate in the nation, 27 percent above the U.S. average. However, the rate for Garrett County in Maryland is 35 percent

below the U.S. average, ranking it in the bottom third of all U.S. counties. Similarly, the rate for the state of Montana is 18 percent below the U.S. average, while Deer Lodge County, Montana, has a rate 71 percent above the U.S. average, ranking it near the top of all U.S. counties. Standardized mortality rates for almost all cancers are higher in predominantly urban than in predominantly rural counties (Table 1.11). Even the county-by-county data may mask large differences. For example, three districts in Los Angeles County with a high concentration of petro-chemical industries, and for which high levels of the carcinogen benzo[a]pyrene have been measured in the air and soil, have lung cancer rates in white males 40 percent above those in the remainder of the country.[18]

There are some apparent exceptions to the overall association between industrialization and excess cancer rates, which reflect a wide range of factors. For instance, there are certain urban counties in the not yet highly industrialized state of Florida that have high cancer rates comparable to those in heavily industrialized New Jersey counties. This most probably reflects migration to Florida of retired senior citizens who have lived and worked for most of their lives in the heavily industrialized northeast. Simi-

---

* The chemical industry has attempted to explain away the high cancer rates in New Jersey on a variety of grounds. The most bizarre of these are contained in a pamphlet, "A Rational View of Cancer in New Jersey," by Harry B. Demopoulos, a pathologist at New York University Medical Center, which was widely circulated by the New Jersey Chamber of Commerce, although apparently never submitted for publication to a scientific journal. Demopoulos argues, with lack of any supporting evidence, that the high cancer mortality rates in New Jersey are the result of average incidence rates coupled with below-average cure rates due to the large number of foreign-trained doctors in the state. Demopoulos also asserts that most workplace exposures in

New Jersey are fully controlled, that asbestos is a "weak carcinogen" (although there is over-whelming evidence that it is one of the most potent known carcinogens), that vinyl chloride is a weak carcinogen (although this produces malignant tumors in animals at the lowest level, 1 ppm, yet tested, and in exposed workers at levels below 10 ppm), that cigarette smoking is the cause of all lung cancer (ignoring substantial evidence that a wide range of occupational carcinogens, including asbestos, are unequivocally incriminated as causes of lung cancer), that high fat diets are the cause of all colon cancer (when the farthest that current hypotheses go is that such a diet may be a contributory or promoting factor in some cases).

Table 1.9 States with the Five Highest and the Five Lowest Cancer Mortality Rates

	Five Highest States		Five Lowest States		Difference between
	State	Mortality Rate*	State	Mortality Rate	Highest & Lowest
Males					
	New Jersey	205.01	Utah	133.13	
	Washington, D.C.	203.75	New Mexico	136.30	
	Rhode Island	203.17	Wyoming	138.93	
	New York	199.24	Idaho	139.02	
	Connecticut	195.68	North Carolina	140.11	
	All five	200.36	All five	138.51	45%
Females					
	New York	148.01	Utah	102.06	
	New Jersey	147.92	North Carolina	106.97	
	Rhode Island	143.37	Arkansas	108.03	
	Washington, D.C.	141.73	Wyoming	109.09	
	Maine	140.46	Idaho	110.15	
	All five	147.37	All five	107.09	38%

Source: Based on T. J. Mason and F. W. McKay, "U.S. Cancer Mortality by County, 1950-1969," DHEW Publication (NIH) 74-615, Washington, D.C., 1973.
* Age-adjusted annual mortality rate for all cancers per 100,000 population.

Table 1.10 Comparison of Cancer Death Rates: New Jersey, Wyoming, and North Carolina, White Females*

Cancer Death Rates	State			Excess Rate for New Jersey (%)	
	New Jersey	Wyoming	North Carolina	Wyoming	North Carolina
Overall	147.9	109.1	107.0	36	38
Lung	7.2	4.4	4.5	64	60
Bladder	2.9	1.6	2.1	81	38
Leukaemia	5.7	4.8	5.6	19	20
Colon and rectum	21.7	12.4	10.9	71	99
Pancreas	6.3	5.1	5.2	24	21
Breast	30.6	21.1	19.3	45	59

Source: Based on T. J. Mason and F. W. McKay, "U.S. Cancer Mortality by County, 1950-1969," DHEW Publication (NIH) 74-615, Washington, D.C., 1973.
* Age-adjusted annual mortality rate per 100,000 population.

Table 1.11 Ratios of Cancer Mortality Rates in Urban Counties Compared to Rates in Rural Counties*

White Males		White Females	
Cancer Site	Ratio	Cancer Site	Ratio
Esophagus	3.08	Esophagus	2.12
Bladder	2.10	Lung	1.64
Lung	1.89	Breast	1.61
All malignant neoplasms	1.56	Bladder	1.58
Stomach	1.45	All malignant neoplasms	1.36

Source: R. Hoover, T. Mason, F. W. McKay, and J. F. Fraumeni, Jr., "Geographic Pattern of Cancer Mortality in the United States," in *Persons at High Risk of Cancer: An Approach to Cancer Etiology and Control*, ed. J. F. Fraumeni, Jr. (New York: Academic Press, 1975), pp. 343-60.
* Based on NCI 1950-69 data in 970 counties (of which 957 were "entirely" rural and 13 entirely urban).

larly, the high cancer rates in the non-industrialized city of San Francisco probably reflects contiguity with the three adjacent counties of Alameda, Contra Costa, and San Mateo, which all have heavy concentrations of petrochemical industries, and steel fabricating plants.

While it is not possible to use cancer maps to determine the precise factors responsible for the striking differences in overall cancer rates and in rates for cancer of specific organs among counties all over the United States, the location of large petrochemical plants in counties with excess rates — with the strong likelihood of pollution of nearby communities — is the most plausible explanation. Calculations based on figures such as those in Tables 1.9 and 1.10 suggest that such industrial pollution may be a cause of 30 to 40 percent of cancers in the general population, but it would be unwise to interpret these figures except in a general way, as they may also reflect an incremental role of non-industrial sources of air pollution. It is clear, however, that industrial chemicals are major causes of cancer

in the general population as well as the workforce.

The New Era of Petrochemical Carcinogens

The recognition that environmental agents are the major cause of cancer, and the identification of the specific causal roles that many of them play, has led to an increased concern about the carcinogenic and other toxic effects of the many new chemicals which are being produced and dispersed into the environment. A measure of this concern and evidence that the petrochemical industry itself can no longer cope with the risks of its own operations is the industry's skyrocketing insurance premiums, with renewals sometimes fifty times higher than old rates. We are living in a new era of organic chemicals, not just familiar ones, but exotic ones which have never previously existed on earth, and to which no living thing has previously had to adapt. Organic chemicals containing carbon, hydrogen, and chlorine (or other halogens) are

Table 1.12 Rate of Increase in Production from 1945 to 1970 of Selected Groups of "New" Chemicals

Chemical	Percent Increase
Synthetic fibers	5,980
Plastics	1,960
Nitrogen fertilizers	1,050
Synthetic organic chemicals	950
Organic solvents	746

Source: Barry Commoner, *The Closing Circle*, N.Y., Knopf, 1971.

Table 1.13 Growth in U.S. Crude Refining Capacity from 1900 to 1960

Year	Capacity (millions of barrels, daily)
1900	0.50
1931	3.91
1952	7.70
1960	10.36

Source: Kirk and Othmer, eds., *Encyclopedia of Chemistry and Technology*, 15:3 (1968); and W. L. Nelson, *Petroleum Refinery Engineering*, N.Y., McGraw-Hill, 1936.

rarely, if ever, found in nature. Organochlorines are non-degradable or poorly degradable, persist in the environment and in the body, and are fat soluble and have accumulated and concentrated in the food chain. As a class, it also contains a disproportionately high number of carcinogens (several of which will be discussed in the case studies that follow). Literally thousands of new organic chemicals are being released into the environment, and not in lots of a few pounds or gallons but by the millions and billions of pounds and gallons. The intricate biochemical defenses that living beings throughout evolution have developed to cope with their environment are now being constantly violated by foreign materials introduced into the environment in petroleum products, synthetic organic chemicals, and organic pesticides (Table 1.12).

Petroleum Products

Petroleum first achieved commercial importance in 1859, but significant quantities were not produced until the development of the internal combustion engine in the late nineteenth century. The growing use of gasoline led to the development in 1913 of large-scale hydrocarbon cracking processes, which for the first time made available large quantities of low-molecular-weight hydrocarbons, the starting material for the production of many organic compounds.[19] After World War II, catalytic cracking made possible yet another dramatic increase in hydrocarbon production from petroleum sources. The age of chemical solvents had begun. The growth of refining capacity is traced in Table 1.13.

Synthetic Organic Chemicals

Prior to 1900, the great bulk of all organic raw materials was derived from coal tar, and, to a lesser extent, from the distillation of wood. In 1931, the U.S. National Bureau of Standards and the American Petroleum Institute began a systematic study of petroleum hydrocarbon synthesis and uses. This culminated after World War II in a fundamental shift of organic chemical production to the petroleum industry, which, along with increased hydrocarbon production from catalytic cracking of petroleum, gave birth to a new petrochemical industry. Petrochemicals are the quintessence of the "process industry," in which a small number of primary constituents from crude oil are converted into a large number of intermediate chemicals and a still larger number of large scale end products.† A disproportionately large number of recognized carcinogens fall into just three families of widely used petrochemicals: aromatic amines, in the form of dyes and synthetic intermediates, particularly epoxy compounds and hydrazines; chlorinated olefins, as monomers and pesticides; and alkyl halides, as solvents and degreasing agents. Benzene provides a good example of the exponential growth of a petrochemical product. Its production in the United States rose from 125 million gallons in 1940 to 410 million in 1955 to 1.5 billion in 1976.

Insecticides

Large-scale use of insecticides began in the 1870s, when the potato beetle was spreading rapidly eastward across the United States. Inorganic pesticides, calcium arsenate and copper sulfate, for example, were used to control pests and fungi, and they dominated these agricultural markets until World War II.

Organic pesticides, which were expensive and variable in supply, were limited to a few natural products, such as rotenone, nicotine, and pyrethrum. The inorganics, however, tended to leave toxic residues which accumulated in the soil until levels were reached which made further growing of crops unprofitable. In 1939, when DDT was developed for widespread use, synthetic organic insecticides began to gain importance. After the war, many other chlorinated organic pesticides were developed, such as chlordane, toxaphene, dieldrin, and aldrin. As will be seen

in chapter 7, many of these compounds, which have been released into the environment in mammoth quantities (DDT at 2.75 million pounds per month in 1945), are highly persistent and carcinogenic.

As is apparent, the end of World War II marked a turning point in the growth of the chemical industry. American enterprise, with its enormous productive capacity, had to create new products at an unparalleled pace in order to keep its large plants and refineries operating. It set to work aggressively developing "needs" for new types of goods and services.‡ As a by-product of this prodigious effort, more new chemicals to be used in making these goods were created, which in turn required the creation of new markets to produce them on a large, and hence economically profitable, scale. Table 1.12 shows the rate of production of a variety of chemical substances which had not existed on the face of the earth until a few decades ago.

This productive spiral continues to accelerate, dipping occasionally only to wait for markets to stabilize, for new products to catch on, or for capital to become available. Figure 1.2 shows the trend in production for various classes of synthetic organic chemicals over the past sixty years. As can be seen, the total U.S. production of synthetic organic chemicals increased from about 1 billion pounds in 1940 to 300 billion pounds by 1976. Annual growth rates of 15 percent or more are not uncommon for the organic chemical industries, at a time when the rest of the economy is advancing

---

† As Barry Commoner stresses, the petrochemical industry is the most capital-intensive of all manufacturing industries, producing only about $.80 of value added per dollar of capital invested, as compared with about $3.64 in the case of a typical natural competitor, the leather industry. The economy of scale in the petrochemical industry allows it to successfully invade large, well-

developed markets, such as the clothing industry, which exhibit a high elasticity of demand.

‡ These innovations supplant pre-existing markets and products, and establish a type of economic imperialism for the petrochemical industry, leaving consumers with little option but to surrender old products, most of them natural, in favor of synthetic replacements.

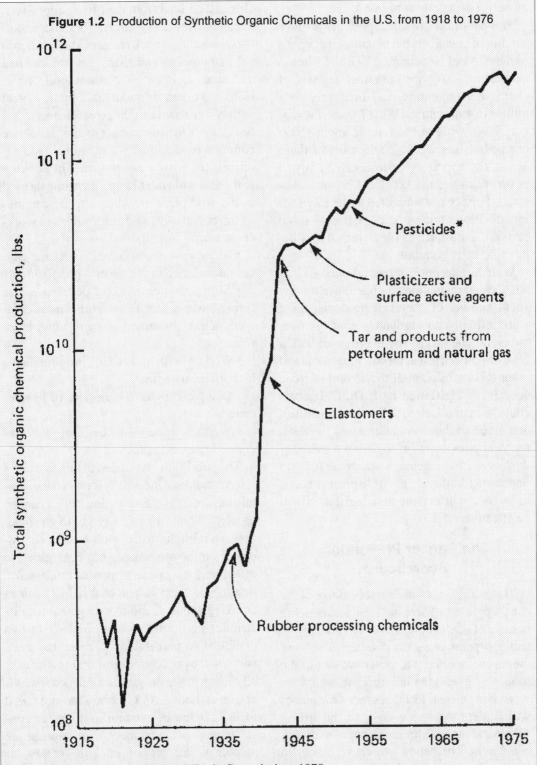

Figure 1.2 Production of Synthetic Organic Chemicals in the U.S. from 1918 to 1976

Source: U.S. International Trade Commission, 1978.

* Arrows indicate year when usage became sufficiently "significant" to be included as specific categories in Commission reports.

by only 4 or 5 percent per year.

This pattern of growth applies not just to a handful of chemicals but to tens of thousands of them. As of November, 1977, the Chemical Abstracts Service computer registry of chemical compounds contained over four million distinct entries. What's more, the registry is growing at the rate of about 6,000 compounds per week. While most of these are exotic laboratory curiosities which will never reach the market, the Chemical Abstracts Service has submitted to the Environmental Protection Agency a list of some 33,000 chemicals in its files which it now believes to be in common use.[20]

With the exception of special-purpose legislation and regulation relating to a relatively small number of chemical products, there were virtually no regulatory controls over industrial chemicals, the majority of which have never been tested for carcinogenesis and other toxic effects, until the advent of toxic substances legislation in 1976. Chemicals could be manufactured in limitless quantities and introduced into commerce and the environment with no effort to discover whether they were carcinogenic or otherwise toxic to humans and other forms of life. (It remains to be seen whether the new legislation will be effective.)

The Cancer Prevention Scoreboard

The public is now undeniably aware of the cancer problem. There has been an unending barrage of media coverage of environmental and occupational cancer disasters involving the air we breathe, the water we drink, the food we eat, and the industries in which we work. Now there is fear that supersonic planes will deplete the ozone layer of the stratosphere and increase the incidence of skin cancer. Chloroform, known to cause cancer in rodents, has been found in drinking water in many major cities. Drinking water in New

Orleans, derived from the Mississippi River, contains over 200 synthetic organic pollutants, including a wide range of known chemical carcinogens and many yet unidentified and untested chemicals. Automobile emissions and urban air pollutants contain a great variety of known carcinogens. Saccharin has been shown to cause cancer in animals. Some common food additives and animal feed additives are proven carcinogens. In addition to these, a still wider range of chemicals used in the workplace are known to be carcinogenic, potentially exposing millions of workers to cancer hazards.

• Asbestos workers have a high lung cancer rate relative to the general population.

• Some plastics workers develop a rare form of liver cancer, besides other more common cancers, from exposure to vinyl chloride.

• Workers with nickel and chromium have high lung cancer rates.

• Dye workers have high rates of bladder cancer.

• Workers exposed to benzene have increased rates of leukaemia.

The public has responded to this assault of information on cancer risks with generally fatalistic reactions: "Everything causes cancer, so why bother?" or "You've got to go somehow, so it might just as well be cancer." Industry on the other hand, has been quick to minimize the scope and extent of cancer risks, to attribute them to personal habits such as smoking and diet, and to exaggerate the difficulties and costs of their control. In this denial of responsibility, industry has been supported by academic consultants who usually speak under the guise of independent scientific authority. And industry has not failed to exploit the awakening anti-cancer consciousness of consumers with appropriate responsive campaigns, such as for low-tar cigarettes.

The cancer prevention scoreboard has low

entries in all categories, except confusion. While there is clearly need for improved understanding of the scientifically complex problems behind cancer, there is an even greater need for corrective political action. The decisions that are made today will have long-lasting effects on our own and on future generations.

> *The human animals that provide the raw material are available in immense numbers; the wild ones are an independent lot and some of them behave in peculiar enough ways to satisfy the demands of the most imaginative investigator.*
>
> Richard Doll, British epidemiologist.

Chapter Two

Cancer: The Human Experiment

Historical Background

From earliest times, it has seemed logical to search for the cause of a disease by examining the characteristics common to those contracting it. The logic of this approach includes studying groups of people who have differing chances or risks of developing the disease, not just those already afflicted with it. The science that encompasses such studies is called epidemiology. Epidemiological studies, by exploiting the "natural experiments" that people perform on themselves or that society or the environment inflict on them, are as close as we can reasonably get to performing actual experiments on humans.

Epidemiology has been much more successful in the study of acute infectious diseases, such as typhoid and cholera, than in the study of chronic diseases like cancer. Most infectious diseases spread rapidly and can be reproduced in the laboratory. Various hypotheses as to cause, effect, and prevention can thus be tested quickly, and once an infectious agent is isolated, it can be comparatively easily shown to cause the disease.

The epidemiology of cancer is more complex. In its broadest sense, cancer epidemiology is the study of the environment of the types of people who do and who do not get a particular type of cancer. Unfortunately, cancer epidemiology is a search for clues to the causes of cancer in a world where clues are both scarce and difficult to interpret.[1] It is a search for factors that differentiate cancer patients from other individuals, pursued in the hope that discovering such factors will lead to the development of preventive methods for those who have not contracted the disease. Epidemiological evidence is often the first clue that a problem exists. Occasionally, it is the only clue as to cause and prevention. The peculiar nature of cancer, especially the long natural history of the disease, in which clinical evidence of illness often occurs several decades after initial exposure to a carcinogen, makes cancer epidemiology frustrating, often controversial, and sometimes a useless exercise.

Some Perspectives and Pitfalls of Cancer Epidemiology

The fundamental problem of epidemiological research is that it is quite difficult to assemble a large enough number of cancer cases of a particular type upon which to draw conclusions about its causes. In numbers of people affected cancer is a major killer, but from a statistical point of view a particular type of cancer is a relatively rare event. For example, the overall incidence of lung cancer in the general population in 1970 was about forty cases for each 100,000 people, although its incidence is much higher in the middle-aged and elderly.[2] As the probability of an individual contracting lung cancer in that year was thus about one in 2,500, an extremely large number of people would have to be observed to ensure that there would be enough cases of the disease to study.

The very task of assembling a sufficient number of persons to satisfy the statistical requirements of such an investigation is often the principal obstacle to the study, demanding as it does access to large population groups and substantial financing for salaries of interviewers, statisticians, and other investigators.

Identifying a sufficient number of cancer cases, together with their medical and exposure histories, is central in the use of epidemiology as a tool for investigating the cause of the cancer. To assist in this undertaking, a number of localities and states have set up cancer registries for the purpose of identifying all new cases of cancer. The nation's oldest such registry is that of the state of Connecticut, which maintains computerized files for use by epidemiologists and statisticians.[3]

Even in the best of circumstances, however, registries cannot predict what types of exposure to ask patients about, so that the "right" type of questions may simply not be asked. Cancer cells are not, after all, labeled for "carcinogen of origin." The clinician discovering cancer at a specific site may not have any useful idea what its cause could have been and what past exposures of the patient should be investigated.

Even when a particular chemical product or process has been shown to be carcinogenic in animals, hence suspect in humans, recognized human cancer cases due to the chemical may, for a long time, be too few to show up above background levels in the general population induced by other carcinogens.* Additional difficulties may be posed by latency, which for some carcinogens is decades (twenty to forty years for smoking and up to fifty years for asbestos).

Quite apart from these intrinsic difficulties in performing adequate epidemiological studies, there are also methodological problems which plague even the best designed ones. The most serious is the inability to obtain adequate data on exposure to carcinogens at times which preceded the finding of cancer by many years. It is nearly impossible to reconstruct industrial exposures to chemicals twenty years or more in the past if specific measurements were not recorded, because in that period the original processes often have changed radically or disappeared altogether. Even for chemicals voluntarily taken by people, such as saccharin, reliable information on how much was ingested or even whether it was taken at all, is difficult to obtain from interviews. This is the case because persons who have a disease which they suspect to be related to a particular chemical may selectively "recall" its use even sometimes when it never took place, and ignore other relevant chemical exposures.

Another major difficulty in most epidemiological studies is sorting out the relevant from the irrelevant and controlling for unknown and unsuspected risk factors. Claims of relationships between certain influences or exposures and disease may be due, not to those particular influences, but to other factors such as diet, location of residence, or lifestyle which the investigator may have overlooked or discounted.

* For this and other reasons, epidemiology is weak at identifying relatively low levels of cancer risk. The lowest clearly identified excess cancer risk, after some twenty years of intensive study, is the 30 percent excess risk for childhood leukaemia following irradiation in later pregnancy.

Basic Epidemiological Techniques

The basic epidemiological techniques used in investigating environmental and occupational causes of cancer can be illustrated by describing their use in the tobacco-cancer problem.

The Informed "Hunch"

The informed hunch is often an important first step in developing a hypothesis about which type of exposure might be linked with a given cancer. It was responsible for early suspicions linking tobacco and lung cancer.

Lung cancer has not always been a major killer. In 1912 a British doctor published a book on the then obscure disease, wondering: "Is it worthwhile to write a monograph on primary malignant tumors of the lung?"[4]

In 1939, however, a German researcher observed that many lung cancer patients he was treating were heavy cigarette smokers.[5] About the same time, a similar observation was made in the United States by the now renowned heart surgeon, Michael DeBakey. These observations stimulated speculation, but without some way of comparing the lung cancer patients to healthy people, there was no way to exclude a host of other factors besides smoking as causes for the cancer. The main problem was that the number of lung cancer cases then seen by any one doctor was relatively small. The epidemic of what is now the most common cause of cancer deaths had only just begun. Only when the number of cases began climbing in the decades after World War II, could scientists begin to check out this hunch further.

Many, if not most, leads for epidemiological studies were developed in just this way, through astute observations by clinicians. The association, for example, between maternal medication with diethylstilbestrol and vaginal cancer in their daughters was developed after a doctor noted a number of similar cases of cancer and began a thorough investigation of use of the drug by obstetricians. This testifies to the importance of close links and communications between clinicians and epidemiologists in the cancer research effort.

Follow-up Studies

By the late 1950s a number of classical epidemiological studies on lung cancer and other disease complexes thought to be due to cigarette smoking were in progress in different countries. Some of these were follow-up or prospective cohort studies, which is to say a large number of healthy people are followed for several years in order to determine which of them contract and die from a specific disease.[6] A follow-up study begun in 1959 by E. Cuyler Hammond of the American Cancer Society is a good example.[7] In a massive effort by volunteers in twenty-five states involving about $1 million of public funds, about one million men and women were questioned about their age and disease and smoking histories. The American Cancer Society managed to keep track of over 90 percent of the initial subjects for a dozen years. Updated questionnaires were supplied every four years or so, or, if a subject died, a death certificate showing the cause of death. The number of deaths observed among people in a specific category was divided by the number expected for people in the category, yielding a value known as the Standard Mortality Ratio (SMR).†

The American Cancer Society found that the SMR from lung cancer increased dramatically with the number of cigarettes smoked and with the inhalation of smoke. It also found that the SMR for ex-smokers decreased as the time since quitting lengthened. More recent

---

† The society regards the tapes containing the raw data of this study as proprietary, and has declined to make them available to outside scientists.

analysis also shows some lessening of the lung cancer death rate among smokers who switched from high to low-tar cigarettes.[8]

A single epidemiological study cannot alone validate or invalidate an assumed link between exposure and disease. However, over the past twenty-five years a parade of other follow-up studies conducted in the United States, England, Japan, and elsewhere, has extended and confirmed the causal association between smoking and lung cancer.[‡]

Case-Control Studies

The logistic problems of follow-up studies, which require enrollment of great numbers of healthy subjects in order to observe a statistically meaningful number of cases of disease, prompted epidemiologists to develop the case-control approach. A case-control (or retrospective) study depends on locating patients with a particular disease (the cases) and another group of people, either healthy or with some unrelated disease (the controls) and asking them the same set of questions. This approach is particularly appropriate for use in hospitals, where most people with serious disease eventually come. (In studies of lung cancer, the questions asked obviously include detailed smoking histories.) A figure called the relative risk is estimated from the replies. Relative risk is

to a case-control study what an SMR is to a follow-up study, namely, a measure of the strength of association between exposure and disease. Both of these are measures of risk relative to the control group. But follow-up studies have an advantage over case-control studies in that they can be used to calculate absolute disease rates as well as relative ones.[*] Thus, one can determine whether the incidence of the disease being studied is unusually large or small in the population being studied. However, this advantage is far outweighed by the enormous logistical difficulties and scale of follow-up studies.

The case-control studies of lung cancer and smoking performed during the last twenty-five years have confirmed the conclusions of the follow-up studies. However, case-control studies have also shown that not all types of lung cancer are affected by smoking to the same extent. A type of lung cancer called adenocarcinoma is much less closely related to smoking than the more usual types, squamous, or oat cell, cancers.[9] Some of the studies also showed that the risk of lung cancer is greater among urban than rural dwellers, thereby supporting the case for an additional role of air pollution in lung cancer. A final important finding was that the risk of lung cancer is lower in smokers

---

‡ However, these studies have generally failed to inquire into occupational histories and have thus neglected a probable role of exposure to occupational carcinogens. Of further interest in this connection is the fact that deaths from pleural mesotheliomas due to asbestos are listed as lung cancers in the International List of Causes of Disease (which is used as the basis for reporting cancer mortality data). Thus, malignant lung disease due to occupational exposure or by such exposure interacting with the effects of tobacco smoke are misrepresented as being exclusively lung cancer deaths exclusively due to tobacco. It is thus likely that the role of occupational exposure to

industrial chemicals as a cause of lung cancer has not been adequately recognized. (For a more extreme expression of this position, see T. D. Sterling, "Does Smoking Kill Workers or Working Kill Smokers, or The Medical Relationship Between Smoking, Occupation, and Respiratory Disease," *International Journal of Health Services*, 8 (1978), pp. 437-52.)

* Additionally, risk estimates in case-control studies are strictly valid only when the disease under study is statistically a rare one. Most cancers satisfy this mathematical restriction. J. Cornfield and W. Haenszel, "Some Aspects of Retrospective Studies," *J. Chronic Diseases*, 11 (1960), pp. 523-34.

of filtered than non-filtered cigarettes.[10]

By 1964, based on the remarkable agreement of seven follow-up and twenty-nine case-control studies, U.S. Surgeon General Luther Terry, in his famous report on smoking and health, could bluntly state: "Cigarette smoking is causally related to lung cancer in men."[11]

Historical Follow-up Studies†

Many of the currently accepted occupational causes of cancer have been verified in human populations through a technique which exploits the follow-up approach, but in which the initial population of exposed workers, known as the cohort, is identified many years after the initial exposure. This is called a historical follow-up or a retrospective-cohort study. This method has been successfully used by NIOSH and other investigators to identify such carcinogens as asbestos, vinyl chloride, and benzene.[12]

In brief, the cohort of workers is defined to be all those engaged in a particular process at some time in the past. In the follow-up, a variety of documents are searched, such as employment, social security, or motor vehicle records, to ascertain the vital status of each cohort member at some later time. Causes of all deaths are obtained from death certificates. Then, based upon actuarial tables the SMR is calculated. The greater the SMR, the stronger is the inference of carcinogenicity.

Epidemiology: Conduct and Misconduct

Epidemiological investigation of a chronic disease, such as cancer, is difficult under the best of circumstances. But because of the major economic impact of a finding that an industrial product or process can cause cancer, industries have often compounded these difficulties by failing to undertake necessary studies or encouraging interpretation or even manipulation of the data to bias the studies in their favor.

Until recently, most industries have been opposed to any epidemiological study of their work force. They have either refused to cooperate in proposed studies, and in many cases have failed to accumulate meaningful records, or even destroyed these records. One reason for this has been their realization that such records could possibly damage the company in prospective Workman's Compensation claims or negligence suits.

Since passage of the 1970 Occupational Safety and Health Act, some companies have agreed to cooperate with government studies or else have hired their own staff or outside consultants to do the job. This apparent willingness to investigate the cancer risk to workers often masks a biased operation in which the preordained outcome is a clean bill of health. Indeed, a collection of statistical devices with built-in biases for handling data have become standard strategy to avoid regulation of carcinogens and other toxic chemicals. The tobacco industry alone has remained stalwart in its assertion that epidemiology, inasmuch as it is entirely statistical, is inappropriate for the study of cancer. This self-serving argument has been abandoned by virtually every other industry in favor of more sophisticated methods of manipulating numbers.

Many studies begin and end with the observation that workers in a given plant have a lower cancer or disease rate than the general population. This may in fact be correct, but it does not prove that workers in that industry are free from cancer or other illness due to occupational exposure, for it is well known that workers in any industry will have a death rate significantly lower than that of people of similar age drawn from the general population.[13] The general population includes disabled and chronically ill individuals, while

---

† Also known as "cohort studies."

the industrial population is at least healthy enough to perform work.‡ Thus, even when a working population develops cancer from an industrial carcinogen, the overall increase in worker death rate may not be great enough to exceed the death rate of a similar age group in the community. The only meaningful comparison group for any given work force under investigation is a control group of workers from other industries where there is no exposure to the suspected carcinogens.*

The most common error in conducting prospective studies is failure to obtain an adequate follow-up. If a large number of persons have been lost to follow-up, serious errors in computing cancer death rates can arise. For example, industry studies on retirees often find living retirees in a far greater percentage than they find the death certificates of retirees who have died. Whether by mischance or by inadequate effort to identify deaths, this means seriously underestimating the death rate for employees of the industry. A related problem is simply attempting to do a study on too few people, known as the "too few" technique. If the cohort size is too small, then even a greatly increased risk of cancer or any other disease cannot be detected statistically.[14]

Another common error of cohort studies is to follow workers for too short a period of time. Since most cancers have a latent period of at least ten years (and many have twenty-year or greater latencies), it is essential to follow workers for at least this much time after their first exposure before a meaningful cancer death rate can be expected. An example of the "short follow-up" technique is the current industry claim of the rarity of leukaemia following occupational exposure to benzene. This claim is, in part, based on an average follow-up of only three years.[15] Another example is the claim for the rarity of cancer in workers exposed to vinyl chloride. In this case the effects of vinyl chloride on workers with long-term exposures have been masked by including in the study many workers only recently exposed and by having a follow-up of only a few years, thereby resulting in a deceptively reduced cancer mortality rate.

Any particular epidemiological study can demonstrate various permutations and combinations of these different statistical devices, as will be illustrated in the various case studies in chapters 5, 6, and 7. For instance, using the "too few" and the "short follow-up" techniques, Shell Chemical Company has claimed that the pesticides aldrin and dieldrin are not carcinogenic, since workers engaged in their manufacture apparently did not have an increased cancer risk. Shell also used this argument as the basis for its claim that the overwhelming data on the carcinogenicity of these pesticides in rodents should be discounted in favor of the allegedly conclusive human evidence of safety.†

Cancer, Geography, and the Environment

What do we know of other factors, besides smoking, that are causes of cancer? Are these factors environmental or genetic? Differences all over the world in the incidence of cancers of particular organs help answer

---

‡ This is sometimes known as the "healthy worker effect."

* This is the major reason why so few industries have yet received any epidemiological evaluation.

† In an attempt to improve the quality and reduce the bias of epidemiologic studies on the basis of which regulatory decisions are made, the Interagency Regulatory Liaison Group has developed guidelines for cohort studies, released in draft form on May 31, 1978, which recommend minimal criteria for the acceptability of such studies, including availability of supporting documentation, definition of follow-up procedures, discussion of potential bias, and disclosure of source of sponsorship and funding.

these questions.

We now know that the incidence of various types of cancer exhibits great geographical variation. For example, in Scotland, the rate of lung cancer among men is the highest in the world, 78 cases per 100,000. In the United States, for white males, the rate is half that of Scotland and in Portugal only one-seventh. The death rate for stomach cancer in Japan is eight times that of U.S. whites, which is now the lowest in the world and still decreasing. The death rate from prostate cancer for U.S. blacks is the world's highest, ten times that of the Japanese."[16]

An almost unbelievable geographical variation exists in a broad belt of central Asia. The Ghurjev district of Khazak in the USSR has an extremely high incidence of esophageal cancer, over 500 cases per 100,000 males. In a small section of Iran near the Caspian Sea, the rate of this disease among women varies by a factor of as much as thirty over a distance of only 100 miles. This high-cancer region has been mapped and inexplicably has a very sharp edge.[17] Similarly inexplicable is the fact that breast cancer also varies geographically by a factor of six, from its lowest national incidence in Japan to its highest in

the Netherlands.[18]

Cancer of the mouth is relatively rare in the United States, representing about 3 percent of all cancers. In parts of Asia, however, it accounts for up to thirty-three percent of all cancers. In this instance, the reason for such a striking difference is known. It results from the habit among many Asians of chewing betel nuts and leaves, wads of which are wrapped around shredded tobacco and lime and held in the mouth for long periods.[19]

The fact that there are such geographical differences in cancer rates does not tell us whether environmental or genetic factors are involved. However, epidemiological studies have shown that when people migrate from one area to another, their disease patterns tend to adjust to that of the country to which they migrate. A 1968 study on the offspring of Japanese migrants to the United States showed that their stomach cancer rate was reduced by two thirds, their colon cancer rates tripled, and their rates of cancer of the pancreas and lung, and of leukaemia increased (Table 2.1). These changes in cancer patterns were all in the direction of matching the comparable cancer rates for the U.S. white population. Since this second-generation

Table 2.1 Mortality Rates of Offspring of Japanese Migrants to the U.S.

Cancer Site	Relative Cancer Mortality Rates		
		Offspring of	
	Japanese	Migrants	U.S. Whites
Stomach	100	38	17
Colon	100	288	489
Pancreas	100	167	274
Lung	100	166	316
Leukaemia	100	146	265

Source: W. Haenszel and M. Kurihara, "Studies of Japanese Migrants. I. Mortality from Cancer and Other Diseases Among Japanese in the United States," *J. Natl. Cancer Inst.* 40 (1968), pp. 43-68.

group tended only to intermarry among themselves or with new migrants from Japan their genetic characteristics as a group remained basically the same. Such studies give strong evidence for the environmental rather than genetic causation of cancer.

The National Cancer Institute has recently published an "Atlas of Cancer Mortality for U.S. Counties: 1950-1969."[20] This is a set of colored maps ranking U.S. counties by cancer mortality rates of white males and females, adjusted for age. A similar study for non-whites was subsequently published.[21]

The "Cancer Atlas" has proved a valuable resource for epidemiologists. Its value lies in its use of 3,056 U.S. counties in forty-eight states as the basic units for the study. These units are sufficiently small to be homogeneous in factors which might influence cancer risk, yet large enough to provide statistically useful estimates of cancer rates at specific body sites. Since the U.S. Census provides basic social and economic information also broken down by counties, it is possible to correlate these with the cancer death rates, and thus to test hypotheses about the association between cancer mortality and suspected socioeconomic variables.

For example, males show a striking variation in distribution of cancer mortality rates, with highest rates of certain cancers in counties with heavy concentrations of petrochemical industries. Salem County, New Jersey, where 25 percent of the men are employed by the chemical industry, has the highest mortality from bladder cancer for white males in the United States.‡ High bladder cancer rates are also found in industrial cities like Buffalo, Toledo, and Chicago. Liver and lung cancer rates are high in the petroleum refinery and shipbuilding areas of the Texas Gulf Coast and Louisiana. Excess lung cancer rates are also correlated with locations of chemical and paper industries. Lung cancer is also high in counties where copper, lead, and zinc smelters are located. Lung cancer rates are consistently higher for both men and women in all U.S. counties in which non-ferrous metal smelters that emit arsenic are located than in non-smelter counties. Deer Lodge County, Montana, has the tenth highest lung cancer mortality rate among all U.S. counties from 1950 to 1969. It also had the world's largest smokestack located at an Anaconda copper smelter plant that emits up to 22 tons of particulates daily, much of it the known carcinogen inorganic arsenic. The fact that the corresponding cancer rates among women in some cases show less striking variations suggests the cancers in the men are substantially occupational in origin.* However, since excess cancer rates are also seen in women living in heavily industrialized states and counties, it is clear that environmental factors are also critically involved (Tables 1.9 and 1.10). Further confirmation of the risks of living near chemical plants has come from a recent NCI study showing higher rates of cancer of the lung in men and women, as well as cancer of the nasal cavity, skin, testis, and other sites in men living in counties with major petroleum refineries.[22]

The nature of these environmental factors involved in geographical clustering of excess cancers in heavily industrialized locations is gradually becoming clearer. Evidence is accumulating of the discharge or escape of a wide range of occupational carcinogens from

---

‡ Interest in the high cancer rates in New Jersey has been recently highlighted by the discovery of a cluster of six cases of acute childhood leukaemia in the 21,000 population of Rutherford over the last five years. On the basis of chance alone, not more than one case should have occurred in this time.

* The present-day cancer incidence reflects exposure perhaps ten or twenty years ago, when the percentage of women in the industrial work force was much lower than at present. Thus, male-female differences in cancer incidence, except of course for sex organs, can give evidence of occupation related cancer.

inside petrochemical and smelting plants into the air and water of the surrounding community, or the dumping of carcinogen-containing wastes in hazardous waste or other undesignated disposal sites. Although only relatively few investigations of this kind have so far been made, carcinogens such as nitrosamines, vinyl chloride, kepone, tetrachloroethane, benzene, benzidine, arsenic, and asbestos, have all been found and measured in nearby communities outside particular industries or hazardous waste disposal sites. Another source of family exposure is the carcinogenic chemicals and dust brought home on workers' skin and clothes.

In tracking down specific industrial and environmental correlations with cancer, the cancer maps are valuable only up to a certain point. At best, the data can be used to obtain clues or leads as to identification of possible high risk groups, which must be further investigated by additional epidemiological methods and chemical monitoring of the industries. For example, the bladder cancer map reveals a clustering of high risk counties for both white males and females in easily delineated industrial locales. Since many different types of industry tend to be located near each other, however, identifying the specific industries responsible can be difficult. Also, other variables known or suspected to cause cancer are more prevalent in urban industrial areas. Explanations for higher cancer rates in these areas should also take other possible urban-rural differences into account.

Epidemiology versus Animal Testing

In conclusion, epidemiology is used to study the incidence of cancer in populations who have already been exposed to carcinogens. While of obvious value in helping to establish causal relationships, particularly for high-risk populations, these studies must invariably rely for their data on people who have already contracted cancer, or who do so during the course of the study. In preventive terms, it is a case of "locking the barn door after the horse has run out," at least for the population being studied.

In contrast, animal testing of new chemicals not yet introduced into commerce allows relatively simple and rapid determination of carcinogenicity, allowing the possibility of subsequent control prior to human exposure.

The major categories of twenty-five known human carcinogens, the majority of which are occupational carcinogens or industrial processes (the remainder being drugs), are listed in Appendix I. In the case of the five industrial processes, the precise chemical identity of the causative agents is unknown. As can be seen, there is very good general correspondence between the human and the experimental animal data.

The bottom line on carcinogenesis testing is this. You can drown an animal in a pool of some substance, suffocate an animal under a heap of it, or beat an animal to death with a sock full of it, but if it isn't carcinogenic, you can't give an animal cancer with it.

William Hines and Judith Randal,
Washington, D.C. journalists.

Chapter Three

Cancer: The Animal Experiment

Whenever it is announced that a chemical has been shown to be carcinogenic in animals, there is usually an accompanying disclaimer that "the chemical has not been found harmful to humans." Every time you read this kind of statement in the press, or hear it announced on the radio or television, you should mentally insert the word "yet." You should ask yourself the question, "If the chemical is carcinogenic to humans, how would we know?" As we have seen, we can only know if the appropriate epidemiological study has been done and its results are conclusive beyond doubt — which is rare — or if the chemical induced an extremely rare tumor.

This chapter explains the rationale for animal experiments, the standard test methods used on animals, and how animal test results should be interpreted. It also deals with some current controversies in interpretation, particularly when major economic interests are threatened.

Some Historical Perspectives

Experiments studying causes of cancer in laboratory animals are not new, but the systematic use of animals to test whole classes of chemicals (e.g., food additives) for the purpose of deciding whether they can be safely used or not is a relatively recent development. This lies at the heart of much of the modern cancer controversy. However, there is now overwhelming agreement by most qualified scientists that if a chemical causes cancer in well-designed animal tests, then there is a strong likelihood that it will also cause cancer in exposed humans.[1] Experience continues to prove that this is, indeed, the case.

Distasteful as it may seem to some to use animals in experimental research, even in accord with standard humane guidelines for the prevention of unnecessary pain and suffering, there is no practical and reasonable alternative to their use. Modern medicine, including vaccines, antibiotics, drugs, and transplants, would not have been possible had it not been for animal studies. The same is also true for cancer research.

During the early 1900s, scientists, familiar with the classic writings more than 100 years earlier of Percival Pott on the role of soot in scrotal cancer among chimney sweeps, tried unsuccessfully to reproduce this in animals using coal tars prepared from soot.[2] Then, in 1916, two Japanese scientists succeeded in inducing skin tumors on rabbit ears by daily application of coal tar for a period of more than six months.[3] This single experiment suddenly opened up the use of animals in cancer research.

It is important to appreciate the difficulty that early investigators experienced in inducing cancers in laboratory animals. First, the time required to produce cancer in an animal was found to be much longer than the time to produce an infection such as rabies or typhus. Such unforeseen delays alone caused many researchers to abandon their experiments. Second, the Japanese scientists were fortunate in their choice of the rabbit as a test animal, for rabbits appear to be particularly sensitive to the effects on skin of this kind of carcinogen. It took three more years before the results of the coal tar experiments were confirmed.[4]

Another reason why work proceeded so slowly was that, in addition to the experimental difficulties in inducing cancer, scientists in the early 1920s didn't believe that cancer could even be caused by a particular chemical. The conventional wisdom of the day was rather that the tumors resulted from a generalized irritation of cells and tissues, irrespective of the identity of the agents causing the irritation.

During the 1930s, the experimental foundation of chemical carcinogenesis was firmly established by a research team led by Sir Ernest Kennaway at the Royal Cancer Hospital in London.[5] In a short period, his team demonstrated the carcinogenicity in mice of tars extracted from pitch and oils. They showed that the cancer-causing activity was greatest in the chemical fractions with the higher boiling points.[6] These chemicals, called polycyclic aromatic hydrocarbons, are found in cigarette smoke and air pollutants, and are the products of incomplete combustion of organic matter.

In their most dramatic experiment, the London researchers produced tumors by applying a pure synthetic chemical, dibenz[a,h]-anthracene, which was also known to be one of the many components of tar.[7] This was the first time it had ever been shown that an individual pure chemical, rather than a mixture such as coal tars, could cause cancer. Finally,

one of the group, J. H. Cook, proceeded to test various chemical fractions extracted from a pitch sample originally weighing two tons, and thereby identified benzo[a]pyrene, another powerful skin carcinogen and also a major component of tobacco smoke.[8]

About the same time, epidemiological studies in the United States and elsewhere were finding a clear relationship between the high incidence of bladder cancer among workers in the dye industry and their exposure to particular chemicals, such as benzidine and 2-naphthylamine.[9] In order to study the basic mechanisms involved here, it was logical to try to reproduce this disease in animals by exposing them to these dye chemicals. Not until 1938 was this successfully performed by the late Wilhelm C. Hueper, one of the great early pioneers of environmental and occupational carcinogenesis.[10] His good fortune was to have chosen the dog as the test subject, rather than the usual experimental animals, rodents. Dogs and humans have similar sensitivity to 2-naphthylamine, which induces bladder cancer in both, whereas rodents are relatively resistant to this carcinogen, and when cancers are induced they are found in organs other than the bladder.

From Mouse to Man

Unless we can relate the occurrence of cancer among other species of animals, however induced, to human cancers, the most elegant animal experiment will have been at best academic.

The legitimate inference that what is found to cause cancer in one species must also be assumed to cause cancer in others (known as the species-to-species extrapolation) is fundamental to cancer research. This inference rests on over half a century of intensive scientific investigation into the biology and chemistry of carcinogenesis and carcinogens in many organisms, including humans. Acceptance of the extrapolation principle is grounded in the fact that fundamental life processes in mammalian and other animals are basically the same as those in humans. Thus information on the origin of cancer drawn from observations of animal experiments can be applied, with appropriate reservations, to man. While the substance of these reservations has often been the source of intense controversy in specific instances, the basic fact that extrapolation is a reasonable undertaking is nearly universally accepted by biomedical researchers and is indeed fundamental to all experimental biology and modern medicine.

By the time a cancer has developed in a test animal, a great many events have taken place at the molecular, cellular, and organ levels. Also, a relatively long period of time, the latency period, has passed since the initiation of the cancer process. Cancer probably begins with a single identifiable event within a cell, such as the breakage of some critical genetic component of the cell by the carcinogen. While such events are probably frequent, and normally handled by cellular repair and detoxification mechanisms, in certain cases they may go unrepaired, and the cancer process begins. The cancer cells grow in an uncontrolled fashion, invade local tissues, and often spread (metastasize) to distant parts of the body.[11]

There are very striking similarities between cancer in humans and other living organisms with regard to the widest possible range of biological characteristics. Cancer is found in multicellular organisms, including insects, fish, and even plants. The probable reason for this is the essential similarity of their cellular ultrastructures, in particular their genetic structure and coding. Carcinogenic chemicals thus tend to be similarly active in many different test animals. However, there are often differences in the susceptibility of various animal species, in differing strains of any species, and in different individuals in any particular strain or sub-strain. Additionally, the target organ affected by the carcinogen may vary from species to species. Neverthe-

less, if a carcinogen is active in any one species, it is likely to also be active in others, including man.

The use of small mammalian animals, particularly mice and rats, has been and continues to be standard practice in routine carcinogenicity testing. Considerations of convenience apart, the key role of these rodents in carcinogenicity testing has been repeatedly endorsed by numerous expert committees and authorities, as illustrated by the following statement from the National Academy of Sciences in 1960:

> The rat and mouse have been shown to be susceptible to the carcinogenic action of a large variety of compounds and, indeed, most of our knowledge of chemical carcinogenesis is based on the use of these species. The hamster and guinea pig are relatively resistant to the carcinogenic action of several compounds which produce tumors readily in the rat and mouse. On the other hand, no known carcinogens for the hamster and guinea pig are inactive in the rat and mouse.[12]

It must be realized that the activity of many known human carcinogens was first recognized in rodent tests. These include 4-aminobiphenyl, bischloromethylether, aflatoxins, vinyl chloride, mustard gas, melphalan, and diethylstilbestrol. Conversely, all chemicals known to induce cancer in man, with the possible exception of arsenic, also do so in experimental animals, generally rodents.[13] In any one instance where a chemical is found to be carcinogenic in a proper animal test, there is no possible way in which absolute assurances can be given that the chemical will also be carcinogenic in humans. However, the general similarity in response to carcinogens of a very wide range of species, including humans, and also the good track record of animals as predictors of human response, afford strong reasons for accepting the results of well-conducted animal experiments as surrogates for human experience.

The predictive value to humans of carcinogenicity tests in mice has been repeatedly challenged by industry.* It has been claimed by Shell Chemical Company and other segments of the chemical industry that the mouse is an unsuitable animal for carcinogenicity testing of products such as pesticides because it is unusually sensitive and because it has a high incidence of spontaneous tumors. These criticisms have been particularly focused on the supposed unreliability of mouse liver tumors as an indication of response to carcinogenic chemicals.† There are just no scientific grounds for these allegations. On the basis of an extensive review of the literature on chemical carcinogenesis, Lorenzo Tomatis of the International Agency for Research on Cancer in Lyon, France, published recent studies which demonstrate that the results of carcinogenicity tests in mice are closely similar to and predictive of those in rats or other rodents.[14] Tomatis found that of fifty chemicals producing liver tumors in mice, all induced tumors of the liver or other organs when adequately tested in rats and hamsters.

A major deficiency in current carcinogenicity tests is their simplistic nature, dictated in part by practical considerations, such as testing the effects of one chemical at a time. Carcinogenicity tests thus do not adequately reflect the realities of multiple concurrent and sequential exposures to a wide range of carcinogens in the general environment and the workplace. Because of the relatively small numbers of animals that can be tested and the impossibility of predicting human sensitivity from animal tests, there is also substantive evidence of interactions between individual carcinogens making the carcinogens together much more potent than either separately. Also interactions between carcinogens and a wide range of noncarcinogenic chemicals may increase the potency of the carcinogens. For example, the incidence of liver cancers induced in trout by feeding as little as 0.4 parts per billion (ppb) of aflatoxin‡ is sharply increased by addition of various noncarcinogenic oils to the diet.[15] Similarly, the carcinogenic effects of low concentrations of benzo[a]pyrene on mouse skin are increased 1,000-fold by the use of the noncarcinogenic n-dodecane as a solvent.[16] Benzo-[a]pyrene and ferric oxide injected in the trachea of adult rodents induce a high incidence of lung tumors, only if the animals are pretreated at birth with a single low dose of another carcinogen, diethylnitrosamine. The quantitative response to a particular carcinogen can be substantially influenced by a wide range of factors, including interaction with other carcinogenic and noncarcinogenic chemicals. Thus, these so-called synergistic effects further confound attempts to find safe levels of carcinogens. Such interaction studies

---

* Few epidemiological studies have been undertaken for carcinogens found active in rodent tests, and industry sometimes equates this absence of epidemiological data with evidence of noncarcinogenicity in humans. Accordingly, industry argues that regulation should primarily, if not exclusively, be directed at those few carcinogens identified by human epidemiologic studies. A reductio ad absurdum of this position has been put forward by Vaun Newill, Medical Director of Exxon Corporation, in Cancer Bulletin 29 (1977): 177-78: "A regulatory program based on experimental screening models to evaluate new chemicals prior to their introduction into the environment, however, will hinder the better documentation of this correlation [between human and animal carcinogenicity data] than we have presently. When a carcinogen is prevented from entering the environment on the basis of screening results, there can be no data regarding that exposure in man."

† Those industries such as Shell which challenge the significance of the induction of cancers in test mice by their products continue to use the failure of other products to induce cancers in mice as proof of their safety.

‡ Allowable limits for aflatoxin contamination of milk and other foods are 0.5 and 20 parts per billion, respectively.

clearly confirm that threshold levels of carcinogens cannot possibly be predicted by calculations based on setting a dose arbitrarily lower than the lowest apparently carcinogenic animal dose in a particular experimental situation. Epidemiology has given important clues on interactive effects between carcinogens, such as smoking and asbestos or uranium, and between carcinogens and noncarcinogenic chemicals, such as arsenic and sulfur dioxide. There are now critical needs for large-scale interactive tests designed to elucidate such additive and synergistic interactions as they occur in daily life, particularly when suggested by epidemiological observations.

Principles of Animal Testing

Test Guidelines

The National Cancer Institute has recently published a set of specific recommended procedures for carcinogenicity testing in rodents.[17] Useful guidelines have existed since the early 1960s, but they are too general for current regulatory needs. As the results of more and more animal tests are now subject to public scrutiny, the proposed NCI guidelines will probably have an increasing influence on carcinogenicity testing.

There is now general acceptance of the need to conduct tests in accordance with accepted humanitarian principles.

Test Animals

Just as the chemist pulls a bottle of chemicals off the shelf and is assured of reasonably standard quality, so does the cancer biologist like to use particular species and strains of animals in which a reasonably standard response can be expected.[18] As noted above, the two species used more than any others are rats and mice. There are various strains of each species available, each with its own characteristic biological properties and sensitivities. There are some important advantages to using highly inbred rodent strains.

Their incidence of spontaneous cancers and of cancers following treatment with various chemical carcinogens is more predictable than is the case with random-bred animals. Additionally, strains can be selected that are either highly sensitive or highly resistant to certain classes of carcinogens.

On the other hand, as human populations represent a genetic smorgasbord, it is more likely that random-bred animals will give results more in line with expected human responses. A compromise, which is now currently favored, is to use a hybrid of two inbred strains which combines the advantages of predictable responses with genetic heterogeneity.

Routes of Tests

Among the many possible methods and routes by which a carcinogen can be administered to an animal are feeding, inhalation, and skin painting. The same carcinogen administered through different routes can produce cancer in either different or in the same organs; there is no way of predicting the type and site of response. The most common test route for tests of food additives and other dietary compounds is by incorporating the test substance in animal feed or administering it directly into the stomach by a tube (this process is called *gavage*). Feeding is also a standard test method for administering many other types of possible carcinogens. Feeding of test animals can be and is also used when the route of human exposure is by the skin or lungs, especially when there is a likelihood that cancers will result in internal organs, such as the liver or kidney.

When exposure on the human skin results in skin cancer (or is suspected to cause skin cancer), as in workers exposed to petroleum and shale oils, then skin painting in animals is the proper method to use. Skin painting, however, is not sufficiently sensitive for investigating carcinogenic effects of chemicals such as amine hair dyes and textile fire retardants, which are absorbed through the skin and induce cancers at distant sites.* A technical background statement in the NCI "Guidelines for Carcinogen Bioassay in Small Rodents" makes this clear:

> Although this type of test (skin painting) might provide useful information on some chemicals, it might be unreliable for measuring the effects of such chemicals on internal organs.[19]

If a chemical is suspected of causing lung cancer when inhaled by humans, the logical way of testing is by inhalation. However, inhalation studies are technically difficult and relatively expensive. They are also complicated by the fact that a rodent, unlike humans, can breathe only through its nose, filtering the chemical being tested through a highly developed defense system and possibly reducing its effects. Despite the obvious importance of inhalation as a major route of human exposure, particularly for air pollutants, industrial chemicals, pesticides, and cosmetics, relatively few chemicals have so far been adequately tested for carcinogenicity by long-term inhalation.[20]

Dosage

In well-designed tests, a range of doses is used. If the dose of a carcinogen is too low, few or no animals in the typically small test groups may get cancer. If it is too high, animals will die quickly from toxic effects of the chemical, well before cancer has had a chance to develop. To determine the proper dosage range for a carcinogenicity study, it is standard practice to perform preliminary toxicity tests to estimate the maximally tolerated dose (MTD). This is defined as the highest quantity or dose of a chemical that can be administered over the lifetime of an animal, during the course of a carcinogenicity test, without producing toxic effects, such as reduction in the life span or weight loss in excess of 10 percent of control animals, other than those directly resulting from the induction of cancers.† In well-designed studies, additional doses, based on one or more fractions of the MTD are also tested. The various dosages used in an experiment are usually expressed as so many milligrams (mg) of chemical per kilogram (kg) of animal body weight, mg/kg. This allows a comparison of the effects of equivalent doses in different animal species with different typical body weights. The duration and periodicity of the dose are also important. Some carcinogens will induce only a relatively low incidence of cancers when given in one large dose, but will produce a higher incidence when broken up into a series of intermittent and lower doses over the course of months.

Use of Relatively Large Dosages. Perhaps the aspect of cancer research most distorted by industry and misunderstood by the public is the necessity to use much larger doses of a substance being tested than humans could possibly be exposed to. The superficial absurdity of a rat consuming the human equivalent of about a thousand cans of diet soda per day from fetus to adulthood has been exploited by industry, misinterpreted by the press, and misunderstood by the lay public, which has come to believe that anything given in large enough doses will cause can-

---

* The insensitivity of skin painting is due to the fact that it is difficult to apply sufficiently high concentrations of test material by this route. For this reason, a positive result is all the more significant.

† Administration of a carcinogen at doses in excess of the MTD, resulting in toxicity and premature death, will generally result in a decreased tumor response (competing toxicity), and such tests cannot be accepted as valid evidence of noncarcinogenicity. Subject to qualified scientific consideration, however, carcinogenic effects induced by doses in excess of the MTD are acceptable.

cer in animals.‡ This simply is not true. The need for large dosages of chemicals (as the highest of a range of doses) in some experiments is a reflection of the facts (1) that some carcinogens are much less potent than others and (2) that animal experiments, no matter how well planned, must make use of finite animal resources. To illustrate this point, let us suppose that humans and rats are equally sensitive to some chemical carcinogen which causes one case of cancer in every 10,000 persons (or rats) to which it is given. If 220,000,000 Americans were exposed to this chemical, 22,000 cases of cancer would occur. On the other hand, if fed to the typical fifty rats used in an experiment, the chances that even one rat would get cancer is one-half of one percent; 10,000 rats would have to be fed the chemical (at human dosages) to observe even one cancer.[21]

Given that a human-level dosage might not produce a detectable result in a small rat population, even for a carcinogen which may be the cause of many thousands of cases in humans, the only alternative is to increase the dose, and thereby increase the probability of inducing a cancer in a particular animal. Once the dosage is increased above real-life levels, scientists must begin to make assumptions about their findings in the following vein. If the equivalent of, let us say, 1,000 cans of saccharin-containing soda per day produces one tumor in 50 rats, then it is plausible to assume that 100 cans will produce one-tenth as many tumors, or one tumor in 500 rats. Continuing the argument, the equivalent of 10 cans per day would produce one-tenth as many as before, that is, one tumor in 5,000 rats. Finally, one can per day would produce one tumor in 50,000 rats. If, as we assume, humans and rats are equally sensitive to this carcinogen, one can of soda per day would produce one tumor in 50,000 people, or about 4,000 cases of cancer in the nation's population.*

Two basic assumptions are involved in the above argument. First, as stated, we assumed humans to be as sensitive as rats. Of course, in any particular situation, humans may either be less sensitive or more sensitive than rodents to the toxic or carcinogenic effects of the chemicals in question. For example, the lowest dose of thalidomide inducing birth defects in pregnant women is 0.5 mg/kg/day; the corresponding values for the mouse, rat, and dog are 30, 50, and 100 mg/kg/day, respectively. Thus, humans are 60 times more sensitive than are mice to thalidomide, 100 times more sensitive than rats, and 200 times more sensitive than dogs.[22] Moreover, certain aromatic amines, such as 2-naphthylamine, are potent bladder carcinogens for man, monkeys, and dogs, but not for rats, mice, and other rodents, in which tumors at other sites are produced.[23] Hence there is no known method for predicting a safe human level or threshold for carcinogens on the basis of experimental animal data, if indeed such safe levels for humans exist at all.[24] Second, we assumed that equal proportions of tumors would occur at all dosages, known technically as a linear dose response extrapolation. This assumption is the least strong, because it is simply not practically verifiable by direct experimentation. As a conservative method for extrapolating animal data from high to low doses, however, it has become standard practice. By conservatism, we mean use of a mathematical method which errs, if at all, on the side of safety to humans. As former

---

‡ In addition to being carcinogenic at relatively high dose levels, saccharin is also carcinogenic in rats at doses in the diet extending down to 0.01 percent, equivalent to the amount of saccharin in one and one-half cans of diet soda.

* This argument has been simply explained in R. W. Rhein and L. Marion, *The Saccharin Controversy* (New York: Monarch Press, 1977), p. 58.

NCI Director Frank Rauscher, Jr., admitted to an American Enterprise Institute round-table on saccharin on April 21, 1977, "In protecting the public's health, there is no choice but to assume that the extrapolation is linear."

The justification for the conservative approach to the absence of a threshold for carcinogens or the inability to determine its existence rests largely on our ignorance of the nature of the lower ends of dose-response curves. There is, in fact, no evidence at all of the existence of thresholds for the irreversible processes involved in carcinogenesis. There is also no evidence of complete repair of DNA damaged by any carcinogen; any residual unrepaired DNA would perpetuate the carcinogenic hazard.†

Finding the Evidence

One of the most poorly conducted areas of animal cancer research is the identification of the cancer in the animals' bodies. The process of finding a cancer in the fresh carcass of a mouse or rat is different from the discovery of cancer in a human by a doctor. The rodent cannot complain of painful symptoms before death. Also, since carcinogens may cause cancer in any of a wide range of organs, the entire body of the animal must be meticulously searched. This is not possible if, through neglect or poor husbandry, the animal has been allowed to die and decompose before an adequate autopsy, as is often the case.

The Statistical Significance of the Evidence

The ideal experiment is one in which either the chemical being tested induces no tumors in the test group with none in controls, in which case the chemical is determined to be noncarcinogenic, or the chemical induces a high incidence of tumors in the test group with none in controls, in which case the chemical is determined to be carcinogenic. Unfortunately, the results are rarely this clear. Typically, the test animals have a certain percentage of tumors, which are considered to be induced, and the controls have a smaller percentage, which are considered to be spontaneous. It is then the job of the statistician to sort out the data and decide whether the difference in tumor yield between the test and control groups is statistically significant or simply due to chance. The statistician is also concerned with the time from the initial dose which elapses before the tumors appear, as not only do carcinogens increase the number of cancers in test animals in contrast with those occurring spontaneously in controls, but they also induce these cancers earlier in the life of the test animals. The statistician thus deals with four factors in a standard carcinogenicity test: the number of animals tested; the number of given types of cancers induced in each animal and in each test and control group; the time required to induce these cancers; and the number of tumors in both the test and control groups. Apart from the individual importance of each of these factors, their effects interact with each other statistically.

A critical factor in these tests is the number of animals tested. The greater the number of animals tested in each of the various dosage groups and in the control group, the

---

† Jerome Cornfield, in "Carcinogenic Risk Assessment," Science 198 (1977): 693-99, proposed a hypothetical model for carcinogenesis which in effect gives a threshold. Cornfield, however, stressed that his model is based on the assumption that all of a carcinogen below a given dose level, administered on a single occasion, could be inactivated instantaneously, by some unknown defense mechanism. The unverifiable and unrealistic nature of Cornfield's assumption invalidates his model. (C. C. Brown et al., "Models for Carcinogenic Risk Assessment," Science 202 [1978]: 1105.) Cornfield has, however, protested that only a "misreading" of his article could have led to the conclusion that he was proposing a threshold model (Science 202 [1978]: 1107-8).

more meaningful is any observed difference. A 20 percent tumor rate among the test group, compared to a 5 percent spontaneous rate among controls, unambiguously indicates a carcinogenic response in a group of 200 animals. But in a group of only 20 animals with the same exposure the difference between 20 percent and 5 percent is not statistically significant and the carcinogenic effects of the exposure cannot be established.

Short-Term Tests

Over the last two decades, some dozen or so short-term tests have been developed for predicting the carcinogenicity of chemicals by methods that, in contrast to conventional animal tests, are inexpensive and rapid, taking a few days or sometimes only a few hours.[25] Short-term tests are based on underlying chemical, physical, or biological properties that are shared, or rather are believed to be shared by carcinogens but not by noncarcinogens. The successive appearance of each short-term test has characteristically been initially greeted with uncritical enthusiasm. This becomes progressively dampened when subsequent studies on more extensive series of chemicals reveal poor correlations with carcinogenicity, at which stage the test gradually falls into more limited use or disuse. For this reason, there is now recognition that the utility of short-term tests must depend on their validation with large numbers of carcinogens and non-carcinogens from a wide range of different chemical classes.

The most recent short-term test was developed in 1975 by Bruce Ames.[26] In the initial validation of this test, about 90 percent of 174 carcinogens from selected chemical classes were shown to induce mutations in bacteria, while only 13 percent of a group of 108 non-carcinogenic chemicals were found to be mutagenic. Besides the rapidity and economy of the Ames test, an additional attraction is that it is based on the detection of types of genetic damage which are thought to be critically involved in the induction of cancer (somatic mutation theory). The test system utilizes bacteria, as indicators of mutagenic damage, combined with rodent liver homogenates to allow activation of the chemicals tested and thus approximate to the major types of metabolic transformations in the human body.

Since its introduction, the Ames test appeared promising and is now being widely used, particularly in conjunction with a battery of other short-term tests. Since it allows large numbers of chemicals to be screened rapidly, the pharmaceutical, pesticide, and other chemical industries are using it routinely in early development phases for screening chemicals for possible carcinogenic activity. Additional applications of the test include looking for carcinogens in complex, ill-defined organic mixtures such as extracts of air and water pollutants of hair dyes, and for carcinogenic metabolites in the urine or blood of workers with suspected exposure to occupational carcinogens. Presumptive evidence of carcinogenicity of several important industrial chemicals has been recently obtained with the Ames test, often in conjunction with a battery of short-term tests. These include the flame retardant Tris (manufactured by Velsicol Chemical Co.), hair dyes, and the Japanese food additive AF2 (furyl furamide).

Apart from responsible uses of the test, it has also been used by some segments of industry to argue that animal tests are too expensive, impractical, and unreliable and, in the absence of conclusive human epidemiological evidence of carcinogenicity, should be replaced by the Ames test. This would create a "no-lose" situation. A negative Ames test would be taken to exculpate any chemical from questions of carcinogenicity and to allow its marketing. Depending on economic considerations, a positive test could either be accepted or rejected in the full knowledge that regulatory agencies would be reluctant (and rightly so) to base regulatory actions exclusively on the results of tests in bacterial systems.

An example of misuse of the Ames test is afforded by the recent controversy surrounding the fire retardant, Fyrol FR-2, which is now used in some polyester children's sleepwear. During attempts to ban the carcinogenic Tris, Stauffer Chemical Company advertised and sold a substitute, Fyrol FR-2, claiming that it was inactive in the Ames test and therefore safe. Suspecting the claim to be in error, since Fyrol is similar to Tris in chemical structure, Fyrol was then independently tested and found to be Ames positive. This then led to the withdrawal of Fyrol which by then had found its way into approximately three million pairs of children's sleepwear (mainly those sold by J. C. Penney Co.).

Although short-term tests are now being widely and successfully used, they do have their limitations. First, several noncarcinogenic chemicals have been found to be mutagenic in one or more short-term tests (false positives). Second, they miss several important classes of carcinogens (false negatives).‡ In fact, about half of the carcinogens discussed in the case studies in this book are inactive in the Ames test. Additional false negatives include most heavy metals; many polycyclic aromatic hydrocarbons; steroids; azonaphthols; antimetabolites; some carcinogens activated by intestinal rather than liver enzymes, such as cycasin; carcinogens of the chloroform class, and major classes of carcinogenic organochlorine pesticides, such as DDT. Third, the correlation between mutagenic effects and carcinogenicity are not as good as 90 percent for every chemical class (particularly for carcinogens with complex metabolic routes). In a recent survey of 273 carcinogens of a wide range of different structures, an overall correlation with mutagenicity of 77 percent was found.[27] While for some classes of carcinogens, the correlation was shown to be excellent, it was poor in others. In fact, correlation was shown to be a function of the structural type of carcinogen selected for test. Fourth, the test has become more complicated as more types of liver activation systems have been introduced in attempts to decrease false negatives. Fifth, the test only picks up a genetic damage at the gene level, and cannot detect chromosomal mutations that are considered to be involved in cancer and other human diseases.* However, it is not clear whether there are many chemicals (other than possibly the drug Griseofulvin) that induce chromosomal but not gene mutations. Finally, recent studies with the carcinogen dimethylbenzanthracene have indicated that different types of molecular interactions with DNA are involved in its effects in the Ames test (using rat liver) and in its carcinogenic effects on the skin of mice.[28] (However, the ability of short-term tests to use activation systems from tissues of different species, including humans, may well be advantageous.)

It is now widely agreed that the Ames test, especially when compared with a battery of other such short-term tests based on mutagenicity, such as neoplastic transformation and DNA damage and repair, and on structure-activity relations have a range of useful applications.[29] A positive result in these tests with a chemical for which no carcinogenicity data are available is clearly a cause for concern, especially if potential human exposure is involved. However, a negative result cannot be taken as presumptive exculpation of carcinogenicity, unless the chemical be-

---

‡ In classic quality-control terminology, a false negative result represents a "consumer risk" (in that it underestimates risk to the consumer), and a false positive a "producer risk" (in that it overstates risk to the producer). Units of producer and consumer risk are not fixed and can be expressed in terms of duration of disease-free life or dollars, and the proper balance between these can be expected to vary according to particular circumstances.

* Furthermore, the Ames test detects only certain types of reverse mutations.

longs to a particular class for which strong correlations with carcinogenicity have already been established. For this reason, particularly, exclusive reliance on data from these tests seems unwise, especially for regulatory purposes. There is just no reliable substitute for animal carcinogenicity tests.

The Practicality of Animal Testing

The practicality of animal testing is often challenged by industry on the grounds that too many new chemicals are being introduced into commerce each year to be handled by conventional animal testing and that the cost of such testing would be prohibitive. In fact, this has been used as one of the main arguments for the need for short-term tests.[30] However, based on various recent estimates including those by the Council on Environmental Quality, it seems that the number of these new chemicals which actually reach commerce is under 700 annually. There is every reason to believe that current facilities could be expanded to cope without excessive strain with this number of chemicals. In addition, there are large potential facilities at the National Laboratories, such as Oak Ridge, Tennessee, and Argonne, Illinois, besides an underutilized facility at the National Center for Toxicological Research, in Arkansas. There seems every reason to believe that the NCI Bioassay Program, given high priority (particularly under its new direction by the National Toxicology Program), could increase its present efforts to handle 700 or so chemicals annually, rather than the 120 which the NCI projected for 1979.

With regard to expense, the annual costs of testing one chemical for carcinogenicity in groups of fifty mice and rats of each sex at two dose levels is under $300,000. Properly conducted carcinogenicity tests also provide information on a wide range of chronic toxic effects, including testicular damage leading to sterility, central nervous system damage leading to paralysis or behavioral changes, and damage to the liver leading to cirrhosis. The maximum $210 million costs for testing 700 chemicals would be unlikely to result in substantial increases in production and retail product costs.† These testing costs should be contrasted with chemical industry 1975 gross sales of $72 billion (of which they represent about 0.2 percent) and after-tax profits in excess of $5.5 billion.

The costs of testing should be further contrasted with the far greater costs of failure to test and regulate, including the majority of the $30 billion recognized annual costs of cancer due to preventable causes and the even greater costs of surveillance of workers exposed to occupational carcinogens. It is clear that the costs of failure to test and regulate are inflationary.

---

† Much of these costs could be redistributed through tax write-offs and price pass-throughs.

Industrial concerns are in general not particularly anxious to have the occurrence of occupational cancer among their employees or of environmental cancer among the consumers of their products made a matter of public records. Such publicity might reflect unfavorably upon their business activities and oblige them to undertake extensive and expensive technical and sanitary changes in their production methods and in the types of products manufactured. There is moreover, the distinct possibility of becoming involved in compensation suits. . . . It is therefore not an uncommon practice that some pressure is exerted by the parties financially interested in such matters to keep information on the occurrence of industrial cancer well under cover.

Wilhelm C. Hueper, the modern pioneer of
environmental and occupational carcinogenesis, 1943.

Chapter Four

Introduction to the Case Studies

In the next three chapters case studies on some twelve individual carcinogens or classes of carcinogens are examined.* These are grouped according to their site of greatest social impact: in the workplace (chapter 5), in consumer products (chapter 6), and in the general environment (chapter 7). While convenient, this grouping is somewhat artificial. Carcinogens such as asbestos, vinyl chloride, and benzene pose major hazards to the exposed work force. However, these same carcinogens also escape or are discharged into the air outside the plants where they are being processed or manufactured and can produce cancer and other disease in people living in the local community. While carcinogenic pesticides are widely recognized as environmental contaminants, they represent still greater hazards to workers engaged in their manufacture, formulation, and application. Concerns about carcinogens in consumer products, such as sex hormones used as drugs

and animal feed additives, have stimulated subsequent concerns about their role as occupational carcinogens.

While discussions of each substance are particular, all the case studies deal essentially with two basic sets of questions:

(1) *What do we know?* What are the patterns of manufacture and use of the product or process? What are the patterns of human exposure? What is the evidence of carcinogenicity from animal tests or epidemiological studies? What will be the economic and social impacts of regulation and of failure to regulate?

(2) *To what use has this information been put?* How has the affected industry reacted? What was the response of the regulating agency? What roles have public interest groups and organized labor taken? Also of concern are the roles of the Administration, Congress, courts, press, professional and scientific communities, and the nature of public perceptions.

---

* The case studies are generally based on information available up to April, 1979.

A few common themes will emerge throughout the case studies. Most of the information we have on the products and processes involved has come from industry itself, either through in-house technical staff or indirectly through commercial consultants and laboratories. Apart from their general poor quality, built into most industry-sponsored studies is a tendency to minimize risks and maximize benefits, and to emphasize the difficulties and costs of regulation. They may fail to ask the relevant questions to assess risks and benefits, and in doing so fail to undertake the necessary studies to answer them. Worse yet, the results are occasionally manipulated or even destroyed.

The most serious effect of this information bias is the inappropriate shift in the burden of proof from the private to the public sector. The consumer or worker who bears the risk from exposure to an untested or poorly tested product then must also bear the burden of raising questions about its safety or proving its dangers or of ensuring that the federal government proves its dangers.

The regulatory role of federal agencies is often complicated by inherent ambiguities and inconsistencies in the statutes under which they operate. Be that as it may, the major problem here is not one of inadequate laws but of unwillingness to enforce the law. The track record of federal agencies in regulating industry and in protecting workers and consumers from carcinogenic hazards reflects extreme laxness often compounded by undue responsiveness to special interests.

Over the last decade, many regulatory actions against carcinogens in the workplace, in consumer products, and in the environment have been developed only at the initiative of public interest groups or organized labor. The scientific community has been largely indifferent. The exceptions are the few independent professionals who have worked with public interest groups and labor, and a small but influential segment of the scientific community working closely with industry in efforts to impede or block attempts to regulate environmental and occupational carcinogens. Over two decades ago, President Eisenhower warned against the growing national threat of the military-industrial complex. The medical-industrial complex now appears to be as serious a threat.

'Tis a sordid profit that's accompanied by the destruction of health. . . . Many an artisan has looked at his craft as a means to support life and raise a family, but all he has got from it is some deadly disease, with the result that he has departed this life cursing the craft to which he has applied himself.

Bernardino Ramazzini, an Italian physician, considered the founder of occupational medicine, 1705.

Chapter Five

The Workplace: Case Studies

The total U.S. work force numbers approximately 100 million.* Various categories of workers are at high risk of exposure to carcinogens. These include approximately 670,000 workers in the petrochemical industry, 365,000 in metallic and non-metallic mining, and 1.1 million in the metal processing and smelting industries.[1] These figures do not reflect the extent of exposure to occupational carcinogens. Estimates by HEW in 1978 indicate that from 8-11 million workers have been exposed to asbestos since World War II. On the basis of a recent National Occupational Hazards Survey, the National Institute for Occupational Safety and Health (NIOSH) estimates that 880,000 workers are currently exposed to just those carcinogens or other toxic substances that are currently regulated by the Department of Labor's Occupational Safety and Health Administration (OSHA).[2] The range of industries involving exposure to occupational carcinogens is shown in Table 5.1.

In general, workers are denied knowledge of what chemicals they are exposed to, and in what concentrations.[3] They are also not in-

formed whether these have been adequately tested, whether they are toxic under conditions of exposure in the plant, or whether they are carcinogenic. This is in striking contrast to chemicals in consumer products, which must be tested in animals before they can be used, and for which there are labeling requirements, however imperfect.

The toxic and carcinogenic chemicals to which workers may be exposed at relatively high concentrations in the workplace also are discharged or escape into the air and water of the surrounding community. The worker may be exposed to the same chemical carcinogens through consumer products and the general environment as in his or her workplace.

What are the conditions of exposure to toxic and carcinogenic chemicals in the workplace and what precautions are taken to protect workers from such exposures? What is the role of government, industry, and the medical community in preventing and regulating such exposures? The British medical journal *Lancet* gives some answers to these questions in a recent editorial, "The Medical

---

* Of these, 41 million are women. The numbers of women in the work force are growing. In 1977, 48 percent of all U.S. women were in the work force, as opposed to 38 percent in 1960.

Table 5.1 Occupations Associated with an Excess Risk of Cancer

Site of Cancer	Carcinogen	Occupations
Liver	Arsenic, vinyl chloride	Tanners, smelters; vineyard workers; plastic workers
Nasal cavity and sinuses	Chromium, isopropyl oil, nickel, wood and leather dusts	Glass, pottery and linoleum workers; nickel smelters, mixers and roasters; electrolysis workers; wood, leather, and shoe workers
Lung	Arsenic, asbestos, chromium, coal products, iron oxide, mustard gas, nickel, petroleum, ionizing radiation, bischloromethyl-ether	Vintners; miners; asbestos users; textile users; insulation workers; tanners; smelters; glass and pottery workers; coal tar and pitch workers; iron foundry workers; electrolysis workers, retort workers; radiologists; radium dial painters; chemical workers
Bladder	Coal products, aromatic amines	Asphalt, coal tar, and pitch workers; gas stokers; still cleaners; dyestuffs users; rubber workers; textile dyers; paint manufacturers; leather and shoe workers
Bone marrow	Benzene, ionizing radiation	Benzene, explosives, and rubber cement workers; distillers; dye users; painters; radiologists

Source: P. Cole and M.B. Goldman, "Occupation," chapter 11 in J.F. Fraumeni, Jr., ed., *Persons at High Risk of Cancer* (New York: Academic Press, 1975), pp. 167-84.

Industrial Complex":

> Involved in this sinister complex are numerous big industrial manufacturing firms who are reluctant to believe that any product they use or manufacture, from asbestos insulation to benzidine or betanaphthylamine, can be harmful. The medical men and scientists directly employed by these firms are chiefly concerned with their employers' and their own profits, and are indifferent to the health of the exposed employees. Some of the firm's employers have, it is alleged, ignored even legal regulations and got away with it. Another alleged tack is for the firm singly or in combination with like firms, to set up supposedly independent research institutes whose scientists seem always to find evidence to support the stance taken by the firm, despite massive contrary evidence. Thus, when some high-sounding institute states that a compound is harmless or a process free of risk, it is wise to know whence the institute or the scientists who work there obtain their financial support. But there are Government agents, Federal and State, to enforce safety measures and draw up others, to see that regulations are in force, and to monitor dangerous processes. Alas, it seems that these people, too, are often involved in the medical/industrial complex, and are reluctant to enforce regulations, to emphasize risks to employees, or to see that measures are taken to warn or protect them against industrial hazards. They also seem, as individual contractors or as members of research organizations, to attract an undue proportion of Federal research grants.
>
> The indictment is a strong one, and is coupled with accounts of factories where employees work in fogs of asbestos dust and beryllium dust, or with beta-naphthylamine and benzidine slopped about. Ever greater numbers of employees are being recognized as suffering from pulmonary asbestosis, berylliosis, bladder and lung cancer, and mesotheliomas. The greatest danger, as far as the numbers exposed go, seems to be asbestos, and the carcinogenic properties of this material are creating general alarm. Large numbers of the general public are exposed to it through the drinking water in one city. The number of industrial hazards and of workers killed or injured by them seems to be increasing, and the public has reason to be worried. The industrial/medical complex is now required to answer the case, and as its credibility has been seriously impugned it had better be a clear answer.[4]

This chapter presents case studies on four substances: asbestos, vinyl chloride, bischloromethylether, and benzene. These are chosen to illustrate some fundamental problems of exposure to carcinogens in the workplace.[5]

Asbestos

Asbestos, known as the "magic mineral,"[1] has been used in one form or another for centuries, dating back to its first recorded use for pottery making in Finland some 4,500 years ago.† Virtually indestructible, it is highly resistant to fire, has high tensile strength, and its fibers can be spun into yarn and woven into cloth. The asbestos industry has grown phenomenally since the first North American asbestos mine opened in 1879 in Thetford, Quebec, with a first-year output of

---

† Asbestosis is a generic name for a group of naturally occurring fibrous mineral silicates, which consist of two major classes: serpentines, largely represented by chrysotile, a relatively pure magnesium silicate that comprises 90-95 percent of the world's asbestos production; and amphiboles, including five main types (actinolite, amosite, crocidolite, anthophyllite, and tremolite) in which the magnesium component is partially or wholly replaced by other cations. Chrysotile is often known as white asbestos, amosite as brown asbestos, and crocidolite as blue asbestos.

300 tons. Johns-Manville was founded in the United States in 1901 and is still the world's largest asbestos company, and Turner Brothers, still the largest British company, in 1916. World production of asbestos in 1920 was only 20,000 tons, about 0.5 percent of present levels (about 4.3 million tons). Of the present world output, 1.7 million tons are mined in Canada (and fabricated largely in the United States) and 2.5 million tons in the Soviet Union. At the heart of this booming industry is a research effort which has led to use of asbestos in cement, asphalt, wallboard, pipes, textiles, insulation, food and beverage processing, brake linings, and countless other everyday products.[2] It has also led to approximately 50,000 deaths per year in the United States from cancer and other diseases.[3]

Occupational Exposure

Occupational exposure to asbestos dust occurs in a wide range of operations from the mining and processing of the ore to its fabrication and use in many industries, particularly construction, shipbuilding, insulation, and textiles.

By 1918 enough was known about the dangers of asbestos to lead to the decision of U.S. and Canadian insurance companies to stop selling life policies to asbestos workers.[4] It was not until the early 1920s that descriptions of a new respiratory disease resulting from exposure to asbestos (asbestosis) first appeared in the medical literature. An often fatal disease, involving progressive scarring of the lungs and leading to respiratory disability and heart failure, asbestosis is akin to black lung and other chronic chest diseases (pneumoconioses) which afflict miners and processors of various kinds of minerals and fibers. In England, where it was first studied and reported in the medical literature, asbestosis was covered under Compensation laws in 1931, after which some efforts were made to improve working conditions and reduce exposure to asbestos dust.[5]

By the 1930s, based on numerous case reports of asbestosis and lung cancer occurring together in asbestos workers, scientists began to suspect that asbestos is carcinogenic. But no full-scale studies were made on asbestos plant workers until the 1950s, when the British epidemiologist Richard Doll investigated employees with at least twenty years exposure in an asbestos textile plant. Doll found that this group experiences ten times the lung cancer deaths of non-asbestos workers of the same age.[6]

Also during the 1950s, Irving Selikoff, now a leading occupational epidemiologist at Mt. Sinai Hospital in New York City, noted that fifteen of seventeen of his patients employed at Union Asbestos and Rubber Company in Paterson, New Jersey, had developed asbestos-related lung disease. By the early 1960s, the disease incidence was climbing at an alarming rate, prompting Selikoff to inquire into the employment records of workers in this and other asbestos plants. After being refused this information by industry, he contacted the New York and New Jersey locals of the International Association of Heat and Frost Insulators and Asbestos Workers, the union representing many of the men. Selikoff then conducted a cohort study based on all men belonging to those locals who had been employed in the asbestos industry over a particular length of time. Starting with 632 workers listed on the union rolls in 1943, he inquired into their fates, checking how many had died and the cause on each death certificate. This type of study is ordinarily difficult because it involves tracing the whereabouts of a worker twenty years after employment in a particular job. In this case the union had kept fairly detailed records of work histories. The union also administered the death benefits for its members, who as retirees had good reason to keep in touch right up to the time of their deaths.

By 1973, 444 of the original 632 workers were dead.[7] Table 5.2 is an epidemiological analysis which shows the number who had died of various causes, compared with the number who would have been expected to die of each cause.‡

Table 5.2 shows that by 1973 this cohort of workers had experienced a death rate 50 percent greater than the average white male. Among these "excess" deaths, lung cancer by far exceeded the expected experience of such a group of men by a factor of seven. The rate of all cancers combined was four times as great for these men, and there were thirty-five cases of mesothelioma, which for non-asbestos workers should not have occurred at all.* Finally, even the rates of cancer of stomach, colon, and rectum were more than three times that expected.

Conditions at the Johns-Manville plant in Scarborough, Ontario, give further insight on conditions of occupational exposure to asbestos. This plant opened in 1946 for the manufacture of asbestos and silica cement pipes and fiberglass insulation. Within a few months, men were working without respirators in dust that was so thick that they could not see more than a few yards ahead of them.† Even after a new ventilation system was installed in 1952, counts of 50 million fibers per cubic meter (m³) of air persisted in some areas. Selikoff visited Scarborough in the mid-1960s and predicted a high incidence of cancer deaths in the coming decade. Management

Table 5.2 Causes of Death in 444 Asbestos Workers

Cause of All Deaths	Number of Deaths, 1943-1973		
	Expected	Observed	Ratio (observed/ expected)
Total deaths, all causes	300.65	444	1.48
Cancer — all sites	51.26	198	3.86
Lung cancer	11.68	89	7.62
Pleural mesothelioma	0	10	. . .
Peritoneal mesothelioma	0	25	. . .
Cancer of stomach	5.10	18	3.53
Cancer of colon-rectum	7.50	22	2.93
Asbestosis	0	37	. . .
All other causes	249.39	209	0.84

Source: I. J. Selikoff and E.C. Hammond, "Multiple Risk Factors in Environmental Cancer," chapter 28 in J.F. Fraumeni, Jr., ed., *Persons at High Risk of Cancer* (New York: Academic Press, 1975), pp. 467-83.

‡ The ratio of observed to expected numbers of deaths is the *standard mortality ratio*. The larger this ratio is than 1, the more likely it is that a particular occupational exposure was the cause of death.
* Mesothelioma is a form of cancer of the lungs (pleural mesothelioma) or abdomen (peritoneal mesothelioma). It should be noted that deaths from

pleural mesothelioma are reported as lung cancer deaths in cancer mortality records (based on the International List of Causes of Disease) and can thus be falsely attributed to smoking rather than asbestos.
† Dust counts were probably about 80 million fibers per cubic meter (m3) of air.

dismissed these concerns as alarmist, and made little attempt to improve working conditions. Since then, over fifty workers of a total work force of approximately 500 have been disabled by chronic respiratory diseases and there have been twenty-seven deaths from lung cancer.

Regulation of Occupational Exposure

The ultimate acceptance of the carcinogenicity of asbestos has not been easily achieved. Even today, the controversy persists, but now the questions are not "whether" but "how much" and "what type." The importance of this issue is directly related to the vast economic stake which industry has in winning its battle with the government over the standard regulating levels of exposure to asbestos in the workplace.

When OSHA began hearings in 1972, the industry fought strenuously against any reduction in permissible exposure levels on the alleged grounds that the dangers of asbestos were minimal.[8] The basis for the industry case was strongly argued by academic consultants, some from medical schools or schools of public health, some of whose research and publications were supported directly or indirectly by grants or funds from the industry or industry-financed foundations.[9]

Regulatory standards for asbestos are based on the number of fibers in a unit volume of air.[10] The current OSHA standard is 2 fibers per cubic centimeter or 2 million fibers per cubic meter, over an eight-hour working day.[11] In the course of an average day, a worker inhales about 8 cubic meters of air, equivalent to an allowed inhalation of 16 million asbestos fibers. Even where the standard is met, total exposure levels are much higher. Current optical microscopic techniques for counting fibers in the workplace only detect those which are relatively long, more than 5 microns in length. Smaller fibers, or fibrils, which can only be counted by electron microscopy and not by optical microscopy, may outnumber the longer ones by as much as 100 to 1.‡ Thus, occupational exposure to asbestos at currently regulated levels of 2 million fibers, may result in the daily inhalation of as many as 1.6 billion short fibers. It should be recognized that these are believed to be more carcinogenic than the long fibers. It should finally be recognized that there are critical needs for the development of practical and sensitive methods for monitoring of total asbestos fibers, both long and short, in the air breathed by exposed workers.

The key issue in the 1972 OSHA hearings was the proposal by NIOSH to lower the then temporary exposure standard of 5 million asbestos fibers per cubic meter of air to 2 million fibers, the 1969 British standard. This lower standard, however, was primarily designed to protect just against asbestosis, without any consideration of the cancer problem.* The asbestos industry argued at the hearings that the 5 million standard exposure level did not cause much disease, and that to lower it further would create severe economic dislocation and unemployment. In spite of the threat of job losses, organized labor fought strongly for the improved standard, pointing out that asbestos is a major health hazard not only for asbestos workers, but also for workers in many other chemical and manufacturing industries which use asbestos in many forms.

---

‡ Asbestos counts in the workplace are invariably counted by optical microscopy and hence reported as fibers per cubic meter of air. In contrast, electron microscopy is the only practical technique for measuring public exposure in the general environment, and these counts of fibrils and fibers are translated into mass and reported in nanograms rather than counts per cubic meter.
* Later, the British standard was subsequently shown by U.S. investigators to be inadequate for protection against asbestosis, let alone against lung cancer.

The involvement of the asbestos industry in health research, and its propagandizing of the public is long-standing. While the asbestos industry takes some pro forma precautions in the open scientific forum, these are not apparent in its public relations literature. Some good examples of this can be found in a recent publication by the Quebec Asbestos Mining Association (QAMA) of a bilingual pamphlet, "Asbestos and Your Health."

Can a little bit of asbestos kill you? No — long-term medical studies of workers who are exposed to asbestos show that low to moderate levels of exposure do not lead to an increased rate of disease. In these studies, a higher-than-normal incidence of disease was found only among employees exposed to extremely high asbestos concentrations for long periods of time.

Note the deliberate omission of the word "cancer." Also, the statement is simply false. Short term and low-level exposures are known to cause disease.

The lung's normal cleaning mechanisms quickly remove the majority of inhaled particles, including respirable-sized asbestos fibers.

On the contrary, the majority of fibers either remain in the lung or move to the gut, where it is suspected they contribute to the development of cancer of the gastrointestinal tract.

Some cases still occur among long-service employees whose exposure began at a time when little was known of the amount of asbestos a human could tolerate . . . . With expanding medical knowledge and today's improved dust control measures, however, there is every reason to believe that these cases will decrease in the future and asbestos-related disease will cease to be an occupational problem.

The controls which industry fought for at the OSHA hearings were sufficient to cause levels of disease among New York insulation workers at which 20 percent died of lung cancer, 10 percent of gastrointestinal cancer, 10 percent of mesotheliomas, 10 percent of other cancer, and 10 percent of asbestosis.

Over the past decade, industry has also supported major scientific studies at McGill University in Montreal, by the Industrial Health Foundation in Pittsburgh and by Tabershaw-Cooper Associates on the West Coast, all of which have minimized the danger of working with asbestos. One of the most controversial of these studies, involving more than 11,000 employees and ex-employees of Quebec asbestos mines, was carried out by J. Corbett McDonald, then in the Department of Epidemiology and Public Health at McGill. In presenting his results to the OSHA hearing officers, McDonald introduced himself as a full-time employee at McGill University, and an independent research worker.

I do not work, nor am I associated with any asbestos producer or manufacturer. The research I shall be describing is supported by grants, not to me but to McGill University, from a number of sources — the Institute of Occupational and Environmental Health, the Canadian government, the British Medical Research Council, and the USPHS [U.S. Public Health Service].[12]

However, anyone glancing at his paper, published in 1971 in the Archives of Environmental Health, would have noticed, in the customary small typeface at the end of the text, the acknowledgment:

This work was undertaken with the assistance of a grant from the Institute of Occupational and Environmental Health of the Quebec Asbestos Mining Association.[13]

McDonald made several claims on the basis of his study. First, he maintained that "the findings suggest that our cohort of workers in the chrysotile [a kind of asbestos] mining industry had a lower mortality than the population of Quebec of the same age." Second, he claimed that while indeed some workers did seem to get more lung cancer than others the "excess" cancer deaths were confined to those workers who had been much more heavily exposed than the rest. Lastly, he concluded that "these findings strongly suggest . . . that chrysotile is less likely to cause malignant disease of the lung and pleura than other forms of asbestos, such as crocidolite."

Criticism came swiftly from independent scientists in the United States. Major objections were directed not only at the overall design of the study, but at the statistical analysis of the data as well. McDonald had selected a method for computing death rates which seemed to ignore the long latency period of lung cancer. This resulted in an underestimate of the excess deaths which occurred among men with a long duration of employment.[14] Faced with mounting criticism and complaining that his "life had been made hell," McDonald resigned his position at McGill.[15] Taking his asbestos-cancer research funds, including continuing support from the National Cancer Institute (NCI),[16] he returned to England, where the London School of Hygiene and Tropical Medicine appointed him to the Trade Union Congress Chair of Occupational Medicine.

Another illustration of the industry position was afforded when a recent NIOSH study demonstrated an increased risk for lung cancer and other lung diseases among South Dakota gold miners exposed to asbestos dust levels even lower than the 2 million fiber standard proposed by NIOSH in 1972.[17] A sharp response from Paul Kotin, the medical director and senior vice president of Johns-Manville, the world's largest

asbestos manufacturer, was subsequently circulated in attempts to minimize the impact of these findings and to persuade the safety of exposure to levels of 2 million fibers.†[18] The NIOSH group prepared a rebuttal which defended their original analysis and demanded:

Why should it surprise Drs. Kotin and Chase that asbestos at concentrations less than 2 million fibers per cubic meter is associated with excessive risk of respiratory cancer? Indeed, it is known that asbestos fibers have been previously demonstrated to be carcinogenic to man at all fiber concentrations studied under adequate epidemiologic method.[19]

On December 15, 1976, John F. Finklea, as Director of NIOSH, communicated with Morton Corn, then Assistant Secretary of Labor for OSHA, pointing out that the 1969 British 2 million fiber standard, which had been the basis of the 1972 proposed NIOSH standard, had since been shown to be excessively high and should be reduced. Finklea referred to studies on exposures as low as 250,000 fibers per cubic meter, at which workers had twice the likelihood of the general population of dying from lung cancer or asbestosis. Finklea further proposed that the standard should be lowered to a maximum of 100,000 fibers. NIOSH clearly recognized that even this proposed lower standard did not represent a safe exposure level. Finklea finally stated:

Because it is not possible to specify a safe exposure level for a carcinogen, only a ban on the use of asbestos can ensure complete protection against this mineral's carcinogenic effect. Therefore, emphasis should be placed on prohibiting the occupational

---

† These and other current positions on chemical carcinogenesis are in striking contrast to views expressed by Kotin when in government employ in 1970 (see Appendix II), and in even more striking contrast to his testimony at the Mirex cancellation proceedings (FIFRA Docket 293, EPA, November, 1973).

use of asbestos in other than completely closed operations and on substituting other products whenever possible. Asbestos should be replaced where technically feasible, by substitutes with the lowest possible chronic toxicities.[20]

NIOSH also pointed out that all forms of asbestos, including chrysotile, amosite, crocidolite, and tremolite, can induce asbestosis and also cancer.

The OSHA standard still rests at 2 million fibers, twenty times in excess of the level that NIOSH now recommends. The stance of industry in fighting even the unsatisfactory OSHA standard is further illustrated by the record of R. T. Vanderbilt Company, Norwalk, Connecticut, which owns a number of talc mines in upstate New York and Vermont.[21] Shortly after OSHA promulgated its 1972 standard, R. T. Vanderbilt belatedly realized that the high asbestos content of its talc threatened its market, as several purchasers of its products had been advised by NIOSH to switch to other, safer materials. Vanderbilt, realizing it had missed its legal chance to comment on the regulations before they became law, put pressure on Congressmen Robert McEwen (R-N.Y.) and Jerry Pettis (R-Cal.) to help out. On June 20, 1973, McEwen wrote OSHA Secretary John Stender, "Should these mines be forced to close, you can readily understand that it would have a serious and adverse economic effect in that area."[22]

Over the objection of his own Health Standards Chief, Standards Director Gerald Scannell encouraged Vanderbilt in December, 1973, to do its own sampling to determine whether or not their talc contained asbestos, and to advise their customers of the results of the tests. Vanderbilt took the hint and immediately redefined tremolite so as to exclude its classification as asbestos, even though it is clearly defined as such in the legal standard. Vanderbilt then notified its customers "that our talc products used in their manufacturing processes are not subject to the asbestos standard."

The illegality of this procedure came to a head after an OSHA inspector cited a Vanderbilt customer, Borg-Warner, for a violation of the asbestos standard on July 9, 1974. This involved a material purchased from Vanderbilt, Nytal, which was accompanied by "self-certification" that it contained no asbestos. The case went to the Occupational Safety and Health Review Commission, the highest arbiter of OSHA cases. On June 28, 1976, Judge Jerry W. Mitchell, ruled against the company.[23] In the lengthy interim, OSHA issued a field directive supporting Vanderbilt's claim that its talc was asbestos-free, but failed to order its field operatives to enforce the directive.

The seriousness of this evasion is emphasized by the results of a NIOSH epidemiological investigation on workers at Vanderbilt's mines. This identified "both respiratory diseases and lung cancers which appear to be significantly above those expected."

Smoking and
Occupational Exposure

Many epidemiological studies have indicated that asbestos workers who smoke have a much greater lung cancer risk than asbestos workers who don't smoke. Industry has argued that these studies prove that smoking and not asbestos is the real problem for asbestos workers, and that the development of lung cancer in these workers was their own fault for smoking. However, recent studies, including one by NIOSH in 1977, indicate that the smoking effect is less clear-cut than earlier reports suggested, and that nonsmoking asbestos workers also have excess risks of lung cancer.[24] Additionally, smoking is unrelated to the risks of developing mesotheliomas which occur with equal and increased frequency among smoking and nonsmoking asbestos workers.

The Asbestos "Pentagon Papers"

A new era in the history of asbestos has dawned with the discovery of a voluminous set of industry documents dating back from 1933 to 1945, dubbed the Asbestos Pentagon Papers.[25] These were obtained during pre-trial discovery proceedings in recently proliferating product liability suits against the asbestos industry. The documents (which were publicly released in San Francisco at the October, 1978, hearings of the Subcommittee on Compensation, Health and Safety of the House Committee on Education and Welfare) include correspondence among senior executives, lawyers, physicians, consultants, and insurance companies of Johns-Manville, Raybestos-Manhattan Inc., and other asbestos industries. According to South Carolina Circuit Court Judge James Price, the only judge to have reviewed the correspondence so far, "it shows a pattern of denial and disease and attempts at suppression of information" that is so persuasive that he ordered a new trial for the family of a dead insulation worker whose earlier claim had been dismissed. Judge Price noted that the correspondence "further reflects a conscious effort by the industry in the 1930s to downplay, or arguably suppress, the dissemination of information to employees and the public for fear of promotion of lawsuits." Judge Price also recognized compensation disease claims filed by asbestos insulation workers against several companies, which quietly settled them, including eleven asbestosis cases settled by Johns-Manville in 1933 to keep them out of a New Jersey court, "all predating the time (1964) when these companies alleged they first recognized the hazard to insulators." Judge Price concluded that settlement of these claims "constitute compelling proof of actual notice to certain manufacturers that asbestos-containing thermal insulation products indeed caused disease in insulation workers."

The Asbestos Pentagon Papers afford unusual and detailed insight as to the mechanics of suppression and distortion by industry of information on the hazards of asbestos, as illustrated in the following series of incidents. By 1932, the British had fully documented the occupational hazard of asbestos dust inhalation.[26] On September 25, 1935, the editor of the trade journal *Asbestos* wrote Sumner Simpson, President of Raybestos-Manhattan, requesting permission to publish an article on the hazards of asbestos, and referred to the magazine's past acquiescence to the American industry's desires that this dirty linen not be publicly aired.

Always you have requested that for certain obvious reasons we publish nothing and naturally your wishes have been respected. . . . [However] discussion of it [the alleged asbestos hazard] in *Asbestos* along the right lines would serve to combat the rather undesirable publicity given to it in current newspapers.

While Simpson was unpersuaded, in a letter (October 1, 1935) to Vandivar Brown, Secretary of Johns-Manville, he praised the magazine for "not reprinting the English articles," and observed that "the less said about asbestos the better off we are . . ." Brown agreed and suggested that if an article on asbestosis had to be published, it should reflect "American data rather than English."

The American data referred to was a study by Anthony Lanza on behalf of Raybestos-Manhattan, Johns-Manville, and the Metropolitan Life Insurance Company, the insurance carrier for both manufacturers. The Lanza study, based on X-rays of 126 workers with three or more years asbestos exposure, was begun in 1929 and completed in late 1931, but the results remained unpublished until 1935.[27]

Brown's confidence in the American (Lanza) data was well founded, as he and other industry officials and lawyers were to serve in an editorial capacity prior to its publication. Lanza submitted his galley proofs to Brown on December 7, 1934. Brown returned the galleys on December 10, 1934, commenting that Lanza had omitted from his final draft a sentence that had appeared in an earlier draft: "Clinically from this study, it [asbestosis] appeared to be of a type milder than silicosis." Hobart, Johns-Manville's New Jersey attorney, further explained in a letter to Brown (December 5, 1934) why Johns-Manville needed to portray asbestosis as a disease milder than silicosis. Referring to pending Workmen's Compensation legislation in New Jersey, Hobart stated that Johns-Manville opposed the inclusion of asbestosis as a compensable disease.

> It would be very helpful to have an official report to show that there is a substantial difference between asbestosis and silicosis: and by the same token, it would be troublesome if an official report should appear from which the conclusion might be drawn that there is very little, if any difference, between the two diseases.

On December 21, 1934, Brown forwarded Hobart's suggestions to Lanza and asked that "all of the favorable aspects of the survey be included and that none of the unfavorable be unintentionally pictured in darker tones than the comments justify." Lanza agreed, and in his eventual publication concluded that asbestosis was milder than silicosis. Presumably in the further spirit of cooperation, Lanza omitted reference in his paper to the findings that 67 of the 126 workers (53 percent) he had examined were suffering from asbestosis.

Seeking ammunition for courtroom use "against ambulance chasing attorneys and unscrupulous doctors" (memorandum Brown, January, 1933), Simpson wrote F. H. Schulter, President of Thermoid Rubber Co., on November 10, 1936, suggesting that several manufacturers jointly fund asbestos experiments at Saranac Laboratories (Trudeau Institute). Simpson allowed that the benefactors "could determine from time to time after the findings are made whether we wish any publication or not." The decision to publish, of course, being a function of the nature of the results of the study. "It would be a good idea to distribute the information to the medical fraternity, providing it is of the right type and would not injure our companies."

Conferences between industry and Saranac representatives culminated in a deal being struck whereby certain experiments would be conducted, with the decision whether or not to publish the scientific results resting entirely with the sponsors. In a letter of November 20, 1936, Brown emphasized to Leroy Gardner of the Saranac Laboratories:

> It is our further understanding that the results obtained will be considered the property of those who are advancing the required funds, who will determine whether, to what extent and in what manner they shall be made public. In the event it is deemed desirable that the results be made public, the manuscript of your study will be submitted to us for approval prior to publication.

In a reply to Brown on November 23, 1936, Gardner agreed to accept the industry sponsors as the sole arbiters of publication of the results of the experiments. "The Saranac Laboratories agree that the results of these studies shall become the property of the contributors and that the manuscripts of any reports shall be submitted for approval of the contributors before publication." Even this arrangement was not watertight. On learning that Gardner was presenting papers which referred to his preliminary asbestos findings, Simpson complained to Brown (letter May 4, 1939): "The reports may be so favorable to us that they would cause us no trouble, but they might be just the opposite which could be very embarrassing."

In a survey of a Johns-Manville Canadian

plant in which seven workers were found to have asbestosis, the medical director, Kenneth W. Smith, deemed it inadvisable that the workers should be warned of their peril.[28]

It must be remembered that although these men have the X-ray evidence of asbestosis, they are working today and definitely are not disabled from asbestosis. They have not been told of this diagnosis, for it is felt that as long as the man feels well, is happy at home and at work, and his physical condition remains good, nothing should be said. When he becomes disabled and sick, then the diagnosis should be made and the claim submitted by the Company. The fibrosis of this disease is irreversible and permanent so that eventually compensation will be paid to each of these men. But as long as the man is not disabled, it is felt that he should not be told of his condition so that he can live and work in peace and the Company can benefit by his many years of experience. Should the man be told of his condition today there is a very definite possibility that he would become mentally and physically ill, simply through the knowledge that he has asbestosis.

The Johns-Manville policy of refusing to advise workers of early evidence of asbestosis was characterized in a sworn statement on January 11, 1978, by Wilbur Ruff, a former plant manager, as a "hush-hush policy" and one that persisted until the late 1960s.

The mid-1950s found the asbestos industry embroiled in Workmen's Compensation litigation with asbestos workers who were lung cancer victims. The escalating cancer claims moved Smith in March, 1956, to request the Asbestos Textile Institute retain the Industrial Health Foundation to conduct a cancer study which would enable industry to "procure information which would combat current derogatory literature." Smith suggested an alliance with the Quebec Asbestos Mining Association (QAMA) which was con-

ducting a similar study. After agonizing over this proposal for over four years, the Asbestos Textile Institute finally rejected it in March, 1957, for the following reasons:

(1) QAMA has a similar program;
(2) There is a feeling among certain members that such an investigation would stir up a hornets' nest and put the whole industry under suspicion.
(3) We do not believe there is enough evidence of cancer or asbestosis in this industry to warrant this survey.

Perhaps the most graphic illustration of the corporate mores of Johns-Manville comes from the testimony of Smith before he died in 1977. In response as to whether he had ever advised Johns-Manville officials to place warning labels on asbestos containing insulation products, Smith replied:[29]

The reasons why the caution labels were not implemented immediately, it was a business decision as far as I could understand. Here was a recommendation, the corporation is in business to make, to provide jobs for people and make money for stockholders and they had to take into consideration the effects of everything they did, and if the application of a caution label identifying a product as hazardous would cut out sales, there would be serious financial implications. And the powers that be had to make some effort to judge the necessity of the label vs. the consequences of placing the label on the product.

In June, 1963, Institute members obtained copies of Selikoff's cancer study of insulation workers,[30] (as described in Institute minutes of June 6, 1963, and October 8, 1964) and braced itself for the 1964 New York Academy of Sciences Symposia on Asbestos by discussing the retention of a "public relations man to get accurate publicity to the public."[31] In minutes of a February 4, 1971, General Meeting of the Institute, an industry medical consultant labelled Selikoff a "dangerous man." To the question as to whether the American Medical Association might be able to control Selikoff, the consultant replied that "pressure" on Selikoff's hospital, Mt. Sinai, might be "effective."[32]

In a report of September 23, 1963, by Thomas Mancuso to Phillip Carey Manufacturing Co., he emphasized that the asbestos-cancer relationship was beyond dispute, and that the company should warn all concerned.

> Internally within the company the question has been raised as to why medical problems, particularly relating to cancer and asbestos were not recognized before. Actually, they were recognized, but the asbestos industry chose to ignore and deny their existence.

Phillip Carey responded by declining to renew Mancuso's contract, and failing to warn its workers and customers.

Legal Impact. These documents are likely to affect more than 1,000 asbestos-related lawsuits, totalling more than $1 billion and involving more than one hundred different law firms all over the nation. Ronald Motley, a South Carolina attorney, who is informally directing these actions, has established an "Asbestos Litigation Group" for the purpose of disseminating information and coordinating this extensive litigation. While most plaintiffs have worked with asbestos for over thirty years, others include spouses who have contracted mesotheliomas from washing asbestos-laden clothes of workers, and a case involving Franklin Brooks, a former Georgia Tech All-American football player, who developed asbestosis although only exposed for three consecutive summers. The largest lawsuit to date was filed in Los Angeles in October, 1978, on behalf of five hundred present and former workers who contracted various asbestos-induced diseases at Todd Pacific Shipyards in San Pedro and the Long Beach Naval Shipyard. The suit asks for general and punitive damages, besides medical expenses and loss of earnings.

In the typical product liability or third-party insulator case (of which Borel v. Fibreboard Paper Products Co., 493 F.2d 1076 [5th Circ. 1973] is precedential), there are often as many as ten defendants because the average worker has used products from that many different companies, such as Johns-Manville, Raybestos-Manhattan, Owens-Corning Fiberglas Co., Celotex, Pittsburgh-Corning Co., and Standard Asbestos Manufacturing and Insulating. Of pivotal importance is the question of whether the companies concerned knew about the hazards of asbestos products prior to the 1964 report by Selikoff on the high incidence of lung cancer, mesothelioma, and asbestosis in insulation workers,[33] when they claimed they were first made aware of this, and what use if any they then made of this information. The primary defense in such cases is that there was no medical or scientific information on risks from asbestos-containing products prior to 1964. Additional lines of defense include statute of limitation exemptions, "contributory negligence" of workers, and their smoking. Johns-Manville's Kotin has been able to persuade the courts in four of five cases in which he has so far testified, that the pre-1964 studies were not definitive, thus absolving the industry from the need to have labelled their products and to have issued warnings. The asbestos "Pentagon Papers" are likely to diminish both the vigor of such arguments and the likelihood of their future success.‡

In September, 1978, at hearings before the Senate Human Resources subcommittee on labor on S.3060 (a bill designed to provide comprehensive reform of workers compensation programs including extended use of

---

‡ In spite of these revelations, Johns-Manville devoted six of the fifty-two pages in its April, 1979, annual report to castigating the news media for its "sensationalized coverage" of asbestos-related

product liability suits to compensate workers or their heirs), Johns-Manville expressed the view that product liability suits were inadequate and inefficient methods of compensation. As an alternative, Johns-Manville proposed that government and labor join with industry to defray the costs of workers compensation through the creation at a state level of a "second injury fund" an alternative that industry, in general, is now vigorously supporting.

Public Exposure

In 1960 an alarming report came from J.C. Wagner in South Africa of sixteen new cases of the rare mesothelioma.[34] While six of these were in asbestos mine workers, none of the other ten had ever worked in the mines. All had lived in the vicinity of the mines, though, many as children. Public or non-occupational mesotheliomas have since been reported from nine other countries, including the United States. These cases are generally thought to be due to exposure of family members to asbestos brought home on the clothes of asbestos workers. Additional sources of exposure include contamination of the air with asbestos from nearby plants or factories. High concentrations of asbestos fibers have recently been demonstrated in communities adjacent to asbestos industries.

The indestructibility of asbestos, its indiscriminate use, and the careless disposal of its waste products make it difficult to predict the extent and level of exposure of the general public. For instance, Certain-Teed Products Corporation, an asbestos-cement pipe manufacturer, has in the past dumped about 2,700 tons each year of crushed asbestos pipe in an open-air landfill site in Ambler, Pennsylvania.

The dump not only snakes diagonally

through the very center of the town, which has a population of 8,000, but it is fifty feet high, anywhere from one to two city blocks wide, and about ten city blocks long. In fact, it is estimated to contain some million and a half cubic yards of waste material . . . Kids play on an asphalt basketball court that has been built smack on top of material from the dump, and is literally covered with loose asbestos fiber and wads of waste material containing (chrysotile) asbestos.[35]

Drinking water is an additional possible source of non-occupational exposure to asbestos. Reserve Mining Company, a subsidiary of Armco and Republic Steel, for years has been dumping taconite mine wastes, rich in asbestos fibers, into Lake Superior at levels of about 67,000 tons a day. Not unreasonably, this gave rise to fears that polluting the drinking water of Great Lakes communities with asbestos would lead to excess cancer rates, especially of the stomach and colon.[36]

In April, 1974, Federal District Judge Miles Lord issued an injunction in Duluth, Minnesota, restraining the Reserve Mining Company from further dumping its taconite mine wastes into Lake Superior. Reserve Mining witnesses attempted to prevent this ruling by testifying that there were no alternatives to this lake dumping, although it appears that the company had developed plans for land disposal sites as early as 1970.

It is not yet known whether the resulting asbestos contamination of drinking water of Lake Superior towns, including Duluth, will lead to cancer. Preliminary studies with laboratory animals have so far yielded ambiguous results. Certainly, it has been established that persons occupationally exposed to asbestos have an increased risk of alimentary tract

---

health problems, which reflected "a very apparent antibusiness bias." In the following month Johns-Manville threatened Congressman George Miller (D-Calif.) with a libel suit if he repeated

outside Congress statements he had made charging the industry with decades of "cover-up and lies" and failing to disclose the other workers' information on compensation settlements.

cancer* as well as lung cancer. Without waiting for answers to these questions, a Federal Appeals Court reversed Judge Lord's decision, on grounds that it was not based on adequate proof of risks to health, and permitted Reserve Mining to resume dumping its tailings into the lake, pending the development of alternate land disposal sites.

In May, 1975, Congress approved $4 million to build a water treatment plant in Duluth to filter out the asbestos fibers from drinking water. The State of Minnesota appropriated $2.5 million in local funds for the project, which became operative in November, 1976. Reserve Mining is now phasing out lake dumping, and is building a land disposal site, in accordance with a court order that dumping is to be terminated by 1980.[37]

In addition to environmental exposure to asbestos in air and water, the general public receives a wide range of further exposures.[38] Particularly important sources are construction operations involving the spraying of asbestos, the use of crushed stone containing unbound asbestos in roads and driveways, and demolition. Exposure to asbestos also results from its use in fireproofing and insulation, air ducts, automobile brake linings, cement water pipes, filter pads for beers, wine, and drugs, cosmetic talcs, and hand-held hair dryers. Resulting levels of public exposure can be high. For example, counts of 10 million fibers per cubic meter of air have been found in the vicinity of construction sites during asbestos spraying, and counts of 3 million fibers have been found in public buildings, and schools treated with asbestos as a fire retardant.†[39]

Regulation of Public Exposures

In an ineffective attempt to protect the general public from asbestos air pollution, EPA developed an emission standard for asbestos as a hazardous air pollutant in April, 1973. The standard, however, is only based on visible emissions and on poorly enforced work practices, and not on asbestos fibril counts.‡

Acting on a petition from a public interest group, the Natural Resources Defense Council, the Consumer Product Safety Commission announced in December, 1977, that patching and spackling compounds containing asbestos would be banned from the $400 million market by June, 1978. Under the commission's order, fifty manufacturers ceased production in January, 1978, leaving retailers the next six months to clear their shelves. While these patching compounds are used primarily by professional builders, about 10 percent of the market is for home hobbyists and craftsmen.

The Future

Realization is gradually dawning that except under the most restrictive conditions all forms of asbestos have become too expensive

---

* These include pharynx, esophagus, stomach, colon and rectum cancers.

† In May, 1979, the House Education and Labor Committee voted to establish a three-year, $330 million program to detect and remove asbestos material from schools, where it had been widely used for soundproof ceilings and insulation from about 1960 to 1973, when its use was banned. Under heavy lobbying, the Committee voted against levying the industry for a $30 million detection fund, but directed the Justice Department to investigate whether the government "should or could" sue the industry to recover all or part of the costs. Johns-Manville, which supplied the asbestos to the manufacturers and construction industries, contends that levels in schools are too low to cause cancer. Also in May, 1979, Gloria Zwerdling, a former school teacher, filed a $2.5 million suit in Manhattan Supreme Court against fourteen corporations including Johns-Manville, claiming that she had contracted lung cancer from asbestos insulation used in schools.

‡ The only effective method of measuring community exposure to asbestos is by counting fibrils using electron microscopy, which in fact is rarely done. Results are expressed as a mass in nanograms per cubic meter.

in terms of human disease for commercial use. Further illustration of this are the individual and class action suits for asbestos cancer and disease, in the multimillion-dollar range now being filed by some of the four and one-half million workers employed in Naval shipbuilding yards during World War II.

The Navy has since abandoned the use of asbestos in shipbuilding in favor of alternative materials, including fiberglass. However, there are also reasons for concern on the use of fiberglass as an asbestos replacement. Experimental studies indicate that fiberglass, particularly the more modern short-fiber products which were introduced into large-scale use in the early 1960s, may produce a type of disease and cancer similar to that produced by asbestos.[40] Epidemiological studies are now only suggestive of an increased cancer risk, probably because exposed workers have not been followed up for the three or so decades it generally takes for asbestos fibers to induce cancer. Industry is attempting to quiet these concerns in moves which reflect the growing shift from asbestos to fiberglass for insulation and a wide range of consumer products, including draperies. An interesting insight into such tactics was afforded by a recent letter to New Times by Johns-Manville's Kotin, bearing no reference at all to his industry employment, protesting that "epidemiological studies show that there is no chronic health effect in humans as a result of exposure to fibrous glass."[41]

Apart from fiberglass, other possible replacements for certain asbestos applications include long inorganic fibers made from aluminum or zirconium, such as those manufactured by Imperial Chemical Industries of England.

Another area of growing concern relates to the emerging trend in the asbestos industry to relocate in lesser developed countries, such as Mexico and Taiwan, where their capital investment is welcomed and not restricted by governmental health and safety regulations.[42]

On April 26, 1978, HEW Secretary Joseph Califano issued the most explicit warning ever made by government on the dangers of asbestos. Califano estimated that as many as half of all workers exposed to asbestos could develop serious diseases such as cancer of the lung and gastrointestinal tract, mesotheliomas, and asbestosis. Califano also estimated that from 8 to 11 million workers may have been exposed to asbestos since the start of World War II. Besides urging exposed workers to have a chest X-ray, HEW has sent a "physician advisory" letter regarding the dangers of asbestos to the nation's 400,000 doctors.* While Califano properly stressed the added danger of smoking to asbestos workers, an impression of "blaming the victim" appears to have been created by the absence of any balancing reference to the more urgent needs for control of exposures in the workplace.

Califano's statement appears to have been prompted by the growing number of lawsuits filed against federal agencies for having failed to notify workers in the past of the known hazards of asbestos exposure.† As such, Califano's statement is also important for what it failed to say. Workers were not informed of their rights to sue the government. Nor were any plans announced for organization of a surveillance program, including con-

---

* The gravity of the Califano statement has been underlined by preliminary findings in May, 1978, of lung abnormalities in 59 percent of 360 workers in northern California shipyards, and by the subsequent report that of 6,640 workers who handled asbestos products for over seventeen years at the Long Beach Naval Shipyard, 31 percent are now suffering from asbestosis. In spite of Califano's warnings, as of January, 1979, neither NCI, NIOSH, nor any other agency has yet developed plans for the surveillance and examination of the millions of asbestos workers at risk.
† So far, about 1,000 asbestos law suits have been filed and some 500 asbestos workers have collected $20 million in damages, including $5 million from the federal government.

tacting and examining former government workers. Nor was any mention made of the long overdue need to implement the recommendation of NIOSH for a 100,000 fiber standard as the only meaningful way to protect against asbestos-induced cancers and disease. Finally, no mention was made of the growing evidence of the hazards to the public-at-large, particularly those living in the vicinity of asbestos plants, quite apart from exposures due to asbestos containing consumer products.‡

In spite of all the problems of omission and emphasis in the Califano statement, its significance is epochal and unique. It opens the door of national health care policies to preventive medicine. Specifically, the statement recognizes in principle that prospective surveillance is needed for groups at high risk of cancer, although how this will be achieved for asbestos workers is still unclear. It is likely that the high costs of surveillance may well act as future incentives to reduce risks of occupational exposure to carcinogenic and other highly toxic agents, forcing the ultimate realization that prevention is cheaper than "cure."

Summary

While the dangers of asbestos have been well recognized for over five decades, the industry was able to largely ignore or suppress these until studies in the 1950s by Doll in England and by Selikoff in the U.S. (sponsored by the asbestos insulators union) established the relationship between asbestos and asbestosis and cancers at various sites. Since then the industry has employed scientific expertise to advocate its position in professional journals and to successfully resist and prevent effective government regulations. With an estimated 8 to 11 million workers

having been exposed since World War II, the toll of asbestos occupational disease and cancer is now reaching epidemic proportions. Workers have begun to exercise legal initiatives, including third-party and medical malpractice suits, resulting in multimillion dollar awards.

Concerns are also mounting on the dangers to the public from "low-level" asbestos contamination of air and water and from asbestos-containing consumer products such as hair dryers.

As the realization is dawning that asbestos is too expensive in terms of disease and death to continue using, the industry is beginning to develop the strategies of relocating in lesser developed countries and promoting the use of fiberglass as an asbestos substitute in the United States. There are serious unresolved questions as to the dangers of fiberglass and there are possibilities that it may be no less hazardous than asbestos.

The massive human toll taken by asbestos is probably the single most important incentive to the development of coherent national policies recognizing preventive medicine as a major future component in the delivery of health care.

Vinyl Chloride

One of the most common pejoratives applied to modern times is "the plastic age." And just as age-old natural materials like wood, glass, and metal have been replaced by cheaper synthetic plastics, this seems to imply, so has the value of our lifestyle been degraded. Many things we now touch or use daily are made of plastic. Yet the plastic transformation of our society has only taken place over the last forty years. The consequences to society of its plasticization, in terms both

---

‡ Effective regulation of the countless asbestos-containing consumer and industrial products must necessitate complete inventorying and material balance audits of all asbestos imported, mined, processed, and fabricated in the U.S.

of high energy and health costs, have only recently been appreciated. One of the major costs is from cancer.[1]

Manufacture

Plastics are the leading product of the modern petrochemical industry. This era of plastics dawned in the 1930s with the realization that petroleum was the cheapest and simplest starting material for the synthesis of the vast array of organic chemicals now used by modern industry. Petroleum then gradually replaced coal, which had been previously used for this purpose, and is now almost the exclusive basis of the organic chemical industry.

Vinyl chloride (VC) lies at the heart of the plastics industry. VC was first discovered in 1837. Large-scale production, however, did not start until the 1930s, when it was synthesized from chlorine and ethylene, largely for the manufacture of synthetic rubber.[2] Production levels increased rapidly after World War II at a rate of 15 percent per year, reaching a total of about 7 billion pounds this year.

VC is a simple chemical consisting of a small single molecular unit (a *monomer*) which is normally a gas but can be shipped and stored as a liquid under pressure. VC reacts under conditions of heat and pressure and in the presence of plasticizing chemicals to form large molecular chains (*polymers*) of polyvinyl chloride (PVC) resins. The polymerization of the VC monomer never proceeds to completion, but always leaves some unreacted VC entrapped in the PVC resin. Depending on the production process, this unreacted VC has concentrations ranging as high as 8,000 parts per million (ppm).[3] This residual VC can be dissolved out of the polymer or released by heating it.[4]

PVC resins are molded, injected, and extruded in the fabrication of a wide array of plastic products. These include phonograph records, wire and cable insulation, floor coverings, garden hose, furniture, upholstery fabrics, car bodies, coating of fabrics and wallpaper, containers, bottles, and food wrappings. It is difficult to get an accurate count of the number of U.S. workers involved in all the various stages of PVC production. There are about seventeen VC manufacturing plants, employing about a thousand workers, and forty PVC plants, employing about six thousand workers.[5] There are no figures available, however, on the number of fabricating plants or on the number of their employees. These must run into the hundreds of thousands.

Suppression by the Industry of Data on the Carcinogenicity of Vinyl Chloride

In May, 1970, an Italian toxicologist, Pier Luigi Viola (employed by Solvar Manufacturing Corporation), reported at an international cancer congress in Houston, Texas, that long-term intermittent exposure of a small group of rats to 3 percent of VC in air (30,000 ppm) resulted in the production of cancers in a wide range of organs.[6]

This first report on the carcinogenicity of VC created little impact because Viola had claimed that the type of tumors induced were peculiar to rats and without human significance, and also because of the very high levels of VC to which the rats were exposed. In fact, Viola had induced tumors at much lower concentrations, extending down to less than 5,000 ppm. These facts were discussed in detail at a Manufacturing Chemists Association meeting in November, 1971, where it was concluded that they should not be published, as this would otherwise "lead to serious problems with regard to the vinyl chloride monomer and resin industry . . . and force an industrial upheaval via new laws or strict interpretation of pollution and occupational health laws."[7] Union Carbide further expressed its concerns that in view of the large stake it had in "areas most likely to be affected, such as food, food packaging, fiber and aerosols [it] would be seriously hurt by arbitrary or panic-induced government restrictions."

Prior to this, there had apparently been no studies in the plastics industry on the possible carcinogenicity of VC, although tens of thousands of workers the world over had been exposed to it for over three decades and at least seven fatal cases of liver cancer had occurred in VC/PVC workers prior to 1970.[8] Disturbed by Viola's public report, a consortium of giant European chemical industries, led by Italy's semi-governmental Montedison, and with contributions from British, Belgian, and French firms, financed a major study initiated in July, 1971, by Cesare Maltoni of the Bologna Cancer Institute.*[9] An extensive series of tests were conducted in which adult, infant, and pregnant mice, rats, and hamsters were exposed to VC in inhalation chambers at concentrations ranging from the relatively low 50 ppm level to the toxic 100,000 ppm (10 percent) level. By late 1972, Maltoni had confirmed and extended Viola's results. VC was shown to be a potent carcinogen, inducing a rare type of liver cancer (called angiosarcoma), as well as more common liver cancers (hepatomas) and cancers of other organs, including kidney, brain, and lung. The cancers were subsequently found even at the lowest level then tested, 50 ppm. The overall tumor incidence was concentration-dependent, with higher doses increasing the incidence and rate of development of the cancers.[10]

In October, 1972, the Manufacturing Chemists Association, the major trade association of the U.S. chemical industry, entered into an agreement with the European consortium to share their information, but not to disclose it without prior consent.[11] In January, 1973, the U.S. industry representatives visited Maltoni and were given full details of his experimental studies. The Manufacturing

Chemists Association (and Maltoni) subsequently failed to disclose this information, in spite of the fact that NIOSH, in the same month, had publicly requested all available data on the toxic effects of VC. In March, 1973, the Manufacturing Chemists Association recommended to NIOSH a precautionary label for VC that made no reference to toxic or carcinogenic effects on animals or humans.

Four months later, however, representatives of the Manufacturing Chemists Association met in secret with Marcus Key, then Director of NIOSH and now Professor of Occupational Medicine at the University of Texas, Houston, and a small group of his senior staff. They were informed that Maltoni had induced tumors in rats exposed to VC levels of 250 ppm. At one stage of the meeting, an industry representative, V. K. Rowe of Dow Chemical Company, adjourned to a separate office for a private meeting with Key.[12] Rowe subsequently commented that "this private discussion of the carcinogen problem was worth the whole effort." Finally, industry concluded that as a result of a meeting "the chances of precipitous action by NIOSH on VC was materially lessened. NIOSH did not appear to want to alienate a cooperative industry or they did not want to know too much unpublished data."

In March, 1973, following complaints of an unpleasant taste, Schenley Distillers found 10-20 ppm levels of VC in their liquors sold in PVC bottles. On the basis of these findings, and still knowing nothing about the carcinogenicity data, FDA then banned the use of these liquor bottles. In December, 1973, the Society of Plastics Industry, the plastics industry trade association, provided the FDA with data on migration of VC from PVC containers to food,

---

* An additional reason for initiating these tests, revealed by Maltoni in 1975, was his hitherto undisclosed finding in 1969 of malignant cells (of a large cell adenocarcinomatous type not seen in smokers) in the sputum of VC/PVC workers, suggestive of early lung cancer or precancerous changes.

but made no reference to problems of carcinogenicity.

On January 22, 1974, B. F. Goodrich announced that since 1971 three PVC workers in their Louisville, Kentucky, plant had died of angiosarcoma of the liver. On that same day, the Manufacturing Chemists Association revealed the by now fifteen-month-old Maltoni data to NIOSH.

According to a recent special committee report of the American Association for Advancement of Science, the Manufacturing Chemists Association "appears to have deliberately deceived NIOSH regarding the true facts. . . . Because of the suppression of these data, tens of thousands of workers were exposed without warning, for perhaps some two years, to toxic concentrations of vinyl chloride."[13]

Distortion by the Industry of Data on the Carcinogenicity of Vinyl Chloride

The first published case reports of angiosarcoma of the liver in VC/PVC workers generated an intensive epidemiological investigation of cancer mortality in the industry in several countries. A British Petroleum Corporation study, published in Lancet in 1975, claimed that the longer one worked in a VC plant, the less was the risk of getting cancer.[14] Closer examination by NIOSH, however, questioned the interpretation of the English data. Expected death rates in workers exposed to VC for fifteen or more years were artificially reduced, and rates in workers with lesser exposures were artificially inflated. Re-analysis of the data by NIOSH, using standard methods, showed a clear excess of mortality from all causes and all cancers, including digestive system and lung cancers, besides angiosarcoma of the liver (Table 5.3).

Exaggeration by the Industry of the Costs of Regulating Occupational Exposure to Vinyl Chloride

As information on the carcinogenicity of VC began to surface, OSHA was prodded into action. On April 5, 1974, OSHA reduced permissible exposure levels from 500 ppm to a new emergency standard of 50 ppm. Under pressure from labor and independent scientists, who insisted that the new standard was too high for safety, on May 10, 1974, OSHA proposed a VC standard "at no detectable level" (in the range of 0 to 1 ppm) to be achieved by the use of engineering controls, rather than worker use of respirators. Faced with strenuous industry opposition and alarming economic impact analyses, OSHA did not proceed to adopt this standard, but on October 4, 1978, instead issued the more lenient final 1 ppm standard.[15] Even at that time, however, it had been shown that exposure of small numbers of rats to 5 ppm VC induced an increased incidence of cancer, and there was no evidence then (or now) of any safe exposure level for VC, or indeed to any other carcinogen.†

Nevertheless, industry objected strongly to the "no detectable level" proposal on the grounds that it was unnecessary, too expensive, and beyond their compliance capability. To bolster these claims, contracts were given out by the Society of the Plastics Industry, Inc. to Arthur D. Little, Inc., of Cambridge, Massachusetts. Also, OSHA gave out a contract to Foster D. Snell, a division of Booz, Allen and Hamilton, for the purpose of estimating the economic impact of the new standard. The consulting firms predicted costs as high as $90 billion and losses up to 2.2 million jobs, persuasive arguments in the depressed economic climate of 1974. However, these estimates were shown by the subsequent experience of the plastics industry to

---

† Later studies by Maltoni and others demonstrated carcinogenic effects, including breast cancer, in rodents following inhalation of VC at levels as low as 1 ppm.

Table 5.3 Comparison of Causes of Death in VC Workers Reported by British Petroleum (BP) and Recalculated by NIOSH

Cause of Death, Reported by BP and Recalculated by NIOSH	Standard Mortality Ratios* for Workers Exposed to VC for Varying Times		
	Years of Exposure		
	9 or less	10-14	15 or more
All causes			
BP	112	107	61
NIOSH	79	137	353
All cancers			
BP	123	58	73
NIOSH	86	76	428
Digestive system cancer			
BP	106	47	121
NIOSH	75	62	702
Lung cancer			
BP	129	101	62
NIOSH	90	133	366

Source: J. K. Wagoner, P. F. Infante, and R. Saracci, "Vinyl Chloride and Mortality." *Lancet* 2 (1975): 194-95.
* Values greater than 100 indicate excessive deaths relative to expected population values.

be gross exaggerations.[16] In spite of massive industry lobbying and pressures, OSHA stood firm on the new 1 ppm standard, which was passed on April 1, 1975.

The Society of the Plastics Industry then petitioned the 2nd Circuit Court of Appeals to review the 1 ppm final OSHA standard stating:

The evidence clearly demonstrates that the Standard is simply beyond the compliance of the industry. . . . The general increase in raw materials costs (an unavoidable result of this Standard), and the costs of monitoring, respiratory protection, medical surveillance and record keeping all militate against the likelihood that the bulk of this segment of the industry would be able to survive economically. The evidence is clear (that these various industries) would at the very least suffer economic disaster if not close down completely.

Within one year, the VC/PVC manufacturing industry had successfully met the new standard, and without any major economic dislocation or plant shutdowns. B. F. Goodrich, one of the industry giants, redesigned its manufacturing technology to enclose VC manufacturing and handling processes and plug possible sources of leaks. Additionally, a "stripping" process was developed to reduce levels of the unreacted VC monomer in the PVC resin and to decrease VC loss in the process. The initial capital costs of the compliance technology were only $34 million. Contrary to the estimates of the industry consulting firms, B. F. Goodrich found that the new cleanup technology actually cut labor costs and could be profitably leased. (In spite of this, B. F. Goodrich increased the price of its PVC products in 1976, claiming higher production costs and blaming these on regulatory standards.) The experience of Union Carbide is similar. In late 1975, R. N. Wheeler, a senior technical official expressed surprise as to how unexpectedly easy it had been for his company to comply with the 1 ppm standard. However, earlier intercompany reports had documented the economic advantages of compliance through recovering and recycling VC which would have otherwise been discharged into the environment. Estimates of the economic impact of compliance had ignored the major costs to industry from losses of VC gas, with resulting air pollution of the plant and adjacent community. They had also ignored or discounted the major costs to society, both direct and indirect, from failure to regulate, with resulting VC-induced disease. Finally, these estimates did not reflect the emergence of a small and booming industry manufacturing the monitoring equipment now required to meet OSHA regulations.

It is clear that, despite uniform and overwhelming protestations and prophecies to the contrary, the industry had no major difficulty in meeting the 1 ppm standard. It is also clear that the industry is flourishing with high production, strong demand, growing capacity, and steady prices. The slump in the PVC market in 1974 and 1975, reflecting the 1973 oil embargo and a general pattern of recession, has been replaced by a boom, well recognized in chemical trade publications since 1976. (See for instance, Chemical and Engineering News, July 24, 1978, p. 12, and September 4, 1978, p. 13.)

Cancer and Other Diseases Due to Vinyl Chloride

Long before the 1974 reports of angiosarcoma in VC/PVC workers, VC was known to be toxic to experimental animals and to humans at relatively high concentrations. Studies on experimental animals in the early 1960s, by Dow Chemical Company and others, established that VC induced toxic effects in the liver and kidney at concentrations as low as 500 ppm, then the U.S. occupational standard.[17] At higher levels skin and bone abnormalities were also noted.

Acute toxic effects, such as headaches, disorientation, dizziness, drowsiness, and loss of consciousness had been noted in VC/PVC workers as long ago as 1949.[18] In the same year, the Russian scientific literature reported the occurrence of chronic gastritis, hepatitis, and skin lesions from VC exposure. In 1957 there appeared the first report of a new occupational disease among vinyl plastic workers called acroosteolysis, characterized by a thickening or clubbing of the fingers and toes, spasmodic contraction of the blood vessels, painful bone changes, and arthritis of the knuckles. Additional cases of acroosteolysis have since been noted from plastic plants all over the world. By 1966, it was recognized that liver damage, hepatitis and cirrhosis, was common among VC/PVC workers and in some cases occurred after only one or two years of employment.

Since 1974, seven independent retrospective epidemiological studies have identified over seventy deaths from angiosarcoma of the liver in VC/PVC plants in the United States and elsewhere.‡ While most have involved polymerization workers, others have occurred in workers exposed to lower concentrations of VC, including four cases in PVC fabricating plants, where PVC levels were probably

---

‡ At least seven fatal cases of primary carcinoma of the liver, subsequently diagnosed as angiosarcoma, had been recognized in VC/PVC workers before 1970. Six of these cases occurred in the United States between 1961 and 1968, and the other in Sweden.

below 10 ppm. Cancers at various other sites including the lung, brain, kidney, and digestive tract, besides lymphomas and leukemias, have also been found in VC/PVC workers.* The lung cancers were mainly of a type (adenocarcinoma and undifferentiated large-cell) not generally associated with smoking, and were found in workers engaged in a wide range of VC/PVC operations, including PVC milling and packaging. While the occupational exposures preceding these various cancers have generally ranged from thirteen to twenty years, there have been four reports of liver angiosarcoma following less than six years of exposure. The true incidence of VC/PVC cancers in exposed workers is still unknown, because of considerations of latency, and also because of the ever-increasing number of cancers reported in organs other than the liver, which can no longer be considered the exclusive or even predominant site of VC/PVC-induced cancers.[19] It should be noted that the wide range of VC cancers found in workers is, in general, similar to the types and distribution of cancers induced in animal tests.

Despite the growing evidence of chronic human disease and the many thousands of workers at risk worldwide, the industry failed for more than thirty years to undertake any carcinogenicity tests in animals. Such tests could as easily have detected the carcinogenic effects of VC in the 1940s as they eventually did in the 1970s.

There are still elements of the academic community who minimize the risks of VC exposure. A recent brochure from the University of Louisville's Vinyl Chloride Project, a multimillion dollar NCI-funded program for the prevention and detection of VC-induced occupational cancer and other diseases, states:

The low incidence of cancer development among people with prolonged exposure to vinyl chloride is a reflection of the body's ability to remove the chemical agent safely without developing cancer. Some individuals do not have this capability and develop cancer after years of exposure.[20]

The brochure makes no reference to the fact that the present apparent "low incidence of [VC] cancer" may simply reflect its long latency period. Additionally, the independence of this University project has been questioned following recent disclosure of its receipt of undisclosed support from the Manufacturing Chemists Association.†

Cancer and Other Diseases Due to PVC

While in the past concerns have focused on VC itself as the major toxic and carcinogenic agent to VC/PVC workers, there is growing realization of other serious hazards posed by PVC dust to far greater numbers of workers in operations involving the packaging and milling of PVC, and its fabrication into innumerable plastic products. These hazards most probably reflect the presence of unreacted VC entrapped at concentrations up to about 1 percent (10,000 ppm) in the PVC resin or products, and which can be released by their beating or processing, or can be dissolved from inhaled PVC dust by tissue fluids. Additionally, VC gas can be absorbed on PVC or on other dusts which may act as inert carriers.

Experimental studies have shown that inhalation of PVC dust or its instillation into the lungs of rodents can induce acute inflammation followed by chronic granulomatous changes. Similarly, a wide range of abnor-

---

* An excessive incidence of brain tumors (glio-bastoma multiforme) has been noted among VC workers in Union Carbide and Monsanto plants in Texas City, Texas, and is now being investigated by OSHA and NIOSH. There have been ten deaths from the brain tumor among workers at the Carbide plant since 1962.

† This was admitted at an NCI site visit meeting at the University of Louisville on September 26 and 27, 1977.

malities has been recognized in the lungs of workers exposed to PVC dust in a variety of operations involving bagging and packaging of PVC resins and their fabrication of PVC products, where dust levels have been found to range as high as 20 mg/m^3, and where the dust may be so fine that most is inhaled deep into the lungs. The lung abnormalities reported include reduction of lung function, radiological changes, and chronic lung disease (pneumoconiosis). "Meat-wrapper's asthma" is a possibly related problem well recognized among supermarket and wholesale meat workers who, in packaging cuts of meat, use a "hot wire" or "cool rod" to cut and seal the sheet of Saran Wrap‡ or other PVC plastic film used for wrapping.[21] In the cutting process, particularly when high temperatures are used, irritant fumes, including hydrochloric acid, are given off. While the industry has readily ascribed the asthma to such irritants, it is not yet known whether there are any carcinogenic hazards posed by unreacted VC, or other related carcinogenic agents, such as vinylidene chloride, which may be liberated from the plastic film by the heat cutting.

More ominous than the inflammatory lung changes, an excess frequency of cancer deaths has been reported in four retrospective epidemiological studies of workers predominantly exposed to PVC dust.[22] These include lung cancer (of the same type as described in VC workers), and cancers of the urinary tract, digestive system, and lymphatic system.

Public Exposure to Vinyl Chloride

The public and the regulatory agencies are now beginning to realize that what goes on in a plant often affects the health of those living nearby in the community. The closer you live to a plant manufacturing VC or PVC or fabricating PVC products, the more VC you

are likely to breathe. EPA has estimated that 4.6 million people live within five miles of VC/PVC plants.[23] No estimates are available for the presumably greater number of people living near the uncounted PVC fabricating plants scattered over the country. Measurements by EPA in 1974 and 1975 indicated that in 90 percent of cases, VC levels in the vicinity of VC/PVC plants were below 1 ppm; EPA estimated that average exposure within a five-mile radius would be about 17 parts per billion (ppb). Higher levels, however, were found in 10 percent of communities sampled — 33 ppm at a distance of one-third of a mile from the center of one plant.

EPA also estimated that VC/PVC plants were losing 220 million pounds of VC into the air annually, mainly from PVC plants. These considerations, together with reports of excess birth defects in Ohio women living near VC/PVC plants, prompted EPA in October, 1976, to propose regulating VC as a "hazardous air pollutant" and to limit plant emissions to 10 ppm. These regulations would be expected to reduce VC emissions by about 95 percent of previous levels and to reduce community exposure by a similar amount. However, no regulations have yet been developed for plants fabricating PVC products nor for municipal incinerators, which discharge VC into the air from thermal processing and combustion of plastic products, respectively.

The results of a June, 1977, EPA investigation of an elementary school in Saugus, California, located across the road from Keysor-Century Corporation, which manufactures PVC and phonograph records, are disturbing.[24] Levels as high as 2.8 ppm VC have been measured in the air in classrooms. This heavy contamination largely results from VC losses during tank car unloading at the plant in the night.

---

‡ Saran Wrap, a product of Dow Chemical, is a co-polymer of VC and the related vinylidene chloride, which has recently also been shown to be carcinogenic in rodents, inducing angiosarcoma of the liver in addition to other cancers.

The occurrence of VC disease in the general population has been suggested by preliminary findings of an incidence of 18 congenital malformations per 1,000 live births in women living in three Ohio communities near PVC plants, in comparison with an incidence of 10.5 per 1,000 in those living at a distance.[25] Most of these malformations were of the brain. In addition, an excessive number of brain tumors in adult males were found in those communities near the PVC plants. A similar excess of birth defects over a period from 1966 to 1974, has been recently noted in Shawinigan, Quebec, where a large VC/PVC plant is located.*[26] These various effects have been associated with the detection of VC in the air of communities adjacent to VC/PVC plants.

Another way in which the public has been exposed to VC is from aerosol propellants in consumer products such as insecticides, hair sprays, disinfectants, and furniture polishes.[27] EPA studies show that during use of hair or insect sprays, users breathed VC in the 100 to 400 ppm range. After much prodding, the FDA banned the use of VC as a propellant in cosmetic products, including hair sprays. However, the FDA did not consider the matter serious enough to order a recall of VC-containing products so that the public could avoid further exposure. The Health Research Group eventually pried out from the FDA the brand names of hair sprays that used VC as a propellant, identifying Clairol as a top selling product. According to a recent survey by Consumer Product Safety Commission staff, no new consumer products containing VC have been manufactured since 1974, and no VC-containing products remain on the market in 1978.

The FDA also showed reluctance in moving against the use of PVC containers for food products, although it was aware that unreacted VC was leached out of the container walls by the foods or fluids inside. By 1974 the FDA knew that VC levels as high as 9 ppm had been found in vegetable oils sold in rigid PVC containers.[28] High levels were also found in other PVC-packaged products, including beverages and cosmetics. While the FDA proposed a ban on the use of rigid PVC containers for food products and beverages, the use of PVC film for wrapping foods is still sanctioned.

Extensive research is now being done by industry with the object of reducing VC levels in PVC products, especially those intended for food packaging and medical applications.[29] However, as indicated in a recent trade journal article, the prospects of success seem slim:

> At present conventional devolatilizing techniques cannot be successfully offered to PVC. . . . It cannot be expected, however, that a completely monomer-free PVC resin will be a commercial reality in the near future.[30]

Summary

Vinyl chloride (VC) is a simple gaseous chemical which can be polymerized to form a wealth of plastic materials. Despite recognition for several decades of a wide range of chronic toxic effects in animals and exposed workers, it was not until 1970 that the carcinogenicity of VC was first established experimentally. A consortium of European plastics manufacturers then funded further carcinogenicity testing of VC which confirmed and extended the earlier findings. These results, which were shared with the Manufacturing Chemists Association, remained unpublished for over eighteen months until the announcement by B. F. Goodrich in January, 1974, of

---

* More recently, five cases of angiosarcoma of the liver have been reported in women who have lived for prolonged periods close to VC polymerizing or PVC fabricating plants, and who have never worked in these plants or been exposed to other carcinogens known to induce angiosarcoma (such as arsenic or thorium dioxide).

the occurrence of three fatal cases of an extremely rare cancer, angiosarcoma of the liver, among its VC/PVC workers. On the same day, the Manufacturing Chemists Association revealed the results of tests showing VC to be a potent carcinogen in rodents, inducing angiosarcoma of the liver and a wide range of cancers at other sites at exposures of 50 ppm and below.

In the absence of available information on the carcinogenicity of VC in animals, its effects in exposed workers were only finally recognized because of the occurrence of the three rare angiosarcomas of the liver. Had VC only induced lung cancer, its carcinogenicity would in all probability have remained unrecognized or ascribed to smoking.

The present occupational standard of 1 ppm was promulgated by OSHA in spite of estimates by industry of grossly exaggerated costs and unemployment. While the standard affords some degree of protection to workers in VC/PVC plants, it is clearly excessive. Furthermore, it does not protect the greater number of workers in PVC packaging and fabricating plants, nor does it prevent exposures to VC of the public-at-large, particularly those living in the vicinity of VC/PVC plants, with attendant risks of cancer and also possibly birth defects.

Quite apart from VC itself, there has been recent recognition of the carcinogenic hazards of exposure to PVC dusts in a wide range of operations involving bagging and packaging of PVC resins, and their formulation into innumerable plastic products.

My own company is very conscientious and careful about the chemicals we use in the manufacturing process.

Ellington M. Beavers
Medical Director and Vice President
Rohm & Haas Company

Bischloromethylether

It is surprising how quickly the scandals of yesterday become today's respectable textbook classics. A standard 1975 medical text, Occupational Medicine, contains the following matter-of-fact account of the discovery of bischloromethylether (BCME) as a potent human carcinogen:

[Dr. William Figueroa] reported on lung cancer found in chloromethylmethylether workers and suggested another occupational hazard that increases the risk of lung cancer. They surveyed and studied a chemical manufacturing plant with approximately 2,000 employees where periodic chest X-ray surveys had been carried out for many years. In 1962, management became aware that an excessive number of workers suspected of having lung cancer were reported in one area of the plant, and promptly engaged consulting services to identify and resolve what appeared to be a serious problem.[1]

Claims of "prompt" action by this company, Rohm and Haas (R&H), one of the world's dozen largest chemical manufacturing companies, have often been reiterated in the medical literature. The facts prove the contrary. As shown, among others, by Philadelphia *Inquirer* reporters William Randall and Stephen Solomon in the award-winning investigative book, *Building Six*, the response by R&H was not prompt.[2] As documented in the book, the company did its best not only to obstruct studies of the lung cancer outbreak, but also to discredit those studies.[3] Finally, R&H tried to block protection of other workers by fighting against adequate exposure standards for BCME and other occupational carcinogens.[4]

Discovery of BCME

BCME was developed in 1948 by R&H chemist Robert Kunin at the company's Bridesburg laboratories in Pennsylvania. Attempts to scale up the laboratory process to a 100-gallon batch, however, revealed that BCME was intensely caustic, so much so that it virtually destroyed the plant machinery. By 1950, BCME was replaced by the closely related chloromethylmethylether (CMME), which in its industrial form contains from 1 to 7 percent BCME as a contaminant. Based on BCME and CMME, R&H chemists developed manufacturing processes for ion-exchange resins and promoted their application in various technologies, including water purification, and fabrication of nuclear weapons and fuel for power plants.

The scale-up of the BCME manufacturing process is typical of the way in which industries move newly developed technology from the laboratory to the production line. BCME is not an end-product chemical, but an intermediate which is produced and used at the production site during synthesis of ion-exchange resins. In 1948, after R&H chemists were convinced they had developed a valuable material, the first stage of large-scale production commenced in the "semi-works," so-called because it was a sort of halfway house for testing chemical processes on a larger scale than the laboratory.

As long as BCME synthesis had been confined to the laboratory, work proceeded under ventilated hoods, which drew toxic fumes up and away from the chemist. At the semi-works, however, there was no such ventilation. And the chemical was prepared not in test-tube quantities but in 100-gallon batches in open kettles that continued to be used after BCME was replaced by CMME in 1950.

In 1954, the process was moved from the semi-works to building 6, a windowless five-story building also used for the manufacture of insecticides such as Rothane, a mainstay of R&H's operations. Randall and Solomon quote an R&H spokesman's description of the CMME process in building 6:

> The operation started at the top floor, where the CMME was actually manufactured by shovelling paraformaldehyde flakes and aluminum chloride into kettles of hydrochloric acid. There were a good bit of fumes from the aluminum chloride, a fine powder, as soon as the air hit it. The kettle had to be charged quickly or it would become gummy. The men would cough, then turn away. . . . Then the CMME would go down a chute to the level below, where agitators would mix it in kettles that men would have to open from time to time so they could check on its progress. When they did lift the lids, vapors came rolling up at them. Then the mixture was dropped to the level below, where water was poured in on top to quench the reaction. This time, when the men hit the switch on the agitator, the fumes billowed out and they would have to run from the building gasping for air, then wait to go back in again.[5]

One of the insecticide workers who shared the building with the CMME process, was quoted:

> When the CMME fumes hit the floor, it was like a London fog. Everybody had to run outside to breathe. It was so goddamn hot in there you couldn't wear a mask. They were old rubber masks and you couldn't get your breath through them and so whenever there was a spill, and it happened a couple of times a day when the foreman pushed the men a little and they added the flakes a little too fast, everyone in the whole building got a shot. And if you tried to smoke after getting a shot of that stuff, it made you puke.[6]

Medical Problems

By 1962 it had become obvious that there was something wrong at R&H. Fourteen BCME workers had died of lung cancer in the preceding seven years. Their average age at death was 50, ten years younger than the average age of death of lung cancer victims. Among these was a woman of 28 and men aged 33, 38, 41, 43, and 49. The national death rate for lung cancer in white males in that age group was then about 15 per 100,000. To have seen even one or two lung cancers in workers under 50 in a 2,000-person plant should have immediately alarmed the company.

R&H claims that it "warned" its employees about the possibility of the cancer risk as soon as it knew. None of the employees has ever recalled any such warning. A memorandum, which the company maintains was read to small groups of its employees in 1962, contains a cryptic reference to "our concern over the cases of cancer that have appeared among building 6 personnel." It is clear however, that the main thrust of the memorandum was different:

> The personnel department is currently in the process of making arrangements for the next chest X-ray survey of the Bridesburg employees ... During several of these surveys, cases of TB (tuberculosis) have been uncovered, and as a result, people who worked around these individuals have been and are now being checked to be sure they have not contracted the disease.[7]

"Making arrangements" refers to the company's consultation with Katherine Boucot Sturgis, a well-known Philadelphia chest specialist, who for several years had been X-raying some Bridesburg employees as part of the Philadelphia Pulmonary Neoplasm Re-search Project. Sturgis' advice came in two parts. First, she agreed to add the entire building 6 and semi-works personnel to her yearly project X-rays, although this was never in fact done. Second, she recommended R&H to contract with Norton Nelson of New York University, to do carcinogenicity tests on BCME. Sturgis agreed to turn over all her findings directly to the company, but none of her patients, the workers, seems to have received any warning from her or the company.†

Animal Experiments

The negotiations between R&H and Nelson over company sponsored carcinogenicity tests on BCME collapsed after two years, apparently over Nelson's insistence on permission to publish any findings. After another year's delay R&H instead contracted with Hazleton Laboratories, a commercial testing company, to do carcinogenicity tests on BCME, CMME, and other chemicals in use at the Bridesburg Plant. By 1966, Hazleton reported that BCME and CMME, as well as some of the other chemicals, were carcinogenic.

Meanwhile, the New York University team had also begun a study of the carcinogenicity of BCME and CMME using government funds. By 1971 they found that BCME was one of the most potent carcinogens ever tested.[8] At 0.1 ppm in the air they breathed, rats developed a high incidence of lung cancers.

Human Experimentation

Between 1962 and 1968, when the screening phase of the Philadelphia project ended and the X-rays stopped, workers continued to die. Although their impending deaths were often picked up on X-rays, too late to save them, no meaningful effort was made to prevent further exposure. The X-ray reports

---

† Recently juries have awarded damages in lawsuits against company-retained doctors who concealed medical findings from employees. They rejected company arguments that, since the company bought the medical service, only they were entitled to know the results of the examinations.

were sent to the R&H medical office and were simply filed away. Even in 1968, one of the Philadelphia project physicians noted an excess of R&H lung cancer deaths, but failed to draw any conclusions, not having been told of worker's exposure to the carcinogenic BCME in the semiworks and building 6.

Then, in 1971, one of the workers with lung cancer was referred to William Figueroa, an internist at the Germantown Dispensary and Hospital near Philadelphia for treatment. Figueroa was surprised to find that this worker had never smoked, since the type of lung cancer he had (oat cell) is rare in nonsmokers. The worker recalled several other men who had previously died of cancer after working at similar jobs in the plant. Figueroa consulted one of his former professors at Hahnemann Medical College, Philadelphia, William Weiss, who had conducted much of the Philadelphia Pulmonary Neoplasm Research Project, to see what information was available for the other men. He also attempted to obtain occupational exposure histories for the group of 125 R&H workers for whom he had X-rays and medical and smoking histories. As he later found out, of the fifty-four lung cancer deaths at R&H, four occurred in the project group during the screening period from 1963 to 1968.[9] R&H, however, insisted, that they had no work histories and exposure records on any of these 125 workers, and that they did not know why these workers had been selected for screening. Subsequently, R&H did manage to produce some of these records at a workman's compensation hearing to show that a particular worker had not been exposed to BCME and was therefore ineligible for benefits.

The importance of knowing which of the 125 workers had been exposed to BCME and which had not was critical to a prospective-type epidemiological investigation of the lung cancer epidemic at R&H. Figueroa had to calculate a death rate among exposed workers and compare it with that of the general population. He knew that 4 of the 125 workers had lung cancer, but without the exposure data, he could not calculate a cancer rate and thus, assess the significance of these findings. In the absence of company cooperation, Figueroa turned to his only available source of information, the lung cancer patient who, in his years of working at R&H, had come to know many of the plant employees. From memory, the man reconstructed the work histories of many of the plant employees on the Pulmonary Neoplasm Project list. The results were astonishing. Of the 125 men screened, only 44 had definite exposure to BCME. (Thus, the death rate was 4 out of 44, or 9 percent.)‡ This excessive rate, coupled with the young age of many of the victims, was remarkable. Figueroa immediately published his findings in the *New England Journal of Medicine*.[10] His paper stands as an indictment of BCME as a potent carcinogen and, more telling, an indictment of R&H.

Simultaneous with the appearance of Figueroa's publication, NIOSH released the results of an investigation at a Diamond Shamrock CMME plant, Redwood City, California, initiated in 1971.[11] This study also showed a high incidence of lung cancers in relatively young workers. A number of other epidemiological studies in the United States and Germany have since confirmed the extreme carcinogenicity of BCME.[12]

Industry Fights Back

In 1972 R&H launched a campaign to discredit the experimental and epidemiological findings on the carcinogenicity of BCME. They informed NIOSH of their position that none of the cases of lung cancer in their plant could possibly have been due to BCME exposure; that instead they were caused by smoking and air pollution.

‡ More recent follow-up of the Pulmonary Neoplasm Project screenees resulted in the identification of seven more lung cancer deaths at R&H.

In the spring of 1973, R&H Senior Vice-President for Health Ellington M. Beavers, who in 1971 had refused to provide Figueroa with exposure data on BCME, was appointed to OSHA's Standards Advisory Committee on Occupational Carcinogens. Beavers urged the committee to reject proposals for minimal regulation of occupational exposure to carcinogens, and argued against the identification of occupational carcinogens by animal tests, recommending instead the need for more convincing human studies.

R&H and the Manufacturing Chemists Association also lobbied strongly against enactment of a workplace exposure standard for BCME, which was finally promulgated in an emasculated form in a package of standards for fourteen occupational carcinogens in January, 1974.

It has recently been discovered that BCME can be formed spontaneously in reaction mixtures containing the common chemicals hydrochloric acid and formaldehyde.[13] This places many thousands of workers in danger of potential exposure to BCME. For example, many textile workers use formaldehyde in making permanent press fabrics, which are then treated with an acid wash.

A Needless Tragedy

Fifty-four workers at R&H have so far died of lung cancer. Yet the deaths due to BCME were unnecessary, as shown by the experience of Dow Chemical Company, R&H's closest competitor in the manufacture of CMME and BCME.

On the basis of findings in the late 1940s that BCME was an intense lung irritant to animals, Dow enclosed the manufacturing process at its Midland, Michigan, facility since its inception in 1949. Dow's Research Laboratory director commented on the cost of providing this type of protection:

At first thought, it seemed to me that such methods would be so expensive that they could not be used in normal chemical manufacture. Actually, this may not be true. The enclosure for the manufacture of chloromethylether need not be a six-foot wall of concrete, but only a normal airtight building . . . If such operation proves impractical, I believe we should abandon large-scale work with chloromethylether.[14]

A 1972 NIOSH field inspection of the Dow facility reported that

the industrial hygiene philosophy employed is to completely contain the product inside the process equipment and to have local exhaust ventilation at points of potential leakage, such as around seals with rotating shafts. This allows the worker to be in the production area without having to rely upon respiratory protection.[15]

In fact, the health record of Dow BCME employees is difficult to evaluate. In its twenty-five years of operation, only about 120 workers were known to have been potentially exposed. Dow claims that only one of the workers, a heavy cigarette smoker, developed lung cancer. R&H had allowed eighteen years to elapse before, in 1967, it finally followed Dow's example of enclosing the CMME manufacturing process.

Summary

Bischloromethylether (BCME) is used to manufacture ion-exchange resins and appears virtually indispensable as an intermediate product in nuclear fuel processing. BCME has been manufactured on a large scale at only two industrial sites during the past 25 years, and by only two chemical companies, Dow Chemical and Rohm & Haas. While Dow engineered its process from the start to reduce human exposure to BCME, Rohm & Haas scaled up production with little regard for its obvious toxicity or emerging information on its carcinogenicity.

Workers in Rohm and Haas started dying

of lung cancer in the early 1960s. The company attempted to conceal this information, and subsequently to ascribe the cancer to smoking. When the need for animal testing became inescapable, Rohm & Haas aborted negotiations with New York University over the issue of open publication of results, contracting instead with a commercial testing laboratory. Even after BCME was shown to be one of the most powerful carcinogens ever tested in animals, and in the face of the increasing lung cancer death toll in its employees, Rohm & Haas resisted paying compensation to its employees' families and vigorously fought attempts by OSHA in 1973 to regulate BCME and other occupational carcinogens.

Benzene

Benzene is one of twelve chemicals used in largest volume by U.S. industries. Both production and manufacturing capacity have increased steadily by about 5 percent per year over the last decade. U.S. benzene production in 1977 was approximately 11 billion pounds, some 90 percent of which was produced in petroleum refining and petrochemical industries, and the remainder in the coke ovens of the steel industry.[1] The manufacture of tires accounts for approximately half of all benzene used. Commercially, benzene is also used as an intermediate in the production of a wide range of chemicals, such as nitrobenzene, phenol, cyclohexane, cumene, maleic anhydride, and detergent alkylate. Another major usage is as an octane booster in gasoline. Further end-products of the use of benzene include nylons, pesticides, adhesives, laminates, coatings, inks, paints, varnishes, and moldings.

Occupational Exposure

The occupational hazards of benzene have long been recognized, although their seriousness has, until recently, been underestimated.

While in the past exposures in the range from 100 to 500 ppm were commonplace, current levels in some workplaces are generally lower, reflecting the 1971 occupational standard of 10 ppm. Workers in petroleum and petrochemical refineries, in chemical plants (especially those manufacturing rubber products and solvents), and in the steel industry are at particularly high risk from benzene exposure. Additional categories of workers exposed include printing pressmen and lithographers, shoemakers, gasoline pump attendants, and professional artists and craftsmen.

A National Occupational Hazards Survey published by NIOSH in 1977, found that nearly 50,000 full-time workers are exposed to benzene, of whom 55 percent work at facilities that have no engineering controls or protective equipment.[2] More than 75 percent of the workers do not receive periodic blood tests to check for benzene toxicity. NIOSH estimates that about 2 million workers are now exposed to benzene.

Public Exposure

While benzene has been well known as an occupational problem for more than eighty years, recognition of the hazards posed to the general public is only recent. Public exposure to benzene falls into three major categories: communities near industries producing, processing, or using the chemical; the general public (from gasoline); and the homeowner (from benzene-containing consumer products).

Based on recent estimates by Stanford Research Institute, it is clear that while these exposures are at much lower levels than occupational exposures, they are virtually unregulated at present and affect much of the U.S. population (Table 5.4).[3] These rough estimates of general population exposure in the vicinity of petroleum refineries and gasoline service stations have, in general, been subsequently confirmed by limited industry monitoring, including that by the American Petroleum Institute.

Table 5.4 Industries Causing Exposure of the General Public to Benzene

Source	Number of People Exposed to Various Concentrations of Benzene ppb*					Total Number of Exposed People
	0.1-1	1-2	2-4	4-10	Over 10	
Petroleum refineries	6,529,000	64,000	4,000	.....	.....	6,597,000
Chemical manufacturing	7,497,000	970,000	453,000	644,000	319,000	9,883,000
Solvent operations	208,000	5,000	2,000	.....	.....	215,000
Coke ovens	15,726,000	521,000	50,000	2,000	.....	16,299,000
Gasoline stations						
People using self-service	.....	.....	.....	.....	37,000,000	37,000,000
People living nearby	87,000,000	31,000,000	.....	.....	.....	118,000,000
Urban exposures from autos	68,337,000	45,353,000	.....	.....	.....	113,690,000

Source: S. J. Mara and S. S. Lee, "Human Exposures to Atmospheric Benzene," Center for Resources and Environmental Systems Studies, Report No. 30, Stanford Research Institute, 1977.

* Based on estimates of annual averages.

Over half the benzene supply in the United States comes from a small number of petroleum refineries in Texas, California, Louisiana, and Illinois.[4] These four states, together with Pennsylvania and New Jersey, account for about 70 percent of the total national refining capacity. It is estimated that more than 6 million people who live in the vicinity of these refineries are being constantly exposed to benzene emissions in the 0.1 to 1 ppb range. An additional 64,000 people living still closer to the plants received exposures up to 2 ppb.[5]

A wide range of chemical manufacturing plants throughout the United States, but particularly concentrated along the Gulf Coast, leak substantial quantities of benzene into the atmosphere.[6] A 1971 study by Mitre Corporation indicated that annual losses are in the region of 260 million pounds, about 2.5 percent of total production. The worst offenders seem to be facilities manufacturing aniline and maleic anhydride. The actual concentrations to which local populations are exposed are highly variable, depending on factors such as height of gas stack, temperature of exhaust gas and wind patterns, but more critically on proximity to the plant. Average benzene levels are estimated to be in the 100 to 3,000 ppb range directly outside some plants, with progressive reduction at increasing distances.

Relatively little is known about the amounts of benzene used in solvent industries, for purposes such as manufacture of tires, natural and synthetic rubber products, adhesives, printing inks, paints, paint removers, leather and leather products, and floor coverings.[7] Limited monitoring data have found benzene levels as high as 700 ppb within a quarter of a mile of a B. F. Goodrich Company solvent operation.[8] There is a gradual trend, particularly in the rubber industry, to substitute toluene as a much safer and effective alternative for benzene.

Sixty million tons of blast furnace coke are produced from coal each year in sixty-five U.S. steel plants, most of which are concentrated in four states: Pennsylvania, Indiana, Ohio, and Alabama.* For each ton of coke, about four gallons of "light oil," most of which is benzene, are produced as a by-product. Most coke ovens are old and "leaky," allowing the escape of benzene and other volatile toxic materials such as carbon monoxide, hydrogen sulfide, and sulfur oxides. Benzene levels are estimated to range as high as 50 ppm inside the plants and 300 ppb immediately adjacent to them, decreasing to a few ppb at twelve miles distance. It is further estimated that about 16 million people are exposed to annual average concentrations in the 0.1 to 1 ppb range and 50,000 in the 2 to 4 ppb range.[9]

By far the most extensive operations resulting in benzene exposure to the general population are gasoline stations, of which there are about 200,000 in the United States. With the gradual phasing out of gasoline lead additives, the use of benzene as an octane booster has doubled over the last four years to current levels from 1 percent to 2.5 percent in most gasoline brands. Most of the vapor liberated during a typical fill-up operation results from the displacement of benzene trapped within the gas tank, and not from the gasoline being pumped. Recent measurements in U.S. self-service stations found benzene levels averaging 250 ppb immediately adjacent to the gas pumps. It is estimated that about 37 million people are intermittently exposed to such benzene levels through the use of self-service facilities. Gasoline attendants, of course, are continuously exposed to them. So are also the 118 million people, more than half the U.S. population, who are exposed to levels between 0.1 to 2.0 ppb by virtue of living near a gas station.[10] And automobiles themselves are mini-dispensers of benzene, both from tailpipe emissions

---

* These plants consist of an estimated 13,000 ovens contained in about 230 coke oven batteries.

and evaporation from the gas tank. Estimates of average benzene levels from these sources range from 1 to 4 ppb in downtown Dallas, Los Angeles, St. Louis, and Chicago, where the highest levels were found. Concentrations in the suburbs of these cities were from two to ten times lower.[11]

Many commonly used consumer products contain benzene. These include solvents, adhesives (including the cement in bicycle tire patch kits), carburetor cleaners, and paint and wood strippers. A popular paint stripper, Red Devil Paint and Varnish Remover, contains over 50 percent benzene. Recent NIOSH measurements in a closed garage after a half-hour of furniture stripping found benzene levels ranging from 75 to 225 ppm.[12] Professional artists, craftsmen, and hobbyists are often exposed under poorly ventilated conditions to benzene in their homes, studios, and workshops from the uses of common materials, such as resin and fluorescent dye solvents, paint and varnish removers, and silk-screen washes. Another NIOSH survey at The Cooper Union School of Art and Architecture in New York, measured benzene levels of 37 ppm in a breathing zone sample on a photoetcher. A 1977 investigation by a New York public interest group, the Center for Occupational Hazards, found the following benzene consumer products readily available.[13] Seventeen of twenty randomly selected hardware stores sold products listing benzene on their label, but with little or no indication of the dangers involved. Paint removers are particularly hazardous since they may be from 15 to 100 percent benzene.

A most dramatic example of community exposure to benzene and other carcinogenic solvents is afforded by the case of the Galaxy Chemical Company, Elkton, Maryland.[14] This company started operations in 1961 for

Brand Name	Products
Red Devil's Paint Products	Red Devil's Paint and Varnish Remover
	Liquid #99
	Liquid #66
	No-Wash #88
	Paste #77
Wilson Imperial Products Products	Imperial Wonder-paste Paint Remover
	Imperial Rapid Brush Cleaner
	Imperial Cleanwood
	Wil-Bond Sanding Liquid
KWIK Products	KWIK Liquid No-Wash Paint and Varnish Remover
	KWIK Semi-Paste Paint and Varnish Remover
Classic	Classic Rubber Repair Cement
Kleen Kutter	Kleen Kutter Paint Remover

Source: Art Hazards Project, Center for Occupational Hazards, Inc., 1976.

the purpose of recovering solvents from the wastes of major chemical industries, such as Du Pont. The company first stored these wastes in tanks vented directly to the atmosphere. Following processing at Galaxy, the "bottoms" or residues were discharged into open drying beds. After evaporation, the final wastes were dumped in nearby landfills. Additionally the company periodically had large spills of carcinogenic and other chemicals.† Complaints of foul odors commenced as soon as the plant opened and became almost constant by 1964. Monitors outside the plant in 1970 found levels of benzene as high as 23 ppm and other solvents such as carbon tetrachloride, at levels of 140 ppm.

---

† According to a deposition of the director and owner of Galaxy, Paul Mraz, the company "spilled" about 1,000 gallons of trichloroethylene in 1965, and several hundred gallons of acrylonitrile in 1971 or 1972. Mraz estimated that the company "spilled" on the average of 1,250 gallons of chemicals each year.

By 1974, a local pathologist, Pietro Capurro, who had himself been involved in the monitoring, noted an excess of lymphoma cases in Elkton. Capurro, after trying in vain to get help from the Maryland State Department of Health, prepared in March, 1974, a preliminary manuscript reporting his findings, but not specifying Galaxy as the source of the pollution. *Medical World News* subsequently interviewed Capurro and printed an article naming Galaxy as the pollution source. The director and owner of Galaxy, Paul Mraz, claimed that Capurro's article was defamatory and resulted in the loss of business, and sued Capurro for over $2 million. The case came to jury trial in December, 1977. Edward Radford, Professor of Epidemiology at the School of Public Health, University of Pittsburgh and consultant to Galaxy, claimed that Capurro was "reckless and irresponsible" in writing the draft of his article, and that Galaxy could not possibly have been responsible for the admitted excess of lymphoma cases in Elkton. On the basis of the scientific and other evidence, the jury found for Capurro.[15] Mraz appealed this verdict to the Maryland Special Court of Appeal.

Galaxy Chemical Company was dissolved in 1975, and has since reopened as Solvent Distillers, again under the ownership of Mraz.‡ In spite of some improvements in the operations of the new company, complaints of odor persisted, as indicated at the trial. Continuous monitoring in 1976 revealed periodic benzene levels in the 200 to 900 ppb range.

Occupational Diseases[16]

Virtually all knowledge of the effects of benzene on humans comes from studies on exposed workers. Benzene is highly toxic, inducing a wide range of acute and chronic adverse effects. Unless contaminated with other more readily absorbed solvents, benzene is poorly absorbed through the intact skin. The primary route of entry into the body is inhalation, with rapid absorption from the lungs into the blood. Benzene accumulates in various organs and sites of the body in proportion to their fat content. Most is rapidly metabolized, primarily by liver enzymes, to water soluble derivatives which are excreted in the urine. One of the early metabolic products of benzene is benzene epoxide, which is highly reactive and may ultimately be responsible for the toxic bone marrow effects noted below.

Aplastic Anaemia. Benzene is a potent marrow poison, inducing a wide range of toxic effects, the best recognized of which is aplastic anaemia, which is characterized by pallor and fatigue and can exist alone or together with a condition known as *pancytopenia*. In this condition, bleeding can occur in the skin and elsewhere in the body, and there also is increased susceptibility to infection.

It is difficult to assess the long-term outcome of aplastic anaemia. While the immediate prognosis of early and mild cases may be good if benzene exposure is discontinued, apparently complete recovery is sometimes followed by the development of acute leukaemia up to twenty or so years later.

Case histories of aplastic anaemia/pancytopenia in benzene-exposed workers have gradually been accumulating in the U.S. and European literature over the last five decades. Cases have been reported in a wide range of occupations, including printers in rotogravure plants, rubber workers, aircraft construction workers, and leather and shoe workers. One of the most important series of studies has been based on Turkish shoe workers, who between 1955 and 1960 started using adhe-

---

‡ Solvent Distillers has been renamed Spectron, Inc. On May 8, 1978, an explosion at the plant involving release of white fumes from barrels containing polyurethane and ink resins resulted in the evacuation of more than fifty residents from Elkton. Mraz characterized the vapors as "nonlethal."

sives containing high levels of benzene, and were exposed to levels in the 150 to 650 ppm range.[17] Individual cases of aplastic anaemia were noted in 1961. By 1977, 46 workers had developed aplastic anaemia, of whom 14 died from the disease. Five of these workers later developed leukemia, from which they subsequently died.

Chromosomal Effects. Since the early 1960s, several European studies have shown that there is a relatively high incidence of chromosome abnormalities in the lymphocytes (white blood cells) of workers, with varying degrees of marrow damage following benzene exposure.[18] These abnormalities were generally found in workers intermittently exposed to benzene levels from 25 to 150 ppm. The literature then was conflicting with regard to chromosome damage at lesser exposure levels.

By the summer of 1977, Dow Chemical Company had completed extensive chromosome tests on some forty workers in its Freeport, Texas, plant exposed to "low" benzene levels, believed to be under 10 ppm. The Dow scientists reportedly found clear-cut evidence of chromosome damage, particularly in men over forty. The Michigan corporate offices of Dow initially decided not to disclose these results.* The news, however, leaked out. NIOSH sent two letters to Dow in late 1977 and another in January, 1978, requesting details of this study, which Dow finally released in March, 1978. This study confirmed the occurrence of chromosome damage in workers with average exposure levels of 2 to 3 ppm.

Unpublished studies from Sweden also seem consistent with the results of the Dow studies, with the findings of chromosome damage in industrial workers and crews of petrol tanker ships, following exposure to benzene in the 5 to 10 ppm range.[19]

The occurrence of chromosome damage in the absence of any other evidence of benzene toxicity is important for several reasons, particularly when found at relatively low exposure levels. First, there are theoretical grounds for associating induced chromosome damage with the subsequent development of leukaemia. Second, similar abnormalities are induced by X-rays, which can also produce leukaemia. Third, these changes can persist long after there has been apparent recovery from benzene poisoning, and well before leukaemia develops. Finally, these changes are commonly found in leukaemic blood cells.

Leukaemia in Humans. Four major types of this fatal form of cancer of white blood cells are recognized: acute myelogenous, chronic myelogenous, acute lymphocytic, and chronic lymphocytic. The association between acute myelogenous leukaemia in humans and benzene exposure is unequivocal. There are three major lines of supporting evidence for this: First, benzene is known to be toxic to bone marrow, producing aplastic anaemia/pancytopenia and also chromosomal abnormalities, both of which are probable precursors of leukaemia. Second, there have been over 100 case reports of acute myelogenous leukaemia following occupational exposure to benzene, many of which first developed as aplastic anaemia. Finally, and most important, various epidemiologic studies have concluded that benzene induces leukaemia and is thus a carcinogen.

For example, an impressive series of studies has been done by Muzaffer Aksoy based on 28,500 shoe workers in Istanbul, Turkey, exposed to benzene levels from 210 to 650 ppm over a period ranging from one to fifteen years.[20] Of these cases, 26 developed acute myelogenous leukaemia from 1967 to 1973; this is an annual incidence of 13/100,000 and about four times that seen in the

---

* This would have jeopardized the industry position of fighting against the 1977 proposed OSHA reduction of the benzene standard to 1 ppm.

general population. Additionally, the average age of these leukaemia cases was 34 years, which is much lower than the 60-year average age of leukaemia deaths in adults.

Similar results have been reported in Italian shoe and rotogravure workers in Milan and Pavia, where the risk of acute myelogenous leukaemia was calculated in 1964 to be approximately twenty times greater than that of the general population. It is of particular interest that no new cases of aplastic anaemia or leukaemia were observed in the rotogravure industry during the ten-year period following the substitution of toluene for benzene in 1964.[21]

In 1974, J. Thorpe, Associate Medical Director, Exxon Corporation, published a large-scale epidemiological study of leukaemia mortality, based on 36,000 employees and retirees of eight European affiliates exposed to "low levels" of benzene from 1962 to 1972.[22] Thorpe found no excess risks of leukaemia. However, there was a wide range of problems in this study, some of which were admitted by the author. These included inadequate follow-up of older employees (who were most likely to develop leukaemia), incomplete exposure histories, inadequate measurement of exposure levels, and suspect diagnosis reporting. As one critic expressed it, "With case finding techniques as apparently relaxed as those in the Exxon study by Dr. Thorpe, one cannot help but doubt the accuracy of the data presented."[23]

A recent epidemiological study by Peter Infante of NIOSH† involved a cohort of 748 men who had been exposed to benzene from 1940 through 1949 at the Akron and St. Mary's, Ohio, plants of the Goodyear Tire and Rubber Company, while engaged in the manufacture of "plio-film," a natural rubber cast film.[24] A virtue of this study was the "purity" of the exposure; that is, the workers were exposed only to benzene, rather than to the

mixture of other organic solvents usually encountered in the rubber industry. Although a 1946 report by the Ohio Industrial Commission indicates that benzene levels in the pliofilm operation were relatively low, ranging from zero to 10 ppm, the value of this study is probably more qualitative than quantitative. Of 140 deaths observed by 1975, 7 were leukaemias, mainly acute myelogenous, while only 1 or 2 would have been expected from U.S. death rates. The risk of workers in this plant dying from leukaemia was calculated to be about ten times that of the general population. Unpublished reports from Lund, Sweden, in 1977 also indicated a high incidence of acute myelogenous leukaemia in gasoline pump attendants.

There is a clear relationship between benzene and acute myelogenous leukaemia, and there is growing information incriminating benzene in other forms of leukaemia and other malignancies. Much of this evidence, however, comes from studies in which there are mixed exposures to other solvents besides benzene, such as in the rubber industry. For instance, a 1963 HEW study reported 54 percent increase in death rates for "cancer of the lymphatic and haematopoietic system," besides excess cancers of other sites in the rubber industry compared with other manufacturing industries.[25] A comprehensive study of rubber workers by scientists of the University of North Carolina showed an excess death rate from all forms of leukaemia, including lymphatic leukaemia, and also lymphosarcoma and Hodgkin's disease. Other studies of the rubber industry have also confirmed the findings of excess lymphatic leukaemia. There have also been scattered case reports on the association between benzene exposure and lymphosarcoma, Hodgkin's disease, multiple myeloma, and reticulum cell sarcoma.[26] For instance, six cases of Hodgkin's disease have been recently reported in Turkish shoe

---

† Now in OSHA.

workers following one to twenty years of occupational exposure to benzene.

Leukaemia in Animals

In 1897, a German physician, G. Santesson, investigating an outbreak of skin haemorrhages in a group of women working with benzene, was able to reproduce these effects in rabbits by injection and skin application of the chemical. Since then, there have been numerous investigations on the effects of benzene in animals. In general, these have shown that benzene is a marrow toxin, depressing marrow function, and producing an aplastic anaemia/pancytopenia-like condition. In more recent studies, chromosome damage, of a type similar to that found in occupationally exposed workers, has been found in circulating lymphocytes.[27]

Attempts to induce leukaemia and other cancers in experimental animals by chronic administration of benzene have on the whole been unsuccessful until very recently. It has been customary to regard benzene as one of two major exceptions to the rule that all chemicals found to be carcinogenic in humans will also induce cancer in animals (arsenic is the other). However, there are grounds for questioning whether benzene is really an exception. First, many claimed negative animal experiments are inadequate in that they used too few animals or observed them for too short a period. Second, there are several animal studies which, while individually flawed, together are highly suggestive of the induction of leukaemias or lymphomas. Examples are a 1932 German study, in which eight out of forty-four surviving mice developed leukaemia or lymphosarcoma, and a 1963 Japanese study, in which fibrosarcomas were induced in five of eight mice surviving chronic benzene administration.[28] Finally, two recent unpublished studies seem to confirm the carcinogenicity of benzene. The preliminary results of one study were presented by Cesare Maltoni at a meeting sponsored by Chemical Week in New Orleans, October 21, 1977. Groups of sixty to seventy rats of both sexes were fed benzene at doses of 50 and 250 mg/kg. Five rare ear gland tumors, five skin tumors and three other tumors were found in the high dose group. No such tumors occurred in 300 controls. The second, still incomplete, study from New York University has established that benzene induces leukaemia in rodents. This study is based on exposure of groups of forty to sixty rats and mice to benzene by inhalation at 100 or 300 ppm for up to two years. So far, one rat and one mouse have died from chronic myeloid leukaemia, another mouse from acute leukaemia, and a third mouse from a leukaemic-like disease. Additionally, most mice at the higher dose level developed severe anaemia.

Regulatory Developments

The year 1977 was a year of regulatory confrontation for benzene, as moves were finally made by federal agencies to limit and control exposures in the workplace, in the general environment, and in the home.

Regulation in the Workplace. The 1977 occupational standard of 10 ppm was originally based on a standard developed by the American Conference of Governmental Industrial Hygienists in 1969.[29] This is one of several industry-oriented organizations in whose hands occupational standards were set prior to passage of the 1970 Occupational Safety and Health Act. The American National Standards Institute is another such organization. Standards set by these organizations are often referred to as "consensus standards," although the consensus did not generally reflect the views of consumers or organized labor. While Section 6(a) of the Occupational Safety and Health Act allows conferring of federal authority on such standards, these have recently come under increasing scrutiny and revision. The consensus standard, adopted as an OSHA standard in 1971, allowed average benzene exposures of 10 ppm, with an acceptable ceiling of 25 ppm, and periodic excursions up to 50 ppm. Both the consensus and resulting OSHA standard were based on the general toxic effects of benzene, without any consideration of risks of leukaemia, in spite of the substantial evidence of this effect which then existed.

The risks of leukaemia could no longer be ignored when the results of the Turkish shoe worker study by Aksoy were published in 1974.[30] Accordingly, NIOSH submitted a criteria document to OSHA on benzene admitting that "the possibility that benzene can induce leukaemia cannot be dismissed."[31] Nevertheless NIOSH recommended retention of the 10 ppm standard. Resentment against this standard surfaced on April 23, 1976, when the United Rubber, Cork, Linoleum and Plastic Workers of America wrote to Secretary of Labor William J. Usery urging that an Emergency Temporary Standard regulating occupational exposure to benzene be issued in order to protect workers from leukaemia. According to the Act, an Emergency Temporary Standard may only be issued if there is a condition of grave danger, and if action by OSHA can mitigate this. Under the Nixon and Ford administrations, OSHA showed extreme reluctance to engage in such emergency rule-making. Usery denied labor's request on May 18, 1976.

In June, 1976, the National Academy of Sciences released an EPA-contracted review on the "Health Effects of Benzene," prepared by its industry-dominated Committee on Toxicology.[32] This emphasized the need for further research and study but admitted that "benzene must be considered as a suspect leukemogen," a conclusion which was, however, sharply qualified:

It is probable that all cases reported as "leukaemia associated with benzene exposure" have resulted from exposure to rather high concentrations of benzene and other chemicals.

This statement has been exploited by the American Petroleum Institute and other industry as the basis for their view that further study rather than further regulation of benzene is needed, and in support of their objections to the 1977 proposed OSHA standard of 1 ppm.

These views of the National Academy of Sciences Committee are also in sharp contrast to the unequivocal statement that benzene was a leukemogen, contained in an updated criteria document submitted to OSHA in August, 1976, by then director of NIOSH, John Finklea, clearly reversing the agency's 1974 assessment.[33] The updated document stated, "It is apparent from the literature that benzene leukaemia continues to be reported, . . . [thus] no worker [should] be exposed to benzene in excess of 1 ppm in air." The document also recognized that the risks of leukaemia were such that no safe level of exposure to benzene can be established. NIOSH followed this move by a letter to OSHA on October 27, 1976, recommending that the standard be revised downwards from 10 to 1 ppm.

The next development was the completion, in January, 1977, of the NIOSH pliofilm industry study by Infante, which clearly confirmed excess leukaemia risks from benzene at apparently relatively low exposure levels.[34] OSHA, already sensitized by the 1976 update of the NIOSH criteria document, reacted promptly to these new studies. In February, 1977, OSHA alerted industry to the imminent and urgent need for reducing exposure levels, by issuing a "guideline" recommending a new standard of 1 ppm and outlining probable requirements for engineering controls, monitoring, and employee medical surveillance. Reaction from the industry was prompt. Without waiting for the formalization of the guidelines into proposed standards, the National Petroleum Refiners Association, in a March press release, attacked the proposal as unnecessary and unjustified, claiming that it would entail a $267 million capital outlay and subsequent annual costs of $75 million.[35]

On April 29, 1977, Secretary of Labor F. Ray Marshall and Assistant Secretary for OSHA Eula Bingham announced an Emergency Temporary Standard of 1 ppm, reducing the 25 ppm ceiling level to 5 ppm and eliminating permissible peaks of 50 ppm.[36] This was scheduled to go into effect on May 21, 1977, and to become a permanent standard six months from then. In announcing the measure, Marshall recognized the historic and critical importance of the proposal by declaring that

> [this] signals a new day for an agency which in the past has been criticized for acting too slowly when lives were at stake. . . . We are going to focus our primary attention in OSHA on major, rather than minor problems. . . . We are going to catch whales rather than minnows.[37]

OSHA made it clear that it did not regard the 1 ppm standard as safe, but rather as the lowest feasible level for the current detection and control of benzene exposure. In fact, practical instrumentation is available which is sensitive down to 0.05 or 0.1 ppm. OSHA pointed out that if this new level was not found to be adequately protective, it would then urge for the large-scale substitution of less harmful solvents for benzene. Of the 2 million workers whom NIOSH estimates are exposed to benzene, only approximately 153,000 workers and 1,200 work sites will be covered by the emergency standard. For the time being, however, gasoline pump attendants and industries using less than 1 percent benzene in any liquids or formulations are exempted. OSHA indicated that the costs of meeting the emergency standard would be of the order of $40 million, and that for the permanent standard a maximum of $500 million. These are fractions of the costs claimed by the American Petroleum Institute and the National Petroleum Refineries Association.

The practicality of the emergency standard and also of a zero exposure standard were further emphasized in May, 1977, by an Economic Impact Statement submitted to OSHA. This stressed that benzene has already been or soon will be replaced by other chemicals in a wide range of processes; that most benzene is already used by large industry in closed systems; and that the price of benzene had quadrupled from 1973 to 1976, providing economic incentives for the further use and perfection of closed systems. The impact statement also quoted the American Petroleum Institute to the effect that since 1970, 90 percent of benzene exposures in the petrochemical industry are under 1 ppm.

The proposed emergency standard came under immediate attack from several quarters, from industry as being too stringent, and from labor and the Health Research Group as being too weak. The Industrial Union Department of AFL-CIO, filed a petition in the U.S. Court of Appeals for the District of Columbia Circuit, on the basis that there is no known safe exposure level for a carcinogen. Labor and the Health Research Group made no secret of their strong support for the OSHA action as a first step in the right direction.

The Manufacturing Chemists Association on behalf of the chemical industry, and the American Petroleum Institute, on behalf of ten major oil companies, strongly protested the proposed standard. On May 29, 1977, the American Petroleum Institute petitioned the Federal Court of the New Orleans Fifth Circuit for a stay of execution of the emergency standard, which was granted. The petition was transferred in June to the District of Columbia Circuit, which denied an appeal by OSHA and continued the stay. The industry's position in the appeals brief was inconsistent and questionable. Shell Oil claimed that the emergency standard would make it necessary for them to monitor about 150 workplaces. A survey by the Oil, Chemical and Atomic Workers Union however, showed that Shell owns only seventeen chemical plants and eight refineries. Standard Oil of Ohio claimed that it had only about ten respirators that it could use for the new regulations, whereas the workers in its Toledo refinery found over 100 cartridge and 32 self-contained respirators in that one plant alone. Union Oil Company of California made similar statements.[38]

Some industry groups, however, were more cooperative. Goodyear Tire and Rubber Company said that it expected to be able to meet the new emergency standard and reported that it was well along in replacing benzene in its operations. Other chemical industries, and also some universities, announced that they were switching from benzene to safer solvents, such as toluene and petroleum ether. A memorandum from Atlantic Richfield to its employees said, "We believe some aspects of OSHA's new standard may be overly restrictive, but intend to comply as quickly as possible with all of its provisions."

Public hearings on the proposed OSHA standard began on July 19, 1977. OSHA's main exhibit, apart from the 1976 NIOSH criteria document, was the Infante study. Also testifying was Louis Beliczky, of the Rubber Workers Union, who called for a stricter standard and for economic protection through "rate retention" of workers found to have toxic effects from benzene exposure. Sidney Wolfe, of the Health Research Group also testified in favor of stricter standards, pointing out that the only safe exposure level for benzene, as for other carcinogens, is zero and that this could be achieved by product substitution and engineering controls. It should be noted that support for the zero exposure standard has been clearly stated by Donald Hunter in 1969 in his internationally recognized standard text on occupational diseases:[39] "The safe concentration of benzene vapor in a factory or workshop is zero parts per million." The Health Research Group also demanded that all employers proposing to use benzene should first be required to obtain a "use permit," which would allow OSHA to

regulate more effectively, to physically inspect the workplace before issuing a permit, and to institute uniform work practices and labeling.

The industry attacks against the standard focused on three major points: They claimed that the Infante study was invalid, that the current 10 ppm standard was a safe threshold against leukaemia risks, and that any possible remaining risks were far outweighed by the benefits to society of the continued use of benzene under currently regulated conditions.

The major criticisms against the Infante study, by then published in *Lancet* (July 9, 1977), were presented by the chief industry witness, Irving Tabershaw, long-time industrial consultant and editor of the industry-oriented *Journal of Occupational Medicine*.[40] Tabershaw attempted to recalculate the Infante data so as to minimize the excess leukaemia incidence in the exposed work force. He did this by the device of computing mortality rates on groups of workers as a whole, in a way similar to that used by McDonald to minimize the cancer risk of asbestos miners, rather than by computing rates on workers at risk for specified periods of exposure time. The latter approach is essential to the analysis of mortality rates for diseases with a long latency period, such as cancer. The Tabershaw argument was published in a letter to *Lancet* on October 22, 1977, together with a counter-rebuttal by Infante.[41]

One of the industry witnesses was Robert E. Olson, Chairman of the Department of Medicine, St. Louis University, whose seventeen-page testimony, a quarter of which was devoted to listing his own academic achievements, attacked the Infante study on the grounds, among others, that none of its authors had an M.D. Olson made it clear that he was under the impression that the literature had established thresholds for carcinogenic effects:

The carcinogen, vinyl chloride, shows clear-cut threshold behavior in both animals and man. The threshold for tumor induction by vinyl chloride in animals is 10 ppm, a concentration at which hepatic glutathione levels were not depressed and no tumors occurred. After 25 years of observation, doses of vinyl chloride in the air of approximately 2,000 ppm in industrial plants have been shown to cause tumors in man, whereas levels below 200 ppm have not.[42]

Stranger still was Olson's belief that benzene could not be regarded as a human carcinogen, because human experience had not been validated in animal experiments. "In my opinion benzene cannot be called a primary carcinogen, because no cancer has been demonstrated in animals after benzene exposure and no mutagenic activity has been demonstrated in mutant microorganisms (Ames test)." Robert Synder, Professor of Pharmacology, Thomas Jefferson University, another industry witness, agreed with Olson on this point: "The major stumbling block to general acceptance of the theory that benzene induces leukaemia has been the inability to produce any form of this disease in mice or rats exposed to benzene." (These statements are reversals of the usual industry position of demanding human validation of carcinogens established in animal tests.)

A leading industry witness was James J. Jandl, Professor of Medicine at Harvard University Medical School and a prominent hematologist, testifying on behalf of Organization Resources Counselors, Inc., a New York-based consulting firm that represents about fifty top national corporations, including Du Pont and Union Carbide. Jandl maintained that leukaemia had been caused only by long-discontinued exposures in the 50 to 100 ppm range. He further reported that of 4,448 case reports of workers exposed to 100 to 1,000 ppm of benzene since 1939, which he had reviewed, "only" 169 (4 percent) had developed aplastic anaemia, and of these 148 (88 percent) had recovered completely. Jandl provided no documentation for these case reports. Apart from the fact that he found eleven deaths from aplastic anaemia or leukaemia, his follow-up period for the aplastic anaemia cases averaged only three years. The literature, however, makes it clear that the latency period for leukaemia can extend for fifteen years or more.

Jandl also supported the industry position of "blaming the victim," claiming that only hypersusceptible workers developed leukaemia following benzene exposure, and that these could be detected by periodic surveillance and screening programs. One of the flaws in this argument, apart from the fact that there was no evidence presented for it, became apparent in a report subsequently submitted by Dow Chemical Company, which found a four-fold excess of leukaemias in employees exposed to benzene in its Michigan plant, in spite of the fact that the company has elaborate pre-employment and blood screening programs for exposed workers.

The Jandl testimony included a critical but poorly substantiated analysis of the Infante study, unfavorable references to the "explosive interest" of Aksoy on "an alleged but undocumented 28,500 Turkish workers in the shoe making industry," and sarcasm directed against OSHA, which he charged with engaging in "self-serving . . . dramatization."

The final argument presented by the Manufacturing Chemists Association at the OSHA hearings summarized the views of its consultants and alleged that "the best available evidence" indicates that there are two thresholds for toxic effects of benzene, 100 ppm for leukaemia and 40 ppm for aplastic anaemia. Anyway, argued the Manufacturing Chemists Association, why worry about aplastic anaemia, especially in view of Jandl's reassurances that the mortality rate for this disease is so low? For these reasons, they protested, why revise the standard downwards, especially as this would involve considerable expense?

Following the public hearings in February, 1978, OSHA promulgated its permanent benzene standard, which prohibited worker exposure to an average concentration above 1 ppm, and which also prohibited skin contact with solutions containing more than 0.5 percent benzene. The new, tougher standard was, however, never enforced, as the American Petroleum Institute, the National Petroleum Refiners Association, and other trade groups immediately petitioned the Fifth Circuit Federal Court of Appeals in New Orleans for a stay, on the grounds that no health hazard had been demonstrated below 10 ppm and that the health benefits of the standard (to the workers) did not justify the costs (to the companies) of implementation.‡ A temporary stay of the standard was granted in March, 1978, by the Fifth Circuit. In October, 1978, the Court permanently overturned the standard, leaving workers subject to the previous 10 ppm standard.

The specific ground for setting aside the 1 ppm standard was OSHA's alleged failure to provide an estimate, supported by "substantial evidence," of expected benefits from the lower limit. The Fifth Circuit Court specifically rejected OSHA's arguments that the benefits of regulating a known carcinogen would be "appreciable," and that regulations should be based on whether industry compliance is feasible. The language of the decision exemplified the Court's belief that economic feasibility and costs of compliance are the prime determinants in standard setting, and that the burden of proving that these costs would be outweighed by the health benefits should be borne exclusively by OSHA. Even as the Court was drafting its final decision, Foster D. Snell released a study for the Manufacturing Chemists Association showing that control of process vents and benzene storage tanks could achieve 95 percent reduction of all emissions for considerably less cost than previous estimates.

The government, clearly unable to allow the Fifth Court's position on economic constraints to determine future policies of the Labor Department, in December, 1978, filed an appeal to the Supreme Court, with the Industrial Union Department of AFL-CIO as an intervenor.

Regulation of Public Exposure. By early 1977, evidence of OSHA's growing concerns on occupational hazards of benzene encouraged the extension of these concerns to similar hazards in the general environment and home.

On April 14, 1977, the Environmental Defense Fund petitioned EPA to list benzene as a "hazardous air pollutant" under section 112 of the Clean Air Act. EPA did so on June 7, 1977, and recommended that industrial emissions of benzene be reduced to the "lowest possible level." This action required the agency to develop appropriate standards and abatement programs within a subsequent ninety-day period.

EPA, meanwhile, was preparing the scientific basis for its proposed action. This consisted of three key documents: "Benzene Health Effects Assessment, an External Review Draft," dated October, 1977, the chief author of which is Bernard D. Goldstein, a hematologist at New York University Medical Center;[43] "Human Exposure to Atmospheric Benzene," a preliminary draft by Stanford Research Institute, dated October, 1977;[44] and "Preliminary Report on Population Risks to Ambient Benzene Exposures," prepared by the Carcinogen Assessment Group of EPA.[45] The first document is a comprehensive literature review up to the summer of 1977, confirming the leukemogenicity of benzene at levels under 100 ppm, confirm-

---

‡ The Fifth Circuit Court is known not to be unsympathetic to the interests of the petrochemical industry. OSHA standards on chemical exposures are now being developed with growing expectations that they may well be litigated in this Court.

ing the occurrence of chromosome damage in levels down to 25 ppm, and dismissing any suggestion that only the "susceptible" worker develops aplastic anaemia or leukaemia from exposure to benzene. The Stanford Research Institute document identified all major industrial sources of benzene emissions into the air, estimated the average and worst-case levels of exposure for various population groups, and concluded that exposure levels of the general population were in the 1 ppb range, although much higher levels could be found in the vicinity of various industries. On the basis of these two documents, the third EPA document estimated that thirty to eighty cases of leukaemia could be anticipated each year in the general population from exposure to estimated average 1 ppb levels. These are minimal estimates, as they ignore the likelihood of synergistic interactions between benzene and other environmental carcinogens, which could result in much greater numbers of leukaemias and cancers.

Flanked by its lawyers and consultants, the American Petroleum Institute, Organization Resources Counselors, the Manufacturing Chemists Association, the American Iron and Steel Institute, and other concerned industries launched into an attack on the EPA position at a meeting of the Environmental Health Advisory Committee, December 12, 1977. The Stanford Research Institute document was attacked as speculative and based merely on estimates, rather than hard monitoring data, which the industry claimed could have easily been obtained from them by the government.

Direct questioning of the industry by members of the advisory committee, however, made it clear that in the summer of 1977, EPA had requested industry to supply it with monitoring data in the general environment, but received virtually no response. Just before the advisory committee meeting the American Petroleum Institute released some limited monitoring data which agreed well with the Stanford estimates. Additionally, EPA had

submitted a draft of the Stanford Report to the industry and had included all their limited comments in the final draft, which the industry subsequently attacked at the advisory committee meeting.

The industry was questioned as to the availability of the Dow study on chromosome abnormalities in workers exposed to levels of benzene believed to be under 10 ppm which NIOSH had repeatedly requested since late 1977. Dow finally made these data available on March 1, 1978. The results of the Dow studies clearly demonstrated the occurrence of a statistically significant incidence of chromosome abnormalities in a group of fifty-two workers exposed to benzene for an average period of fifty-six months, ranging from one month to twenty-six years, at estimated time-weighted average levels of 2-3 ppm.[46]

Shell Oil submitted a written statement which chided EPA for failing to differentiate between a carcinogen and a leukemogen. The statement reflected puzzlement that thresholds for benzene could not be found for the general public, since "they can be determined for workers." Finally, Shell dismissed the Stanford document as based largely on estimates rather than on hard monitoring data when, like the rest of the industry, Shell had failed to supply such information requested by EPA.

Jandl attacked the EPA position which he claimed was unscientific. However, he was unable to explain why he based his claims for the high recovery rate from benzene-induced aplastic anaemia and the rarity of leukaemia on an average of only three years follow-up.

In February, 1978, the Advisory Committee concluded that available scientific evidence strongly supported the proposed EPA action to regulate benzene as a "hazardous air pollutant." The scientific basis underlying the proposed regulation was confirmed by a subsequent report prepared for EPA by Pedco Environmental of Cincinnati. In addition to stressing the occurrence of chromo-some damage at benzene exposure levels of 2 to 3 ppm, the report describes two other significant toxic effects at exposure levels of 3 to 15 ppm — reduction in serum complement levels, and interference in the synthesis of heme, the oxygen-carrying blood pigment of hemoglobin, manifested by the accumulation of a precursor (delta-aminolevulinic acid).

Consideration of the health risks both to the general population and the work force from exposure to benzene is clearly going to be influenced by the costs of achieving reduction in emissions. It is likely that there will be increasing emphasis on the important fact that steps taken to reduce benzene emissions will also result in concomitant reduction of emissions of a wide range of other toxic and carcinogenic chemicals. This is certainly the case for coke oven emissions, as well as for emissions from petrochemical plants.

The NCI maps on cancer mortality have already focused attention on excess cancer rates in counties with heavy concentrations of petrochemical industries. In October, 1977, William J. Blot of the NCI published a further study based on thirty-nine counties where at least 100 persons and at least 1 percent of the population work in petroleum refining plants.[47] Blot found a 6 percent higher overall cancer death rate in petroleum counties than in matched non-petroleum counties. Much higher excesses were found for cancers of various sites: nasal cavity, 48 percent higher; lung, 15 percent higher; skin, 10 percent higher; testes, 10 percent higher; stomach, 9 percent higher; and rectum, 7 percent higher. Excess lung cancer rates were also found in female residents of the petroleum counties, clearly suggesting the role of carcinogenic emissions from industry into the surrounding community. The NCI study suggested that some of the excess cancers could also be due to other classes of carcinogens emitted by refineries or other chemical indus-tries located nearby.

While OSHA, NIOSH, and labor were moving to reduce occupational exposure to benzene, and EPA, prodded by the Environmental Defense Fund was moving to control industrial emissions to the general environment, concerns were growing that the home and arts and crafts schools are major sources of exposure, particularly for artists, craftsmen, and hobbyists. The only current regulatory restriction for such products is a requirement under the Federal Hazardous Substances Act for special labeling if they contain 5 percent or more benzene. In May, 1977, two public interest groups, the Health Research Group and the New York Center for Occupational Hazards, petitioned the Consumer Product Safety Commission to ban benzene-containing household products, including paint strippers and adhesives.[48] The petition noted the poor or nonexistent labeling practices of the manufacturers of these products and concluded that "there is no safe way for artists, craftspeople, hobbyists or children to work with benzene in their home or studio." The Commission has not yet taken action on this petition.

Summary

Literally millions of Americans are exposed to benzene, in many instances almost continuously, from sources including coke ovens, petroleum refineries, petrochemical plants, gasoline stations, auto exhaust, and a variety of consumer products including rubber cement and paint remover. While exposure to benzene has been known for nearly 100 years to cause blood diseases, growing epidemiological evidence over the last two decades has shown that it also causes aplastic anaemia and leukaemia, as well as chromosomal damage.

Following initiatives by organized labor and public interest groups, steps were taken in 1977 by OSHA, EPA, and the Consumer Product Safety Commission to regulate benzene exposure in the workplace, general environment, and the home. Industry, led by the Manufacturing Chemists Association and the American Petroleum Institute and with the support of their academic consultants, attacked EPA estimates on environmental levels of benzene, while having failed to previously supply such information on request and in spite of the fact that the government estimates agreed well with industry findings. Industry also attempted to discredit the epidemiological evidence on the leukaemogenicity of benzene and to assert that there was a "threshold" below which it was safe to expose workers to benzene, in spite of the overwhelming rejection of the threshold concept by the informed and independent scientific community. Industry also argued against accepting human evidence on the carcinogenicity of benzene because earlier studies had failed to produce these effects in animals, while at the same time rejecting more recent animal studies which appear to confirm the carcinogenicity of benzene.

Out of the industry experience in mobilizing support to attack proposed federal regulations of benzene, a new organization, the American Industrial Health Council, was spawned from the Manufacturing Chemists Association to fight current attempts by OSHA to develop "generic" standards for carcinogens in the workplace.

Chapter Six

Consumer Products: Case Studies

Consumer products represent the most direct way in which the consumer is exposed to industrial chemicals. Regulatory responsibility for different classes of consumer products is shared by various agencies, including the Food and Drug Administration (FDA), for food and animal feed additives, cosmetics, and drugs; the Consumer Product Safety Commission, for household products, including cleaning agents, flame retardants, refrigerants, and paints; the Environmental Protection Agency (EPA), for pesticides; the United States Department of Agriculture (USDA), for grading and labeling of meat, poultry, fruits, and vegetables; and the Federal Trade Commission, for advertising of all classes of consumer products, including tobacco which is otherwise virtually unregulated. Requirements for testing and labeling of the various classes of consumer products, and for evidence of their efficacy, are inconsistent. The ways the consumer is exposed to chemicals in these products are highly varied.

Smoking is generally regarded as a voluntary action, although it is usually initiated in adolescence and in response to massive advertising campaigns and peer pressures. However, smoking also exposes nonsmoking bystanders involuntarily. Similarly, the use of certain food additives, such as saccharin, is also generally considered voluntary, especially in the case of adults deliberately taking it in various beverages such as diet sodas and foods or as drugs. However, exposure of the embryo to the carcinogenic effects of saccharin, and other carcinogenic food additives, is clearly involuntary. Many classes of additives, such as the food dye Red #40, are so ubiquitous and poorly labeled in the food supply that the consumer, wishing to avoid

them, has only limited options to do so. Consumer options are similarly limited for a wide array of chemicals, including: flame retardants in fabrics and textiles; chemical additives to cattle or poultry feed, residues of which are found in meat products; pesticide residues in food; and residues of chemicals that migrate from plastic food packaging. Drug taking, especially prescription drugs, is essentially involuntary and often without informed consent of the consumer-patient. The pharmaceutical industry and prescribing physicians usually do not make available to the patient full information on risks.

This chapter presents a series of five case studies: tobacco, Red dyes #2 and #40, saccharin, acrylonitrile, and female sex hormones.

A custom lothsome to the eye, hateful to the nose, harmful to the braine, dangerous to the lungs, and in the blacke stinking fume thereof, neerest resembling the horrible Stigian smoke of the pit that is bottomelesse.

James I, 1604.

Tobacco

Within 24 hours of setting foot on the soil of the New World, Christopher Columbus picked up the tobacco smoking habit from American Indians and later introduced it to Europe. The habit spread like wildfire, being particularly popularized in England by Sir Walter Raleigh, whose smoking, like his politics, was offensive enough to James I to eventually have him beheaded.

A century later, the Italian physician, Bernardino Ramazzini, one of the great pioneers of industrial medicine, noted that Italian tobacco workers, who prized their jobs, did so in spite of headaches and stomach disorders from tobacco dust.[1] "The sweet smell of gain," Ramazzini commented, "makes the smell of tobacco less perceptible and less offensive to those workers. . . . This vice will always be condemned and always clung to." Emotional and other considerations apart, this clinging is now seen to be the result of physiological habituation or addiction to nicotine.

Many people feel that the book on tobacco has been closed, that we know as much as we need to about its cancer-causing properties, and that whatever lessons need to be learned about the prevention of tobacco-related diseases have already been learned. But the continued study of the relation between tobacco smoking and disease is still necessary for several reasons: first, to provide further understanding on how tobacco smoke causes cancer, respiratory, cardiovascular, and other diseases; second, to provide information on the interaction of tobacco smoke with other environmental and occupational carcinogens and toxic chemicals; third, to further educate the public on the hazards of smoking in order to better pressure the government and voluntary health agencies, such as the American Cancer Society, to develop more aggressive approaches to regulating tobacco sales and advertising; and finally, to provide surveillance of the tobacco industry, including monitoring the effects of constantly changing tobacco products and markets.*

The pattern of cigarette smoking in the United States is changing.[2] The total number of adult smokers, particularly in the upper socioeconomic groups, has been declining since 1970. However, the number of smokers among teenagers and pre-adolescents, particularly young girls, is on an alarming rise. In 1977, 27 percent of all teenage girls smoked cigarettes, compared to 22 percent in 1964. This is happening despite a growing awareness among all age groups that smoking is a serious health hazard.[3] Because of the long time from the first cigarette puff to the appearance of cancer, current trends will not affect disease rates for many years to come. Even so, the male lung cancer rate is increasing at a lesser rate than previously. The rate for women, however, continues to climb as sharply as before and may eventually reach that of men.[4]

The Chemistry of Tobacco Smoke[5]

The chemical composition of tobacco smoke is quite complex, which probably comes as a surprise to most smokers, who tend to think of smoke only in terms of nicotine and "tar." Tobacco is a cured, dried plant leaf. When burned in a paper wrapper, it produces a variety of products from incomplete combustion of the leaf, the wrapper, and the many curing agents, additives, fillers and a wide range of pesticide contaminants also present in cigarettes. These combustion products are either completely vaporized or are released as a suspension of microscopic particles in the smoke. The gas phase of the smoke contains a great variety of toxic and carcinogenic gases, some of which are listed in Table 6.1. These include several nitrosamines, such as dimethylnitrosamine (DMN), nitrosopyrrolidine, nitrosopiperidine, and N-nitrosonornicotine (found exclusively in tobacco smoke), which are all potent carcinogens.

The gas phase of cigarette smoke also contains a number of other chemicals which are either tumor promoters, such as formaldehyde, or impair the lung's natural defenses by dis-

---

* Further research would be largely unnecessary if the government were to ban tobacco advertisement and mount a massive campaign to persuade people to give up smoking. An even more effective curtailment of the industry would result if it were forced to accept financial responsibility for each tobacco-related death.

abling the cilia, as nitrogen oxides do, thereby permitting carcinogens from tobacco smoke and polluted air to penetrate and remain in the lungs.

When the gas phase is separated from tobacco smoke by filtration, a moist substance called total particulate matter is left behind. When the moisture and nicotine are then removed, a dry condensate known as tar remains. The tar contains literally innumerable chemicals, at least 1,200 of which have been identified. Many of them are known carcino-

gens and tumor promoters.

The Epidemiology of Lung Cancer[6]

Many factors are involved in the association between tobacco smoking and lung cancer.

Type of Tobacco Product Smoked. Cigarette smokers have a higher lung cancer rate than cigar or pipe smokers.[7] This is probably due to the fact that the smoke of cigars and pipes is more alkaline than that of cigarettes and is not likely to be inhaled so deeply. Al-

---

Table 6.1 Quantities and Concentrations of Some Gaseous Components of Cigarette Smoke

Substance	Quantity (μg/cigarette)	Concentration (ppm)	TLV† (ppm)	Activity‡
Acetaldehyde	770	3,200	100	CI
Acetone	578	1,100	1,000	....
Acrolein	84	150	0.1	CI
Ammonia	80	300	25	....
Benzene	67	....	....	CA
Carbon dioxide	50,600	92,000	5,000	....
Carbon monoxide	13,400	42,000	50	....
Dimethylnitrosamine	0.08	....	....	CA
Formaldehyde	90	30	2	P
Hydrazine	0.03	....	....	CA
Hydrogen cyanide	240	1,600	10	CI
Hydrogen sulfide	....	40	10	....
Nitric oxide	....	250	5	....
Nitrosopiperidine	0.01	....	....	CA
Nitrosopyrrolidine	0.1	....	....	CA
Toluene	108	....	....	....
Vinyl chloride	0.01	....	1	CA

Source: E. L. Wynder and D. Hoffmann, *Seminars in Oncology, 3* (1976): pp. 5-15; and I. Schmeltz, D. Hoffmann, and E. L. Wynder, in *Trace Substances in Environmental Health,* D.D. Hemphill, ed., 7 (1974): pp. 281-95.

† Threshold limit value, maximum concentration permitted for workers exposed to the same substance in the air of their workplace.

‡ CA=Carcinogen, CI=ciliotoxic agent, P=promoter.

kaline nicotine is more toxic than its neutral form and is more readily absorbed through the mouth and nose. Because of the rapid absorption of nicotine, cigar and pipe smokers need to smoke less to maintain a given nicotine level. Additionally, cigar and pipe smokers usually inhale less than cigarette smokers.[8] Among those few cigar and pipe smokers who inhale, lung cancer and coronary heart disease rates are as high as for cigarette smokers. Additionally, cancers of the lips, tongue, mouth, and esophagus are as high if not higher among pipe and cigar smokers, irrespective of the degree of inhalation.

Quantity Smoked. Nearly every epidemiological study has found a dose-response relation. The more cigarettes, cigars, or pipes smoked per day, the greater is the cancer risk.[9]

Duration of the Habit. The longer a smoker continues to smoke, the greater is the risk of cancer.[10]

Inhalation. Most recent studies confirm the obvious notion that inhalation increases the risk of cancer.[11] An interesting sidelight comes from studies of smoking in France, where the lung cancer rate is the lowest in the Western world, yet cigarette consumption is among the highest. This is probably due to the fact that French smokers inhale less than Americans. One reason for this is that French smokers favor the government-distributed brand. Gauloises, made with a black variety of tobacco rather than the blond Burley blends of American and English cigarettes; black tobacco smoke is highly alkaline, while blond smoke is acidic.*

Smoking Cessation. There is ample evidence that stopping smoking decreases the cancer risk, and also the risk of heart disease, even for long-term smokers.[12] However, the extent of relief is still unclear (see Table 6.2).

Tar Yield. It has long been assumed that the major carcinogens in tobacco smoke are found in the particulate rather than the gas phase. Tar condensates have been measured annually by the Federal Trade Commission for over a decade and the results must now be displayed in advertisements.

When filter cigarettes first became popular in the mid-1950s, their major role was the reduction of tar. This single step has led to lower death rates from lung and larynx cancers among smokers of filtered cigarettes, compared with smokers of high-tar cigarettes.[13] However, death rates among filter cigarette smokers are in excess of those in nonsmokers.

Only half the cigarettes smoked in the United States in 1960 were filtered. Today over 90 percent are filtered and have tar levels less than 20 mg per cigarette. Federal Trade Commission ratings have also shown a very marked increase of cigarettes with tar levels under 10 mg, as many as 28 brands being available by June, 1977.

One problem with low-tar cigarettes is that they have a lower nicotine/tar ratio than unfiltered cigarettes. To compensate for this lower nicotine content, smokers of filtered cigarettes may inhale more and use more cigarettes than would be the case if they smoked unfiltered cigarettes. Thus filter cigarette smokers may end up inhaling more tar than they would from high-tar cigarettes. Low-tar cigarettes also produce relatively higher levels of carbon monoxide, due to relatively incomplete combustion, and increased carbon monoxide inhalation appears to promote heart disease. Additionally, there may well be unrecognized risks from the extensive use of hundreds of secret and untested flavor additives used to restore flavor lost in the high

---

* The nicotine from alkaline smoke is more easily absorbed through the mouth and tongue, allowing the smoker of French cigarettes to satisfy the craving for nicotine without inhaling the carcinogenic smoke.

filtration process in low-tar cigarettes. From all points of view, there is absolutely no better way to deal with these problems than to stop smoking.

Histology of Lung Cancer. There are several different types of lung cancer. The most common type, *squamous carcinoma,* comprises cancers of the epithelial cells lining the trachea and bronchi and is caused by smok-

ing. A second type, called *oat cell carcinoma,* is also strikingly related to cigarette smoking. Smoking probably causes a third type, *adenocarcinoma,* but much less frequently than the other types.

Worldwide Data. Many countries now either support limited epidemiological surveys on smoking or participate in programs developed by international health agencies. The

Table 6.2 Comparison of Relative Lung Cancer Death Rates for Men Aged 50-69 for Cigarette Smokers, Ex-Smokers, and Nonsmokers

Smoking Habits	Death Rates Relative to Nonsmokers
1.0	
Current smokers (cigarettes/day)	
1-9	3.5
10-19	8.8
20-39	13.8
40 or more	17.5
Current smokers with different inhalation practices	
None or slight	10.6
Moderate	11.7
Deep	13.9
Ex-smokers of 1-19 cigarettes/day who had quit for specified number of years	
1 or less	7.2
1-4	4.6
5-9	1.0
10 or more	0.4
Ex-smokers of 20 or more cigarettes/day who had quit for specified number of years	
1 or less	29.1
1-4	12.0
5-9	7.2
10 or more	1.1

Source: E.C. Hammond, "Smoking in relation to death rates of one million men and women," National Cancer Inst. Monogr. *19*: pp. 129-204, 1966.

British Tobacco Research Council, an industry trade association, publishes reports on the use of tobacco products by Britons, as does the Verband der Cigarettenindustrie in Germany.

Recently, a high degree of correlation has been demonstrated between the present lung cancer mortality rate in nineteen different countries and their per capita cigarette consumption thirty years ago.[†][14] Three countries that did not fit this correlation well were France, Ireland, and Japan. The French data can be explained by the fact that smokers in that country tend to inhale less than Americans. The Japanese anomaly was thought due to the Japanese custom of *kazami,* in which the cigarette is puffed, but not inhaled. The Irish data are largely unexplained, but may reflect lesser concomitant exposure to occupational carcinogens.

Differing Cancer Rates in Various Groups.
Until about 1950, few American women smoked. The rapidly rising cancer rate among women today reflects the smoking habit established about thirty years ago and continued since then. The cigarette-smoking habit is now increasingly common among adolescents of all classes and working people, while the white-collar classes, particularly professional men, are giving it up in increasing numbers. Also, a greater proportion of black men smoke than whites and they are more likely to use non-filters than whites. The lung cancer incidence rate among black males in this country is about one-third greater than that for white males.[15]

Smoking and Air Pollution. Various surveys in England and the United States have indicated that smokers of a given age, sex, and level of tobacco consumption have a higher lung cancer rate if living in urban areas with high air pollution levels, than if living in the relatively unpolluted suburbs. It seems likely that there is a synergistic interaction between smoking and urban air pollution.[‡]

Lung Cancer among Nonsmokers and in Workers. About 20 percent of lung cancer deaths occur in nonsmokers, and the incidence of lung cancer in nonsmokers is on the increase. While there is a marked increase in the incidence of lung cancer in asbestos workers and uranium miners who smoke, there is also an increase, though a lesser one, in nonsmokers who work in these industries. An important role of exposure to occupational carcinogens in lung cancer deaths previously exclusively attributed to smoking is likely. It must be recognized that the role of work history and occupational exposures to carcinogens was ignored in the classical epidemiological studies relating smoking to lung cancer. This has led to a possible overestimate of the risks of smoking compared to the risks of exposure to occupational carcinogens or interaction between the two.[*] (This has been compounded by the fact that lung cancer mortality rates based on the International List of Causes of Disease fails to distinguish between lung cancer of different histologi-

---

† The thirty-year lag reflects the long latency period for lung cancer.
‡ According to Schneiderman *Preventine Medicine* 7 (1978) pp. 424-38), there has been a decline in cancer rates in England since their Clean Air Program was initiated in the mid-1950s. Schneiderman also points out that from 1947 to 1970 there has been an increase in U.S. lung cancer rates in the order of 10 to 20 percent which cannot be accounted for by smoking.

* Echoing Wilhelm Hueper's earlier warnings, Joseph Wagoner of OSHA has recently stated that overemphasis on smoking has been a major barrier to research into occupational causes of lung cancer. (For a more detailed discussion and confirmation of this viewpoint, see J. G. French et al., NIOSH, "Interactions Between Smoking and Occupational Exposures," The Surgeon General's Report on Smoking and Health, January 11, 1979.)

cal types, some of which, such as adeno-carcinoma, are unlikely to be due to cigarette smoking and other forms of malignant disease of the lung, such as pleural mesothelioma, which is due to asbestos and not smoking.) As Schneiderman of the NCI has recently pointed out (see statement to OSHA, Docket 090, April 4, 1978), "We are unable to say how much of the risks attributed to cigarettes is a 'pure' cigarette risk and how much is cigarette times another, possibly on-the-job hazard."

It should be noted that these various epidemiological studies proving the tobacco-cancer relationships were all based on analysis of groups of individuals with varying smoking habits as compared to nonsmokers. In the absence of population groups with such differences in exposure, epidemiology cannot readily establish causal links between disease and exposure. (This is why epidemiology is of limited value for the detection of such environmental carcinogens as food additives and pesticides to which the population-at-large is extensively exposed.) One possibility that has not been adequately recognized is that some cancer cases identified in these epidemiological studies derive from exposure to occupational carcinogens, such as asbestos, as well as or instead of tobacco smoke.

This epidemiological summary would be incomplete if it left the impression that lung cancer is the only type of cancer caused by smoking. Tobacco smoking is also incriminated in cancers at other sites, including the lip, tongue, mouth, larynx, pharynx, esophagus, urinary bladder, pancreas, and possibly kidney and liver.† In addition to cancer, smoking is the major cause of chronic bronchitis and emphysema in the United States. Smoking also has a striking relationship to coronary heart disease, stroke, aortic aneurysm, and other diseases, including peptic ulcers.

Astoundingly enough, industry claimed for some time that the association between tobacco and all of these diseases showed that their product could not possibly be at fault. In this they were supported by academic consultants, including the well-known statistician, Joseph Berkson,[16] of the Mayo Clinic, who protested in 1958, "I find it quite incredible that smoking should cause all of these diseases. It appears to me that some other explanations must be formulated." In view of the fact that tobacco smoke contains hundreds of identifiable chemical components, it is now surprising that smoking causes so few diseases.

Involuntary Smoking

Passive or involuntary smoking is the inhalation by nonsmokers of the secondhand products of cigarette smoking, usually in situations not of their own choosing. This type of exposure is potentially serious, because the toxic and carcinogenic chemicals released from the burning tip of a cigarette enter the atmosphere totally unfiltered. This so-called sidestream, smoke contains high concentrations of tar, carbon monoxide, nicotine, and nitrosamines. (The smoker thus breathes the double load of mainstream and sidestream smoke.) Many nonsmokers are highly sensitive to cigarette smoke, the most noticeable effects of which are eye and throat irritation. In poorly ventilated enclosed areas, such as bars, automobiles and conference rooms, allowing one pack of cigarettes to burn has produced levels of nitrosamine carcinogens ten times higher than in inhaled smoke itself, a tar concentration of 17 mg/m^3 and carbon monoxide levels of 70 ppm.[17] In such an environment, the carboxyhemoglobin level of a nonsmoker, a measure of carbon monoxide inhalation, has been found to double. Such studies have shown that this environment for the passive smoker, especially the elevated

---

† The attributable risk (the proportion of a disease to a given cause) of lung cancer due to smoking has been estimated as 0.8 to 0.85 (80-85 percent); for bladder cancer, 0.4-0.5; for pancreas cancer, 0.3-0.4.

carbon monoxide, is particularly dangerous for people with cardiovascular disease, and can aggravate or bring on anginal symptoms.[18] It is not yet known what effect such exposure has on lung cancer risks, although on theoretical grounds it is likely that they are increased.

A second category of involuntary smoker is the fetus. Many studies have found a marked decrease in birth weight of infants born to mothers who smoked during the second half of pregnancy, even as little as one cigarette per day.[19] The immediate effect of maternal smoking on the health of the child can be seen in the poor survival rate for these infants with a lower birth weight. The 1974 surgeon general's report estimated that of 87,000 perinatal deaths in the United States, 4,600 were a direct result of the mother's smoking. The smoking mother is also 80 percent more likely than the nonsmoker to have a spontaneous abortion. Other effects also occur, such as the increased carbon monoxide in the mother's blood causing a more rapid heartbeat in the fetus. In addition, both nicotine and the carcinogen benzo[a]pyrene cross the placental barrier and reach the fetus, which at that stage in development is particularly sensitive to carcinogens. Children of smoking parents also have a higher incidence of bronchitis and pneumonia than the children of nonsmokers. Finally, the role parents play as models for their children should not be overlooked; children of smokers are probably more likely to smoke than children of nonsmokers. In spite of such evidence, the Tobacco Institute,‡ supported by the NCI's Gori, says that there is no hazard in involuntary smoking and that there is no need for regulatory controls to protect the nonsmoker.

Financial Costs of Smoking

While it is difficult to properly calculate the financial costs of smoking, it seems clear that these are much greater than the $6 billion annual tax revenues generated.[20] Annual costs in the United States include treatment and deprivation of earnings of the 80,000 or so tobacco-associated lung cancer victims and the approximately 200,000 victims of respiratory and cardiovascular diseases caused by smoking. The costs of passive smoking have not yet been adequately recognized, let alone estimated. Other direct costs include the millions of public research dollars spent on tobacco-induced diseases, income loss from tobacco-induced diseases, and excess fire protection costs. In the latter category for example, fire protection and fire damage costs from smoking in Massachusetts alone are estimated to be $18 million and $26 million, respectively. Recent estimates of total annual costs from smoking are in the $20 billion range.

The Role of Government in "Prevention" of Tobacco-Related Cancer

What is the government doing to reduce the number of cases of tobacco-related can-

---

‡ The Tobacco Institute was created in 1958 to handle the industry's lobbying and image-making. Its current budget of about $5 million is largely derived from tobacco company dues, half of which can be deducted from taxes as the institute is chartered as a nonprofit trade association. The institute's legal bill (for lawyers including former Kentucky Senator Marlow Cook and former North Carolina Representative Henderson) topped $1 million in 1977. Over the last two decades, the institute has spent about $74 million on "independent research" on to-bacco and health. The institute encourages new legislators from tobacco states to seek seats on key committees. The president of the institute is Horace B. Kornegay, former North Carolina congressman, and its chief lobbyist is Jack Mills, former Republican party power-broker. The Tobacco Institute is probably one of the most powerful trade associations in its ability to mold the legislative and regulatory process to the advantage of the industry. The American Cancer Society provides virtually no effective opposition to these activities.

cers? The only major effort now federally funded is a coordinated set of projects administered by the NCI, known as the Smoking and Health Program. The program's fundamental premise is that since an outright ban on cigarettes is not possible now, the best compromise is to develop a "less harmful cigarette."[21] However, it is inappropriate for the taxpayer to fund this research through the NCI, especially when it is clear that the industry will profit from apparent successes in the research program. The most serious criticism of the Smoking and Health Program, apart from its token budget, is its lack of anti-smoking education activities. Instead of opposing smoking as its main goal, the government program merely seeks to reduce the risks entailed in smoking, thereby supporting the industry efforts to persuade smokers to persist in their habit but switch to "less harmful" cigarettes.

The avowed goal of the Smoking and Health Program is to attempt to reduce the risk for the smoker who refuses to or allegedly cannot quit. The project consists of a range of activities with this common theme. The major current tobacco blends are analyzed to identify their chemical constituents. These are then tested in animal models to determine their individual roles in tobacco cancer. On the basis of these results, an experimental cigarette is "built," which contains a minimum of toxic products. Flavor agents or additives are then added to this "less harmful cigarette" to make it more palatable to the average smoker. The possibility of toxic or carcinogenic effects from these tobacco additives does not seem to have been adequately investigated.

To oversee the smoking program, the NCI set up the Tobacco Working Group, consisting of health and industry experts, including vice presidents and research directors of Liggett & Myers, the Brown & Williamson Tobacco Company, R. J. Reynolds Industries, Lorillard Research Center, and Philip Morris, not to mention representatives of major consulting firms, such as Hazleton Laboratories and Arthur D. Little, Inc. Apart from the industrial domination built into the Tobacco Working Group, research and educational activities were trivial in relation to the importance of smoking as the number one cancer killer. The Tobacco Working Group, which was disbanded in 1977,* funded only a single large-scale epidemiological study on smoking and cancer and failed to fund studies on interactions between smoking and industrial chemicals in the workplace and in the general community. Additionally, the pattern of research support awarded by the Tobacco Working Group has demonstrated clear conflicts of interest in that much of the support was awarded to the members of the Group or to the institutions to which members of the Group belonged.

An example of how similar were the perspectives of the Tobacco Working Group to those of industry is the allegation by its recent director, Gio Gori (deputy director of the NCI's Division of Cancer Cause and Prevention and now on leave of absence as a student at Johns Hopkins' School of Public Health), that a so called "practical threshold" exists for each popular brand of cigarette, constituted by the number that can be smoked daily without leading to a detectable increase in risks of lung cancer.[22] An immediate rebuttal was issued by Arthur Upton, NCI Director, and Robert Levy, Director of the National Heart, Lung and Blood Institute, in a joint statement of August 10, 1978.

> We fear Dr. Gori's paper may mislead the public. We are even more concerned about his assertion that the risk involved with low-tar-and-nicotine cigarettes is "tolerable."

This was followed by a similar disclaimer from Assistant HEW Secretary Julius B. Richmond.[23]

---

* Since then, there do not appear to have been any major changes in NCI policies on tobacco.

No one should be misled by Dr. Gori's study into the belief that there is some way that one can adjust one's smoking habits and the cigarettes one smokes and thus avoid all health risks.

NCI statisticians John Gart and Marvin Schneiderman (in an unpublished but widely circulated letter to *Science)* attacked Gori's methods as "so seriously in error that we find the conclusions based on the statistical analysis . . . to be invalid."[24] Correcting for errors, Gart and Schneiderman showed that recalculation of Gori's own data proved that smoking as few as one cigarette every five days, considered by Gori to be "tolerable," produced as much as a 10 percent increase in risks of lung cancer. Other critics pointed out that Gori had considered only six components of cigarette smoke (tar, nicotine, carbon monoxide, nitrogen oxides, hydrogen cyanide, and acrolein), quite apart from ignoring hundreds of other known toxic components; that he had not considered potential toxic or carcinogenic effects of newer untested cigarette additives; and that he had not dealt adequately with the behavioral problem of "compensation," whereby persons who switch to lower tar cigarettes often smoke more cigarettes or inhale more deeply to adjust for the lower nicotine level of their adopted brand. The tobacco lobby, however, was jubilant. Senator Paul Huddleston of Kentucky remarked that the NCI study "indicated our efforts to produce a safer cigarette and reduce potential hazards are drawing some beneficial results."[25] *The Wall Street Journal* reported that at least 10 percent of the nation's 63 million

smokers would try Carlton, the lowest-tar brand, as a result of the Gori report.[26]

The NCI, with a current annual budget of over $900 million, last year spent less than $9 million on all its tobacco research projects, most of which went to the Smoking and Health Program. Much of this research support is channelled through a prime commercial contractor, Enviro Control, of Rockville, Maryland. Less than $2 million a year is spent by the NCI on educational programs, in contrast with the $400 million the industry now spends annually on cigarette advertising in magazines and newspapers.

The Role of the Government in the Increase of Tobacco-Related Cancer

The extent of federal support of the industry is not generally appreciated. This support is more than amply compensated by massive revenues from tobacco sales. Federal, state, and local governments collect about $6 billion in tobacco taxes annually. In 1977, $97 million was spent by the government in direct assistance programs and in indirect support of the industry. This includes a $50 million USDA research program studying better ways to grow and process the crop, and contract-supported research at the universities of Kentucky and North Carolina. Other federal subsidies include inspection and grading of domestic crops, administration of tobacco price support programs, and loans for sales abroad under the 1954 Food for Peace program.† In December, 1977, President Carter pledged continued federal support for tobacco growers, expressing the view that the

---

† Federal tobacco "subsidies," established by President Roosevelt in the 1930s as a means of stabilizing a market of thousands of small farmers and only a few large conglomerates who purchased their crops, are more accurately described as price support programs. Some justification for their retention, in the absence of effective regulation of tobacco, is provided by a 1978 Con-

gressional Research Service Report (to Congressman Andrew Maguire) "Information on Tobacco Production, Marketing and Government Programs." This report contends that removal of "subsidies" would result in the decline of tobacco prices, increase domestic consumption, and increase the consolidation of small farms into large conglomerates.

assistance programs and health dangers of tobacco should be considered as separate issues.

In a speech on January 12, 1978, HEW Secretary Joseph Califano announced, on the occasion of the 14th anniversary of the surgeon general's classic report on smoking and health, an anti-smoking campaign particularly aimed at the nation's youth.[27] Calling smoking "slow-motion suicide," he asked the major broadcasting networks to increase anti-smoking commercials; called for a ban on smoking in most public areas of HEW buildings; endorsed the Civil Aeronautics Board proposal to ban cigarettes on commercial airliners; urged an increased tax on cigarettes; asked insurance companies to give premium discounts to nonsmokers; and asked the FDA to amend labeling on oral contraceptives to indicate the even greater risk of strokes and heart attacks for smokers.‡

Asked to comment on the apparently contradictory thrusts of the Carter and Califano statements, White House Press Secretary Jody Powell commented:

> The Administration does not feel that there is any logic in asking thousands of families and communities to bear the burden of economic ruin which would result if we abolished the part of the farm program because of the habits of an entire nation.[28]

The reaction of the tobacco industry to Califano's speech was summarized by Raymond J. Mulligan, President of the Liggett Group, Inc., who called the Secretary "a silly ass."[29] The Kentucky state legislature went further and demanded Califano's resignation. It is clear that an administration attack on tobacco price supports would be damaging to the base of Carter's political support in the South. It is not clear how the administration weighs political expediency against 300,000 American deaths each year.

The Role of Industry

The tobacco industry did not welcome the early reports of the adverse health effects of smoking. During the 1950s, when many of these studies were just getting under way, the industry did its best to discredit them by sponsoring their own studies in search of contrary results and by supporting highly publicized and unproductive forays into improbable areas of research. These strategies were relatively successful for many years, as the few independent scientists who devoted their careers to tobacco and health research were repeatedly forced to enter public forums to respond to industry challenges.

It is important to understand the claims of the tobacco industry, because many of them are being echoed in the present-day debates over other environmental carcinogens. The standard gambit then, as now, was that the health research implicating smoking was based only on statistics and not on medical observations. If a real cause and effect sequence from cigarette smoking inhalation to cancer could be shown, the industry cried, rather than all these statistics, that indeed would constitute proof.

Another favorite industry fallback was, and still is, the genetic, or constitutional issue. This claims that some people, predestined by their genes to get cancer, are also by nature predisposed to smoke cigarettes. In simpler terms, cancer causes smoking![30] The logical conclusion of this argument is that "susceptible" people somehow should be identified and discouraged from smoking so that the rest of the population can continue to be exposed

---

‡ While these proposals are to be welcomed, they are merely proposals to other agencies, without any regulatory force and without any preventive economic measures, such as increased tobacco taxation or incentives to tobacco farmers to develop other crops (for a recent discussion of nonregulatory approaches to decrease tobacco consumption, see M. A. Schneiderman, "Legislative Possibilities to Reduce the Impact of Cancer," *Preventive Medicine 7, 1978, pp. 424-38).*

"safely." This line of reasoning is sometimes applied to the debate on exposure standards in the workplace, where other industries talk of finding and screening out "hypersusceptible" workers.

In terms of funding research, the tobacco industry remains at consultant's length from the NCI smoking program, as it would not do to have government money paid directly to tobacco companies for health research. On April 12, 1977, the industry launched its own Tobacco and Health Research Institute on the University of Kentucky campus.* In a three-day conference held in Lexington to mark the dedication of this institute, the thrust of research to be undertaken there was revealed. Of nineteen talks given by well-known speakers invited from academia, ten were devoted to the genetic factors and immune response involved in "hypersusceptibility" to tobacco smoke. Indeed, the title of the program, "Pulmonary Disease: Defense Mechanisms and Populations at Risk," only hinted at the reality. The institute appears to have adopted the tobacco industry's tactic of shifting the burden of proof away from themselves and onto the victims.

Early efforts at regulating the sale of tobacco, based on health reports in the 1950s, inspired massive counter-lobbying by the industry and tied up the Federal Trade Commission for years in administrative logjams.[31] Even when the writing at last appeared on the wall with the famous 1964 warning of Surgeon General Luther Terry that smoking presents "a health hazard of sufficient importance . . . to warrant remedial action," industry decided to dig its heels in still more firmly.[32]

The biggest blow against cigarette smoking was initiated in 1970 by John Banzhaf II, Director of a public interest group known as Action on Smoking and Health. Banzhaf petitioned the Federal Communications Commission to use the Fairness Doctrine to require TV and radio stations that broadcast cigarette ads also to give equal time to anti-smoking ads. The commission and the courts agreed with Banzhaf. Tough anti-smoking spots began giving the public the other side of the smoking story. So strong were the spots that the cigarette industry decided to remove their ads from the airwaves, which had the effect of removing the anti-smoking spots also.

The tobacco industry's voluntary withdrawal from TV and radio advertising was one of the most successful gambles in the history of mass marketing. The industry thus saved hundreds of millions of advertising dollars, which were then used to strengthen its printed advertising, which would continue unthreatened by anti-smoking commercials. Advertising revenues to newspaper and magazine publishers have increased nearly seven-fold since 1970, reaching a current annual total of approximately $400 million. Also, to get further media exposure, the industry sponsors athletic contests, such as the Virginia Slims Tennis competition.† A new organization of health professionals called "Doctors Ought to Care" has filed a request that the U.S. attorney general forbid televising the Virginia Slims Tournament under that name on the grounds that such advertising is against Federal Communication Commission regulations.

The latest marketing gimmickry is the introduction by R. J. Reynolds of a new brand of cigarettes called Reals. Reals were launched in 1977 with a $50 million promotional campaign described in the press as "the most heavily advertised cigarette introduction of all time," and as "the biggest marketing

---

* The Institute is an operation of the Commonwealth of Kentucky, and is entirely supported by an allocation from the state cigarette tax.

† In 1975, the Florida Chapter of the American Cancer Society offered to cosponsor the tournament. The offer was abruptly withdrawn when the national office in New York found out what was happening.

campaign in the history of consumer packaged goods." The industry itself promised that "before long you won't be able to turn around out there without having Reals hit you over the head."[33] The thrust of this advertising campaign, which bombed because it failed to stress low tar strongly enough, was that Reals are "natural" cigarettes containing no synthetic flavoring or other additives. The clear and misleading inference is that Reals are safer than other cigarettes and should be favored by health-conscious consumers.

Senator Edward Kennedy (D-Mass.) is currently exploring new initiatives designed to deter adolescents from smoking. These are based on the use of HEW funds to support private and public educational programs on TV and through other media. Additional approaches also being considered by Senator Kennedy include mandating the use of more effective and explicit labels on cigarette packs.

The Role of the American Cancer Society

Much of the early work on the causal association between smoking and cancer was supported by the American Cancer Society. In fact, the society was one of the few major health groups to request President Kennedy in 1961 to take action against tobacco. Having made this important contribution, the society took the position that the matter was out of its hands. In its own words, the society "had used [its] resources to uncover the health risks of smoking. Now it was up to the government to take a stand and to respond accordingly."[34]

This attitude has typified subsequent policies of the American Cancer Society. Following publication of the 1964 surgeon general's report, the society expressed disappointment at the failure of government to act. However, when Banzhaf petitioned the Federal Communications Commission in 1971 for equal time against tobacco ads, the society refused to support him, let alone defend the subsequent FCC ruling in his favor.‡

Since the Banzhaf episode, the record of the society has remained mixed. It has supported ordinances to prohibit or restrict smoking in public places, to request more stringent warnings on cigarette packs, including use of the word "death," and to establish a graduated federal excise tax on cigarettes based on their tar and nicotine content.

In October, 1976, the society created a National Commission on Smoking and Public Policy, under the direction of Victor Weingarten (an experienced public relations consultant), with Philip R. Lee (University of California School of Medicine, San Francisco) as acting chairman. The Commission was asked to assess the effectiveness of current anti-smoking activities and make appropriate recommendations for new strategies. The Commission held extensive hearings, took testimony from over three hundred individuals, and examined voluminous published and unpublished data, including industry files. The Commission reported back to the society in January, 1978, recommending the development of strong legislative action, and endorsing earlier recommendations to this effect by Nutrition Action (a Washington-based public interest group). The Commission further recommended that the Society set up a powerful anti-tobacco lobby in Washington, D.C., and spend the maximum amount of money permitted by law for legislative activities. The American Cancer Society rejected these recommendations, but, in an apparent compromise move, published a report critical of its own past performance,

---

‡ According to Banzhaf, the society "has never participated in a judicial, regulatory, or legislative petition related to smoking . . . [their usual response being] We don't want to get involved in anything controversial." (Frank Greve, "Cancer Society's Efforts Found Wanting," Philadelphia *Inquirer,* April 30, 1978.)

and pledged to support HEW Secretary Califano's new anti-smoking initiatives.

The "Target 5," five-year program of the society, designed to reduce the number of young people and adults who smoke and to reduce the toxicity and carcinogenicity of tobacco smoke, stands little chance of success without a well-organized lobbying activity. The society still has not announced plans to lobby Congress or to file petitions with the Federal Trade Commission and other concerned agencies. The society has a part-time lobbyist in Washington, D.C., Tanny Pollster, whose major activity seems to be protecting the NCI budget, and who views his role primarily as a "collector of information for the society," rather than as a lobbyist. It is widely rumored that Pollster's salary is defrayed by a direct pass-through to the society from Mary Lasker. In early 1978 the society hired the late Marvella Bayh, wife of Senator Birch Bayh and a breast cancer victim, as a full time lobbyist.* It would not seem unreasonable to expect that the society should develop strong lobbying activities in order to secure legislative and regulatory support for its anti-smoking programs and objectives.†

The Role of the Press

The press is now the almost exclusive medium of major advertising for the tobacco industry. The massive coverage given the Vietnam War, with some 40,000 U.S. deaths in all the war years combined, and the violent crime deaths of some 20,000 per year contrasts with the virtual silence of the press on a single agent incriminated in about 300,000 preventable deaths a year. The enormous revenues generated probably account for the apparent lack of interest of the press in devoting proportionate space to tobacco health hazards.

There are, however, some notable exceptions. The *Reader's Digest,* which does not accept cigarette advertisements, has published a series of authoritative articles on the dangers of smoking over the last two decades, and *The New Yorker* has published several outstanding articles by Thomas Whiteside on the political and advertising strategies of the tobacco industry.

The Role of the Courts

The courts have not been helpful in the past in gaining legal redress for victims of tobacco cancer. At least fifty such suits have been filed, but none has ever resulted in an award. During the 1950s and 1960s, the main argument of the plaintiffs was that the producers had failed to supply a product of marketable quality and that they had not fulfilled their responsibility to make sure that cigarettes were harmless, while implying such in their advertising. The successful defense of industry was that there had been no way to foresee the harm their product might do a consumer.

The farthest such a case has ever gone was *Green v. American Tobacco Co.* Edwin Green of Miami contracted lung cancer in 1956, after smoking Lucky Strikes for thirty years. A jury found in favor of the company at first, but the Court of Appeals, acting on an appeal by the heirs of the by then deceased Green, directed a new jury trial. The second jury found that Luckies were indeed "reasonably fit for general public consumption," since as one juror later told reporters, if it took twenty

---

* The society appears to have placed Mrs. Bayh in a position of potential conflict of interest. Senator Bayh, as a member of the subcommittee on Labor and HEW of the Appropriations Committee, has considerable influence on the NCI budget. He has, however, failed to persuade Senator Kennedy that the "War on Cancer" be made an integral part of proposed National Health insurance plans.

† Under the Tax Reform Act of 1976 (Sec. 4911, Tax Code Amended, 1976), tax exempt organizations such as the American Cancer Society are allowed to spend up to $1 million annually on lobbying.

to thirty years to affect the plaintiff, they must be reasonably safe. This juror, however, gave up smoking after the trial.[35]

A new appeal by the heirs against this adverse decision resulted in a temporary reversal, in which the Court stated:

> We are now left in no substantial doubt that under Florida law the decedent was entitled to rely on the implied assurance that the Lucky Strike cigarettes were wholesome and fit for the purpose intended and that under the facts found by the jury [his widow is] entitled to hold the manufacturers absolutely liable for the injuries already found by a prior jury to have been sustained by him.[36]

But this consumer triumph was short-lived. In April, 1969, thirteen years after the case had been started and with Edwin Green long in his grave, the U.S. Fifth Circuit Court reversed the decision and found in favor of American Tobacco.[37] Shortly afterward, the universal labeling of cigarette packages with health warnings seemed to virtually close the door on this type of law suit. The smoker now stands warned with every pack he buys and with every advertisement he reads, that cigarette manufacturers do not claim their product to be entirely harmless. The main impact of this warning, advocated by many to help discourage smoking, may in the end be to release tobacco companies from liability and further shift the burden of smoking-induced disease to the victim.

On December 20, 1976, Donna Shimp, an employee of New Jersey Bell Telephone Company, obtained a court injunction ordering Bell to provide a workplace free of cigarette smoke for its nonsmoking employees.[38] The court took into account expert testimony that carbon monoxide, nitrogen oxides, tar, and nicotine given off by cigarette sidestream smoke can aggravate lung and heart disorders, and that up to 10 percent of the population may be allergic to the smoke. The court ruled that smoking was not necessary to the operation of Bell's business, and that no employee should have to assume the risks of inhaling smoke as a condition of employment. The court also noted that, considering that smoking is prohibited near certain telephone equipment because "delicate parts" may be damaged, a human being should be entitled to at least as much protection.

Probably one of the most effective ways of decreasing the tobacco death toll would be to make the industry pay for tobacco-associated cancer and other diseases, as well as other national costs. Cigarette companies have in the past successfully defended themselves against lawsuits by claiming an "assumption of risk" by the victim or his or her family. This claim could be countered by the fact that the industry advertises widely to entice people, including minors, to start smoking. Such advertisements create "an attractive nuisance," often with fatal consequences. Perhaps what is needed now is a series of large successful lawsuits against the industry, still a distant hope.

The Role of Consumer Groups

The rights of the nonsmoker to breathe air unpolluted by tobacco smoke have been vigorously asserted recently by a number of public interest groups created especially for this purpose. Recent information on the dangers of passive smoking have lent further emphasis to these rights. Prominent among these is the Washington-based Action on Smoking and Health. This public interest group has appeared before the Federal Trade Commission in hearings to beef-up warnings on cigarette packages, and to impose stricter advertising rules; before the Federal Communications Commission to get "little cigar" commercials off the air and more anti-smoking ads on; and before the FDA to provide labels on birth control pills warning women about higher disease risks among pill takers who smoke. At the instigation of Action on

Smoking and Health, the Civil Aeronautics Board voted on November 23, 1977, to authorize banning of all cigar and pipe smoking on commercial airlines and took steps that could eventually prohibit cigarette smoking as well. In January, 1979, the Board moved to further tighten anti-smoking restrictions including avoidance of "sandwiching" nonsmokers between groups of smokers, special segregation of pipe and cigar smokers, and the prohibition of all smoking whenever the airplane's ventilation system is not fully operating.

Environmental Improvement Associates, the New Jersey-based group set up by Donna Shimp after her court victory against Bell, is demanding smoke-free working conditions for the nonsmoker. The first "Nonsmoker's Guide to Washington," produced by Washingtonians for Nonsmokers Rights, a project of the Washington, D.C., Lung Association, lists restaurants and hotels which offer nonsmoking areas, besides tips on handling smokers tactfully and effectively. The guide also gives a good rundown on the legal rights of nonsmokers.

Future Trends

The facts speak for themselves. There is a steady and progressive overall increase in tobacco sales in the United States.[39] The smoking habit is extending to younger and younger ages. An HEW survey in April, 1979, found that about 12 percent of 3.3 million adolescents between the ages of twelve and eighteen are smokers. The administration has made it clear that it opposes effective regulation or further taxation of the industry and that it intends to continue subsidies. NCI expenditures on tobacco research are not only trivial but indirectly support the industry by focusing on "less harmful" cigarettes, rather

than on an aggressive anti-smoking campaign. The American Cancer Society's efforts are weak where it really counts, at the legislative and regulatory levels.

It is true that cigarettes in the United States and other developed countries, have 50 percent less tar and nicotine and that the carcinogenic activity of the remaining tar has been decreased.‡ It is also true that filters are becoming more effective at removing selected gases, such as volatile phenols. However, the possible benefits, in terms of reduced cancer risks, are likely to be counterbalanced by increased tobacco consumption and inhalation in some smokers due to the lowered nicotine content of low-tar cigarettes and due to consumers being misled by the illusion of safety of the low-tar cigarettes. Additionally, smokers of low-tar cigarettes are likely to have increased risk of heart disease from the proportionately higher carbon monoxide content of these cigarettes.

More hopeful trends, however, are that the middle class are giving up smoking, and that vigorous public interest groups are carrying the battle into the legal and political arenas.

An important recent development has been the adoption of tough public smoking regulations, effective July 1978, by the New Jersey Public Health Council under the state sanitary code. The council acted following refusal of the New Jersey legislature to address this problem. According to the new regulation, smoking is restricted in restaurants seating more than 50, and prohibited except in areas designated as "smoking permitted," which may not exceed 75 percent of the total area. The nonsmoking area must be equally attractive and convenient and have ventilation adequate to prevent build-up of levels of carbon monoxide above those outside the restaurant. The New Jersey legislature, under pressure from the hotel and

---

‡ The industry's continued insistence on their product's safety contrasts with their aggressive marketing strategies on low-tar cigarettes, reflecting sensitivity to the public's cancer concerns.[40]

Low-tar cigarettes are the only growth segment of the industry, inspiring the biggest and most competitive advertising and marketing campaigns since filters were introduced in the mid-1950s.

restaurant lobby, is threatening to override these new regulations.

A similar move to restrict smoking in restaurants and other public areas in New York was recently proposed by Assemblyman Alexander B. Grannis (D-Manhattan). In May, 1978, Grannis charged that the Retail Tobacco Dealers of America, Inc., which had failed to register under the state's lobbying law, had illegally generated over 30,000 postcards — the largest outpouring of public opinion in this year's legislative session — protesting the proposed bill. Regardless of the success or failure of the New Jersey and New York initiatives, they clearly presage the likelihood of increasing controls and restrictions on smoking by local government.*

As the anti-smoking campaign is beginning to gain ground among professionals and upper socioeconomic classes in developed countries, the tobacco industry is intensifying its promotional campaign in the Third World. British American Tobacco, Inc., is moving aggressively to exploit these newer markets unrestricted by government regulation or social pressures.† Efforts by international organizations, such as the World Health Organization and the International Union Against Cancer to counter this dangerous trend in the Third World are effectively neutralized by actions of the U. N. Development Program and the Food and Agriculture Organization to encourage investment in tobacco as a cash crop.

Summary

Tobacco plays a central role in the modern subculture, fulfilling emotional and physical "needs" which are assiduously and skillfully promoted and nurtured by the industry, with increasing emphasis on the enticing of adolescents. Smoking is the single most important cause of lung cancer, as well as cancers at other sites, chronic bronchitis and emphysema, and cardiovascular diseases. There is growing evidence that switching to filter cigarettes may not necessarily reduce cancer risks and may actually increase the risks of cardiovascular disease. There is also growing evidence on potential hazards to nonsmokers from "secondhand smoke." Finally, there is now firm evidence on the interaction of smoking and other carcinogens, particularly occupational, in the induction of lung cancer. All these adverse effects were emphasized as key findings of the Surgeon General's January 11, 1979, report on "Smoking and Health"‡ (released on the fifteenth anniversary of the first Surgeon General's report on the same subject). Conservative estimates indicate that the costs of smoking approximate 300,000 deaths and $20 billion annually.

The response of government to this national disaster is fragmented and contradictory, reflecting the $6 billion annual tax revenues and the political influence of the Southern congressional network. The USDA openly subsidizes the tobacco industry and, with the blessing of President Carter, sponsors research to improve crop yields. Educational and research activities of the NCI are weak. They include programs to develop "less harmful cigarettes" which are made palatable by chemical additives. Congress has banned cigarette advertising from broadcasting, but not from

---

* A proposed ordinance to ban or severely restrict cigarette smoking in a wide range of indoor public places was defeated by only 835 votes of 190,000 ballots cast in a referendum in Dade County, Florida, in May, 1979. The narrowness of the defeat, in spite of a massive lobbying effort by the tobacco industry, signals the possible early success of future anti-smoking ordinances.

dinances.

† Philippine Kent cigarettes have about three times as much tar as British Keats.

‡ The report, which is an encyclopedic compilation of the published literature, avoids taking stands on the dangers of passive smoking and on the needs for more vigorous federal anti-smoking policies and regulation.

print.* Sensitive to $400 million advertising revenues, the press has engaged in a "conspiracy of silence" to ignore or minimize the human death toll from tobacco. While the American Cancer Society played an important role in the early 1960s in proving and drawing attention to the dangers of smoking, its more recent activities, particularly at the legislative and regulatory levels, have been weak and diffuse. Although the courts are beginning to uphold the rights of nonsmokers to unpolluted air, they have failed to take the only single effective step of controlling smoking, that is finding the industry liable for the costs of disease due to tobacco.

Recent trends that may have powerful impact on the tobacco market include regulatory initiatives being developed at the state and local levels, and industry attempts to counter the possible slowing of tobacco consumption in the United States by opening up massive new markets in lesser developed countries, where the population is poorly informed on the dangers of smoking.

Artificial colors are highly objectionable on ethical grounds because they deceive, and on hygienic grounds because they injure.

Harvey Wiley, Chief
Bureau of Chemistry, USDA, 1907.

Red Dyes #2 and #40

Food is the single most important route of exposure for humans to synthetic chemicals. In a year the average American eats about 1,500 pounds of food containing about 9 pounds of chemical additives (other than sugar and salt). Several thousand chemicals are added to food for a wide range of purposes.[1] These include preservatives, flavoring agents, stabilizers, and colors and are known as *intentional food additives*. An additional class of chemicals, which become incorporated in food during some phase of processing, packaging or storing (such as pesticide residues or chemicals migrating from packaging materials) are known as *indirect food additives*.

Chemicals added to foods and beverages solely for the sake of improving their appearance are popularly known as *cosmetic food additives*. Since antiquity, foods and beverages have, to some extent, been artificially tinted to make them look more appealing and appetizing. Until the relatively recent development of synthetic colors, "natural" pigments such as lead, chromium, and arsenic compounds, were popular additives, although somewhat unpredictable in their coloring — as well as their toxicity. More sensibly, natural plant dyes have also been used for the same purpose.

The use of cosmetic additives often entails consumer deception, in that they make a food look better and more appealing than it really is, or than its condition really warrants.[2] Current labeling laws do not require that the consumer be given explicit information on the presence or concentration of these artificial colors in foods, which are instead labeled "artificial colors," FD&C (Food, Drug and Cosmetic) or U.S. certified colors. Additionally, many colored foods, such as cheese, butter, and ice cream, are exempt from even these minimal labeling requirements. This taken with absence of alternative, uncolored foods and beverages hardly allows the consumer to exercise free choice in the marketplace. To make matters worse, there is mounting evidence of the toxicity and carcinogenicity of synthetic colors, and this is in no way indicated on the labels of beverages or foods containing them.

Natural plant dyes were the cornerstone

---

* A similar ban on print advertising would appear to present grave first amendment problem.

of the industry until the latter part of the last century, when they were ousted by synthetic dyes based on coal tars.[3] The coal-tar dye industry had its origin in 1856, when an English college student, William Henry Perkin, attempting to synthesize quinine, succeeded only in obtaining a dirty reddish-brown precipitate. Intrigued, he repeated the reaction using a simpler starting material, aniline sulfate, and from the resulting black residue extracted a purple compound which was lightfast and stuck to textile fibers. Within the year, this new compound, which he dubbed mauve, appeared so useful that the Perkin family began manufacturing it on a large scale. Similarly, in 1897, a German company, BASF, discovered a highly profitable technique for the synthesis of indigo from a derivative of coal tar, naphthalene. Indigo, long one of the most important dyes, had for centuries been manufactured from plant extracts.

The burgeoning synthetic dye industry was initially a closed German enterprise, stimulated by their expertise in organic chemistry and favorable tariff and financing laws. This lucrative industry got a sudden boost in the United States during World War I, when, deprived of German products, the American chemical industry developed its own synthetic methods and new dye products.

The largest single class of dyes are chemical derivatives of coal tars. These compounds are used for coloring beverages, food, cosmetics, and textiles, as well as paints and inks.

The largest single user of FD&C colors is the beverage industry. At least two of the colors, tartrazine and amaranth, you probably ate or drank recently. Their common names are Yellow #5 and Red #2, respectively. According to FDA estimates, some children eat as much as one quarter of a pound of coal-tar dyes each year.

Many coal-tar derivatives and dyes are also known carcinogens, among them 2-naphthylamine and benzidine, which induce bladder cancer in occupationally exposed workers.[4] As knowledge of the carcinogenicity of so many coal-tar dyes is well established, why should it come as any surprise that some dyes used by the food industry have also been shown to be carcinogenic? According to a recent analysis of FDA data by the Health Research Group, most of the seven coal-tar dyes (currently used as food additives) have not been adequately tested for carcinogenicity, although requirements for updating these data have been imposed by the FDA.†[5]

However, there are pressures from industry to continue using "coal-tar" food dyes. In this, they have been abetted by the past regulatory laxness of the FDA. The Food Protection Committee of the National Academy of Sciences, with close ties with the food industry, from which it received about 40 percent of its funding, has taken the position that use of these dyes is "legitimate."[6]

A ban on the use of all cosmetic food additives would not cause undue marketing

---

† As an example, the Center for Science in the Public Interest petitioned the FDA on February 15, 1976, to ban Orange B, an azo dye similar to Red #2 and used mainly in hot dogs sold in the southeastern United States, on the grounds that its safety had not been demonstrated. In May, 1970, in the absence of any FDA action, the manufacturer of Orange B, the Stange Company of Chicago, announced it would "voluntarily" withdraw the product from the market, as it had been shown to be contaminated with the potent bladder carcinogen 2-naphthylamine, thereby preempting an anticipated FDA ban. In November, 1978, the FDA rejected the Health Research Group's petition to ban various coal-tar food colorings, including Citrus Red #2, Blue #1 and Yellow #5 on grounds of their carcinogenicity. In their notice of rejection, the FDA imposed unscientific and onerous criteria for carcinogenicity, including insistence on monotonic dose response relationships and denial of analyzing responses by individual sex. This general position appears consistent with that adopted by the FDA in allowing continued use of Red #40, pending conclusive resolution of substantial questions as to its carcinogenicity.

problems. As established in a Gallup poll commissioned by *Redbook* in March, 1976, 59 percent of all women surveyed favored banning all additives used only to improve the appearance of food. Banning cosmetic additives might also discourage the fad for non-nutritious "junk foods" such as soda pop, candies, and cookies, in which food colors are extensively used. Instead this might encourage use of more expensive natural dyes, such as beet juice. It should be noted that support for such a ban has not come from the FDA or from scientific and nutrition communities, but largely from public interest groups, such as the Health Research Group, the Center for Science in the Public Interest, and the Consumer Federation of America.

Red #2

The Congress probably did not consider cancer when it passed the Pure Food and Drug Act of 1906, which approved an initial seven "coal-tar" food colors, including Red #2, or amaranth. This was done over the strenuous objections of Harvey Wiley, chief of the Bureau of Chemistry, USDA, the agency then responsible for enforcing the Act. In the wake of Upton Sinclair's 1906 expose of the meat industry in his classic book, *The Jungle,* food law reformers were more concerned with preventing people from dropping dead from bacterial contamination and poisonous adulterants than from long-term risks such as cancer. Not surprisingly, therefore, the government permitted color manufacturers to have their products registered as safe, a procedure made mandatory by the 1939 Federal Food, Drug, and Cosmetic Act. This registration was supposed to be the public's guarantee that food additives were harmless. The burden of proof, however, was then on the government to demonstrate that a given additive was harmful. Nevertheless, sixteen previously "approved" coal-tar colors were tested and banned by the government before 1960, when a new set of Color Additive Amendments to the 1938 Act shifted the burden of proof, now requiring industry to prove new products to be safe. Far from being onerous, however, the new laws were actually beneficial to industry, as they allowed continued use of unsafe and inadequately tested additives by registering them provisionally.

The recent history of Red #2 is a saga of past regulatory incompetence coupled with preoccupation with industry interests.[7] Between 1960 and 1975, the FDA extended the provisional registration of the dye fifteen times. Meanwhile, Red #2 was becoming one of the most widely used cosmetic food additives, accounting for over $14 million in direct annual sales, and being incorporated in $10 billion worth of food.

In 1970 the FDA learned of some new Russian studies in which the dye was shown to induce birth defects and cancer in laboratory animals. One of these studies concluded that "chemically pure amaranth possesses carcinogenic activity of medium strength and should not be used in the food industry."[8] FDA scientists meanwhile had become convinced, on the basis of their own and the Russian studies, that Red #2 should be banned. On November 18, 1971, an internal FDA memorandum from scientists of the Bureau of Foods recommended:

It would be prudent to limit FD&C Red #2 only to indirect or incidental applications involving food; that is, limit use of the color to such applications as food packaging where migration to food is nil, color marking of animal food additives, and to external uses in drugs and cosmetics.

The FDA, however, still refused to take any regulatory action, claiming that it could not examine the Russian data or check the purity of the dye used in their tests. In the wake of publicity about its procrastination, the FDA decided to pass the problem to the National Academy of Sciences, which initially rejected the request as too routine. However, under pressure from its Industry Liaison Panel, the academy subsequently conceded and set up an ad hoc subcommittee of its Food Protection committee. The subcommittee produced a report in June, 1972, favorable to the industry, finding "insufficient reason" to ban Red #2 or reduce its use.[9]

About the same time, the FDA decided to undertake on its own an extensive series of tests designed to finally resolve all the safety problems of Red #2. The first set of FDA tests showed that the dye is metabolized in all major organs in the body. A second group of studies explored the question of whether Red #2 causes adverse inheritable genetic mutations. Initial results were inconclusive, but the results of another set of experiments, begun in 1972, remained unanalyzed for over three years through "administrative oversight." A third set of studies showed that the dye would kill rat embryos at daily doses in excess of 15 mg/kg. Applying the standard 100-fold margin of safety used by the FDA for such toxic effects, this would result in setting a "safe level" of 0.15 mg/kg in humans, equivalent to less than one can of cherry soda daily. The FDA attempted to "resolve" this problem by proposing an unprecedented 10-fold reduction in the safety factor for Red #2 thus setting "safe levels" of 1.5 mg/kg.[10]

The big news, however, was the fourth set of FDA tests, those on carcinogenicity. These were initiated in March, 1972, using five groups of fifty male and fifty female rats each, four of them to be given different dosage levels and one to act as a control group. In January, 1973, only nine months into the two-year study, a technician noticed that one rat's identification tag did not match its cage number. Subsequent investigation revealed a fiasco.[11] There was widespread mixing of animals among assigned dosage groups, and a general neglect of husbandry that had left many rats dead and decomposed in their cages. Of the original 500 animals, 231 were unusable

and 71 more had only a few of the necessary organs available for examination, leaving only 198 intact animals. Enough data were salvaged, however, to demonstrate that at the highest dose, at least, the dye induced a large number of malignant tumors in female rats surviving to two years. That was enough to finally force FDA Commissioner Schmidt to ban the food color in January, 1976, though not enough to motivate recall of colored foods from grocers' shelves.

In spite of the fact that industry could conceivably have continued its fight for years to come, particularly in view of the obvious inadequacies of the FDA carcinogenicity tests, Red #2 seems to have been allowed to die a natural death, largely because of forceful protests by consumer and public interest groups, especially the Health Research Group. Allied Chemical, one of the six major U.S. manufacturers of Red #2, also holds the patent on what is claimed to be the best — in fact, the only — available substitute, Allura red, or Red #40.

Red #40

In 1965, Allied began to introduce Red #40 into the profitable food coloring market, and contracted with Hazleton Laboratories to do the required testing. The mainstay of the Hazleton studies was a planned two-year carcinogenicity test, using a total of 300 rats fed various concentrations of the dye. However, after only six weeks of testing, an epidemic of respiratory disease killed many young animals. To halt the infection, survivors were treated with antibiotics. The total mortality was so high that the test had to be terminated prematurely at twenty-one months, leaving only 59 of the original 300 rats available for examination. Clearly, this study has very limited value as a chronic toxicity or carcinogenicity test.[12] The only finding of note admitted by a Hazleton pathologist was kidney damage in some of the higher-dosed animals that died at six months. This diagnosis was subsequently discounted by senior Hazleton staff in a "retrospective histo-pathological analysis," and all references to toxic kidney effects were omitted from the final FDA report.‡[13] On the basis of their Red #40 study, Hazleton scientists nevertheless concluded that Red #40 was noncarcinogenic. Other Hazleton tests, including studies on birth defects in rats and rabbits, gave suspicious or marginal results. These findings were transmitted by Allied to the FDA in 1970, which accepted the Hazleton data and approved the dye for use in foods and drugs in 1971 and for cosmetics in 1974.

The FDA approval allowed Allied to go ahead with aggressive marketing and claims of safety. In early 1971, Allied claimed:

> Allura red has undergone one of the most extensive batteries of testing ever used for a food colorant. The screening included two series of feeding tests — one lasting two years, another lasting five years.[14]

In fact, no five-year study was ever reported to the FDA.

The permanent approval given Red #40 by the FDA in 1971 contradicted its own guidelines, endorsed by several worldwide health organizations, that food additives should be tested for carcinogenicity in at least two animal species. In 1974, an expert committee of the World Health Organization refused to grant even temporary approval for the dye, "as only very limited information is available."[15] Not surprisingly, the dye has not been approved for use in Canada, Sweden, Norway, Japan, Italy, Israel, France, Austria, United Kingdom, or Australia. The FDA has since claimed that they gave approval for the dye in 1971 because they were under the impression that it would be used only for mara-

schino cherries.[16]

Meanwhile, use of Red #40 was growing in the United States. It has become the standard coloring agent in a great many common beverages, processed foods including meats, "junk" foods, such as imitation fruit drinks, soda pop, hot dogs, jellies, candy and ice cream, and even cosmetics and pet food. With more than a million pounds certified by the FDA in 1976, Red #40 has grown in six years from zero sales to the second most prevalent food coloring agent in the U.S., behind only Yellow #5.* It is now virtually impossible to eat most normal meals uncontaminated by the dye. At the current rate of consumption, a child of today will consume one-third of a pound of this "coal-tar" dye in his or her lifetime.[17]

Faced with an urgent need for new test data to unblock foreign markets, Allied again contracted with Hazleton in late 1974 for further studies on rats and mice. About a year into this study, the results to date were presented to FDA. Nothing of particular interest had been observed in the rat experiment. However, early in the mouse test animals started developing cancers of the lymphatic system (lymphomas). Furthermore, the incidence of these cancers seemed related to dosage. An FDA advisor recommended that a large number of apparently healthy mice be sacrificed ahead of schedule — at 42 weeks — in order to see whether there were any undetected lymphomas in either controls or test animals.[18] This action nearly wrecked the study, because it markedly reduced the number of mice in each group remaining at risk, that is, who could survive to develop cancer later in their lives.

On February 25, 1976, the Center for Science in the Public Interest petitioned FDA to

---

‡ On April 8, 1976, then Commissioner Schmidt testified before congressional hearings that the FDA had found major deficiencies in Hazleton testing, which it intended to investigate, stating that the firm did not examine many animals with gross lesions histologically, reported on nonexistent slides, and rewrote their own pathologists' reports.

* Red #40 is used in almost all artificially colored red, orange, and brown foods.

prohibit the use of Red #40 on the grounds that it had been originally allowed into the food supply on the basis of crude studies that did not establish the dye's safety. On the same day, Allied Chemical was meeting with FDA to inform them of "ambiguous findings" in the 1974 mouse feeding study: six of a small group of dye-fed mice had died of cancer, whereas all controls had survived. However, as the experiment proceeded the controls eventually began developing tumors.[19] The FDA responded by asking Allied to undertake a further study, but did not ban the dye. Allied agreed and contracted again with Hazleton in spring of 1976. The refusal of FDA to take any regulatory action at this stage seems contrary to its own guidelines, as spelled out by its own 1969 panel of experts. The guidelines define carcinogens not only in terms of an increased production of tumors in test animals, but also in terms of "an earlier occurrence of tumors in the treated animals than in the controls, the incidence being the same in both."

Apparently sympathetic to the position that Red #40 was industry's last good, cheap synthetic food color, the FDA convened in December, 1976, a special working group of senior researchers and statisticians, together with the NCI and the National Center for Toxicological Research. This group receives monthly reports on the mouse studies, and undertakes independent analysis of the results. In the group's own words:

> Consideration of the results of these studies by the working group will ensure that any decision subsequently reached by FDA regarding the safety and use of FD&C Red No. 40 are legally sound and scientifically supportable . . . The completion dates for the two mouse studies cannot be precisely ascertained.[20]

In April, 1978, on the basis of one completed mouse test and another then in its sev-

enty-sixth week, an interim report by the working group concluded that "experiments provide no evidence at this time" that Red #40 is carcinogenic. This conclusion was made in spite of the fact that mice on the lowest dose of color in the incomplete study have a higher incidence of tumors than in controls, and in spite of the fact that Adrian Gross, a senior scientist in FDA's Division of Scientific Investigations (now senior toxicologist in the EPA), on the basis of a statistical analysis of the latest carcinogenicity data, had warned the agency on February 8, 1978, that Red #40 was carcinogenic. In a forty-eight-page memo to FDA Commissioner Donald Kennedy, Gross responded to the report of the working group by criticizing their statistical techniques and conclusions. To resolve this dispute, Kennedy requested three outside consultants reevaluate the data. The consultants agreed with Gross, stating that the working group's statistical procedures "weren't well suited" for a determination of carcinogenicity. Kennedy then sent a warm note of appreciation to Gross, and reconvened the working group with Gross as a full member.

The comment of Sidney Wolfe, of the Health Research Group, that the working group is "playing a very deadly statistical game," seems apt.[21] It is now over five years since questions of carcinogenicity of Red #40 were first raised. The FDA's refusal to have taken and to now take regulatory action, with continuing involuntary exposure of almost the entire U.S. population to the probably carcinogenic food color, constitutes an inappropriate shift in the burden of proof from industry to the public.

Summary

Red #2 and #40 are "coal-tar" dyes without any nutritional benefits which are added to foods, particularly junk foods, for cosmetic purposes, and in the general absence of explicit labeling which would allow the consumer the exercise of free choice. A recent

Gallup poll established that about 60 percent of women surveyed favored the banning of all such cosmetic food additives.

Many coal-tar derivatives, including some previously used as food additives and since banned, are human carcinogens. There are serious questions as to the carcinogenicity, besides other chronic toxic effects, including birth defects, of those dyes in current food use. It is estimated that some children eat as much as one quarter of a pound of "coal-tar" dye additives each year.

The history of Red #2 and Red #40 reflects regulatory sluggishness of the FDA and the continued sacrifice of the interests of the consumer to the special interests of the food and chemical industries. Between 1960 and 1975, the FDA extended the provisional registration of Red #2 annually for a total of fifteen times, pending the submission by industry of the required toxicological data, meanwhile, allowing the dye to insinuate itself into an $11 billion food market.

In face of mounting evidence of carcinogenicity, including that derived from one of its own bungled tests, the FDA refused to take regulatory action against the dye until it finally acceded to pressure from consumer and public interest groups and in 1976 reluctantly banned the dye.

Red #40 was approved for food use by the FDA in 1971 on the basis of tests by Hazleton Laboratories, under contract to Allied Chemical Company, the manufacturer, which were so inadequate that they were rejected by the World Health Organization and most countries. With the banning of Red #2, the use of Red #40 has expanded and it is now the second most commonly used food dye in the United States. Subsequent tests have raised further and still unresolved questions on the carcinogenicity of Red #40.

The FDA, in permitting the burden of proof to be shifted from industry to the public, is allowing continued use of the dye pending final resolution of these questions.

Anyone who says saccharin is injurious to health is an idiot.

Theodore Roosevelt, 1907.

Saccharin

Saccharin was discovered in 1879 by Ira Remsen, then professor of chemistry and later president of Johns Hopkins University, and also a good friend of President Theodore Roosevelt.[1] Remsen, though a good chemist, was a poor businessman. Constantin Fahlberg, the student who had helped him develop saccharin, took out a patent on its synthesis in his own name and made a fortune. Remsen did not make a nickel.

Manufacture and Current Usage

The method by which Remsen originally synthesized saccharin, known as the Remsen-Fahlberg method, was its major source for many years.[2] A superior method, known as the Maumee synthesis, was later introduced to get rid of the bitter after-taste caused by an impurity in the process, *o*-toluenesulfonamide.

Saccharin is a non-nutritive and non-caloric artificial sweetener, about 350 times sweeter than sugar. The current saccharin market is large and profitable. The foods and beverages in which it is used have a net annual value of about $2 billion.[3] SherwinWilliams is the only domestic producer of saccharin, although some is imported from Japan and Korea. In 1976, about 7 million pounds of saccharin were used in foods, 75 percent in diet sodas (a can of pop contains about 150 mg of saccharin), 15 percent in dietetic foods, and 10 percent in "table top" sweeteners. The relatively minor non-food uses of saccharin include flavoring of mouthwashes, toothpaste, cosmetics, cigarette paper, and animal feeds. Saccharin is also used as a non-prescription drug and as a flavoring agent in prescription drugs, especially antibiotics for pediatric use.

Saccharin is consumed by about 14 percent of the general population, largely by teenagers. In comparison, and contrary to popular belief, saccharin is used regularly by only about one-third of all diabetics.

Efficacy or Benefits

Saccharin is currently approved by the FDA as an intentional food additive. The current food additive law requires proof of safety and "function," but not of "efficacy" or benefit. This means that an additive must perform its registered function. For instance, a sweetener must sweeten food or a color must color food, but this function does not necessarily have to serve any useful purpose.

Claims have been made by the Calorie Control Council[4] an industry trade lobby, and a variety of other groups such as the American Diabetic Association, the American Weight Watchers Association, and the Grocery Manufacturers Association of the value of saccharin in the treatment of diabetes, obesity, dental caries, and other disorders. None of these claims, however, has been backed up by any published studies. In fact, the relatively scant available literature seems to indicate the contrary. The first clue to this came in 1947, when it was shown that as little as 50 mg of saccharin, equivalent to about one-third of a can of diet soda, decreases blood sugar in humans by about 16 percent.[5] Since appetite and hunger can be triggered by a drop in blood sugar, ingestion of saccharin may induce a person to eat more, hardly a good prescription for a low-calorie sweetener. These effects were subsequently confirmed in animal studies, in which it was also shown that rats fed low doses of saccharin actually ate more and gained more weight than saccharin-free controls.[6]

In 1956, a cooperative study by the nutrition department of the Harvard School of Public Health and the dietary department at the Peter Bent Brigham Hospital, Boston, on the use of saccharin and cyclamates in the management of diabetics and the obese concluded:

> No significant difference was apparent when the weight loss of users and non-users of these products was compared. No correlation was found between the length of time these products were used and weight loss, nor was the degree of overweight associated with the use of these products.[7]

In 1974 a report by an expert subcommittee of the National Institute of Medicine of the National Academy of Sciences chaired by Kenneth Melmon, concluded:

> The data on the efficacy of saccharin or its salts for the treatment of patients with obesity, dental caries, coronary artery disease, or even diabetes has not so far produced a clear picture to us of the usefulness of the drug.[8]

More recently, eminent diabetes and dietetic experts, including Jesse Roth, Director of Endocrinology and Diabetes at the National Institutes of Health, the late Max Miller, Chief of the Diabetic Clinic at Case Western Reserve Medical School, and Ann Galbraith, Chief Dietician at the Massachusetts General Hospital and past-president of the American Dietetic Association, have all endorsed this particular conclusion of the Melmon subcommittee. Further confirmation on the lack of any substantive evidence on the medical efficacy of saccharin was presented at hearings before Congressman Paul Rogers (D-Fla.) on March 22, 1977, by Sidney Wolfe, of the Health Research Group,[9] and before Senator Gaylord Nelson (D-Wisc.) on June 7, 1977, by Donald Fredrickson, Director of the National Institutes of Health and Donald Kennedy, FDA Commissioner.[10]

Carcinogenicity Tests

Saccharin has been extensively tested for carcinogenicity in rodents over the last three decades. The majority of these studies are still unpublished, having been sponsored by industry or government, and until recently never subject to independent scrutiny. The quality of these studies is variable in regard to design, execution, and interpretation.

Approximately a dozen conventional feeding tests, one dating back to 1948, have shown that saccharin is carcinogenic in both rats and mice.[11] While each of these individual studies may be criticized on some grounds or other, taken together the weight of evidence proving the carcinogenicity of saccharin is overwhelming. The dietary concentrations of saccharin tested and found to be carcinogenic have ranged from as low as 0.01 percent, equivalent to a daily consumption of about one and a half bottles of diet pop, to 7.5 percent, equivalent to daily consumption of about 800 bottles.

In addition to cancer of the urinary bladder in rats, the predominant tumor induced in these tests (Table 6.3), saccharin also induced cancers in female reproductive organs, and lymphomas or leukaemias (Table 6.4) in both mice and rats.

Three of the most important studies were those by WARF (the Wisconsin Alumni Research Foundation) in 1973, the FDA in 1973, and Arnold, *et al.*, in Canada's equivalent of the FDA, the Health Protection Branch, in 1977. The WARF study confirmed that saccharin over a dose range from 0.05 to 5 percent, induced cancer of the bladder, the uterus, and the ovary. The 1973 FDA study involved groups of forty-eight male and female rats fed saccharin over a dose range from 0.01 percent to 7.5 percent. This study confirmed the induction of bladder cancer and also found breast cancer. The 1977 Canadian study was a crucial one because it was based on feeding pure saccharin, produced by the newer Maumee synthesis, to large numbers of rats over the course of two generations. A higher incidence of bladder cancer was produced in the second generation, warning of the in-

creased sensitivity of the embryo to the carcinogenic effects of saccharin. Ortho-toluenesulfonamide (OTS), a common contaminant in most commercial saccharin,[12] was also tested and shown to be noncarcinogenic. The details of this study have been reviewed and confirmed by a panel of ten independent pathologists.

An extensive FDA analysis of the Canadian study concluded:

> The upshot of the Canadian study is that the feeding of a "pure" sodium saccharin to rats for their lifetime, when either exposed from weaning or from time of conception, resulted in a significant incidence of urinary bladder tumors. The results confirm the findings of the earlier FDA and WARF studies. Further, the Canadian study showed that OTS was not the responsible agent, that urinary pH was not a factor, and that urinary calculi are likely not a factor. Therefore, the conclusion must be drawn that there are now at least three studies that show saccharin to be a urinary bladder carcinogen in the rat.[13]

David Rall, Director of the National Institute of Environmental Health Sciences, commented, "It's absolutely a superb scientific study — it was very well done. I think the data are pretty convincing that saccharin is carcinogenic."[14]

The Calorie Control Council has repeatedly attacked the Canadian carcinogenicity test, which precipitated the FDA ban, as being unscientific.[15] However, prior to initiating the saccharin test in 1973, the Canadian government sent the council a full plan of its intended study with a request for suggestions and comments. The council returned the plan without criticism. In October, 1976, the council invited Harold Grice, of the Canadian Health Protection Branch, to report on the progress of the study at its annual meeting in Ottawa. At that stage, Grice was able to report that *o*-toluenesulfonamide was not car-

Table 6.3 Tumors of the Bladder in Rats Fed Saccharin

Study	% Saccharin in Diet	Sex of Rat	Number Animals with Bladder Tumors (%)	
			Control	Treated
Lessel, 1959	5	F	0/20	2/20 (10%)
Litton, 1972	5	F	0/2 0	1/2 6 (4%)
FDA, 1973	5	F	0/2 4	0/28
	5	M	0/25 (4%)	1/21 (5%)
	7.5	F	0/24	4/31 (13%)
	7.5	M	1/25 (4%)	7/23 (30%)
WARF, 1973	0.05	F	0/17	1/17(6%)
	5	M	0/16	7/16 (44%)
Munroe et al. (Canada),1973	0.2	F	0/56	1/56(2%)
	0.2	M	0/57	1/51(2%)
	2	M	0/57	2/52 (4%)
Arnold et al. (Canada),1977	5	M	1/78(1%)	19/83 (23%)
	5	F	0/85	2/89 (2%)

Source: Based on a table prepared by Melvin Reuber, included in testimony of Public Citizen's Health Research Group, before the Subcommittee on Health, House Commerce Committee Hearings on Saccharin, March 21, 1977.

Table 6.4 Tumors Other Than of the Bladder in Rodents Fed Saccharin

Study	% Saccharin in Diet	Equivalent Pop "Bottles/Day"	Animal (Sex)	Number Animals With Tumors (%)		Type of Tumor
				Controls	Treated	
FDA, 1948	0.01	1.6	Rats (M)	0/20	8/14 (57%)	Lymphosarcoma
	5	800	Rats (F)	0/2 0	9/17 (53%)	Lymphosarcoma
Schmähl (Germany), undated	0.2	32	Rats (M)	4/104 (4%)	6/104 (6%)	Lymphoma
	0.5	80	Rats (F)	4/104 (4%)	8/104 (8%)	Lymphoma
WARF, 1973	0.05	8	Rats (F)	0/17	1/17 (6%)	Malignant tumors of the uterus & ovary
	0.5	80	Rats (F)	0/17	2/15 (13%)	
	5	800	Rats (F)	0/17	4/20 (20%)	
FDA, 1973	0.01	1.6	Rats (F)	6/20 (23%)	14/30 (47%)	Breast
	0.01	1.6	Rats (M)	6/29 (21%)	14/25 (56%)	Breast
NIHS (Japan), undated	0.2	32	Mice (F)	0/14	3/18 (17%)	Ovary
	1	160	Mice (F)	0/14	7/11 (64%)	Ovary
Bio-Research, 1973	1	160	Mice (M)	9/19 (11%)	14/29 (48%)	Lung

Source: Based on a table prepared by Melvin Reuber, included in testimony of Public Citizen's Health Research Group, before the Subcommittee on Health, House Commerce Committee Hearings on Saccharin, March 21, 1977.

cinogenic, although the results of the saccharin test were not yet complete. The council seemed delighted by this news, and expressed no critical comment on the design of the study. Only after the subsequent findings of the carcinogenicity of saccharin did the council attack its scientific credibility.[16]

In addition to the findings of carcinogenicity in the Canadian and other conventional feeding tests, saccharin has also been shown to induce bladder cancer in various other types of studies, including one in which pellets were implanted in rodent bladders, and another for "promoting activity," in which rats were fed saccharin after their bladders had first been primed by local instillation of very low doses of a nitrosamine-type carcinogen.[17]

Quite apart from problems of carcinogenicity, a metabolite of saccharin isolated from the urine of saccharin-fed rats, has recently been shown to induce bacterial mutations.[18]

Human Studies

A series of studies have been made on human populations consuming saccharin, with a view to determining whether this is associated with an excess risk of bladder cancer. The majority of these studies have either compared national bladder cancer rates with the patterns of saccharin usage[19] or studied patients with bladder cancer to determine if they had been heavy saccharin users.[20] Other studies have examined the incidence of bladder cancer in diabetics,[21] on the reasonable assumption that diabetics are more likely to be saccharin users than the general population. In general, these studies have not identified an excess bladder cancer risk in saccharin users, or presumed saccharin users. These apparently negative findings have been widely hailed by the industry as conclusive evidence that saccharin is noncarcinogenic, and that the extensive findings of carcinogenicity in animal tests should hence be disregarded.

Closer examination, however, reveals that the quality of these data does not support the claims of safety. The inherent limitations of epidemiology are particularly applicable in the case of saccharin. First, there may be a latency period of decades between exposure and disease, as with bladder cancer induced by occupational exposure to aromatic amine carcinogens. Second, the success of epidemiology depends on the availability, for comparative studies, of large populations of exposed and unexposed individuals. None of the studies done so far have identified and contrasted a large number of patients with bladder cancer who used and who did not use saccharin. Third, epidemiology, even under ideal conditions, is unlikely to be able to detect relatively small increases in cancer incidence. Yet, increases of this order could still result in a large number of excess cancer cases in the U.S. population. Viewed against these general limitations, it is clear that none of the apparently negative human saccharin studies can be used to give it a clean bill of health with regard to bladder cancer. Large-scale usage of saccharin commenced in the 1960s, so that judging from what is known of other known bladder carcinogens, not enough time may have elapsed for any significant excess of saccharin-induced cancers to have appeared in the general population.† With regard to the diabetic studies, the number of cases involved are inadequate to detect any but the grossest increase in cancer incidence. Additionally, diabetics are more likely to die at a relatively young age from complications of their disease, rather than from cancer. Finally, there is no reason at all for the epidemiological studies on saccharin to have focused exclusively on bladder cancer, to the exclusion of cancer at other sites. Not only is

---

† The Connecticut Tumor Registry has found a large increase in bladder cancer over the past four decades (150 percent for men and 50 percent for women) which cannot be entirely accounted for by smoking and in which a causal and/or synergistic role for artificial sweeteners seems likely.

there no necessary correspondence between the sites of action of carcinogens in different species, such as rodents and humans, but also the rodent studies clearly show that saccharin induces cancer in many sites other than the bladder.

In the fall of 1977, *Lancet* published a paper entitled "Artificial Sweeteners and Human Bladder Cancer," by a team of government and university scientists written under the auspices of the Canadian National Cancer Institute, a voluntary fund-raising agency.[22] This study was based on recent interviews of all patients with newly diagnosed bladder cancer in three Canadian provinces. Each case was then matched to other individuals of similar characteristics living nearby, so-called neighborhood controls, who were also asked the same questions. It was found that men who used saccharin had a 65 percent greater risk of developing bladder cancer than those who didn't. It was also found that this risk increased with both duration and amount of use.‡

Regulation and Politics

Questions on the safety of saccharin are long-standing. In 1911 saccharin was declared "a poisonous and deleterious substance" and banned from general food use on the basis of digestive disturbances and other evidence of toxicity in human studies. Until 1959 the use of saccharin was restricted to those with special medical needs who took it as a prescription drug or used it as a "table top" sweetener or in diet foods in preparations labeled:

Warning: to be used only by those who must restrict intake of ordinary sweets.

Saccharin was first suspected of being carcinogenic in 1948 on the basis of an FDA chronic toxicity test. The questions of carcinogenicity were raised again in 1959 when, with the explosion of the soda pop market, saccharin first came into widespread general use, initially as a one-tenth mixture with cyclamates, another artificial sweetener. These questions became more pressing in 1969, when cyclamates were banned on grounds of carcinogenicity, leaving saccharin the entire diet pop market.

In 1972 saccharin was removed from the GRAS (Generally Recognized as Safe) food additive list on the grounds of the WARF study. This action had the legal force of allowing a future ban on saccharin if there was any question of safety, irrespective of the provisions of the Delaney Amendment to the 1938 Federal Food, Drug, and Cosmetic Act which requires an automatic ban on food additives causing cancer in animals or man.

A recent report to Congress by the General Accounting Office, identified twenty-three studies since 1970 which indicate potential carcinogenic hazards of saccharin.[23]

On March 9, 1977, Acting FDA Commissioner Sherwin Gardner announced a proposal to ban the use of saccharin in foods and beverages. The FDA press release stated that this action was based on the results of a recently completed Canadian carcinogenicity test in which rats developed bladder cancer after being fed daily the equivalent of 800 cans of diet soda. The press release, however, hastened to reassure that "saccharin has been in use for more than eighty years and has never been found to harm people." The press release also stated that this action was unequivocally required by the terms of the Delaney Amendment.

This FDA press release was misleading. It implied that the Canadian carcinogenicity test was an isolated experiment. It questioned the value of the Canadian study by empha-

---

‡ These results were confirmed in a preliminary U.S. study by E. Wynder, reported to the NCI in November, 1977, and presented to the Senate Subcommittee on Health and Scientific Research by Commissioner Kenney in May, 1979, which found that the risks of bladder cancer were doubled in men using saccharin.

sizing the high doses of saccharin inducing carcinogenic effects, while ignoring the fact that this is standard practice in carcinogenicity tests. It cast doubt on the value of the study by ignoring the dozen or so other carcinogenicity studies known to the FDA, including its own 1948 and 1973 studies. In contrasting the Canadian study with the alleged human experience of safe use, the FDA press release in no way indicated the limitations of the human studies, which are so serious as to invalidate any inferences of safety. Finally, in invoking the Delaney Amendment as the legal basis for the proposed ban, the FDA showed an apparent ignorance of its own laws, which anyway require a ban on the basis of safety requirements of general food law.

The way the FDA handled this matter has been regarded by some as inept, and by others as a deliberate attempt to provoke a consumer and congressional backlash against the Delaney Amendment, which was implied to be both inflexible and unscientific. It was well known that many upper-level agency officials, including previous commissioners, notably Charles Edwards,* were openly sympathetic to the industry position that the Delaney Amendment was an unnecessary and unfair restriction to their freedom to add known carcinogens, at supposedly safe levels, to the American food supply.

Not unexpectedly, the FDA press release provoked a sharp reaction from the industry. The Calorie Control Council barraged Congress with cables and letters in protest, and took out full-page advertisements in leading national newspapers complaining about the unreasonable and unscientific proposal of the FDA.[24] These advertisements went so far as to equate the proposed ban with an attack on democracy and freedom of choice of the consumer. The American Diabetic Association claimed that saccharin was necessary for the treatment of diabetes. The American Cancer Society attacked the ban on the grounds that the animal carcinogenicity data should be disregarded because saccharin was of great medical benefit and safe on the basis of human experience. The past president of the society, R. Lee Clark, protested that "banning saccharin may cause great harm to many citizens while protecting a theoretical few."[25] While the American Cancer Society cannot be necessarily faulted for this ill-considered statement, it has yet to retract or modify this position.†

Even the apparently informed scientific community joined in the attack. At hearings before Congressman Rogers on March 2, 1977, Guy Newell, Acting Director of NCI, Kurt Isselbacher, Professor of Medicine at Harvard and chairman of the Harvard University Cancer Committee, and Arnold Brown, Professor of Pathology at the Mayo Clinic (now dean of the University of Wisconsin Medical School at Madison) and then candidate for the NCI directorship, vigorously attacked the proposed FDA ban. Isselbacher, a well-known physician (although not a recognized authority on carcinogenesis or epidemiology), asserted:

> I would submit to you that in the case of saccharin, the available data indicates, in my view, that the risk to humans for de-

---

* Edwards' career is a classic case of the "revolving door" between industry and Government. Prior to becoming FDA Commissioner he was a Senior Executive at Booz, Allen & Hamilton, a major management consulting firm. After a stint in the FDA, he returned to industry as Senior Vice-President for Research at Becton-Dickinson Medical Supply Home. Edwards is now president of the Scripps Clinic and Research Foundation, San Diego, California.

† Ignorance aside, questions have been raised as to the propriety of this position in view of the fact that the society had previously accepted a substantial grant from Coca-Cola, the manufacturers of diet soda, to defray the costs of travel expenses for a delegation of society staff and volunteers to attend a conference in Russia in June, 1976.

veloping cancer from saccharin in the amounts ingested by the average individual is remote, while the harm, I believe, which may occur to millions in the absence of a non-nutrient sugar substitute, is great.[26]

Brown recommended that the admittedly unequivocal animal carcinogenicity data be ignored, because of the alleged evidence of safe human use, and also that the *Delaney Amendment* be relaxed.‡ A lone voice on the side of the FDA at the Rogers hearings was that of Sidney Wolfe, of the Health Research Group, who ably marshalled the scientific evidence supporting the ban.[27]

This was then the background of events confronting the incoming FDA commissioner, Donald Kennedy, who within a few days of assuming his new post in April, 1977, issued a press release in which he made a determined effort to set the record straight. Commissioner Kennedy confirmed the proposed ban of saccharin in foods, beverages, and cosmetics, but also proposed in the Federal Register of April 15, 1977, that saccharin should be made available as an over-the-counter, non-prescription drug to diabetics and others requiring it for medical reasons. The hooker in this was the legal requirement that the industry would have to show evidence of efficacy, in accordance with the Kefauver-Harris amendments to the Federal Food, Drug, and Cosmetic Act. Kennedy also explained that the basis for the proposed saccharin ban was the general safety requirements of food law, quite apart from the Delaney Amendment. He endorsed the scientific merits of the Canadian cancer tests as confirming earlier carcinogenicity studies and

explained that the relatively high test doses used were in accordance with standard test practices. He also explained that there was no valid basis for concluding that human experience had demonstrated the safety of saccharin, and quoted FDA estimates that lifetime ingestion of saccharin by the general population could lead to 1,200 excess cases of bladder cancers annually.

Finally, Kennedy dismissed claims for the medical benefits of saccharin:

> I know of no other drug whose only use is to change the taste of food. I know of no other drug which is to be taken not for what it can accomplish in itself, but because the only alternative — in this case sugar — must be avoided.

Kennedy's actions could not, however, diminish the growing anti-ban and anti-Delaney sentiment, which was supported by the Calorie Control Council, the food chemical industry, and its extensive cadre of consultants. The council launched a massive lobbying campaign in the general press and in Congress protesting that the FDA ban was undemocratic and an outrage depriving millions of Americans of an important and useful additive, besides being unscientific: "We find it incredible that the new Commissioner would move to propose an action of this significance on less than scientifically supportable data."* However, in spite of all the strident rhetoric on the importance of saccharin to the American consumer and on its alleged medical efficacy, the industry has not, so far, produced any scientific evidence to support these claims.

More than 100 senators and representa-

---

‡ Brown's highly qualified position on the predictive value of animal carcinogenicity tests also raised serious questions as to his fitness for the NCI directorship, as subsequently expressed in a letter of May 17, 1977, from Congressmen Andrew Maguire (D-N.J.) and Henry Waxman (D-Cal.) to HEW Secretary Califano. These questions are thought to have been instrumental in

Brown's failure to gain the NCI post. Brown is still chairman of the Clearinghouse on Environmental Carcinogens, an advisory committee to the NCI bioassay program dealing with carcinogenicity testing in animals.

* Congress received more mail opposing the saccharin ban than it did on any day in opposition to the Vietnam War.

tives have backed over a dozen bills to amend the Delaney Amendment or exempt saccharin from the ban. Congressman James Martin (R-N.C.) gathered vocal support for a bill allowing industry to continue using a carcinogen in food for economic reasons. Congressman Andrew Jacobs (D-Ind.) in the words of a recent article in *Consumer Reports,*" hit a comedic high and a know-nothing low" with a bill† calling for saccharin to be labeled "Warning: the Canadians have determined that saccharin is dangerous to your rat's health."[28]

The voices of sanity and restraint in Congress were few and far between, notably Senator Gaylord Nelson and Congressman Paul Rogers, Richard Ottinger (D-N.Y.), and Andrew Maguire (D-N.J.). Senator Kennedy attempted to dampen the hysteria by referring the saccharin problem to the Office of Technology Assessment (OTA), which issued a well-balanced report on June 7, 1977, concluding:

1. The doses of saccharin used in the rat cancer tests were admittedly high, but were valid.
2. The most convincing animal cancer tests indicate that saccharin is a weak carcinogen in rats.
3. Saccharin is also likely to be a relatively weak carcinogen in people.
4. Though weak, for several important reasons saccharin should be regarded as having the potential of posing a significant health hazard to humans.[29]

Accepting the position of the OTA that neither the risks nor the alleged benefits could be adequately expressed in terms of the expected number of human cancer cases, Senator Kennedy stated in a June 10 conference:

I believe that, because of the division in the scientific community, because of the division in the OTA Panel, because of the genuine uncertainty on each side of the risk/benefit equation, the individual ought to be fully informed and then allowed to make a personal decision.

While this statement seems reasonable, it does not reflect the fact that the informational process is largely proceeding via full-page ads taken out by the Calorie Control Council and other partisan groups, and that the majority of saccharin users, adolescents, are hardly likely to be able to make reasoned decisions on the risks and benefits of saccharin. These considerations are still more cogent for the unborn generation exposed prenatally to saccharin.

Senator Kennedy also announced his intent to support legislation to suspend the FDA ban on saccharin for eighteen months to allow a detailed study of food additive law by the National Academy of Science. Kennedy proposed that saccharin-containing foods be labeled with a warning during this interim period. In his press release, Senator Kennedy appeared to rely on unsupported advice that the carcinogenic hazards from saccharin were remote and that its benefits were real.

The subsequent decision by Congress on October 17, 1977 (P.L. 95-203), to postpone the FDA ban for eighteen months (until May 13, 1979) was understandable in the circumstances. While heading off the concentrated industry attacks on the Delaney Amendment, quite apart from the proposed saccharin ban, the decision offered an opportunity for more deliberate examination by Congress of the underlying facts on risks and benefits. In an attempt to limit further public exposure to saccharin during this interim period, Senator Nelson introduced legislation on September 14, 1977, to restrict usage of saccharin to those with a specific medical requirement and to require that saccharin products be labeled with a cancer warning. Senator Nelson, moreover, warned Congress of the unwise precedent it was setting by interfering with the

---

† Uncrazying of Federal Regulations Act of 1977, H.R. 6685, March 28, 1977.

specifics of the regulatory process and by legislating special treatment on a product-by-product basis:

> By delaying a regulatory restriction on the use of saccharin in the food supply, Congress is risking the public health for the benefit of large economic interests. Saccharin is one of 2,100 food additives approved for use directly in food. Approximately 10,000 are approved for indirect uses, such as in packaging. Does Congress expect to react to every request for special consideration of food additives?[30]

Nevertheless, Congress subsequently passed the eighteen-month moratorium, which was signed into law on November 21, 1977, by President Carter. Subsequent to this, the Canadian government, however, banned the use of saccharin in beverages and foods on the grounds of its carcinogenicity. Saccharin is still available in drugstores in Canada as a non-prescription drug.

The voices of reason have been belatedly raised in the scientific community. At a September 16-17, 1977, Washington conference on saccharin organized by the Society for Occupational and Environmental Health, leading protagonists discussed available data on carcinogenicity testing, epidemiology, and the efficacy of saccharin. There was a clear scientific consensus that the animal carcinogenicity data were sound and created a strong presumption of human cancer risk; that the earlier human studies provided no indication of safety; and that indeed the 1977 Canadian epidemiological study raised further serious questions as to the carcinogenicity of saccharin. In short, participants other than industry concluded that the use of saccharin entails significant risks and provides no matching benefits for the general population nor for those alleged to have special medical needs.

In accordance with the provisions of the Congressional moratorium, the National Academy of Sciences established two panels, one to study and report on risks and benefits of saccharin, and the other to examine general food safety policy.‡ In November, 1978, the first panel issued its report confirming the validity of the animal tests on saccharin and concluding that saccharin had been demonstrated to be both a carcinogen and a promoter, and hence a potential carcinogenic hazard to humans.[31] The panel further concluded that saccharin itself and not any potential impurities was the carcinogen. After thorough review of possible benefits, the panel agreed that "Essentially, there is no scientific support for the health benefits of saccharin." Finally, the report warned:

> The observation that young children are becoming increasingly greater consumers of saccharin suggests that public health officials should take a prudent course of action since there has been insufficient time for the possible effects of this greater consumption to be manifest. This may be particularly important because of the anticipated long latent period between exposure to the potential carcinogen and the manifestation of cancer, and because of the recently recognized promoter effects that

‡ The second panel report, issued on March 2, 1979, proposed revamping food safety laws to reflect benefit-risk considerations, including relaxation of the Delaney Amendment and the classification of additives into low, moderate, and high risk. A minority report strongly objected to these recommendations, particularly the concept that the adult or child consumer of all educational and cultural levels (quite apart from the fetus) is willing and able to make informed and appropriate benefit-risk calculations for every item of food purchased. This report makes it unlikely that saccharin will remain on the market until the Ninety-sixth Congress grapples with the broader issues of rewriting food safety laws (see R. J. Smith, "Institute of Medicine Report Recommends Complete Overhaul of Food Safety Laws," *Science* 203 [1979], pp. 1221-24).

have been exhibited by saccharin in laboratory tests.*

Summary

Saccharin is a 100-year-old non-nutritive, non-caloric sweetening agent. Formerly popular mainly among diabetics, its use has exploded over the last twenty years as a staple of the diet food and drink craze. Its major current consumption is in diet pop by teenagers, and not by diabetics and the obese. The public now firmly believes that foods containing saccharin are effective in weight control, and has been persuaded by the soft drink industry (through the Calorie Control Council) that these benefits outweigh any possible health risks.

The Calorie Control Council has also carefully cultivated the popular but mistaken belief that animal tests using large doses of a weak carcinogen are absurd, and has in this way undermined the public's trust in the use of standard animal tests for carcinogenesis, and their predictive value to humans. As a result, a powerful industry lobby backed up by popular sentiment has prompted Congress to take the extraordinary action of suspending the FDA's power to regulate saccharin until May, 1979, pending further scientific study.

In fact, there is no available evidence that saccharin is in any way effective in the treatment of diabetes and obesity. Some published studies indicate just the contrary. More than a dozen animal tests over the last thirty years have demonstrated the carcinogenic effects of saccharin in the bladder and other sites, particularly female reproductive organs, and in some instances at doses as low as the equivalent of one to two bottles of diet pop daily. Additionally, recent epidemiological studies have shown that saccharin usage is associated with an increased risk of bladder cancer.

The mishandling of the proposed saccharin ban dealt a serious setback to the whole field of environmental regulation. It brought to focus the failure of regulators to adequately inform the public about the underlying issues, the uncertainty that appears to exist in the informed scientific community, and the ability of concentrated industry interests to manipulate decision-making processes. In its unique preemption of the FDA's regulatory authority, by placing an eighteen-month moratorium on the saccharin ban, Congress forced an evaluation of the Federal Food and Delaney Law and the use of risk-benefit analysis in environmental regulation. In this, they were supported by the administration, which, through the Council on Wage and Price Stability, opposed the ban on economic grounds. Pending final resolution of the broader issues, the Congressional action has resulted in the continued exposure of some 14 percent of the U.S. population to a carcinogen added to their diet more for its market than nutritional or medical value.

Acrylonitrile

The old Talmudic saying, "Don't be concerned by the look of a bottle, but rather by what's inside it," doesn't seem to apply to modern experience with acrylonitrile. Monsanto, Inc., found this out at great expense, when the contents of its newly marketed plastic bottles were shown to contain the potent carcinogen, acrylonitrile.

Plastic Bottles

It all started about 1972, when Pepsi-Cola and Coca-Cola carried their rivalry into the search for a plastic bottle that would be lighter

---

* The first panel concluded that there was no meaningful way of developing quantitative assessments of the cancer risks of saccharin (see Table 9.11). This is at variance with the unsupported contention of the second panel that the risks can be defined, providing a rationale for benefit-risk approaches to continued usage of saccharin.

than glass, but tough enough to stand the pressure of carbonation. Each of the soft drink giants went to a chemical giant for help — Pepsi to Amoco Chemical Corporation, and Coke to Monsanto. Engineers at both Amoco and Monsanto then set about finding suitable plastic bottles for their respective clients. Amoco came up with a bottle for Pepsi made from a polyester, polyethylene terephthalate (PET).† Monsanto developed its bottle made from another widely used acrylonitrile (AN) plastic, a co-polymer of styrene and acrylonitrile.

Then came the test-marketing period. While both companies initially had a tough time interesting the public in their new products, the Pepsi PET bottle seems to have caught on well, and has since generated orders for about 50 million pounds, most being supplied by Goodyear Tire and Rubber Company.[1] Goodyear claims that its bottles have exceptional clarity, that they can be safely incinerated without giving off toxic fumes, and can be compacted for landfill and recycled. During this time, the rival AN, marketed by Monsanto under the name Cycle Safe, started running into problems of carcinogenicity, which the company had failed to anticipate in the earlier developmental stages.

Carcinogenicity and Other Problems

In a series of carcinogenicity tests sponsored by the Manufacturing Chemists Association in the laboratories of Dow Chemical Company, AN was administered to rats by feeding and inhalation.‡ A high incidence of cancers of the breast, brain, and stomach were found in test animals.[2] Other studies showed that AN induced a wide range of birth defects in pregnant rats[3] and mutations in bacterial (Ames) systems.[4]

Evidence on human effects was quick to follow. On May 23, 1977, the medical director of Du Pont reported, on the basis of preliminary epidemiological studies, that he had identified sixteen cases of cancer, with eight deaths occurring between 1969 and 1975 among 470 workers exposed to AN from 1950 to 1956 in the company's textile fibers plant in Camden, South Carolina.[5] This was nearly three times the incidence of cancers that would have been expected in a similar group of unexposed workers. Six of these were lung cancers, three were colon cancers, and seven were in various other organs.

These findings should not have come as a complete surprise to anyone. There is an obvious similarity of chemical structure between VC, known by the industry since 1970 to be carcinogenic, and AN, which should at least have triggered earlier questions.

vinyl chloride	acrylonitrile or vinyl cyanide
$CH_2 = CH — Cl$	$CH_2 = CH — CN$

Relevance of Carcinogenicity Data to Safety of Coca-Cola Bottles

AN, like VC, is a small gaseous monomer, which under the influence of heat, pressure, and plasticizers can be reacted to form long-chain polymers, and then fabricated into solids or films. As with VC, the polymerization reaction never proceeds to completion, and there is always some unreacted AN monomer in the final polymeric product. The unreacted monomer will dissolve or leach out of bottles made from the polymer into the fluid it contains. The amounts leached out will vary widely, depending on the conditions in which the bottle was fabricated, its thickness and

---

† Coincidentally, this polyester was selected by Hoechst Chemical Co. as a replacement for the fire retardant Tris, which the Consumer Product Safety Commission banned because of its carcinogenicity and mutagenicity.

‡ Requirement for these tests was imposed by the FDA, under interim food additive regulations, following the marketing of Cycle Safe bottles.

size, and the duration and temperature of storage of the product. This problem of leaching and migration of toxic or carcinogenic monomers or other chemicals from plastic bottles or food wrappings into their contents is a problem of major importance in the food, cooking oil, beverage, and cosmetic industries. It is not just unique to AN and VC.

Monsanto at first contended that there was no detectable migration of AN into the contents of the bottles, and that the bottles met the migration limits of 50 ppb (0.05 ppm) set by the FDA for food-contact or wrapping materials. Monsanto has since admitted, however, that it did not have test methods sufficiently sensitive to back these claims. In fact, FDA food-simulating extraction tests indicate that significant migration does occur, as confirmed by the finding of 13-20 ppb AN levels in Coke bought in retail stores.

Regulatory Developments on the Plastic Bottle

In January, 1977, on the basis of interim results of the still incomplete Dow carcinogenicity tests, the Natural Resources Defense Council petitioned the FDA to set a zero tolerance for AN migration, and to ban the plastic beverage bottles. In face of sharp protests from Coca-Cola, the FDA acted on this request on March 11, 1977, and announced a ban on the sale of the bottles after they had been marketed for little over a year. The ban was made final in September, 1977. Monsanto was left with 20 million bottles worth $2 million, and with lost 1977 sales exceeding $30 million. The FDA ban also extended to the use of AN bottles manufactured by Borg-Warner for apple juice.*

Following the final September ban, J. Virgil Waggoner, Monsanto's executive vice president complained, "We do not agree with these findings. We believe that our Cycle Safe bottles are safe and that this action is unwarranted."[6] In October, 1977, Coca-Cola decided not to wait out the predictably lengthy appeal by Monsanto, filed in November in the U.S. Court of Appeals, but switched instead to the rival Amoco's PET bottles. These bottles were described by their producer, Goodyear, as producing an extraction level 1,000 times lower than the FDA 50 ppb limit, requiring less energy to manufacture than any other soft drink package, and recyclable.†

Regulatory Developments in the Workplace

Current production of AN is approximately 1.6 billion pounds, and involves about 125,000 workers, 10,000 of whom are exposed to AN on a regular basis.[7] Besides the planned use of AN in Coca-Cola bottles, it is widely used in the manufacture of acrylic and other synthetic fibers, such as Orlon, Acrilan, Creslan, synthetic rubber, and other plastics.

In the wake of unfavorable publicity, following disclosure of excess cancers among AN workers at Du Pont, the company voluntarily reduced its exposure limits from the then OSHA 20 ppm standard to 2 ppm in June, 1977.

In January, 1978, on the basis of the experimental and epidemiological carcinogenicity data, OSHA concluded that AN constitutes "A potential carcinogenic risk to humans." Accordingly, OSHA issued an emergency temporary standard of 2 ppm for workplace exposure to AN. Countering industry's

---

* This prompt FDA action on the basis of incomplete test results contrasts sharply with its foot-dragging on Red #2 and more recently on Red #40.

† A recent editorial in *The Wall Street Journal* ("A Low Growth Microcosm," October 10, 1978) was critical of the FDA ban on grounds includ-

ing the fact that the 13-20 ppb level found in Coke were equivalent to only one molecule per bottle of Coke. In a letter to the *Journal* of October 23, H. P. Pohlmann, Director of Amoco Chemicals Corporation, corrected the estimate to about 100 quadrillion molecules (10^{17}) of AN per bottle, or about 10^{14} molecules per cubic centimeter.

argument that the lengthy induction period of cancer makes such an emergency standard unnecessary, OSHA director Eula Bingham stated:

> As a carcinogen, AN can pose its life-threatening danger in a very brief period of exposure. Without this emergency temporary standard, employees would continue to be exposed to this threat during the period of time necessary to complete normal rule-making procedures.[8]

Bingham also explained her reluctance to issue an absolute-zero exposure level. Noting that even though OSHA clearly recognizes that no safe level exists for carcinogens, she explained, "In this case a level was chosen to immediately minimize the hazard to the greatest extent possible within the confines of feasibility." The emergency standard was promptly challenged in the Cincinnati Circuit Court by the manufacturers of AN, including Monsanto, American Cyanamid, Borg-Warner, and Vistran Company, a subsidiary of Sohio, on the grounds that the danger was not grave enough to warrant emergency measures. In March, 1978, the appeals court denied the request for a stay. Meanwhile, President Carter's newly created Council on Wage Price and Stability, which had been examining case histories of specific standards as a means of exploring economic and other considerations involved in the standard setting process, selected acrylonitrile as a test case. Following a meeting on May 4 with Grover Wrenn, who heads health standards at OSHA, the Regulatory Analysis Review Group of the Council criticized the standard on the grounds that OSHA had failed to adequately weigh the anticipated benefits to workers health against the high costs of compliance. The new OSHA standard of 2 ppm, which became effective November 2, 1978, applies only to about 5,000 employees of nineteen major producers and users of AN, but not to the unknown but much larger numbers of workers in fabricating plants. This standard gives industry two years to install engineering controls, while requiring submission of plans for compliance, including a schedule for implementation. It is clear from the reaction of industry that the new standard poses few if any problems. The Society of the Plastic Industry, which had vigorously opposed the emergency standard a few months previously, now commended OSHA for setting "a performance-based standard that will protect workers health." Monsanto called the standard "strict but realistic." While the new standard clearly provides an increased measure of protection to a limited number of workers, it is excessively high and should be revised downwards and extended to cover polymer fabricating operations and end users of AN fibers, who are currently unprotected.

Summary

The case of acrylonitrile (AN) is a clear-cut example of inadequate premarket testing of a major ingredient of a food and soft drink container. It is also a paradigm of the larger problem society faces as industries rush to market new products or, without regard for the deliberate process of testing needed to exclude possible public health hazards.[‡]

Following the original and unwise decision by Monsanto and Coca-Cola to market AN bottles, evidence of the substance's carcinogenicity was found in test animals by Dow Chemical and in exposed workers by Du Pont. The subsequent banning of AN bottles by the FDA and regulation of AN in the workplace by OSHA have been challenged in the courts by Monsanto, the same company that has recently launched a massive national advertising campaign to prove to the public that synthetic chemicals are essentially safe unless misused, and to assert that regulatory con-

---

‡ This further typifies, at least with regard to health and pollution considerations, the conven-tional industry position of "shooting first, then drawing the bull's-eye around the hole."[9]

trols such as the Delaney Amendment are "unscientific." The 2 ppm occupational standard is excessively high and should be revised sharply downward, and extended to fabricating, besides manufacturing plants.

Nobody has shown a cause-and-effect relationship between Premarin and cancer. It does not cause cancer. It just accelerates it.

A vice president, Ayerst Laboratories
November 23, 1977.

Female Sex Hormones

Hormones are low-molecular weight chemicals secreted into the bloodstream by the endocrine glands which influence most biochemical and metabolic processes in the body.[1] The group that regulates all aspects of reproductive development and function are the steroidal sex hormones, of which three major classes are recognized: estrogens and progestins, both female hormones, and androgens, male hormones. Natural estrogens are a mixture of three related hormones, estradiol, estrone, and estriol.* The balance between the levels and functions of the different sex hormones is exquisitely sensitive and imbalance, occurring spontaneously or following their administration for therapeutic or other purposes, seems to be associated with excess risks of cancer.

In addition to natural estrogens, diethylstilbestrol (DES) is a synthetic chemical which has high estrogenic potency, although it is chemically unrelated to steroids.

Uses

Second to tranquilizers, female sex hormones are the most commonly prescribed drugs in America today.[2] They are also extensively used as feed additives that stimulate growth in poultry, cattle, and hogs.

Oral Contraceptives. During research on progestin fertility drugs in the mid-1950s, it was found that contamination with small amounts of estrogens reversed their effects, and instead effectively prevented pregnancy. Starting in 1956, large-scale trials of oral contraceptives in Puerto Rican and Haitian women, based on combinations of estrogens and progestins, demonstrated the nearly complete effectiveness of the "combination pill," which is now used commonly throughout the world.[3] A second type of oral contraceptive is the "sequential pill," so-called because its three phase cycle consists of two weeks on estrogen, one week on estrogen and progesterone, and one week off.

In June, 1960, the FDA approved the first oral contraceptive pill, Enovid, marketed by G. D. Searle Company. This was rapidly followed by competitive products from other pharmaceutical companies, including Syntex, Ortho Pharmaceutical, and Eli Lilly. This enormous experiment, in which a non-medicinal drug was mass-marketed without adequate prior safety testing, took place with the approval of the FDA and an uncritical medical establishment. In this they were aided by a "diplomatic immunity" extended by the press to the pill for nearly a decade after its introduction.[4]

About eight million U.S. women now regularly use oral contraceptives, representing a pharmaceutical market in excess of $100 million annually. The industry is highly protective of this market and, while enthusiastically promoting the unchallenged effectiveness of the pill, has shown extreme reluctance to admit or investigate any possible hazards involved. Searle, for example, set up a "Bad Press Committee" designed to counter any

---

* While estradiol is the main secretory product of the ovary, the liver readily interconverts these hormones.

bad publicity in the medical and popular literature on Enovid.[5] In fact, until quite recently, national preoccupation with the effectiveness of the pill has been so great as to virtually repress the alarming information which has gradually accumulated on its dangers.

Estrogen Replacement. Tantalized by promotional campaigns of "Feminine Forever," five million menopausal U.S. women regularly use estrogens for "estrogen replacement therapy," with an annual market over $80 million, a market which has approximately quadrupled over the last decade.[6] The object of estrogen replacement therapy is to "replace" the dwindling supply of estrogens secreted by the ovaries as the menopause approaches and menstruation ceases.

Since Victorian times, the medical profession has tended to view the menopause and some of its discomforting symptoms as an illness to be treated, rather than as a natural process.[7] The symptoms for which estrogen replacement therapy is recommended in a standard medical text include

hot flashes alternating with chilly sensations, inappropriate sweating, paresthesias [tingling], formication [sensation of crawling ants], muscle cramps, and myalgias and arthralgias [muscle and joint soreness]. There is an unbearable uneasiness that gives rise to manifestations of anxiety, overbreathing, palpitation, dizziness, faintness, and syncope. Untreated, a few women become chronic invalids, some experience years of ill health, and most feel genuinely miserable and understandably lack vigor and initiative.[8]

In spite of this impressive plethora of symptoms, there is a growing body of informed opinion, particularly among younger, pro-feminist physicians, that what gynecologists label as estrogen-deficient illness in large measure reflects societal attitudes toward loss of fertility, as well as other social and family pressures to which middle-aged women are often subject.[9] While it is true that a small proportion of women do experience severe postmenopausal problems, these are usually only temporary. Many women, however, are untroubled by their menopause, and continue to secrete reduced but significant quantities of estrogens from their ovaries and adrenals.

Why, then, do doctors prescribe estrogens to such an extent? For one thing, treatment is immediately satisfactory in those few women with disabling problems, such as persistent hot flashes, drenching sweats, and vaginal atrophy:

Replacement-therapy is probably the most gratifying use of hormones both to patient and physician . . . The physician can achieve brilliant clinical results with small doses of hormones.[10]

A more important reason, however, is the reliance of the medical profession for guidance on the sales-representatives and promotional literature of the pharmaceutical industry. The most popular formulation for estrogen replacement therapy is Premarin,† a brand of natural estrogens which until very recently was prescribed for about 13 percent of all women in the 45 to 64-year age bracket.

The synthesis of DES in Britain in 1938 made available a cheap estrogenic drug which was widely used from 1940 to 1960 for replacement therapy in over three million women. Unlike natural estrogens, DES can be taken by mouth without loss of effectiveness. Based on the belief that habitual miscarriage and other complications of late pregnancy are due to estrogen deficiency, DES was widely used from 1945 to 1970 for the treatment of threatened miscarriages and for preventive purposes in women with a history of habitual miscarriage. The DES dosage var-

---

† So named because it is manufactured from the urine of *pregnant mares*.

ied widely from 2.5 to 150 mg per day, and the duration of treatment from 3 to 212 days, most women being treated with 50 mg daily for 150 days. Apart from being ineffective, this treatment has resulted in vaginal cancer in the daughters of the treated women and sterility and congenital genito-urinary defects in their sons, apart from excess breast and other cancers in the treated women themselves.

Other Medical Uses.[12] Estrogens are prescribed for various gynecological problems, such as menstrual cramps and irregularity and genital itching, for some of which they appear effective. They are also extensively used for many other purposes for which the evidence of their usefulness seems slender. These include: acne and hirsutism, probably reflecting an assumption that feminine hormones can "soften" or neutralize these "masculine" conditions; "feminizing" ingredients in cosmetics; and, osteoporosis or thinning of bones, which normally occurs with aging and sometimes results in fractures and collapse of vertebrae, particularly in the upper back, producing the familiar "dowager's hump." An unquestionably effective but relatively minor use of estrogen is as a component in the treatment of advanced prostate cancer.

Another common use of estrogens is in the postcoital contraceptive, or "morning-after pill"[13] for preventing the risk of pregnancy resulting from unprotected intercourse. DES is still prescribed for this purpose at many university health clinics, although not authorized for this purpose by the FDA. It is also made available to rape or incest victims by some agencies, at an approximately 250 mg dosage over a five-day period, equivalent to the estrogen content in about a two-year supply of oral contraceptives.‡ There are, how-

ever, questions as to how effective DES really is as a postcoital pill. Quite apart from possible risks of cancer to any young woman from this massive dose of estrogen, there are also carcinogenic and other hazards to her infant if she is pregnant and the DES fails to terminate the pregnancy.

Feed Additives. In late 1954, DES was approved by the USDA for use as a growth stimulant in poultry, hogs, and cattle. Its estrogenic effects make animals grow to marketable weight faster and on less feed. Poultry farmers found the increased growth and fat content of young roosters gave them the appearance of capons without the trouble and expense of castration, and, in advancing the feminine characteristics of young hens, yielded a product that according to one feed manufacturer was "juicier, more tender, and with better flavor." This effect, however, was largely achieved by increasing the conversion of feed to fat, rather than protein. Similar effects were achieved with DES fed to or implanted as pellets under the skin of cattle, two million head of which were put on DES-treated feed within three months of its availability. It has been estimated that a beef animal given DES reaches market weight of about 1,000 pounds approximately thirty-five days sooner than an untreated animal, saving about 500 pounds of feed per animal. The direct savings to the cattle and feedlot industry were estimated in 1974 as over $90 million a year. These advantages are, however, achieved at the expense of meat quality, which is reduced. A Department of Agriculture meat inspector, John S. White, made attempts in 1963 to draw attention to the inferior quality of DES-beef. Following threats of disciplinary action and dismissal if he attempted to pursue his concerns and findings, White re-

---

‡ The FDA will approve use of DES for such emergency situations if a manufacturer provides patient labeling and special packaging. The FDA has not given approval for any manufacturer to market DES as a postcoital contraceptive, and has withdrawn from the market the 25 mg DES tablets formerly used for this purpose.

signed and subsequently published his conclusions in a farming journal in 1966.[14]

Interestingly enough, the original research on the basis of which DES was first introduced as a feed additive was conducted at Iowa State University, in Ames, which had a licensing agreement with the manufacturer, Eli Lilly, and received a royalty from its sales.[15] This research was of questionable quality, being characterized in a 1972 report of the Agribusiness Accountability Project as "an example of land grant [college] research at its worst — it is at once a service to industry and a disservice to consumers — DES has produced a royalty of $2.9 million for ISU, which means that the taxpayer has helped Eli Lilly . . . to sales of $58 million."[16]

Carcinogenic Effects of "Estrogens"

There is overwhelming evidence of the carcinogenicity of sex hormones in both experimental animals and humans.[17] The pharmaceutical and feed additive industries have attempted to minimize or explain away these findings on the grounds that natural hormones or chemicals based on them cannot possibly be carcinogenic, and that even if they are the risks involved are more than outweighed by the massive benefits. There is no question that the balance between the normal production and levels of sex hormones is delicate and sensitive, and that imbalance occurring naturally or following hormone administration to humans and experimental animals is associated with excess risk of cancer. This carcinogenic effect appears to involve some interaction between the steroid sex hormones and other hormones produced by the anterior pituitary gland, particularly prolactin. We will examine separately the animal and human studies:

In Experimental Animals. Natural and synthetic estrogens and progestins have been found to induce cancer in animals in experiments dating back thirty years.[18] Estradiol has been extensively tested in several rodent species, in which it produces a wide range of cancers both in reproductive and other organs. These include cancers of the breast, uterus, cervix, vagina, testes, pituitary, and lymph glands in mice; breast and pituitary in rats; uterus, stomach, and spleen in guinea pigs; and kidney in hamsters. Progesterone, the main progestin hormone, induces cancer of the ovary, uterus, and breast in mice, and precancerous ovarian changes in dogs. It also increases the incidence of various tumors in mice, rats, and rabbits that have been pretreated with other carcinogens.

When DES was first synthesized in 1938, it was also found to be carcinogenic, inducing breast cancer in male mice. Subsequent studies showed that DES was approximately ten times more potent as a carcinogen than natural estrogens. Experiments in 1964 showed that daily feeding of mice with 6.25 ppb of DES in their diet, equivalent to a daily dose of about 0.02 μg, produced breast cancers in female mice. Doubling this dose produced similar cancers in castrated male mice.*

In addition to breast cancer, experiments in 1959 and 1962 showed that feeding dogs with DES induced a high incidence of ovarian cancers. Injection of DES caused cancer of the cervix and leukaemia in mice, and kidney cancer in hamsters. Feeding hamsters with DES in late pregnancy resulted in tumors and other abnormalities in the reproductive tract of their female offspring and abnormalities in the testes of the males.[19] Implantation of DES pellets under the skin of rodents, a standard route for administration to poultry and cattle, induces cancers of the testes in mice, breasts in rats, kidney in hamsters, and uterus in monkeys.

In Humans. Administration of female sex hormones has been shown to induce cancer

---

* These doses are in the same order of magnitude as those prescribed for menopausal women, 10 pg/kg.

of the uterus, cervix, vagina, breast, and ovary in women, and of the breast in men.[20]

Many independent epidemiological studies have established that administration of Premarin increases the risks of cancer of the endometrial lining of the uterus from four to fourteen times.[21] These and other studies also showed that the risk is proportionate to dose and duration of dosage, but was unaffected by the particular type and brand of estrogen prescribed, whether natural, such as Premarin (Ayerst Laboratories), or synthetic, such as Genesis (Organon, Inc.) and Estrace (Mead Johnson Laboratories).[22] There seems little question that the recent dramatic increase in the incidence of uterine cancer is due to the large-scale use of estrogen replacement therapy, which started in the early 1940s and nearly tripled between 1965 and 1975. In some parts of the United States the incidence of uterine cancer has been increasing at a rate of 10 percent per year, an increase that has rarely if at all been paralleled in the whole history of cancer research.[23] The maximum incidence has occurred in women over fifty in high socioeconomic groups, those most likely to be given estrogen replacement therapy.

In November, 1978, two Yale physicians published a case control study alleging that the risk of uterine cancer from the use of estrogen replacement therapy was low.[24] The study maintained that previous contrary reports were biased by the fact that estrogen usage produces symptoms, particularly vaginal bleeding, in many women which bring them to medical attention earlier, and that this results in "finding" more cancers than would otherwise be detected. To counter this so-called "detection bias," they conducted a study on endometrial cancer patients as usual, but the controls were women hospitalized for a dilation and curettage (D&C) or hysterectomy. With this particular control group, the cancer risk appeared to be increased by only 70 percent (not quite double relative to the

controls), as compared to a 1,000 percent increase in risk (ten-fold), when controls in previous studies were chosen in a standard way. The Yale study has been roundly criticized as utilizing "a method that was abandoned by others precisely because it introduced a large selection bias into a research design in which selection bias was not inherently an important feature."[25] While the alleged "detection bias" would scarcely affect the rate of diagnosis of endometrial cancer, it would probably increase the number of cases of various benign conditions, such as uterine polyps, atrophy, and hyperplasia, which made up the majority of the Yale controls. If, as is generally accepted, these conditions are actually caused by exogenous estrogens and may, in fact, be pre-cancerous, then the Yale study used the worst possible set of controls, namely, a group of women also characterized by relatively high usage of Premarin or other estrogens. Compared to such a highly biased control group, the cancer cases then would not appear to have an unusually high estrogen intake. Furthermore, the Yale study failed to analyze their data by duration of estrogen administration; long term users would be expected to have the greatest risk, as other studies have shown. The Yale study was paid for by a grant from Ayerst Laboratories, the manufacturer of Premarin.

A more recent case-control study (H. Jick, *et al. New England Journal of Medicine*, February 1, 1979) suggests that the risk of uterine cancer declines rapidly after discontinuation of estrogen replacement therapy. The relatively brief duration of follow-up, however, suggests that conclusions on this study should be deferred for at least a further decade.

Premarin has also been recently incriminated as a cause of ovarian cancer, generally a rapidly developing and fatal disease which attacks about 10,000 women each year in the United States.[26] A 1977 NCI study has found that while there has been a gradual decrease in the incidence of ovarian cancer in younger women, this has been balanced by an increase in older women, the ones most likely to be given estrogen replacement therapy. The NCI study also found evidence of a strong relationship between Premarin dosage and the incidence of ovarian cancer. Besides uterine and ovarian cancer, risks of breast cancer seem to be approximately doubled by replacement therapy, this being particularly marked among those women receiving high and prolonged dosage and developing benign breast disease during treatment.[27]

Worldwide use of birth control pills, in spite of conclusive evidence of carcinogenicity of estrogens in experimental animals, constitutes the largest uncontrolled experiment in human carcinogenesis ever undertaken. This reflects the failure of both industry and government to develop any large-scale system designed to detect and report long-term adverse effects, particularly cancer. While many scattered investigations of cancer and the pill have been undertaken, their results have been somewhat ambiguous or negative. The number of women studied generally has been too few, not enough time has yet elapsed for an increased incidence of cancer to become apparent, and little or no attention has been directed to identifying subsets of susceptible women defined in terms of other risk factors (such as benign breast diseases). Nevertheless, suggestive evidence of a relationship between oral contraceptives and excess breast and cervix cancers has appeared periodically. A study involving a total of 34,000 women by New York researchers concluded that pill users had a higher cervical cancer rate than diaphragm users. While there are possible objections to the significance of these findings, including the fact that pill users tend to belong to lower socio-economic groups, who are known to have a higher risk of cer-

vix cancer, than diaphragm users, and that use of the diaphragm could block a possible sexually transmitted cancer virus, the study nevertheless merited publication. When an article based on the study was submitted to the *Journal of the American Medical Association,* which is heavily supported by advertisements from the pharmaceutical industry, the editors insisted that it could be published only if accompanied by a rebuttal statement in the same issue. Faced with these unusual demands, the authors instead published their findings in the *British Medical* Journal.[28]

An extensive follow-up (or prospective) study has been under way for some time among nearly 18,000 female patients of the Kaiser Foundation Health Plan in the San Francisco Bay region. By 1977, thirty-five cases of cervix cancer and an additional thirty-one new cases of a possible pre-malignant condition, cervical dysplasia, were reported. A dose-response for cancer was found, with a cancer rate 5.4 times as great among long-term pill users (over four years) than among non-users.[29] In another recent investigation (known formally as the Kaiser-Permanente Contraceptive Study or informally as the Walnut Creek study after the location of its headquarters), elevated risks of malignant melanoma and skin cancer were found in long-term users of oral contraceptives.[30] This study is ongoing and, as its participants pass beyond the latent periods of other cancers, may well yield further information on cancer risk of the pill.

Another condition associated with pill usage over the last decade is *benign hepatic adenoma,* a proliferative liver tumor the incidence of which is now sharply increasing. These can prove fatal by eroding large blood vessels, with subsequent massive abdominal hemorrhages, and can also progress to frank liver cancers.†

---

† This association was first suggested in 1973 by a clinician who reported seven cases of the liver disease.[31] Further cases were subsequently published, and a number of liver tumor registries were established. However, because liver cancer is so rare that studies in individual hospitals are diffi-

In April, 1971, the Massachusetts General Hospital reported seven cases of a rare form of cancer of the cervix and vagina in young women aged fifteen to twenty-two. In most cases, these women had first consulted their doctors because of irregular or heavy periods, and were treated with hormone therapy on the assumption that this was due to irregular ovulation. Only after treatment had proved ineffective were thorough pelvic examinations performed, including direct microscopic inspection of the cervix, using an instrument known as a colposcope. Vaginal cancers were found, in addition to other possibly pre-malignant lesions of the cervix and vagina called adenosis. One of these seven women died eighteen months later, after unsuccessful surgery. A common thread was found linking the victims. Their mothers had been treated with DES during pregnancy for habitual or threatened miscarriage some two decades ago.[33]

It is variously estimated that between 500,000 and 2 million young women have been exposed to DES *in utero* in the United States since its first clinical use in 1946, and that between 20,000 and 100,000 pregnancies were treated each year from 1960 to 1970. While the incidence of vaginal cancer so far recorded is still relatively rare, estimated by HEW to range between 0.14 and 1.4 per 1,000 involved, vaginal adenosis occurs in 30 percent to 90 percent, the incidence depending more on how early DES was given in pregnancy rather than on dosage. There is, however, no way of telling how many adenosis cases will in time progress to cancer. All these women will require careful and regular follow-up for the rest of their lives.

Some women who took DES in the early 1950s did so apparently unwittingly as part of a large-scale clinical trial, the object of which was to investigate the value of DES in the prevention of complications of late pregnancy, including threatened miscarriage. These events took place at the Lying-In Hospital of the University of Chicago, where about 2,000 women were each given about 10 to 12 g DES, and an equal number received a control placebo.‡ The explanation given to these women was summarized in a 1953 publication by W. J. Dieckmann of the Department of Obstetrics and Gynecology of the University of Chicago and the Chicago Lying-In Hospital:

> Each patient was told that previous reports indicated that the tablets were of value in preventing some of the complications of pregnancy and that they would cause no harm to her or to the fetus.[34]

Not only were the women treated with a carcinogenic drug — evidence for which had been established over a decade prior to the test — but according to some they were told that the pills they received were vitamins.* The initial tests produced somewhat ambigu-

---

cult, the National Cancer Advisory Board requested that the American College of Surgeons' Commission on Cancer to estimate the scope of the problem nationwide. Results of the national survey of 477 hospitals revealed that while over 90 percent of all liver tumors found in men were malignant, over half of those in women were benign. Three fourths of the cases in women (with either of the two main types of benign liver tumors, hepatic cell adenoma and focal nodular hyperplasia were found to be pill users, though fewer than 40 percent of U.S. women in the same age bracket are users. The investigators concluded: [These findings] strongly support the association between use of oral contraceptives and some types of benign liver tumors, specifically hepatic cell adenomas and focal nodular hyperplasias.... the problem of the malignant potential of benign hepatic tumors should be addressed. There are case reports of an adenoma progressing to a malignant neoplasm and of hepatocellular carcinoma coexisting with focal nodular hyperplasia.[32]

‡ The DES and placebos were supplied by Eli Lilly Company, a leading DES manufacturer.

* It should be recognized that medicinal ethics as then practiced did require "informed consent" of a patient for experimental treatment.

ous results and were forgotten until the discovery in 1970 and 1971 of vaginal cancers in the daughters of DES-treated women.†

The vaginal cancer scare brought many of these DES-treated mothers into contact with each other. One of the original mothers was Assistant Secretary of State Patsy Mink, former Congresswoman from Hawaii. Ms. Mink filed a class action suit against the University of Chicago and Lilly on behalf of herself and about 1,000 other mothers in the experiment. In this she has been joined by the Health Research Group and the Citizen Litigation Group (both Nader affiliates). A motion by the University of Chicago to dismiss this case was rejected by the courts in March, 1978. Other such cases which are also pending include the $100 million damage suit and a $1 billion class action for punitive damages filed in March, 1976, by three Long Island mothers against a score of major pharmaceutical companies and five physicians.

Fuel has been recently added to the fire of the University of Chicago-Eli Lilly lawsuit by preliminary data indicating an approximate doubling of the incidence of breast, besides an increase in other hormone-related cancers in the women given DES in the 1950s.[36] These data, based on an August, 1977, progress report to the National Institutes of Health by the University of Chicago, were obtained by the Health Research Group under the Freedom of Information Act. Additionally, these breast cancers occurred in younger women than in untreated controls. While the University of Chicago has challenged the statistical significance of these conclusions, they seem consistent with the results of the 1977 NCI study which found a higher incidence of breast cancer in women treated with estrogen replacement therapy. In October, 1978, HEW Secretary Califano released a report of an NCI task force, set up in response to initiatives of the Health Research Group, which concluded that the risk of breast or gynecological cancer for DES mothers is "not established (although) sufficient cause for serious concern."

DES, used in the past for estrogen replacement therapy, has been incriminated, together with Premarin, as a cause of ovarian cancer. Cancer of the breast in elderly men has developed following treatment with DES and other estrogens for prostate cancer. Similar cancers have developed in young transvestites taking large doses of estrogen to promote female secondary sexual characteristics. While there is little in the way of substantive epidemiological evidence on the carcinogenicity of progestins, recent studies have incriminated progesterone as a cause of ovarian cysts.

Other Toxic Effects of Estrogens

Apart from cancer, various studies from all over the world over the last twenty years have focused suspicion on the pill as a cause of premature heart disease and stroke.[37] The FDA decision to market the first oral contraceptive in 1960 was based on tests with only 132 women for only 38 months. On this basis was begun the first mass prescription in medical history of a non-medical drug. Early studies suggesting blood clotting *(thromboembolic* disease) and other dangers of the pill were countered by authoritative FDA reassurances, such as those by Joseph Sawdusk, FDA's top physician and later vice-president of Parke Davis, that the pill is "safe when given under a doctor's supervision." The FDA was joined in these assurances by the medical journals, the medical establishment, leading physicians such as John Rock and Alan Guttmacher of Planned Parenthood, and the promotional literature of the industry.

In January, 1966, when the long-compliant

---

† Subsequent studies have also shown that sons of the DES-treated women have not escaped and have been found to suffer from a wide range of congenital genito-urinary defects, and a high incidence of infertility and sterility.[35]

FDA Commissioner George P. Larrick was replaced by James L. Goddard, an advisory committee warned of possible blood clotting problems due to oral contraceptives. The press, which had for years been silent on the dangers of the pill, belatedly and slowly started covering the growing information on this problem. In May 1968, a study published in the *British Medical Journal* clearly implicated the pill with excess thromboembolic disease, in which a blood clot forms within the vein and if dislodged can lead to a fatal stroke.[38] The FDA obtained agreement from the manufacturers to include a warning about blood clotting in the package labeling given to the pharmacists, but without any direct warning to the patient. In August, 1969, the FDA Advisory Committee on Obstetrics and Gynecology confirmed the thromboembolic risks of the pill and summarized the data on experimental carcinogenicity of estrogens, but nevertheless concluded that the pill was "safe."[39]

In January, 1970, Senator Gaylord Nelson held widely publicized hearings on the safety of oral contraceptives before his Subcommittee on Monopoly. The hearings summarized the known hazards of the pill and made it clear that users were not being adequately informed of these. It was also emphasized that the pill had not been adequately tested prior to its massive use. Industry, the FDA, and the medical establishment, including family planning and birth control organizations, on the other hand, insisted that the pill was perfectly safe and that users were being told all they needed to know. Nevertheless, after the hearings, about 19 percent of pill users quit.[40] Critics of Nelson claimed 100,000 unwanted pregnancies resulted and dubbed them "Nelson babies," an allegation which has never been substantiated.

These issues came to a climax in a 1977 publication of two British studies in *Lancet,* one conducted by the Royal College of General Practitioners on 46,000 women, and the other on 17,000 women by the Oxford Family Planning Association.[41] Both studies concluded that death from coronary heart disease, hypertension, and stroke were five times more common among pill users than controls, and ten times as frequent among pill users who had been on the pill for over five years. The excess death rate among pill users was also further increased by cigarette smoking. Both studies recommended that all women over thirty-five years should stop taking the pill, that women between thirty and thirty-five should consider changing to different contraceptives, but that women under thirty need not worry. These findings supplemented previous knowledge that estrogen usage increases the risk of thromboembolic disease. Pill usage also affects fat metabolism, increasing serum triglycerides and thereby increasing the risk of coronary artery disease, especially in the presence of other risk factors such as smoking or hypertension. Both the pill and estrogen replacement therapy increases the risks of gall bladder disease by two to three times.

Several reports have also suggested a marked association between intrauterine exposure and congenital birth defects of the heart and limbs. The use of hormonal tests for pregnancy has also been incriminated as a cause of congenital defects of the central nervous system.‡

Recent Occupational Problems

In 1966, the Oil, Chemical, and Atomic Workers Union organized the Dawes Laboratories in Chicago Heights, Illinois, an agricultural products and DES manufacturer.[42] Ventilation was practically nonexistent and

---

‡ As recently reported (*London Times*, June 7, 1978), responding to complaints of the newly formed "Association of Children Damaged by Hormonal Pregnancy Tests," an Ombudsman has been asked to investigate why the British Committee on Safety of Medicines had failed to warn doctors and the public of the dangers of birth defects of hormonal pregnancy test tablets until 1975, since their danger was first demonstrated in 1967.

the whole interior of the plant, including the cafeteria and toilets, was covered by dust containing as high as 10 percent DES by weight. From 1968 to 1971, many workers complained of sexual impotence and some men developed enlarged breasts, in one case requiring surgical removal.

In their subsequent contract negotiation, in 1971, the union demanded and obtained full medical examinations of all workers, provided by the company, as well as a commitment to improve working conditions. The union also requested an independent evaluation program of the effects of exposure to DES. On this program, eight male employees were admitted in 1973 to the National Institutes of Health Hospital in Bethesda, Maryland, where they were given testosterone therapy to relieve some of the symptoms. Following this evaluation, medical consultants of the union explained to the workers the effects of DES, and the workers renewed their demands for improved working conditions.

The years passed by without the plant being cleaned up. The recommendations for improved industrial hygiene made by Dawes' own insurance company were ignored. Then, in March, 1977, the Oil, Chemical, and Atomic Workers Union again inspected the plant and confirmed that conditions had not materially changed since 1971. This was followed by an OSHA inspection which resulted in a citation for willful negligence and a fine of $46,000, one of the largest ever imposed for a health violation. Dawes will probably never pay the full amount, as the Act permits appeal of the dollar value of fines based upon subsequent cleanup or even a mere show of "good faith." The company has since appealed and the fine was lowered to $21,000. An interesting legal sideline is that OSHA was obliged to cite the "General Duty Clause" of the Occupational Safety and Health Act as authority for these actions, since there is no occupational standard for DES.[43]

A similar recent incident occurred at an oral contraceptive plant in Puerto Rico. Following complaints of enlarged breasts in male employees and menstrual disorders in females, NIOSH investigated the plant in May, 1976, and found evidence of excessive estrogen exposure. In this case, management instituted the necessary dust control measures and improved work practices, which appear to have resolved the problem.[44] In April, 1973, similar complaints were reported in male and female employees of a plant manufacturing birth control pills in Sao Paulo, Brazil. Following intervention by the Ministry of Labor, ventilation of the plant was improved, and the problem reportedly controlled.

Regulatory Developments

The large-scale use of female sex hormones as both feed additives and human drugs poses two sets of regulatory problems which, however different, are linked by the common theme of cancer risk.

Feed Additives. It is currently the responsibility of the feed additive and animal drug manufacturers, when submitting an application for approval, to provide "a description of practicable methods" for the specific analysis and routine monitoring of animal drug residues in foods. The FDA has responsibility for approving the registration and use of human drugs and feed additives, besides other animal drugs, and for setting tolerances for permissible residues of animal feed additives and drugs in meat and other dairy products.*

Although the carcinogenicity of DES was established in tests as early as 1938,[45] the USDA in 1947 approved the fattening and caponizing of chickens by implanting 15 mg pellets under the skin of the necks. Warning signals of trouble came quickly. Within three

---

* From a regulatory standpoint, there are three kinds of residues: first, *permissible residues* of

noncarcinogenic drugs below prescribed tolerance levels; second, illegal residues of noncar-

years the USDA was sued by mink ranchers whose animals had become sterile after eating the heads and necks of chickens containing DES residues. The USDA still allowed the use of DES in chickens. In 1954 permissible uses of DES were extended to cattle, which could be fed with 5 to 10 mg daily, providing treatment was stopped forty-eight hours prior to slaughter in order to prevent residues occurring in the meat. Highest residues levels are found in liver, and these are about ten times greater than in muscle meat.

Concerned by the mounting evidence on the carcinogenicity of DES, which the FDA seemed to be ignoring, Congressman James Delaney (D-N.Y.) introduced a statement to this effect in the Congressional Record in February, 1957.[46] The FDA immediately denied that DES was a carcinogen. Ensuing congressional concerns with DES were one of the main factors leading to the passage of the 1958 Delaney Amendment to the Federal Food, Drug, and Cosmetic Act which flatly prohibited the introduction to food of additives found to be carcinogenic in either animals or humans. At that time, the amendment made no distinction between chemicals added directly to food as food additives, and those which might enter human food indirectly through the diet of food-producing animals. This amendment, however, did not prevent the continued use of DES, as the FDA argued the technicality that it could not be applied retroactively to DES but could only be used for future applications on carcinogenic food additives.[47]

Using improved analytic techniques, residues were found in poultry in 1959, each carcass containing about 25 µg DES, about a thousand times greater than daily doses found to induce breast cancer in mice. The situation was only resolved with the decision to ban the use of DES in chickens and the willingness of the USDA to buy and remove from the market an estimated $10 million worth of treated poultry. The poultry ruling did not affect the use of DES for cattle and sheep, as residues had not apparently been found in their meat. Alarmed by the poultry ban, the industry lobby introduced the Kefauver-Harris 1962 Drug Amendment to the 1938 Federal Food, Drug, and Cosmetic Act. This is known as the Feed Additive Amendment or the DES Clause, and it specifically exempted DES and other carcinogenic feed additives, such as dinestrol diacetate, from the Delaney requirement. Their use was allowed, provided that the manufacturer made available a "prescribed and approved" monitoring method for the detection of prohibited residues, and that no residues were left when the additive was used according to "label directions that are reasonably certain to be followed in practice." The clear implication here was that any DES subsequently found in meat would be considered the result of bad feeding practices and not due to any inherent properties or danger of DES. In shifting the burden of responsibility from the legislative to the executive branch of government, Congress seemed willing to gamble on the regulatory discretion of the FDA and USDA.[48]

The USDA and FDA rarely checked on compliance. They sampled only a relatively small number of carcasses with biological assay techniques which were impractical, non-specific, and sensitive only to 10 ppb, in spite of the fact that DES was known to produce breast cancer in mice at levels down to 6.5 ppb. The agencies took the additional precaution of keeping results of these samplings confidential. Meanwhile, use of DES was

---

cinogenic drugs above tolerance levels, or *excessive residues;* third, illegal residues of any detectable level of carcinogenic drugs, *prohibited residues*. The USDA has authority to prevent the occurrence of illegal, prohibited, and excessive residues by monitoring meat and products from food-producing animals and birds, generally at the time of slaughter, using FDA-approved methods.

growing. By 1970, 75 percent of all beef produced in the United States, 30 million head per year, were fed with DES. Responsive to the growing DES market and to a request of Eli Lilly Company, the FDA in 1970 doubled permitted dosage levels to 20 mg per day per animal. The FDA, however, did not then take the opportunity to enforce the 1962 DES Clause requiring the manufacturer to provide a sensitive monitoring method for residues.

With the 1971 discovery of vaginal cancer in the daughters of DES-treated women, the USDA-FDA position on DES came under scrutiny and attack. Agency information was discovered proving that DES residues had been found in beef liver as far back as 1966, when 1.1 percent of 1,023 samples tested were positive, and again in 1967 when 2.6 percent of 495 samples were positive.† As typically found, DES residues of 2 ppb are equivalent to about 0.3 µg in a 150 gm serving of liver, an appreciable addition to natural hormonal levels.[49]

In August, 1971, using a newly introduced chromatographic technique sensitive to 2 ppb, the USDA found high DES residues in the livers of twelve cattle and sheep, in one case as high as 37 ppb.[50] These findings, while initially concealed, created a furor, especially since the USDA had previously denied finding any residues at all. Senator William Proxmire (D-Wisc.), introduced legislation to ban DES as a feed additive, and Representative L. Fountain (D-N.C.) held extensive hearings in November, 1971. DES critics pointed out that the additive had already been banned in over twenty foreign countries, that most Europeans would not buy U.S. meat because of its DES content, that any use of DES must obviously lead to residues in meat, and that there was an overwhelming scientific consensus that there was no known way for setting safe levels for carcinogens. The industry, supported by Agriculture Secretary Earl L. Butz

and FDA Commissioner Charles C. Edwards, fought against a ban, claiming that this would cost from $300 to $400 million a year, and that DES residues in meat were so small as to be toxicologically insignificant.

In January, 1972, the USDA attempted to answer growing criticism by extending the 48-hour withdrawal period to 7 days, cattlemen being put on their honor to sign a "certificate of compliance" to this effect. The belief of the safety of a seven-day withdrawal seems to have been based on a single FDA experiment with one cow fed one dose of DES.[51] Furthermore, such withdrawal periods are not only unenforceable, but unresponsive to the standard practice of slaughtering and selling just when the market prices are highest.

Following the finding of DES residues in nearly 2 percent of all cattle tested (in spite of the seven-day withdrawal period), the FDA announced its intent to hold further hearings in June, 1972. The meat lobby objected that the hearings were unnecessary, and public interest groups claimed that more than enough was known to ban without hearings. When asked, the American Cancer Society declined to take any position on the matter. By August, the FDA changed its mind and decided to cancel the hearings. The indecision continued until March, 1973, when the Senate Commerce Committee held hearings on the Federal Food Inspection Act of 1973, largely addressing problems of DES and other animal drugs, in which concerns on the deficiencies in Federal monitoring programs for carcinogenic residues in meat and diary products were vigorously expressed. These concerns were heightened by the discovery that the FDA was also in violation with regard to a wide range of other carcinogenic animal drugs, as it had no practicable test methods for detecting and measuring prohibited residues of seventeen of nineteen drugs then in

---

† The number of cattle sampled continued to dwindle and by 1970 was down to 192.

widespread use.‡ Such regulatory casualness was all the more serious in view of the burgeoning market in new animal drugs and feed additives, which by 1971 had increased to 1,372, including approximately twenty carcinogenic additives, a gain of nearly 25 percent over 1970 figures.[52]

Still further concerns at the 1973 Commerce Committee hearings were provoked by a report of the National Academy of Sciences which found that there was only clear-cut evidence of efficacy for 18 percent of 706 animal drugs in current use. The highlight of the hearings, however, was the introduction of an internal FDA memorandum from K. R. Johnson, Director of the Division of Veterinary Medicine, in which, on September 27, 1972, he warned the FDA that "unless FDA resolves this drug residue problem, we will soon be in direct confrontation with Congress and the consumer, defending an untenable position. For the FDA to ignore this problem would be disastrous."[53]

The FDA capitulated and following the hearings announced a partial ban on DES as a feed supplement from January, 1973, but still permitting its use in implants, which were later disallowed on April 25, 1973, when the ban became complete. A coalition of the meat and drug industries, including Dawes Laboratories of Chicago, appealed to the U.S. Court of Appeals in December, 1973, claiming that the ban would cost the country $1.8 billion, a figure some 450 percent in excess of the 1971 estimates. The appeal was sustained on the grounds that the manufacturers had not been afforded adequate opportunity for a public hearing. Thus the ban was reversed, and DES was officially returned to the market on January, 1974. How did the industry cope during the nine months total

ban on DES? They simply switched to substitute implants of other carcinogenic estrogens which had not been included in the DES ban, such as Synovex (Syntex Pharmaceutical Inc.) and Ralgro and Zeranol (Commercial Solvents Corporation), which were about six times as expensive as DES, although similarly effective.

Caught between the legislative mandate of the 1962 DES Clause and escalating consumer concerns, the FDA then decided to try to move against DES on two fronts, by attempting to ban its use and by attempting to regulate its residues. On January 12, 1976, the FDA proposed a total ban on all remaining feed additive uses of DES, this time allowing ample opportunity for public hearings. The chemical manufacturers, including Dawes and American Home Products, were the leading opponents of the FDA at the hearings which dragged on until January, 1978. On September 21, 1978, Administrative Law Judge Daniel Davidson ruled that feed additives were not safe, and upheld the FDA ban on their use. During the subsequent mandated fifty-day comment period, the DES manufacturers appealed the decision to Commissioner Donald Kennedy. Regardless of Kennedy's final decision, a further lengthy court battle is a certainty. In the meantime, public exposure continues.

In February, 1977, the FDA moved to tighten control of the uses of all carcinogenic feed additives within the framework of the 1962 DES Clause.[54] Their proposals emphasized the long-standing requirement for manufacturers to provide reliable, practical, and sensitive analytic methods for measuring residues, and also required the use of the most sensitive methods to become available at any time in the future. The required withdrawal

---

‡ Dinestrol diacetate, for example, had been incriminated as a cause of vaginal cancer in young women whose mothers were given it in early pregnancy. In August, 1972, the FDA belatedly requested the manufacturer to provide an appropriate test method, as this drug had been illegally registered in the absence of such a method. Although the manufacturer failed to respond, the drug was still in extensive use in chicken and turkey feed at the time of the hearings seven months later.

period prior to slaughter would be that time, under normal conditions of livestock management, which would be necessary to reduce residues to below the lowest level of reliable measurements.

The proposed regulations were promptly challenged in the District of Columbia Federal District Court by the Animal Health Institute, not an animal producers' lobby but an organization with links to the pharmaceutical industry. In January, 1978, the Court ruled in favor of the drug companies, but the FDA appealed and the issue will probably not be resolved for several years.

Human Drugs. In spite of repeated warnings from the scientific literature and from its own advisory committees, the FDA took no regulatory action against oral contraceptives for over a decade after they were first marketed in 1960.[55] On March 4, 1970 the last day of Senator Nelson's hearings on dangers of the pill, Commissioner Charles Edwards testified announcing an explicit proposed statement, "What You Should Know about Birth Control Pills," that the FDA was considering for package warnings. The American Medical Association and the pharmaceutical industry protested strongly and the FDA backed off, revising out most of the warnings and all mention of cancer. The modified statement provided the basis for package warnings ordered by the FDA in September, 1970.

By December, 1972, after the FDA had announced a ban on DES as a feed supplement, it had become public knowledge that DES was being dispensed by major university health clinics as post-coital contraceptives, in spite of the fact that it had never been approved for such use. The usual DES dosage of 250 mg was approximately a million times greater than a dose of 0.3 μg in a 100 gm serving of liver containing 2 ppb residues and equivalent to the estrogen content in about a two-year supply of oral contraceptives. The FDA has recently withdrawn from the market the 250 mg DES tablets formerly used for this purpose and has not given approval for any manufacturer to market DES as an oral contraceptive. The FDA, however, will approve use of DES in emergency situations, such as rape or incest, if a manufacturer provides patient labeling and special packaging. In view of the alarming outbreak of DES-related cancer, a special DES Task Force was set up in 1978 under the NCI's Division of Cancer Control. In the Task Force's summary report, women who had taken DES were advised to avoid any further estrogen usage. The report concluded that, while a further link with breast cancer had not yet been established, continuing studies were critically needed. In addition, Surgeon-General Julius Richmond issued a "Physicians Advisory/ Health Alert" to all U.S. doctors discussing the known DES-related cancer risks, and recommending thorough follow-up for all women known to have taken DES, as well as their children of both sexes.

By 1976, evidence had accumulated that the sequential pill was not only less effective than the combination pill, but also even more dangerous in terms of clotting disease, besides being incriminated in excess risks of uterine cancer. At the FDA's request, the manufacturer "voluntarily" withdrew sequentials from the market.

With mounting evidence on the carcinogenicity of Premarin and other forms of estrogen replacement therapy, and following the recommendations of its Advisory Committee on Obstetrics and Gynecology in December, 1975, the FDA finally took firm steps to control the burgeoning use of estrogens and replacement therapy. In October, 1976, the FDA ordered the pharmaceutical manufacturers to insert explicit patient package warnings in formulations of natural and synthetic estrogens in addition to DES. Patients had to be informed and warned against uterine cancer and a wide range of other risks, including other cancers, particularly of the breast and liver, and cardiovascular and thromboem-bolic diseases.

The ruling on labeling of estrogens used in replacement therapy was unusual for the FDA, which in the past has only required a mandatory "patient package insert" for oral contraceptives, intrauterine devices, and isoproteronol drugs used by asthmatics. The Pharmaceutical Manufacturers Association, joined by the American College of Obstetricians and Gynecologists and supported by the American Cancer Society, protested that information on drugs should be withheld from patients, and challenged the constitutional authority of the FDA to require such informative labeling. In September, 1977, the Pharmaceutical Manufacturers Association and the American College of Obstetricians and Gynecologists filed suit in the U.S. District Court in Delaware against the FDA proposal, claiming

> that it interferes with the practice of medicine by physicians according to their best professional judgment and by dictating the way in which they may practice their profession. . . . The regulation will discourage patients from accepting estrogen therapy when prescribed by their doctors which will impair the reputation of estrogens and reduce the sale of the drug and others.[56]

The Center for Law and Social Policy and Consumers Union have intervened against the suit on behalf of the FDA. The case is still pending. A successful outcome to the suit could well open up the Pharmaceutical Manufacturers Association and the American College of Obstetricians and Gynecologists, quite

apart from individual gynecologists, to malpractice liability actions by women developing uterine cancer, as well as cancer of other sites, from the continued use of estrogen replacement therapy.

The FDA followed up their move to label estrogens used in replacement therapy by a request to Congress in October, 1977, for authority to order patient package inserts when necessary.* Of particular interest is the recent announcement by FDA that manufacturers of oral contraceptives must supply physicians and patients with revised labeling, by April, 1978, warning of the dangers of heart attack and cardiovascular disease from the combined effects of smoking and contraceptives.† The labels also warn that estrogens can cause cancer in certain animals and may, therefore, also cause cancer in humans, although it is stated that studies to date of women taking currently-marketed oral contraceptives have not confirmed this.

Finally, in October, 1978, the FDA withdrew approval for the use of estrogens to relieve "postpartum engorgement" (to dry up the milk supply in newly delivered mothers), on the basis that the known risks of estrogens exceed the benefits.

Summary

Worldwide use of the contraceptive pill, dating back to 1960, constitutes the largest uncontrolled experiment in human carcinogenesis ever undertaken. This was only made possible by the importunity of the drug industry; in its massive marketing and heavy promotional campaigns for a poorly tested product and its unwillingness to face sub-

---

* The FDA estimates that such warnings on adverse drug effects will be required in 50 percent to 75 percent of all prescription drugs.
† One of the unique elements of these new warnings is the information provided on the relative effectiveness and risks of oral contraceptives compared with other forms of contraception. However, the statistical basis for the association

between the combined effects of the pill and smoking with excess cardiovascular disease has been recently challenged by Tobacco Institute staff and consultants (Hearings of the House of Representatives Intergovernmental Relations and Human Resources Subcommittee of the Committee on Government Relations, October 3, 1978).

stantive questions on risk of cancer and cardiovascular disease that subsequently developed; by the FDA's allowing the marketing of a poorly tested drug and refusing for years to take minimal regulatory action, and by the silence of the press on the growing evidence of dangers of the pill. Not surprisingly, the public accepted assurances of the pill's safety and abandoned other forms of contraception in its favor.

The carcinogenicity of estrogens and other female sex hormones has been repeatedly demonstrated in animal experiments begun as long ago as fifty years. Use of the contraceptive pill is associated with excessive risks of rare liver tumors, and there is also suggestive evidence of increased risk of cervix and breast cancers. Additional and major risks of the pill include heart disease and stroke, these being particularly marked in women who also smoke. The large-scale and common estrogen replacement therapy of menopausal women with Premarin, which is largely restricted to the upper socioeconomic brackets, is not only generally unnecessary but has also resulted in a virtual epidemic of uterine cancer. In spite of this, the Pharmaceutical Manufacturers Association and the American College of Obstetricians and Gynecologists, joined by the American Cancer Society, have challenged the legality of the FDA's recent label warning on the grounds that this will reduce the sale of the drug, and that it interferes with the doctor-patient relationship.

Evidence for the carcinogenicity in animals of DES, a synthetic chemical with estrogenic activity, dates back to 1938. Nevertheless, DES has been widely prescribed in attempts to prevent the complications of late pregnancy, although there is no substantive evidence to support such efficacy. This has resulted in an excess of breast cancer in the women themselves, vaginal cancers and the more common vaginal adenosis in the daughters of these women, and infertility and genito-urinary abnormalities in their sons. In spite of all the evidence on its dangers, DES is also still commonly prescribed as a post-coital contraceptive, in the absence of clear evidence as to its effectiveness, although the FDA is now attempting to regulate this.

DES was introduced as a feed additive in 1947. Extreme regulatory laxness by both the USDA and FDA, coupled with 1962 legislative exemption, at the urging of the industry, of DES from the Delaney Amendment, has resulted in the extensive and increasing use of DES and other carcinogenic estrogens as feed additives. In spite of the requirement for withdrawal periods prior to slaughter, residues of these additives continue to be found in meat products. A powerful coalition of the meat and drug industries has now effectively blocked FDA attempts to regulate the use of these carcinogenic additives in animal feeds.

Chapter Seven

The General Environment: Case Studies

This chapter deals with two sets of case studies: the pesticides aldrin/dieldrin and chlordane/heptachlor, and nitrosamines, a large group of organic chemicals now found throughout the environment, many of which have been shown highly carcinogenic in animal tests. These are chosen to illustrate some basic problems of exposure to chemical carcinogens that are so widespread in the general environment as to be ubiquitous. While these particular pesticides are synthetic, nitrosamines, in contrast, can be produced by interactions between different classes of chemicals which may be common and naturally occurring.

Pesticides

Pesticides are chemicals that are intended to kill pests such as insects (insecticides); mites (miticides); weeds and unwanted vegetation (herbicides); fungi (fungicides); and rats and other "vermin" (rodenticides).*

Historical Background[1]

We are now entering what is generally recognized as the "third generation" of pesticide use. The first generation of pesticides, which were developed and used until the 1940s, included naturally occurring organic chemicals such as pyrethrum and rotenone, and inorganic compounds, such as copper, zinc, mercury and lead salts, and arsenates. The inorganic pesticides created significant problems of toxicity, carcinogenicity, and environmen-

tal contamination (though these effects were generally confined to the area of application). Another problem with first generation pesticides was that they were relatively expensive and variable in supply. The second generation was based on synthetic organics, the large-scale production of which commenced about 1940 with the advent of DDT and related organochlorine pesticides. The use of other major classes of synthetic organic pesticides which entered production about this time, including organophosphate insecticides and phenoxy herbicides, has substantially increased over the last decade. The third generation of pesticide use is based on an appreciation of fundamental ecological principles and on the maintenance of pests at economically acceptable levels rather than on futile and counterproductive attempts at eradication. Third generation strategies are based on integrated use of biological control, pest-resistant crop varieties, crop rotation, insect predators, insect hormones, viruses, and sterilizing agents, either alone or in combination with minimal application of highly selective, "narrow spectrum" pesticides. Such programs of pest control, known as "integrated pest management," are still in their infancy, due largely to industrial indifference and scanty federal support, but they have shown great promise in agricultural and urban pest control, including home lawn and garden applications.[2]

In March, 1977, Secretary of Agriculture Bob Bergland announced that the USDA

* Fumigants are another class of pesticides used to kill a variety of pests by volatilization in confined spaces such as grain elevators and other food storage facilities.

would work to move farmers away from their dependence on chemical pesticides and encourage greater emphasis on integrated pest management. There is, however, no material evidence yet of this intent.

The Toxic Effects of Pesticides

The second generation of pesticides was initially greeted with uncritical enthusiasm, as a triumph of modern synthetic chemistry, heralding a new era of agricultural efficiency. In nature, however, there are no "free lunches," and problems soon began to surface. First, it was noted that insects can acquire resistance to a particular insecticide or class of insecticides, necessitating progressively greater, more costly applications, and resulting in progressively smaller agricultural yields, until the infestation eventually becomes uncontrollable.[3] This is known as the "pesticide treadmill." Second, many pesticides produce "broad spectrum" effects, damaging various forms of insect, animal, and plant life other than the intended target.[4] Third, many classes of pesticides, particularly organochlorines, are highly stable, resist degradation, and accumulate in the food chain at levels often more than a million-fold in excess of those found in the environment. Fourth, many pesticides have been found to induce a wide range of toxic effects in experimental animals, including birth defects, sterility, and cancer, thus posing grave public health hazards, especially in view of their widespread environmental dissemination and persistence. Finally,

some of the more stable pesticides become widely dispersed in the environment, air, food, water, and the human body, at locations far distant from their initial application. Pesticides are thus now one of the most important classes of general environmental pollutants, and result in extensive involuntary exposure and contamination of human populations.

Many of these concerns were lucidly and cogently expressed by Rachel Carson in her 1962 classic *Silent Spring*, with particular and illustrative reference to DDT.[5] Reaction from the agrichemical community — including the Manufacturing Chemists Association, chemical industry equipment manufacturers, farm organizations, land grant colleges, industrial organizations such as the Nutrition Foundation,† industry consultants or grant recipients in university departments of nutrition, and state and federal departments of agriculture — was immediate and strident.[6] Carson was attacked as unscientific and hysterical. Typical of the misleading criticisms leveled against Carson were the self-interested statements by William Darby,‡ then nutritionist at Vanderbilt School of Medicine:

> Her ignorance or bias on some of the considerations throws doubt on her competence to judge policy. For example, she indicates that it is neither wise nor responsible to use pesticides in the control of insect-born diseases.[7]

Darby, like most of Carson's critics, made

---

† The Nutrition Foundation was incorporated in 1941 to support "fundamental research and education in the science of nutrition." Its membership consisted of fifty-four companies in the food and chemical industries, the president of whose companies served on the Foundation's Board of Trustees. The foundation funneled industry money, as research grants, to nutrition departments of many prestigious universities, whose recipients were among Carson's most vociferous critics. As part of its educational activities, in 1963 the foundation published a "fact kit" attacking

Silent Spring and defending large-scale use of chemical pesticides.

‡ Darby is a veteran member of the Food Protection Committee of the National Academy of Sciences, long dominated by industry, and now the director of the Nutrition Foundation. He is also member of the EPA Science Advisory Board and was recently appointed to a special subcommittee to review EPA policies on pesticide tolerances in food in response to continued grave Congressional charges of mismanagement.

Table 7.1 Organochlorine Pesticides: Production, Use, and Carcinogenicity

Class and Name of Pesticide	Manufacturer	1972 Production, Million Pounds	Major Use	Carcinogenicity
Oxygenated compounds				
Chlorobenzilate (Acaraben)	Geigy	1–4	Miticide	+
Dicofol (Kelthane)	Rohm & Haas	1–4	Miticide	No data
Dieldrin	Shell	Under 1	Insecticide	+
Endosulfan	FMC	1–4	Insecticide	–
Endrin	Shell; Velsicol	1–4	Insecticide	+
Kepone (Chlordecone)	Allied	No data	Insecticide	+
Methoxychlor	Multiple	5–14	Insecticide	+
Ovex (Chlorfenson)	Dow	No data	Miticide	+
Sulfenone	Stauffer	No data	Miticide	No data
Tetradifon (Tedion)	FMC	No data	Miticide	–
Benzenoid non-oxygenated compounds				
Benzene hexachloride (BHC)	Diamond; Hooker	1–4	Insecticide	+
Dichlorobenzene (PDB)	Multiple	50–99	Fumigant	No data
Dichloropropene-propane (DD)	Dow; Shell	15–29	Fumigant	No data
DDT	Multiple	30–49	Insecticide	+
Lindane (Gamma BHC)	Diamond; Hooker	1–4	Insecticide	+

Table 7.1 (continued)

Class and Name of Pesticide	Manufacturer	1972 Production, Million Pounds	Major Use	Carcinogenicity
Pentachloronitrobenzene				
(Quintozene)	Olin	1–4	Fungicide	+
Perthane	Rohm & Haas	No data	Insecticide	+
TDE (DDD)	Allied; Rohm & Haas	Under 1	Insecticide	+
Non-oxygenated, non-benzenoid compounds				
Aldrin	Shell	5–14	Insecticide	+
Chlordane	Velsicol	15–29	Insecticide	+
Ethylene dichloride				
(Dichloroethane)	Multiple	5–14	Fumigamt	+
Heptachlor	Velsicol	5–14	Insecticide	+
Mirex (Dechlorane)	Allied	Under 1	Insecticide	+
Strobane	Tenneco	No data	Insecticide	+
Toxaphene (Terpene polychlorinate)	Multiple	50–99	Insecticide	+

Source: Epstein, S. S. "The Carcinogenicity of Organochlorine Pesticides," pp. 243-65, in *Origins of Human Cancer;* Book A. ed. by H. H.Hiatt, J. D. Watson, and J. A. Winsten, Cold Spring Harbor Laboratory, 1977.

a great show of reporting what she had never said. What in fact Carson had questioned were the overall methods of combatting insect-borne diseases which relied almost exclusively on massive pesticide use. Carson summarized her position as follows:

> It is not my contention that chemical insecticides must never be used. I do contend that we have put poisonous and biologically potent chemicals into the hands of persons largely or wholly ignorant of their potential for harm —. I contend, furthermore, that we have allowed these chemicals to be used with little or no advance investigation of their effect on soil, water, wildlife, and man himself. Future generations are unlikely to condone our lack of prudent concern for the integrity of the natural world that supports all life.[8]

The book, however, made a deep impact on the independent scientific community and on the nation.[9] President Kennedy requested his Science Advisory Committee to create a special Panel on the Use of Pesticides to review the charges against pesticides. Both the Kennedy Committee and another Science Advisory Committee appointed by President Johnson in 1965 reported that the charges were indeed scientifically well founded. They concluded that organochlorine pesticides were dangerous, quite apart from often being ineffective, and that their production should be phased out as soon as possible. The importance of these recommendations has been more recently emphasized by growing information on the carcinogenicity of organochlorine pesticides as a class (Table 7.1).

Of the twenty-five organochlorine pesticides listed, nineteen have been shown to be carcinogenic in animal tests. There are no data available on four of the remaining six pesticides, while data on the other two (endosulfan and tetradifon), which are claimed to be noncarcinogenic, are still incomplete. Indus-

try has repeatedly attempted to dismiss these finding by such tactics as selective interpretation of the data, challenging their human relevance, and asserting that alleged human experience of safe manufacture and use has vindicated their products. In fact, there are no published human epidemiological studies on carcinogenicity and other chronic toxic effects for the majority of organochlorine and other pesticides. Recent review of twelve organochlorine pesticides by an expert committee of the World Health Organization International Agency for Research on Cancer concluded that there are no valid human data which can possibly justify the conclusions of safety claimed by industry.[10]

The Pesticide Market

There are approximately 1,400 active ingredients currently used in some 40,000 different pesticide products. A relatively small number of these products dominate the pesticide market, twenty basic ingredients accounting for 75 percent of total sales of agricultural formulations. Table 7.2 shows that about half of all pesticides are used in agriculture, while remaining uses are divided between industry (for purposes such as moth-

Table 7.2 Estimated Average U.S. Use of Pesticides

Use	Percent of Sales
Agriculture	55
Industry	20
Home, lawn and garden	15
Federal, state, and local government	10

Source: Environmental Protection Agency, Office of Water Programs, "Patterns of Pesticide Use and Reduction in Use Related to Social and Economic Factors," Washington, D.C., 1972.

proofing carpets and fabrics and clearing rights-of-way), government (for brush and pest control on public grounds), and the general public (for home lawn and garden purposes).

Synthetic pesticides are one of the top classes of synthetic chemical products in the United States, with current annual sales in the region of $4 billion, about 6 percent of the 1975 gross sales ($72 billion) of the chemical industry.* From 1950 to 1975 overall pesticide production increased by about 15 percent per year, from an estimated 200,000 pounds to 1.4 billion pounds. The increase in production of herbicides and organophosphate insecticides was even greater during the same period. The only class of pesticides whose growth rate has declined are the organochlorines, particularly those belonging to a subclass known as cyclodienes, which include aldrin and dieldrin (A/D), chlordane and heptachlor (C/H), Endosulfan, and Endrin.

Support for the pesticide market comes from a politically and economically extremely powerful consortium of diverse interests.[11] In addition to the major agrichemical industries, this consortium includes pest control operators; aircraft applicators; agribusiness concerns such as banks, utility companies, and farm equipment manufacturers; food processors; key politicians, particularly from the corn and cotton belts; elements in federal agencies, particularly the USDA; elements in state agencies, particularly state departments of agriculture; segments of the media, such as the chemical and farm journals, rural newspapers, and chemical company house organs; professional societies such as those represented in the Council for Agricultural Science and Technology (CAST);† elements in land grant universities; and consultants in other universities.

At the bottom of this conglomerate of interests are the pesticide salesmen, who are generally ignorant of the efficacy as well as the hazards of their products.‡

---

* In 1975, approximately 588 million pounds of pesticides were exported, of which it is estimated (by the Natural Resources Defense Council) that approximately 15 percent were not registered for use in the U.S. Exporting unregistered pesticides is big business for U.S. manufacturers.

† CAST is a consortium of agricultural science societies claimed to be an "educational" rather than a lobbying organization, and as such is tax exempt. The major spokesman for the organization is its Executive Vice President, Charles A. Black, Professor of Agronomy at Iowa State University, where CAST is presently located. In 1978, about 50 percent of the CAST's $293,000 budget was directly contributed by agribusiness (including fifty chemical, twelve seed, eleven manufacturing, twelve feed/processing, and other corporations totalling ninety-six). Ten of the world's twelve leading agribusiness firms, accounting for about 76 percent of total world sales, are supporting CAST members, as are six of the top twelve U.S. firms (Dow Chemical, Du Pont, Eli Lilly, Monsanto, Stauffer, and Union Carbide). CAST is a major resource for the industry, issuing a wide

range of publications, including "consensus" Task Force reports on regulatory issues of critical interest to the industry, which it publishes by the thousands (about 8,000 copies of Report #77 on phenoxy herbicides were recently printed). CAST also employs a full-time Washington "liaison," who visits Congressmen, appears at regulatory hearings, and engages in a variety of related quasi-lobbying activities. CAST is also reputed to maintain a "hit list" of journalists, such as Jack Anderson, Lauren Soth, and Daniel Zwerdling, who have published articles unfavorable to agribusiness (Unpublished Report, 1978, Charles Benbrook, University of Wisconsin, Madison; for further discussion of the pro-industry bias of CAST, see E. Marshall, "Scientists Quit Antibiotic Panel at CAST," *Science* 203 [1979], p. 723; and M. Burros, "The CAST Controversy: Impartial Scientific Research Group or Industry Advocate," *Washington Post*, March 8, 1979).

‡ Their role in the proliferation of pesticides has been questioned by many, including the late Robert Van den Bosch, the world's leading expert on integrated pest control: "The greatest absurdity

Profits and Losses
from Pesticide Use

What have been the agricultural returns for the recent massive uses of pesticides in agriculture? In spite of the fact that the total U.S. harvested acreage has remained steady over the past two decades, expenditures on pesticides for agriculture have increased about tenfold, an increase well above the inflationary rate and disproportionately greater than increases in crop value (Table 7.3).

According to estimates by David Pimentel of the Department of Entomology at Cornell University, the harmful recognized effects of pesticides represent a cost to the nation of at least $3 billion annually, including

hospitalization costs for 6,000 human pesticide poisonings; costs of about 60,000 days of work lost from the pesticide poisoning hospitalizations; additional medical costs for 8,000 human pesticide poisonings treated as outpatients; and costs of about 30,000 days of work lost from humans not ill enough to be hospitalized.*[13]

To these estimates can be added further losses from toxicity to domestic animals, livestock, fish, and wildlife; from losses of crop products; from seizure of food containing pesticide residues above tolerance levels, from the approximately 200 people estimated by EPA to die annually from acute pesticide poisoning; and from an unknown number of deaths due to the carcinogenic and other chronic toxic effects of pesticides, alone or

Table 7.3 Increasing Costs of Pesticides, 1955 to 1975

	1955	1975
Number of harvested acres	335 million	340 million
Farmers' expenditure for pesticides	$184 million	$1.96 billion
Cost of pesticides per acre	$0.55	$5.76
Cost of pesticides in relation to farm production value	1 percent	4.4 percent

Source: Statistical Research Service, United States Department of Agriculture, 1978.

in contemporary pest control is the dominant role of the pesticide salesman who simultaneously acts as diagnostician, therapist, nostrum prescriber, and pill peddler. It is difficult to imagine any situation where society entrusts so great a responsibility to such poorly qualified persons. (This characterization also seems generally apt for drug salesmen.) Pesticides rank with the most dangerous and ecologically disruptive materials known to science, yet under the prevailing system these biocides are scattered like dust in the environ-

ment by persons often utterly unqualified to prescribe and supervise their use."[12]

* Most cases of poisoning by accidental carelessness are due to the use of highly hazardous pesticides instead of less hazardous available alternatives. An important example is the widespread use of the highly toxic organophosphate Parathion. By replacing Parathion with Sumithion (a related but much safer insecticide not available for patent reasons in the United States), the Japanese have reduced their accident rate.

in combination with other carcinogenic and toxic chemicals. In sum, the total national losses from use of synthetic pesticides are probably in the same order of magnitude as the $8.7 billion estimated by Pimentel as the cost of annual crop losses due to pest attacks.

I mean there is no fooling around, the major issue is cancer.

Herbert L. Perlman
EPA Administrative Law Judge

Aldrin/Dieldrin

Aldrin and dieldrin (A/D) are two closely related organochlorine pesticides. The former is naturally converted to the latter by an oxidation process both in the field and in the body.

Sales and Uses

Aldrin and dieldrin were first developed in 1947 and, from 1952 to 1977, were manufactured exclusively in the United States by Shell Chemical Company, a subsidiary of Shell Oil. At first they were chiefly used on cotton, but the increasing resistance of the boll weevil to A/D in the late 1950s caused these uses to decline. With growing concern about insect resistance and its toxicity, A/D sales declined from a peak of 22 million pounds in 1966 to about half that amount in 1972. Even then, A/D ranked sixth in sales among all U.S. insecticides, with registration for about 1,300 products handled by some 350 firms. Apart from termite control, which constituted about 15 percent of total sales, the major use of A/D was on corn. In the eight-state corn belt, where over 70 percent of the nation's five to six billion bushels of corn is grown, A/D were used prophylactically on approximately 8 percent of the crop as insurance against possible future infestation by the corn soil insect complex (root-

worms, wireworms, and cutworms), rather than for treatment of actual infestations.

Environmental Contamination[1]

Until about 1970, A/D were applied by aerial spray, even in the vicinity of lakes and streams, causing high levels of contamination of air and water. This contamination was found to persist, although at lower levels, even after use was restricted to direct soil application in accordance with recommended agricultural practice. The routes of this contamination by A/D were threefold: volatilization; transport on dust particles; and agricultural runoff of treated soils and dusts into waterways.

Dieldrin was found in 85 percent of air samples monitored by the EPA from 1970 to 1972, with average national values of 2 ng/m^3 (nanograms per cubic meter), resulting in daily human intakes in the order of 0.1 µg (100 ng). Household dust levels in the corn belt averaged about 2 ppm. An additional and generally unrecognized source of household exposure comes from woolens and rugs which have in the past been routinely mothproofed with dieldrin. Dieldrin was found more often in surface waters than any other insecticide, in average levels as high as 0.4 µg per litre.

Aldrin and dieldrin are highly persistent, and more than 50 percent of an original application of dieldrin can be recovered from soil after four years. Contamination of corn and forage grown on A/D-treated soil was the major source and route of residues in meat and dairy products, and ultimately also the major source of human contamination. Average residues of 10 ppb were found in soybeans rotated with corn in the corn belt. EPA monitoring programs from 1972 to 1974 found dieldrin residues in virtually all human body fat samples analyzed, with average levels of about 0.3 ppm and sometimes ranging as high as 15 ppm.[2] Levels in blacks were about twice those in whites. These residues are relatively stable and persistent: an average of 50 percent of initial residue levels are still present at about nine months.† Further, these residues are of the same order of magnitude, and in some cases greater, than levels in rodents which developed cancers after feeding with A/D.

Economic Losses

The profits Shell made by selling A/D have been at the expense of the national economy, which suffered major direct losses from the extensive environmental contamination caused by agricultural uses of A/D.[3] In 1972, about half the catch of chub and trout from Lake Michigan had to be seized by the FDA, because they were found to contain residues over the permissible levels of 0.3 ppm. This came as a surprise to many, because dieldrin levels in Lake Michigan waters were "only" in the ppt range. However, the persistence and fat solubility of A/D allowed them to accumulate and concentrate in the food chain at levels nearly a billion times greater than those of the lake.

In the whole class of organochlorine pesticides, A/D are second only to Endrin in toxicity to lower species. A/D have been responsible for major kills, a single application resulting in the extermination of one million fish of thirty different species in a Florida marsh. Some fish show toxic effects at 2 ppb levels, and oysters are damaged below 1 ppm, a level which killed 100 percent of quail chicks exposed. Egg shell thinning and breakage, induced by very small body burdens of dieldrin, has been particularly destructive for predators at the top of the food chain, and it has been estimated that A/D are responsible for about 10 percent of all bald eagle deaths.

Destruction of livestock and poultry due to excessive dieldrin levels has been commonplace since 1969, when the extent of this contamination was first appreciated. In February, 1974, a routine test by USDA inspectors discovered unusually high residues in a batch of

chickens being processed by a Mississippi broiler farm. Within days, more lots of contaminated birds were identified from five poultry plants. As the residues in each chicken exceeded the allowable standard, they were ordered destroyed. By the end of March, more than eight million chickens had been gassed and buried, at a cost approaching $10 million. The source of contamination was thought to be low-grade soybean oil containing dieldrin levels as high as 58 ppm and originally intended for industrial use but diverted instead into more profitable use in poultry feed.[4]

On March 26, 1974, a network of Southern senators headed by Senator James O. Eastland (D-Miss.), and supported behind the scenes by the Nixon administration, then anxious for sympathetic Southern votes against the pending impeachment charges, tried to rush through a bill indemnifying the poultry and egg producers and processors for the losses they had suffered. In fact, the major beneficiaries of this bill would have been five large conglomerates, and not the individual family farmers who serve as their sharecroppers. Senator William Proxmire (D-Wisc.) managed to put a last-minute hold on the bill, until the measure could be finally debated, when it was overwhelmingly rejected.

Are such economic losses, quite apart from questions of excess cancer risks, an inevitable and necessary penalty for maintaining the corn yield so vital to the national food supply? The answer seems to be no.[5] There are, in fact, real questions as to whether A/D are of any actual agricultural value against the corn soil insect complex, the major use. A 1972 USDA survey of corn crops found that of all acres treated with A/D, 60 percent were for rootworms, 16 percent for wireworms, and 24 percent for cutworms. However, rootworms and wireworms had by then become largely resistant to A/D. More important, rootworms and wireworms can be effectively controlled by other measures including crop rotation with soybeans. While

---

† The measure of this persistence is known as the biological half-life of a pesticide.

Shell admitted this by labeling its products "Do not use in areas of suspected rootworm resistance," the pesticide salesmen countered this caution by aggressive sales pitches. As far as cutworms are concerned, infestation is relatively rare, occurs only in limited areas, and can then, if necessary, be treated by acceptable alternative pesticides, rather than by routine preventive application of A/D.

Most farmers are dependent on advice from salesmen for principles and details of pesticide use. Farmers also rely on university entomologists and economists, much of whose research is funded by the industry. There seems little doubt that A/D had been oversold by Shell and pesticide salesmen to farmers as an insurance against the entire corn soil insect complex, against most of which it was ineffective. Even for cutworms, recommended application levels seem to have been more than twice that actually needed for effective control.

A wide range of independent experts, including Robert Metcalf (University of Illinois), the late Robert Van den Bosch (University of California), and Donald Chant (University of Toronto), are agreed on the major ecological disruption caused by A/D and organochlorine pesticides.[6] Many state entomologists are also agreed that A/D were unnecessary in the treatment of the corn soil insect complex. There is also a consensus that crop rotation is not only a more effective, but also a cheaper method of control.

Carcinogenicity of A/D

While information on the ineffectiveness of A/D and on its extensive environmental pollution was becoming increasingly appreciated, it was the question of carcinogenicity that finally influenced EPA to commence regulatory proceedings against these insecticides in 1971. The major issue in the subsequent agency hearings was the validity of the experimental carcinogenicity data, and the relevance of such data to human risk.

Animal Tests. By the time the proceedings started, A/D had been tested for carcinogenicity in several feeding studies in mice and rats by the FDA, Shell, and other laboratories under contract to Shell. In general, these studies had either reported negative findings or that A/D induced allegedly non-neoplastic liver nodules or "benign liver tumors" in mice (Table 7.4). In spite of these conclusions, however, the Mrak Commission in 1969 had concluded that A/D were carcinogenic on the basis of the 1962 FDA study.[7]

In an effort to explore these studies further, besides explaining fundamental principles of carcinogenesis to the court, EPA assembled a small team of independent experts that included Melvin Reuber, then of the University of Maryland, Umberto Saffiotti of the NCI, Arthur Upton, then from the State University of New York at Stony Brook and now Director of the NCI, and Adrian Gross of the FDA.‡

Apart from evaluating the specific findings of the various carcinogenicity studies, the EPA team made substantial contributions in broader areas of carcinogenesis. These were subsequently summarized and formulated by EPA as the following "nine cancer principles," and were of great importance in the final stages of the regulatory battle to ban A/D:*[8]

1. A carcinogen is any agent which increases tumor induction in man or animals.
2. Well-established criteria exist for distinguishing between benign and malignant tumors; however, even the induction of benign tumors is sufficient to

---

‡ The author was a member of this team.
* These cancer principles have broad general applicability. They summarize the overall conclusions of many national and international committees on environmental carcinogenesis. (See, for example, Appendix II, the 1970 Surgeon General's Report on Environmental Carcinogens.) In the EPA brief the principles were followed by 29 pages of citations from reports and testimony.

Table 7.4 Summary of Carcinogenicity Tests on Aldrin/Dieldrin in Mice

Authors	Strain	Concentrations (ppm)		Carcinogenicity		Comments
		Aldrin	Dieldrin	Author's conclusion	Conclusion in subsequent independent re-evaluation	
Davis & Fitzhugh, 1962 (FDA)	C$_3$H	10	10	"Benign liver tumors"	Liver cancer	Liver cancer
Davis, 1965 (FDA)	C$_3$H	10	10	"Benign liver tumors"	Liver cancer	1. Liver cancer 2. Study still unpublished
Song & Harville, 1964	Swiss	15	15	Liver "neoplasia" in unspecified groups	None	Unacceptable
MacDonald et al., 1972		...	3-10	"Non-neoplastic" liver lesions	Liver cancer	1. Liver cancer 2. Study still unpublished
Walker et al., 1973 (Tunstall 1)	CF$_1$	...	0.1-20	"Type A and B" liver tumors	Liver cancer	1. Liver cancer with no apparent threshold at 0.1 ppm, and follow-ing only 1-2 months treatment at 10 ppm. 2. Multiple site tumors at low doses. 3. Submitted to FDA 1968, but unpublished till 1973.
Thorpe & Walker, 1973 (Tunstall 2)	CF$_1$	...	10	"Type A & B" liver tumors	None	Liver cancer, with high incidence pulmonary metastases

Source: S. S. Epstein, "The Carcinogenicity of Dieldrin, 1," *Science of the Total Environment*, (4) 1975, pp. 1-52.

characterize a chemical as a carcinogen.

3. The majority of human cancers are caused by avoidable exposure to carcinogens.

4. While chemicals can be carcinogenic agents, only a small percentage actually are.

5. Carcinogenesis is characterized by its irreversibility and long latency period following the initial exposure to the carcinogenic agent.

6. There is great variation in individual susceptibility to carcinogens.

7. The concept of a "threshold" exposure level for a carcinogenic agent has no practical significance because there is no valid method for establishing such a level.

8. A carcinogenic agent may be identified through analysis of tumor induction results with laboratory animals exposed to the agent, or on a post hoc basis by properly conducted epidemiological studies.

9. Any substance which produces tumors in animals must be considered a carcinogenic hazard to man if the results were achieved according to the established parameters of a valid carcinogenesis test.

In an effort to resolve some questions on the interpretation of the pathology findings of the various carcinogenicity tests, Reuber reexamined most of the original liver sections, and found that where "benign tumors" or "non-malignant" nodular liver lesions had been claimed, these, in fact, were often unequivocal cancers.[9] In some instances, confirmation of the malignant nature of these tumors was obtained by other independent pathologists, and by the fact that some of the tumors spread or metastasized to the lungs and were also transplantable. Following Reuber's reevaluation, G. McDonald, a pathologist who had previously reported one of the industry-sponsored studies as negative, reexamined his original sections and was then obliged to admit that Reuber was substantially correct.

The available information, particularly as modified by the EPA reevaluation, clearly established that A/D were carcinogenic in five separate feeding tests involving three different strains of mice and at concentrations as low as 0.1 ppm and following only two months feeding. Simultaneous administration of the carcinogen DDT markedly enhanced the carcinogenicity of A/D in excess of an additive effect. During the proceedings, evidence of carcinogenicity in two additional strains of mice was revealed. While the major cancer site was the liver, cancers were also found in various other organs, including the lung, particularly at relatively low dose levels.[10]

The rat data were less extensive, largely because the tests had generally been conducted at such high A/D concentrations that the animals died relatively early from toxic effects. Nevertheless, two studies, FDA 1964 and Tunstall 1, confirmed the carcinogenicity of A/D in rats, finding a wide range of multiple site tumors, particularly at lower doses. Reevaluation of the histology of one of these studies also confirmed the occurrence of liver cancers in treated rats.[11]

How then could Shell contest the carcinogenicity of A/D, dragging out the proceedings over 1,700 days, the written record of which occupied nearly thirteen feet of shelf space? The answer is simple. The studies which were largely generated or contracted for by Shell were either handled in such a way as to discount, dismiss, or interpret away any findings of carcinogenicity, or alternatively were so inept as to invalidate the claimed conclusions of noncarcinogenicity. These tactics were facilitated by the practice of not publishing the reports but submitting them in confidence to a then uncritical FDA.

At the hearings, Shell further bolstered its claims that A/D were noncarcinogenic by developing, with the aid of an apparently impressive array of academic consultants, a novel approach to carcinogenesis based on an imaginative set of myths which were used in attempts to explain away the results of the animal tests. The Shell case largely rested on the claim that the liver tumors induced in mice were not real cancers, but only "hyperplastic" nodules or, using a newly invented terminology, benign "Type A" tumors. As a fallback position, Shell also argued that the mouse was an unsuitable animal for carcinogenicity tests, although for over a decade it had used negative data in mouse carcinogenicity tests as proof of safety of its products. The basis for this argument was that the mouse liver is "labile," and that all that A/D did was to somehow "augment" the induction of liver tumors, which were really due to an "unknown oncogenic stimulus."[12]

The tumors at sites other than the liver in A/D-treated mice were an obstacle to this set of propositions that had to be explained. What better way to do this than to produce some fresh information discounting them? This is just what Shell did. In the middle of the proceedings, when discussion on extra-hepatic tumors had become critical, Shell suddenly produced some "missing" data sheets going back to the 1967 studies at its Tunstall Laboratories in England purporting to prove that sixty additional test mice had no extra-hepatic tumors, and that statistical analysis of the new and old data combined proved that the incidence of these tumors was insignificant.[13]

The lengths to which Shell's consultants were willing to go is illustrated by the testimony of Paul M. Newberne, Professor of Nutritional Pathology, MIT, who said, "It is my feeling that mice as a species . . . should not be used for safety testing," and agreed with Shell scientists that all the extensive

mouse data on carcinogenicity should be ignored.[†14]

The rat carcinogenicity data were sharply contested by Shell, particularly Reuber's finding of an excess incidence of liver cancer in treated rats in his reevaluation of the 1964 FDA study. In an effort to discredit this, Shell created an Ad Hoc Committee of Pathologists headed by Stephen Sternberg, a pathologist at the Sloan Kettering Institute, New York, who had written the section on carcinogenesis in the report of a 1972 advisory committee appointed by the National Academy of Sciences claiming that A/D were noncarcinogenic. The ad hoc committee examined slides from twenty-two treated rats (among whom Reuber had found twenty carcinomas) and reported two carcinomas, one borderline carcinoma, and eleven animals with "hyperplastic nodules." This does not seem to constitute a substantive difference of opinion, particularly as it is generally agreed that nodules are premalignant, and are in fact now classified as neoplastic nodules, and particularly as liver carcinomas and nodules are exceptional in rats other than those treated with carcinogens.[15]

Shell and its witnesses adamantly insisted on a progressive escalation of the standards of proof for the carcinogenicity of A/D, which were so extensive and difficult to meet that their compliance would exclude almost every known chemical carcinogen. These standards included:

1. Induction of carcinogenicity must be statistically significant at all dose levels.
2. A uniformly positive dose-response relationship must be found at all doses, even if there is competing toxicity and high mortality at high doses.
3. A causal association between A/D treatment and carcinogenic effects cannot be sustained unless the mechanism of ac-

---

† Newberne is also an advisor to the NCI bioassay program for carcinogenicity testing, which was and still is largely based on the use of mice.

tion of the carcinogen can be demonstrated.

4. Conclusions on carcinogenic effects of A/D cannot be accepted until the possibility of unknown "augmenting factors" has been excluded.
5. A carcinogenic effect must be consistent and reproducible in a series of different tests before it can be accepted.
6. The induction of liver tumors in mice is no indication of carcinogenic effects, even if they are unequivocally malignant.
7. Tumor production in mice, even in various different organs and even when replicated, cannot be accepted as evidence of carcinogenicity.
8. Even the finding of carcinogenic effects in two or more animal species is unacceptable proof in the absence of evidence in humans.‡[16]

Human Evidence. The final fallback position of Shell was that the animal tests should be discounted, whatever their findings, because epidemiological studies on workers exposed to "high levels" of A/D had conclusively established that there was no excess of cancers. This claim was based on a study, published by K. W. Jager in 1970, of a cohort of 826 full-time male workers, including maintenance crew and operators, employed between 1954 and 1967 at a Shell insecticide plant in Pernis, Holland.[17] Some of them had additional exposures to unrelated pesticides. During the proceedings, the study was updated to 1973 by a Shell witness. There was a high turnover rate at the plant, as the largest number of workers at any one time, 1962, was only 230, and there was also "more or less frequent movement of workers between units" in the plant. Of the 826 workers, only

166 had more than four years exposure and fifteen years observation, and there were only 69 workers with more than ten years exposure and fifteen years observation. Finally, no worker had been exposed for more than nineteen years.[18] Although a leading Shell witness admitted that this study "cannot be considered as statistical proof of noncarcinogenicity," other industry witnesses repeatedly cited it as proving that A/D were noncarcinogenic. Sternberg, for example, made the proposition that if A/D were really carcinogenic, then pre-cancerous symptoms should by now have developed in the exposed workers.[19]

The Pernis study was reviewed in detail by leading independent epidemiologists, including Marvin Schneiderman of the NCI, and Herbert Seidman of the American Cancer Society, who unanimously agreed that the study was so flawed and inadequate that it was not possible to draw any conclusion at all from it. The International Agency for Research on Cancer also agreed, stating that the study "does not allow any conclusions on the existence of an excess risk of developing cancer."[20] Not only was it based on too few workers, exposed and observed for too short a period for any significant excess of cancer other than a catastrophic one to be noted, but it was also clear from blood analyses that over 30 percent of the workers never had any substantial exposure to A/D in the workplace. Additionally the study had failed to follow up hundreds of other exposed employees.

Three studies in the general population have developed suggestive evidence of an association between excess human residues of dieldrin and cancer.[21] A 1967 New Zealand study has shown that dieldrin levels in the lungs of patients with lung cancer are significantly higher than in noncancerous controls. A 1968

‡ This position was unequivocally reiterated more recently by M. J. Sloan, director of the Regulatory Division of Shell Chemical Company, at a discussion of a paper on "The Carcinogenicity of Organochlorine Pesticides," which the author gave at a conference on "The Origins of Human Cancer" at Cold Spring Harbor Laboratories in September, 1976.

study in Hawaii found that dieldrin levels were highest in patients with a variety of cancers. Another 1968 study reported higher dieldrin fat levels in patients dying in Florida with various malignant diseases, including leukaemia and Hodgkin's, than in normal controls.

Other scattered cases of association between A/D exposure and malignant disease have been noted. In 1970 a federal court in Missouri *(Burke v. Stauffer Chemical Co.)* ruled that a case of Hodgkin's disease had been caused by prior exposure of a worker to dieldrin.[22] Since then, there have been several other product-liability suits, most of them brought by pesticide operators involved in termite proofing with A/D formulations, which Shell has settled out of court, presumably to avoid the possibility of creating a legal precedent.

The Battle to Ban A/D

The battle to ban A/D has been long and bitter. In this, Shell was aided by powerful friends in Congress, headed by Senator Eastland and Congressman Jamie Whitten (D-Miss.), and in the USDA, which intervened in support of Shell's position. Useful behind-the-scenes support came from staff of the EPA Office of Pesticide Programs, particularly those who had transferred from the Pesticide Regulation Division of the USDA when EPA was created in 1970. Final and enthusiastic support came from Shell's university consultants and the land grant colleges.

The first round of the battle began in May, 1963, when a special panel of President Kennedy's Science Advisory Committee published a review on "Use of Pesticides," which called for reexamination of FDA tolerances for seven pesticides, including A/D. The review concluded that "elimination of the use of persistent toxic pesticides should be the goal."[23] The panel also noted with concern a 1962 FDA study which had shown that liver

tumors were induced in mice by feeding them with 10 ppm of A/D. On the basis of this review, the FDA appointed an Advisory Committee which in 1965 recommended that the tolerances for dieldrin in foods should be reduced, and that further carcinogenicity tests be undertaken on A/D, as it found that the existing information was inconclusive. Accordingly, Shell withdrew some of its A/D registrations, including foliar application to corn, and initiated further extensive carcinogenicity studies, known as the Tunstall 1 tests, in its Tunstall Laboratories in England. The results of these tests, which were completed by June, 1967, and transmitted to the FDA in 1968 though not published until 1973, confirmed the carcinogenicity of A/D contrary to the conclusions earlier claimed by Shell.[24] The FDA, however, took no action and did not seem anxious to share the information with anyone, including a blue ribbon HEW advisory committee appointed by Secretary Robert Finch in 1969 to examine the relationship between pesticides and health and to consider whether DDT should be banned (the Mrak Commission). At one meeting of the Carcinogenicity Panel of the Commission, a senior FDA scientist, O. Garth Fitzhugh, jocularly remonstrated with some members of the panel,* "I don't know why you should be so concerned about the carcinogenicity of DDT, you should see what we have on dieldrin." When asked what the FDA "had" on dieldrin, the answer was, "That's confidential," presumably referring to Shell's mouse data, the publication of which was withheld for six years.

The Mrak Commission was nevertheless able to conclude, on the basis of the 1962 FDA test in which Fitzhugh had been involved, that A/D were carcinogenic and should be banned.[25] Under pressure from the environmentalists, armed with this fresh support for their position, USDA reluctantly agreed in March, 1970, to cancel "non-essential" uses of A/D,

---

* Including the author.

including its application in aquatic environments.

EPA came into existence by order of President Nixon on December 2, 1970. The next day, the Environmental Defense Fund filed a petition to ban all uses of A/D on the grounds of its adverse ecological effects and its carcinogenicity. One month later, EPA Administrator William Ruckelshaus received the decision of the D.C. Circuit Court to ban DDT and to develop policies for cancellation of other toxic pesticides, whenever their use raised "substantial questions of safety." It was against this background of events that the regulatory struggle on A/D began in earnest.

In March, 1971, EPA announced its intent to move to the cancellation of A/D registrations for agricultural purposes by hearings before an administrative law judge. This action was taken under the authority of the 1947 Federal Insecticide, Fungicide, and Rodenticide Act, which allows the agency to move against pesticides by cancellation or suspension.†

Like all compromises, the cancellation decision did not please anyone. The Environmental Defense Fund promptly appealed, arguing that the cancer risks of A/D posed an "imminent hazard." The industry demanded their rights, under the terms of the 1947 Act, to have the matter referred to an advisory committee appointed by the National Academy of Sciences-National Research Council, which based on the past track record of such committees could have been expected to be sympathetic to the industry position.‡ The NAS advisory committee released its report in March, 1972, endorsing the continued major uses of A/D.[26] The section of the report dealing with carcinogenicity written by Sternberg, who was later to appear as a principal witness for Shell, is puzzling. Sternberg only discussed the then unpublished Tunstall 1 study, which had concluded that A/D were not carcinogenic, and ignored the published 1962 FDA study, on the basis of which the Mrak Commission had previously concluded that A/D were clearly carcinogenic. Sternberg concluded that "if there is a carcinogenic action in dieldrin, it is likely a weak one at a level much like DDT."

In response to a ruling of the appeals court, EPA reaffirmed the cancellation decision in June, 1972, and requested public comment as to whether the agency should proceed to suspension. Shell responded by demanding a public hearing, again its right under the terms of the 1947 Act. Preparation for the trial began. On the government side, the litigation team was headed by Anson Keller and John Kolojeski of the Office of General Counsel. This team started work in virtual isolation, as the Office of Pesticide Programs, where the supposed scientific expertise on pesticides was located, was and still is highly sympathetic to agrichemical interests, quite apart from resenting the Office of General Counsel's apparent policy-making trends and ease of ac-

† Cancellation proceedings are often protracted over several years, while suspension, which is more rigorous and resembles a preliminary injunction in that it bans continued manufacture and distribution during the proceedings, is much more expedited, and can be justified only on the grounds of "imminent hazard." Suspension orders are, however, only temporary bans, pending the final outcome of more definitive cancellation proceedings.

‡ See also discussion on the National Academy of Sciences Committee on Toxicology 1976 report on "Health Effects of Benzene," the Food Protection Committee 1972 report on Red #2, and reports on a wide range of other topics. It should be noted that membership of many such NAS committees has often reflected dominance by industry representatives or their consultants, who are appointed by NAS staff. Scientific members of the academy have not been commonly involved in these committees. It must, however, be recognized that the NAS, prompted by vigorous external criticism, now recognizes these problems and over the last two years or so has instituted various internal reforms which have improved the quality and independence of some of its reports.

cess to the administrator. The Office of Pesticide Programs was actually hostile to the proceedings. While this office was largely staffed by transfers from the FDA and the Pesticide Regulation Division of the USDA, the Office of General Counsel was staffed by young, environment-minded lawyers. The bitter schism which developed, known as the "scientists v. the lawyers," largely reflected the fundamental political ambivalence between environmental activism and traditional pro-industry conservatism, which had existed in the agency since its inception, rather than focusing on specifics of the A/D proceedings.

The failure of the Office of Pesticide Programs to provide scientific assistance in the proceedings opened the door for the Office of General Counsel to go outside the agency for help. This, however, turned out to be not so easy. Most university agricultural economists and entomologists receive research support from the industry and were unwilling to help the government position. The majority of experts on toxicology and carcinogenesis who were approached were either in a similar position or unwilling to take the time to help. The government case had then to rest on the efforts of the small litigation team and a handful of independent outside scientists. These were pitted against the resources of one of the largest and most powerful law firms in Washington, Arnold and Porter, under the direction of William D. Rogers, supported by a profusion of consultants from universities all over the world. In the government case against Shell conducted by EPA, Shell was supported in court by another branch of government, the USDA. The legal fees of Shell amounted to approximately $1 million. These were more than amply repaid by their annual profits of $10 million from continued sales of A/D during the proceedings, which it was to Shell's advantage to protract.

After months of unsuccessful negotiations, the cancellation hearings began on August

7, 1973. News of the Mississippi chicken massacre of February, 1974, interrupted the leisurely pace of the proceedings.[27] This triggered an EPA announcement that it was again considering suspension. It asked Shell to agree to discontinue its intended A/D manufacture for the 1975 crop year, scheduled to begin around September, 1974. Shell refused. EPA then dropped its plans for suspension, presumably out of deference to Congressman Whitten, whose House Appropriations Subcommittee was then reviewing the EPA budget.

The reluctance of EPA to proceed more aggressively on the suspension of A/D was beginning to draw unfavorable comments from the press. On August 2, 1974, the new EPA administrator, Russell Train, announced his decision to suspend on the grounds of "imminent hazards," noting that production and use of A/D had recently increased, that environmental and body burdens of A/D were also increasing, and that further evidence of carcinogenicity had developed. In spite of the acknowledgment of "imminent hazards" in the suspension order, Train allowed the continued sale of existing A/D stocks. It was no secret that EPA had little option but to permit this or be faced with the statutory requirement of indemnifying Shell for unused stocks.

The cancellation record, consisting of about 24,000 pages of transcript and 950 exhibits comprising another 11,000 pages, was then incorporated into the suspension proceedings, which began on September 1, 1974. Because of the urgent nature of the suspension hearings, only fifteen days were allowed for opposing arguments. The final EPA brief was submitted on September 16,[28] and Judge Perlman submitted his decision to the administrator on September 20, recommending suspension.[29] This was subsequently confirmed by the administrator on October 1, 1974.[30]

Of particular importance was the incorporation of the "nine cancer principles" in the final EPA brief as "established principles of carcinogenicity which can be applied to individual substances to determine their human cancer hazard." These principles, which were similar to the "seven cancer principles" used by EPA in the DDT cancellation proceedings, were developed by Kolojeski of the Office of General Counsel, based on the testimony of its "acknowledged cancer experts," Umberto Saffiotti of the NCI in particular. These nine principles, which were backed up by extensive supporting documentation and references and also by refutation of contrary Shell evidence, were implicitly incorporated in both the recommended decision of Judge Perlman and the subsequent decision of the administrator. These principles were also to become the salient point of contention in the subsequent C/H hearings.

The principles aroused the strident opposition of industry. Industry objections were largely channelled through a task force of CAST composed of seventeen trade and largely captive scientific associations. The CAST task force consisted of thirteen scientists, including Newberne, the Shell witness, and Jesse L. Steinfeld, Professor of Medicine at the University of California and previously U.S. Surgeon General. The task force reports reaffirmed the industry position that the burden of proving the safety of a pesticide was the responsibility of the public, and recommended that rodents were too sensitive for carcinogenicity tests and should be replaced by monkeys.[31] Not only is the latter suggestion economically prohibitive, but given the longer life span of monkeys it would also mean that any carcinogenicity test would take over ten years, rather than the two years required with rodents.

Both sides appealed the administrator's decision, the Environmental Defense Fund on the grounds that the suspension order still allowed use of existing A/D stocks, and Shell and USDA on the grounds that it objected to the basis of the ruling. There was considerable jockeying as to where the appeal should be heard, the Environmental Defense Fund favoring the D.C. Circuit Court, and Shell favoring the more sympathetic climate of the Fifth Circuit in New Orleans. The case was heard in D.C., and the decision of the administrator was affirmed in a unanimous decision of the court. In April, 1975, Shell announced that it would no longer manufacture A/D for use in the United States. A West Coast firm now manufactures aldrin for those relatively small uses exempted in the original cancellation order, including domestic termite treatment and "closed-system" mothproofing of fabrics. It is difficult to comprehend why such uses have not also been banned, as they pose at least equal "imminent cancer hazards to man" as agricultural applications which were banned. As Shell not unreasonably asked: "How did the agency decide that 1½ pounds of aldrin under an acre of corn in the Midwest . . . leads to an unacceptable cancer hazard for man, when a rate of up to several hundred pounds per acre in the soil under a human dwelling does not."[32]

Dieldrin, meanwhile, continues to be sold and used for agricultural purposes in most countries outside the United States. The EPA decision banning A/D was rejected in Britain on the grounds that "experts not trial judges were competent to judge the issue" of carcinogenicity. The British experts who concluded that dieldrin is not carcinogenic are members of a Pesticide Safety Precaution Scheme committee of the Ministry of Agriculture and Fisheries, which meets behind closed doors. The ministry is closely linked with industrial and agricultural interests.*[33]

---

* Such linkages, which permeate the scientific establishment, industry, and government, are commonplace in Britain where the opportunity for independent inquiry is restricted by a parliamentary system devoid of any public forum where civil servants can be held accountable (such as

Summary

Aldrin/dieldrin (A/D) are highly persistent organochlorine insecticides which have been used mainly for the prevention and treatment of corn infestation, in spite of evidence that the complex of insects involved have become largely resistant. Use of these insecticides has resulted in extensive environmental contamination of air, soil, water, fish, wildlife, and meat products, resulting in major economic losses to the agricultural and fishing industries, and also contamination of the human body.

The carcinogenicity of A/D was established in animal tests by the FDA in 1962 and subsequently confirmed in tests by the manufacturer, Shell Chemical Company, in spite of their claims to the contrary. In regulatory proceedings against these insecticides by EPA, beginning in 1971, Shell and an extensive array of its academic consultants attempted to argue away the findings of carcinogenicity in its own and other tests by developing a set of scientific myths, escalating to the assertion that mice are unsuitable animals for carcinogenicity tests. Shell's confidence in these positions did not seem shaken by the fact that they had regularly used negative results in mouse carcinogenicity tests as proof of the safety of a wide range of their other chemical products, and also by the fact that A/D were carcinogenic in rats, besides mice. As a fallback position, Shell argued that even if the animal tests were positive, these should be discounted, as there was no evidence of carcinogenic effects in workers involved in the manufacture of A/D. However, the number of workers exposed was so few and the period of time over which they were observed was so brief that any possibility of detecting even a powerful carcinogenic effect was virtually excluded.

The success of the regulatory proceedings against A/D, resulting in their 1975 ban on the grounds of imminent carcinogenic hazard, was due to the combined efforts of a public interest group and the EPA's Office of General Counsel aided by a small team of independent experts. These were pitted against the massive legal and scientific resources of Shell and the USDA, which supported Shell's position, aided by the politically powerful Southern congressional network and the EPA's own Office of Pesticide Programs, which was hostile to the proceedings.

Chlordane/Heptachlor

Chlordane and heptachlor (C/H) are two closely related organochlorine pesticides of the same general cyclodiene subclass as A/D. Both chlordane and heptachlor are transformed in the environment and in the body to persistent and stable epoxide derivatives, oxychlordane and heptachlor epoxide, respectively. Technical formulations of chlordane contain about 7 to 12 percent heptachlor, besides various other related impurities.

Sales and Uses

Chlordane and heptachlor have been sold since the late 1940s and are exclusively manufactured by the Chicago-based Velsicol Chemical Corporation, a subsidiary of Northwest Industries Inc. (Chlordane is manufactured at Marshall, Illinois and heptachlor at Memphis, Tennessee.) Their major agricultural uses have been as corn soil insecticides. They have also been used for treatment of termite infestation and as general insecticides

the U.S. Congressional committee system). Additional restrictions include a draconian "Official Secrets Act," which can be invoked to protect information held to be "secret" by industry (such as levels of discharge of toxic pollutants into surface waters), crippling libel laws which inhibit investigative journalism, and the virtual absence of an effective public interest movement.

around the home, lawn, and garden. Even prior to their suspension in 1975, the agricultural uses of C/H were on a gradual decline due to increasing insect resistance and the emergence of alternatives, particularly organophosphate and carbamate insecticides, which are more effective and do not pose comparable problems of environmental contamination. This decline was, however, temporarily arrested between 1973 and 1975, when the regulatory proceedings against A/D created demands for alternative corn soil insecticides.

Environmental Contamination[1]

Chlordane and heptachlor and their principal derivatives are highly persistent, mobile, and fat soluble. Like A/D, their use in accordance with recommended agricultural practice has led to widespread environmental dissemination and the pollution of soil, air, and water. This, in turn, has led to accumulation and concentration of C/H in the food chain and resulted in substantial human contamination.

Residues of C/H are found in soil more than ten years following application.[2] Although the highest levels occur in agricultural areas of the corn belt states, residues are also high in urban soils, with average recorded values in the early 1970s of 0.16 ppm resulting from use around the home and garden. C/H are also highly volatile and escape into the air, whether applied to the soil surface or injected into the subsoil.[3] In addition, C/H are transported as dust, particularly in areas where soil erosion is high. Dust levels of chlordane ranged up to 135 ppm in homes of pesticide formulators, and to about 40 ppm in homes of people who have no occupational exposure. Based on EPA monitoring data, the daily respiratory intake of an average adult would be in the order of 0.6 µg chlordane and 0.2 µg heptachlor, levels of the same order of magnitude as those from food.

Residues of C/H are found in surface waters all over the United States. Stream sediments containing chlordane residues as high as 800 ppb have been found in corn belt states. Chlordane residues are also found in fresh and saltwater fish, with levels reaching as high as 24 ppm. Laboratory experiments have shown that even very low levels of C/H cause mortality and reproductive failure in fish. Significant residues of heptachlor epoxide and oxychlordane have been found in eggs of many birds, including fish eaters. Much wildlife has been killed as a result of using C/H to control fire ants.

Diet is probably the most important source of human contamination by C/H.[4] Once applied to soil, these insecticides begin a continuous movement up the food chain. Root crops grown on land treated with C/H as long as ten years ago absorb measurable quantities of these insecticides. FDA market basket surveys in 1973 and 1974 have shown that C/H, and particularly heptachlor epoxide, are found in the majority of dairy products, meat, poultry, and fish; the data on oxychlordane, while more recent and limited, also indicate extensive food contamination. The calculated total daily intake of heptachlor and its epoxide in the diet of a normal adult, excluding other environmental sources, is about 0.7 µg.

Residues of heptachlor epoxide and oxychlordane are found in virtually all body fat samples, each at levels from 0.1 to 0.2 ppm but ranging as high as 10 ppm for the former and 2 ppm for the latter.[5] Levels in the United States are lower than in France and Italy, where agricultural use of C/H is more intense. Residues are also found in umbilical cord blood and in mothers' milk. It is important to note that human fat residues of heptachlor epoxide are roughly the same magnitude as levels in rats following feeding with the lowest level tested and found to be carcinogenic (0.5 ppm).

Nearly all available information on environmental contamination with C/H is related to agricultural use. It is remarkable that there seem to be no published reports on contamination of air, dust, drapes, textiles, food, and the human body following home and garden use, especially following treatment for termite infestation.

Carcinogenicity of C/H

As was the case with A/D, the regulatory battle to ban C/H largely focused on questions of carcinogenicity. C/H have been extensively tested for carcinogenicity in rats and mice in a total of some eleven studies, most of which have never been published.[6] One exception is a 1965 FDA mouse study on the basis of which the Mrak Commission in 1969 concluded that heptachlor and its epoxide were carcinogenic.[7] Apart from this study and more recent ones by the NCI, the results of which first became available in 1975,[8] the main body of information on the basis of which C/H were claimed to be noncarcinogenic and safe was generated under contract to Velsicol by two commercial testing laboratories, the Kettering Laboratories of the University of Cincinnati, Ohio, and the International Research Development Corporation, Mattawan, Michigan. Studies in the latter laboratory were based on feeding C/H and heptachlor epoxide to mice and concluded that these insecticides were noncarcinogenic, although they noted a dose-related incidence of "liver nodules" in treated animals. Similar negative conclusions were reached in the Kettering rat studies.

In view of the uncertain validity of the conclusions of these various carcinogenicity tests, particularly those of the Kettering and the International Research Development Corporation, EPA decided that the liver sections should be reexamined by a team of independent pathologists headed by Melvin Reuber. Reuber undertook an extensive examination of most available liver sections, and these were spot-checked by four other pathologists in the team, who in general confirmed Reuber's findings.[9] Where the International Research Development Corporation and Kettering had reported either normal conditions or non-malignant nodular liver lesions in C/H-treated mice and rats, Reuber and his team found a high incidence of unequivocal liver cancers. Reuber's results in many cases were statistically analyzed, showing that the incidence of liver cancers induced by C/H were highly significant. An honest difference of opinion, you might say, but for the fact that there were no discrepancies between the diagnoses of the industry laboratories and the EPA team in untreated control animals. Nor were there discrepancies in diagnoses of the positive control animals treated with the known potent carcinogen acetylaminofluorene, as a check on their sensitivity, which resulted in a high incidence of liver cancers. An additional obstacle to the "honest difference of opinion" theory is that two Velsicol consultants who reviewed the liver sections of the International Research Development Corporation concluded that these showed cancers in the C/H-treated animals. They informed Velsicol of this by letter in December, 1972.[10]

C/H were also tested in the NCI bioassay program, the preliminary results becoming available in 1975 and the final published results in 1977. These studies confirmed the carcinogenicity of C/H in mice, although the results in rats were less clear-cut.[11]

Taken together, the results of all these tests, particularly following independent re-evaluation of the industry-generated data, clearly proved that C/H and heptachlor epoxide were carcinogenic in mice. These conclusions were subsequently confirmed by a 1977 Pesticide Committee report of the National Academy of Sciences, which agreed that there was unquestionable evidence of carcinogenicity in mice, and that accordingly, C/H represented a carcinogenic hazard to humans.[12] The rat data, while less extensive, again proved the carcinogenicity of heptachlor and its epoxide. While the results of chlordane testing in rats were equivocal, all the positive data on heptachlor and its epoxide are also applicable to technical chlordane, since heptachlor is a major component of technical chlordane.

As was the case in the A/D hearings, the industry minimized the human relevance of the carcinogenicity findings in rodents.†

Industry further asserted that great weight should be attached to the human epidemiological studies which had failed to demonstrate the carcinogenicity of C/H. Three such unpublished studies have been recently conducted on behalf of Velsicol, two on pest control operators, and one on workers involved in the manufacture of C/H.‡[16] All these studies suffered from the major defects of inappropriate methodology, too few workers exposed, too brief duration of follow-up, lack of exposure records, and lack of appropriate controls. As a result, it is impossible to make any valid inferences on safety or carcinogenicity.

Over the last twenty years there has been an accumulation of scattered reports of aplastic anaemia and leukaemia, besides other malignant disease, in humans exposed to C/H, under a wide range of conditions. There have also been recent reports of cancer and leukaemia in infants and young children born to mothers exposed to chlordane during pregnancy following house-proofing for termites.[17] Recent product liability suits filed by workers who have developed cancers of various sites against Velsicol and exterminating companies have been settled out of court, presumably to avoid the possibility of a successful legal precedent.

The "Banning" of C/H

On November 18, 1974, EPA announced its intent to cancel all agricultural and domestic uses of C/H, excluding termite control, on the basis of carcinogenicity and widespread environmental contamination.

In the agency's first pretrial brief of April 1, 1975, the "nine cancer principles" developed during the A/D suspension hearings, were presented as "the most advanced research findings and policy of both national and international cancer experts and agencies," in support of the proposed cancellation.[18] Velsicol objected on a broad overall basis, particularly challenging principle number two, which deals with the essential similarity of benign and malignant tumors following administration of carcinogens, and number seven, affirming scientific inability to set thresholds or safe levels for carcinogens.[19] Velsicol attempted to have the validity of these principles referred to a commit-

---

† The scientific and emotional demeanor of some industry witnesses was unusual. William J. Butler, an English pathologist, in response to a question as to whether the induction of liver cancer in rats by C/H in the NCI Tests constituted evidence of carcinogenicity, responded, "This would slightly raise my suspicions."[13] Another consultant, John Rust of the University of Chicago Medical School, responding to a question on the occurrence of metastases in the lungs of rodents from liver cancers induced by C/H, expostulated, "I would like to say right now [gesturing towards respondent's counsel] that Judge Perlman ought to throw you bastards out for bringing this to Court."[14] Other industry consultants, such as Klaus Stemmer and Frank Cleveland of the Kettering Laboratories, who had undertaken carci-

nogenicity tests for Velsicol purporting to show that C/H were not carcinogenic, admitted in court that they had no training or expertise in chemical carcinogenesis.[15]

‡ Typical of these studies was one presented by a Velsicol consultant, Brian MacMahon, Professor of Epidemiology at the Harvard School of Public Health, in testimony at the cancellation proceedings (FIFRA Docket 33, EPA, 1977). Based on a preliminary study of about 16,000 males with some occupational exposure to C/H during 1967-76, MacMahon concluded that there was no evidence of increased cancer mortality, while admitting the relatively short duration of follow-up of this study. The small number of workers who had been exposed for more than five years also invalidates the conclusion of noncarcinogenicity.

tee of the National Academy of Sciences for review. EPA opposed this motion on the grounds that "benign" and malignant tumors have synonymous scientific and regulatory implications in carcinogenicity testing. The appeal was denied by Judge Perlman, as was a subsequent appeal by Velsicol on more narrowly defined grounds. In these exchanges, Velsicol took the position that any burden of uncertainty in the carcinogenicity data should be borne by the agency and the public, not by industry.

On June 27, the EPA litigation team, led by Jeffrey H. Howard, Frank J. Sizemore III, and William E. Reukauf, moved to have some thirty-eight facts officially noted and incorporated in the hearing record. The first seventeen facts were an amplification of the nine cancer principles and were developed with the assistance of Umberto Saffiotti, on whose testimony the original nine principles had been largely developed in the A/D hearings.

On July 29, 1975, Administrator Train issued a further notice of intent, this time to suspend all uses of C/H other than those exempted in the cancellation order. Train cited new confirmatory evidence on carcinogenicity based on reevaluation by the EPA team of independent pathologists of previously claimed negative carcinogenicity tests, and declared an "imminent hazard of carcinogenicity" as the basis for his ruling. In his order, the Administrator discussed the seventeen cancer principles as "the basis for evaluation" of cancer risks, and thus ensured their adoption in the suspension proceedings.*

In a move apparently intended to neutral-

ize the seventeen principles, William M. Upholt† wrote to NCI, then under the directorship of Frank Rauscher, asking for their reevaluation. This matter was handled in NCI by Gary Flamm.‡ Flamm referred the matter to the Subcommittee on Environmental Carcinogenesis of the National Cancer Advisory Board chaired by Philippe Shubik, Director of the Eppley Cancer Research Institute, of the University of Nebraska. Shubik, then and still a member of the National Cancer Advisory Board, is a well-known industrial consultant who has recently faced charges including mishandling federal funds and conflict of interest.[20]

The Shubik Committee discussed the seventeen cancer principles at a meeting on November 10, 1975, and in principle was sympathetic to them. The transcript of the meeting also makes it clear that the committee was anxious to avoid reversal or criticism of the principles. Shubik, however, prepared an unsigned "working draft," which had neither been reviewed nor approved by his committee, and released it through Flamm to Judge Perlman.[21] The draft not only gave the impression that the NCI committee had rejected cancer principles, but also perpetuated the alleged distinctions between "benign and malignant tumors."* The draft report was immediately picked up by the trade journals and publicized as a formal NCI rejection of the cancer principles.†[22]

The draft report had its presumably intended impact on Judge Perlman, who had been saturated by argument and counter-argument on questions of the carcinogenicity of C/H. Not unnaturally, Perlman was in-

---

* The author was involved in these proceedings as an EPA expert witness.

† Senior Science Advisor to the acting administrator for Water and Hazardous Materials, EPA, previously of the Pesticide Regulation Division of USDA and now an EPA consultant on pesticides.

‡ Then assistant director of the Division of Cancer Cause and Prevention, a geneticist recently

recruited to the NCI from FDA and noted for his public speeches on the need to develop tests to "exculpate chemicals from carcinogenicity, rather than to indict them."

* This and other current positions of Shubik on chemical carcinogenesis are in contrast to the views he previously expressed in a government document in 1970 (See Appendix II).

† The final report of the NCI Subcommittee on

clined to give weight to the findings of what appeared to be a top-level NCI report.[23]

As news of this intervention leaked out, Shubik and Flamm sent a telegram to Perlman in late November asking that the draft should "not be misinterpreted or used prior to its completion." Additionally, Flamm has since claimed that they were forced to release the draft under the requirements of the Federal Advisory Committee and Freedom of Information Acts. However, there is no record of any such demand for the document under the terms of these Acts.

On December 12, 1975, Judge Perlman submitted his conclusion to EPA, that he was "hesitatingly unwilling at this time to find that heptachlor and chlordane are conclusive carcinogens in laboratory animals . . . [and that he could] not find an 'imminent hazard'."[24] This decision was rejected on December 24 by Administrator Train, who emphasized that while Judge Perlman did not find the evidence on imminent hazard from use of C/H to be conclusive, it certainly was not the agency's burden to establish risks, but rather the registrant's burden to establish safety, and this Velsicol had clearly failed to do.[25] Velsicol appealed the decision to the D.C. Circuit Court of Appeals, which upheld the EPA suspension ruling on November 10, 1976. The suspension created the authority for a temporary ban, pending the final outcome of the cancellation proceedings. These began in June, 1976, and opposing briefs were filed in January, 1978.

The three years of administrative litigation ended on March 6, 1978, with the announcement by EPA that a settlement had been reached between the litigants, including the Environmental Defense Fund, to phase out all agricultural uses of C/H over a five-year period ending in September, 1982, to allow agricultural users to shift to alternative crops and pest control technologies.[26] The settlement allows the production of no more than 7.25 million pounds of C/H annually, compared to the 20 million pounds prior to the EPA restrictions. All uses during the phaseout are restricted to certified applicators and commercial seed-treating companies.

The settlement is no victory for public health. It was apparently forced on a reluctant Environmental Defense Fund by the alliance of industry and EPA, whose Office of Pesticide Programs has been clearly adversarial to the objectives of effective pesticide regulation since its inception and to the efforts of the public interest movement in this regard. The settlement allows continued public exposure to excessive amounts of these carcinogenic and widely disseminated pesticides. Additionally, the language of the settlement clearly underestimates the human health hazard posed by the continued use of C/H. The settlement contains no legal finding of fact that C/H are carcinogenic and is thus open to subsequent challenge by industry other than the litigants.‡ Finally, the settlement in no way limits continued domestic use of C/H for termite control.

Criminal Indictment of Velsicol

On April 4, 1977, it was reported that a special grand jury in the Federal Court of Chicago was investigating Velsicol on charges that the company had criminally conspired to conceal information on the carcinogenicity of C/H. Specifically, Velsicol was charged with withholding the findings of carcinogenicity arrived at by its own consultants in

---

Environmental Carcinogenesis, issued in June, 1976, is however, essentially consistent with the 17 cancer principles.

‡ Velsicol's position on this is understood to reflect their intent to limit the scope of future legal actions brought against the company by pest control operators or householders developing cancer following use of C/H for termite control. This position is further strengthened by the language of the settlement, which asserts that the previous suspension decision by the EPA against C/H should not be considered as findings of fact under federal rules of evidence — an assertion of questionable legality.

1972 on the basis of their review of the liver sections in tests done by the International Research Development Corporation. In announcing the indictment, EPA general counsel stated:

> Velsicol Chemical Co. may have violated the reporting requirements of #6(a) (2) of the Federal Pesticidal Statute [which states that] "if at any time after the registration of a pesticide the registrant has additional factual information regarding unreasonable adverse effects on the environment of the pesticide, he shall submit such information to the Administration."

In December, 1977, the federal grand jury handed down an eleven- count felony indictment, naming six present or former company executives, all of whom face prison terms, charging:

> From August 1972 to July 1975 the defendants . . . conspired to defraud the United States and conceal material facts from the United States Environmental Protection Agency by failing to submit data which tended to show that Heptachlor and Chlordane induced tumors in laboratory animals and thus might pose a risk of cancer to humans.[27]

A series of motions to dismiss the indictment were filed by Velsicol in March, 1978. These included technical pleadings and allegations of conflict of interest and prosecutorial misconduct based on the fact that an EPA attorney, Bingham Kennedy, had worked on the case with the grand jury on behalf of the Department of Justice. Following an evidentiary hearing in the fall of 1978 with respect to the motion to dismiss the hearing record was closed. Oral arguments were presented to Judge George Leighton in January, 1979. The case was dismissed on procedural grounds on April 20, 1979, without reaching the merits of the original issues of conspiracy raised by the indictment.

Summary

Chlordane and heptachlor (C/H), like aldrin and dieldrin (A/D), are highly persistent organochlorine insecticides used on corn, around the home as general lawn and garden insecticides, and also for treatment of domestic termite infestation. Like A/D, their use in accordance with recommended agricultural practice has resulted in extensive environmental contamination.

The carcinogenicity tests on C/H were made under contract to their manufacturer, Velsicol Chemical Company, by a commercial and a university laboratory, both of which reported negative results. During subsequent EPA proceedings against C/H, samples of the histological sections from these tests were reviewed by an independent team of experts who proved that these insecticides were in fact carcinogenic and had induced a high incidence of liver cancers. The impact of these findings was, however, blunted by the intervention of Philippe Shubik, chairman of a National Cancer Advisory Board subcommittee, and a well-known industrial consultant who at this writing faces major charges, including conflict of interest; Shubik sent EPA a working draft of his subcommittee's report, which challenged the nature of the carcinogenic effects induced by C/H but which had not been seen or approved by committee members. The subsequent refusal of the administrative law judge to suspend the insecticides was, however, reversed by Administrator Train.

Bowing to congressional and industry pressures, EPA subsequently reorganized its internal policies to exclude the possibility of initiation of further litigation against pesticides by its Office of General Counsel and to place this responsibility, instead, largely in the hands of its Pesticide Regulation Division, which has been hostile to the proceedings against both C/H and A/D. (Since this reorganization, EPA has failed to initiate and conclude successful regulatory actions against any pesticides, and has developed regulations allowing the provisional registration of pesticides which have not been tested for carcinogenicity and other chronic toxic effects.)

Faced with an EPA now apparently hostile to pesticide regulation, a settlement to phase out major agricultural uses of C/H over the next five years has been developed between Velsicol, EPA, and the Environmental Defense Fund, which had prompted the original proceedings against C/H. The settlement excludes any legal "finding of fact" as to the carcinogenicity of C/H, and also permits their continued use for termite treatment. Termite treatment results in exposure of pest control operators and also householders to C/H. Case reports on the development of aplastic anaemia, leukaemia, and cancers following such exposures are now accumulating.

Nitrosamines

Although several classes of agents, including synthetic organic chemicals, metals, fibers, and radiation, have been shown over the past few decades to induce a wide range of human cancers, there are many types of cancers for which no such carcinogenic agents have been identified.

Over the last decade, there has been growing interest in the possibility that nitrosamines and other N-nitroso compounds may be a major class of universal carcinogens responsible for a substantial number of human cancers and cancers in other forms of life, under the widest possible range of conditions and circumstances, including pre-industrial societies.[1]

Nitrosamines are a large group of chemicals, many of which are found in air, food, and water, and most of which are highly carcinogenic to a great range of organs in all animal species tested.[2] A more important reason why nitrosamines qualify as prime candidates for human carcinogens is that they can be simply and rapidly synthesized by a process called nitrosation, both in the environment and in the body, from two types of common and extensively distributed compounds, amines and nitrites or nitrogen oxides.[3] In addition to naturally occurring amines, a wide range of consumer products, drugs, pesticides, and industrial chemicals are also amines, and can thus be nitrosated to form nitrosamines.

Basic Chemistry

Nitrosamines are characterized by a terminal N-nitroso, N-N=O, group. They are typically formed by the interaction of amines and nitrites or oxides of nitrogen, which are therefore called *precursors* of nitrosamines.[4]

Chemical analysis and measurement of nitrosamines, particularly at environmental levels in the ppm to ppb range, has until recently been difficult and time-consuming, thus limiting progress in investigating their presence in the environment. These problems have been resolved with the introduction of a highly specific and sensitive instrument, the Thermal Energy Analyzer, developed by the Thermo Electron Cancer Research Center, Waltham, Massachusetts, which is capable of rapid routine analysis of nitrosamines below the ppb level.[5]

$$\begin{array}{c} R_1 \\ \diagdown \\ \diagup \\ R_2 \end{array} N\text{-}H \ + \ H\text{-}O\text{-}N \ = \ O \ \rightarrow \ H_2O \ + \ \begin{array}{c} R_1 \\ \diagdown \\ \diagup \\ R_2 \end{array} N\text{--}N{=}O$$

| Secondary Amine | + Nitrous Acid | Water | + Nitrosamine |

Carcinogenicity

Of about 130 different nitrosamines so far tested, 80 percent have been shown to be carcinogenic.[6] Nitrosamines are carcinogenic in more than twenty different animal species tested, and no species has been found to be resistant. Individual nitrosamines produce various types of tumors in many organs of various animal species. Among nitrosamines are some of the most potent known carcinogens: dimethylnitrosamine (DMN), diethylnitrosamine, nitrosopyrrolidine, and dipropylnitrosamine, all of which produce cancers in test animals following administration at the ppm level in food, water, air, or by other routes. The lowest daily level of DMN which has been so far tested in rodents and found to be carcinogenic is 50 µg/kg, which is equivalent to an entire lifetime dose of less than 30 mg.

Formation of Nitrosamines in the Environment[7]

The growing realization that nitrosamines are ubiquitous environmental carcinogens largely reflects the widespread distribution of amines and nitrites or nitrogen oxides. Amines are chemical derivatives of ammonia, and are classified as primary, secondary, tertiary, or quaternary, depending on their increasing degree of chemical substitution. Amines, particularly dimethylamine and diethylamine, are well known constituents of many foods, particularly meat and fish, in which they are found at the 10 ppm range. Many common drugs and pesticides are also amines. Other important sources of amines include nicotine in tobacco smoke, ethanolamines, used as emulsifying agents in cosmetics, detergents and pesticides, and air and water pollutants. Finally, amines are a major class of industrial chemicals and are used, for example, as catalysts in the manufacture of plastics, antioxidants in the manufacture of rubber, and fuel additives.

Nitrites are the reduction products of nitrates, the most common form of inorganic nitrogen in the environment. Nitrate/nitrite are present in a wide variety of foods, particularly leafy vegetables, and are also common food additives. Nitrate/nitrite are also normal constituents of drinking water and human saliva. Oxides of nitrogen, often referred to as NO_x, are major air pollutants emitted from all combustion sources, including incinerators and automobiles, and are present at high concentrations in cigarette smoke.

Amines can be nitrosated by nitrite or NO_x to form nitrosamines. These reactions occur in the test tube, air, food, and water — even in the stomach or other organs. A wide range of factors can alter the rates of synthesis of nitrosamines. Rates are increased in acidic conditions, such as those found in the stomach, by bacterial enzymes, and by salts such as thiocyanates, levels of which are particularly high in the saliva of smokers. On the other hand, some chemicals, such as vitamins C and E in high doses, can retard but not block nitrosamine synthesis.

Air

Nitrosamines have been detected by use of the thermal energy analyzer in the air of several American cities, particularly in the vicinity of chemical plants manufacturing or handling amines. In the summer of 1975, levels ranging up to about 0.05 ppb DMN were found in the downtown areas of Belle and Charleston, West Virginia.[8] These were traced to a large Du Pont Chemical complex in Belle, which manufactures a wide range of chemicals and is the largest alkyl amine producer in the United States. Du Pont subsequently reported that they had isolated and plugged the source of the leakage.

DMN levels of about 0.1 ppb have been found in downtown Baltimore, originating two miles away at an FMC Corporation plant which manufactured dimethylhydrazine as a rocket fuel for military purposes. Plant levels were over 300 times higher, ranging up to 36 ppb; levels in an adjacent residential community were about 1 ppb. The rocket fuel production section of the FMC plant was ordered closed in February, 1976.*

It is difficult to translate air levels of DMN into daily human exposures. Making some reasonable assumptions on the average volume and rate of breathing, an atmospheric concentration of approximately 1 ppb DMN in air corresponds to a daily intake of about 14 µg or 0.21 µg/kg for an average adult male; this is only about one hundredth of the lowest dose of DMN which has been shown to be carcinogenic in conventional rodent tests. Such intake levels are in excess of DMN concentrations in tobacco smoke and in nitrite-preserved meats.

Among the significant potential sources of amine air pollutants is automobile exhaust. Of approximately seventy registered fuel additives, more than half are amines. These can be nitrosated by NO_x in automobile exhaust or subsequently in the air to form nitrosamines; another common air pollutant, ozone, has been recently shown to catalyze the rate of nitrosation. NO_x are a major class of air pollutants, originating from a wide range of stationary sources, such as municipal incinerators, industrial furnaces and domestic space heating units, besides mobile sources, such as automobiles. Levels of atmospheric NO_x are steadily increasing. According to a recent report of the Council on Environmental Quality, they are the only major pollutants whose concentrations in air have increased since the passage of the Clean Air Act in 1970. Relatively high levels of NO_x, ranging up to 0.4 ppm, are found in the air of large U.S. cities. In a non-industrial city, mobile and stationary sources contribute about equally to atmospheric levels of NO_x, with the relative proportion from mobile sources increasing during rush hours. In an industrialized city, the contribution of stationary sources is proportionately greater. It may

be noted that a current EPA standard regulates automobile emissions of NO_x to levels of 1.5 g/mile, with the goal of reducing emissions to below 0.4 g/mile after 1981. EPA also regulates atmospheric levels of NO_x to an average annual standard of 0.1 ppm, based on short-term acute irritant effects, and without reference to problems of possible long-term effects, including nitrosamine formation. The importance of these problems is further indicated by two recent epidemiological studies, suggesting an association between high atmospheric levels of NO_x and excess cancers of all sites, including breast and lung. Commenting on one of these studies, the National Academy of Sciences concluded:

> The consistent relation postulated by Hickey between cancer death rates and nitrogen dioxide are of enormous potential importance. Hickey reported an association in 38 metropolitan areas for breast, lung and total cancer over a nitrogen dioxide concentration range of 0.08-0.116 mg/m^3 (0.04-0.06 ppm), concentrations that are frequently encountered in the ambient air of large cities.[9]

It should be appreciated, however, that such attempted correlations between a single pollution index, NO_x, and several types of cancer may be simplistic, and not necessarily implicate that specific pollutant. Rather, the correlations may reflect an overall increased exposure to a wide range of environmental pollutants. Regardless of possible limitations in these epidemiological studies, recent evidence on environmental synthesis of nitrosamines, and on high levels of atmospheric nitrosamines, lends still further urgency for a long-term NO_x exposure standard reflecting these considerations.†

Water

There has been relatively little work on the

---

* There is no information available as to where this operation was relocated.

† Recent studies in the author's laboratories have

demonstrated biosynthesis of nitrosamines in rodents following inhalation of NO_2 at levels below 10 ppm.

detection and measurement of nitrosamines in water. High concentrations have been found in a limited number of samples of sea and river water, and effluents from sewage plants treating wastewater from industries using or manufacturing amines or nitrosamines. DMN levels as high as 9 ppb have been detected in effluents from sewage treatment facilities handling wastewater from the FMC plant in Baltimore and the Du Pont plant in Belle, West Virginia. The intake for the drinking water supply of the Du Pont plant was about 500 feet downstream from where it discharged its effluents into the Kanawha River.

Food

Since time immemorial, nitrate has been used to preserve and cure meat. In fact, early European cave paintings show the use of saltpeter for this purpose by the Cro-Magnon man. The typical pink red color of cured meat is due to the interaction of nitrite, formed by the reduction of nitrate, with myoglobin — a muscle protein related to the blood pigment hemoglobin — to form colored derivatives.

Nitrite has a general antibacterial action, besides being particularly effective in inhibiting the outgrowth of spores of *Clostridium botulinum.*

For these reasons, nitrite is used to prevent the production of the heat-labile toxin responsible for botulism (which is deactivated by heating to 185° for about 15 minutes). Botulism is a rare and often fatal "food poisoning" mainly occurring following production of the toxin under anaerobic conditions, such as in cold cuts and other processed meats, and particularly in home canning of low acid foods such as beans.

Over the years, the meat packing and processing industries have found that certain nitrate/nitrite ratios were ideal both for preserving meat and also producing the reddish color which consumers have grown to expect as visual proof of so-called "freshness." As the necessity for preservation has diminished,

largely owing to modern refrigeration methods, the "cosmetic" use of nitrite has assumed greater importance to the meat industry and involves a $12.5 billion cured meat market. Until recently, USDA and FDA standards have allowed addition of nitrite to meat and fish up to residual levels of about 200 ppm, regardless of whether its use is preservative or, as is mainly the case, cosmetic.

Nitrosamines have been found in many different meat and fish products, as expected from their content of natural constituent amines and nitrite food additives.[10] The highest concentrations of nitrosamines in food are found in cooked bacon, with DMN levels as high as 10 ppb, and nitrosopyrrolidine levels as high as 50 ppb. Nitrosamine carcinogens have also been found in various other foods such as cheese, salami, hot dogs, nitrite-cured sable fish, salmon, and shad.

Nitrosamine formation in food can largely be avoided by banning the use of nitrite as a food additive for all purposes except when otherwise required by proven risks of botulism. Even then, minimal levels should be used, and whenever feasible nitrite should be replaced by other effective preservatives, including common salt.

On September 19, 1977, a USDA advisory committee on nitrosamines recommended that the meat industry be given up to three years to find replacements for nitrite in all circumstances where addition of nitrite leads to formation of nitrosamine in meats. However, Carol Tucker Foreman, Assistant Secretary for Food and Consumer Services, USDA, in a statement of October 18, 1977, requested the industry to develop information within six months on the prevention of formation of nitrosamines in cooked bacon, either by finding suitable replacements for nitrite, or by reducing nitrite to levels at which no nitrosamine synthesis can be detected. It must be understood that the USDA proposals are based on prevention of nitrosamine formation in the meat itself, and not in the human stomach, a more difficult and possibly a still more important problem.

As a further move to encourage the sale of nitrite-free meat products, on April 28, 1978, USDA announced plans to propose new rules that would allow use of the name "bacon" on bacon-like meat products that differ from traditional bacon in that they contain little or no nitrite or nitrate. The same new rules will apply to corned beef, frankfurters, ham, and similar products. USDA also proposed the elimination of nitrite and nitrate in baby, toddler, and junior meat foods. Foreman followed this up by another proposal on May 15, 1978, reducing levels of nitrite which may be added to bacon to 120 ppm (together with 550 ppm of ascorbate or erythorbate), effective June 15, 1978, and to 40 ppm by May, 1979. These requirements were intended to reduce to less than 10 ppb the levels of nitrosamines in cooked bacon.[11]

Foreman has been criticized by the industry for wanting to ban bacon. Her intent, of course, is to ban nitrosamine formation in bacon. How this objective is reached is clearly up to the industry.

In August, 1978, the FDA released a report by Paul M. Newberne of MIT (Final Report on Contract FDA 74-2181, "Dietary Nitrite in the Rat," May 18, 1978), which claimed that feeding nitrite to groups of rats, at levels ranging from 250 to 2,000 ppm, induced a low incidence of lymphomas.‡ For reasons which Newberne did not explain, he maintained that these carcinogenic effects were due to the nitrite itself, rather than to the possibility of nitrosamines being synthesized from nitrite in the diet or in the stomach of the rats. In spite of the considerable publicity which this study received, its significance is questionable. Informal review by NCI scientists in December, 1978, challenged the accuracy of the histological diagnoses, and concluded that there was no statistically significant increase in the incidence of tumors in the test animals over controls which had an unusually high incidence of spontaneous tumors. Following the May, 1978, reduction in bacon nitrite levels to 120 ppm, the USDA initiated a series of tests in about ninety plants to check on nitrosamine levels in the product (the tests were based on the use of the thermal energy analyzer, positive results being checked by mass spectroscopy). While the USDA has indicated that the results of the tests were generally consistent, in that the substantial majority of the plants were in compliance (with nitrosamine levels under 10 ppb), on January 8, 1979, the agency nevertheless refused a request under the Freedom of Information Act from consumer groups and the news media for their specific findings. The agency based its decision on the grounds that the act allows investigatory records to remain private (and requested confirmation of this by the Department of Justice), and on the grounds that disclosure "could be misleading and result in erroneous conclusions."

Pesticides

Many common pesticides can be nitrosated to form nitrosamines. This happens either if the pesticide is formulated as a basic salt, dimethylamine or ethanolamine, or if the pesticide itself contains amine groups. In either

---

‡ In the wake of the ensuing publicity, HEW and USDA developed plans for a gradual phasing out of the nitrate additives. At Secretary Califano's request, the plan was submitted to the Justice Department for approval, which ruled it illegal in March 1979. As an alternative to a politically vulnerable immediate ban, HEW and USDA drafted legislation for Congress that would delay regulatory action until at least May, 1980, and would schedule a timetable for complete phasing out of nitrates by May, 1982, as acceptable alternatives are developed. The basis for these proposals, however, rests on concerns over nitrosamines, rather than on the validity of the questionable Newberne study.

circumstance, the common practice of coating metal containers with nitrite to inhibit rusting further contributes to nitrosation.

Very high concentrations of nitrosamines have been recently found in randomly selected commercial samples of pesticide formulations commonly used around the home and garden, as well as for agricultural purposes. These include Trysben (or Benzac), manufactured by Du Pont as an herbicide designed for use on highways and rights-of-way but also generally available to home owners, and Treflan, the commercial formulation of Trifluralin, manufactured by Eli Lilly, one of the nation's most commonly used herbicides with an annual market of $230 million, mainly used on cotton, vegetables and soybeans. Trysben was found to be contaminated by DMN in concentrations up to 640 ppm, and Treflan was found to be contaminated by dipropylnitrosamine up to 154 ppm.

At hearings on September 20, 1976, before Congressmen John Moss (D-Calif.) and Andrew Maguire (D-N.J.), the industry admitted to these high nitrosamine levels in their products.[12] Du Pont had already recognized the problem and discontinued the practice of adding nitrite to Trysben containers. Lilly agreed to modify their manufacturing process, thereby reducing nitrosamine levels in Treflan approximately tenfold.

The industry, however, attempted to minimize the public health significance of the contamination of their products.[13] Du Pont insisted that Trysben was not used on food crops nor by homeowners, but only by "professional applicators." In fact, Trysben can be purchased in most hardware stores. Lilly asserted that the "trace levels" of nitrosamines in Treflan posed "no hazard to human health" because they are unstable and rapidly "dissipated and degraded in air" and because "the average farm applicator comes in contact with far less nitrosamines [from Treflan] than from other sources" such as eating bacon and smoking cigarettes. Du Pont gave similar assurances, quoting the views of the Haskell Laboratory of Industrial Toxicology that "there was no imminent hazard." This prompted Congressman Maguire to ask, "Who pays their salary?" The reply was, "Du Pont Corporation."[14]

Farm workers were also not impressed by these assurances. In the spring of 1977, the Migrant Legal Action Program filed suit demanding the banning of Treflan and Trysben on the grounds of imminent hazard to field workers using agricultural sprayers and field cultivators. The suit included statements from several workers, presumably considered by the industry as "professional applicators," complaining that they had been heavily exposed to herbicide spray during application and that they were not warned of possible hazards nor given protective equipment.

In addition to the few pesticides tested and found to contain high concentrations of nitrosamines, EPA admitted at the hearings that similar contamination was probable in as many as 1,000 pesticide products on the market.[15] Exposure to these levels of nitrosamines, by routes including inhalation, ingestion, and skin contact, poses major carcinogenic hazards to occupational groups involved in their manufacture, formulation, and application. Hazards are also posed to the general public using such pesticides around the home and garden. These exposures are avoidable. First, industry should discontinue the practice of formulating pesticides as basic salts, and instead formulate them as acid salts. Second, industry should take precautions to avoid nitrosation of amine-containing pesticides, during both manufacture and application. Third, the use of nitrite rust inhibitors should be abandoned whenever there is any possibility of nitrosation. Fourth, pesticides labeled for use by "professional applicators" should not be made available to unskilled operators or to the general public. Finally, greater control should be developed to prevent hazardous occupational exposure at manufacturing, formulating, and application stages.

Drugs[16]

Many common over-the-counter and prescription drugs contain amine groups which can be nitrosated, particularly under acidic conditions in the stomach, to produce high levels of nitrosamines. Many of these drugs are prescribed or taken voluntarily at high doses for prolonged periods: aminopyrine, an analgesic, chlorpromazine, a tranquillizer extensively used to treat psychoses, and methadone, the heroin "substitute" distributed free to addicts in many cities, all of which yield DMN upon nitrosation; Disulfiram, or Antabuse, used to treat alcoholism, which yields diethylnitrosamine; and phenmetrazine, an amphetamine-type drug prescribed to control obesity, and Tolazamide, an oral hypoglycaemic agent used in the treatment of diabetics, both of which yield nitroso derivatives.

Various recommendations have been made to cope with this difficult problem. These include incorporation of high doses of vitamin C in drug formulations, and the use of encapsulated time-release formulations, from which the active amine-containing ingredient will be released in the small intestine rather than in the stomach. At best, these can only reduce nitrosamine yields, but not prevent nitrosation. The ideal solution would be the development of new classes of drugs containing no amines for use in all except life-threatening or terminal diseases. The ingenuity of the pharmaceutical industry can surely meet this challenge.

Cosmetics

Lotions and shampoos are major classes of cosmetics whose function is in part to moisten and soften skin. Many cosmetics contain ethanolamines as wetting agents, which emulsify the oily ingredients and increase their retention and absorption on the skin. Nitrosation of these amines to form the carcinogenic nitrosodiethanolamine has been recently demonstrated. Nitrosamine levels up to 48 ppm have also been identified in common commercially available cosmetics, including baby lotions (Table 7.5).

Table 7.5 Nitrosodiethanolamine Levels Reported in Common Cosmetics

Product	Concentration, ppb
Max Factor, Ultralucent Whipped Creme Makeup	48,000
Revlon, Moon Drops	3,700
Helena Rubinstein, Silk Fashion	1,200
Clairol, Herbal Essence Shampoo	260
Scholl, Rough Skin Remover	140
Johnson's Baby Lotion	100
Avon, Topaz	100

Source: "N-Nitrosamines Found in Toiletry Products," *Chemical and Engineering News*, March 28, 1977, p. 7.

Excess risks of cancer, particularly of the lung and bladder, and leukaemia have been suggested by recent epidemiological studies on beauticians, who would be expected to be heavily exposed to a great variety of cosmetics. Whether these are related to exposure to nitrosamines or to other carcinogens in cosmetics, such as oxidative hair dyes or VC (used until recently as an aerosol propellant) has not been determined. In any case, it is clear that cosmetics should be formulated without ethanolamines, possibly using non-nitrogen-containing glycerol derivatives instead, and certainly without known carcinogens.*

* In April, 1979, the FDA asked for "voluntary industry action" to reduce nitrosamine levels in cosmetics by product reformulation, failing which the possibility of future regulation was implied.

Tobacco Smoke[17]

Tobacco smoke contains high concentrations of NO_x, at levels from 240 to 1,600 ppm, which are acutely irritating to the lung and which are almost completely absorbed during inhalation. Additionally, NO_x can nitrosate the wide range of amines present in smoke to form nitrosamines. The smoke from a typical American cigarette contains various nitrosamine carcinogens, particularly DMN and N-nitrosonornicotine; the mainstream smoke from twenty U.S. blended cigarettes contains about 2 μg of the former and 3 μg of the latter. French cigarettes are likely to contain still higher nitrosamine levels because of their greater nitrate content.

A recent study has shown that the concentration of DMN in the sidestream smoke emitted from the glowing tip of a cigarette is much greater than the mainstream smoke directly inhaled by smokers.[18] A nonsmoker at a crowded, smoke-filled bar inhales in one hour approximately the same amount of DMN as that inhaled by the smoker of about sixteen non-filter or twenty-five filter cigarettes.† These facts lend urgent emphasis to the assertion of the rights of nonsmokers to breathe air unpolluted by tobacco smoke, which could be accomplished by the segregation of smokers in restaurants, bars, and other public places.

The Workplace

Countless organic chemists, technicians, and students, in industry and universities, have been involved in the synthesis and use of nitrosamines. Such exposure is a suspected cause of the excess cancer rates, especially pancreatic and lymphatic, found by the NCI in a 1969 survey on organic chemists.

Several nitrosamines have been used extensively as accelerators and antioxidants in the manufacture of various types of rubber. Approximately a million and a half pounds of nitrosodiphenylamine, involving exposure of up to 1,000 workers, are now synthesized each year in the United States. This is used as a retardant in the rubber curing process, involving exposures of an additional 5,000 workers. Preliminary studies on the rubber industry have recently revealed marked excesses of cancer of the stomach, prostate, and lymphatic system. What role nitrosamines play in these excess cancers has not yet been determined.‡ This may well prove difficult, since workers in this industry are also exposed to benzene, a known ieukemogen, as well as other carcinogens such as benzo[a]pyrene.

Levels of up to 10,000 ppm (1 percent) nitrosodiethanolamine have been recently reported in commercial cutting oils, used by machine operators in innumerable industries for purposes including cooling, grinding, and lubricating.[19] According to NIOSH estimates, approximately 750,000 workers are exposed to cutting oils. Exposure to nitrosamines from these oils occurs via skin contact and inhalation of mists and vapors. The nitrosamines are formed from nitrite and triethanolamine, which are normal constituents of cutting fluids. NIOSH has recommended the omission of these nitrosamine precursors from cutting fluids and introduction of engineering controls and protective equipment.

The finding in August 1975 of relatively high DMN levels in the air of Belle, West Virginia, in proximity to the Du Pont chemical complex stimulated concerns as to possible hazards from occupational exposure to nitrosamines.[20] In December, 1975, Thermo Electron, working under an EPA contract, sampled the workplace air and found DMN levels

---

† One commercial 85-mm. non-filter cigarette, for example, produced 680 ng of DMN in its sidestream smoke.

‡ Recent findings on nitrosamines as occupational carcinogens include high levels of nitrosomorpholine in the rubber curing areas of tire factories, where a high incidence of lung cancer has been observed, and high levels of DMN in leather tanneries, which have not as yet been investigated epidemiologically (D. Fine et al., in press, 1979).

comparable to those found outside the plant. Du Pont subsequently challenged these findings. Thermo Electron repeated the tests in February, 1976, but this time found no nitrosamines in the plant except in one unrepresentative location. The mystery was apparently solved when Du Pont explained that the earlier findings of nitrosamines resulted from a side reaction in a small-lots manufacturing operation which management had subsequently recognized and controlled.

These events led to congressional hearings in New Jersey on May 28, 1976, which were filmed by CBS. Du Pont representatives were invited to testify, but declined to do so on grounds of "short notice." Du Pont management quietly attended the hearings as spectators, however, and were obliged to testify when they were found passing notes to the press offering to "field questions . . . at the noon recess."[21]

An additional issue raised at the hearings was the occurrence of an excess risk of cancer in the Du Pont plant in Belle, particularly cancer of the eye and the kidney, and to a lesser extent the lung.[22] Cancer of the eye is exceptionally rare. The occurrence of five cases in a relatively small group of fifty workers, some of whom had cancers of other sites, is of sentinel importance. Based on Connecticut tumor registry data, this is about forty-four times higher than the incidence of cancer that would be expected in a matched control population. Whether the eye cancers are due to a nitrosamine-like carcinogen such as ethylnitrosourea, which induces similar cancers in experimental animals, has not yet been determined.

Du Pont has denied the existence of an excess cancer risk in its workers, but refused to make available to NIOSH the necessary records to substantiate its claims, alleging a need to protect the privacy of its workers. In December, 1977, the courts upheld the rights of NIOSH to these records.

In addition to problems of excess cancer risk in Du Pont employees, it should be noted that Kanawha County, where the Belle Du Pont plant is located, is among the highest in the United States in incidence of lung cancer and leukaemia. The same county also has a high rate of central nervous system birth defects.

The Nitrosamine Balance Sheet

It is difficult to compare the relative amounts of all major possible sources of exposure to nitrosamines. Table 7.6 attempts to give some idea of the relative orders of potential exposures involved.

There are many problems involved in such comparisons, including the fact that some exposures occur by eating, others by inhalation, and by skin contact. Perhaps a more important limitation still is the fact that, with one exception, all the exposures listed are based on levels of nitrosamines found in the product itself, rather than on the higher levels that can be expected to be synthesized in the body. In the case of the bacon and spinach meal, the exposure level is based on expected yields of DMN formed by interaction of precursors in the stomach. As can be seen, DMN levels in the stomach are higher than in cooked bacon itself.

A recent preliminary report (based on six volunteers), highly publicized by the meat industry, demonstrated substantial synthesis of nitrite and nitrate in the intestine (presumably by nitrification of ammonia or organic nitrogen compounds).[23] Based on this report, the industry claimed that levels of dietary nitrite are insignificant compared to the available body pool. These claims ignore the fact that dietary nitrites, particularly in cured meats, react with amines to form nitrosamines in the food, and that such levels will be further increased in the stomach. They also ignore the fact that there is no evidence that fecal nitrite is available for interaction with

Table 7.6 Possible Daily Human Exposure to Nitrosamine Carcinogens

Exposure	Nitrosamines*, µg					
	DMN	NDEA	NPYR	NNN	NMOR	Other
Cooked bacon, 100 g	1	...†	5	...	...	...
Tobacco smoke, 20 cigarettes	2	...	...	3	...	...
Bacon and spinach meal, with synthesis of nitrosamines in the stomach	7	...	...	...	...	...
Drinking water, New Orleans	...	...	...	...	...	8
Air, Baltimore residential community, 1975	10	...	...	...	...	...
Cosmetics, Max Factor, 10 g	...	480	...	...	...	...
Herbicide spill, Trysben, 1 ml	640	...	...	...	...	...
Leather Tannery	630	...	...	...	...	...
Tire Factory	...	...	...	...	92	...

Source: Based on D. H. Fine et al., "Human Exposure to N-nitroso Compounds in the Environment," pp. 293-307, in *Origins* of *Human Cancer*, Book A., eds. H. H. Hiatt, J. D. Watson, and J. A. Winsten, Cold Spring Harbor Laboratory, 1977; J. M. Fajen et al., Paper 78, Air Pollution Control Association Annual Meeting, Houston, Texas, June 26, 1978.
* DMN=dimethylnitrosamine; NDEA=nitrosodiethanolamine; NPYR=nitrosopyrrolidine; NNN=nitrosonornicotine; NMOR=nitrosomorpholine.
† No data.

intestinal amines to form nitrosamines.

The ubiquity of nitrosamines makes it imperative that environmental levels be reduced to the smallest limit possible. Methods for achieving this goal depend almost exclusively on rigorously restricting the further introduction of nitrosamine precursors into the environment, especially under conditions of potential interaction.

Summary

Nitrosamines are a large group of chemicals, most of which are carcinogenic, producing tumors in a wide range of organs of a wide range of test animals. Although there is no direct epidemiological evidence, nitrosamines are considered to be major human carcinogens in both non-industrialized and industrialized countries, particularly because of their ubiquity in the environment. This is due to the fact that they can be easily and rapidly synthesized by the interaction of common precursors, nitrites or oxides of nitrogen and amines, in a process called nitrosation.

Regulatory control of nitrosamine formation can be achieved by avoidance of the use of amine-containing products, such as pesticides, drugs, detergents, cutting oils, and cosmetics, and avoidance of adding nitrite to amine-containing materials, including foods such as bacon, particularly under conditions in which nitrosation can occur.

> *Cancer in its many forms is undoubtedly a natural disease. It is probably one of nature's many ways of eliminating sexually effete individuals who would otherwise, in nature's view, compete for available food resources without advantage to the species as a whole.*

F. J. C. Roe
Consultant to the American Industrial Health Council
February, 1978

Chapter Eight

How To Improve Industry Data

The overwhelming bulk of benefit and risk data, on the basis of which most regulatory decisions are based, comes from the industries being regulated. These data are either generated and interpreted by in-house scientists or by commercial laboratories and universities under contract. In-house scientific staff are not immune to pressures from research and development and marketing departments anxious to hurry their product or process into commerce. Industrial contracts with commercial laboratories and universities are usually awarded secretly, without bids having first been solicited on the open market, a practice hardly consistent with the ethos of competitive capitalism. The contractee, anxious about the award of future contracts, is also not immune to unspoken pressures to produce information or interpretations consistent with the perceived interests of the contracting industry. Consultants, generally from prestigious universities or research institutes, provide data with an additional mantle of authority. The industrial interests of these consultants, often unknown to the public and to their own institutions, are either not disclosed to the agencies they advise, or, if disclosed, are usually kept confidential. A similar tendency operates in testimony before law courts and congressional committees.

Faults with Industry Data

Constraints on data, from gross inadequacy, biased interpretation, manipulation, suppression and outright destruction, are commonplace, especially when profitable products or processes are involved.[1] Evidence of such constraints now justifies *a priori* reservations about the validity of data developed by institutions or individuals whose economic interests are affected, especially when the data base has been maintained as confidential at industry's insistence.

Decision-making at all levels of government presupposes the availability of a body of information, on the basis of which the merits of alternate policies can be analyzed. If this data base is constrained or invalid, resulting decisions will also be constrained or invalid. This threatens the very fabric of democratic government.

Constraints in the information base will be illustrated in three general areas relating to its generation, interpretation, and suppression or destruction, with particular reference to problems of occupational and environmental cancer.

Constraints in the Generation of Data

The most common problem with industrially generated data is its poor quality. Complementing this are faults of design and performance consciously or unconsciously built into toxicological and epidemiological studies. These tend to produce results influenced or predetermined by short-term marketing considerations.[2]

Deeply concerned by the inadequacy of data submitted in 1967 to the FDA by industry in support of food additive petitions, Commissioner Herbert Ley complained:

Almost half of the food additive petitions originally submitted to the Food and Drug Administration have been incomplete or have not adequately supported the regulation requested and, therefore have required subsequent supplementation, amendment, withdrawal or denial.[3]

There is substantive evidence that the situation has not improved over the last decade.

Problems related to improper initial design of animal cancer tests include:

1. Using too few animals
2. Exposures in excess of the maximally tolerated dose, resulting in premature animal deaths before onset of cancer
3. Doses too low for the size of the animal test group, resulting in failure to obtain a statistically significant incidence of tumors
4. Deliberate premature sacrifice of animals for other "studies" during the course of the main test, thus depleting the number of animals remaining alive and at risk for cancer
5. Premature termination of the test before sufficient time has elapsed for the animals to develop tumors.

A second set of performance problems relates to husbandry. These include:

1. Poor housing, diet, and care, resulting in infections, sickness, and premature death
2. Failure to insure that each test and control group receive appropriate prescribed treatments as originally intended
3. Failure to inspect cages regularly so that dead animals become decomposed, resulting in the possibility that tumors may be missed at autopsy
4. Inadequate autopsies
5. Failure to examine appropriate tissues and organs for histological (tissue) study
6. Poor record keeping
7. Alteration, falsification, and even destruction of records.

The following examples illustrate common patterns of experimental deficiencies and misconduct. A 1969 review of seventeen industry-sponsored studies on the carcinogenicity of DDT by consultants to the Carcinogenicity Panel of the Mrak Commission on Pesticides concluded that fourteen of these studies were so inherently defective as to preclude any determination of carcinogenicity.[4]

Having spent $500,000 on the carcinogenicity and toxicological testing of the cosmetic food additive Red #40 by Hazleton Laboratories, which concluded that it was safe, Allied confidently submitted these data to the FDA in 1970 and embarked on an ambitious advertising and marketing program. Not only had Hazleton failed to perform the customary mouse carcinogenicity test, but their rat test was of little value, as most animals died early in the test from intercurrent infection, not leaving enough alive to have revealed any but a massive carcinogenic effect.[5]

Carcinogenicity tests in rats of aldrin/dieldrin sponsored by Shell and of chlordane/heptachlor sponsored by Velsicol produced results that were claimed negative by the sponsors. In fact, these results were hardly interpretable because such high and toxic doses of both pesticides were fed the animals that many died early in the experiments, before they could have developed cancer.[6]

Other data submitted by Shell and Velsicol were used to claim that their pesticides were not carcinogenic in mice, and that the liver lesions induced in them were not really cancers, but just non-malignant nodules. Review by independent experts, however, proved just the contrary.[7] Faced with such major discrepancies and under pressure from Senator Kennedy's Subcommittee on Administrative Practice and Procedures, EPA finally reviewed other industry data on pesticides. Twenty-four currently used pesticides were selected on the basis of their highest permissible residues (tolerances) on common foods. Their extensive toxicological files, which had been previously submitted to EPA by a variety of manufacturers, were then independently reevaluated. In an EPA report of April 9, 1976, it was concluded that with one possible exception these data were so inadequate that it was not possible to conclude whether any of the pesticides were safe or whether there would be any hazard in eating common foods with now legal residues.[8]

These and other grave deficiencies in the EPA data base on pesticides were discussed in a recent Congressional Staff Report:

> EPA almost exclusively rules upon data submitted by the pesticide companies. This data is the informational linchpin in the Agency's regulatory program. Yet in spite of repeated warnings, beginning at least 5 years ago, EPA has failed to take corrective action designed to discover and supplement further data.[9]

More serious than inadequacies of data are the numerous examples of fraud, such as those described in the *Congressional Record* of July 30, 1969.[10] Manipulation of data has been established with such drugs as MER/29, for which officials of Richardson-Merrill Company were criminally convicted; Dornwall, for which Wallace and Tiernan Company were found guilty of submitting false data; and Flexin, about which McNeil Laboratories omitted toxicity data on drug-related liver damage, including eleven deaths, in their submissions to the FDA.

On January 20, 1976, then FDA Commissioner Schmidt testified before Senator Edward Kennedy (D-Mass.) that Hazleton Laboratories (Vienna, Va.), under contract to G. D. Searle Company, reported on nonexistent histological findings in carcinogenicity tests on the drug Aldactone.[11] Hazleton was also charged with falsifying data on the artificial sweetener Aspartame.*

Schmidt further testified on April 8 that investigation of Hazleton tests revealed a wide range of problems including ". . . large numbers of autolyzed tissues; failure to assay test substances; failure to assay treatment-diet mixture; failure to adequately review records and verify their accuracy; the use of a statistical method that included autolyzed tissues, on which no observation had been made in the denominator for determining the number of lesions found; lesions reported at necropsy for which slides had not been made; tumors reported microscopically for which slides have never been made."†

A striking example of inept design is the fiasco of nitrilotriacetic acid (NTA).[12] In 1970, Monsanto and Procter and Gamble

---

* Following approval of Aspartame in July, 1974, FDA issued a stay after questions were raised on the reliability of the data. In May, 1979, FDA rejected a request by Searle to remove the stay on marketing approval pending an adjudicatory hearing.

† Following similar statements by the author in a recent article, "Polluted Data" *(The Sciences,* July/August, 1978, pp. 16-21), despite the written Congressional record, Roy M. Dagnall, Vice President and Director of Research Hazleton Laboratories, wrote to the editors of *The Sciences* protesting that "this is not true and at no time have any such charges been made by anyone except Epstein in the article in question," *The Sciences,* May/June, 1979, pp. 2-28.

were poised to launch a new type of detergent onto the market, based on NTA instead of phosphates. This would have resulted in the annual discharge of approximately five billion pounds of the new detergent into the surface waters and ultimately into the drinking waters of the United States. The industries concerned had spent about ten years investigating the toxicological and ecological effects of NTA, concluding that it was non-carcinogenic and that it degraded in water into harmless constituents. In fact, the industries had not done a single test to determine the mechanism of degradation of NTA in water, nor of the possible interaction of such degradation products in water with other water pollutants. The industry had also failed to appreciate that degradation was incomplete over a wide range of operating conditions with the resulting likelihood that drinking water could become contaminated with the detergent. These and other considerations led to the "voluntary" withdrawal of NTA from the market with a loss of some $300 million to the industries concerned.‡ The detergent was subsequently shown in studies sponsored by the National Cancer Institute and the National Institute of Environmental Health Sciences to produce cancer of the kidney and ureter in mice and rats.

There are similar examples throughout the field of safety testing, whether of drugs, pesticides, food additives, industrial chemicals — even motor cars. For instance, in 1972 Ford Motor Company manipulated emission control certification tests on their new fleet of cars. With approval of the Nixon administration and Department of Justice, the industry managed to ward off a subsequent criminal prosecution and jail sentence by paying a $7 million fine.[13]

Industry has manipulated economic as well as scientific data. It is now common practice for an industry "threatened" by an impending regulation or standard designed to protect against occupational cancer, environmental pollution, or some other adverse effect to protest first that the measure is unnecessary and then that it is so expensive it will put them out of business. In this they are supported by economic consultants whose analyses apparently confirm the industry contention. For example, the economic impact analyses of the anticipated costs of meeting the proposed "no detectable level" vinyl chloride standard in the workplace, undertaken by Foster D. Snell and Arthur D. Little in the summer of 1974, estimated costs of up to $90 billion and job losses of 2.2 million, supporting the industry claim that the standard would be too expensive and impractical.[14] These estimates have turned out to be grossly exaggerated, quite apart from neglecting savings to industry from recovery of VC that would otherwise be lost to the outside air, and also major costs to society from VC-induced cancer and other diseases in the workplace and surrounding communities.

Spearheaded by the Manufacturing Chemists Association and Dow Chemical Company, an essential strategy in the industry attempt to block toxic substances legislation, which had been languishing in Congress for six years prior to its passage on October 11, 1976, was the claim that it would cost too much. In 1975, industry asserted that these costs would be in the range of $2 billion a year. In contrast, EPA and the General Accounting Office estimates ranged from $80

---

‡ The major precipitating event to the withdrawal of NTA from the market was the report that the author prepared as a consultant to the Senate Committee on Public Works which raised substantial questions on safety of the new detergent, besides challenging the claim that its use would prevent eutrophication in lakes, which was the main basis for its proposed large-scale use as an alternative to phosphate detergents.

to $200 million.

Constraints in Interpretation of Data

Explaining away awkward data is part of the now familiar scenario of constraints. Over the years, the industry position on carcinogenicity data has crystallized into a set of five defensive propositions.

These have been aired on two major occasions:[15] at the 1973 meetings of the Department of Labor Advisory Committee on Occupational Carcinogens, by industries including Dow, Du Pont, Rohm and Haas, and Esso Research, in addition to the Manufacturing Chemists Association and the Synthetic Organic Chemical Manufacturers Association; and at the cancellation/suspension hearings on aldrin/dieldrin, by Shell Chemical Company, and on chlordane/heptachlor, by Velsicol Chemical Company. These five propositions are:

1. *"Tumorigens are less dangerous than carcinogens."* This argument was used at the pesticide hearings to explain away the allegedly "benign liver tumors" induced by DDT, aldrin/dieldrin, and chlordane/heptachlor which were hence claimed by industry to be "tumorigens," not carcinogens. Independent review established that these "tumors" are in fact cancers, which in some cases metastasized to the lungs; it was also shown that they produced cancers in a wide range of sites other than the liver and hence are clearly carcinogens. There is no conceivable basis for drawing any scientific and regulatory distinctions between allegedly "benign tumors" and cancers induced by administration of carcinogens.

2. *"Animal carcinogens are less dangerous than human carcinogens."* In other words, the results of animal tests must be validated by deliberate and continued human exposure before instituting rigorous controls. This argument was vigorously pro-

posed for occupational carcinogens such as dichlorobenzidine and ethyleneimine, for which there are as yet no human data, and is still pressed, even though the activity of most recently recognized "human" carcinogens, such as diethylstilbestrol and vinyl chloride, was first demonstrated in animal tests.

3. *"Most chemicals are carcinogenic when tested at relatively high concentrations."* This is not consistent with available information. Mice or other animals can be fed with massive doses of most chemicals and they will not develop cancer. For instance, in an NCI contract study by Litton Bionetics from 1963 to 1969, approximately 140 industrial compounds and pesticides, selected because of strong suspicions of carcinogenicity, were tested at maximally tolerated doses in two strains of mice. Less than 10 percent of these chemicals were found to be carcinogenic.[16]

Further, of a total of some 7,000 compounds listed in the NCI's "Survey of Compounds Which Have Been Tested for Carcinogenic Activity" only about 1,000 have been reported to be carcinogenic. By current standards only half of those tests are estimated to be valid, and a total of about 700 compounds are now accepted as carcinogenic. The compounds on the NCI list were selected on the basis of known similarity to proven carcinogens.

4. *"Safe levels of exposure to carcinogens can be determined."* It is alleged that no or negligible risks result from exposure to "low levels" of occupational or environmental carcinogens. These low levels are generally determined on the basis of the sensitivity of available monitoring techniques, technical expediency, or other poorly articulated concepts. The American Conference of Governmental Industrial Hygienists has in the past assigned acceptable "threshold limit value" levels for carcinogens such as asbestos, BCME, and nickel carbonyl, but expert na-

tional and international scientific committees and regulatory agencies are agreed that there is no mechanism for setting thresholds or safe levels for any chemical carcinogen.

5. *"Human experience has demonstrated the safety of occupational exposure to 'animal carcinogens' or to 'low' levels of human carcinogens."* These claims are generally based on a lack of positive evidence of excess cancer deaths, or on the basis of undisclosed or partially accessible records covering small working populations at risk, with undefined turnover rates and short periods of follow-up. Clearly, such data do not permit development of valid inferences, and fail to recognize inherent limitations of epidemiological techniques.

Dow and Du Pont were insistent at the 1973 Department of Labor Advisory Committee meetings on occupational carcinogens that their own experience had proved the safety of three widely used "animal carcinogens," ethyleneimine, 1-naphthylamine, and methylene-2-bischloroaniline (MOCA).* After repeated challenge to produce the underlying epidemiological data, the industries finally admitted that they had destroyed the workers' records after ten years exposure as a matter of company policy, thereby making it almost impossible to detect a human carcinogenic effect.[17]

While these assertions cannot withstand elementary scientific scrutiny, they have nonetheless been vigorously and effectively asserted in various public forums and adjudicatory proceedings. They are myths, spawned by pressures on industry scientists and academic consultants to develop and interpret safety data on chemical carcinogenesis consistent with short-term marketing interests, and are calculated to minimize the significance of the effects of human exposure to occupational carcinogens.

Apart from explaining away carcinogenesis, attempts have also been made to explain away other chronic toxic effects, including birth defects (teratogenicity). An example of this is a 1971 Dow publication on the teratogenicity in rats of the herbicide 2,4-D.[18] The summary and text of the publication state that it was tested in pregnant rats and found to be non-teratogenic while tabular data indicates the production of a wide range of congenital defects of the skeleton. However, since some of the affected progeny were shown to be capable of surviving in early infancy, Dow decided that the defects were of no particular consequence and could be dismissed. To bolster this position, Dow redefined the standard term teratology as congenital defects that are fatal or preclude optimal function. If generally applied, this definition would exclude thalidomide-type defects and most congenital heart defects.

Suppression or Destruction of Data

Occasionally data that can't be designed out of existence or interpreted away are suppressed or even destroyed. Known instances of this are legion. The carcinogenicity of the organochlorine pesticide kepone, besides its toxic effects on the reproductive and central nervous systems, were discovered by studies sponsored by the manufacturer, Allied Chemical Co., in the early 1960s.[19] Allied suppressed this information for about a decade, until workers at Life Sciences in Hopewell, Virginia, an Allied spinoff corporation, developed crippling neurological and other diseases from exposure to very high levels of kepone in grossly deficient working conditions.

---

* In September, 1978, Du Pont announced its intent, based on economic and safety considerations, to phase out the manufacture of MOCA by the end of the year.

In December, 1972, Velsicol was informed by its own consultants that chlordane/heptachlor were carcinogenic.[20] However, the company suppressed this information, resulting in their criminal indictment by a Chicago federal grand jury in December, 1977.[21]

Reserve Mining Company testified in court in the early 1970s that there were no alternate sites which could be used for the daily disposal of 67,000 tons of asbestos-laden taconite tailings into Lake Superior. In fact, the company had previously developed detailed plans for land disposal sites.

The carcinogenicity of vinyl chloride in the liver of rats was discovered in late 1972, but the Manufacturing Chemists Association (and Maltoni) withheld this knowledge for more than eighteen months, until the human evidence could no longer be ignored.[22]

In the course of meetings of the Department of Labor's 1973 Advisory Committee on Occupational Carcinogens, Dow and Du Pont admitted routine destruction of workers' records, including those exposed to occupational carcinogens.[23]

Industrial Biotest Labs, Northbrook, Illinois, a subsidiary of Nalco Chemical Company, faced with federal investigation in April, 1977, for fraud and submission of questionable test data, destroyed files dealing with toxicological and carcinogenicity testing of thousands of federally approved products including drugs, pesticides, food additives, and industrial chemicals.[24] The president of the company, A. J. Frisque, has admitted that he ordered the shredding of laboratory documents immediately prior to the initiation of the investigation, but claimed that this was due to a "misunderstanding."

FDA and EPA investigators have established that Industrial Biotest submitted falsified data on potential carcinogens to the government. It has also been established that at least four unidentified major pesticide manufacturers were aware of this fraud when they submitted the test data in product registration applications.[25]

Industrial Biotest has also been charged by Rep. Thomas Downey (D-N.Y.) with having mismanaged toxicological tests by "shoddy amateurish" laboratory practices on irradiated food in a U.S. Army project dating back to 1953, which has so far cost the taxpayer about $51 million.[26] More recently, Industrial Biotest and Nalco have been sued by former industrial clients, including Syntex Pharmaceutical and Wesley-Jesson, Inc., for alleged breach of contract and misrepresentation of test data.† On September 23, 1978, the Swedish EPA banned eight pesticides, including captan and metabromuron, that had been registered on the basis of tests conducted at Industrial Biotest. According to Miljöcentrum, the major Swedish public interest movement headed by Björn Gillberg, the Swedish EPA had been aware for many years of problems of misconduct at certain American laboratories, but failed to take action until finally forced to do so by the Ombudsman in response to a complaint of a coalition of environmental groups. The EPA and other concerned U.S. regulatory agencies have not yet revealed the identities of the pesticides and other products registered on the basis of tests at Industrial Biotest Laboratories, nor has there yet been any indication as to whether or when such registrations will be revoked or cancelled.‡

As recently divulged in the asbestos "Pentagon Papers," the asbestos industry, under the leadership of Johns-Manville, has for decades successfully suppressed and manipu-

---

† Nalco has been attempting to sell the Industrial Biotest facilities in Northbrook and Wedges Creek, Illinois, since June, 1978. The third IBT facility in Decatur has been purchased by Whittaker Corporation and renamed Toxigenics.

‡ In July, 1978, IBT established a Validation Assistance Team (VAT) in cooperation with EPA, FDA, and its industry sponsors in attempts to salvage possibly-useful data from remaining records of past studies.

lated information on the carcinogenicity and other hazards of asbestos. Involved in this conspiracy network were senior industry executives, their medical staff, attorneys, insurance companies, trade associations, scientific consultants, and commercial laboratories. Apart from detailing the mechanics of data suppression, these documents are the most revealing insight of corporate mores yet.

Extremely grave questions are being raised about the moral standards or ethical behavior of the business world today.

W. Michael Blumenthal
ex-President Bendix Corp.,
Treasury Secretary
May 25, 1975

How to Improve Industry Data

What Not to Do

The reaction of industry to recently escalating evidence on the constraints of their data base has been one of angry denial followed by grudging acceptance of the possibility of an occasional unfortunate "slip-up." The present response, from which we can probably expect only "more of the same," is to increase their own toxicological and carcinogenicity testing capabilities. One of the earliest manifestations of this approach was the creation in 1974 of the Chemical Industry Institute of Toxicology, supported by the leading chemical industries. The Institute has recently moved to a new $10 million facility in Raleigh, North Carolina. The institute is headed by Leon Goldberg, a long-time industrial consultant dedicated to such standard myths as the "benign" nature of liver tumors induced by carcinogenic pesticides.

Goldberg, asserting that the institute is oriented toward the "public good," is highly critical of EPA for their "crisis approach" to toxic chemicals and of the NCI because their carcinogenicity testing procedures are "likely to produce false positives."[27] The institute's current research activities are being done by outside consulting laboratories, prominent among whom has been Industrial Biotest Laboratories.

Industry is responding to the recent passage of toxic substances legislation with a massive expansion of its facilities.[28] Du Pont recently enlarged its toxicological capabilities in Newark, Delaware, by about 70 percent. Dow increased its Midland, Michigan, facility by 50 percent, and Monsanto, which until now has contracted out its testing to independent laboratories, is building a new facility in St. Louis. Shell recently announced the creation of a new toxicology laboratory in Westhollow, Houston, to be headed by Donald Stevenson, the leading figure of the Shell toxicology team who attempted to discount the liver cancers induced by mice by aldrin/dieldrin at the 1974 EPA hearings.

There is no apparent basis for assuming that any of these new ventures will be less constrained by their direct linkage to industry than any of their predecessors, or any less a threat to long-term industrial interests.

What to Do

Approaches now being considered and developed by FDA, EPA, NCI, and other agencies include formalization of protocols or guidelines, formalized inspection, selective auditing and monitoring, licensing of testing laboratories, and unannounced sample testing, with increased penalties for manipulation or suppression of data.* Congress has recognized this problem by allo-

---

* A recent move in the direction of providing guidelines for epidemiologic studies has been made by the Guidelines Committee, Epidemiology Work Group, of the Interagency Regulatory

cating an extra $16.6 million to the FDA in 1977 to insure quality control of the data submitted to the agency in support of the products it regulates. But contracts still seem to be awarded to laboratories found guilty of such practices, and products registered on the basis of their prior tests have not been banned or otherwise restricted. These approaches, however helpful, do not address the inherent conflict of interest, which remains unchanged. Another useful approach developed by Senator Gaylord Nelson (D-Wisc.) with particular reference to drug testing is based on the concept of "third party testing" by federal laboratories at cost to the industry concerned.

Radical approaches are clearly required to free testing from the crippling constraints of corporate influences. One possible approach is based on the introduction of the following type of neutral "buffer" between those who test and those whose product is being tested:

> There is a growing consensus of opinion on the need for legislation to ensure impartial and competent testing of all synthetic chemicals for which human exposure is anticipated. The present system of direct, closed-contract negotiations between manufacturing industries and commercial and other testing laboratories is open to abuse, creates obvious mutual constraints, and is thus contrary to consumer, and long-term industrial interests. One possible remedy would be the introduction of a disinterested advisory group or agency to act as an intermediary between manufacturers and commercial and

> other testing laboratories. Various legal and other safeguards would have to be properly developed to avoid or minimize potential abuses and conflicts of interest in the operation of this intermediary group. Manufacturers would notify the advisory group or agency when safety evaluation was required for a particular chemical. The advisory group would then solicit contract bids on the open market. Bids would be awarded on the basis of economics, quality of protocols, and technical competence. The progress of testing would be monitored by periodic project site visits, as routine with Federal contracts. At the conclusion of the studies, the advisory group would comment on the quality of the data, make appropriate recommendations, and forward these to the regulatory agency concerned for appropriate action. . . . Additionally, quality checks during testing would ensure the high quality and reliability of data, and minimize the need to repeat studies, and thus also reduce pressure on involved federal agencies to accept unsatisfactory data and post hoc situations. This approach would not only minimize constraints due to special client interests, but would also serve to upgrade the quality of testing in commercial and other testing laboratories.[29]

Industry could be protected from the possibility of incompetent work by requiring a contractee to post an indemnifying bond, should tests have to be repeated because they were bungled or for any other reason. Some form of limited liability provisions could

---

Liaison Group. The committee issued a draft "Documentation Guidelines for Epidemiologic Studies: Cohort Studies," on May 31, 1978. These guidelines, while flexible, recommend minimum criteria for satisfactory epidemiologic studies to be used in investigating environmen-

tal and occupational health hazards. These include availability of full supporting documentation and definition of follow-up procedures and methods of statistical analysis, discussion of potential bias, and disclosure of sponsorship and source of funding.

also be built into a buffer system. This could insure that industry complying with these requirements would be protected from possible open-ended future testing needs, and also from legal responsibility for future adverse effects not predicted by properly conducted tests.

These proposals seem more consistent with the avowed industrial practice than is the present practice of secret award of unbidded contracts to commercial testing laboratories.† It would also free top-level corporate management from the influence of those in the lower corporate structure who are over-responsive to short-term marketing interests at the expense of long-term stability and growth.

Finally, there must be greater appreciation of the enormity and public health consequences of the manipulation or suppression of toxicological, epidemiological, and other data on health, safety, and exposure. Mechanisms should be developed for banning products registered on the basis of tests by commercial or other laboratories indicted of malpractice. Medical malpractice suits are now commonplace; the strong threat of laboratory malpractice suits is clearly needed to police the practice of industrial toxicology and safety assessment. Homicide or assault by toxic chemicals is a serious variant of white-collar crime. The recognition and social stigmatization, including maximum criminal penalties, of those involved in these crimes is long overdue.

Future Trends

With increasing recognition of the questionable validity of the scientific data base of industry, it is likely that their future strategies will become more sophisticated (such as performing carcinogenicity tests with low test doses on the grounds that this is "realistic," and challenging the significance of carcinogenicity results in mice and of allegedly "benign" tumors). However, there has been a recent, more fundamental shift in industry tactics. It has now become less useful to minimize (in various ways) scientific evidence of hazardous effects, than to argue for the acceptance of these effects on the basis of economic and cost/benefit considerations (such considerations generally reflect exaggerated compliance costs, while failing to adequately, if at all, recognize externalized costs of failure to regulate). Industry has found massive support for this new strategy of economic manipulation in the recent anti-inflation policies of the administration, whose Council on Wage and Price Stability depends largely on industry economic analyses as a basis for policy. Further support for the industry position has also come from the October, 1978, Fifth Circuit Appeals Court decision, overturning the new OSHA benzene standard, largely on economic grounds.

Industry is now better equipped to play the economics game rather than the science game, particularly as there is very little expertise on industry economics outside of industry. The ability of federal agencies to estimate compliance costs of abatement technologies is poorly developed. Academic economists, with traditional myopic preoccupations with the GNP, and often with close consulting ties to industry, have little comprehension of or interest in the concept of externalized costs. A new breed of economic

---

† This problem has been clearly recognized in a November, 1978, Congressional report on "Cancer-Causing Chemicals in Food" (Subcommittee on Oversight and Investigations of the House Committee on Interstate and Foreign Commerce):

EPA should develop a system for pesticide safety testing which removes testing from the manufacturers' own labs and places it in the hands of independent, impartial laboratories.

activists oriented toward disease prevention and public health has yet to emerge, although there are isolated spokesmen for these considerations.‡

‡ See the recent exchange on cost-benefit analysis between Murray L. Weidenbaum (Center for the Studies of American Business, Washington University, St. Louis), expressing traditionalist industry positions, and Nicholas A. Ashford (Center for Policy Alternatives, MIT), expressing broader societal concerns.[30]

Chapter Nine

Governmental Policies

Environmental and occupational cancer are now becoming prime topics of national concern. Their underlying political and economic determinants are at last becoming appreciated. The data base of past decision-making is now known to have been massively distorted, or constrained, and responsive to narrowly defined special interests. Accordingly, policy and decision-making are at last moving from closed discussions between the executive branch of government and industry into the open political arena.

Congress

Congress is both initially and ultimately responsible for all agency policies and priorities. Congressional control is exercised in the Senate and in the House through committees serving three basic types of functions. *Legislative committees* hold hearings on a particular bill and report out the bill, which is voted up or down on the floor. If voted up, the bill becomes law and provides overall authority to research and regulatory agencies. The *appropriations committees* decide how much money and staff each agency will receive each year. And both types also have an *oversight function:* they examine the administration of a law by the agency concerned and otherwise monitor its performance to see whether the Congressional intent is being met.

The most concrete generalization that can be made about the government policy on carcinogens is that there is no single such policy yet. Rather, policies and responsibilities are distributed over many diverse agencies and institutes, with widely differing philosophies, priorities, and practices and often with overlapping and poorly defined jurisdictions.

While these differences reflect such factors as external pressures, historical background, and personalities, the most substantive determinants are the confused and often inconsistent authorities governing regulatory controls over air, water, food, drugs, cosmetics, industrial chemicals, and the workplace. These authorities have been created piecemeal by Congress over the last few decades and now form a legislative patchwork quilt. Rather than resolving legislative ambiguities and stalemates, such as those allowing the continued use of carcinogenic cattle feed additives, Congress has often abdicated its authority and relegated it to regulatory agencies, using vague, value-laden terms such as "unreasonable risks" or "feasibility." The subsequent actions of the regulatory agencies are then open to challenge in the courts, as is failure to take any action. Congress has thus allowed decision-making to evolve into an uneasy triangular relationship, involving besides itself the executive and the courts.

Federal Agencies

Broadly speaking, there are two types of federal agency: those primarily engaged in research, and those primarily engaged in regulation and enforcement.

Legislative inconsistencies aside, federal priorities in research on cancer prevention and on the regulation of environmental and occupational carcinogens have been, and still are, low. This has been reflected in administrative failure to ensure that the various environmental programs of federal agencies function in an effective and coordinated manner, and in the personnel ceilings imposed by successive recent administrations. These ceilings, even more than budgetary limitations, have had and still have a crippling effect on the functions of both research and regulatory agencies.*

In contrast with personnel limitations, there has been major growth in federal expenditures on environmental and occupational health during the last decade. A 1972 congressional report contrasted the then $215 *million* total federal effort in environmental health with the $82.5 *billion* value of products regulated in 1970 by one agency alone, the FDA.[1] But even the $215 million figure was misleading, for it included biologic agents such as vaccines. When these are eliminated, the total shrinks to a $96 million effort for chemical and physical pollutants, of which only about $24 million was spent for carcinogenesis research. By 1976, however, federal expenditures in environmental health and carcinogenesis research had more than doubled, totaling $485.7 million and $76.8 million, respectively (Table 9.1); nevertheless they are still small compared to the value of the products and processes regulated by federal agencies. As reflected in 1979 budgetary figures, this rate of growth has been sustained, over and above inflationary increases. It is, however, also clear that these expenditures are relatively trivial compared to the overall costs of environmentally induced disease and cancer, and to the 1978 total national health care expenditures of $185 billion. In this connection, HEW Secretary Califano, in his September, 1978, address to

the national AFL-CIO conference on occupational safety and health, stressed that of the $48 billion federal expenditures on health care, fully 96 percent is directed at treatment, and only 4 percent (under $2 billion) is earmarked for programs to prevent disease.

The National Cancer Institute

The National Cancer Institute (NCI) is the lead agency for cancer research.

Early History. Created in 1937 under the National Cancer Act, the NCI is the only federal institution with exclusive responsibility in cancer research.[2] Although incorporated into the National Institutes of Health in 1944, the NCI has always been considered by Congress and the public as a semi-autonomous agency. This sense of independence was further consolidated by the 1971 National Cancer Act, which assigned managerial responsibility to the director of the NCI, who reports to the President, through the Office of Management and Budget, bypassing the director of the National Institutes of Health and the HEW Secretary.[3]

When the first annual NCI budget of $400,000 was established in 1937, scientific interests in cancer largely focused on problems of treatment, with little concern for prevention. Congressional and public opinion then reflected this attitude. Although considerable research was being conducted in the United States and elsewhere on chemical carcinogenesis, this was largely viewed as basic science, with little relevance to prevention of

---

* Since the Johnson administration, in a series of running battles with Congress, the executive has imposed ceilings on the numbers of personnel that can be hired by federal agencies. This has not, in fact, reduced the size of government, but instead has forced agencies to contract out federal work to nonfederal employees. This has created overwhelming administrative problems for federal agencies, particularly those concerned with environmental and occupational health. In the fiscal 1979 Appropriations Bill for the Departments of Labor and HEW,

Congress specifically mandated personnel increases in specific program areas, including environmental and occupational health. The administration is challenging that action and refusing to lift the personnel ceilings. It is anticipated that the General Accounting Office (GAO) will make a final determination on this matter in the spring of 1979 which, if unfavorable to the administration, will be implemented by sending Congress a notice of impoundment, on the basis of which the Courts could force the ceilings to be lifted.

Table 9.1 Federal Expenditures in Environmental Health and Carcinogenesis Research

Agency	Total 1976 Research Budgets ($ million)	
	Environmental Health	Carcinogenesis Research*
Department of Health, Education, and Welfare (total)	301.1	70.3
National Cancer Institute	(149.5)	(47.5)
National Institute Environmental Health Sciences	(49.1)	(8.4)
National Institute Occupational Safety and Health	(48.8)	(8.4)
National Center for Toxicological Research†	(12.9)	(6.0)
Other agencies		40.8)
Environmental Protection Agency	51.4	1.0
Department of Energy‡	60.7	5.5
National Science Foundation	4.7	NA
Army	14.1	NA
Department of Labor	16.8	NA
National Aeronautics and Space Administration	1.6	NA
Department of Transportation	18.0	NA
Department of Housing and Urban Development	1.8	NA
Department of Interior	7.1	NA
Department of Defense	8.4	NA
TOTAL	485.7	76.8

Source: NIEHS, Report to the Senate Appropriation Committee on Federal Support for Environmental Health Research, 1977.

* NA (not available) means there is no line item on cancer research in the agency's budget.
† Excludes $4 million from EPA.
‡ Excludes radiation carcinogenesis.

human cancer. This background is important to understanding how NCI priorities have evolved over the subsequent four decades.

Attempts were made to challenge these priorities, particularly by the late Wilhelm C. Hueper, a German-born physician and distinguished researcher on the carcinogenic effects of radioactive agents and aromatic amine dyes at the Haskell Laboratories of Du Pont, who was appointed chief of the Environmental Cancer Section of the NCI in 1948. Hueper's outstanding research on environmental and occupational carcinogenesis was matched by his integrity, obduracy, and the energy of his advocacy. Although he was supported by Rod Heller, then NCI director, Hueper ran afoul of the federal establishment, particularly the Atomic Energy Commission and the FDA, quite apart from drawing the concentrated wrath of the chemical industry.[4] Attempts were made to silence him, to censor his reports and block his research. In 1952, Hueper was refused clearance to testify before Congressman James J. Delaney's (D-N.Y.) Select Committee Investigating the Use of Chemicals in Food and Cosmetics, a move that Hueper countered by testifying as a private citizen. In the same year, he was ordered to discontinue his epidemiologic studies on occupational and community cancer.[5]

To Hueper, harassment came early and recognition late. Hueper is now widely appreciated as the leading pioneer in the concept of cancer prevention.[6] Among other recent distinctions, Hueper was presented with the first Annual Award of the Society for Occupational and Environmental Health in March, 1975.[†] The concluding remarks of the citation read:

To Wilhelm C. Hueper, M.D., Head of the Environmental Cancer Section, National Cancer Institute, Department of Health, Education and Welfare, in recognition of his role in pioneering and fostering the study of occupational and environmental cancer and in establishing the scientific and public awareness that most human cancers are caused by environmental factors and can be prevented.[7]

Hueper, in fact, had little visible impact on NCI priorities. The annual budget of the NCI in 1948 was $14.5 million, of which Hueper's section received $90,000, a sum which had not materially increased when he retired sixteen years later, despite a tenfold increase in the NCI's total budget.[8]

By the late 1950s, research in the treatment of cancer had produced some interesting leads, particularly the finding that drugs inhibiting folic acid metabolism could produce remissions in childhood leukaemias and other forms of malignant disease. The significance of these findings was exaggerated and hailed as the dawn of a new era when cancer could be cured by the "magic bullet" of chemotherapy. In fact, the basis for such optimism was slender. The "cancer cure lobby," headed by cancer clinicians, notably Solomon Garb of the American Medical Center in Denver, and the late Sidney Farber, politically astute director of the Children's Cancer Research Foundation, Boston, and including the American Cancer Society and Mary Lasker,[‡] a New York philanthropist who had close contacts with the administrations of successive Presidents, exerted a powerful influence on Congress and the public. Both were exhorted and persuaded by hard-sell techniques that the cure for cancer was just around the corner, and only needed more support and funding

---

† The award was made by the author, then president of the society.

‡ Mary Lasker is the widow of Albert D. Lasker, the multimillionaire advertising tycoon, who handled American Tobacco's Lucky Strike ac-

count and who coined what has been called the most successful slogan in American salesmanship "Reach for a Lucky Instead of a Sweet," aimed at inducing women to smoke.

for the American Cancer Society and the NCI. In the optimistic search for "magic bullets" the NCI financed a huge Cancer Chemotherapy Program for mass-screening of hundreds of chemicals for anticancer activity in tissue culture and animal tumor systems.

The National Cancer Program. The 1971 National Cancer Act (42 U.S.C. 282), embodying the Senate Conquest of Cancer Bill and the House National Cancer Attack Bill,[9] had as its principal objective the launching of the National Cancer Program to cure cancer.[10] The Act reflected a Senate report of the National Panel of Consultants on the Conquest of Cancer, of which Farber and Garb were leading members, which sounded a clarion call to attack and eradicate cancer. In a full-page advertisement entitled MR. NIXON, YOU CAN CURE CANCER in *The New York Times* of December 9, 1969, paid for by the "Citizens Committee for the Conquest of Cancer," whose leaders included Farber, Garb, and Lasker, Farber is quoted as follows: "We are so close to a cure for cancer. We lack only the will and the kind of money and comprehensive planning that went into putting a man on the moon . . . Why don't we try to conquer cancer by America's 200th birthday."[11]

The Consultants' Report which was presented to the Senate Committee on Labor and Public Welfare on December 4, 1970, effectively misled the Congress into believing that the cure for cancer was imminent, needing only a massively funded national effort.* The report also insisted that NCI had to be removed from the "bureaucracy" of NIH and

be given autonomy in order to find the cure for cancer.[12]

The 1971 legislation itself is poorly drafted and naive. It reflects the bias of the Consultants' Report and emphasizes immediate possibilities for the cure of cancer without attaching any significance to prevention. The Act also authorizes the establishment of National Cancer Centers "for clinical research, training, and demonstration of advanced diagnostic and treatment methods relating to cancer." The centers were not assigned any responsibility for establishing carcinogenesis or epidemiological programs, nor for any other problem-solving activities relating to cancer prevention.

The National Cancer Advisory Board and Panel. The 1971 Act mandates major changes in the NCI by establishing strong links with the President and giving it virtual autonomy, while formally retaining it within the parent National Institutes of Health. This move was consistent with the general policy of the Nixon administration in obtaining direct control over Federal agencies.

The NCI Director is authorized to submit his annual budget for approval to the Office of Management and Budget, thereby bypassing the National Institutes of Health and HEW.† In addition to personally appointing the NCI Director, the President also appoints a National Cancer Advisory Panel of three which meets monthly and establishes NCI priorities and policies.‡ Executive functions for the panel is provided by a Presidentially appointed advisory board of twenty-three

---

* Only a few members of Congress were not persuaded by the cancer lobby, particularly Sen. Gaylord Nelson and Cong. Paul Rogers who tried to fight the separation of NCI from the NIH.
† While the national policy-making influence of OMB was formally pivotal, it is becoming increasingly supplanted by an enlarged White House staff and by a resurgent and restive Congress that has created its own budget office to do much of the analytic work once performed ex-

clusively by OMB.
‡ The lack of checks and balances in Presidential control of the executive and advisory functions of the NCI were periodically emphasized by Benno Schmidt's transmittal of White House policy positions (during Republican administrations) as a means of influencing Board decisions. The nature of these past policy linkages between Schmidt and the White House is yet to be revealed.

members, five from government and eighteen from the public sector, which meets quarterly. The National Cancer Advisory Board is executive, in contrast to its Advisory Council predecessor, which had only advisory functions.

The chairman of the Cancer Panel was and still is Benno Schmidt, a New York investment banker and a friend of the Nixon and Ford administrations, with ties to the oil, steel and chemical industries through J.H. Whitney and Co., of which he is managing partner. Schmidt has, with substantial success, attempted to dictate NCI policies over the last eight years. Membership of the Advisory Board has also included industry representatives, such as the late Elmer Bobst, Warner Lambert, and Clark Wescoe of the drug industry, but no representatives of labor or the public interest movement. Scientific membership of the board largely reflected expertise in basic science, cancer diagnosis, and treatment. The National Cancer Advisory Board and Cancer Panel have had close interlocking relationships with the leadership of the American Cancer Society.*[13]

Conflicts of Interest on the National Cancer Advisory Board. One long-time member of the board is Philippe Shubik, an accomplished carcinogenesis researcher. In November, 1975, as chairman of the Subcommittee on Environmental Carcinogenesis, Shubik played a major role in attacking the "cancer principles," leading to the refusal of

the EPA administrative law judge to suspend the registrations of chlordane and heptachlor.[14]

Shubik's influence on the Advisory Board has further weakened the regulation of environmental carcinogens. Apart from attacking the cancer principles, Shubik in November, 1975, argued successfully for abandonment of the system of Memoranda of Alert, by which the NCI warned the community of early findings in its bioassay program (designed for large-scale carcinogenicity tests on chemicals to which humans are likely to be exposed).†

Shubik worked closely with then NCI Director Frank Rauscher and roadblocked the bioassay program over the objections of the associate director of the Carcinogenesis Program, Umberto Saffiotti. On some occasions, Shubik attended NCI meetings representing his personal industrial interests. At a 1971 meeting to discuss the carcinogenicity of Procter and Gamble's detergent ingredient nitrilotriacetic acid, Shubik argued for the continued use of the product. When asked by Saffiotti, "Would you for the record identify what capacity you are here under?" Shubik replied, "Procter and Gamble."[16]

Shubik's membership on the board poses problems of conflict of interest with respect to his involvement in NCI policy-making while being a major recipient of NCI research funding.‡ Shubik's list of consulting clients was

---

* Some of these relationships have been fruitful, such as the NCI-ACS 1974 Conference on "Persons at High Risk of Cancer," and its subsequent publication (ed. J. F. Fraumeni, 1975).

† General Foods, to whom Shubik consults, is known to have been particularly incensed by the results of a bioassay program test on trichloroethylene, used to decaffeinate coffee, which was found to be carcinogenic and which resulted in claimed losses to the company of $20 million.[15] Methylene chloride, now widely used as a substitute for trichloroethylene with permissible levels of 10 ppm in roasted beans, is currently under

test in the NCI Bioassay Program. However, since January, 1979, Coffex Ltd. of Switzerland has been marketing coffee decaffeinated by a hot-water process, using no chemical solvents.

‡ Shubik's potential for conflict of interest is not unique on the NCI Advisory Board. In this, he has been joined by Frank J. Dixon, a consultant for Eli Lilly and Co., and Jonathan E. Rhodes, then Chairman of the Board and Director of Penwalt Corp., a chemical manufacturer, quite apart from the industry representatives on the board.[17] (Henry Pitot is current chairman of the Advisory Board.)

first disclosed in the 1976 NCI budget hearings when Congressman David Obey (D-Wisc.) asked Rauscher who his chief advisor on environmental cancer was. Rauscher replied that it was Shubik. Obey then asked Rauscher if Shubik also consulted for industry. Rauscher replied in the affirmative, while expressing ignorance as to which industries were involved. When pressed further, Rauscher agreed to supply the list of industries, but, following the hearings, asked that this be excluded from the public record. Rauscher's request was denied. It was then revealed that Shubik consulted for Royal Crown Cola, Abbott Laboratories, Miles Laboratories, General Foods, Procter and Gamble, Colgate Palmolive, the Flavor and Extract Manufacturer's Association, and the Calorie Control Council.*[18] It has since been discovered that Shubik's Eppley Cancer Research Institute operation in Omaha has numerous other industrial clients, including the cosmetic industry, and oil and chemical companies.

Shubik is also involved in a direct conflict of interest over multimillion-dollar contracts from the NCI to the Eppley Cancer Research Institute, University of Nebraska, Omaha, which he directs.† As a member of the National Cancer Advisory Board, Shubik had considerable influence over NCI staff, and normal review mechanisms were waived for his contracts which, apart from being awarded non-competitively, were instead handled by special *ad hoc* procedures (contracts, unlike grants, are monitored by staff of the agency concerned).[19] In spite of what in July, 1977, Congressman Obey said were "strongly negative comments by a number of reviewers," Shubik's contracts continued to be renewed.[20] Shubik has been the subject of a Congressional inquiry and a GAO investigation which raised serious questions about poor administrative practices and accounting of $12 million of contract expenditures dating back to 1973, including the use of federal funds to support industrial research.[21] The GAO investigation also questioned the scientific value of this multimillion-dollar contract, as evidenced by "NCI's inability to cite more than a few notable accomplishments." According to an article in the Omaha *World-Herald*,‡ based on the results of a more recent HEW investigation, the government is demanding refund of $1 million from the University of Nebraska for NCI contract funds which it is claimed that Shubik "used for unauthorized purposes." The Eppley Institute, however, claims that only $85,000 of federal funds are unaccounted for. An HEW audit released in November, 1978, repeated the demand for the $1 million refund. Simultaneously, it was announced that the Office of Investigators of the HEW Inspector General was pursuing an inquiry on a "non-audit matter," which, it was stressed, does not necessarily mean that criminal charges will be pressed. In December, 1978, it was revealed that the University of Nebraska was conducting its own investigation of Shubik, following the request of Senator Larry D. Stoney (D-Omaha) who presented the administration with a "list of concerns" by Eppley employ-

---

* Shubik is also president of the Toxicology Forum, an industry-sponsored colloquium. The secretary of the Forum is David B. Clayson, Deputy Director of the Eppley Cancer Research Inst., principal investigator of the NCI contract to the Eppley, and executive member of the NCI Clearinghouse on Environmental Cancer.

† In the last 10 years the Eppley has received about $23 million in grants and contracts from NCI. The major project officer for these contracts was Gio B. Gori, proponent of the "practical threshold" concept for cigarettes, now on leave of absence from the NCI.

‡ Prior to this article, all criticisms of Shubik and his conflicts of interest which have appeared in the national press were ignored or toned down in the Omaha *World-Herald,* the leading Nebraska daily, and in other Nebraskan press in general. This may possibly reflect recognition of the substantial federal research dollars Shubik has brought into the state.

ees, including allegations of misuse of state funds.*[22]

Shubik continues to exert considerable influence through various channels, including membership on the National Cancer Advisory Board, which in the absence of his prior resignation will extend until 1982.†

The NCI Budget and Priorities. Over the years, the NCI budget has climbed by leaps and bounds from a 1938 level of $400 *thousand* to a 1958 level of $56 *million,* and to a 1968 level of $183 million. Passage of the National Cancer Act, with its strong emphasis on cure rather than prevention, led to a 1971 budget of $223 million, which by 1979 quadrupled to almost $1 *billion* (See Table 9.2). The rapid rate of growth of the NCI budget from 1971 through 1975, however, has

now leveled off. For the last seven years the NCI budget has accounted for about 30 percent of the total NIH budget. It is, however, clear that the early rapid growth of the NCI budget was achieved largely at the expense of basic research in other NIH institutes, particularly the National Institute of General Medical Sciences, rather than by an increased overall federal commitment to biomedical research. This has not unnaturally polarized the biomedical scientific community into pro- and anti-NCI camps. This polarization has been further compounded by the growing recognition of the questionable track record of the NCI in overall administration and fiscal management.

Under the control of the Cancer Panel and Director Rauscher, the budget of the NCI was

Table 9.2 Growth of NCI Budget from 1971 to 1979 in Comparison with that of NIH

Year	Budgets ($ millions)		NCI Budget As a Percentage of NIH Budget	Percent Increase NCI Budget over Previous Year
	NCI	NIH		
1971	$223	$1,183	18.9	29
1972	379	1,467	25.8	70
1973	492	1,713	28.7	30
1974	527	1,745	30.2	7
1975	692	2,044	33.9	31
1976	762	2,201	34.6	10
1977	815	2,500	32.6	7
1978	872	2,828	30.8	7
1979	937	3,197	29.3	7

Source: National Institutes of Health, 1979.

---

* Shubik was placed on leave of absence from Eppley in July, 1979, and Norman Cromwell (Professor of Chemistry at the University of Nebraska), who had been involved in recruiting Shubik in 1968, was appointed acting director.

† On March 3, 1978, Shubik was given the 27th Annual Bertner Award by the University of Texas M.D. Anderson Hospital and Tumor Institute for

"distinguished contributions to cancer research" for scientific work done jointly with Israel Berenblum about thirty years ago. In receiving the award, Shubik acknowledged the warm support of Lee Clark, President of the M.D. Anderson Hospital and University of Texas Cancer System, and then President of the American Cancer Society and member of the NCI Cancer Panel.

skimpy on prevention. In testifying before Congress in 1976, Rauscher admitted that only 20 percent of the NCI budget went to environmental carcinogenesis, while agreeing that 85 percent of cancers are environmental in origin. But even this low figure of 20 percent was inflated. To be sure, the budget of the Division of Cancer Cause and Prevention was about 18 percent of the NCI total, but this included programs such as virology, constituting almost half the entire budget of the division, which apart from their intrinsic scientific importance have only limited, if any, relevance to environmental carcinogenesis (Table 9.3). Thus the percent of the NCI budget devoted to chemical carcinogenesis, comprised by the programs in Carcinogenesis and Field Studies and Statistics, amounted to about 12 percent of the total NCI budget of $762 million, rather than the 20 percent claimed by Rauscher.

What have been the returns for all the billions of dollars spent on cancer treatment? In the last four decades there has been little overall improvement in our ability to treat and cure most cancers. The modest improvement from the 20 percent overall five-year survival rates in the mid-1930s to about 33 percent in the mid-1950s reflects advances in surgery, blood transfusion, and antibiotic treatment, rather than specific advances of cancer treatment. Over the last two decades, there has been

Table 9.3 Analysis of the NCI 1976 Budget

Division	Amounts ($ millions)	Percentage of Total
Cancer Research, Resources and Centers	332.0	43.6
Cancer Biology and Diagnosis	57.8	7.6
Cancer Treatment	119.2	15.7
Cancer Control and Rehabilitation	56.5	7.4
Cancer Cause and Prevention	135.3	17.8
Office of Division Director	(13.0)	(1.7)
Virus Cancer Program	(62.0)	(8.2)
Task Forces Program	(5.4)	
Field Studies and Statistics		(0.7)
Program	(12.3)	(1.6)
Carcinogenesis Program*	(42.6)	(5.6)
Office of NCI Director	37.7	4.9
NIH Management Fund	23.0	3.0
TOTAL	761.5	100.0

Source: National Cancer Institute, 1976.
* This figure reflects institute-directed research (intramural, contracts, and Cancer Research Emphasis Grants), but excludes investigator-initiated extramural grants.

little or no further significant improvement In overall cancer survival rates, nor in survival rates, for major cancer sites such as lung, stomach, pancreas, and brain, which are still virtual death sentences, nor for breast, colon-rectum, cervix, and uterus, whose five-year survival rates continue to range from 45 percent to 75 percent, with little or no change as yet (Table 1.4).[23] These facts in no way diminish the critical importance of recent striking improvements in treatment and survival of some relatively rare cancers, especially Hodgkin's disease, Wilm's tumor, choriocarcinoma, and childhood leukaemia.

In 1976, an Environmental Epidemiology Branch with a budget of $2.6 million was created in the Field Studies and Statistics Program. Funding has approximately doubled in 1978, now representing about 20 percent of the overall epidemiology program budget.

Of the 1976 Carcinogenesis Program budget of $40.1 million, only some $11 million, less than 2 percent of the total NCI budget, was spent on the bioassay program, which was formally initiated in 1968 to undertake large-scale carcinogenicity tests on industrial and consumer product chemicals to which populations are currently exposed.‡ Most testing since 1974 was done by subcontractors under the management of a prime contractor, Tracor Jitco, Inc. (on a cost-plus-award fee basis), thereby diffusing the responsibility of the NCI. Rauscher neglected this program, and with the approval of the Advisory Board and

---

Table 9.4 Analysis of the NCI Bioassay Program

	Number of Compounds in Bioassay Program		
Year	Entered	Terminated	In Print or Preparation
1969	30	0	0
1970	2	1	0
1971	34	14	0
1972	83	17	0
1973	71	2	0
1974	14	73	0
1975	19	71	0
1976	7	52	1
1977	40	25	17
1978	76	9	156†
Total	376*	264	174

Source: National Cancer Institute, 1978.

* Excludes a few assays judged to be "incomplete."

† Includes all Technical Reports in print or in preparation, but excludes about fifty compounds yielding "insufficient data." Also excludes about 223 Bioassays not reported to Congress (G. J. Ahart, G.A.O. Report to Congressman H.A. Waxman, March 30, 1979).

---

‡ However, a wide range of carcinogenesis testing activities, such as the Litton Bionetics contract, preceded the bioassay program.

its Subcommittee on Environmental Carcinogenesis, chaired by Shubik, gave it low priority for manpower and resources, gradually bringing its activities to a near halt. In 1973, about seventy new compounds were tested each year, but within three years this number had declined to only seven (Table 9.4). In spite of a major increase in the overall NCI budget during this period, there was no parallel increase in the bioassay budget.* In fact, in 1976, a total of only five professional staff were allotted to select test chemicals, define test protocols, oversee the contractors, analyze the data, and prepare technical reports. Additionally, the limited bioassay program staff were subjected to bureaucratic roadblocks, including frequent temporary reassignments to other responsibilities. As a result, only one report was published up to 1976, and a backlog of over two hundred bioassays, over half of which had been completed more than twelve months previously, had accumulated.

Criticisms of Rauscher. Criticisms of Rauscher's administration, low NCI priorities on environmental carcinogenesis, and the gross inadequacy of the bioassay program gradually surfaced. These were expressed in a report by the Comptroller General of the United States[24] and by Congressman Obey in House Appropriations hearings in 1976.[25] Rauscher was given additional appropriations and instructed to increase emphasis on environmental carcinogenesis. Specifically, he was told by Congress to create sixty new positions in the Carcinogenesis Program and seventeen new positions in the newly formed Epidemiology Branch in 1977.† He was also

instructed to make $3 million NCI funds available to NIOSH to support a projected $8 million program on occupational carcinogenesis, an instruction ignored in 1976. The criticisms of Rauscher received further dramatic support on April 14, 1976, with the resignation of Saffiotti from the associate directorship of the Carcinogenesis Program, and his transfer to the Experimental Pathology Branch of the program, a position in which (as of May, 1979) he continues to serve. In a memorandum subsequent to his letter of resignation, Saffiotti protested against NCI policies in the following terms:

> (1) Lack of manpower to operate a rapidly expanding program of major national importance; (2) Inadequate support for carcinogen bioassay operations and for cancer prevention; (3) Inadequate participation offered to staff scientists in the development of NCI policies in this field; (4) Removal of integral components from the program with resulting fragmentation of program direction; and (5) Administrative action and managerial policies.[26]

Saffiotti's resignation was shortly followed by the resignation of other staff from the Carcinogenesis Program. The program was further emasculated in July, 1977, by being split into two administratively distinct units, the Carcinogenesis Testing Program and the Carcinogenesis Research Program. This move essentially deprived the bioassay activities of needed scientific backup.

In an effort to further diffuse responsibility and head off burgeoning criticisms of the Bioassay Program, Rauscher, in February, 1976,

---

* Deficiencies of these early bioassays include the failure to have an adequate number of matched controls and the failure to make proper initial determination of the maximum tolerated dose (MTD) so that in many bioassays test animals died prematurely from acute toxicity and dosages had to be lowered during the course of the tests. However, it must be borne in mind that NCI devoted paltry resources to these activities, and that such

large-scale tests must necessarily go through developmental phases. (For a critique of the inadequacies in Tracor Jitco's management, see G. J. Ahart, G.A.O. Report to Congressman H. A. Waxman, March 30, 1979.)

† About twenty-eight of these positions have been eliminated as a result of the freeze on federal employment instituted in October, 1978.

proposed the formation of an extramural Clearinghouse on Environmental Carcinogens. Its main function was intended to be the cleaning up of the backlog of unpublished bioassay reports, and to serve as a standing peer review group for their evaluation. Additional proposed functions were the nomination of chemicals for test, improvement of the scientific base and methodology of the Bioassay Program, and increasing the public understanding of the issues involved. Membership of the Clearinghouse, which first met in November, 1976, under the Chairmanship of Arnold Brown (who a few months later opposed the FDA saccharin ban on the grounds that the positive animal carcinogenicity data should be negated by the alleged negative human data), was selected from a wide range of interests in academia, industry, labor, and public interest groups, and represented a heterogeneous amalgam of scientific and social perspectives and adversarial viewpoints, which were nevertheless expected to decide by vote on largely scientific issues. In spite of such maneuvers, it had become clear that Rauscher was not only crippling any possibilities for using the vast resources of the NCI to prevent cancer, but that he also failed to understand why he should do so. Criticisms against Rauscher escalated, and he resigned from the NCI on November 1, 1976, to assume his present position as Vice President for Research of the American Cancer Society.‡ His deputy, Guy R. Newell, became acting director of NCI and continued to perpetuate previous policies of low priorities for environmental carcinogenesis, and to starve the Bioassay Program of essential resources.

In spite of its earlier failure to take a leading role in shaping federal research programs on cancer prevention, NCI in the past few years has made some limited but notable achievements. Its contributions have included: supporting research programs on chemical carcinogenesis; developing criteria for application of animal carcinogenicity data to human experience; funding the International Agency for Research on Cancer in Lyon, France, for the production of an excellent series of monographs summarizing the carcinogenicity and related data on major classes of industrial compounds;* the publication of guidelines on carcinogenesis testing in rodents; and providing advice and guidance to regulatory agencies and congressional committees. Saffiotti has served the latter advisory functions with major distinction.

Recent Developments. Present NCI Director Arthur Upton was appointed in July, 1977, with the backing of the scientific community and with the support of labor and public interest groups. Upton, a scientist with particular expertise in radiation carcinogenesis, expresses deep concerns on problems of environmental cancer, and on the urgency of needs for the NCI to institute more effective programs for the prevention of cancer, which

---

‡ Rauscher attributed his resignation to financial needs. His salary at the American Cancer Society is substantially more than he received in government.

* These monographs which have been produced on an ongoing basis since 1971 by the secretariat of the agency, under the direction of Lorenzo Tomatis, supported by *ad hoc* teams of international experts are the best available compendia of comprehensive carcinogenicity data (see Lorenzo Tomatis et al., *Cancer Research* 38 (1978), pp. 877-85). So far, 368 chemicals selected on the basis of evidence of human exposure and suspicions of carcinogenicity, have been evaluated, the results of which are published in the first sixteen volumes of the IARC Monographs. For 26 chemicals, there is both epidemiological and experimental evidence of carcinogenicity (Appendix I); for 221 chemicals, evidence of carcinogenicity is found in at least one species of experimental animal; and for the remaining 121 chemicals, available human and experimental data are inadequate for the evaluation of carcinogenicity.

Table 9.5 Analysis of NCI Budgets in terms of Research Grant and Contract Support

Year	Budgets ($ million)	Research Grants*		Research & Resource Contracts†	
		Total ($ million)	Percentage of Budget	Total ($ million)	Percentage of Budget
1976	762	312	41	221	29
1979	937	409	44	236	25
1980‡	1,055	492	47	234	22

Source: National Cancer Institute, 1979.
* Excludes construction, training, and cancer control (educational and demonstration) grants.
† Excludes construction and cancer control contracts.
‡ Based on January, 1979, projections.

he maintains is, or should be, the primary function of the NCI.

So far, Upton's main achievement has been to establish a climate of integrity and openness at the NCI. Upton has initiated a review of the entire range of NCI programs and activities, and has established the reasonable policy that contracts, particularly large ones, should generally be restricted to supporting applied mission or service needs, rather than basic research. To this end, there has been a substantial shift in research support from contracts to grants (Table 9.5).

Upton has shown sensitivity to problems of conflict of interest within the NCI. A vexing problem has emerged over the past few years among certain NCI branch chiefs and division heads with regard to the award of research contracts in the millions of dollars range to commercial laboratories, particularly in virology and immunology programs.† This practice had its genesis in the early days of the National Cancer Program, when the NCI's newly increased budget outstripped the

size of its scientific staff. These "captive contracts" allowed some NCI scientists to build up large research empires in outside laboratories, which were then closely directed to pursue research goals consistent with the career objectives of the scientists concerned. In some instances, the award of captive contracts, particularly in virology, appears to have been accompanied by the restriction of competitive contract awards to outside scientists in universities or research institutes. Upton has essentially resolved this issue by reorganizing the Division of Cancer Cause and Prevention into administratively separate intramural and extramural activities, and by strengthening external peer review for contracts. This separation has also created a mechanism whereby extramural services and resources, such as animal facilities and histology, can now be made available to intramural scientists. Upton has also moved to resolve another internal problem in the NCI with regard to policy positions. Hitherto, ill-informed statements and publications by NCI

† An outside review of the Special Virus Program in 1974 (the Zinder report) characterized it as "a self-serving bureaucracy, full of conflicts of interest. . . . [Those running it come] from a

narrow section of the scientific community." The leadership of this program is now well represented among the senior scientific staff of the Division of Cancer Cause and Prevention.

Table 9.6 Bioassay Results Recently Announced by the NCI

Use Category	Positive	Negative	Inconclusive	Total Tested
Dyes and Dye Intermediates	13	3	1	17
Chlorinated Hydro-carbons, Solvents, and Intermediates	7	2	1	10
Other Industrial Chemicals	3	5	1	9
Pesticides and Agricultural Chemicals	13	7	2	22
Drugs	11	11	2	24
Food Components and Natural Toxins	1	1	1	3
Total	48 (56%)	29 (34%)	8 (9%)	85

Source: NCI Press Release, June, 1976, to September 1978 (not based on draft or final reports).

staff minimizing the dangers of environmental cancer, on topics ranging from carcinogens in drinking water to saccharin, have been presented to the public under the mantle of NCI authority, rather than as individual opinions. Only the office of the Director is now authorized to issue such policy statements. (Marvin Schneiderman's recent appointment to Upton's office as Associate Director for Science Policy is likely to be of further help in this regard.) Upton's awareness of the cancer prevention concerns of the public interest community has also been strengthened by the appointment of Charles Wurster, Professor of Biology at Stonybrook University, New York, and founder of the Environmental Defense Fund, as consultant to the Director's office.

NCI has finally become responsive to the needs of regulatory agencies. Upton strongly endorsed the EPA's proposal for regulation of carcinogens and other organic pollutants in drinking water, and OSHA's proposal for "generic" standards for occupational carcinogens. Upton was also a prime mover in the establishment of the NCI-NIEHS-NIOSH task force that produced the September 15, 1978, report on "Estimates of the Fractions of Cancer in the United States Related to Occupational Factors" that has led to more clear understanding of the full impact of occupational carcinogens.

In December, 1977, James Sontag, Assistant to the Director of the Division of Cancer Cause and Prevention and Executive Secretary of the Clearinghouse (in an internal NCI memorandum), expressed dissatisfaction with the performance of the Clearinghouse and recommended its dissolution. Sontag made it clear that the Clearinghouse had outlived any possible useful original purpose (of wiping out the bioassay program backlog and compensating for the meager resources allocated by Rauscher to the program). Sontag pointed out that there was no longer any need to "bolster the scientific base of the program." Other criticisms by Sontag included: the Clearinghouse discussions "have tended to obfuscate issues rather than clarify them"; the Clearinghouse has nominated only one chemical for test; the Clearinghouse has "made few, if any, concrete suggestions on improvement in testing methodology"; and the Clearinghouse has cost the NCI about $150,000, for little if any returns other than possibly increasing the openness of the program operation. Additionally, Sontag pointed out that the heterogeneous composition of the Clearinghouse resulted in confusion between scientific and societal problems, in that societally adversarial groups are obligated to vote along "party lines" on scientific issues, such as the definition of a carcinogen. Other problems that Sontag failed to discuss include substantive questions of conflict of interest affecting several senior members of the Clearinghouse. An outstanding example is David B. Clayson, Shubik's Deputy Director at the Eppley Cancer Research Institute, who is a member of the executive committee of the Clearinghouse and Chairman of a key committee deciding on the selection or rejection of chemicals for test. Clayson is also principal investigator of a major NCI Bioassay Program contract, in which the Eppley uses test methods that still fail to conform to standard procedures and guidelines long established by the NCI. Results of the Eppley bioassay activities also come under review of the Clearinghouse. Finally, Clayson is a consultant to various industries including the Calorie Control Council, and has testified for industry on repeated occasions with regard to environmental and occupational carcinogens.

Upton rejected Sontag's recommendation, and the Clearinghouse is still operational. In May, 1978, the Clearinghouse issued a report on the "Review of the Bioassay Backlog and Data," which factually reported recent progress in eliminating the backlog (Table 9.4), but without any reference to Sontag's criticisms.‡ Additionally, Upton has improved the overall operation of the program, systematized the basis for future compound selection, and has planned to increase the testing to about 120 compounds in 1979. (The practical importance of the Bioassay Program is illustrated by reference to the types of chemicals tested in Table 9.6.) In spite of these recent improvements, it nevertheless had become clear that the bioassay program was proving an embarrassment to the NCI. In January, 1978, congressional testimony, Upton raised questions on what should be the future role and responsibility of the NCI in the Bioassay Program:

> The role of government will need to change over the next decade from one of providing major support for chronic toxicity testing to one of primary concern with the development and validation of new test methods and quality control of testing conducted by industry.[27]

Meanwhile, discussions at top HEW levels to coordinate federal toxicology programs culminated in November, 1978, with the creation of the National Toxicology Program

---

‡ For a recent critique of the Bioassay Program, see G. J. Ahart, G.A.O. Report to Congressman H. A. Waxman, March 30, 1979. This report emphasizes that (as of March, 1979) only 139 of the 207 backlogged assays have been published. G.A.O. identified at least 223 additional bioassays, including those performed by Frederick Cancer Research Center, the Eppley Institute, and NCI's in-house programs, that have not been reported to Congress and published.

(NTP) under the program directorship of David Rall, Director of the National Institute of Environmental Health Sciences. While NCI continues to be fiscally liable for the Bioassay Program to up to $22 million for its first year of operation, its scientific direction is now the responsibility of the TP.* A future role for the Clearinghouse, as presently constituted, appears questionable.

In April, 1978, Gregory T. O'Connor, a pathologist with expertise in geographical influences on cancer, was appointed Director of the Division of Cancer Cause and Prevention, a post he had held on an acting basis since September, 1977. O'Connor abolished problem-oriented programs in carcinogenesis and virology, and reorganized the division on fiscal lines into intramural and extramural programs, in neither of which is there now clear program identification with cancer cause and prevention. The intramural program is a collection of separate laboratories and branches without overall focus on cancer prevention, and the intramural scientists have little opportunity for shaping the overall thrust of extramural activities. O'Connor is on record as stating that the main function of his division is good basic research, rather than good research on the scientific basis for cancer prevention, and he directs major emphasis on virology and molecular biology research programs. Intramural and extramural resources are now divided into three major program areas: biological carcinogenesis or viral oncology; epidemiology; and chemical and physical carcinogenesis. In the fall of 1978, NCI appointed a board of fifteen scientific counselors, representing a wide range of interests and expertise in areas including immunology, virology, and molecular biology, as an outside review group for the Division. Less than five of the group, however, have any identification with chemical carcinogenesis or with problems of cancer prevention.

Unresolved Dilemmas. Historically, the NCI has operated as a collection of semi-autonomous programs, each with its own set of objectives, priorities, loyalties, and outside peer pressure groups, and often working in conflict with each other in the virtual absence of overall coordination and integration. Outside of government, the basic science and clinical communities regard the NCI as their fiscal and political territory, and believe that the prime responsibility of the NCI is to support and promote their respective interests. The basic science and clinical communities, and their committee representatives on the National Cancer Advisory Panel and Board, generate strong pressures to further influence already sympathetic senior NCI staff to support these narrowly defined professional perspectives.†

It must be recognized that the low priority which the NCI has accorded to research on environmental carcinogenesis in the past has been an important factor in limiting possible regulatory initiatives for cancer prevention and control. The absence of adequate information on carcinogenicity testing of suspect carcinogens and on epidemiological investigations on environmental and occupational carcinogens is one of the most common arguments used by industry to oppose regulatory controls. Notwithstanding Upton's sincere protestations that

---

* Administratively, NTP appears to be in a state of limbo between NCI and loosely defined interagency collaborative mechanisms.

† The continued retention of Guy R. Newell as Deputy NCI Director helps to foster, at least, the perception that NCI is not primarily committed to problem-solving. Newell has a key role in Upton's office and acts as a filter between Upton and division heads. Newell bears a large measure of responsibility for the bioassay backlog, and his track record is of indifference, if not hostility, to environmental concerns. Newell's responsibilities were further extended in December, 1978, by his assignment as Program Director of the Program on Nutrition and Cancer, budgeted for $18 million in 1979.

Table 9.7 Analysis of the NCI 1979 Budget*

Division	Amounts ($ millions)	Percentage of Total
Cancer Research, Resources and Centers	72.9	7.8
Cancer Biology and Diagnosis	169.4	18.1
Cancer Treatment	236.3	25.2
Cancer Control and Rehabilitation	70.3	7.5
Cancer Cause and Prevention	240.5	25.7
Office of Division Director	(20.1)	(2.1)
Virus Cancer Program	(54.9)	(5.9)
Task Forces Program	(5.8)	(0.6)
Field Studies and Statistics Program	(23.1)	(2.5)
Carcinogenesis Program†	(56.2)	(6.0)
Research Grants	(80.5)	(8.6)
Office of NCI Director	45.3	4.8
Cancer Center Support	67.1	7.2
NIH Management Fund	35.0	3.7
Total	936.8	100.0

Source: National Cancer Institute, 1979.
* These budgetary categories are not comparable with those in Table 9.3 as they reflect recent NCI reorganization involving transfer of the grants programs from the Cancer Research, Resources and Centers to other respective divisions.
† This figure reflects institute-directed research (intramural, contracts, and Cancer Research Emphasis Grants), but excludes investigator-initiated extramural grants.

he believes that the prime function of the NCI should be to prevent cancer or reduce its incidence, it is clear that he has so far been unable to summon the necessary aggression to translate this into operational practice by appropriate budget and personnel allocations at division levels. The 1979 NCI budget (Table 9.7) still reflects the major imbalance of Rauscher's 1976 budget (Table 9.3), with regard to the paucity of definable allocations for carcinogenesis and prevention activities, in contrast with disproportionately high expenditures in areas including treatment, cancer centers, and virology.‡ In fact, there has not been any pro-

‡ The 1979 Carcinogenesis Program Budget ($56 million) is approximately 30 percent greater than the 1976 level ($43 million), while the total 1979 NCI budget ($937 million) is 23 percent greater than the 1976 equivalent ($762 million). This proportionate decrease, from 1976 to 1979, in Car-

portionate increase in fiscal or personnel allocation in the Division of Cancer Cause and Prevention, or any definable shifting of funds for this purpose within the division.*

The pressures on Upton not to increase NCI resources on cancer prevention at the expense of other program areas are complex and come from powerful and well focused constituencies. These include: the "cancer cure lobby," particularly outside clinical research scientists, cancer centers, and the American Cancer Society; the outside basic science community; and the NIH establishment, as expressed by the position of Director Donald Fredrickson that NIH has little responsibility for problem-solving, but only for excellent basic research; and indirect pressures from the industry lobby. These influences are in no way balanced by the "prevention lobby," represented by the diffuse and relatively weak activities of public interest groups and labor, and Congressional concerns, now expressed mainly by Congressmen Obey and Maguire. The absence of a powerful national cancer-prevention constituency, in the final analysis, is probably the major constraint on Upton. Meanwhile, it is unlikely that there will be major shifts in NCI priorities without an explicit and detailed congressional mandate.

The ability of the NCI, as of any other federal agency, to function effectively depends critically on its ability to attract and retain competent scientists, besides administrators, willing to cope with the problems of the bureaucracy for the sake of participating in critical national research programs. Whether the sense of purpose and direction of the NCI is sufficiently defined for this goal seems questionable. The shrinking availability of outside research funds may, however, aid future recruitment plans.

Future Policies. Upton has already expressed the intent that the NCI should exercise a major role in problem-solving approaches to cancer prevention, over and above preserving excellence in basic and clinical sciences. Just as the primary role of the entire USDA is to encourage the production of food and fiber, so should the primary role of the entire NCI be to reduce the incidence of cancer. It is, however, clear, that this intent has not been reflected at division levels in the NCI by appropriate fiscal and personnel allocations.

It is likely that the next major reauthorization of the NCI budget will be enacted by May 15, 1981, for fiscal years 1982 and beyond. This review will provide a timely opportunity for critical review of the first decade of the National Cancer Program, and an accounting of its approximately $8 billion expenditures.

It is clear that the hard-sell of the 1970 Senate Panel of Consultants has now been replaced by more somber appreciation of the realities. In Benno Schmidt's 1977 report to the President, he stated, "We are still far away from being able to put either a date or a price tag on the ultimate conquest of cancer."[28] A full accounting of the accomplishments of the National Cancer Program is overdue. This could be undertaken by one or several of the appropriate Congressional committees aided

---

cinogenesis Program funds (which in part reflects a shift from contract to extramural grants) should be further contrasted with a 92 percent increase in Division of Cancer Cause and Prevention funding over the three years (which in part reflects transfer of the grants programs from the Cancer Research, Resources and Centers).

* For a recent critique of the National Cancer Program, see G.A.O. Reports to Congressman H. A. Waxman of July 26, 1978, and March 30, 1979.

According to the 1979 report, the proportion of NCI resources allocated to "carcinogenesis activities" has remained virtually unchanged since 1972. See also testimony of the author at the Oversight Hearings of the Senate Subcommittee on Health and Scientific Research, March 7, 1979, for an analysis of NCI priorities and a discussion of the claimed NCI expenditures on obligations of $175 million on environmental carcinogenesis in 1979.

by a special staff established for the review, with additional support from the General Accounting Office. The programs of the NCI should be examined, using a wide range of criteria, in relation to its achievements in cancer prevention, cancer treatment, and basic sciences. Its programs should also be examined in relation to other research agencies and to regulatory agencies.

On a more immediate level, a series of substantive policy changes should be implemented that would improve the responsiveness of the NCI to the need for cancer prevention. For the purpose of illustrating how such changes could be reflected at the operational level in NCI, the following changes in policies may be considered:

1. *Amendments to the National Cancer Act.* First, consideration should be given to the need to insulate NCI from direct Presidential influence, and to restore it to administrative control of NIH. Second, the dictatorial authority of the Senate Panel of Consultants and the executive role of the National Cancer Advisory Board should be replaced by a more conventional advisory function of a council of committees that would be subject to the public checks and balances of the Federal Advisory Committee Act,[29] including attention to needs for disclosure of special interests of its members.† Third, senior NCI appointments should be upgraded by recruiting qualified scientists with commitment to problem-solving and cancer prevention, in addition to basic and clinical sciences. Fourth, strong emphasis should be given to the development of high priority programs designed to identify causes of cancer and its prevention. An NCI division with an exclusive commitment to environmental carcinogenesis should be authorized, which should have a clearly defined budget commensurate with its importance.‡ Finally, legislative provision must be created for the reimbursement of NCI by industry for costs of testing profitable chemicals incurred in the bioassay program.

A useful initiative in the attempt to focus NCI priorities on problem-solving has been provided by Congressman Andrew Maguire's (D.-N.J., and member of the House Health and Environment Subcommittee) 1978 Cancer Prevention Act (H.R. 10190), an amendment to the National Cancer Act of 1971. Key elements of the Maguire bill were incorporated into Chairman Paul Rogers' (D.-Fla.) (House Health and Environment Subcommit-

---

† As presently constituted, the National Cancer Advisory Board is top heavy with clinicians and basic scientists. Prior to 1979, there were no problem-oriented epidemiologists or statisticians on the Board or Panel, let alone recognized authorities with activist reputations in environmental and occupational carcinogenesis. (However, new appointees to the Board in April, 1979, include Irving Selikoff and Sheldon Samuels.) There are also critical needs on the Board for representation from the Department of Energy. Public members of the Board are appointed as political payoffs rather than as a reflection of deep commitment to cancer prevention; industry is well represented, unlike labor and public interest groups. Board or Panel membership should exclude those scientists who receive, or whose institutes receive, major NCI contracts. Although Benno Schmidt's tenure expired in March, 1978, as of January, 1979,

he still serves as Panel Chairman in spite of a long record of disinterest in cancer prevention. (In spite of the fact that his credibility as a senior science advisor is in question as in view of his track record at the NCI, in December, 1978, Schmidt expressed interest in membership of the Senior Advisory Committee of NIH. According to a July 26, 1978, G.A.O. Report to Congressman H. A. Waxman, "Since the first meeting of the President's Cancer Panel in 1972, there has been minimal discussion of cancer prevention and carcinogenesis research at its meetings."

‡ At hearings on the National Cancer Program before Senator Kennedy on March 7, 1979, Upton announced intent to create a new formal division of environmental carcinogenesis. Upton also claimed that NCI obligations for environmental carcinogenesis in 1979 totalled $175 million, although this was not supported by the budgetary

tee) Biomedical Research and Training Act. The essence of this bill became law in November, 1978 (P.L. 95-622).

The Maguire amendments (which received strong support from the Industrial Union Department of the AFL-CIO and the Oil, Chemical and Atomic Workers Union) are a major and unique contribution to the drive to refocus NCI's attention on the occupational and environmental causes of cancer. They direct the NCI to conduct "an expanded and intensified research program for the prevention of occupational or environmental exposure to carcinogens." They also require the HEW Secretary to publish an annual report containing a list of all substances known, or reasonably anticipated to be carcinogens; an estimate of the number of people exposed to each of these carcinogens; a statement identifying those carcinogens for which there is no effluent, ambient, or exposure standard; and a statement on the extent to which existing standards will decrease the cancer risk from such exposures.* This provision, designed to assess the effectiveness of existing regulatory standards, drew last minute fire from Benno Schmidt, who (during the House-Senate Conference between Chairman Rogers and Senator Ted Kennedy, who heads the Senate Subcommittee on Health and Scientific Research) engaged in unsuccessful lobbying to have the annual report requirements stricken from the bill. Schmidt admitted that this represented "a head-on defeat."

The Maguire amendments also require the NCI to develop demonstration programs designed to protect occupational and other groups at high risk, and to insure that cancer centers develop an emphasis on prevention. Another amendment requires that at least five of the eighteen-member National Cancer Advisory Board be "individuals knowledgeable in environmental carcinogenesis," and that the heads of all concerned regulatory agencies be *ex officio* members.

2. *Comprehensive cancer centers.* Continued funding of the nineteen centers should be made explicitly contingent on their developing strong programs in cancer prevention, with particular emphasis on carcinogenesis and epidemiology, in addition to their present, almost exclusive, emphasis on treatment. Centers should also be required to establish tumor registries, with particular interest in identifying environmental and occupational carcinogens, and with special emphasis on the surveillance of occupational populations at high risk of cancer.

3. *The bioassay program.* This should be singled out as a high priority in the NCI and NTP, with adequate budget and personnel. Besides selecting compounds and supervising their testing in contract and subcontract laboratories, with particular emphasis on industrial chemicals, the program should emphasize critical evaluation of the test data and early development of reports, which should also summarize information relevant to problems of human exposure. The bioassay program should be closely related to programs in epidemiology and biostatistics in the NCI, and in all agencies involved with the NTP, as well as to basic research in carcinogenesis, and should be extended to cover problems of synergistic and other interactions, especially when clues on such interactions are afforded by epidemiology. Consideration should also be given to requiring the contract laboratories, with appropriate supervision, to prepare bioassay reports rather than maintaining this as a direct NCI responsibility. Some system of interim cancer alerts should be restored to

---

details. It may thus be reasonably anticipated that the proposed new division will be funded at a minimal annual level of $175 million.

* While Maguire originally proposed that the NCI be directed to prepare the annual carcinogen re-

port (the first of which is due before the end of 1979), in deference to Upton's wishes the Secretary of HEW has assumed this responsibility which will be implemented through the NTP.

give public warning pending publication of the reports.

Careful thinking and planning are needed for the conduct of future bioassay tests. These should be designed as chronic toxicity tests, in which the discovery of carcinogenicity is a major but not exclusive end. Tests should more clearly recognize other important manifestations of chronic toxicity (including toxic effects on the central nervous and reproductive systems, liver, and kidney) by observation and functional studies during the test and histological studies following its conclusion. Methods exist to elicit a wide range of neurobehavioral effects in animals during routine handling. Chromosome and some reproductive studies can be made in animals without prejudicing the two-year bioassay test. There are a wide range of such possibilities for improving the quality and quantity of information that can be derived from the standard two-year bioassay test, leads from which can be followed up by more specialized procedures.[30]

4. *Tobacco research programs.* The major emphasis should be placed on meeting the needs for aggressive epidemiological and other research on smoking and cancer and to develop explicit anti-smoking educational campaigns. NCI programs on smoking and cancer must be commensurate with the role of tobacco as a major cause of cancer.† Future programs must be segregated from the dominant influence of industry (exercised in the past through the NCI Tobacco Working Group) and protected from past patterns of conflict of interest in its award of research support. There must also be increased emphasis on problem-oriented research, including development of improved test methods, analytic and monitoring procedures for environmental and occupational carcinogens, and carcinogenesis research at the cellular level.

5. *Environmental cancer research programs.* NCI should, with the highest possible priority, develop active, large-scale internal programs on environmental and occupational carcinogenesis research and also fund such research by outside scientists, to whom all appropriate internal resources of NCI should be made available. These activities should encompass experimental carcinogenesis, epidemiology, surveillance of high risk groups, and analytic and monitoring techniques for chemical carcinogens. Basic scientists should be encouraged to develop interest in these problem-solving activities. NCI should also fund the training of scientific investigators in these various fields.‡

6. *Relation of NCI and regulatory agencies.* NCI should preserve its primary function as a research agency, with emphasis on problem-solving, and should not become directly involved in regulatory specifics. NCI should, however, develop special formalized large-scale resources for providing guidance and counsel to regulatory agencies on all scientific matters relating to chemical carcinogens in the general environment and workplace.

A critical resource which NCI should develop is a documentation and analysis center, to collate and systematize available carcinogenicity data from sources including the Bioassay Program with particular reference to potential environmental and occupational exposure. Such a center should be directed by a scientist with recognition in chemical car-

---

† NCI tobacco program expenditures in all areas including research and education were under $7 million in 1977, $8.9 million in 1978, and are projected to be $12.8 million in 1979. Thus, approximately 1 percent of the NCI budget is allocated to an agent associated with up to about 20 percent of total U.S. cancer deaths.

‡ Although NCI recognized the need to establish training programs in toxicology and veterinary pathology in testimony before the Senate Appropriations Committee in 1977, no such programs have yet been established in spite of appropriate legislative authority.

cinogenesis and with experience and sensitivity to the needs of regulatory agencies, and should be adequately staffed with biometricians, statisticians, and epidemiologists so that it can also be capable of performing risk estimates. Finally, the center should be capable of analyzing the impact of failure to regulate a particular carcinogen in terms of total costs from induced or associated cancers and other diseases. The current failure of NCI to have developed such a resource was critically noted in a recent United Nations document (*International Register of Potentially Toxic Chemicals Bulletin* 1, June, 1978, p. 4):

> The National Cancer Institute of the National Institutes of Health, U.S. Department of Health, Education and Welfare, has certain program elements that relate directly or indirectly to concerns about exposure to specific agents that are environmental carcinogens. However, there is currently no identifiable program that assesses, on a holistic basis, the potential hazard from the carcinogenic insult of air and water pollutants, diet contaminants, and other composite stresses.

7. *Overall management.* Questions have been raised by Congressman David Obey (D-Wisc.) and others as to whether the administrative skills of the NCI are adequate to sustain its expanded budget, especially in the absence of adequate personnel and an adequately defined sense of mission and priorities. The apparent relief of the NCI in recently surrendering scientific direction of the Bioassay Program to NIEHS may well express tacit admission of NCI's desire to further divest itself of mission research and other problem-solving activities relating to cancer cause and prevention. This seems to be resulting in a perpetuation of the Rauscher era of predominant emphasis on clinical research and basic science programs unrelated to cancer prevention which could more appropriately be handled in other NIH Institutes. However,

it is unlikely that such a pattern of activity would exert adequate appeal to Congress, besides to the broad scientific biomedical community, to justify anything like the approximately $1 billion NCI budget.

Other Research Agencies

The National Institute for Occupational Safety and Health (NIOSH). This institute was created within the Department of HEW by the 1970 Occupational Safety and Health Act (P.L. 91-596), and incorporated the previous Bureau of Occupational Safety and Health. Organizationally, NIOSH was originally located in DHEW's Health Services and Mental Health Administration but, following the dissolution of that Administration in 1973, was transferred to the Center for Disease Control (CDC), a HEW agency with primary responsibility for infectious diseases within the Public Health Service, where it remains today. The NIOSH Director, headquartered in Rockville, Maryland, thus reports to the CDC Director, headquartered in Atlanta, Georgia, who in turn reports to the Assistant Secretary for Health, HEW, headquartered in Washington, D.C. Most of NIOSH's personnel are located in Cincinnati, Ohio, and Morgantown, West Virginia. From a budget of $26 million and a complement of 745 positions in 1972, NIOSH has grown to a 1978 budget of $64 million with 913 positions.

NIOSH has exclusive responsibility for research into all aspects of occupational health and safety. This research is designed to provide a critical basis for the development of regulatory standards by OSHA. A critical activity of NIOSH is its conduct of epidemiological surveys, and its development of Health Hazard Evaluation Reports for industries, where major problems of occupational health and safety are suspected. Apart from the fact that NIOSH has only carried out about 150 of these evaluations each year, their quality, in general, has been unsatisfactory. Until recently, they seemed to be falling under the increasing operational control of CDC, especially in politically "sensitive" situations.* NIOSH is also responsible for funding outside research activities, administers a program for establishing Educational Resource Centers at major universities throughout the country, and has developed educational and training programs for industrial hygienists and other professionals. NIOSH periodically issues Current Intelligence Bulletins to alert the occupational health and safety communities to emerging critical problems, and it publishes an annual Registry of Toxic Effects of Chemical Substances, which in 1976 listed 25,000 different chemicals. Included in this is a list of about 2,000 suspect carcinogens.

The major objective of the various research functions of NIOSH is the development of criteria documents recommending new updated and revised standards to OSHA. The development of these documents is the responsibility of the Division of Criteria Documentation and Standards Development, one of NIOSH's eight divisions. The proportion of the NIOSH budget allocated to criteria documents doubled from 1972 to 1973, but has remained constant at about 10 percent since then. Currently, the division employs about 80 people, and while no major increase in personnel is planned for activities under the Occupational Safety and Health Act in 1979, an increase has been requested to meet the requirements of the 1977 Federal Mine Safety and Health Act.

The criteria documents, some 85 percent of which are developed by outside contractors at a cost of about $300,000 each, review and summarize the toxicological, epidemiological, industrial hygiene, and control technology information on specific chemical and physical agents and industrial processes. The documents make recommendations on regulatory standards, work practices, and medical surveillance.[31] By April, 1979, over one hundred documents had been transmitted to OSHA. These were generated at an average rate of eleven a year since 1972, and about double that number since 1976. Only in one case, arsenic, was a NIOSH criteria document the initial stimulus for OSHA action, although in four other cases (asbestos, benzene, cotton dust, and vinyl chloride), OSHA issued standards for hazards described in criteria documents. Even before promulgation as regulatory standards, criteria documents are widely distributed and used by industry and labor as a basis for control practices.

The quality of these documents, in general, has been unscientific and unsatisfactory, and their conclusions appear to have been improperly influenced by undefined economic and feasibility considerations.† With the notable exceptions of the asbestos and coke oven documents, few other documents, many of which were prepared by outside contractors with clear conflicts of interest, have survived the OSHA hearing and standard-setting process. To some extent, the NIOSH track record on criteria documents reflects difficulties imposed on agencies that bridge research and regulatory functions. Responsive to these criticisms and with a view to improving the process, in September, 1978, CDC initiated an in-depth review of the criteria documentation program, including the validity of its data base and its utility to OSHA (Policy Research Inc., Baltimore, Md., "Evaluation of the NIOSH Criteria Documentation Program,"

---

* An example of this is the usurpation by CDC of a 1976 request to NIOSH for evaluation of a Becton-Dickinson plant in Puerto Rico, where workers making thermometers were found to be suffering from mercurial poisoning (Charles Edwards, formerly FDA Commissioner, was then a Senior Vice President at Becton-Dickinson).

† The documents fail to reflect quantitative consideration of health benefits that could be reasonably anticipated from reduction in exposure levels envisaged in the proposed standard, and fail to consider the range of available control technologies.

CDC Contract #210-78-0048).‡ In addition to criteria documents, Current Intelligence bulletins and Health Hazard Evaluation reports, NIOSH also produces two other emergency-type documents, Special Hazard Reviews and Recommendations for an Emergency Temporary Standard.

The NIOSH budget for carcinogenesis programs had increased from $1.8 million in 1975 to $6.9 million in 1976, reaching $10.7 million in 1977, including $3 million in "pass-through" funds from the NCI.[32] Carcinogenesis funding thus represents approximately 20 percent of NIOSH's total budget. The occupational carcinogen program includes laboratory studies, field surveillance, and industry-wide epidemiological studies.* The surveillance studies, which focus on groups at high risk of developing cancer, have been particularly important. The groups to be studied are identified on the basis of industrial practices, epidemiological data, and information from labor and other sources. Industries recently surveyed by NIOSH include printing, milling and mining, coal gasification, plywood, pulp and paper, steel, metal smelting, and pesticide formulation. NIOSH has also undertaken epidemiological investigations on industries using various carcinogens, including benzene, trichloroethylene, VC, vinylidene chloride, chloroprene, styrene-butadiene, epichlorhydrin, polychlorinated biphenyls, and asbestos-containing talcs.[33]

An important undertaking of NIOSH has been the National Occupational Hazard Survey from 1972 to 1974,[34] covering nearly 5,000 plants and close to one million workers, the results of which were later summarized in a document entitled, "The Right to Know."[35] The survey spelled out the extent and potential costs of exposure of workers to carcinogens:

> One in every four American workers (approximately 21 million) currently may be exposed on either a full or part-time basis to OSHA-regulated hazardous substances. Upwards of 40 to 50 million persons or 23 percent of the general population in the United States may have had exposure to one or more of OSHA-regulated carcinogens or hazardous substances during their working lifetime.

> The annual costs to society of monitoring workers with either full or part-time exposures to all OSHA-regulated hazardous substances including carcinogens could range between $675 million and $2 billion.[36]

> Besides monitoring, it was estimated that lifelong, surveillance costs for just those few carcinogens currently regulated is in the region of $8.5 billion.† Such cost estimates ignore possible additional employer liability resulting from discovery of compensable impairment during examination, entitlement under various federal and state programs, recovery for damages under third-party legal action brought by workers, and even greater costs from past exposures to carcinogens not regulated by OSHA.

"The Right to Know" also confirms the fact that a substantial number of workers in industry are exposed to chemicals the identification of which the industry has refused to

---

‡ In March, 1979, NIOSH announced plans to direct future emphasis to the production of criteria documents dealing with control technology, encompassing across-the-board processes at the expense of traditional single-agent documents.

* Probably the most successful of these were directed by Joseph K. Wagoner (ex-chief of the Division of Field Studies and Clinical Investigations by NIOSH and now Special Assistant for Occupational Carcinogenesis at OSHA), who has pioneered a wide range of important epidemiological investigations on occupational carcinogenesis. Wagoner has also been an articulate and well-informed witness at various Congressional hearings.

† Additionally, the cost of physical examinations would be about $230 million a year.

disclose; over 70 percent of all exposures were found to arise from trade name products of undisclosed composition. According to the document, "A major stumbling block to identifying exposed workers is the failure of chemical re-packagers and primary producers to show the chemical composition of their product."[37] Beyond knowing who has been exposed to what, "There is currently no effective mechanism for locating and notification [of workers]."

Concerns have been growing over the inability to identify workers today who have been exposed to carcinogens in the past. Responding to these concerns and to an amendment to the Internal Revenue Service Code offered by Senator Gaylord Nelson (D-Wisc.), President Carter authorized NIOSH in November, 1977, to obtain from the Internal Revenue Service addresses of workers whom it suspects of having been exposed to carcinogens. Among the first workers targeted for notification are the many who may have been exposed to asbestos, arsenic, benzene, and benzidine.

The previous administration did not give NIOSH high priority. President Ford's request for the 1976 NIOSH budget was $32 million, the same amount as appropriated by Congress in the previous year. His Office of Management and Budget eliminated a proposed line item for occupational carcinogenesis, a move that was countered by Congressman David Obey (D-Wisc.) of the House Appropriations Committee, resulting in an increase in total NIOSH appropriations to $48 million. (Obey has played a major role in overseeing carcinogenesis and related programs and priorities in NCI as well as NIOSH.)

One of the major problems of NIOSH, apart from critical shortages of funds, has been and still is its relatively low political visibility and stature. Since NIOSH reports directly to CDC, the NIOSH director has no direct access to the HEW secretary (in contrast to the Assistant Secretary of Labor for Occupational Safety and Health, Eula Bingham, who reports directly to the Secretary of Labor). In spite of these and other problems, NIOSH has made significant strides in its research, epidemiological surveys, training programs (including establishment of Educational Resource Centers), and development of criteria documents.

The previous director of NIOSH was John F. Finklea, who resigned in January, 1978. Prior to Finklea's NIOSH tenure, he was in charge of air pollution biomedical research activities at EPA, where he made important contributions. While at NIOSH, Finklea had to struggle against crippling fiscal limitations imposed by unsympathetic Republican administrations, a Department of Labor more responsive to interests of commerce than health and safety, and the low bureaucratic status of NIOSH. Finklea's resignation resurrected latent questions as to the future of NIOSH and its appropriate position within the Federal bureaucracy. Possibilities, each of which had proponents, included upgrading of NIOSH within HEW to an agency level (reporting directly to Secretary Califano or Julius Richmond, HEW Assistant Secretary for Health), a move endorsed by organized labor; the transfer, intact, of NIOSH to the Department of Labor; and, the preservation of the NIOSH *status quo* as advocated by CDC. These speculations, fueled by the protracted failure of HEW to replace Finklea, were eventually resolved with Califano's announcement at the September, 1978, AFL-CIO convention in Washington, D.C., of the appointment of Anthony Robbins, Director of the Colorado Health Department and Labor's candidate, to head up NIOSH, an appointment formalized by the Civil Service Commission in December, 1978.

Reflecting still unresolved ambiguities, and possibly foreshadowing events to come, in November, 1978 (pending ratification of the Robbins appointment), CDC moved to appoint W. Clark Heath, a staff epidemiologist, to a key NIOSH position.‡ In view of Robbins' known opposition, this move appears to reflect undue CDC influence in NIOSH policies, and also insensitivity to the concerns of labor, by whom Heath is viewed as ultraconservative, if not hostile.* Responsive to labor's protest and Congressman Obey's intervention, Califano blocked Heath's appointment. (Instead, Philip J. Landrigan, another CDC epidemiologist was appointed in April, 1979.)

The tensions between NIOSH and CDC appear to reflect territorial, rather than conceptual, considerations. CDC can no longer justify its present budget and personnel levels on the basis of its anachronistic mission of infectious disease control, but only by subsuming the occupational health and safety missions of NIOSH.† Forcing the NIOSH tail to wag the CDC dog may well ensure continued low federal priority for the missions of NIOSH. However, it is also possible that Robbins' personal contacts at HEW and elsewhere in Washington may be adequate to counterbalance bureaucratic formalities. It also seems likely that NIOSH could benefit from the recognized professionalism and administrative skills of CDC.

A series of initiatives, now under consideration, would develop greater consistency in the interpretation and discharge by NIOSH and OSHA of their respective mandates under the terms of the 1970 Occupational Safety and Health Act. In October, 1978, the Department of Labor requested the cooperation of HEW in improving the relationships between OSHA and NIOSH, and in the creation of a NIOSH "Planning Group Activity" within the Labor Department, under the direction of Assistant Secretary Eula Bingham, but including representation from the Mine Safety and Health Administration and the Employment Standards Administration, both of which have close working relationships with NIOSH. The Department of Labor, in order to ensure appropriate priority for its research needs, also requested authority from the Office of Management and Budget to participate in NIOSH budget-setting for fiscal 1981. Irrespective of the precise outcome of these initiatives, it is clear that the primary and explicit function of NIOSH must be to undertake research that will more effectively enable OSHA to discharge its responsibility in improving occupational health and safety.

Robbins appears to have a good grasp of the more pressing problems of NIOSH. His well-attuned political instincts coupled with integrity and dedication should enable him to cope with the bureaucratic ambiguities and complexities he has inherited. Within a few days of his appointment, Robbins expressed intent to upgrade the quality and quantity of Health Hazards Evaluations, to improve the quantity, quality, and utility of criteria documents and synchronize them better with OSHA's needs, and to improve professional skills at NIOSH, particularly in clinical and engineering areas.‡

---

‡ This position, Director of the Division of Surveillance, Hazard Evaluation and Field Studies in Cincinnati, had just been vacated following the unrequested transfer by CDC of Bobby Craft, the previous Division Director, to the Educational Resource Center at the University of Utah.

* As an example, contrary to established NIOSH policy of open joint involvement of management and labor in planning and undertaking field investigations, in 1974, unbeknown to NIOSH and labor, CDC met privately with management of a Union Carbide plant in South Charleston, West Virginia, to discuss the medical examination of workers exposed to vinyl chloride. Following discovery, protests by the Industrial Union Department of AFL-CIO forced cancellation of the CDC plans, and NIOSH was authorized to conduct the evaluation elsewhere (at the Firestone, Pottstown, Pennsylvania, facility).

† This motivation was admitted at a private discussion between a senior CDC official and Labor in July, 1978.

‡ A recent expression of this perception is the Control Technology Program, budgeted for $4.2

The National Institute for Environmental Health Sciences (NIEHS). Created in the fall of 1966 and located in Research Triangle Park, North Carolina, this is the only NIH Institute located away from the Bethesda, Maryland, Campus.* NIEHS supports basic research on the toxic effects of environmental pollutants and on ways to predict such future crises.

Although one of the youngest and smallest NIH Institutes, NIEHS has taken the lead in several major areas of research, particularly mutagenesis, which is important because of the promise of mutagenesis as a short-term test for carcinogenicity, quite apart from intrinsic public health problems of mutagenicity. A second major field is the development of improved statistical methods for extrapolating from animal tests to humans, and from high-dose to low-dose responses. (Institute statisticians have been prominent in reaffirming the scientific basis of the Delaney law, and the inability of science to determine threshold levels for carcinogens.) An additional area has been study of the rate of absorption, distribution, metabolism, and excretion of toxic and carcinogenic substances in the body. The Institute has also served as a major supporter of a number of critical areas of extramural research, including Selikoff's pioneering work on asbestos, and the studies of Norton Nelson's group at New York University, which led to the identification of BCME, dimethyl carbamoyl chloride, and epichlorhydrin as major industrial carcinogens.

Probably the most important contributions of NIEHS have been in the development of national recognition of toxicology as a major field of scientific endeavor, and in the organization of a broad forum for discussion of the scientific basis of important regulatory issues. Such activities have included the establishment of two Task Forces on research planning in environmental health, which focused the attention of policy makers and scientists on research and manpower needs in this field, and the creation of a new journal, *Environmental Health Perspectives,* which has served as a key instrument in the rapid communication of proceedings of conferences convened by the Institute.

The NIEHS budget has grown from $49 million in 1977 to about $69 million in 1979.† Of the current budget, approximately $19 million is allocated to "Disease Prediction," $11 million to "Disease Mechanisms," $15 million to "Manpower Development," and $21 million to "Intramural Research." Research funds are evenly divided between intramural and extramural activities.

There are clearly some ambiguities and areas of jurisdictional overlap between the functions of NIEHS on the one hand and NCI and NIOSH on the other. This is illustrated by the recent shift in scientific responsibility for the NCI's Bioassay Program to NIEHS by the creation of the National Toxicology Program (NTP) on a two-year experimental basis. NTP was set up as an interagency department-wide cooperative program (including NCI, NIEHS, CDC/NIOSH, FDA, and other members of the Interagency Regulatory Liaison Group) under the direction of David P. Rall, Director of the NIEHS, who will report to the Assistant HEW Secretary for Health. The avowed objective of the NTP is "to strengthen the Department's activities in the testing of chemicals of public health concern, as well as in the development and validation of new and better integrated test meth-

million in 1979, in which selected industries involving carcinogenic exposures are being assessed from the standpoint of control and process technology. Similar control technology programs are being developed at EPA.

* Long an occupant of limited rental laboratory space, NIEHS will be moving into adequate research facilities in Research Triangle Park in 1980.
† Congressman David Obey (D-Wisc.), in particular, has recognized the contributions and potential of NIEHS, and has been a key supporter of its sustained growth.

ods." In its first year, the approximately $41 million budget of the NTP is comprised of the following contributions: NCI $22 million; NIEHS $10 million; FDA $7 million; and CDC/NIOSH $2 million.

Rall is both skilled and enthusiastic, and has emerged as one of the leading scientific protagonists of the hazards of toxic and carcinogenic environmental pollutants. He has also been involved in critical public issues, such as defending the Delaney Amendment from industry attacks and in backing the proposed FDA ban on saccharin. Rall additionally serves as Chairman of the DHEW Committee to Coordinate Toxicology and Related Programs, which draws together the DHEW agencies (and observers from non-DHEW agencies) for the purpose of improving information flow and program coordination of toxicology research.

The National Center for Toxicological Research (NCTR). This center, in Pine Bluff, Arkansas, was established in 1971 by President Nixon, is administered by the FDA, and is jointly funded by the FDA and EPA. Its stated objectives are the development of methodologies for chronic toxicity and carcinogenicity testing, studies on exposure to low levels of carcinogens, and extrapolation of carcinogenicity data from animals to humans. The track record of the NCTR illustrates how research functions are subverted by political considerations. From its inception, senior FDA officials made it clear that they intended using the center to develop data for the purpose of challenging the scientific basis of the Delaney Amendment so as to allow the FDA to set tolerances for carcinogens deliberately added to food. At hearings before Congressman Whitten's Subcommittee on Agriculture

and Related Agencies of the House Appropriations Committee in April, 1971, then Commissioner Edwards stated in congressional hearings that "the Pine Bluff testing facility will provide FDA with the scientific basis on which the Delaney anti-cancer clause may be changed," reiterating his view that the agency is "locked into an all or nothing" position because of the Delaney box. "The FDA didn't want to make it more difficult by recommending changes until it has the scientific data to justify a modification."[38] Four years later FDA made it clear that it had not changed its position of fundamental hostility to the Delaney anti-cancer clause.[39]

The research programs developed by the NCTR were poorly conceived. The most widely touted of these was the "Mega Mouse" experiment, in which hundreds of thousands of mice were to be tested in attempts to find safe levels for profitable chemical carcinogens, such as DDT, that had been or were about to be banned. Not only did this approach suffer from major statistical problems, but there were not enough personnel available to undertake the necessary autopsies. The center (apparently seriously) suggested instead that they would spot-check animals at the end of a carcinogenicity test, rather than autopsying them all.‡

Responding to mounting criticisms and at the request of HEW, NCI Director Rauscher appointed an expert committee under the chairmanship of the distinguished pathologist, Harold L. Stewart to evaluate the center's programs. The committee's unanimous report in August, 1973, concluded:

The program will not contribute materially to progress toward its stated objective, viz., improved capability for assessing the carcinogenic hazard for man on the basis of

---

‡ In spite of these problems, results of recent large-scale NCTR tests on the potent carcinogen acetylaminofluorene are consistent with the no-threshold concept of carcinogenesis, as evidenced

by a linear extrapolation through zero. In other words, they confirm the extreme difficulty, if not impossibility, of setting "safe levels."

data obtained in laboratory animals.[40]

Morris F. Cranmer, then director of the center, reacted hostilely, asserting that the critics were not familiar with his programs and had failed to understand his objectives. Apparently interested in avoiding embarrassment to the FDA, Rauscher rejected his committee's report. Four years later, however, a National Academy of Sciences committee came to essentially the same conclusions.[41] The immediate problem was resolved in December, 1977, when Cranmer was relieved of his post following investigations by the General Accounting Office and the FBI resulting in charges of conflict of interest and major mishandling of federal funds.[42] As of May, 1979, completion of formal action to terminate his FDA appointment is still pending and Cranmer is contesting the charges.

The Energy Research and Development Administration (ERDA). ERDA was created in 1974 by the Energy Reorganization Act and is now part of the Department of Energy. Its Biomedical and Environmental Research Program, budgeted at $122 million in 1977, is responsible for investigating the public health and environmental effects of developments in energy technology, including nuclear power and coal gasification. Most of ERDA's health effects research is on radiation, but $5.5 million is budgeted for other aspects of environmental carcinogenesis. Ruth C. Clusen, past president of the League of Women Voters, is Assistant Secretary for Environment of the Department of Energy.

Office of Technology Assessment (OTA). Following years of deliberation and public debate, Congress passed the Technology Assessment Act creating OTA in 1972. The bill was guided through Congress by Representative Emilio Daddario (D-Conn.) and Senator Edward Kennedy (D-Mass.). OTA began operations in late 1973 with Kennedy as the first Board Chairman and Daddario (by then no longer in Congress) as the Office's first Director, to be succeeded by Russell W. Peterson in January, 1978.* From initial funding of about $2 million in 1974, the OTA budget increased to about $8 million in 1978, with an estimated 1979 projection of $11.2 million.

The Office of Technology Assessment is intended to serve Congress as a nonpartisan think tank on issues relating to science and technology, and to assess the impacts of technological change on society. The concept of "technology assessment" first originated with the House Committee on Science and Astronautics in the mid-1960s, as Congress wrestled with scientific and technical issues whose consequences were unclear or on which there was sharply polarized opinion. These include the impacts of supersonic transport, new transportation systems, anti-ballistic missiles, and toxic chemicals. While the original perception of OTA was that of Kennedy's "Brain Child" and answer to Nixon's Office of Science and Technology (currently transformed into the Office of Science and Technology Policy), Congress now appears to accept it as a useful resource for "scientific foresight." It is, however, questionable whether Congress interprets "technology assessment" in terms of secondary and tertiary impacts, rather than as merely assessing the soundness of a particular technology.

OTA currently operates in eleven principal areas: energy, food, genetics and world population, health, materials, national security, oceans, R&D policies and priorities, technology and world trade, telecommunications and information systems, and transportation. Within these areas, OTA studies involve consultants, contractors, and citizen advisory panels to augment the in-house professional staff

---

* Peterson resigned on March 31, 1979, and was replaced by John Gibbons, a physicist from the University of Tennessee.

Table 9.8 Standards Promulgated by Regulatory Agencies to Control or Ban Carcinogens

Legislative Authority	Carcinogen	Agency Action	Action Initiated by Public Interest or Labor Groups*
Occupational Safety and Health Act (Section 6, Workplace standards)	Asbestos	OSHA, 1972	AFL-CIO, 1972
	Package of 14 carcinogens	OSHA, 1973	OCAW and HRG, 1973
	Vinyl chloride	OSHA, 1974	AFL-CIO and URW, 1974
	Coke oven emissions	OSHA, 1976	....
	Benzene	OSHA, 1978	URW, 1976
	Acrylonitrile	OSHA, 1978	....
Clean Air Act (Section 112, Hazardous Air Pollutants)	Beryllium	EPA, 1973	....
	Asbestos	EPA, 1973–1976	....
Federal Water Pollution Control Act (Section 307, Toxic Pollutants Effluent standards)	Vinyl chloride	EPA, 1976	....
	DDT	EPA, 1977	EDF, NRDC, CBE, etc.
	Endrin	EPA, 1977	....
	Aldrin/dieldrin	EPA, 1977	....
	Benzidine	EPA, 1977	....
	PCB	EPA, 1977	....

(continued on following page)

Table 9.8 (continued)

Act	Chemical		
Federal Insecticide, Fungicide, and Rodenticide Act	DDT	EPA, 1972	EDF, 1969
	Cyanamide	EPA, 1972	....
	Aldrin/dieldrin	EPA, 1974	EDF, 1970
	Vinyl chloride (aerosols)	EPA, 1974	HRG, 1974
	Chlordane/heptachlor	EPA, 1975	EDF, 1974
	Mirex	EPA, 1976	EDF, 1973
	Kepone	EPA, 1976	....
	Octamethyl-phosphoramide	EPA, 1976	....
	Safrole	EPA, 1977	....
Federal Food, Drug, and Cosmetic Act	Violet #1	FDA, 1973	CSPI
	Vinyl chloride (aerosols)	FDA, 1974	HRG
	Chloroform (cosmetics)	FDA, 1976	HRG
	Red #2	FDA, 1976	HRG
Consumer Product Safety Act	Vinyl chloride (aerosols)	CPSC, 1974	HRG
	Asbestos	CPSC, 1977	NRDC
	Tris	CPSC, 1977	EDF

Source: S. M. Wolfe, "Standards for Carcinogens: Science Affronted by Politics," in *Origins of Human Cancer*, Book C, eds. H. H. Heath, J. D. Watson, and J. A. Winsten, (Cold Spring Harbor Laboratory, 1977) pp. 1735-48.
* OCAW=Oil, Chemical, and Atomic Workers Union; HRG=Health Research Group; URW=United Rubber Workers; EDF=Environmental Defense Fund; CSPI=Center for Science in the Public Interest; NRDC=Natural Resources Defense Council; CBE=Citizens for a Better Environment.

of scientists, engineers, lawyers, and policy analysts. In the past, OTA responded principally to requests from congressional committees or OTA Board members. However, during 1978, OTA launched a broad outreach effort to determine the general perception of the most important issues warranting OTA study, on the basis of which new priorities were established.

In the health area, OTA reports have addressed issues such as drug bioequivalence (the first report issued by OTA), the need for assessing the safety and efficacy of medical technologies such as the computerized axial tomography (CAT) scanner, the carcinogenicity of saccharin, and methods for carcinogenicity testing. While past reports have been restricted to assessment of the benefits and risks of various policy alternatives, OTA is considering moving in the direction of making specific recommendations which, subject to approval by Board majority, are authorized by the enabling legislation of the Technology Assessment Act. OTA reports have often been the basis for congressional action, or for programmatic changes by Federal agencies, besides serving as a useful resource for the scientific and technical community and the general public.

The Council on Environmental Quality (CEQ). The first official act of President Nixon was the signing of the National Environmental Policy Act, dedicated to improving environmental quality.[43] The Act also established CEQ in the executive office of the President, where its primary duty is to give Congress an Environmental Quality Report each year, setting forth the status and conditions of the nation's environment.† Under the successive leadership of Russell Train and Russell W. Peterson, the council has played an important role in developing critical analyses of environmental pollution problems, in emphasizing the urgent need to develop preventive approaches to environmental problems, particularly cancer, and in stressing the importance of interagency collaboration in meeting these objectives. Under the chairmanship of Charles Warren, who was appointed in March, 1977, the council is living up to the promise of past performance. Warren came from the California State Assembly, where he built up a sound record on energy and environmental concerns. The second member of the three-person council is Gus J. Speth, appointed in April, 1977, an attorney who was one of the original founders of the Natural Resources Defense Council and who has strong interests in problems of nuclear power, water pollution, and corporate policy.

Regulatory Agencies

The function of regulatory agencies is to regulate. This entails not only developing standards but enforcing them as well. The former is cosmetic without the latter. The regulatory function of every agency is mandated by statutory legislative authority, and confusion or ambiguity in the mandate will be reflected in agency practice.[44]

As illustrated in the various case studies in chapters 5, 6, and 7, the track record of federal agencies in regulating carcinogens in the workplace, in consumer products, and in the general environment has been unsatisfactory. Of the few regulatory actions that have been undertaken against carcinogens in the past decade, the great majority have been formally initiated or instigated by public interest or la-

---

† The Act requires environmental impact statements when proposed projects within the jurisdiction of federal regulatory agencies may significantly affect "the quality of the human environment." CEQ has recently proposed extending the requirements of the Act to the international activities of agencies. Hearings on this proposal were held in June, 1978, by Senator John Culver's Resource Protection Sub-Committee of the Environment and Public Works Committee.

bor groups (Table 9.8).‡ (See Appendix III for a comprehensive list of substances regulated as carcinogens.) It is clear that the fundamental problem with the regulatory agencies has not been a shortage of laws or ambiguities in the laws, but an unwillingness or inability of the agencies to enforce them.*

Statutory Authority. There are two major types of statutory authority governing control of toxic agents and environmental and occupational carcinogens: *product legislation* and *media legislation* (Table 9.9). Product legislation governs the manufacture, distribution, and use of particular products, such as pesticides, food additives, cosmetics, and drugs. Media legislation governs quality of envi-

Table 9.9 Legislation Conferring Regulatory Authority for the Control of Environmental Carcinogens

Type of Legislation	Specific Authority	Regulatory Agency*
Product	Federal Insecticide, Fungicide, and Rodenticide Act	EPA
	Federal Food, Drug, and Cosmetic Act	FDA
	Consumer Product Safety Act	CPSA
	Safe Drinking Water Act	EPA
	Toxic Substances Control Act	EPA
Media	Federal Water Pollution Control Act	EPA
	Federal Clean Air Act	EPA
	Occupational Safety and Health Act	OSHA
	Federal Mine Safety and Health Amendment Act	MSHA

* EPA=Environmental Protection Agency; FDA=Food and Drug Administration; CPSC=Consumer Products Safety Commission; OSHA=Occupational Safety and Health Administration, Department of Labor; MSHA= Mine Safety and Health Administration, Department of Labor.

‡ It is possible that Table 9.8 does injustice to regulatory agencies which, in some instances, were developing the legal basis for action when labor or public interest groups intervened. For a recent discussion of "Chronic Indecisiveness" in regulatory agencies and their inadequate track records, see R. J. Smith, "Toxic Substances: EPA and OSHA are Reluctant Regulators," *Science*

203 (1979), pp. 28-32.
* An important exception to the adequacy of current legislation is its failure to require the retention of exposure and employment records in the absence of any known or suspected environmental or occupational hazards. This deficiency is all the more critical in view of the prolonged latent period of many cancers.

ronmental "media," such as air, water, and the workplace.

Product legislation arises from recognition of the basic obligation of a manufacturer to provide a product of "merchantable quality" which has no harmful effects on the consumer other than those explicitly stated on the label.[45] Over the years, the government's authority has extended from simple labelling to the entire composition and manufacture of a product. More important, the burden of proof has gradually been shifted to the manufacturer, who now must prove the safety of his products rather than demanding that the government or public prove it harmful.

Media legislation attempts to regulate the discharge or emission of toxic and carcinogenic pollutants into the community and workplace environment, as recognized by the subsequent identification of those agents. As such, media legislation is retrospective rather than anticipatory in nature. It says, "By all means use the carcinogen, but don't let any of it or too much of it escape into the environment." Media legislation is specifically addressed to one particular environmental component, air, water, or the workplace, without consideration of the essential unity of the environment. In contrast, toxic substances legislation, while generally considered to be product rather than media in type, insofar as it relates to specific chemicals, is unique in that it can exercise multimedia control over chemicals in air, food, and water in the general environment, home, and workplace.

There is considerable overlap and inconsistency between the authorities of the various regulatory agencies. As an example, VC in 1975 by FDA in food and drug products; and in 1976 by EPA as a hazardous air pollutant.

While regulatory agencies depend on research institutes, such as NCI or NIOSH, for providing the essential data base and advice on which standards are developed, most regulatory agencies also have backup research and scientific resources of their own.

Burden of Proof. The ability of an agency to regulate carcinogens and other toxic agents effectively is substantially influenced by whether or not the burden of proof has been determined by statute to be its responsibility as opposed to that of the manufacturer, who may be required to provide the regulatory agency with information on safety prior to marketing and to update such information after marketing. Exceptions to such requirements in product-type legislation are chemicals in consumer products, regulated by the Consumer Product Safety Commission, and cosmetics, regulated by the FDA, where the onus is on government.

In media-type legislation, the burden of proving hazard for carcinogens and other pollutants, in community air and water and in the workplace is placed on the government. Toxic substances legislation offers EPA the discretionary authority to shift the burden of proof to the manufacturer. An exception to the general burden of proof rule can be made when an agency is petitioned to regulate, for instance, a particular carcinogenic chemical. Then the burden rests not with government or the manufacturer, but with the petitioner, almost invariably a public interest or labor group.

The Occupational Safety and Health Administration. OSHA was created in 1970 as an agency within the Department of Labor after considerable lobbying by AFL-CIO and other labor organizations to create an Act that would "assure so far as possible every working man and woman in the nation safe and healthful working conditions" (P.L. 91-596).†

---

† A major deficiency in the Act is its failure to provide transfer and wage retention (rate retention) rights for workers whose health has been impaired or who are at increased risk from exposure to

After the establishment of OSHA, it was delegated additional responsibility for a variety of health and safety programs within the Department of Labor (including the Walsh-Healey Public Contracts Act of 1936; the Service Contract Act of 1965; the Construction Safety Amendments of 1969; the Maritime Safety Amendments of 1958; the National Foundation on the Arts and Humanities Act of 1965; and the Federal Safety Program). Unlike its predecessor, the Bureau of Labor Standards which had mostly advisory power, OSHA has major regulatory authority, extending to about 2 million workplaces and 75 percent of the U.S. work force. Federal, state, and local government workers, and some other non-federal employees already regulated by the government, are excluded from OSHA jurisdiction. However, the Act allows individual states to administer their own occupational safety and health "state plans," provided these set standards and enforcement levels at least as stringent as the federal, and provided their administration is evaluated and approved by the OSHA Office of Federal State Operations.

In addition to its Washington, D.C., headquarters within the Department of Labor, OSHA has several directorates and regional offices through which it exercises local authority. From 1972 to 1979, OSHA's staff grew to an approximate total of 3,000, with a commensurate budgetary increase from $37 million to $163 million. Of the 1979 budget, about $9.3 million are allocated to Safety and Health Standards, $745,000 to the Occupational Cancer Information and Alert Program, and $178,000 to the Experimental Technology Incentives R&D Program. In October, 1978, OSHA announced award of "New Direction" training grants totalling $6.4 million (divided approximately equally between fiscal 1978 and 1979 funds) to 86 business, employee, and educational organizations for developing institutional competence in job safety and health.

The Occupational Safety and Health Act authorizes OSHA to establish and enforce three types of standards.[46] The first type are the approximately 400 initial (interim) consensus standards, established under Section 6(a) of the Act, previously developed as threshold limit values by industry or quasi-industry organizations, such as the American National Standards Institute. These were largely designed to protect against immediate toxic effects rather than delayed toxic and carcinogenic effects. In 1974, NIOSH and OSHA developed in a collaborative effort a "Standards Completion Process" to supplement and update the original 400 consensus standards (with the exception of carcinogens and certain other selected substances for which NIOSH is preparing individual criteria documents), which can all be covered by a single HEW standard.

The second type are the new permanent (complete) standards, or modification of old ones, which are authorized under Section 6(b) of the Act and designed to assure "to the extent feasible that no employee will suffer material impairment of health." This is the language of compromise which reflects industrial determination of technological and economic feasibility, rather than the goals of health protection. Although NIOSH supplied OSHA with about one hundred criteria documents, the agency, burdened by fiscal constraints and intense political pressures under the Nixon and Ford administrations, has so far passed only ten new final standards of which eight deal with carcinogens: asbestos in 1972; vinyl chloride in October, 1974; a package of fourteen carcinogens without monitoring requirements in January, 1974; coke oven emis-

---

OSHA-regulated substances. Consequently, workers may hesitate to seek medical care or to remove themselves from dangerous exposures unless they are prepared to risk job loss or demotion. (This is in striking contrast to the Coal Mine Health and Safety Act which guarantees rate retention.)

sions in 1976; and benzene, acrylonitrile, DBCP, and arsenic in 1978 (See Table 9.10).‡

The third type of standards are the Emergency Temporary Standards, authorized under Section 6(c) of the Act, which may be imposed without the formal hearing requirement of the Administrative Procedure Act for a maximum of six months on grounds of "imminent hazard." Also embodied here is the ability of OSHA to abate these hazards without feasibility considerations. Emergency standards must be followed by proceedings to establish new standards or they are voided. Six sets of emergency standards, all based on carcinogenicity, have been developed over the last six years: in 1972, a standard for asbestos of 2 million fibers per cubic meter of air; also in 1972, regulation of a group of fourteen carcinogens without monitoring requirements, the permanent standard of one of

Table 9.10 Final Standards Issued by OSHA

Standard	Date Issued	Number of Exposed Workers	In Effect
Asbestos	6/7/72	1,600,000	Yes
Carcinogens (14)	1/29/74	11,000	Mostly*
Vinyl chloride	10/4/74	10,000	Yes
Coke oven emissions	10/22/76	30,000	Yes
Benzene	2/10/78	600,000	Vacated
DBCP†	3/17/78	2,000	Yes
Arsenic	5/5/78	12,000‡	Yes
Cotton dust	6/23/78	600,000	Stayed
Acrylonitrile	10/3/78	125,000**	Yes
Lead	11/14/78	835,000	Effective 2/79

Source: T. B. Clark, "Cracking Down on the Causes of Cancer," *National Journal* 10 (1978): pp. 2056-60.

* Regulation vacated for the most widely used of the fourteen carcinogens. There is no requirement for monitoring, nor are there any prescribed analytical techniques for this package of fourteen carcinogens, in contrast to the other carcinogen standards.

† This standard was issued primarily to protect against sterility, rather than carcinogenicity.

‡ Exact numbers unknown; 660,000 workers are involved in the "commercial cycle of arsenic."

** 10,000 are "most directly exposed."

‡ Probably the most important, precedential, and technology-forcing standard promulgated by OSHA was the November, 1978, lead standard, reducing permissible exposure levels from 200 $\mu g/m^3$ to 50 $\mu g/m^3$. (Major responsibility for drafting the standard belongs to John Froines, who in January, 1979, was appointed Deputy Director of NIOSH.) The Steelworkers Union immediately sued OSHA in the Philadelphia Third Circuit Court of Appeals on the grounds that the standard does not provide an ample margin of safety, that the lead time for compliance is excessive, and, presumably, to preempt the exclusive jurisdiction of the standard in the Fifth Circuit court in New Orleans, where it was known that the Lead Industry Association had planned suit.

which, MOCA, being subsequently success-fully challenged on procedural grounds; a standard of 50 ppm for VC in April 1974; a 1 ppm standard for benzene in May, 1977; an emergency standard for dibromochloro-propane in September, 1977; and an emer-gency standard for acrylonitrile in January, 1978.

Under the Nixon and Ford administrations, OSHA was subverted in a number of ways, including an inducement by Assistant Secre-tary of Labor George Guenther to stall stan-dards-setting procedures in exchange for busi-ness support of the 1972 presidential elec-tion campaign.

The past record of OSHA has been one of extreme inactivity.[47] Inspections concentrated on such trivia as misplaced ladders and split toilet seats rather than seriously attempting to assess blatant health hazards from such sub-stances as lead and asbestos. Fines averaged around $50 per inspection, were often sus-pended on the company's promise of even-tual abatement, and provided little economy incentive for compliance.

Under the leadership of Secretary Ray Mar-shall, and Assistant Secretary Eula Bingham, appointed to head OSHA in March, 1977, there has been considerable improvement in the activities of the Department of Labor for protecting workers against occupational car-cinogens and other toxic agents. The standard-setting process has been strengthened and speeded up, and new policies on carcinogens and other health hazards have been proposed.* Inspectors have been instructed to overlook trivia and instead pursue obvious health haz-ards. Bingham has launched an aggressive recruitment campaign to secure committed and capable specialists, and is transforming OSHA into an effective agency.

Bingham has assigned top priority to pro-mulgating "generic" standards for occupa-tional carcinogens, drafted by Anson Keller, now Special Assistant for Regulatory Affairs at OSHA, during the latter part of the tenure of the previous OSHA Director, Morton Corn.[48] These standards lay down procedures for categorical rule-making to be followed once a chemical is shown to be a carcinogen, and are designed to obviate the virtually im-possible task of separate rule-making for each individual carcinogen — an effort character-ized by Secretary Marshall as "trying to put out a forest fire one tree at a time." While determination of carcinogenicity in these pro-posals is generic, as in the Delaney Amend-ment, subsequent rule-making for each car-cinogen is, however, clearly individualized and not generic and likely to remain a pro-tracted and difficult process. Public hearings and informal rule-making on the proposals commenced on May 16, 1978.†

Broadly speaking, three categories of car-cinogens are recognized in the OSHA propos-als. Category I substances are unequivocal carcinogens, as proven by human evidence, or two independent animal tests, or in one animal and one short term test. Category I clas-sification must be accompanied by the issu-ance of an emergency temporary standard. Exposure to Category I carcinogens would be allowed only at the lowest levels technically feasible, under controlled conditions with sen-sitive monitoring procedures, and with due warnings to all concerned. If safe substitutes

---

* The very low rate of promulgation of OSHA stan-dards has been a critical rate-limiting factor in the control of occupational carcinogens. However, in addition to specific workplace exposure standards, other regulations which can be used to limit car-cinogen exposure include standards requiring the removal of exposed workers and product-safety standards; besides OSHA, EPA and the Consumer Product Safety Commission are involved in the lat-ter. Although only eighty carcinogen exposure stan-dards have so far been promulgated, it is likely that these are beginning to influence the overall ap-proach of big industry to the handling of other car-cinogens and highly toxic substances.

† The author testified on behalf of OSHA on May 26.

are available, then continued use of the carcinogen could be banned completely. While emphasizing the goal of zero exposure, the OSHA proposals are flexible and include a wide range of regulatory options. These include continued use of the carcinogen with add-on pollution control devices, closed-system technologies, personal-control devices (in restricted conditions), product or process substitution, or ban.

Category II "suspect" classification is extended to chemicals found to be carcinogenic in a single animal test, in suggestive epidemiological studies, or in short term tests.‡ Continued use of these carcinogens will be allowed in the workplace subject to standards designed to limit but not prevent exposure. Category III is for chemicals about which there is suspicion but insufficient evidence of carcinogenicity. These will not be regulated, but will be listed in government documents for public information. Category IV is for any chemicals not used in the American workplace.

Preliminary review by OSHA of the 2,415 chemicals on the NIOSH list of suspect carcinogens indicates that about 270 fall into Category I. These include some exotic laboratory curiosities which are unlikely ever to be used in industry, and other various derivatives of the same carcinogen, such as various nickel salts. It is, however, likely that the number of carcinogens which will require regulation will be in excess of 100. It must be appreciated that workers are being currently exposed to such carcinogens in the absence of substantive regulatory controls. It is also estimated that there are about 196 carcinogens in Category II, many of which will require permanent standards, and about 300 chemicals in Category III.

While the proposed OSHA regulations are clearly a move in the right direction, not only for the protection of workers, but also the general public, they clearly do not go far enough. The burden of proof for elucidating the status of Category II carcinogens appears to fall on government and the worker, and continued exposure is permitted during the interim period. Additionally, the proposals contain broad "rebuttal" powers that allow OSHA to decide on a wide range of poorly defined grounds whether the carcinogenicity data are appropriate and relevant.*

Industry has reacted negatively to these proposals, criticizing the scientific basis of the standards and invoking the familiar specter of impossibly high costs. Industry reaction, however, has been far from uniform. Rohm and Haas and Hardwicke Chemical Company have both agreed that the policy is generally "feasible and workable."[49]

In a concerted effort to fight these proposals, the Manufacturing Chemists Association has set up a special task force, the American Industrial Health Council, that represents some hundred and twenty companies and sixty trade associations and has raised funds in excess of $1 million.† In January, 1978, the council produced a misleading and anonymous

---

‡ OSHA is given discretion as to how results from short-term tests can be used.

* The latitude allowed by the regulations is so wide that, in reality, few issues can be totally excluded from rule-making. Additionally, OSHA plans to conduct an individual notice and comment procedure for each of the 270 Class I carcinogens prior to the issuance of emergency temporary standards.

† Approximately one quarter of the Council's budget has been directed to "scientific" activities, and about one third to an economic impact analysis

(by Booz, Allen, and Hamilton) of the "generic" regulations. Dow Chemical Company is exercising a role of leadership in the Council's activities similar to that it assumed on behalf of the chemical industry in attempts to defeat Toxic Substances legislation. The Council is chaired by Dow's Orrefice, and the treasurer, Keith McKennon, is also a Dow executive. The Council has made no secret of its intent to fight any attempt by EPA and the Consumer Product Safety Commission to establish "generic" type cancer standards.

document which minimizes the significance and extent of cancer due to industrial chemicals (ignoring the fact that the majority of industries have not been evaluated for carcinogenic hazards), backed by voluminous statements from other industry and its academic consultants, attempting rebuttal of the OSHA position.[50] The apparent intent is to preclude effective regulation of occupational carcinogens and to play down the public health impact of carcinogenic industrial chemicals in the workplace and general environment.

On September 15, 1978, HEW Secretary Califano released a blue ribbon HEW draft document, "Estimates of the Fraction of Cancer in the United States Related to Occupational Factors," prepared by ten internationally recognized and leading scientific authorities in chemical carcinogenesis, epidemiology, and biostatistics in the NCI, NIEHS, NIOSH, and the International Agency for Research on Cancer. The document concludes:

1. The estimates that only 1-5 percent of total cancers in the United States are attributable to occupational factors have not been scientifically documented and have little meaning for estimating even short-term future risks.

2. Most cancers have multiple causes: It is a reductionist error and not in keeping with current theories of cancer causation to attempt to assign each cancer to an exclusive single cause.

3. Because cancer incidence is strongly dependent on age and duration of exposure, and because most cancers occur late in life, many industrial epidemiological studies detect only a small fraction of cancers (i.e., those developing early).

4. Past exposure to asbestos is expected to result in up to 2 million excess cancer deaths in the next three decades: This would correspond to roughly 13-18 percent of the total cancer mortality expected in that period.

5. Reasonable projections of the future consequences of past exposure to established carcinogens suggested that at least five of them (benzene, arsenic, chromium, nickel oxides, and petroleum fractions) may be comparable in their total effects to asbestos.

6. These projections suggest that occupationally related cancers may comprise as much as 20 percent or more of total cancer mortality in forthcoming decades. Asbestos alone will probably contribute up to 13-18 percent, and the data (on the other five carcinogens) suggest at least 10-20 percent more. These data do not include effects of radiation, or effects of a number of other known chemical carcinogens.

7. Although exposure to some of the more important occupational carcinogens has been reduced in recent years, there are still many unregulated carcinogens in the U.S. workplaces; a number of occupations are characterized by excess cancer risks that have not yet been attributed to specific agents.

8. There is no sound reason to assume that the future consequences of present-day exposure to carcinogens in the workplace will be less than those of exposure in the recent past.

9. Patterns and trends in total cancer incidence (and mortality) in the U.S. are consistent with the hypothesis that occupationally related cancers comprise a substantial and increasing fraction of total cancer incidence.

10. The conclusion that a substantial fraction of cancers in the United States are occupationally related is not inconsistent with conclusions that a substantial fraction of cancers are also associated with other factors, such as cigarette smoking and diet.

11. Occupationally related cancers offer

important opportunities for prevention.

The HEW document (whose publication in final draft form is anticipated in 1979), is the first scientifically supported and detailed estimate of the importance of occupational carcinogens. This is in contrast to the undocumented earlier "guesstimates" of others, including the American Industrial Health Council, which have consistently failed to supply any data base on the numbers of carcinogen-exposed workers in U.S. industries. The statistical basis for the exposure calculations in the HEW document is derived from the NIOSH 1972 National Occupational Hazards Survey, based on a sample of 4,700 establishments out of an approximate 5 million total.

The document fully recognizes the importance of known non-occupational carcinogens (especially tobacco). The document also clearly recognizes the following considerations: that the major impact of occupational carcinogens is still in the future; that multiple factors (such as asbestos or uranium and smoking) may be involved in certain occupational cancers (and therefore the document analyzes associations between carcinogens and cancer, rather than necessarily implying exclusive causality); that relatively few epidemiological studies on cancer risk have been undertaken on an industry-wide basis; and that of the few epidemiological studies that have been done and published, the majority underestimate cancer risk as their cohorts have been followed for relatively short periods (as opposed to workers' lifetimes). However, the HEW document itself clearly underestimates the cancer risk from occupational carcinogens. It fails to take into account radiation; carcinogenic exposure of agricultural workers; a wide range of epidemiologically known occupational chemical carcinogens other than just the six considered, quite apart from a wider range still of carcinogens identified in animal tests; and cancer in the general public (community cancer) occurring as a result of discharge or escape of occupational carcinogens into the air, water, and hazardous waste disposal sites of the surrounding community.

Another important action by OSHA has been the proposal of a labeling standard which would require industry to identify by trade and chemical name, hazardous chemicals to which workers are exposed. A chemical would be considered hazardous that appears on any list such as the NIOSH list of suspect carcinogens. However, identification would not be required for untested chemicals, to which exposure could continue without the workers' knowledge. NIOSH has estimated that 90 percent of the chemicals in trade-name products to which workers are exposed are not identified by the industries concerned. The chemical manufacturers have "fought tooth and nail" to insist that this is the concern of industry and nobody else.[51] There is, in fact, ample basis in the General Duty Clause and other sections of the 1970 Occupational Safety and Health Act to mandate disclosure and to develop appropriate safeguards in those rare instances in which trade secrets may be involved.

The failure of the Occupational Safety and Health Act to fully address the issue of access to proprietary data (on product ingredients and process technology), although several provisions of the Act such as the record-keeping requirements relate to it, is compounded by a longstanding body of state and federal law which impedes efforts at disclosure. Furthermore, while NIOSH may by subpoena require disclosure of product ingredients during hazard investigation,‡ it is unclear whether these data can be made available to OSHA for regulatory purposes. In an effort to resolve these ambiguities, in July, 1978, OSHA issued a "Proposed Rule of Access to Employee Exposure and Medical Records"

---

‡ See *E. I. Du Pont de Nemours and Co. v. Finklea* (S.D.W. Va., December 20, 1977), 6 OSHC 1167.

which requires that the employer shall make available to each employee, former employee, or designated representative all relevant exposure and medical records. Such information should enable more clear recognition of the nature and identity of particular occupational hazards, and thus allow OSHA and labor to attempt their control. Industry has protested on several grounds, including that the rule will involve them in excessive paper work and that making the required information available will create confusion and alarm. Irrespective of OSHA initiatives, Toxic Substances legislation, once fully implemented (particularly in its pre-market notification and testing requirements), is likely to be the major regulatory method for identifying occupational carcinogens, though not necessarily in tracking them through the pipeline from manufacture to trade name products.

Bingham has also developed close working relationships with EPA, FDA, and the Consumer Product Safety Commission with whom, in October, 1977, she set up an interagency agreement to develop consolidated approaches to the regulation of toxic chemicals, including sharing resources and instituting compatible testing and compliance procedures.

In May 1978, Bertram Cottine, former attorney for the Health Research Group and assistant to Eula Bingham for the last year, won Senate confirmation as one of three members of the Occupational Safety and Health Review Commission following prolonged debate and vigorous opposition from national industrial organizations.

Outstanding problems which OSHA still has to resolve include the major difficulties in enforcing the Occupational Safety and Health Act in small businesses, as well as problems of employee-initiated inspections in non-unionized shops. Industry has fought hard to penalize employees who invoke their OSHA rights, docking their pay for time spent accompanying inspectors or firing them outright. An additional problem that OSHA must now contend with is posed by the Supreme Court (Barlow) decision of May 23, 1978, requiring OSHA inspectors to obtain search warrants before making "surprise" inspections in those instances where an employer does not voluntarily agree. However, OSHA will not have to show "probable cause" when it suspects that an employer is guilty of some violation. Surprisingly enough, the Barlow decision has not yet had any impact on plant inspections. From May 23 until September 15, 1978, only about 612 of 59,171 inspections (1 percent) initiated by Federal and state health and safety compliance officers have been refused entry, presumably because of a lack of warrant. The decision has, however, imposed an increased administrative burden on the Solicitor's office.*

Another major problem posed to OSHA is the recent Fifth Circuit Court's decision (now under appeal to the Supreme Court) overturning the 1 ppm benzene standard, that economic feasibility is a prime determinant in standard setting, and that the government must make a specific "estimate of benefits supported by substantial evidence," before any standard can be promulgated. This ruling is in conflict with a wide range of previous legal decisions in which the courts have sustained standards even though OSHA had been unable to determine the precise effect of low-level exposure and thus to make the finding required by the Fifth Circuit (but not by

---

* The American Conservative Union, which paid more than $100 thousand in legal fees for Ferrol G. Barlow (a master plumber from Pocatello, Idaho) in his battle to bar OSHA inspectors, has contacted 170,000 employees previously inspected by OSHA in their *Stop OSHA* project, suggesting that they demand warrants before allowing inspections. In May, 1979, Melvin Booher, owner of a small lead-recycling company in Toledo, Ohio, was jailed for seven days for refusing entry to inspectors; three of his twenty employees had blood lead levels over 118 μg/ 100 ml.

the other Circuits) as to the extent of benefits that will result from reducing exposure to the lowest feasible level. The conflict created by the Fifth Circuit's decision requires immediate resolution. As of January, 1979, there are pending before Courts of Appeals three challenges to OSHA standards: inorganic arsenic (Ninth Circuit); cotton dust (Fifth and Third Circuits); and lead (D.C. Circuit). The validity of these standards, affecting hundreds of workplaces and thousands of workers, is at stake. Additionally at stake is the future of OSHA's proposal for "generic" regulation of occupational carcinogens. If the Supreme Court fails to resolve this conflict in OSHA's favor, industry by filing first with the Fifth Circuit will be able to use the benzene decision to defeat any new OSHA standard. Industry, however, will be unable to do this if the first petition is filed in other Circuits upholding the right of government to set standards without first proving benefits. As pointed out in the December, 1978, Industrial Union Department, AFL-CIO, benzene petition to the Supreme Court:

> The mischief created by this situation was recently highlighted by a courthouse race which ended in a dead heat when those who thought the new standard governing occupational exposure to lead (50 μg/m³) went too far filed in the Fifth Circuit while those who felt the standard did not go far enough simultaneously filed in the Third Circuit.

OSHA's ability to implement the Occupational Safety and Health Act is also critically limited by a shortage of trained personnel (particularly industrial hygienists, epidemiologists, and clinicians). Of a total of 1,000 OSHA inspectors, only 250 are trained occupational hygienists capable of conducting full-scale safety and health inspections; 85 percent of all 1977 inspections were for safety, and 17 percent for health. This contrasts with the approximately 4,500 trained hygienists working

for industry (approximately one tenth of which number work for organized labor). Personnel problems aside, OSHA also lacks adequate instrumentation to monitor carcinogens effectively in any but a very small number of the numerous workplaces covered by OSHA regulations. OSHA's compliance and enforcement abilities are similarly restricted by lack of intramural resources in industrial technological innovation (such as product and process substitution), and by inadequate allocations for R&D in new technologies for carcinogen control ($178,000 in 1979). The New Directions Program does, however, offer OSHA the possibility of developing extramural resources in pollution control R&D. NCI's contribution to this critical area is similarly meager, and is restricted to a few contracts on pollution control R&D (Stanford Research Institute has produced three documents on carcinogens (DES, vinyl chloride, and asbestos) under contract to NCI, which include analyses of control strategies for occupational and non-occupational exposures). EPA, however, does support considerable research on pollution control technology, some of which is relevant to occupational exposures. It is, however, clear that (for reasons that include limited federal resources, the concentration of such resources in industry, and the large number of workplaces to be regulated) OSHA must rely on voluntary compliance and the affirmative duties of industry, both under the Occupational Safety and Health Act and Toxic Substances legislation.

The Environmental Protection Agency (EPA). The current administrator, Douglas M. Costle, was appointed on March 11, 1977. Costle, formerly a member of the Congressional Budget Office staff and head of the Connecticut Department of Environmental Protection, also served in 1969 on the Presidential Ash Committee, which had a major role in designing the EPA.

EPA has extensive legislative authority to control carcinogens under six separate statutes. This includes three media-type laws, the Clean Air Act, the Federal Water Pollution Control Act, and the Resource Conservation and Recovery Act, and three product-type laws, the Federal Insecticide, Fungicide, and Rodenticide Act, the Safe Drinking Water Act, and the Toxic Substances Control Act.

1. *The Clean Air Act.* This 1970 Act provides broad authority for establishing primary ambient air quality standards for dispersed pollutants from stationary and mobile sources, performance standards for stationary sources, regulations for fuel additives, and emission standards for hazardous air pollutants. Section 112 of the Act is designed for the strict and uniform regulation of hazardous air pollutants, those which pose risks of serious adverse effects, particularly cancer, at relatively low exposure levels.[52] While EPA has discretionary authority for listing an air pollutant as hazardous, it has shown a strong reluctance to do so, as opposed to achieving controls through more flexible provisions of the Act. Once a substance is designated as a hazardous pollutant, mandatory rule-making procedures are put into effect within one year. (This is the shortest time required by any pollution legislation, involving preparation of a criteria document and proposing and promulgating a standard.)

Emission standards have been developed for only four hazardous air pollutants including mercury, and three carcinogens, beryllium and asbestos in April, 1973, and VC in October, 1976. In addition, EPA proposed a benzene standard in 1977. However, it is questionable how meaningful these standards really are. That for asbestos is based only on visible emissions and the use of work practices, such as wetting down buildings during demolition, and tends to be more honored in the breach than in the performance. The VC

standard is supposed to limit emissions from all sources to the limits of best available technology, but excludes the innumerable PVC fabrication plants scattered all over the country. Recognizing these various problems, the Environmental Defense Fund petitioned EPA in June, 1977, for more stringent standard setting, with the goal of zero emissions for carcinogenic hazardous pollutants.

2. *The Federal Water Pollution Control Act.* This 1948 law, amended in 1972 and 1977, is one of the most complex and extensive pieces of environmental legislation ever passed, and perhaps the most difficult to administer.[53] Its philosophy is that all water pollution is undesirable and should be reduced to the extent technology allows, rather than to the extent dictated by health considerations alone. Like the Clean Air Act, the Water Pollution Control Act contains a wide range of provisions: new source standards (Section 306), oil and hazardous substances regulation (Section 311), water quality standards (Section 303), water quality related effluent standards (Section 302), and toxic effluent standards (Section 307).

Toxic effluent standards are aimed primarily at limiting the industrial discharge of toxic pollutants that can induce cancer and other serious effects.† The standard takes into account problems of persistence and pollutant degradability in water. However, there is a built-in contradiction in a standard which must be set, regardless of economic considerations, at a level which provides an "ample margin of safety," knowing full well that there is no known safe level for any carcinogen.

In 1973, EPA listed nine pollutants under Section 307 and, following a consent agreement stemming from extensive litigation with public interest groups and industry, promulgated standards for six carcinogenic toxic water

---

† Industrial discharge from point sources are regulated by the National Permit Discharge Elimination System. This system, however, cannot be used to regulate non-point sources of pollution such as agricultural runoff of pesticides and fertilizers and municipal stormwater runoff.

pollutants in 1977: DDT, aldrin, dieldrin, toxaphene, endrin, PCBs, and benzidine. Zero effluent limits were set for DDT and aldrin/dieldrin, which EPA had already banned, while numerical limits were set for effluents of benzidine and PCB. Under the consent agreement, EPA has designated about 140 other toxic pollutants subject to control by "best available technology" in 21 priority industries.

3. *The Resource Conservation and Recovery Act.* This 1976 Act, which amends the Solid Waste Disposal Act, creates a regulatory framework to control hazardous wastes. The Act is designed to comprehensively regulate hazardous wastes, particularly those contaminated by carcinogens, from generation through transport to disposal, and management of disposal sites. The Act does not, however, consider proximity of these sites to inhabited areas or potential adverse effects of toxic runoff to water. The Act aims to systematize the chaotic and inconsistent regulation of hazardous waste-disposal sites at a state level. Currently, forty-six states have some regulatory authority over hazardous waste disposal, although only California fully implements a hazardous waste program. Only fourteen states have designated hazardous waste-disposal sites, of which there are estimated to be over 1,000 nationwide, and only one of these sites (in Massachusetts) is located in an eastern state, where over 40 percent of the nation's hazardous wastes are generated. The

proposed regulations containing minimal criteria for determining which solid waste land disposal facilities shall be classified as having no reasonable probability of adverse effects on health or the environment were published by EPA in the Federal Register on February 6, 1978, followed by a notice of proposed rule-making on December 18. EPA was required by the Act to have promulgated these standards by April 1978. However, it is unlikely that they will be issued prior to January, 1980.‡

A November, 1978, EPA study was undertaken for an interagency task force created to investigate the Love Canal crisis (R. P. Whalen, New York State Commissioner of Health, "Love Canal: Public Health Time Bomb." A Special Report to the Governor and Legislature of the State of New York, September, 1978). This reported that there are more than 30,000 sites, many of which since abandoned by their owners, where toxic wastes may have been improperly dumped. EPA also identified 103 specific sites, including municipal landfills, industrial dumps, and abandoned mining sites, where potential health hazards have already been documented. The agency report concludes that improper disposal of hazardous and carcinogen-containing wastes may be widespread and "constitutes an extremely serious environmental problem." Administrator Costle further commented that such improper disposal affects as much as 90 percent of all hazardous wastes.*

‡ In September, 1978, Illinois Attorney General William J. Scott filed suit against EPA for having failed to issue these regulations, asking that EPA be required to develop these within the next 30 days. ("Wilsonville Battles a Landfill." Special Staff Report, Illinois Issues, August, 1977, pp. 4-6.) In his suit, Scott stated that disposal of toxic wastes in Illinois, which he has repeatedly called the "dumping ground of the nation," is going to become one of the biggest problems in the country in the near future unless it can be controlled.
* Stimulated by the Love Canal disaster, two bills to amend the Resource Conservation and Recov-

ery Act were introduced in October, 1978, by Rep. John L. LaFalce (D-N.Y.): H.R. 14338, which establishes a program for identification and reclamation of abandoned hazardous waste sites and provides for a process for the selection of future sites for hazardous waste disposal; and H.R. 14301, "Toxic Pollution Compensation Act," designed to provide non-exclusive Federal relief to all persons injured as a result of toxic pollutants and to ameliorate the burden of proof and statute of limitation requirements, while retaining the fault concept that will enable recovery of compensation payments from individuals or industries responsible.

4. *Federal Insecticide, Fungicide, and Rodenticide Act.* Passed in 1947, this Act was designed to protect consumers from ineffective products and to warn with appropriate labels against toxic effects, without consideration of carcinogenic and other chronic toxic or ecological effects. The Pesticide Regulation Division of USDA failed to enforce even these minimal requirements. This contributed to the decision to transfer regulatory authority for pesticides to EPA after its creation in 1970.[54] The thrust of this move was, however, blunted by the simultaneous transfer to EPA of USDA Pesticide Regulation Division personnel. These personnel were regrouped in the EPA Office of Pesticide Programs, where they have perpetuated USDA traditions of excessive protection of agrichemical interests at the expense of other considerations. In this, they have been further aided by the USDA, which has supported industry against EPA in all major proceedings to ban carcinogenic pesticides.

An additional serious problem which has adversely influenced EPA pesticide policies was and is the congressional jurisdiction which the House and Senate agriculture committees continued to exercise after the transfer of regulatory authority for pesticides from USDA to EPA.[55] The agriculture committees have traditionally been preoccupied with narrowly focused agrichemical interests and have failed to grasp the need to regulate pesticides to protect public health and the environment. On occasions when EPA seems about to deal decisively with a pesticide problem, the agriculture committees threaten to cancel its authority over pesticides and to transfer it back to USDA.

An example of the power exercised by the House Agriculture Committee is the 1976 bill H.R. 8841, amending the 1947 Act, which, as passed in a somewhat modified form by Congress, severely restricts the authority of EPA to regulate pesticides. The thrust of H.R. 8841 is to give the Secretary of Agriculture

virtual veto power over EPA's suspension and cancellation decisions. EPA is required to notify USDA at least sixty days prior to proposing any pesticide regulations and also to similarly notify the House Committee on Agriculture and the Senate Committee on Agriculture and Forestry. EPA is further required to publish any comments of the USDA in the Federal Register at the same time of publication of final regulations. These seemingly harmless provisions carry the implicit threat of political reprisals if EPA ignores unfavorable comments by USDA on proposed pesticide regulations.

The exclusive jurisdiction of the agriculture committees over pesticide regulation by EPA is further anomalous in view of the fact that about half of all pesticide usage in the United States is for non-agricultural purposes (See Table 7.2). Strong public support is needed to ensure that the House and Senate commerce committees, which represent more broadly based interests, be given a share in the congressional authority over pesticides.

The 1947 Act was substantively amended in 1972, by the Federal Environmental Pesticide Control Act (FEPCA).[56] The amendments express the intent of protecting against "unreasonable adverse effects on man or the environment," and place the burden of producing evidence of safety on the manufacturer. The manufacturer is required to produce evidence of safety and effectiveness when petitioning EPA for registration of products. Pesticides can then be classified for general use or for restricted use by trained applicators only. Registrations are automatically cancelled after five years, unless the manufacturer reapplies with updated information. EPA has the power to suspend manufacture on an emergency interim basis if "imminent hazard" can be proven. Otherwise, banning is by a protracted adjudicatory hearing that can stretch over years, during which the pesticide can be used without hindrance. EPA also has responsibility for setting tolerance levels of pesticide residues on foods, which are then enforced by the FDA.

Over the past eight years, EPA has taken regulatory action against only a handful of pesticides. Some of these were no longer in production at the time of the action, such as octamethylphosphoramide, and some of these actions were initiated at the manufacturer's request, as was the case with safrole (also used as a flavoring agent in root beer). The agency has undertaken successful proceedings only against DDT, aldrin/dieldrin, Mirex chlordane/heptachlor, and VC (used as a propellant in pesticide aerosols). However, all these latter actions were only initiated under threat of legal action by public interest groups (Table 9.5).

These limited regulatory actions taken by the EPA aroused intense opposition from industry, supported by the congressional agriculture committees. In July 1975, EPA announced new regulations for re-registration of all currently used pesticides and for registration of new pesticides.[57] This move coincided with an internal reorganization of pesticide policy in EPA in November, 1974, which effectively wiped out any authority for the Office of General Counsel and gave almost exclusive authority to the Office of Pesticide Programs. The new regulations defined EPA's understanding of "unreasonable adverse effects on man or the environment" in terms of chronic toxic, mutagenic or carcinogenic effects. Pesticides producing these effects are subject to a "Rebuttable Presumption Against Registration" (RPAR). The manufacturer is given ninety days to rebut this presumption on grounds that include the risks being outweighed by the benefits, following which EPA is required to take final action within six months. While in principle this approach may be sound, the agency's implementation of the new regulations can only be regarded as public window dressing. So far, EPA has initiated RPARs against about forty-five pesticides, none of which however, has yet been brought to final action.† In three instances, the pesticides concerned, endrin, chlorobenzilate, and chloroform (an "inert" pesticide ingredient) are carcinogenic.

EPA's record on regulation of pesticide residues in food is as gravely deficient as its record of pesticide regulation.[58] EPA is responsible for establishing all tolerances for pesticide residues on the basis of data submitted by industry as to the nature, level, and toxicity of the residue. Any residue on food is considered unsafe unless a tolerance has been established and the remaining residue is within the limits of tolerance. Authority is shared with

---

† With the exception of voluntary cancellations of kepone and DBCP, EPA has initiated no cancellation proceedings against any pesticide since November, 1974. An illustrative example of non-action on an RPAR candidate is the case of the herbicide 2,4,5-T, a chemical with a tortuous regulatory history. In 1969, the Mrak Commission recommended that this (and its related derivatives, including 2,4-D), be banned because it induced birth defects (teratogenic). Even though a petition for suspension (followed by a law suit) was subsequently filed with the USDA in 1970 by Nader's Center for the Study of Responsive Law, it was not until 1974 that the EPA canceled most uses of 2,4,5-T. However, the day before the adjudicatory hearing was to have begun, EPA withdrew the cancellation notice and postponed the hearing indefinitely on the grounds that they did not have adequate monitoring data for TCDD, the toxic contaminant of 2,4,5-T, in the environment and human tissues. While EDF denounced this move, as the EPA's assumption of the legal burden of proof which should properly rest with the manufacturer, EPA has continued the stance of not being able to take action on this herbicide until indisputable evidence of human contamination exists. However, every time monitoring programs reveal TCDD residues, be it in beef fat or in human breast milk, industry takes exception to the findings and EPA announces that it will perform yet another test, a procedure that takes one or two more years. While independent scientists and environmentalists claim there is currently more than adequate evidence to suspend,

the FDA, which is responsible for enforcing pesticide tolerances by testing food samples. FDA can remove from interstate products any food containing residues in excess of established tolerances.

A 1975 report to Congress entitled "Federal Pesticide Regulation Program: Is It Protecting the Public and the Environment Adequately from Pesticide Hazards?" showed that EPA established many tolerances without sufficient test data to determine levels of pesticide residues on crops and the potential of the pesticide to induce carcinogenic and other toxic effects.[59] Further, EPA registered pesticides for use on food and feed crops without setting tolerances.

As of May, 1976, EPA had examined about 890 of the approximately 1,400 active ingredients of over 40,000 pesticide products.‡[60] Only about 419 ingredients examined had sufficient backup data to allow any assessment of risk, and of these, about 238 fell in a high risk category, 80 percent of which were "suspect carcinogens." These suspect carcinogens are incorporated in about one-third of all pesticide products currently on the market.

In 1976, an EPA consultant reviewed carcinogenicity test data on twenty-four pesticides with the highest tolerances on common

foods. His report concluded that, with the possible exception of data on one pesticide, all other data which EPA had used to set tolerances were so inadequate and defective that no reasonable conclusions could be drawn from them.[61]

EPA seems to have effectively eliminated oversight of its pesticide policies at the agency level by disbanding the Federal Working Group on Pesticides and the Pesticide Policy Advisory Committee. However, in April, 1977, EPA informed the General Accounting Office that its Science Advisory Board had been asked to study the tolerance-setting program. A subcommittee appointed for this purpose met first in February, 1978, and submitted a sharply critical preliminary report in October, 1978.*

Meanwhile, EPA has made little serious attempt to rectify the deficiencies in its tolerance setting programs as indicated in a 1978 General Accounting Office report which concluded "that the American public had not been adequately protected from the potential hazards of pesticide use because of inadequate efforts to implement existing Federal laws."[62]

During the 1977-78 congressional proceedings to reauthorize EPA's pesticide authority, the Office of Pesticide Programs, with enthusiastic industry support, formulated and suc-

---

2,4,5,-T under the RPAR procedure and hence eliminate exposure to TCDD (the most potent carcinogen known to man, one hundred million times more potent than saccharin and ten times more potent than aflatoxin), EPA seems to be waiting for further indisputable evidence of human toxicity. Following disclosures of excess numbers of miscarriages in Alsea, Oregon, women who had been exposed to repeated spraying with 2,4,5-T and 2,4-D by the Forestry Service, on March 1, 1979, EPA announced emergency suspension of 2,4,5-T and Silvex, but not of 2,4-D, for major agricultural uses, excluding rice fields and cattle rangelands. While emphasizing the hazards of TCDD as a contaminant of 2,4,5-T and Silvex, EPA, however, failed to make any reference to 2,4-D and the probability of its incrimination in the miscarriages. On April 2, a fed-

eral court in Flint, Michigan, denied a request by Dow Chemical to delay the suspension.

‡ Twenty-five basic ingredients account for about 75 percent of total agricultural sales. The Office of Pesticide Programs, in a misleading numbers game, has claimed that as many as 40,000 pesticides (formulations) will need to be reviewed for the registration process, rather than just the few hundred (active ingredients) properly requiring review.

* At this meeting, the author (as a member of this subcommittee) raised questions as to the validity of the industrial data based on pesticide toxicology. In a private letter of November 30 to EPA Administrator Costle, Jack Early, President of the National Agricultural Chemicals Association, complained that this was insulting and harassing to industry scientists.

cessfully advocated a series of weakening amendments to the 1972 Pesticide Act (the Federal Pesticide Act of 1978, P.L. 95-396). EPA now has authority to grant three types of conditional registrations: to pesticides identical or substantially similar to current registered pesticides (many of which have been previously registered on the basis of inadequate or defective data); to pesticides with new ingredients not contained in currently registered pesticides; and to pesticides that are registered, but for which new uses are sought. Public health concerns on "conditional registration" largely reflect the broad and virtually unrestricted authority given the agency.† As such, this amendment could effectively negate the registration requirements of the 1972 Act in that it permits potentially hazardous and extensive public exposure from continued or new uses of pesticides for which safety and related data have not yet been generated or, if on file with the agency, have not yet been reviewed for adequacy and validity. "Minor Use Registration" is another weakening amendment that allows considerations of "economic factors" relating to costs of providing safety, residue chemistry, and related data to influence the agency's requirements for registration of pesticides for "minor uses." Such registration would subsidize the industry at the expense of potential public health costs, particularly for those segments of the population with heavier than average consumption of minor crops. Perhaps the most dangerous of all amendments are those that grant new powers to states to register pesticides with minimal EPA supervision, and to enforce their regulation.

Even taking into account legislative ambiguities and pressures from industry and the congressional agriculture committees, the record of EPA on pesticides has been and continues to be unacceptable. The strictures of an earlier congressional report seem at least as apt now as when they were written:

> . . . pesticide regulation in the United States is fundamentally deficient. Pesticide regulation has failed to include many obvious and prudent steps to better protect public health and the environment. Moreover, the severe inadequacies of pesticide regulation are not attributable in any significant way to deficient legislation. Rather, the principal cause lies with EPA's poor administration of the program, including its failure to recognize and correct serious program deficiencies as they arose.[63]

5. *The Safe Drinking Water Act.* While the Federal Water Pollution Control Act is media-type legislation designed to limit the discharge of toxic pollutants into surface and other waters and to control pollutant levels, the Safe Drinking Water Act is a product-type legislation specifically designed to regulate the purity of treated drinking water. As pollutants discharged into surface water are likely to eventually find their way into drinking water unless they are unstable or infinitely diluted, it is unfortunate that there is not a greater consistency in the language and intents of the two laws.

The Safe Drinking Water Act was passed in 1974 in response to pressures by the Environmental Defense Fund and public alarm at the high levels of carcinogens and organic pollutants found in the drinking water of New Orleans. According to the Act, every community water supply serving twenty-five or more people must meet certain minimum standards of purity, thus involving a national total of about 40,000 community water supply systems. "National Interim Primary Drinking Water Regulations" went into effect in 1977, and cover ten chemicals, including the car-

---

† For an effective critique of conditional registration, see "Statement of the Environmental Defense Fund and the National Audubon Society at the November 6, 1978, Public Hearings on EPA's Interim Final Regulation of FIFRA as Amended, September 30, 1978."

cinogens arsenic, cadmium, chromium, endrin, lindane, toxaphene, and methoxychlor. Strangely, EPA's current informational pamphlet "Is Your Drinking Water Safe?" claims that "radioactivity is the only contaminant for which standards have been set that has been shown to cause cancer."

Concerns have been expressed about the finding of high levels of the carcinogenic chloroform in drinking water treated by chlorine. Chloroform and much higher levels of other related (trihalomethane) compounds, most of which are toxicologically active though still unidentified, are produced following chlorination of water heavily contaminated with organic pollutants.‡ The answer is not necessarily to stop chlorination, but to limit discharge of toxic and carcinogenic pollutants into surface waters, which ultimately reach drinking water supply systems, and also to effectively treat drinking water by passage through activated carbon filtration systems prior to its chlorination.

Responding to further pressures from the Environmental Defense Fund, in January, 1978, EPA proposed to regulate four of the main trihalomethanes, of which chloroform is typical, produced from organic pollutants by the chlorination of water, in order to reduce total levels of trihalomethanes to below 100 ppb.[64] EPA also proposed that all cities with more than 75,000 people should be required to design and operate a treatment system which uses granular activated carbon filters or an equivalent technology in order to reduce levels of synthetic organic pollutants to the maximum extent feasible. Variances can be granted only if it can be demonstrated that such treatment is unnecessary. Estimated

household costs for treatment range from $7 to $26 a year.

These proposals are part of a phased implementation program which, over time, will be expanded to cover all public water supplies in the United States. The proposals represent the most significant advances in drinking water treatment since passage of the 1976 Act. They represent the first serious attempt to control contamination of drinking water with synthetic organic contaminants.* It should be recalled that over 700 synthetic organic chemicals, including many carcinogens such as chloroform, carbon tetrachloride, benzene, vinyl chloride, lindane, aldrin, and bischloroethylether, have been identified in drinking water. The organic chemicals so far identified represent only a small fraction of total organic material in drinking water.

Illinois and some other states, backed by the American Water Works Association, are opposing these regulations on various grounds.[65] These include questioning the significance and public health relevance of the carcinogenicity of chloroform and other organic contaminants in water and asserting that the costs of carbon treatment are exorbitant. The position of the states reflects lack of appreciation of fundamental principles of environmental carcinogenesis and of the fact that failure to regulate creates costs greatly in excess of those of regulation.

6. *Toxic Substances Control Act.* Passage of the Act on October 11, 1976, culminated six years of bitter struggle during which a powerful industry lobby pulled out all stops to defeat this legislation.[66] The resistance was spearheaded by Dow Chemical Company and the Manufacturing Chemists Association,

---

‡ Resulting levels of chloroform and trihalomethanes in drinking water in general far exceed concentrations of other synthetic organic pollutants. Chloroform levels are approximately correlated with total organic carbon levels in water.

* Apart from chloroform and other trihalomethanes which are often found in the 100 ppb range, the other organics most commonly found in the low ppb range are pentachlorophenol, dichlorobenzene, trichloroethylene, carbon tetrachloride, and 1,2-dichloroethane.

which formed a semi-autonomous standing committee empowered to lobby without checking back to individual industries approval. This striking change from previous practices indicates the mood of crisis within the industry.

The legislation authorizes the EPA administrator to require information necessary for standard-setting on new chemicals and for chemicals in current use, with the exception of chemicals covered by other legislation.†[67] The legislation, while not authorizing the routine need for information, shifted the burden of proof away from the government and public and placed it firmly on the manufacturer. While the legislation is specifically directed to chemicals, it reflects patterns of use and distribution in the environment, water, air and the workplace, and is thus multimedia as well as product in type. Key provisions of the law are:

• Industry must give EPA ninety days notice before marketing a new chemical, including proposing "significant new uses" of existing chemicals. Data must be provided on structure, composition, uses, quantity to be produced, by-products of manufacture, health or environmental effects, and numbers of workers expected to be exposed. While some guidelines are offered on data that may be required on health effects, no such information is provided in the Act for environmental effects.

• EPA must draw up an inventory of existing chemicals to be exempted from pre-marketing notification requirements, but not necessarily from later challenges.‡

• Each year, an intergovernmental agency group (known as the Committee of Eight) will select no more than fifty potentially hazardous chemicals, particularly chemicals suspected of being carcinogens, and recommend priority for their testing to the administrator.

• Industry must keep records of significant adverse health effects caused by any chemical for thirty years and of environmental damage for five years.

• Chemicals produced in small quantities for research and development will be exempted from pre-market notification. So also will be small businesses, i.e., those with fewer than thirty employees at any one time.*

• Pesticides, tobacco, drugs, cosmetics, food additives, and nuclear materials are exempt from the law, since they are covered by other regulations.

• The Act allows petitions and suits from citizen and public interest groups who wish to challenge EPA decisions.

The main thrust of the law is that if, based on pre-market data, EPA believes a new chemical to be hazardous, within forty-five days the agency must give industry notice of intent to ban. EPA can also seek a court injunction restricting or banning chemicals it believes are "imminently hazardous," and can also take appropriate action against chemicals it considers "unreasonable risks."

This legislation is potentially the most important single preventive public health measure of the century.[68] For the first time, there is the opportunity of controlling industrial chemicals and anticipating carcinogenic and other adverse effects, rather than reacting to

---

† As consultant to the Senate Committee on Public Works, the author developed the first draft of a bill, "The Environmental Protection Act of 1971," which formed the basis of subsequent toxic substances legislation.

‡ Import of toxic chemicals is covered by the law, but inadequately so.

* This exemption allows the license to small business to handle toxic and carcinogenic chemicals and products with virtually no control other than that theoretically available under the Occupational Safety and Health Act. This highest risk group in the chemical industry is generally non-unionized and often transient and ethnic labor.

their occurrence.† However, there is little indication yet as to how well this potential for control will be exercised.

Congress initially allocated a first-year budget of $10 million for the Office of Toxic Substances in EPA, created to implement the new legislation. About 10 percent of the 1979 EPA budget ($5.63 billion) is allocated to the Toxic Substances program ($56.7 million), of which $4.2 million is for "Abatement and Control," $10.5 million for R&D, and $4.6 million for Enforcement. Even this increased figure is small compared to the $150 million budget of the first year of the Clean Air Act.

The costs to industry of toxic substances legislation were estimated in 1975 by EPA and the General Accounting Office to range from $80 to $200 million. These estimates contrast strikingly with estimates of $2 billion by the Manufacturing Chemists Association and Foster D. Snell. The maximal government estimate of $200 million, based largely on costs of carcinogenicity and chronic toxicity testing, represents about 0.3 percent of the chemical industry's total 1975 sales of $72 billion and 3.6 percent of its net profits after taxes of $6.5 billion.

Enforcing toxic substances legislation is probably the most complex and ambitious task any regulatory agency has ever had to face.‡ EPA has been slow to respond, and its toxic chemical program is still embryonic, although it is now attempting to scale up recruiting efforts for much needed professional personnel. So far, EPA has failed to encourage adequate public participation in its planning and activities.

The administration's concerns with inflation, together with the apparently waning interest of Congress, are now emerging as possible threats to the toxic chemical program, particularly in view of the legislative requirements of the Act to consider the costs and benefits of proposed regulation. Illustrative of the administration's position are the emphasis by Commerce Secretary Juanita M. Kreps and Robert Strauss, Special Presidential Counsel on Inflation, on the high costs of regulation to industry. Recent estimates by Chase Econometrics concluded that total costs of EPA programs add less than 0.4 percent annually to the consumer price index. However, as Costle recently pointed out, such estimates do not take into account improvements to public health, reduced property damage by air pollutants, increased crop yields, and many other benefits that result from pollution control spending.

Consumer Product Safety Commission. The Commission was established in 1973 by the Consumer Product Safety Act (CPSA), incorporating the Federal Hazardous Substances Act, the Flammable Fabrics Act, the Poison Prevention Packaging Act, and the Refrigerator Safety Act. The Commission was given responsibility for some 10,000 consumer products, excluding those (such as tobacco, drugs, pesticides, cosmetics, and foods) over which other agencies have jurisdiction. The Commission does not have authority to require pre-market registration of consumer products, and must therefore meet the burden of proving hazard due to "unreasonable risk of injury" before it can regulate.

Prior to the CPSA, Congress enacted product safety legislation haphazardly, reacting to specific hazards rather than adopting a broad product safety statute. With the passage of CPSA, responsibility for overall product

---

† For instance, this legislation affords a comprehensive basis for control of industrial uses of toxic and carcinogenic chemicals by setting occupational standards, with the concurrence of OSHA, and also regulating their emission into the surrounding community.

‡ A further example of the unresolved complexity of the legislation is the problem of alleged trade secrets and the interagency sharing of such secrets. Invoking trade secrecy is a key element in evolving industry strategies to fighting the legislation.

safety was consolidated within a single agency and many more consumer products became subject to regulatory authority than were previously covered by safety legislation. The Commission is specifically mandated by the CPSA to protect the public against unreasonable risks of injury from consumer products, to assist consumers in evaluating product safety, to develop standards for consumer products, to minimize conflicts of these standards at the Federal, state, and local level, and to promote research into the causes and prevention of product-related deaths, illnesses, and injuries. However, the Act is a poorly conceived attempt to fill in legislative "cracks." It is anachronistic in shifting the burden of proof from the manufacturer to the government, which must prove hazard before it can regulate. Statutory limitations aside, the Commission, in its early phases, has not been an aggressive regulator.

The Commission has become increasingly involved in the regulation of chronic, as well as acute, hazards posed by consumer products. In 1974, the Commission was petitioned by the Health Research Group to ban VC propellants in household aerosol products. However, the final order effectively banning such products was delayed until March, 1978, because an earlier order was successfully challenged in court on procedural grounds. In April, 1977, following a petition from the Environmental Defense Fund, the Commission banned the use of Tris as a flame retardant on children's sleepwear. While a court ruled against this action on procedural grounds, the Commission, however, proceeded against Tris garments in individual enforcement actions, and a federal appeals court has sustained this approach in an October, 1978, decision. The court additionally affirmed the Commission's authority to seize without first having a formal hearing in the district court, and also affirmed that the statute does not authorize post-seizure export. In December, 1977, the Commission issued a

final regulation banning consumer patching compounds and artificial emberizing materials (embers and ash) containing respirable freeform asbestos. Reacting to a May, 1977, petition from the Health Research Group and the Center for Occupational Hazards, in the following year the Commission proposed a ban of benzene-containing consumer products, except gasoline and laboratory benzene. The public comments on the proposal are currently being analyzed by Commission staff prior to a possible ban.

In June, 1978, the Commission issued an interim cancer policy statement based in general on the OSHA "generic proposals" concerning the classification, evaluation, and regulation of substances that, if present in consumer products, pose a carcinogenic risk to consumers. A court decision in November, 1978, however, enjoined the implementation of the classification aspect of the proposal, pending issuance of a final policy.

The Commission had come under substantial criticism from consumer groups and from some Congressmen for its regulatory tardiness. In December, 1977, the General Accounting Office issued a report criticizing the Commission for dragging its feet in developing and issuing safety standards and in setting priorities, and for keeping inadequate records on product-related injuries.[69] On February 8, 1978, the embattled chairman of the five-member Commission, S. John Byington, announced his resignation effective June 30, charging that he had been a victim of political harassment by the Carter administration.* His resignation was applauded by Rep. John E. Moss (D-Cal.) as "a very significant public service," and by Senator Wendell E. Ford (D-Ky.) as "in the best interests of the Agency."[70]

On July 1, 1978, Susan B. King succeeded Byington as Chairman, declaring her commitment to make the Commission a fair, but tough and effective regulatory agency. Chairman King has emphasized the need for the

---

* Byington was appointed chairman by President Ford in June, 1976.

Commission to focus its efforts on carcinogenic and other such hidden hazards to which populations are involuntarily exposed in consumer products. In addition to a new Chairman, two of the other four sitting Commissioners were appointed in 1978, and another vacancy will be created early in 1979. One indication of the Commission's new stance was the 1978 reversal (with respect to Tris-treated sleepwear) of its previous statutory interpretation that it lacked authority to ban export of hazardous substances.

Speculations as to the Commission's future were cut short on November 10, 1978, when President Carter signed into law a bill reauthorizing the Commission for three years. The Congress and the Administration have thus indicated their support for the new Commission leadership. A key test now facing Chairman King is her ability to attract quality talent to senior openings in her health sciences program.

Food and Drug Administration. The major regulatory authority of the FDA is mandated by the 1938 Federal Food, Drug, and Cosmetic Act, which gives the FDA authority over food additives, cosmetics, and drugs, all of which are regulated with distinct and differing philosophies and practices. The Act prohibits the marketing of food that contains a "natural or added substance which may render it injurious to health." The Act permits the addition of toxic substances to food within prescribed tolerance levels, but shifts the burden of proof to the manufacturer to show that the additive is safe under the conditions of proposed use.[71]

The 1938 Act was extended by the 1954 Pesticide Amendments, the 1958 Food Additive Amendments, including the Delaney Amendment, the 1960 Color Additives Amendments, and the 1962 Animal Drug or Feed Additive Amendments. The overall laws resulting from these various amendments are complex and inconsistent, especially with regard to the regulation of carcinogens.[72]

The 1958 Delaney anticancer clause is a straightforward piece of legislation, stating that

> no additive shall be claimed to be safe if it is found to induce cancer when ingested by man or animal, or if it is found after tests which are appropriate for the evaluation of safety of food additives to induce cancer in man or animal.[73]

This law reflected the then and currently prevailing scientific consensus that there is no known method for setting safe levels for human exposure to carcinogens.[74] The FDA is given authority only to determine whether the carcinogenicity tests are appropriate, then after these limits of bureaucratic discretion are reached an automatic set of rule-making procedures are invoked leading to a ban of the carcinogenic additive. The requirement for appropriate test methods can be used to exclude carcinogenic effects induced in animals from subcutaneous or intravenous injection of food additives. However, it would seem inappropriate on these grounds to try to exclude carcinogenic effects of additives administered to animals by gastric intubation, a standard practice in carcinogenicity tests, rather than in diets. Nevertheless, the FDA concluded in 1975 that such exemption could be valid.

Although invoked on several occasions, the Delaney anticancer clause has only been formally used twice or so for the purpose of banning a carcinogen: in 1967 for Flectol H and in 1969 for MOCA, both used in food packaging adhesives. The FDA has, however, used the broad statutory authority of general safety provisions of food law to ban several other carcinogens, including: the sweetener dulcin in 1950; coumarin, in Tonka Bean Extracts, in 1954; safrole in 1960; oil of calamus in 1968; the sweetener cyclamate in 1969; diethylpyrocarbonate in 1972; the animal drug DES in 1972; mercaptoimidazoline in 1973; Violet #1 in 1973; and FD&C Red #2 in 1976.

There are many loopholes in the legislative

definition of a food additive that exempt a wide range of carcinogens from the requirements of the Delaney Amendment.†

1. Pesticide residues: These are not defined as food additives. EPA has authority to set tolerances in food for carcinogenic pesticides.

2. Unavoidable or unintentional contaminants: Like pesticides, these are exempt. Most common examples are PCBs, benzo[a]pyrene and other such polycyclic compounds formed during broiling, and chemicals migrating from food packaging materials. Additionally, FDA does not require carcinogenicity testing of unintentional additives derived from packaging materials, some 10,000 of which have been approved for use, unless they are present in concentrations over 1 ppm, and unless the FDA believes there is valid reason to suspect carcinogenicity.

3. Prior-sanction additives: By a "grandfather clause," additives sanctioned by the FDA prior to September 6, 1958, are exempt.

4. GRAS additives: Additives "generally recognized as safe" by experts prior to January, 1958, are not regarded as additives from the Delaney standpoint.

5. Color additives in use before July, 1960: Under a "grandfather clause" of the 1960 Color Additive Amendments, color additives in prior use can be provisionally listed for a period of two and a half years to allow completion of tests. The FDA is allowed to extend this period "in good faith" if necessary. Using this stratagem, FDA extended the provisional listing of Red #2 fifteen times from 1960 to 1965, before its final ban in January, 1976.

6. Animal drugs without prohibited residues: The 1962 Feed Additive Amendment (or the DES clause) allows administration to cattle of carcinogenic drugs or feed additives, such as DES, provided no residues can be detected in meat or animal food products. This special-interest legislation was exploited to the utmost by successive FDA commissioners to allow continued use of DES even though residues were consistently detected from the late 1960s until its ban in 1973, a ban which was, however, overturned on procedural grounds.

The 1938 Act created a specific exemption for coal-tar dyes, provided they are appropriately labeled. The FDA cannot now ban them, even though their carcinogenicity has been recently proven. However, congressional moves which will probably abolish this exemption are now pending.

FDA also has authority for enforcing tolerances on foods set by EPA for pesticides and toxic chemicals. It accomplishes this by testing samples of food to determine if there are residues exceeding tolerance levels, in which case the food can be banned and penalties on violators can be imposed. However, a 1975 General Accounting Office Report criticized the FDA tolerance program for failing to test food for residues of 179 out of 233 pesticides for which tolerances were set.[75] A subsequent General Accounting Office Report in 1978 demonstrated that the FDA had failed to rectify these serious deficiencies.[76] Of 268 pesticides with a total of 5,872 individuals' tolerances on various foods, only 38 percent can be detected by currently used FDA multi-residue techniques. Also, 940 of these 5,872 tolerances are for pesticides which are either carcinogenic or suspected of being carcinogenic. About 70 percent of these carcinogens or suspect carcinogens cannot be detected by FDA monitoring techniques. FDA Commissioner Kennedy in subsequent testimony on February 24, 1978, recognized various of these deficiencies in FDA's moni-

---

† In spite of such regulatory flexibility, the FDA announced in February, 1979, that it plans to seek relaxation of the Delaney Amendment and other federal food safety laws to allow the setting of "acceptable low levels of (carcinogenic) risk (in a) very small" number of cases on the basis of benefit-risk considerations.

toring program. He indicated his intent to institute various reforms, including more effective coordination with USDA and EPA.

Cosmetics are treated differently from food additives under the Federal Food, Drug, and Cosmetic Act. The burden of demonstrating carcinogenic or other hazards is placed on the FDA. Following petitions by the Health Research Group, the FDA banned the use of VC as a propellant in cosmetics in 1974 and of chloroform as an ingredient in cosmetics in 1976, both on grounds of carcinogenicity. While there is no requirement for manufacturers to undertake toxicological testing of cosmetic ingredients prior to marketing, current labeling laws of the FDA require untested products to be clearly labeled as such.[77]

Drug law is as different from food law as is cosmetic law.[78] Unlike food law, which is based on hazard alone, drug law allows consideration of matching benefits. The 1938 Act requires that drugs be "adequately tested to show that they are safe for use under conditions of use prescribed in their labeling." The 1962 Kefauver-Harris Amendments require formal proof of effectiveness and authorizes banning on grounds of "imminent hazard." There are, however, no formal requirements for carcinogenicity testing of drugs before clinical trials are undertaken. Carcinogenic drugs can be used for both medical purposes, such as Flagyl for trichomonas vaginal infections and griseofulvin for athlete's foot and other superficial fungal infections, and for non-medical purposes, such as oral contraceptives.

The current commissioner, Donald Kennedy, was appointed to the FDA on April 8, 1977. Kennedy, a Stanford University biologist, has already made significant impact on an agency whose past record of protection of consumer interests has been grossly deficient.‡ Under Kennedy's direction, FDA moved in the direction of greater concern for consumer safety and interests. Kennedy has taken sound positions on various issues such as dangers of saccharin and nitrite, promoting the use of lower-priced generic drugs, and the labeling of alcoholic beverages (with warnings to pregnant women that too much alcohol may cause birth defects). In May 1978 the FDA announced plans to launch a "cyclic review" of food additives by December. This would include a priority list of about 2,300 substances (some 350 direct additives, 620 natural flavors and spices, and 1330 synthetic flavors) that FDA wants tested now or in the near future.

U.S. Department of Agriculture. The regulatory authority of the USDA over carcinogenic and other contaminants in agricultural products and meat is limited.* The Food Safety and Quality Service conducts programs to protect wholesomeness of meat and poultry products for human consumption. USDA is responsible for preventing the marketing of adulterated raw meat and poultry, including that containing residues in excess of tolerances set by FDA and EPA. As part of this program, USDA samples and monitors meat and poultry, generally at the time of slaughter, for illegal residues. These illegal residues include excessive residues of noncarcinogenic animal drugs, pesticides, and environmental contaminants above tolerance levels, and prohibited residues of any detectable level of carcinogenic drugs such as DES. Apart from these, tolerances or action levels have been set for residues of pesticides and other carcinogenic environmental contaminants, even though a safe level cannot possibly be scientifically established for them. These include the banned carcinogenic DDT and dieldrin, residues of which persist in meat and poultry as a result of their agricultural

---

‡ On April 17, 1979, Kennedy announced his resignation to take a top administrative position at Stanford University, effective August 1, 1979.

* This authority is granted by the 1906 Federal Meat Inspection Act, the 1967 Wholesale Meat Act, and the 1968 Poultry Products Inspection Act.

uses several years ago.†

According to a recent congressional report, the USDA monitoring program is seriously deficient.[79] There are at least 143 known drugs and pesticides, including 40 carcinogens and 18 teratogens, besides an unknown number of environmental contaminants which may leave residues in food-producing animals.‡ USDA's monitoring program tests for only 46 drugs and pesticides, and 8 environmental contaminants. Using USDA data, on the basis of which an overall estimated rate of 2 percent violation with illegal residues was claimed by USDA, the General Accounting Office report showed that from 1974 to 1976 the violation rate may have ranged from 2.6 percent in sheep and goats to almost 16 percent in swine. The actual violation rate is probably very much higher, as USDA fails to test for most drugs and pesticides likely to leave residues. Among pesticides and drugs which are not included in USDA monitoring programs are the carcinogenic drug furazolidone, ethylene-bis-dithiocarbamate fungicides, which break down to the carcinogenic ethylene thiourea, chlorophenoxy herbicides such as 2,4,5-T and Silvex, which are teratogenic and contain the highly persistent and carcinogenic tetradioxin contaminant and 2,4-D which is teratogenic.

High violation rates of carcinogenic and other contaminants in meat and poultry are further compounded by the fact that most illegal residues are discovered only after the meat and poultry have been marketed. Furthermore, FDA and EPA fail to follow up on most residue violations and to take appropriate corrective action.

USDA authority for inspection of illegal and potentially harmful residues in raw meat and poultry is shared with FDA and EPA. Cooperation on enforcement policies has been reached by administrative agreements between these agencies. FDA is responsible under the Federal Food, Drug, and Cosmetic Act of 1938 (as amended) for ensuring the safety of drugs given to food-producing animals, setting tolerances for animal drugs or environmental contaminants allowable in food, and preventing the marketing of raw meat and poultry containing residues that exceed established tolerance levels. EPA is responsible for regulating the introduction of pesticides and toxic substances into the environment. Under the Federal Insecticide, Fungicide, and Rodenticide Act of 1947 (as amended), EPA must approve pesticide products for safety and effectiveness before they can be marketed. Additionally, under the Federal Food, Drug, and Cosmetic Act, EPA must establish safe tolerance levels for pesticides likely to leave residues in food. Finally, under the 1976 Toxic Substances Control Act, EPA regulates the introduction of toxic substances into the environment which can contaminate meat and poultry. Both FDA and EPA are responsible for requiring manufacturers to provide suitable, practical, and sensitive test methods for the detection of chemical residues.

USDA also sets tolerances for nitrate and nitrite in meat, though not in fish, which is an FDA responsibility. The authority of the USDA over nitrate and nitrite in meat is due

---

† DDT has an official tolerance (5 ppm), which by legal definition is a "safe" level. The current dieldrin action level (0.3 ppm) was agreed upon as part of the EPA ban on agricultural uses of aldrin/dieldrin. In both instances, human exposure levels and the rate of decline of residues reflect environmental factors that, apart from determination of action levels, are beyond regulatory controls. In 1976, USDA tests showed that 82 percent of about 900 poultry tested for DDT and 52 percent of 1800 cattle tested for dieldrin had measurable residues, which in most instances, however, were below tolerance levels.

‡ These inadequacies generally reflect the lack of appropriate analytic methods that FDA and EPA should have required from manufacturers prior to their original registration of the animal drugs and pesticides, respectively.

to a legislative quirk by which these two additives were given a prior sanction under the 1907 Meat Inspection Act and were thus exempt from the 1958 Food Additive Amendments.

Assistant Secretary for Food and Consumer Services of the USDA, Carol Tucker Foreman, has taken steps to ensure that the meat industry reduce nitrite in bacon to levels at which no nitrosamines can be detected. In congressional testimony on February 24, 1978, Foreman endorsed the general criticisms of USDA's monitoring program contained in the 1978 General Accounting Office report. Foreman also announced plans of the USDA to improve its sampling and monitoring programs.[80]

It is clear that USDA procedures for meat inspection and monitoring are out of date and inadequately responsive to the grave problems of the modern petrochemical era. Additionally, the fragmentation of authority and responsibility for setting tolerances and food inspection between the USDA and the FDA and EPA is an anachronism which leads to regulatory complexity and diffusion of authority.* In a limited effort to resolve this problem, in December, 1977, the Senate Governmental Affairs Committee recommended that the regulatory function of the USDA over chemical contaminants in food be transferred to the FDA.

Secretary of Agriculture Bob Bergland has shown an apparent sensitivity to toxic and environmental problems of pesticide uses. In March, 1977, he expressed the intent of USDA to wean farmers away from dependence on pesticides and to encourage integrated pest management instead. USDA has not yet implemented such intent.

Other Regulatory Agencies

The Federal Trade Commission, through the 1964 Federal Cigarette Labeling and Advertising Act, requires cigarette packages to be labeled with the familiar warning that smoking "is dangerous to your health." The FTC spends about $125,000 annually to measure the tar and nicotine content of commercial domestic cigarettes, requiring the findings to be printed on the packages. Without this modest pressure, the tobacco industry would have no incentive to reduce the tar and nicotine yield of its products. As it is, the industry has cashed in on the low-tar concept with massive media campaigns to win smokers to the lower-tar brands. Industry efforts to move the testing from the FTC to private concerns were thwarted in 1977. Similar attempts will, however, probably be made in the future. Efforts to regulate the tobacco industry now seem futile in view of its strong support by the administration and a powerful network of Southern congressmen. If there are any possible remedies, they seem to rest in the courts.

The current FTC commissioner, Michael Pertschuk, former chief counsel of the Senate Commerce Committee, is a dedicated consumer activist. He has brought in new staff and has overnight transformed the FTC into an agency aggressively dedicated to protect the interests of the consumer.†

Under the 1974 Hazardous Materials Transportation Act, the Department of Transportation has authority to regulate transportation of various categories of materials, such as flammable liquids or explosives, but not specifically carcinogens.

The Bureau of Mines of the Interior Department has authority under the Federal Coal

---

* OMB is formulating plans for investigation of current national food policies with regard to production, distribution, nutrition, and safety. This project, will also examine the authorities of concerned federal agencies, FDA, EPA, and USDA, for overlap and consistency.

† In May, 1978, Pertschuk was charged with bias in his regulation of TV advertising for children by the Toy Manufacturers of America, the American Association of Advertising Agencies, the American Advertising Foundation, and the Association of National Advertisers.

Mine Health and Safety Act of 1969 and the Federal Metal and Nonmetallic Mine Safety Act of 1966 to enforce federal health and safety in mining operations. The bureau has adopted the 1972 OSHA standards for asbestos and the 1973 threshold limit values for other airborne pollutants.

The Federal Mine Safety and Health Amendments Act of 1977 supersedes the 1966 Mine Safety Act. The 1977 Act established a Mine Enforcement Safety Administration, separate from OSHA, in the Department of Labor.

The "New Look"

The last two years have witnessed the emergence of significant new trends in federal agencies. An important element is the over all and explicit emphasis of the Carter administration on integrity and openness.‡ This has also put new teeth into recent laws governing agency conduct. These laws include the 1973 amendments to the 1967 Freedom of Information Act, making it possible for concerned citizens to obtain copies of documents on the basis of which agencies make decisions and regulatory policies,[81] and the 1972 Federal Advisory Committee Act, governing the conduct of these committees, with particular reference to the needs for balanced representation, disclosure of special interests, and public announcement of meetings.*[82] The administration has also introduced new policies designed to limit conflicts

of interest and the "revolving door" between industry and federal agencies.[83] Senior agency officials are now forbidden to accept positions in those industries they have regulated for one year after resignation from government. A bill approved by the Senate in 1977 mandates an even stricter two-year ban in certain cases.

There is no question that the overall quality of new appointments of agency heads under the Carter administration has been outstanding from the point of view of their past records. While it is too early to make definitive assessments, it is possible to observe some emerging trends in performance. In general, these trends are favorable. Bingham at OSHA, Foreman at USDA, Claybrook at Transportation, Kennedy at FDA, and Pertschuk at the Federal Trade Commission, have all transformed their agencies much for the better. As part of their reforms, they have recruited much needed fresh and skilled new personnel into senior positions. Additionally, Upton at NCI, Costle at EPA, and King at the Consumer Product Safety Commission have also made a substantial impact at their agencies by virtue of their integrity and openness.

Problems of overlapping jurisdictions and regulatory inconsistencies are now being recognized.[84] Attempts are being made to correct this and to develop better coordination of efforts at the fact-finding and regulatory levels. Among the more important cooperative moves that have been made are the forma-

---

‡ While there is no evidence that the Carter administration, which came to Washington pledging "open government" and protection for "whistleblowers," has taken measures similar to those used in the Nixon administration, it has mounted a range of internal inquiries, tightened the National Security Council regulations on interviews, opened the prosecution of an espionage case, filed a breach of contract suit against a former CIA employee who wrote an unauthorized book, and required Justice Department lawyers to sign affidavits about their contacts with reporters as a part of leaking inquiries. Attorney General Griffin Bell has taken

still stronger positions on news leaks, and his department had conducted most of the investigations on unauthorized disclosures, including a recently closed investigation on the *Washington Star*, which refused to disclose its sources of information about alleged corruption in the Interstate Commerce Commission.

* It should be recognized, however, that the National Academy of Sciences, major source of technical advice to Congress and regulatory agencies, has so far successfully resisted legal challenge to require compliance with the Freedom of Information Act.

tion of an Interagency Regulatory Liaison Group (IRLG), involving EPA, OSHA, FDA, and the Consumer Product Safety Commission, the formation of an EPA Toxic Substances Strategy Committee, an overall coordinating group which reports directly to the President, an HEW Committee to coordinate toxicology and related programs, and more recently the National Toxicology Program.

The likelihood for success of these new cooperative ventures is increased by the close contacts and understanding that have developed between Bingham, Costle, and Kennedy, which have been reinforced by similar contacts with heads of research agencies, particularly Upton and Rall. Some of these cooperative moves, particularly the IRLG and the NTP, may well foreshadow the emergence of more extensive and formalized consolidation, probably within HEW, of the functions of the several different agencies now dealing with various aspects of environmental pollution and public health.

Economic Policies
of the Administration

In March, 1978, President Carter issued executive order 12044 requiring regulatory agencies to develop "regulatory analyses" of all major proposed standards with particular attention to their economic impact on business.† The order was promptly endorsed by the U.S. Chamber of Commerce. Since then, the administration has imposed increasing restrictions on health and environmental regulation, particularly through the Regulatory Analysis Review Group of the Council on Wage and Price Stability (COWPS).‡ As an agent of the President, COWPS is now

pitted against the regulatory agencies in their discharge of Congressionally mandated policies.

As OSHA was concluding review of the post-hearing comments on its "generic" cancer policy, COWPS issued a report in October, 1978, sharply critical of the proposal on both economic and scientific grounds. COWPS, which draws freely on affected industries for staff work, cited the economic impact analysis prepared for the American Industrial Health Council by Booz, Allen & Hamilton, admitted by the Council to be "seriously flawed," as its authority for stating that the total costs of the proposed regulations will be well over $1 billion annually. The Council was equally critical of the OSHA benefits analysis for its failure to address the cost-benefit question on a carcinogen-by-carcinogen basis, and for failing to determine incremental benefits over and above those achievable by alternate methods of regulation. This criticism was buttressed by reference to the October, 1978, decision of the Fifth Circuit Court overturning the benzene standard on grounds including economic feasibility, and cost-benefit considerations. The Council was also critical of OSHA for disregarding potency and risk assessment in their essential classification of chemicals into carcinogens and non-carcinogens.

On October 24, 1978, President Carter announced his new anti-inflation program, concluding that inflation is the nation's No. 1 problem, and that prompt remedial action, including round-the-board austerity measures, must be immediately taken.* However, the program embodies budgetary cuts, which are likely to increase unemployment, and further

---

† This order replaced President Ford's Executive Order 11821, which required "inflationary impact statements"; the name of this requirement was changed to "economic impact statements"; on December 31, 1977.

‡ The inequity of these restrictions is further emphasized by reports of soaring corporate profits

in the first quarter of 1979.

* Current inflation is poorly understood. Neither classical nor Keynesian economic theory can explain the combination of unemployment or stagnation and inflation (stag-flation) that has characterized the 1970s. In the absence of firm theory, inflation fighters are groping with traditional em-

restrictions on regulations designed to protect workers and the environment. The new measures, however, fail to protect consumers from runaway price increases in the four basic necessities of life-food, energy, housing, and medical care — those areas where inflation hits hardest.

Following preliminary skirmishing between the Office of Management and Budget and the heads of the major regulatory agencies, President Carter created a Regulatory Council, headed by EPA Administrator Costle, to implement the new regulatory policy. The Council held its first meeting in November, 1978, with twenty-five attendees representing all Cabinet and thirteen independent agencies. The Council established five work groups — health and safety, finance and banking, economics, social justice, and resource development. Federal agencies were asked to submit an immediate list of all planned major regulations with an impact of over $100 million on industry. Besides economic impact, each regulation lists eleven descriptive items, including title, legislative authority, alternatives to regulation, background documentation for the standard, an analysis of the needs for regulation, and an agency contact. The Council was required to submit this to President Carter by February 1, 1979, before publication of the Calendar (containing about 200 regulations), which is intended to provide a regulatory cost-benefit analysis.

The Regulatory Calendar concept has come under vigorous attack, particularly from consumer and minority groups and organized labor, the basic constituency that elected Carter.

Congressman Rogers, (D-Fla.) in a November 15, 1978, speech to the newly formed National Coalition for Disease Prevention and Environmental Health, characterized the Calendar philosophy as saying, "if getting sick is cheaper, then maybe we should not try to prevent illness." The AFL-CIO Executive Council criticized the proposal as "inequitable and unfair."

A portent of the new economic policies of the administration appears to be reflected in the January, 1979, decision of EPA Administrator Costle to weaken the Clean Air Act by allowing reduction in the ozone (smog) standard from 0.08 to 0.12 ppm (which is routinely exceeded in many large cities, such as Houston and Los Angeles). EPA claimed that the new standard will save industry approximately $1.5 billion annually. While Costle acknowledged talking to White House economists before announcing his decision, he insisted that the new standard is justified by "careful re-evaluation of medical and scientific evidence" (although no details of this re-evaluation were provided), and would not lead to adverse health effects in the general population, nor in hypersusceptible groups such as asthmatics. Richard Sinsheimer, president of the American Lung Association, however, called the new standard "dangerous" and warned, "we're playing Russian roulette with our health."

The new administration initiatives raise important constitutional and legal issues, particularly as they appear to represent direct executive usurpation of legislative authority. (This usurpation is over and above the per-

piricism for possible solutions and scapegoats, a role that regulation seems to fit well, especially as it also appeals to the national mood of resurgent conservatism. The issues have been further clouded by the action of the administration in terminating monopolistic airline practices by their deregulation, the success of which has been exploited by both administration economists and industry as further argument for environmental deregulation. Environmental regulation is claimed to be inflationary on various grounds including: It makes technology prematurely obsolete; it fails to promote productivity of future new standards; the regulations are especially hard on small business who may be driven out of the market, resulting in industry concentration; and it is difficult to prove benefits from a regulatory action.

sonnel ceilings imposed by the administration which have prevented agencies from functioning adequately within approved budgetary limits.) Regulatory responsibilities have been created by Congressional Acts to implement specific programs under specific legislation. The Occupational Safety and Health Act, for example, mandates "safe and healthful working conditions" without reference to economic and technical feasibility or cost-benefit considerations. The intervention of White House staff in the regulatory process, in the name of fighting inflation, is not authorized by statute.† Constitutional and legal issues aside, there are serious problems and flaws inherent in the administration's approach to regulation from myopic and narrowly defined cost-benefit perspectives.

First, most cost-benefit analyses do not adequately reflect the economic and other costs of deregulation or failure to regulate in terms of disease and death, and environmental degradation. This is especially so in view of the substantial uncertainties involved in such costing. Quantitative risk costing or assessment is a premature science fostered by pressures to express public health hazards in economically simplistic terms. The uncertainties inherent in this approach are illustrated by the 10 million-fold range in current estimates of the carcinogenic hazards of saccharin (Table 9.11). Additionally, such estimates ignore even greater uncertainties due to potential synergisms and multiple exposures that, in general, cannot be anticipated let alone quantitated.‡

Quite apart from these uncertainties, costings based on medical treatment and income or productivity losses, seem inadequate or inappropriate estimates for pain and suffering and loss of life. For instance, the recognized annual costs of cancer are in the region of $30 billion, and particularly with occupational cancer, there are still larger currently unrecognized and externalized costs. As the burden of environmentally induced cancer and disease has progressively increased, total national health expenditures have soared from $30 billion in 1960 to $185 billion in 1978, and are expected to reach $230 billion by 1980. Health-care costs in 1978 were roughly 9 percent of the G.N.P., and $55 billion more than the defense budget. Health care leads the nation's inflationary spiral, and has been growing at the rate of 15 percent or more for the last five years. The contrast between runaway health-care spending and the resistance of the administration, besides industry, to invest in environmental health protection is striking.[85] Apart from recognized health-care costs, there are related costs that can no longer be externalized, such as the pending multimillion dollar law suits on asbestos. As recently pointed out,[86] even the conservative economist Paul Samuelson warns that conventional estimates on the impact of regulation on economic growth and the gross national product are meaningless, unless —

we adjust for any such "bads" that escape the G.N.P. statistician whenever society is both failing to prevent pollution and failing to make power [or water or air or cotton] users pay for the full costs of the damage they do. [Once we make these adjustments]

---

† In November, 1978, the Environmental Defense Fund sent to the White House a forty-page legal memorandum, arguing that the President has no more authority to intervene in regulatory proceedings after the public comment period has closed than anyone else, unless that authority is explicitly granted by the statute under which the rule is written. The extent to which Congress is likely to resist legislative moves further extending Presiden-

tial authority in this direction remains to be seen.
‡ These grave limitations do not appear to be recognized by the chemical industry and the proponents of deregulation, who are proposing that quantitative risk assessment should be used as a basis for regulation (See, for instance, Cong. J. G. Martin, "Where Does Science Fit In?" address to the Manufacturing Chemists Association, Washington, D.C., September 12, 1978).

Table 9.11 Estimated Human Risks from Saccharin Ingestion of 0.12 g/day

Method of high- to low-dose extrapolation	Lifetime cases/ million exposed	Cases per 50 million/yr.
Rat dose adjusted to human dose by surface area rule		
Single-hit model (Hoel, 1977)	1,200	840
Multi-stage model (with quadratic term) (Hoel, 1977)	5	3.5
Multi-hit model (Scientific Committee of the Food Safety Council, 1978)	0.001	0.0007
Mantel-Bryan probit model (Brown,1978)	450	315
Rat dose adjusted to human dose by mg/kg/day equivalence		
Single-hit model (Saccharin and Its Salts, 1977)	210	147
Multi-hit model (Scientific Committee of the Food Safety Council, 1978)	0.001	0.0007
Mantel-Bryan probit model (Brown, 1978)	21	14.7
Rat dose adjusted to human dose by mg/kg/lifetime equivalence		
Single-hit model (Brown, 1977)	5,200	3,640
Multi-hit model (Scientific Committee on the Food Safety Council, 1978)	0.001	0.0007
Mantel-Bryan probit model (Brown, 1978)	4,200	2,940

Source: "Saccharin: Technical Assessment of Risks and Benefits," Report No. 1, Committee for a Study on Saccharin and Food Safety Policy, National Academy of Sciences, Institute of Medicine, November, 1978.

we see that net economic welfare grows more slowly than [conventionally measured] G.N.P.

Second, there are similar problems in evaluating the costs of regulation.* Compliance strategies involve large degrees of uncertainty and generally ignore treatment of positive externalities arising from innovation associated with add-on devices (as interim measures) and product or process substitution, or alternative technologies. Compliance may achieve substantial economies by recovering and recycling valuable chemicals otherwise lost as air and water pollutants. Cost analyses also rarely reflect the creation of new pollution-control industries which provide employment besides goods and services. According to a November, 1978, report prepared for EPA by Arthur D. Little, Inc., the air-and-water-pollution-control industry (manufacturing equipment, instrumentation, and chemicals for pollution control from industrial plants, and for municipal solid-waste recycling plants) had record sales of $1.8 billion in 1977, accounting for about 36,000 jobs. These new industries are growing about twice as fast as the rest of U.S. industry, and are projected to grow even faster over the next decade. Another important consideration is the fact that industry has a virtual monopoly on data needed to assess costs of compliance. Industry estimates on the cost of regulation are often exaggerated, sometimes by several orders of magnitude, as was shown to be the case for the vinyl chloride occupational standard. OSHA does not have adequate resources to scrutinize such alleged costs and must often rely on consulting firms with close industry ties for economic and technical advice.

Finally, there is the question of equity. The penalties of failure to regulate carcinogens are usually long delayed and impact on different sets of people than those who profit from the manufacture or processing of the carcinogen and who resist bearing the immediate costs of compliance (recognizing also that much of these costs could be redistributed through tax write-offs and price pass-throughs). It would seem reasonable to require that the interests of a worker exposed to hazardous conditions receive substantially more protection than now afforded by the regulatory process, and still more than that envisaged by regulation further attenuated in the name of inflation fighting.

Constraints on Agencies

The performance of Federal agencies, both research and regulatory, is influenced by an interplay of technical and political considerations of such complexity as to discourage simplistic assessments. Besides attempting to resolve inherited legislative ambiguities, agencies must deal with a growing range of constraints.† The most limiting include those imposed by the administration, such as long-standing personnel ceilings, and the new anti-inflationary policies, particularly the narrowly defined cost-benefit analyses demanded by COWPS as a prerequisite to the discharge of congressionally mandated regulatory action. These constraints have been reinforced by the October, 1978, decision of the Fifth Circuit Federal Court of Appeals in New Orleans (now under appeal before the Supreme Court) overturning OSHA's new benzene standard on economic grounds, and placing on government the burden of proving that the costs of compliance are outweighed by health benefits.

---

* These costs, which are immediate, are weighted heavily, while delayed health benefits of regulation are almost invariably discounted.

† According to R. J. Smith, *Science* 203 (1979), pp. 28-32, "chronic indecisiveness" or "chronic avoidance" has emerged as the most recent characteristic of regulatory agencies, accounting for the extreme paucity of their regulatory actions. However, both OSHA and EPA are now attempting to build public constituencies to counterbalance pressures from regulated industries.

The unique preemption by Congress of the FDA's regulatory authority on saccharin, reflects manipulation of the public perception of public health issues by powerful special interests exploiting poorly restricted control of the media, coupled with the failure of regulators to adequately inform the public as to the underlying realities. Notwithstanding the recent impact of organized labor and public interest groups, perhaps the most crippling of all constraints on agencies is the lack of a disease- and cancer-prevention national constituency to balance the pressures of industry and the indifference or hostility of the "cancer cure lobby" and the medical establishment or industry.

Future Trends

Future events will be critically shaped by the outcome of an emerging power struggle between Congress and the administration, not only with regard to the new economic policies of the President, but also with regard to the personnel restrictions imposed on federal agencies. Another critical determinant is the ability of agencies to attract established scientists into key positions in the bureaucracy, besides recruiting lower rank professionals.

Past Republican administrations have achieved more effective environmental regulation with weak agency heads than has been or is likely to be achieved by the present Democrat and liberal administration aided by strong and progressive agency leadership. Determinants of this paradox include emerging fiscal conservatism, increasing pressures by the administration and industry for deregulation in the name of anti-inflation, the public and congressional perception of major uncertainties or confusion in the scientific base of environmental decision making (as illustrated in the mishandling of saccharin) and in risk assessment, and the false issue of freedom of choice being pitted against regulation. Inflation forces are clearly in control in the executive. There is a strong decline in the environment and anti-cancer forces in Congress, with the recent retirement of Congressmen James Delaney (D-N.Y.), John E. Moss (D-Calif.), and Paul Rogers (D-Fla.), and with the emergence of the new fiscal conservatives.‡ The future role of labor has been made uncertain by recent wage limitations imposed by Carter, and it is unclear whether organized labor will make wage or environmental controls their main priority. The likelihood of success of the deregulation trend seems enhanced by the absence of an effective national environmental and anti-cancer constituency.

Initiatives emerging at the state government level represent additional new trends of major potential importance which are being pioneered by California.[87] The 1976 California Occupational Carcinogen Control Act (SB 1678) requires that all industries using designated carcinogens register with the newly created Occupational Carcinogen Control Unit, which has the authority to inspect facilities and levy civil penalties for violation of standards. Other bills introduced to the Califor-

‡ Exemplified by Congressman James Martin (R-N.C.), whose Ph.D. in chemistry seems to have invested him with a role of scientific authority in environmental and health issues. Martin is a strong advocate of the revocation of the Delaney Amendment on the grounds that it is "unscientific," and of the saccharin ban on the grounds that it is only "a weak carcinogen," whose (alleged) benefits outweigh the risks he seems to feel that the consumer is or should be willing to bear. However, Rogers and Moss have been succeeded as chairmen of the key House Commerce Committee's Subcommittee on Health and the Environment and Oversight and Investigation by the liberal Henry A. Waxman (D-Calif.) and Bob Eckhardt (D-Tex.), respectively. Eckhardt has established priorities in agency decision making and in the role and limitations of cost-benefits analysis. Waxman, who does not command a majority on his subcommittee, can be expected to strongly defend the Clean Air Act and retention of the Delaney Amendment, to oppose export of hazardous products, and to advocate a comprehensive national health insurance.

nia legislature in 1978 include AB 3249 on Workers' "right to know" of the identity of chemicals to which they are exposed; AB 3413, which would create a repository of information on toxic chemicals; AB 3414, which would create a University of California training center for occupational health professionals in the north and south of the state; and SB 1530, which would investigate the regional distribution of cancers in Bay Area counties. The 1977 New Jersey "Cancer Control Act," introduced by Senator John M. Skevin, proposing a ban on the manufacture of sixteen known carcinogens and offering the most comprehensive state legislation on control of public exposure to industrial carcinogens, was withdrawn in response to massive industrial opposition and failure to generate adequate public support.

I hope we shall crush in its birth the aristocracy of our monied corporations which dare already to challenge our government to a trial of strength, and bid defiance to the laws of our country.

Thomas Jefferson, 1816

Chapter Ten

Non-governmental Policies

Until recently, industry and labor have been the only major non-government influences on Congress and regulatory agencies in all areas of public health and safety, whether relating to the general environment, consumer products, or the workplace. In the last decade a new element has emerged, the public interest movement, which, in spite of trivial material resources compared to those of industry, has begun to transform the climate of decision making. A discussion of the three — industry, labor, and public interest groups — and also of additional influences with respect to environmental and occupational carcinogenesis follows.

Industry

American industry early gained a reputation for innovation and flexibility. These are among the qualities that established international preeminence for the U.S. free enterprise system. Nowhere has this flexibility been better seen than in the major chemical industries, which have learned to deal with shifting supplies of raw materials and shifting demands of the market.

In spite of this, industry has failed to adequately comprehend the magnitude of health and safety problems entailed in the manufacture and handling of hazardous, particularly toxic or carcinogenic, chemicals. Industry has also failed to comprehend the enormous costs to society of the cancer and other diseases resulting from the use of toxic and carcinogenic chemicals. Industry is not alone in this failure of comprehension, which must also be shared by government and the public. Such failure of comprehension, coupled with historic imbalances reflecting industrial dominance of decision making with regard to its own products and processes, appears to be the major determinant of current industry policies. In analyzing industry policies and problems of constraints in their data, these considerations appear preferable to alternate simplistic theories based exclusively on machiavellianism.

Top management has also failed to be aware of the shortcomings in its own modes of developing health and safety information. As a result, marketing decisions and all-but-irreversible economic commitments are often made on the basis of information that subsequently proves to be defective or based solely on short-term marketing considerations. The conflicts inherent in this tend to limit the interests and incentives of industry to develop equally effective but less hazardous alternative products and processes — hence to stifle needed innovation.

Big industry faces two distinct types of problems in developing control technology. First, there are the difficulties of effectively refitting old plants with add-on devices to allow them to handle toxic chemicals more safely. It is now generally recognized that in many instances this just may not be practical. This does not exclude the possibility of materially decreasing risk by improving work practices. Part of the problem here is the fact that some industries, particularly steel, have in the past failed to plow back profits into renovating old plants.* This problem of old plants with old technology must be dealt with on an industry-by-industry basis. There are no simple solutions or general formulae. It is clear, however, that old plants cannot be allowed to function as before at the continued expense of human health. While they are being phased out, at a pace influenced by industrial economics and public health concerns, improved work practices and engineering controls must be instituted on an interim basis.

The second (and relatively easier) set of problems faced by big business are those involved with the design of new plants. This is where industry can be expected to exhibit bold innovation. Health and safety considerations must be designed into plants at the earliest possible stages. The substitution of safer products and processes must be exploited to the fullest to avoid the use of carcinogenic chemicals. If it can be proven that there are no practical alternatives to the use of a carcinogen, then closed systems must be devised and engineered with all possible precision and safeguards, including constant monitoring with highly sensitive instrumentation. Costs of such controls are a useful incentive to the innovative development of safer alternatives.

The problems of small industry are probably the most difficult and complex. Many of these operate marginally and cannot afford to install expensive engineering controls.† Many also employ poorly educated and tran-

sient, non-unionized labor. While some improvement in work practices to reduce risks is feasible, there are clearly practical limitations as to what can be done in the small plant. To add to these pressures, large corporations have historically sided with government in efforts to regulate and destroy competition from small business. It is clear that small business must be gradually weaned away from handling hazardous chemicals. It is also clear that they should be encouraged in this direction and in the direction of improved work practices by special treatment, including tax subsidies and interim variances.

Industry, like labor, represents a heterogeneous array of interests and objectives. Such diversity, however, tends to be replaced by a common front of intransigence in response to proposed regulation of toxic and carcinogenic chemicals. A complex of interrelated factors seems involved in this posture. These include the near-automatic rejection of federal controls (without a parallel rejection of tax subsidies and other forms of corporate protectionism); preoccupation with short-term marketing interests (often in conflict with needs for hazard controls) rather than consideration of long-term growth and stability; excessive reliance on narrowly based, self-interested recommendations of in-house marketing and scientific staff and their consultants on problems of health and safety; and a tendency to wait for health and safety problems to arise (which they then deal with defensively) rather than developing anticipatory strategies based on long-term considerations.

Strategies

In support of the status quo, industry has evolved a complex set of strategies to use individually or in concert to meet the needs of

---

* The 1976 OSHA hearings on coke oven emissions made it clear that the newer Japanese coke ovens are better designed than their U.S. equivalents.

† It must be stressed that most epidemiological

investigations that have so far demonstrated carcinogenic hazards in the workplace, have been undertaken in large chemical corporations that have some degree of protective controls, as opposed to small industry.

any particular circumstance. These are illustrated by the various case studies discussed in this book. The essence of all of them is to minimize the reality of risks due to a particular product or process, to maximize the social benefits, and to exaggerate the costs and difficulty of regulation. The elements of these strategies are sometimes presented frankly as industry positions, but they often come to us from industry spokesmen and academic consultants as "professional" viewpoints, with no hint of who employs the professionals.

Minimizing the Risk. This standard ploy is exemplified by the Quebec Asbestos Mining Association's position. The association has publicly asserted that asbestos disease is a reaction of poor working conditions in the past which have been so improved that there is now little or no risk. Similarly, the Manufacturing Chemists Association and the academic consultants of industry have testified that benzene-induced leukaemias and other toxic effects reflect high exposures in the past and that now, based on the relatively low exposures encountered under modern working conditions, there is no cause for concern. As a further example, Rohm and Haas, as recently as 1974, denied that exposure to BCME has caused any worker deaths following exposure at their plant. Other illustrative positions include the claim, by such organizations as the Nutrition Foundation and the Council on Agricultural Science and Technology, that there is no risk in being exposed to "relatively low levels" of chemicals found to be carcinogenic in humans, and that there are no substantive risks of exposure to chemicals found to be carcinogenic in animals and for which

there are as yet no human data.‡

Diversionary Tactics. These are generally based on insistence on degrees of precision and legal definition that cannot possibly be met in carcinogenesis tests or in epidemiological studies. Such a demand is often coupled with rejection of experimental carcinogenicity test data and alternative proposals for long-term prospective human studies over the next few decades, pending which, it is claimed, regulatory action should be suspended.

On January 11, 1978, the day HEW Secretary Joseph Califano announced a new "war on smoking," Senator Wendell Ford (D-Ken.), on behalf of his tobacco-producing state, told a news conference that Califano should instead direct the earmarked anti-smoking funds "into well-founded scientific research. The American people can make their own decisions," implying that still more research was needed and that government should do this research but should not set policy based on its results.

A December 13, 1977, meeting of the Toxicology Forum, an industry-sponsored group of toxicologists and geneticists, decided that saccharin should be given top priority for new studies. These new studies, the group concluded, should be directed to identify "impurities" in commercial saccharin, which members apparently had convinced themselves were responsible for the carcinogenic and mutagenic activity of saccharin.

Propagandizing the Public. The media blitz orchestrated by the Calorie Control Council following the FDA's proposal to ban saccharin was unprecedented in regulatory history. The payoff obviously was worthwhile, for the

---

‡ Paralleling the attempts of the petrochemical industry to minimize the hazards of its products and processes are the skyrocketing insurance premiums and the growing difficulty of the industry in obtaining product liability insurance. Some industry trade associations are now considering establishing their own insurance companies in the Bahamas. Another proposed solution, especially favored by the asbestos industry, is the establishment of a no-fault insurance, possibly based on federal subsidies and akin to the limited liability secured for the nuclear power industry by the Price-Anderson Act. Such a move would perpetuate for the consumer the double indemnity of contracting cancer from industrial chemical carcinogens and paying for its costs.

unexpected and tumultuous public response led to a moratorium on its regulation. The council's use of such high-priced public relations firms as Hill and Knowlton reflects the determination of an industry faced with potential control. The council's propaganda is an outgrowth of an evolving media campaign, in which the chemical and oil industries are striving to improve their public images with all the techniques of modern mass advertising.

"Assuming a leadership role" on behalf of the chemical industry, Monsanto Chemical Company has recently launched a major public advertising campaign directed to the importance and safety of synthetic chemicals. Synthetic chemicals, it is claimed, are no different from all other naturally occurring chemicals to which mankind has been exposed for millions of years, and are essentially harmless in the absence of massive exposure or careless misuse. More specifically, the campaign consists of attacks against standard uses of maximally tolerated doses, against the Delaney Amendment, and against other regulatory controls of carcinogenic chemicals, all of which are categorized as irrational and emotional. A Monsanto pamphlet called "The Chemical Facts of Life" explains that the purpose of the campaign is "to explore the benefits and risks of chemicals — to find a clear path through the labyrinth of information and misinformation about chemicals which may help or harm health and the environment."[1]

Monsanto is spending about $5 million this year and is planning to spend similar amounts annually over the next five years on spots on national television, newspaper ads, and pamphlets. Some 500,000 pamphlets have been distributed so far, even to high school children. The campaign has been well planned and seems to limit possibilities of asking for equal time under the Fairness Doctrine. Following protest by the Environmental Defense Fund, Monsanto initially agreed to limit somewhat the scope of its campaign. One sixty-second national television spot features a speaker identified as an agricultural chemist drinking from a glass of water and asserting the dependence of the modern farmer on chemicals such as di-hydrogen oxide — water. He then goes on to discuss the herbicide Vegadex,* explaining that while one would never drink this, it benefits crop growth in several ways. The screen flashes images of weeds being killed and healthy crops growing. The speaker allows that "no chemical is totally safe all the time," but maintains that chemicals such as Vegadex are necessary in circumstances of worldwide food shortages, and concludes that without chemicals life would not be possible.

The Monsanto campaign is not a public service. The company would do better to stress concerns that the chemicals they plan to produce should be well tested to avoid future problems such as those posed by the tox-

---

* Vegadex, or sulfallate, is a chlorinated dithiocarbamate derivative used as a selective pre-emergence herbicide on vegetable crops. It is structurally similar to a number of other pesticides which were shown to be carcinogenic more than nine years ago. In January, 1978, Vegadex was shown to be positive in the Ames test,[2] and in the following March the NCI bioassay program published a report showing that the herbicide is carcinogenic to rats and mice, inducing breast cancers in females of both species, tumors of the stomach in male rats and of the lung in male mice.[3]

Recent production data for Vegadex are unknown, as this is considered proprietary information. However, a 1971 report estimates U.S. production as about 500,000 kg annually. As the NCI report points out, "The potential for exposure to sulfallate is greatest for agricultural workers, but may also be considerable for workers in sulfallate production facilities. Residents of agricultural communities may be exposed to airborne residues following spraying operations. The herbicide is readily taken up by plant roots . . . and the general population may be exposed via ingestion of residues in food crops."

icity and carcinogenicity of its products, such as Vegadex and nitrilotriacetic acid. Monsanto should also consider the judgment of its executives and consultants, on the basis of whose advice this mass campaign was presumably authorized.

Blaming the Victim. Simply stated, the argument is, "Modern industrial working conditions are so safe that if a worker gets hurt or sick it must be his or her fault and not the fault of the industry." The culprit is either the worker's bad habits, such as smoking, or the worker's genetic susceptibility to effects which any normal person would shrug off. Applications of this perspective have taken many forms. Perhaps its latest variant is the stance of Johns-Manville's Paul Kotin, in shifting attention from what *chemicals* cause cancer to what *people* get cancer. Kotin has helped resurrect the notion of the "hyper-susceptible worker," one who, by his own constitutional or genetic makeup, is at higher risk for occupational disease than fellow workers. Starting from the plausible premise that all biological organisms, including humans, vary in their response to external stimuli such as toxic substances or carcinogens, he then advances the following proposition:

> The workplace, no matter how elegantly controlled, cannot assure uniformity of protection to all workers because of susceptibility variation. . . . A safe, acceptable workplace for hypersusceptible workers is as much a cultural concept as it is a scientific one. . . . It is still the responsibility of management to deny the worker the "right" to place himself at increased risk.[4]

Kotin jumps from the variability premise to the assertion of management's "right" to assign sturdier individuals to riskier jobs, overlooking the difficulty, if not impossibility, of making such judgments on scientifically sustained grounds, especially regarding carcinogenesis. However, the viewpoint has superficial appeal, as it rationalizes management's right to make arbitrary work assignments, and leaves open the possibility that management will somehow attempt to predict or decide in advance which workers are cancer-prone.

Another blame-the-victim ploy tries to shift the responsibility for workplace disability from uncontrolled exposure to lifestyle. Thus, industries (other than the tobacco industry, of course) are quick to blame lung cancer on smoking and in so doing try to absolve dusts and chemicals in the workplace from any role in the disease.

There is no question that smoking markedly increases the susceptibility of asbestos workers to lung cancer, but the risk of the nonsmoking asbestos worker is also significantly greater than that of the person who does not work with asbestos. Also, smoking has no relation to other malignant diseases caused by asbestos such as pleural or peritoneal mesotheliomas.

Similarly, alcoholism programs in industry focus almost solely on family and marital problems as a cause of drinking, rather than looking into frustrations on the job as a possible factor. Recent studies on heart disease are focusing on so-called Type-A behavior (characterized by a hard-driving, aggressive, competitive personality), which is considered to predispose to coronary disease. An employer may thus be provided with a rationale for blaming the disease solely on the employee, without considering that the behavior itself may also be influenced by stresses inherent in the work.

An equally insidious blame-the-victim scheme, characteristic of the cosmetic approach of some industry to occupational hazards, involves exaggeration of the known problems of small numbers of people with genetic or enzyme deficiencies. It would be useful to industry to have it proven that those workers who contract occupational illness were genetically defective and thus hypersusceptible.† A deficiency in the respiratory enzyme alpha-1-antitrypsin, for example, is claimed to be associated with chronic obstructive lung disease:

> if susceptible subjects can be identified during pre-employment screening and are effectively excluded from hazardous occupations, some cases of chronic bronchitis may be prevented.[5]

However, a 1975 University of Arizona study demonstrated no association between deficiency of the enzyme and symptoms of chronic obstructive pulmonary disease or reduced lung function, and furthermore, found the frequency of this deficiency in the population to be trivial.[6]

Controlling Information. The overwhelming majority of decisions made by regulatory agencies is based on information provided by the industries themselves being regulated. In retrospect, it seems strange that this practice has persisted so long, and that in fact it still persists. In every case study documented in this book, the relevant data base is inadequate or constrained by incompetence, biased interpretation, or even manipulation and suppression. There is no basis for believing that such examples are uncommon.

Influencing Policy. The methods by which industry influences the legislative and regulatory processes, both in the passage and enforcement of standards, are legion. Even after scientific evidence can be developed which shows that a chemical is carcinogenic, the ensuing regulatory process and development of exposure standards are strongly influenced by industrial lobbyists and trade associations. Throughout the last stages of the writing of toxic substances legislation, lobbyists from the Manufacturing Chemists Association were in daily conference with con-

gressmen and their staffs.[7] Out of that experience emerged a semi-autonomous lobbying group which promises to challenge the environmental legislative and regulatory process for many years to come.

Exhausting the Agencies. Once an agency has determined to regulate, or has been obliged to regulate by concerns of labor or public interest groups, a common tactic of industry is to resort to protracted legal action. This is done in the full knowledge that legal proceedings on one particular chemical product or on one standard alone may extend over years, during which no regulatory control can usually be imposed. The legal costs incurred by the industry during such proceedings are usually small compared to the continued sales profits. One or two cases such as aldrin/ dieldrin can exhaust the legal resources of an agency, which are small compared to the virtually limitless legal and other resources that industry can muster.

Insistence on the case-by-case approach has been a favored industry tactic. Basic questions on carcinogenesis have to be argued over again and again for every separate proceeding (such as for the chlordane/heptachlor case, which revived all the same set of problems settled before in the aldrin/dieldrin hearings). This seems the basis for industry's vigorous opposition to the "cancer principles" and to the generic approach to regulation of carcinogens proposed by OSHA.

In late 1977, the Manufacturing Chemists Association spun off the American Industrial Health Council to "assist" OSHA and other agencies in developing policies on carcinogens.[8] Convinced that "OSHA may be developing the national standard for the identification and regulation of carcinogens" in the environment as well as the workplace, the council provides technical and economic

---

† Another example is the genetically determined condition of hyperinducible aryl hydrocarbon hydroxylase, affecting 10-40 percent of the general population, which appears to increase susceptibility to lung cancer.

analysis on behalf of its member industries. Its counterproposal to OSHA's "generic" carcinogens standard would set up two major categories of carcinogens: "human carcinogens" (Category I) and "animal carcinogens" (Category II). Within each category, it would differentiate high, intermediate, and low-potency agents. More tellingly, it would require OSHA to establish apparent no-effect levels for carcinogens, to assess both risks and benefits before setting workplace exposure levels, and to emphasize the use of controls based on personal protective equipment. This is in contrast to OSHA's and labor's policy favoring stricter work practices. The council's proposals would lay the foundation for unending legal challenges to future attempts to regulate any occupational carcinogen.

The position of the American Industrial Health Council rests on claims that there is no evidence of any recent increase in cancer incidence, that most cancer is due to smoking and diet, that the incidence of occupational cancer is low, only in the region of 5 percent,‡ that the role of industrial chemical carcinogens in occupational cancer is small, and that the costs of regulation as proposed by OSHA are excessive. These cost estimates were developed by Foster D. Snell Inc., Division of Booz, Allen & Hamilton (in a report released on February 27, 1978), whose earlier cost analyses on meeting the "no detectable level" vinyl chloride standard were shown to be grossly exaggerated. The study claimed that the cost of controlling suspect carcinogens could range between $9 billion and $88 billion in capital investment, and between $6 billion and $36 billion in annual operating expenses. However, HEW Secretary Califano, in his September 11, 1978, address to a national AFL-CIO conference on occupational health, commented:

> It is in my judgment myopic to argue that programs to protect workers are inflationary . . . if we do not count in our calculations what those programs buy: safety, health, and often greater productivity.

Apart from the inherent distortions in these claims, they ignore the growing evidence of the occurrence of cancer in the general community due to discharge or release of carcinogens from the workplace to the external environment. They also ignore the likelihood of inducing cancer in the children of exposed pregnant workers, besides in the workers

---

‡ The scientific quality of the testimony of industry and its consultants is not impressive. Union Carbide's Browning, in response to a question as to whether his company had a regular ventilation inspection and maintenance program, whether they just awaited complaints of workers, or what else they waited for, jocularly answered: "Well, we pick up the bodies." James J. Jandl, Professor of Medicine at Harvard (who testified in earlier OSHA hearings to the effect that only hypersusceptible workers develop leukaemia following benzene exposure), when asked to comment on the value of carcinogenicity tests in rodents took a somewhat moderate view from Browning and responded:

> . . . this is a very faulty system. First of all, these are bad seed animals. They are inbred in the most obscene way, mother and son, father and daughter, brother and sister, and this is done by people who enjoy that, for many, many gen-

erations. . . . there has to be some equity achieved by the amount of dose given to these poor little critters to compensate for their short life span. . . .

Richard Wilson, Professor of Physics at Harvard, expressed his view that "compensation or hazard pay" is a preferable alternative to government regulation of occupational carcinogens. Harry B. Demopoulos of New York University Medical School recommended that OSHA could more effectively prevent cancer by controlling smoking, besides alcohol, in the workplace (Demopoulos is author of an unpublished document "A Rational View of Cancer in New Jersey," widely circulated by the New Jersey Chamber of Commerce, which contains unsupported statements such as "only a small number of cancers are industrially related," and "asbestos is a weak carcinogen . . . handled with precautions that lead to low exposures of workers such that cancers will not develop").

themselves. Finally, apart from inherent questions on the validity of economic impact analyses by industry, they ignore the much greater costs to society of failure to regulate industrial chemicals in the workplace, let alone in the general environment.

The debate as to the overall importance of occupational carcinogens as a cause of cancer was, to all intents, effectively settled with the release of the September 15, 1978, HEW report, "Estimates of the Fraction of Cancer in the United States Related to Occupational Factors." In an anonymous October document, AIHC attempted a rebuttal on undocumented grounds including that the HEW exposure estimates were based on past exposures that were much higher than allowed in current "more responsible" industrial practices. Fred Hoerger of Dow Chemical Company and an AIHC spokesman told a news conference on October 26 that "The whole [HEW] paper is exaggerated speculation [with] erroneous assumptions in elementary statistics and elementary epidemiology." In a subsequent interview, David Rall, one of the senior authors of the report, commented, "In general, this is what you'd expect from industry, we're comfortable with our study" (*Washington Post*, October 26, 1978). The American Petroleum Institute (API), however (in a supplemental post-hearing brief of December 19, 1978), adopted a more progressive stance:

> API has always viewed the "cancer epidemic" question as irrelevant, since API supports the general goals of OSHA in improving its ability to regulate carcinogens. Whether occupational sources are partly responsible for 1 percent or 40 percent of all human cancer makes no difference in the context of developing regulatory procedures to control occupational carcinogens.

The inability of the industry during and after the hearing process to substantively chal-

lenge the scientific basis of the OSHA proposals, has become generally apparent.* This inability led to the decision by industry to shift the focus of debate from science in OSHA to economics in Congress, where the issues are clouded by other considerations including the national mood of deregulation. This reflects a more broadly based strategy that industry has recently evolved in opposition to environmental regulation.

The industry position on the allegedly heavy costs of regulation in general and occupational carcinogens in particular has gained the sympathy of the present administration. A Regulatory Analysis Review Group, with representation from the Council of Economic Advisors and the Council on Wage and Price Stability, is now requiring agencies to justify all proposed regulation that is perceived to be inflationary, even if this is unproven. The Group chaired by Council of Economic Advisors Charles L. Schultze, in September, 1978, selected the "generic" carcinogen policy as one of the handful of "very expensive regulations" it would study. On October 24, the Group issued a report criticizing OSHA for proposing too inflexible a regulatory scheme, and one that did not pay adequate attention to the costs of regulation. As yet, OSHA and other regulatory agencies have failed to develop and present a sufficiently strong case for the opposing position: that the costs of regulation are trivial in relation to the costs of failure to regulate, which are highly inflationary though still largely unrecognized.

The Flight of the Multinationals. In the past, when faced by the prospect of local regulatory controls, industry has moved or has threatened to move to Southern states, which have traditionally been more receptive to industrial interests and less concerned with occupational health and environmental consid-

---

* The overall conclusions of the HEW report were supported by two AIHC consultants, Revel A. Stallones and Thomas Downs (of the University of Texas School of Public Health). AIHC failed to include the Stallones Downs review in its posthearing submissions to OSHA.

erations. With the passage of the 1970 Occupational Health and Safety Act, the opportunity for such evasions in the United States became more limited.† U.S. industry with multinational connections then shifted tactics to exporting their hazardous industries abroad. "Runaway" shops were created in lesser developed countries such as Brazil or Taiwan, where there are virtually no regulatory controls and where cheap and unorganized labor is amply available. More surprising, however, is the increasing flight of segments of the chemical industry to runaway shops in eastern Europe, where regulatory controls and opportunities for public protest are minimal compared to the United States.

The growing flight from regulation poses major threats to foreign workers, and to the environmental quality outside the United States, besides reflecting on the corporate ethics of the industries involved. It also poses two sets of threats to the U.S. economy: loss of jobs and unfair advantage in competition with those segments of industry complying with pollution control regulations in the United States. In some industries, the flight from regulation is already established.[9] In others, it appears imminent. The greatest flight is seen in the asbestos textile industries, which are being increasingly located in Mexican border towns and in Taiwan and South Korea. There are also indications that other asbestos manufacturers, particularly of friction products such as brake linings and disc pads, will follow this course. Other flights involve arsenic-producing copper smelters and the plastics, benzidine dye, and pesticide industries.‡

Vigorous legislative initiatives, such as federal chartering of giant multinational corporations, are urgently needed[10] Federal chartering would impose specific restrictions on giant industries where four or fewer firms account for over 50 percent of sales in some major markets, and would restructure them internally to prevent such corporate abuses as bribery, illegal domestic and foreign political contributions, price-fixing, monopolistic practices, regulatory violations (including manipulation or suppression of data), and the export of hazardous products and processes. The broad objectives of the proposed federal corporate chartering would be to achieve corporate accountability to the U.S. government and people

> to assure more corporate democracy by giving greater voice or authority, for example to shareholders over the decision of managers; to require greater disclosure of the social and financial performance of companies; to deconcentrate industries and restore competition; to assure employees their civil rights and liberties by a bill of rights for employees.[11]

The recent proposal of the Council on Environmental Quality to require industry to file environmental impact statements before exporting hazardous products and processes is also an overdue approach to this problem. Patterns of flight need to be carefully monitored by federal groups and other concerned interests, including organized labor and responsible industry.* Assistance should also be requested from international organizations such as the World Health Organization and international labor groups.

An issue related to the flight of the multinational corporations is the common practice

---

† However, the chemical industry in New Jersey, is threatening to move elsewhere if the state perseveres in attempts at regulation, with particular reference to limiting the discharge of carcinogenic chemicals into the environment of the surrounding community.

‡ Following legal action by a coalition of environmental groups, the Agency for International Development announced in 1976 that it would no longer sponsor the export of pesticides banned in the U.S.

* The information available on hazard export is extremely scanty, though the trend is already well established.

of export of products whose use is not permitted in the United States, such as the pesticide leptophos, or products whose use has been banned in the United States, such as the pesticide dieldrin and children's sleeping garments treated with the flame retardant Tris. In January, 1978, Senator Gaylord Nelson (D-Wisc.) called for a ban on export of pesticides whose use is prohibited in the United States, after samples of imported agricultural products show residues of these pesticides. This whole area needs comprehensive legislation to prevent exposure of foreign workers and consumers to products manufactured by the U.S. industry but considered too hazardous for use here.† A critically related issue which demands vigorous international initiatives is the growing promotional campaign of the tobacco industry in the Third World.

Technological Innovation and Regulation

Some segments of industry have repeatedly expressed concerns that the mounting tide of federal regulation over the last two decades is impeding or stifling technological innovation. The Manufacturing Chemists Association and Dow Chemical Company have claimed that requiring chemicals to be tested prior to their introduction into commerce, in accordance with current requirements of toxic substances legislation, is acting as an obstacle to industrial innovation. (These claims have particularly involved the manufacture of pesticides and contraceptive drugs.) Such claims ignore costs to society of the failure to regulate and they do not bear critical scrutiny even on narrowly defined economic grounds. Costs of carcinogenicity and other chronic toxicity testing and costs of toxic substances legislation are small in relation to the profits of the chemical industry.

Ever sensitive to changing national moods, industry demands for deregulation have recently become more clamorous and linked to concerns on Proposition 13, inflation, alleged free-spending by runaway regulation agencies, and growing big government intrusion into free enterprise. Industry has taken out full-page advertisements in leading national newspapers complaining that "the spiraling costs of regulation," both compliance and administrative, are inflationary and are stifling innovation.‡ The industry position is buttressed by articles and letters in leading journals and newspapers from prominent academic spokesmen, and by restrictions on health and environmental regulations newly imposed by the Regulatory Analysis Review Group of COWPS.[12] Apart from the self-serving nature of industry demands for deregulation, these reflect the myopia of traditional economists preoccupied with immediate costs of compliance, rather than with the usual heavier and externalized costs of failure to regulate, such as the recognized $30 billion annual costs of cancer (apart from its much greater unrecognized costs), the multibillion dollar costs of impending law suits on asbestos, and the costs of environmental degradation.[13]

In an address to the Third National Con-

---

† Banned products, being exported include Tris, DDT, cyclamates, and Red #2.

‡ Organizational inertia and vested interests in existing technology are likely to be rate-limiting factors in the development of new technologies. Additionally, it must be recognized that the immediate *costs* of compliance may be disproportionately great for small business which cannot usually capture the economies of scale available to big business adopting control technologies, and may thus exert monopolistic influences. It is, however, clear that advancing information on hazards of occupational carcinogens has not been paralleled by advances in process and compliance technology. (For a critical analysis of the impact of regulation on technological innovation, see N. A. Ashford, *et al.* "The Implications of Health, Safety and Environmental Regulations for Technological Change," Department of Commerce Contract No. NB-79-SAC-A0030, January 15, 1979.)

ference on Health Policies on May 22, 1978, Congressman Rogers (D-Fla.) commented on the dichotomous attitude of industry to costs:

> Yet the contrast is startling between the runaway spending for health care and the resistance of most of American business to spending for environmental health protection. At a dizzying pace, hospitals race to build new beds and new wings, acquire CAT (computerized axial tomography) scanners, open-heart surgery units, and cardiac catherization units — all to treat disease once it occurs.
>
> On the other hand, last year's total environmental control expenditures for all American industry totalled less than $40 billion, that is, less than 20 percent of the Nation's total health care spending. And American industry fought every inch of the way against every environmental health requirement. Every dollar invested to reduce deadly coke-oven emissions, to control arsenic and lead from copper smelters, to block unnecessary radiation exposures, to capture chemical plants' carcinogenic discharges, to curb toxic sulfates and nitrate particles from coal combustion, has come only after protracted political and legal struggles.

Industry demands for deregulation in pollution and preventive health areas are in interesting contrast with their insistence on continued economic regulation to protect monopolistic practices.[14] In spite of all the praise lavished by industry and its public-regula-

tions machinery on the concept of free competition in a deregulated market, industry fights vigorously to foster "economic socialism" whenever its interests are threatened, as illustrated by the opposition of the trucking industry to proposed deregulation by the Interstate Commerce Commission, and the American Medical Association (on behalf of the medical industry) to advertising. As Chairman Michael Pertschuk of the Federal Trade Commission commented in October, 1978:

> Such regulations are not sanctioned by law, but rather are carried on in defiance of the law — not as *government* regulation of business, but as anti-competitive and inflationary *business* regulation of business. And where these forms of business-inspired regulation do remain imbedded in the law, it is because those businesses and professions regulated have stoutly defended their ancient right to be shielded from the discomforts of free competition.

In recent Congressional testimony, Secretary of Commerce Juanita Kreps emphasized that every industry leader agitated by "government intrusion" should understand that industry cannot responsibly demand less regulation without also addressing those social issues that prompted the need for regulation.

> To the extent business helps [through improved corporate social performance] to deal with issues that might otherwise prompt government regulation, it serves its own economic interests.*

---

* However, a December 20, 1978, draft report on "Environmental Health and Safety Regulations" of a Department of Commerce Advisory Subcommittee (of the Advisory Committee on Industrial Innovation) demonstrated lack of comprehension of Secretary Kreps' warning. The committee (which in its exclusive composition of industry appears to violate at least the intent of the Federal Advisory Committee Act) claimed that federal regulations have a severe negative impact on in-

dustrial productivity and industrial innovation on grounds including: diverted capital expenditures from productive to non-productive areas; increased cost of product development; increased product development cycle; uncertain standards; the special problem of small business; inadequate protection of trade-secret information; excessive reporting requirements; and growing costs of product liability loss protection and prevention. The report also calls for consensus standards as a pref-

What we are involved in is a simple but mean-
ingful thing, the commandment that in civi-
lized society thou shall not kill. The propo-
nents of cost-benefit analysis would have us
believe that it is all right to kill if killing is
not too expensive.

James Smith, United Steelworkers
of America economist
OSHA testimony, 1978.

Labor

A 1970 University of Michigan survey sponsored by the Department of Labor found that American workers rated health and safety a higher priority than increased wages.[15] This helped explode the common belief that workers relegate health issues to a minor role compared with bread-and-butter and job-security issues. In fact, workers have placed a high premium on safe working conditions throughout the hundred-year history of trade unions.

Organized labor's support of child labor laws and its insistence on an eight-hour working day led to considerable industrial strife in the 1870s. The March 25, 1911, fire at the Triangle Shirtwaist Company in New York City drew public attention to the atrocious working conditions of many young girls, and led to the enactment of corrective legislation.[16]

One of the unions that has long been involved in health and safety issues is the United Mine Workers, whose members are employed in the most hazardous industry in America. The record of the union on health and safety is mixed.[17] During the late 1940s and early 1950s, frustrated by its inability to obtain minimal compensation for disabled

workers and urged on by Lorin Kerr, Assistant to the Executive Medical Officer of the Union's Welfare and Retirement Fund (Director of the Department of Occupational Health of the United Mine Workers of America since 1969), the Fund paid for the establishment and operation of ten hospitals in mining regions of rural Appalachia and recruited its own doctors and staff.† By 1962, affected both by mismanagement and severe recession in the industry, the hospitals were sold to the Presbyterian church and the experiment ended. One of the staff physicians, Donald Rasmussen, also led an effort to have black lung recognized as a compensable illness. The union leadership, while initially hostile to the pressure which quickly developed in its ranks around the black lung issue, was ultimately forced to support federal legislation. It took a disaster, however, the 1968 explosion at a Farmington, West Virginia, mine which killed seventy-four miners, to bring about enactment of the 1969 Federal Coal Mine Health and Safety Act.

The modern era of labor concerns over health and safety and occupational carcinogenesis is a striking tribute to a handful of labor leaders who have had to overcome crippling problems. Not only have they had to emancipate themselves from the self-serving authoritarianism of industry physicians and other professionals, and to educate themselves in the relatively recent area of adverse health effects due to chemical exposures, but they have also had to develop rank-and-file support. To do this, they have sought out advice and guidance from a few independent professionals in the academic community. On a limited scale, they have also developed their own expertise and resources, particularly in industrial hygiene. Additionally, they have

---

erable alternative to mandatory government regulations. As illustration of the potential of innovation if not fettered by excessive regulation, the health panel of the subcommittee opined "the 'penicillin' for cancer . . . may be just around the

corner if development is encouraged."
† The Fund was established in 1946 under a wage agreement between the Union and Coal Mine operators, and is financed by a royalty paid by the operators per ton of bituminous coal.

had to contend with economic blackmail and threats of job loss by industry whenever they advocate or support attempts to regulate unsafe exposures. Not surprisingly, most of the focus of labor concerns on problems of chemical exposures has so far been expressed in Washington, D.C. rather than at the grass-roots level.

Most prominent among these labor leaders is Anthony Mazzocchi, Vice President of the Oil, Chemical, and Atomic Workers Union (OCAW). One of Mazzocchi's many contributions has been to extend the arena of concerns on health issues to the rank-and-file of union membership. The president of the union, Al Grospiron, has also made important contributions, particularly as chairman of the Standing Committee on Safety and Occupational Health, AFL-CIO. Another labor leader who has taken consistently strong positions on needs to regulate chemical hazards is George Taylor, executive secretary of the Standing Committee on Safety and Occupational Health. Taylor has exerted a powerful influence on the development of a wide range of occupational standards, particularly through his chairmanship of the Staff Subcommittee of the Standing Committee. Another important figure is Peter Bommarito, president of the United Rubber Workers, assisted by his industrial hygienist, Louis Beliczky. Bommarito is chairman of the Executive Committee on Occupational Health and Safety of the Industrial Union Department, AFL-CIO, and has pioneered the development of joint labor — management contracts to universities for research on problems of carcinogenesis in the rubber industry.

The Industrial Union Department of the AFL-CIO, established after the 1954 AFL-CIO merger (the current president is the labor veteran Jacob Clayman), plays a critical role in the whole area of occupational health and safety. The director of the department's Division of Occupational Safety and Health and the Environment is Sheldon Samuels, who has functioned primarily as a policy analyst and technical consultant to the industrial unions. He also monitors the performance of OSHA, NIOSH, NCI and other agencies.‡ Additionally, Samuels has developed educational programs for organized labor on occupational hazards.

Major credit for the development of the 1970 Occupational Safety and Health Act belongs to Jack Sheehan, legislative director of United Steelworkers of America. Sheehan is an accomplished lobbyist whose influence has been felt on most recent major occupational standards.

George Perkel, Director of Research of the Amalgamated Clothing and Textile Workers Union, and Larry Ahern, Research Director

---

‡ An interesting sideline on Samuels was his recommendation in July, 1978 (on behalf of organized labor), that NCI withdraw its invitation to Hans Weill, Professor of Medicine at Tulane University in New Orleans, to cochair a conference on lung-cancer surveillance. Labor's objections were based on the fact that Weill was unlikely to be neutral in view of his close relationship with the American Textile Manufacturer's Institute and with the Asbestos Information Center who had contracted with him to attack the OSHA proposal to reduce to 500,000 the current 2-million-fiber-per-cubic-meter asbestos standard. Weill's position, that the current standard "should be given a reasonable trial while further epidemiologic investigation estab-lished its safety or lack of it" (submission of the Asbestos Information Association on Proposed Revision to the OSHA Asbestos Standard, April 8, 1976, Docket H-033, p. 24), is consistent with his earlier prospective studies of accelerated silicosis among poorly protected sandblasters, during which time workers dying after one and a half years exposure were observed in order to assess "rational occupational environmental standards" (National Heart and Lung Institute Grant Application, September 4, 1975). The latter studies effectively excluded OSHA inspections under an agreement reached between the industry and Weill (see S. W. Samuels, "NCI Disinvitation," *Science* 202 [1978], p. 694).

of the International Chemical Workers Union, have both contributed materially to expressing labor's informed concerns on standards. Perkel also exercised an important influence as Chairman of the Industrial Union Department *Ad Hoc* Committee on Occupational Carcinogens on the precedential 1973 OSHA standards proceedings for fourteen occupational carcinogens.

The International Association of Heat and Frost Insulators and Asbestos Workers, whose president is Andy Haas, has also been prominent in the struggle to protect workers from exposure to carcinogenic dusts and fibers. The successes that the union has achieved in this regard reflect the important collaboration they have developed with Irving Selikoff.

AFL-CIO is now developing closer collaboration with unions outside the Federation, particularly the International Brotherhood of Teamsters and the United Auto Workers Union. In this they have been materially aided by R. V. Durham, Research Director of the Teamsters, and Dan McLeod and Frank Mirer, Industrial Hygienists of the Auto Workers.

Recent labor concerns on occupational carcinogenesis have been largely spearheaded by OCAW, whose members operate many of the nation's largest refineries and chemical plants. Throughout 1969 and 1970, many of the union's nine district councils, covering much of the United States and all of Canada, sponsored workshops entitled "Hazards in the Industrial Environment." At these conferences, Mazzocchi discussed with union members the basic facts underlying health and safety problems in OCAW plants. For many, it was the first realization that problems arising from workplace chemicals could be recognized and dealt with.

Mazzocchi sought out and developed close personal contacts with a handful of professional scientists who helped him increase awareness in labor, Congress, and elsewhere in the government of the major hazards posed to workers by uncontrolled exposure to toxic and carcinogenic chemicals. Mazzocchi also sponsored the formation in 1971 of the Scientists Committee for Occupational Health, which, jointly with the United Auto Workers and other New Jersey labor groups, taught several courses at the Rutgers University Labor Education Center. Their students were workers who, instead of hearing just about ladders and fire extinguishers, found out about cancer-causing chemicals in their own workplaces, many for the first time.

In 1973, 4,000 OCAW workers went out on a five-month strike against Shell Oil in California and in four other states, demanding that their new contract embody specific measures to protect health and safety on the job. The union made four key demands:

1. Establishment of a joint union — management health and safety committee in every plant.
2. Periodic inspections of plants, by independent consultants jointly approved by labor and management, to determine whether workers are being exposed to hazards.
3. Medical examination of workers, at company expense, when indicated by plant inspections.
4. Availability to the union of all company records on worker's sickness and death.[18]

Impressed by the importance of the strike, a group of about twenty-five leading scientists and educators signed a statement, published by the union as a full-page advertisement in *The New York Times* on May 3, 1973.* This statement recognized that the strike was unique in labor history and prompted exclusively by concerns for occupational health:

Workers have long served as unwitting guinea pigs, providing useful toxicological data which helped to protect the public. The effects of most environmental pol-

* The author wrote this statement.

lutants, such as carbon monoxide, lead, mercury and also of most human carcinogens were first detected in workmen; the in-plant environment is a concentrated toxic microcosm of that outside. Additionally, many toxic agents disperse beyond the plant and pose public hazards.

The success of the OCAW strike is critical both to labor and the public. This has already been recognized by ten major environmental and public interest groups who have endorsed the Shell strike and boycott. The demand of labor to participate actively in protecting the health and safety of workers is basic and inalienable and cannot be sacrificed to narrow economic interests. It is hoped that Shell will adopt a posture more consistent with the public interest and the intent of the 1970 Occupational Safety and Health Act . . .[19]

Shell, which at first refused to bargain on "management prerogative" issues, was eventually forced to give in. However, the subsequent enforcement of contract terms continues to be an uphill struggle.

A key labor issue which has been strongly championed by OCAW is the guarantee of full economic protection of a worker in the event he or she is removed from a job classification on the basis of medical examination results. This is known as "rate retention" and means that the worker would, upon transfer, retain the same rate of pay allowed by the previous job classification, as well as all pay increases, seniority, and other benefits accruing to the former position. Another critical area pioneered by the union is the use of the Review Commission of OSHA to protect its members in situations where management contests citations by OSHA for violations against health and safety standards.

Over the recent years, management has encouraged hostility between labor and environmentalists by threatening to close plants when there are major attempts to control in-plant pollution. In 1972, responding to de-

mands to improve working conditions, Union Carbide threatened to shut down its Alloy, West Virginia, plant, elected one of America's ten dirtiest factories by *Business Week* magazine. OCAW President A. F. Grospiron refused to knuckle under to "environmental blackmail," and Union Carbide was eventually forced to improve work practices.[20] In an address to the Union convention in 1973, Sierra Club Executive Director Michael McCloskey commented, "Your Union has been preeminent in recognizing that many environmental threats originate in the workplace and affect the workers first and foremost, before they escape into the community-at-large."

Labor has gradually developed working relationships with NIOSH and OSHA. Representatives of labor, as well as management, now participate in various advisory committees of these agencies. In addition to the more long-standing association of labor with Selikoff (particularly by the International Association of Heat and Frost Insulators and Asbestos Workers), and other such associations of labor as those with Thomas F. Mancuso, occupational physician at the University of Pittsburgh, who contributes an excellent monthly health column in the newsletter of the International Union of Electrical, Radio and Machine Workers, labor has recently developed contractual arrangements with a few universities to investigate specific occupational health problems. Unions that have been prominent in this regard include OCAW, the United Auto Workers, and the United Rubber, Cork, Linoleum, and Plastic Workers of America. A major recent resource for labor besides management and government, is the Society for Occupational and Environmental Health, whose meetings and conferences have created an opportunity for independent and expert analysis of health-related issues.

Realizing the critical importance of developing its own internal scientific and technical resources, several unions have created health and safety departments or units, which are at present largely staffed by industrial hygienists.† OCAW and the United Auto Workers have set up Health and Safety Offices which administer nationwide programs for their members, coordinate activities of individual locals (particularly in testing provisions of the Occupational Safety and Health Act), and help extend the parameters of the collective bargaining agreement. The only union that has had a medical director for any period of time (Lorin Kerr) is the United Mine Workers of America.

AFL-CIO for several years has been considering the creation of its own resource in occupational health and safety. Recent occupational health crises have lent further urgency to these plans and to the realization that, in the final analysis, labor must rely on its own resources.‡ Accordingly, in December, 1977, the AFL-CIO Executive Committee authorized creation of its own "institute or appropriate structure . . . [as a] permanent means of more adequately meeting our responsibilities to protect the health and safety" of workers. With the guidance of OCAW's Grospiron, this proposal was transformed from an earlier concept of an academy-like institution to a department with the on-line function of providing staff services to AFL-CIO as part of its secretariat. The department was formally created in August, 1978, with George Taylor as its head. Taylor reports directly to AFL-CIO President George Meany through his assistant Tom Donahue. It is expected that the department will hire scientific and technical staff in addition to consultants, and that its initial priorities will focus on the standard setting process in both NIOSH and OSHA.*

Another major and overdue development has been the growing awareness in labor that there is an inevitable built-in conflict of interest in the present system of direct employment of occupational physicians by industry. Results of physical examinations on individual workers can thus be directly transmitted to management, with ensuing risks of job transfer or loss.

The role of industry epidemiologists, industrial hygienists, and other professionals involved in occupational health and safety demands critical evaluation. These needs are emphasized by the growing body of information on the existence and extent of constraints on health and safety data, ranging from inadequacy and biased interpretation to manipulation and fraud.

Clearly the salaries of health and safety professionals is the exclusive responsibility of industry as an essential part of the costs of doing business. This should not mean that the loyalty of these professionals must necessarily be directed to their employers. While the salaries of meat inspectors and grain elevator inspectors are in the final analysis paid for by the industries concerned, these inspec-

---

† These include OCAW, United Steelworkers of America, United Rubber, Cork, Linoleum and Plastic Workers of America, and United Auto Workers.

‡ In three recently publicized occupational catastrophes (involving kepone, a carcinogenic pesticide producing neurotoxic and sterilizing effects in workers at Life Sciences Products Corporation in Virginia; leptophos, a pesticide producing neurotoxic effects in workers in a Velsicol Plant in Bayport, Texas; and DBCP [dibromochloropropane], a carcinogenic soil fumigant producing sterility in workers involved in its manufacture at Oc-

cidental Chemical Company in California), it was the workers themselves who first recognized the problem, not the plant physicians and not OSHA. It must be clearly recognized that plant health and safety committees are still the exception in the U.S. and that hygiene and occupational health services are still not available or utilized by most U.S. industries.

* Additionally, an AFL-CIO Workers Institute for Safety and Health, headed by Charles Warren, Secretary-Treasurer of the Ohio AFL-CIO, was incorporated in Columbus, Ohio, in April, 1979, with a satellite office in Washington, D.C.

tors are primarily responsible to USDA. Similarly, health professionals in industry must be primarily responsible to the worker-patient, rather than to industry. It should be a felony for an industrial physician to divulge to management the results of a physical examination. Such information is the exclusive property of the concerned principals, the physician and the worker-patient, and must not be shared with management. This is the only way by which a worker can be protected against economic penalties which management may invoke if a worker is found to be suffering adverse effects from conditions at work. Otherwise, the worker will be forced to choose the Russian roulette of exposure to occupational hazards, rather than risk job loss or transfer to a lower-paid job.

Confidential physician-worker relationships would in no way decrease the ability of an occupational physician to disclose to management and to labor the gross and anonymous results of physical examination and biological monitoring of groups of workers in specific job situations in order to allow necessary corrective action to be taken. Labor has begun to realize that the development of further occupational standards is of limited value, possibly even counterproductive, unless workers can be assured of the independence of the professionals whose responsibility is, or should be, the protection of the workers' health. The worker also must be protected against economic penalties by guarantees of equal pay and seniority rights in the event he is moved from a job with a high level of exposure to one with a lower level.

The Public Interest Movement

The public interest movement, as a modern expression of social ethics and as an instrument of political reform, is now about a decade old. Public interest organizations have generally evolved from the initiatives of young activist lawyers and other professionals, and also from expressions of citizen and consumer concerns. In this, they have been supported by a small number of independent scientists and engineers who have helped bridge the gap between technical and societal considerations.

Public interest organizations embrace a wide spectrum of heterogeneous objectives and styles. While the most influential and best-known groups are Washington-based, citizen and consumer groups more "grass roots" in nature are found in most major metropolitan centers. Student public interest research groups are a nationwide effort. They are autonomous, student-run organizations to be found on most campuses and have a record of local activism. Such groups were inspired in large part by Ralph Nader.

The public interest movement expresses the conviction that the "common good" is inadequately represented in decision making at federal and local levels, where narrow economic and political interests are joined, often at the expense of social equity. The movement also expresses the conviction that the public health and environmental costs of modern technology are poorly perceived and too readily discounted in regulatory decision making, and that the burden of proof for such "externalized" costs is too readily accepted by government, or inappropriately shifted from the private to the public sector. As recently stated:

In almost every judicial, legislative or administrative conflict or policy-making process, the law provides either implicitly or explicitly that the burden of proof rests on one of the parties. The criteria are quite simple. The burden of proof rests on the party that initiates the risk, that profits from the risk, and that has the greatest resources to do something about the risks.[21]

The public interest conviction of the imbalanced and unrepresentative nature of governmental decision making has been supported by evidence of major conflicts of interest in senior staff of regulatory agencies, by their unwillingness to involve qualified citizen and consumer representatives in decision making, by restrictions on public access to data on the basis of which important decisions on health and safety are based, and by evidence of major constraints and deficiencies in this hidden data base.

Broadly speaking, public interest groups are either "resource" or "activist" in nature. The resource function is well illustrated by the activities of the Rachel Carson Trust in gathering, organizing, and interpreting information on pesticides and toxic chemicals, and in disseminating this to other concerned groups and the public.† Activist functions include lobbying, attempting to institute regulatory reforms, monitoring agency performance, and filing legal action as a last resort. Each public interest group tends to specialize in a particular area: drugs, food additives, pesticides, air, and water pollutants, or occupational health and safety, to name a few. While in the past labor has tended to resent the "intrusion" of public interest groups into the arena of occupational health, particularly because of the alleged conflict between job security and safer working conditions, informal accommodations, such as the supportive relationship between the Health Research Group and OCAW, have recently developed.

Public interest groups have faced difficulties in establishing themselves and making an impact on public perceptions and government policies, already sensitive and responsive to the massive and well-focused and financed industry lobby. The most limiting of these problems have been financial.‡ Public interest groups largely depend on voluntary contributions from the general public. Other problems stem from the understandable tendency of the groups to move on to other areas of concern after initial resolution of a particular issue, with resulting inadequate follow-up and the possibility of "winning the battle, but losing the war." Public interest groups have also tended to work in relative isolation from each other, for reasons which include their strong sense of independence and preoccupation with their own immediate aims, sometimes to the exclusion of broader objectives. Recognition of these limitations, in addition to the need to develop closer contact between public interest groups and concerned professionals and labor, led to the creation in 1974 of the Commission for the Advancement of Public Interest Organizations.* Current activities of the commission focus on the development of loose, ad hoc coalitions of public interest groups and labor around critical generic concerns, particularly relating to preventable cancer. These activities include supporting New Jersey citizen and labor groups in their efforts to reduce the high incidence of environmental cancer in their state; nominating qualified professionals to serve on the NCI National Cancer Advisory Board and advisory committees of other agencies with prime responsibility in control of environmental carcinogens; supporting the nomination of qualified scientific and legal professionals to senior positions in federal agencies (for example, the present NCI di-

---

† The author is president of the Rachel Carson Trust.

‡ An important recent development is the "Public Participation in Federal Agency Proceedings Act," sponsored by Senators Edward Kennedy (D-Mass.) and Charles Mathias, Jr. (R-Md.), and Congressman Peter Rodino (D-N.J.), now pending before Congress. The bill would allow public interest groups to participate in agency proceedings and also to file suit against agencies for unlawful acts. It would create a special treasury fund of $15 million annually for three years which would be available for these and related purposes.

* The author chairs this commission, which is an arm of the Monsour Medical Foundation, Jeanette, Pa.

rector, Arthur Upton); and holding "round-tables," where heads of agencies are invited periodically to interact with the public interest and labor communities on such critical questions as environmental and occupational cancer.

The past impact of public interest groups on national perspectives and on the legislative and executive branches of government has been profound and disproportionate to the small size and resources of these groups. In no area of public interest activity has this been better exemplified than in that of preventable cancer. As illustrated in the case studies cited in this book, the great majority of all standards on environmental and occupational carcinogens developed over the last decade have been initiated by petitions and lawsuits of public interest groups and labor against the government (see Table 9.8). The past successes of public interest groups in these actions have been all the more remarkable in that they have generally had to fight on two fronts, against both industry and the regulating agency. Groups that have taken a lead role in these actions are the Environmental Defense Fund, Public Citizen's Health Research Group and Litigation Group, and the National Resources Defense Council. Important contributory roles have also been played by other groups, including the Sierra Club, Consumers Union, Consumer Federation of America, Center for Science in the Public Interest, Federation of Homemakers, Action on Smoking and Health, Migrant Legal Action Programs, Friends of the Earth, the Rachel Carson Trust, the National Audubon Society, and the National Wildlife Federation.

Recent Trends

Past contacts between public interest groups and regulatory agencies and industry have necessarily been adversarial. Adversarial tactics, whether in committee meetings or the courts

and Congress, have been helpful in defining positions on environmental priorities and posing critical environmental and public health problems. Tentative moves are now being made by a few public interest groups to explore the alternative that non-adversarial dialogue with industry may prove to be mutually beneficial in defined circumstances, such as assuring industry of the essential consistency between long-term industrial growth and protection of the environment and public health.

An interesting example of these exchanges is the National Coal Policy Project, the environmental caucus of which is headed by Laurence I. Moss, former president of the Sierra Club.[22] Another is the Business-Environment Project created by the Conservation Foundation in attempts to suggest improved guidelines for toxic substances testing.† A draft document of the Business-Environment Project dated January 16, 1978, entitled "Approaches for the Development of Testing Guidelines Under the Toxic Substances Control Act" reveals an apparent lack of comprehension of the basic toxicological issues involved. The document has been criticized by an industry scientist as "being more concerned with birds and bees than humans." The document places major emphasis on short-term tests as indirect indicators of carcinogenicity. As a final criterion of carcinogenicity, the document recommends the "heritable translocation test," which is a highly specialized procedure that has so far only been applied to fewer than a dozen compounds.

Questions of expertise apart, there are needs to consider whether the public interest movement now has the necessary scientific resources to develop and sustain the type of rapprochement with industry envisioned in these new exchanges. There is a growing likelihood of an increase in these dialogues be-

---

† This project is co-chaired by Karim Ahmed of the Natural Resources Defense Council and George Dominguez of Ciba-Geigy, and is headed up by Sam Gusman, just retired as Washington representative of Rohm & Haas.

tween industry and the public interest movement, which is encouraged by the possibility of foundation and agency funding. It seems possible that premature moves of this type may blunt the limited impact of the public interest movement, even to the point of possible co-option.

An important development has been the recruitment of some key leaders of the public interest movement to senior positions in federal agencies. These include Joan Claybrook, former director of the Public Citizen Congress Watch, currently Administrator of the National Highway Traffic Safety Administration; Carol Foreman, former executive director of the Consumer Federation of America, currently Assistant Secretary of Agriculture; Harrison Wellford, formerly of the Center for the Study of Responsive Law and chief legislative assistant to the late Senator Philip A. Hart (D-Mich.), currently Executive Associate Director for Management and Regulatory Policy, Office of Management and Budget; Gus J. Speth, formerly of the Natural Resources Defense Council, currently a member of the Council on Environmental Quality; David Hawkins, also of the Natural Resources Defense Council, currently Assistant Administrator Air and Waste Management, EPA; Peter Shuck, formerly of Consumers Union, currently Deputy Assistant Secretary of HEW; and Cynthia Wilson, formerly of the National Audubon Society, currently Assistant to the Secretary of Interior.

It is premature to assess the impact of this "move to government." While it is generally welcomed as a potential infusion of "new and honest young blood," a caution has been raised to the effect that not only have the slender ranks of the public interest movement been seriously depleted, but also that its unique strength lies in keeping a distance from government. Nader has been more explicit in his criticism of consumer advocates who have joined the administration.

> . . . I think they've been too cautious. I think they've been too defensive, and I think to some degree they've even been apologetic about prior careers as consumer advocates. They won't admit it, but their behavior has been such that they're leaning over the other way to compensate for it.[23]

The public interest movement is now at a critical juncture. It has lost some of its best leaders and most informed lobbyists to government. In the absence of new initiatives, the future financial base of the movement is precarious. Competition for public funds among the estimated 2,500 public interest organizations is now becoming keener. Direct mailing lists soliciting support for public interest groups have become so overgrazed that they are now of questionable value. Foundation support for public interest groups has sharply declined, consistent with usual foundation policies of initiating but not sustaining. This growing financial crisis has been compounded by the election of a liberal President, who has taken the steam out of left-wing social protest, which in the past has been an important source of public interest support. There has not yet been adequate articulation of this shift of the winds of fortune by public interest groups to the executive branch, Congress, foundations, or the public at large.

The public interest movement has not yet adequately shifted focus from emphasis on specific individual issues, such as a particular carcinogen, pesticide, or feed additive, to broader approaches which will embody a wider set of generic concerns. More critical still is the absence of a grassroots consumer movement which is clearly the only practical way consumers will be able to exercise effective political influence to protect their interests.‡ Industry, on the other hand, has mobi-

---

‡ The absence of such a grassroots base, together with strong pressures from big business on the House of Representatives, were critical factors in the defeat in February, 1978, of the long-em-

lized on a massive and well-financed scale to propagandize the government and an already apathetic or even antipathetic public against the need for regulatory controls and to assert, on the basis of tenuous or misleading evidence, that their costs would be inflationary, while completely ignoring the much higher costs to society from failure to regulate. Industry has launched a new range of well organized and financed cooperative initiatives, such as the Business Round Table, corporate Political Action Committees,* and the American Industrial Health Council, which threaten the future effective control and regulation of industry.

The combination of well-focused intensive legislative pressures from a small army of highly paid lobbyists in Washington, national grassroots support mobilized through Chambers of Commerce all over the country, and lavish advertisements in the press (such as those of the Calorie Control Council in opposition to the proposed FDA saccharin ban), have created major and unparalleled threats to the whole process of democratic decision making as well as to the public interest movement. It is now more urgent than ever the public interest groups address this crisis of imbalance in national policies. This is the critical message that must be intensively disseminated on a grassroots level if public interest groups are to survive, let alone maintain their effectiveness.

The possibility of stronger public interest input into federal agencies was created by a memorandum of April 27, 1978, by President Carter, outlining new functions for the White House Office of Consumer Affairs, headed by Esther Peterson. It is proposed that this office should become actively involved in executive policy making on consumer problems. Existing public interest participation programs in federal agencies will be reviewed. Peterson will also be able to evaluate public interest programs in federal agencies — and other actions that impact on the public interest — and to make necessary recommendations how these may be improved.

Additional Influences on Policy Making

Independent Professionals

Among other groups influencing national policies, a handful of independent professionals of recognized expertise in fields such as toxicology, carcinogenesis, and epidemiology has been particularly important. Over the last decade, these people have been instrumental in providing a critical data base and scientific guidance to leading labor reformers, and to public interest groups and members of Congress concerned about preventable cancer and other environmental and occupational problems. These professionals have also become

---

battled bill to establish a new federal consumer protection agency.

* Political Action Committees, authorized by recent changes in federal election laws, now number about six hundred, while their labor counterparts have leveled off at about 250. Massive expansion of the corporate committees is being organized and stimulated by a consortium that includes the National Chamber of Commerce, the National Association of Manufacturers, the National Federation of Independent Business, and the Center for the Study of Free Enterprise of the University of Southern California's Graduate School of Business. The avowed major objective

of these new committees is to reduce government regulation and bureaucratic paper work. However, as pointed out in a recent OMB report, "Paper Work and Red Tape," much of the paper burden has been created by Congress and the courts, and most complaints mask an opposition to a particular federal program. (Also, major needs for paper work are the necessity to protect the public against fraud and to evaluate government programs.) In fact, despite a large number of new programs with reporting requirements, OMB has shown that there has been a 10 percent reduction in the time spent on report filing since January, 1977.

an important resource to leading press and science writers.

Professional Societies

On the whole, the professional community-at-large and professional organizations and societies have been indifferent, if not hostile, to environmental and occupational problems and needs for controls. The main reason for this is a not unnatural preoccupation with professional concerns, which is often compounded by conservatism, ignorance of the problems, or special interest. The role of the American College of Obstetricians and Gynecologists in joining with the Pharmaceutical Manufacturers Association in opposing the FDA's action on labeling of Premarin with a carcinogenicity warning is illustrative. Other examples include the Society of Toxicology, which has served as a professional base for the protection of industrial interests, such as by fighting against the Delaney Amendment. In a similar class, the American Conference of Governmental Industrial Hygienists has generated so-called safe exposure levels or "threshold limit values," exposure levels for a wide range of chemical agents without adequate consideration of long-term effects, particularly cancer.

On the other side of the coin, organizations such as the Medical Committee on Human Rights have exercised a useful role in informing socially conscious clinicians of needs for safe working conditions. From such activities have sprung a series of Committees on Occupational Safety and Health (so-called COSH groups) many of which continue to play an important long-term role in their communities, such as those in Chicago (CACOSH) and Philadelphia (PHILAPOSH). The Environmental Mutagen Society, created in 1969, has performed and continues to perform a useful service by interesting geneticists in practical

problems of genetic hazards from toxic chemicals in the general environment and workplace, and in educating the scientific and regulatory communities on such problems. The American Public Health Association is also developing a contributory role in environmental and occupational areas. The American Association for the Advancement of Science has developed programmatic coverage of major environmental and occupational problems and their social implications in its annual meetings, and in 1976 formed a Committee on Scientific Freedom and Responsibility to examine underlying ethical considerations.

The Society for Occupational and Environmental Health, founded in November, 1972, represents an important milestone in the history of professional societies.† The society was created to provide a mutual context for dialogue between government, labor, industry, and academia on scientific problems and information underlying regulatory decisions in the workplace and general environment. The uniqueness of the society stems from its broad-spectrum and staunchly independent approach to problems of critical concerns on health and safety, and its promotion of occasions for focusing independent expertise on these concerns. Society meetings and workshops on such topics as occupational exposure to beryllium, lead and arsenic, occupational carcinogenesis, and reproductive hazards in the workplace provide opportunities for unusually frank discussions of scientific and regulatory problems. This is in sharp contrast to conventional practices in the usually self-congratulatory climate of industry and establishment-dominated professional societies dedicated to preserving and defending the status quo. Recognizing these particular qualities, then-Senator Walter Mondale stated in an address at the annual society meeting on

---

† The past presidents of the society were Irving Selikoff (1972-74), Samuel S. Epstein (1974-76), and Joseph Wagoner (1976-78). The current president is Umberto Saffiotti.

December 4, 1973:

> You represent — more than anyone else — the best skills and experience necessary to the accomplishment of the national objective declared by the Occupational Safety and Health Act.

Another important independent organization is the Federation of American Scientists, known as "The Voice of Science on Capitol Hill." The federation is a unique lobbying group of 7,000 natural and social scientists and engineers concerned with problems of science and society. It was first organized in 1946 as the Federation of Atomic Scientists, but its current interests are now broader. It has recently taken an active and informed stand on urgent needs for control of environmental cancer. While the federation is a high-caliber professional society, it also functions as an activist public interest organization.

Cancer is one of the most curable of the major diseases of this country.

American Cancer Society, 1976

The American Cancer Society

The American Cancer Society is the largest private philanthropic institution in the country (besides being the world's largest nonreligious charity), and is devoted exclusively to cancer. It was founded as the American Society for the Control of Cancer in 1913, and incorporated in 1922, by a small group of concerned clinicians and laypersons (mainly industrialists) in order to educate the public in the need for early diagnosis and proper treatment of cancer. Fund raising for the society was undertaken by the Women's Field Army, an association of national women's organizations with no representation on the board, which was composed exclusively of cancer clinicians and hospital administrators.

Mary Lasker's involvement in the society began in 1943, when its budget was $356,000. She recruited Emerson Foote, a senior executive of Lord and Thomas (a Chicago advertising agency whose previous president was Albert D. Lasker), and Elmer Bobst, head of the U.S. arm of the international Hoffman La Roche drug company and honorary chairman of Warner-Lambert Pharmaceutical Company. The triumvirate transformed the society from a voluntary amateur-type organization into a highly efficient and aggressive fund-raising operation, which by 1946 had raised the budget to about $4 million. The name of the society was changed to the American Cancer Society, the bylaws and constitution were rewritten, and the board was reconstituted with 50 percent lay representation. The society then rapidly grew to its present strength to include 2,800 local units (organized in fifty-eight major divisions), with headquarters in New York, a paid staff of over 3,000, and an active volunteer staff of some 300,000. Of a $176 million fund balance in 1977, $114 million came from public contributions at the state level, largely from legacies and the annual April crusade of the society involving over two million solicitors. Direct contributions from industry were in the region of 3 percent of total donations. The national headquarters survives by taking 40 percent of each division's fund. About 60 percent of the society budget goes for staff salaries, office supplies, and other expenses; the 1977 travel budget of the society was about $7 million. Less than 15 percent of the budget is spent on assisting patients (for purposes such as driving them to doctors' appointments, loaning wheelchairs, and donating bandages made by volunteers, rather than paying for treatment costs).

The overall governing group for the American Cancer Society is the 194-member House of Delegates, which in 1977 included one labor representative and one black, but no representative of public interest or citizen organizations. The 116-member National Board of Directors is recruited from the House of Delegates. Of the ninety-four delegates, eighteen are senior officers or directors of banks, seven are members of investment firms, and thirteen are business or industrial executives. Board members have recently included the late Elmer Bobst, and Frank J. Dixon, a consultant to Eli Lilly and Company and member of the NCI Advisory Board. At least eighteen members of the Board and delegates are executive officers or directors of banks which, as of August, 1976, held about 42 percent of the society's cash and investment, totalling $75 million. The major decision making of the society seems to be shared between senior staff, members of the board, and a select group of thirty-two Life Members.‡ The new president of the society (elected November, 1978) is LaSalle D. Lefall, Jr., a black surgeon from Howard University. Among the life members, the banking, insurance, advertising, and pharmaceutical industries are well represented, in the absence of representation from labor or public interest groups. These lay representatives share leadership almost equally with clinicians and research scientists.

Since its inception, the society has been preoccupied by problems of cancer diagnosis and treatment, not unnaturally reflecting viewpoints which generally prevailed until relatively recently. While the society made important contributions to the smoking-cancer problem prior to 1964, its subsequent efforts to control smoking have been weak and diffuse. In fact, it has refused to endorse meaningful activist approaches such as those developed by Action on Smoking and Health, and has yet to develop any effective legislative programs.

Research programs, which are the major emphasis of the fundraising appeals of the society, accounted for about 26 percent of its 1976 budget. Of about $13 million spent on new research projects in 1976, $394,000 was allotted to chemical carcinogenesis, while no new awards were made on problems of environmental carcinogenesis. Society fund raisers have routinely told the public that the society could not finance promising research "due to insufficient funds." This claim was challenged in 1976 by a report of a charity-monitoring service, the National Information Bureau, on the grounds that the society then had over $31 million in uncommitted reserves. The society responded to this criticism by withdrawing their claim, and substituting it with the statement that it "will now place research in perspective as part of overall program needs." The audit further revealed that the research budget of the society declined from 36 percent in 1967 to the 1976 level of 26 percent, while the share given to management and fund raising increased proportionately during this time. There also seems to be evidence of conflict of interest in the award of research funds. Those same board members who decide which research projects should be funded themselves receive support. About 70 percent, $26 million, of the 1976 research budget was awarded to individuals or institutions with whom board members were affiliated.*

The society has supported major experimental and epidemiological research on smok-

---

‡ Bylaws of the society require that laymen fill half the positions on its policy-making boards. These tend to be conservative and mistrustful, if not hostile, to "big government" and federal regulations. Professional representation comes from about 50,000 surgeons, radiologists, and chemotherapists heavily concerned with treatment. As constituted, the power base of the society is overwhelmingly oriented to the diagnosis and treatment, rather than to the prevention, of cancer.

* Pat McGrady, for twenty-five years the science editor of the society and the organization's main liaison between cancer researchers and medical and science writers, recently resigned in embar-

ing, and also some on occupational problems. These include studies on carcinogenesis and other hazards among printers, in collaboration with the Printing Pressmen's and the International Typographical Union, and studies on asbestos by Selikoff in collaboration with the Papermakers Union.

The educational programs and publications of the American Cancer Society emphasize the importance of early detection of cancer, even for those cancers with known low cure rates. The society has issued the widely publicized Seven Warning Signs of Cancer (see below). Apart from smoking, however, no reference is made to any other causes of cancer, such as Premarin as a major known risk factor for uterine cancer. By emphasizing individual responsibility for early detection, without providing information on environmental or occupational carcinogens other than tobacco, the American Cancer Society has implicitly created an impression that it endorses industry's "blaming the victim" perspective.

The Seven Warning Signs of Cancer

1. Change in bowel or bladder habits.
2. A sore that does not heal.
3. Unusual bleeding or discharge.
4. Thickening or lump, especially in the breast.
5. Indigestion or difficulty in swallowing.
6. Obvious change in a wart or mole.
7. Nagging cough or hoarseness.

The Cancer Lobby. Subsequent to her transformation of the society, Lasker's interests grew to encompass the NIH. Over the ensu-

ing decades, her close associations with successive White House administrations and with powerful political figures, such as Representative John Fogarty (D-R.I.) and Senator Lister Hill (D-Ala.), House and Senate Appropriations subcommittee chairmen, respectively, facilitated her activism and contributions to the growth of biomedical research. The death of Fogarty and retirement of Hill in 1967, together with decelerated federal support for the NIH, made her unduly receptive to the overtures of a group of cancer clinicians who had persuaded themselves that just given more funds they could cure cancer. Typical of these was Solomon Garb, a University of Missouri Medical School clinician (support for whose activities had been terminated by the NCI in 1966), whose 1968 book *Cure for Cancer: A National Goal,* with extravagant promises for an early cancer cure, made a deep impact on Lasker. (Garb is now "scientific director" of a thirty-two bed cancer hospital at the American Medical Center, Denver, and still without personal support from the NCI.) Lasker forged a powerful "cancer-cure lobby," including clinicians such as Garb and Farber, hospital administrators such as Lee Clark, and industrial philanthropists such as Foote (most of whom were already actively involved in the American Cancer Society), whose object was to force massive expansion of federal funding for cancer diagnosis and treatment.† To this end, Lasker enlisted the particular support of Senator Ralph W. Yarborough (D-Tex.), Chairman of the powerful Senate Health subcommittee. With Lasker's active involvement, in 1971

---

rassed protest over these and related issues. Of the society slogan: "Control Cancer With a Check-up and a Check," McGrady remarked:

It's phoney, because we are not controlling cancer. That slogan is the extent of ACS's scientific, medical, and clinical savvy. Nobody in the science and medical departments there is capable of doing real science. They are wonderful pros who know how to raise money.

They don't know how to prevent cancer or cure patients; instead they close the door on innovative ideas. (P. B. Chowka, *East/West Journal,* July, 1978.)

† The success of the "cancer-cure lobby" in increasing NCI appropriations has been achieved largely at the expense of other NIH institutions, particularly the National Institute of General Medical Sciences.

Yarborough appointed a National Panel of Consultants on the Conquest of Cancer, whose sixteen members were equally divided between laypersons and cancer clinicians (with virtually no basic scientists), distinguished by a complement of over 60 percent millionaires and its predominant representation of the American Cancer Society. The Panel's recommendation to create a National Cancer Program, with vastly expanded funds and an autonomous NCI, aroused substantial opposition in the scientific community and Congress. This was, however, successfully muted by the propaganda machinery of the society. The society initiated a large-scale letter-writing campaign, buttressed by full-page advertisements in daily newspapers, to pressure Congress to accept the Panel's recommendations. Garb took matters further by exerting direct but counterproductive pressure on Congressman Paul Rogers (D-Fla.), one of the few congressmen who had not been persuaded by the lobby's hysteria, and who favored retaining NCI within NIH. Passage of the 1971 National Cancer Act, with massively increased financial appropriations for the NCI, but without parallel increases in personnel slots, whether an error of omission or commission, virtually ensured dependence of the NCI on the American Cancer Society for direction of its programs and priorities. Rep. David Obey (D-Wisc.) has more recently charged that the society "wants to keep the Cancer Institute strong in bankroll and weak in staff, so that it can direct its spending without too much interference."

The close links that have developed between the NCI and the society have been cemented by the personal relationships between members of the same lobby that supported both organizations, including the late Sidney Farber, Benno Schmidt (Chairman of the NCI Advisory Panel), and Mary Lasker. These interlocking relationships have also helped create a fiscal pipeline from the NCI to clinicians in leadership roles in the American Cancer Society. Certainly, the interlocking relationships between members of the NCI National Cancer Advisory Panel and Board and the American Cancer Society leadership have been important factors in maintaining high NCI priorities on problems of treatment and low priorities in problems of prevention. When Frank Rauscher recently resigned from the NCI directorship, he moved to his present position of Senior Vice President for Research of the American Cancer Society, an appointment apparently reflecting endorsement by the society of Rauscher's policies at the NCI.

In the Spring of 1978, in an effort to increase NCI appropriations, Lasker took out full page advertisements in leading newspapers in every district represented by members of the House Labor HEW subcommittee. Lasker's influence in the Senate was exerted primarily through her friends Senators Warren Magnuson (D-Wash.), Edward Brooks (R-Mass.), and Birch Bayh (D-Ind.), whose late wife was also hired as a society lobbyist. Garb assisted these efforts by direct personal attacks in Wisconsin against Congressman David Obey (D-Wisc.) in response to his criticisms of NCI's maladministration and low priorities on cancer prevention.‡

Apart from being uninvolved in cancer prevention, other than to a limited extent tobacco, senior officials have developed for the society a reputation of being indifferent if not actively hostile to regulatory needs for the prevention of exposure to carcinogenic chemicals in the general environment and workplace. In early 1977, the past president of the society, Lee Clark, joined by Frank J. Rauscher, attacked the FDA for its proposed ban on the carcinogenic saccharin. This apparent position of the society has not yet been modified or retracted. Sidney Arje, Vice President for Professional Education, objects to the FDA proposal for inserting cancer warnings in Premarin packages. The society also

---

‡ Garb's strategy was developed with the initial connivance of the society's Pollster.

objects to FDA requirements for reporting adverse drug reactions in humans receiving experimental anti-cancer drugs in NCI programs, and has demanded legislation to abolish FDA authority in this area. Over the past decade, the society has refused to endorse critical public health legislation and moves such as the Clean Water and Air Acts, and regulation of Red Dye #2, Aldrin, Tris, and the proposed FDA ban on DES in cattle feed.* Its support of the Toxic Substances Act, probably the most important single piece of legislation of the century designed to prevent exposure to carcinogenic and toxic chemicals, was perfunctory and too late to be effective. The American Cancer Society, together with the American College of Radiologists, has insisted on pursuing largescale mammography screening programs for breast cancer, including its use in younger women, even though the NCI and other experts are now agreed that these are likely to cause more cancers than could possibly be detected. While the traditional explanation for the position of the society on cancer prevention lies in an amalgam of conservatism and ignorance, a recent series of critical articles in the press have raised questions as to the possible influence of the wide range of industries in which society directors have financial interests.

On March 9, 1978, Rauscher told a Rutgers University audience that New Jersey's high cancer rate may be a result of personal habits rather than industrial pollution.

> People are talking about a cancer hot spot here. They are blaming industry. They are blaming everybody but themselves.[24]

Rauscher further stated that there is clear evidence that New Jerseyans smoke more than the national average, thus accounting for their excess cancer rates. However, in response to a subsequent question by Congressman Andrew Maguire (D-N.J.), Rauscher admitted that he had no evidence to support his claim.

The problems with the American Cancer Society are largely a function of its history and structure and reflect clinical bias and

---

* In spite of Cuyler Hammond's negativism to the Clean Water and Air Acts, based on his failure to find increased cancer rates in epidemiology studies on Holland and Lincoln tunnel workers, the society initially indicated willingness to support this legislation. This position was reversed when Lee Clark was subsequently told by Texas auto dealers that it would wreck their business. Hammond has also testified on the side of industry in hearings on saccharin and hair dyes, and has been openly critical of the Delaney Amendment. In some such positions, Hammond, and other society officials, such as Lee Clark and Rauscher, claim to be representing themselves and not the society.

This negativism to critical preventive health legislation, which has generally been enacted in spite of rather than because of the society and other voluntary health organizations, aroused the unfavorable comments of Congressman Paul Rogers (D-Fla.) in an address to the Third National Conference on Health Policies on May 22, 1978:

> I regret that this legislation was adopted with little or no help from groups or individuals involved with health care. I can think of no better example of the serious consequences of the organized health interests non-involvement than last year's Congressional battle over the Clean Water and Air law. A key part of this struggle was the auto industry's push to relax automobile pollution standards. The sweeping relaxation of standards proposed by the industry would have posed a very real threat to the health of millions of Americans over the next thirty years. Despite the obvious health implications of the auto industry's proposal, we had to work just to get the American Cancer Society and the Heart Association to take a look at the question. Eventually, after long delays, their entire political activity consisted of one letter of support. It could only be considered too little, too late. The Lung Association and the American Public Health Association were somewhat more active. While they took strong supportive positions early in the battle, and they testified in behalf of strong health protections, their support was never translated into political organization and clout.

stodgy conservatism, coupled with a basic failure to comprehend the importance of environmental and occupational causes of cancer.[25] The society has declined to harness its considerable political clout to support legislation and regulation designed to prevent cancer.[26] The hostility or indifference it has further expressed to particular moves in this direction has been an important determinant in the failure of Congress to act more decisively on cancer prevention and even more seriously, in public apathy and confusion. Equally grievous and damaging are the society's misrepresentation of government cancer statistics as indicating that cancer death rates "are leveling off and in some cases dropping off,"[27] rather than in fact increasing (see for instance, Tables 1.7 and 1.8).

While the overall response of the society to emerging criticisms from quarters including the press, public interest groups, labor, and some key Congressmen, is defensive in the extreme, there are nevertheless limited indications of responsiveness, such as the recent creation of a "public-issues committee." The tempo of such responses is likely to increase further only if the society feels that its public image and fund raising ability is threatened. In the final analysis, it no longer seems possible to avoid the overall conclusion that, since 1964, the American Cancer Society, spearheading the cancer cure lobby, has exercised an essentially negative if not detrimental influence on cancer prevention.

Chapter Eleven

What You Can Do to Prevent Cancer

By now, you will have a grasp of the basic political and scientific problems of cancer cause and prevention. Both are problems, though for different reasons. First, the objective scientific data are often not clear-cut. Second, even when they are, their interpretation is usually distorted by economic and political pressures, which have influenced or shaped regulatory policies. In the final analysis, such policies are based on some kind of risk-benefit equation whose elements are usually concealed or poorly articulated, and whose benefits are not necessarily enjoyed by those who bear the risk.[1] Understanding the risk-benefit equation should help reduce the sense of frustration which often overwhelms lay people when faced with technical discussions on cancer. Understanding should also result in shifting public focus on the cancer problem away from the narrowly scientific to the open political arena, where it clearly belongs.

It is perfectly true that we can make changes in our personal lives and habits that may significantly reduce our chances of getting cancer, but the possibilities here are limited. An asbestos worker with a growing family may well have a true grasp of the dangers he is exposed to, but in all probability he is firmly locked into his particular work situation. Modern industrial society offers most people little opportunity to choose freely where to live, where to work, what air to breathe, what water to drink, what food to eat, and what advertisements to read or see. We must be willing to accept the fundamental reality that a *significant* reduction in exposure to environmental carcinogens will result only from organized political action. The system of checks and balances leading to decision-making must protect the overall interests and welfare of the public. This is the essence of democratic practice. Until very recently, congressional decisions and regulatory policy have too often reflected the overwhelming pressures and influences of industry without significant balance by consumer and labor interests.

Depending on your personal circumstances, you have two major realistic options for effective political action: by working with public interest and citizen groups or by working with organized labor. Review all the case studies presented in this book. Try to analyze the relative roles of government, labor, and public interest groups in protecting against industrial abuses and irresponsibility. Virtually every major action designed to protect consumers or workers against cancer has been initiated by public interest groups or labor (see Table 9.5). There is little basis for assuming that this pattern will change in the future. This is where we must focus our energies and efforts if we are to reduce the massive national toll of cancer. Over the last decade, Senator Edward Kennedy has repeatedly warned that democratic decision-making processes have become increasingly subverted by special interests. Cancer is a visible manifestation of such subversion.

What You Can Do on the Political Level

In order to take meaningful action, become as well informed as possible. Many books, periodicals, and newsletters of various groups dealing with occupational, consumer, and environmental concerns are available.*

Public Interest Groups

Public interest groups have taken a key role in forcing improved regulation of environmental and occupational carcinogens. Some groups function purely in an educational or resource capacity, while others are oriented toward legislative, regulatory, legal, and community action. While the larger groups are based in Washington, most large cities now have their own local citizen or consumer groups. They generally specialize in different areas, such as food additives, occupational hazards, drugs, and radiation, but there is usually overlap between these various categories. Get in touch with these groups, find out how you can become actively involved, which of them is most suitable for your particular interests and purposes, and how you can best support them with your time, energy, and money. Finally, one of the best legacies you can leave your children and society is the inclusion in your will of public interest groups dedicated to the prevention of cancer. The future of the public interest movement depends on its developing adequate financial support and a national grassroots base. Help as much as you can on all these levels.

Needs for a National Anti-Cancer Constituency

A major constraint to the development of effective political action is the virtual absence of a defined national constituency for the prevention of disease, in general, and cancer, in particular. The booming medical industry, euphemistically called "the health care system," has little if any incentive to prevent, as op-

---

* The references given in this book should be a useful beginning. Your librarian should be able to help you further. Most universities now have adult or continuing education courses in these areas. This is, or should be, a function of the university extension service or labor education center. Make sure, by checking with others in your labor or public interest group, that your lecturer is both bona fide and well informed. For a valuable resource, see *Public Policies for the 80's: Perspectives and Resources for State and Local Action,* published by the Conference/Alternative State and Local Public Policies, 1978 (1901 Q Street, N.W., Washington, D.C. 20009). This lists federal agencies and departments; Congressional committees; state legislative committees (where information on pending legislation can be obtained); National Association of State and Local Officials; state associations of municipalities; national labor unions; state Public Interest Research Groups; state and local consumer organizations; national public interest groups based in Washington, D.C.; and Washington-based environmental groups. For a listing of environmental groups based outside of Washington, D.C., see the *Conservation Directory,* published by the National Wildlife Federation (1412 16th Street, N.W., Washington, D.C. 20036). For a listing of public interest publications, see *A Catalog of Periodicals and Newspapers of Public Interest Organizations, 1979,* published by the Commission for the Advancement of Public Interest Organizations. This briefly describes about 100 periodicals and newspapers under 13 major categories, including health and nutrition; environment; public interest law; energy; and appropriate technology. See also R. Nader, "A Seasonal Salute to Crusaders and Their Causes: Nonprofit Civic Literature Available on Many Issues," *Washington Star,* December 27, 1978.

posed to treat, cancer. Further, it has successfully resisted increasing recognition of the importance of disease prevention and the proportionate expenditures of federal funds for this purpose. It is questionable whether the insurance industry would profit from disease prevention as their decreased payments to the sick would be more than negated by increased payments for long-term pensions and retirement policies. While public interest groups and organized labor have emerged as the only coherent anti-cancer lobby, they have yet to impact significantly on a national grassroots level.

Recognizing these problems, Paul Rogers, who retired last year from Congress and the chairmanship of the House Subcommittee on Health and Environment, in November, 1978, announced the creation of a National Coalition for Disease Prevention and Environmental Health, stating that "we have learned that a preventive approach is necessary in light of the spiraling human and economic costs of disease." The coalition, which has attracted the support of about 120 groups (including consumer, public interest, labor, health providers, health planning and voluntary health organizations, pollution control equipment manufacturers, and religious bodies), is hiring a small permanent staff and has set up a Washington-based information center as the focus of its activities.

An untapped potential constituency (besides the church) are senior citizens, pensioners, and retirees, whose numbers are growing disproportionately to the remainder of the population, and who, for considerations of latency, represent the highest cancer risk group, and one on whom the financial burdens of cancer are the heaviest. "Gray Power" could well emerge as a new and potent anti-cancer lobby.†

Organized Labor

Encourage your union to fight to strengthen OSHA. While working for tougher standards, persuade your union to follow the lead of some of the more health-conscious unions, particularly the Oil, Chemical, and Atomic Workers (OCAW) and the United Auto Workers, in lobbying for better laws, developing their own professional resources and skills, including hiring full-time industrial hygienists and trustworthy consultants, demanding OSHA inspections, and educating their own members.

The ability of your union to protect you and your fellow workers ultimately depends on your self-education and understanding of health and safety problems, particularly in high-risk industries. Work collectively with your union leadership to produce a work environment free of added cancer risk. If you feel that your union leadership is ignorant or not interested in these problems, then lobby and campaign to vote them out of office and replace them with more responsive leadership.

The OCAW has a double-barreled strategy of working within and without OSHA. On the one hand, OCAW makes maximum use of both the "general duty" clause of the Occupational Safety and Health Act, guaranteeing a safe and healthful workplace, and the "imminent danger" clause, demanding action when life-threatening situations occur.‡ On the other hand, recognizing that OSHA has had a poor track record for rectifying dangerous health conditions, OCAW has written into many of its contracts specific health and safety language, providing for monitoring of workplace hazards, with results acces-

---

† Leading senior citizen national organizations include the Washington, D.C.-based American Association for Retired Persons (202-872-4700) and the Urban Elderly Coalition (202-857-0166), and the more activist, Philadelphia-based, Gray Panthers (215-382-6644).

‡ The Act has been crucial in supporting union demands that health and safety standards be included, as is now usual, in collective bargaining contracts.

sible to the union's representatives as well as management, and for receiving health statistics compiled by companies. The union has also won an important settlement from the National Labor Relations Board affirming its right to information on the working environment under the representation clause contained in every collective bargaining agreement. The representation clause establishes the union as the sole collective bargaining agent for the employees on matters of "wages, hours, and working conditions." Never before has this clause been used to extract health and safety data. Winning the settlement is an important victory for all organized workers. Thus, even in the absence of specific health and safety clauses, a labor bargaining unit is able to act aggressively on health and safety.

If you are a member of a union which is not health-conscious, seek assistance from any of a number of professional and public interest organizations devoted to labor education on health and safety, or from the new University Labor Educational Centers, such as Rutgers in New Jersey, Cornell in New York, and the University of Wisconsin in Madison.

One area in which an otherwise apathetic union can make an inroad is through its publications.* Ralph Nader has recently pointed out that most union newspapers or periodicals are little more than photogalleries for their officers.

> The feeble state of the labor press means that 30 million union members are left in the dark about some major issues, never review or discuss them, and cannot really come to grips with many of the problems that beset labor . . . [2]

A number of labor publications, on the other hand, do run regular or occasional columns written by health and safety specialists, some of which should be syndicated and run nationwide.

Even the most optimistic estimate of cancer-consciousness in U.S. labor must deal with the fact that three out of four are not organized and so can have very little to say about their working conditions. While every worker is entitled in principle to OSHA protection, the non-union individual who complains may be ignored or, at worst, fired.

State Initiatives

Regulatory and legislative initiatives at a state level which are being pioneered in California and New Jersey are emerging trends of major importance to cancer prevention.† These initiatives provide a focus for education and for well directed political pressure by public interest and citizen groups.

Other Action

Encourage your local media to cover environment-related events, and to run regular columns on topics ranging from congressional legislation on toxic substances to water pollution, particularly as they impact on cancer. During the early 1970s, great sport was made of Boy Scouts bravely paddling up stinking creeks to trace the source of noxious effluents. But it was efforts such as these, particularly because of the television coverage they received, that caught the public's interest and have to some extent sustained it. Aggressive media action may also be the quickest way to uncover hidden relationships between the industrial interests of legislators and of university scientists. It is also worthwhile asking your newspaper editor or publisher some hard-hitting questions, such as why coverage of violent crimes and road accidents is so

---

* The U.S. labor press is comprised of some 800 publications and reaches some 30 million workers.

† Important examples of these include recent ac-

tivities of the California Campaign for Economic Democracy, in collaboration with the California Public Policy Center, and the New Jersey Chapter of the Sierra Club.

complete but coverage of tobacco-related cancer and other diseases and of suppression or manipulation of health and safety data is nonexistent or disproportionately low. Also, look for hidden influences of advertising interests on the coverage of environmental issues. Is this why your local newspaper won't run the Nader column?

Find out the position of your state representative and Congressman on key environmental issues. Let them know of your interest and that you expect them to take vigorous action on the prevention of cancer, if they want your future vote. Pressure them to run on a ticket in which cancer prevention ranks high, if not number one. Remember that President Johnson was forced out of office by his failure to extricate the U.S. from the Vietnam war, the total U.S. death toll of which over all the war years combined was only a fraction of the annual number of cancer deaths. Cancer prevention should be made, at least, to rank with inflation in the next presidential campaign.

If you are a professional, such as a doctor, lawyer, chemist, engineer, physicist, or social scientist, you have a wider range of options. These include working actively with public interest groups and organized labor, testifying at Congressional, State, and Municipal hearings, lobbying at the local or federal levels, supporting responsible regulatory agency officials, criticizing irresponsible or indifferent officials, and pressuring voluntary health agencies, particularly the American Cancer Society, to develop more aggressive preventive programs, if they hope to retain your financial support.

What You Can Do on the Personal Level

You can reduce your own chances of getting cancer by making changes in three major personal areas:[3] your lifestyle and personal habits; your choice and use of consumer products; and your work. These areas obviously overlap, as your work may be an integral part of your lifestyle. In all these overlapping areas, you have only limited options for making decisions that will affect your exposure to environmental and occupational carcinogens and decrease your risks of getting cancer. The major public interest groups publish useful reports dealing in further detail with these various problems, such as carcinogens in food and water. You are recommended to contact them.

Depending on your particular circumstances, some of the recommendations offered here may possibly be impractical. But you should at least know what are your available options, even if you are unable or unwilling to exercise them.

In addition to your efforts to prevent cancer in yourself and your family, you should appreciate the importance of early detection and treatment, particularly of the curable and manageable cancers. Finally, you should be aware of possible legal remedies if you do contract cancer and have reason to believe that someone else is responsible.

Lifestyle and Personal Habits

1. *Smoking.* The most effective single action you can take is never to start smoking or, if this advice comes too late, to stop smoking as quickly as possible. Smokers develop lung cancer at about thirty times the rate of nonsmokers, and about one out of ten smokers of a pack or more a day will develop lung cancer. Smoking also increases risks of cancer of the larynx, esophagus, mouth, and bladder. The additional benefits of quitting extend beyond cancer to chronic heart disease, the incidence of which becomes markedly reduced in the ex-smoker.

While many people can quit "cold turkey," most smokers are so physically and psychologically habituated that they need help. Two well-known organizations (there are others) offer structured help in classes or group therapy, and seem to have good success rates: Smoke-Enders is a private group, that charges a reasonable fee to get smokers to give up the habit in a few weeks; the American Cancer Society also conducts smoke cessation clinics in many cities for a nominal fee.

There can be no argument about the cost-effectiveness of quitting smoking. The current direct medical cost of each lung cancer case is about $10,000, which excludes lost wages and other costs borne by the family of the patient, who rarely survives even a few years.‡ The cost of quitting through a program such as Smoke-Enders is under $200. At current cigarette prices, a one-pack-a-day smoker would save, on the cost of cigarettes alone, enough money to pay for the program in one year. To get ten heavy smokers to quit, and thereby prevent one case of lung cancer, would cost about $2,000, compared to about $10,000 to treat the one who would get lung cancer.

There is no alternative to quitting. Switching to low-tar cigarettes is no substitute for not smoking. Regardless of how low the tar, if you smoke cigarettes your risk will be greater than if you don't. A major danger in changing brands rather than completely cutting out cigarettes is that some smokers compensate for the low nicotine levels in low-tar cigarettes by smoking or inhaling more. An additional problem is that levels of carbon monoxide are relatively higher in low-tar cigarettes, probably increasing the risk of heart attack.

It has been suggested that a cigarette smoker who cannot quit should instead switch to cigars or pipes, since cigar and pipe smokers have lower lung cancer rates than cigarette smokers. However, while lifetime cigar and pipe smokers inhale little of the bitter, alkaline smoke, former cigarette smokers who switch to cigars tend to inhale nearly as much as when they smoked cigarettes. This is not an effective method of preventing cancer.[4]

If you are a nonsmoker, avoid smoke-filled, poorly ventilated places, particularly crowded bars. Also become more aggressive about your rights to clean air in elevators, restaurants, airplanes, and other public places.* Insist, as far as possible, that your employer provide you with a smoke-free workplace.

2. *Alcohol.* While there is no direct evidence that alcohol is itself a carcinogen, heavy drinking, particularly of hard liquor, increases the risk of developing cancer of the mouth, throat, esophagus, larynx, and liver.[5] These risks, particularly for cancer of the mouth and esophagus, are still further increased by heavy smoking; cancer of these sites is about fifteen times higher in heavy smokers and drinkers than in abstainers.

The type of alcohol consumed also seems to influence the cancer risk. Esophageal cancer is highly correlated with both chronic alcoholism and cirrhosis of the liver in certain regions of France, particularly Brittany and Normandy, where Calvados brandy and apple-jack are popular. The death rate from cancer of the esophagus in France is highest in the four contiguous brandy-producing areas of Calvados, Manche, Mayenne, and Orne.[6]

The mechanism of these alcohol-related cancers is unknown. It may be due to the nutritional deficiencies which are common in

---

‡ From the time of diagnosis of lung cancer, the median survival for men and women is about six months.

*Among many examples of the nonsmoker's decreasing reticence to demand clean air is the use of the anti-smoker's spray can. Developed by Paul L. Wright, a Denver management consultant who has so far sold 30,000 cans, it drenches offending smokers with a lemon-scented mist.

heavy drinkers and which may increase susceptibility to tobacco or other environmental carcinogens. Additionally, alcohol may act as a solvent for tobacco or other environmental carcinogens and may, thereby, increase their access to tissues.

The influence of chronic alcoholism on cancer is difficult to evaluate, since heavy drinkers tend to die early of other causes, including accidents and diseases related to malnutrition. However, a 1977 study of Veterans Administration hospital patients with cirrhosis of the liver, commonly associated with chronic alcoholism, found a greatly increased risk of the otherwise relatively rare liver cancer. Additionally, patients with cirrhosis developed cancer at other sites at earlier ages than non-cirrhotic and non-alcoholic patients did.[7] This would seem to suggest that alcoholism may increase susceptibility to cancer in general, besides also increasing liver cancer.

3. *Food.* Your dietary choices and habits are clearly important. Some diets may reduce your cancer risk, while others may increase it. This is, however, an area where caution and common sense must be exercised, especially as the facts are incomplete, and the consumer is caught between opposing viewpoints. Industry, on the one hand, dismisses as hysterical any questions on the safety or carcinogenicity of food,[8] while on the other hand public interest groups emphasize the carcinogenic hazards of many food additives and contaminants.†[9]

These problems are aggravated by the fact that it is difficult for the concerned consumer to know where to go to obtain reliable information on the hazards of food additives and contaminants.[10]

With a few possible exceptions, university departments of nutrition are probably the last place to go. Quite apart from the fact that most such departments have no expertise in toxicology and carcinogenesis, many of them are recipients of major support from the food industry or from industry-sponsored organizations such as the Nutrition Foundation. A joint 1976 report by Congressman Benjamin Rosenthal (D-N.Y.) and the Center for Science in the Public Interest detailed the close ties between academia and the food and chemical industry. While a dozen other universities were mentioned, Harvard's nutrition department was singled out as "riddled with corporate influence."[11] Particular reference was made to the intimate relationships between Harvard's previous department chairman, Fred Stare, and the cereal, sugar, and food industries. Less well known is the case of Jean Mayer, President of Tufts University and previous professor in Harvard's nutrition department. Mayer, a responsible nutritionist who writes a widely read, nationally syndicated column on nutrition, has publicly rebuked Stare for being among those "favorable to the sugar interests" who have distorted nutritional evidence, but has himself advocated the use of textured vegetable protein without mentioning that (prior to 1979) he was director of the product's manufacturer, Miles Laboratories.[12] (Mayer is also a director of the Food and Nutrition Board, which represents interests of the food industry, and a director of Monsanto, which has recently mounted an aggressive campaign to persuade the public of the essential safety of synthetic chemicals.)

Much has been made of the relationship between modern eating habits — particularly high caloric intake, high consumption of animal fats, cholesterol, dairy products, and

---

† Unequivocal support for these concerns is detailed in a November, 1978, report on "Cancer-causing Chemicals in Food," by the Subcommittee on Oversight and Investigations of the House Committee on Interstate and Foreign Commerce, which castigates the EPA, FDA, and USDA for failing "to protect the public from dangerous chemical residues in food." The report also made specific recommendations for the immediate correction of these deficiencies in the regulatory practice of the three agencies.

meat; and low consumption of grain and fiber — and the twentieth century cancer epidemic.‡ On the basis of indirect evidence, it has been suggested that a low-fiber, high-fat diet increases the risk of cancer of the colon and possibly of other cancers, including breast, while a high-fiber, low-fat diet protects against these.* As far as dietary fat is concerned, there is no question that a very wide range of environmental carcinogens, particularly pesticides and industrial chemicals, are fat-soluble and are likely to accumulate in the food chain. So the more animal, dairy products, and other fats you eat, the greater will be your intake of these fat-soluble carcinogens.† It is also known from carcinogenicity experiments that high total fat and high-calorie diets increase the incidence of cancers in animals fed known carcinogens, and that low-fat diets seem to protect against cancer. The apparent protective effect of low-fat diets may, however, merely reflect a reduced intake of the carcinogenic contaminants found in animal fats.

Many claims have been made for the protective effect of "dietary fiber," although this term describes a variety of different foods with substantially different properties. The fiber craze in America culminated in two popular recent books, one by David Reuben[13] and the other by Carlton Fredricks,[14] which advocate the consumption of greatly increased quantities of fiber. The underlying theory,[15] popularized by Denis Burkitt, a British surgeon originally known for his research on childhood lymphomas in Africa, that since fiber increases fecal bulk and thereby decreases "transit time" in the colon, this will reduce the contact times of dietary carcinogens in the intestines. Fiber has also been claimed to promote growth of favorable intestinal bacterial strains, which are said to produce fewer carcinogens or promoting agents than is the case when the diet is low in fiber.

In spite of the lack of evidence supporting the cancer-preventing effects of low-fat, high-fiber diets, there is certainly no evidence that they are in any way harmful. Cancer risks apart, any diet such as the American Heart Association Prudent Diet is likely to reduce your risk of coronary and other diseases.[16]

The principles of low-fat, high-fiber diets are to emphasize vegetables, beans, grains, and fruits, and to decrease intake of dairy products, meat, saturated animal fats, and cholesterol. Animal protein should be obtained from fish,‡ veal, and poultry, rather than from high-fat beef, lamb, and pork. If at all possible,

---

‡ Bread, the high-fiber staple, has been considered the staff of life since time immemorial. Now, only 5 percent of all grain consumed in the United States is eaten by people; the remainder is fed to DES-treated cattle in feed lots, producing high-fat meat.

* There is generally a high degree of correlation between mortality from colon cancer and also from coronary disease, and high consumption of animal fats and low consumption of grains and fiber. This, however, by no means constitutes proof of causality. Berg, for example, concludes that, "Epidemiologically the case against fat is weak because there are populations that have a high fat-intake and little bowel cancer, and there is no case-control study pointing to fat as a risk factor." Berg, J. W., "Diet," in J. F. Fraumeni, Jr., ed., *Persons at High Risk of Cancer: An Approach*

to Cancer Etiology and Control (New York: Academic Press, 1975), pp. 201-24.

† Human breast milk provides a good measure of the amount of fat-soluble carcinogens retained in body fat. A recent study has shown that vegetarians have lower levels of chlorinated hydrocarbon pesticides, particularly DDE, in breast milk than their matched meat-eating controls, and that the more high-fat dairy products eaten by vegetarians, the higher the level of pesticides in their breast milk (T. Page and S. Harris, "The Role of Diet in Breast Milk Contamination," in press, 1979). From this standpoint, a lowfat vegetarian diet, provided it is carefully balanced, would be the diet of choice for a nursing mother.

‡ Deep-ocean fish are less likely to be contaminated by fat-soluble carcinogens (such as chlorinated hydrocarbons, pesticides, and PCBs) than

buy the lean meat of range or grass-fed cattle rather than cattle fattened in feed lots. Lean cuts of meat should be selected, trimmed of fat, the remains of which should be drained off during cooking, and baked or stewed, rather than deep-fat fried. Soups and stews should be refrigerated after cooking, and the surface fat layer skimmed off before reheating. Egg consumption should be kept down to one or two a week, and skimmed milk and low-fat cottage and hard cheeses, margarine, and corn or soybean oils should be used in preference to whole milk, high-fat soft cheeses, and butter.

Nutritional deficiencies can cause cancer. The best-known example of this is the Plummer-Vinson Syndrome, characterized by painful difficulty in swallowing, associated with iron-deficiency anaemia and vitamin B deficiency, in which the subsequent incidence of cancer of the esophagus and pharynx is high. The disease, which used to be common in northern Sweden, where winter diets were deficient, has virtually disappeared since flour has been supplemented, in Sweden and elsewhere, with iron and vitamin B.[17]

Food is the most important single source of exposure to a very wide range of synthetic chemicals, either as direct additives or as accidental contaminants such as pesticides and industrial chemicals. Many of these are carcinogens, and food and beverages containing them or suspected to contain them should be avoided to the greatest possible extent.*

Avoid all highly processed "junk" foods, which are rich in additives and poor in nutrients. Hot dogs, potato chips, sugary breakfast cereals, and soda pop contain the greatest concentrations of synthetic additives. Exclude as much as possible known or suspected carcinogenic food additives, such as saccharin and Red #40, and all other synthetic coal tar dyes. Don't buy any foods or beverages containing cosmetic food additives, labeled FD&C (Food, Drug, and Cosmetic) or U.S. Certified Colors. Another major cosmetic food additive is nitrite, which combines with amines in meat and fish to form the highly carcinogenic nitrosamines. Levels of nitrosamines tend to be particularly high in bacon,† and they are present in lower quantities in sandwich meats, salami and bologna, hot dogs, and smoked meats and fish. All of these should be avoided, especially bacon. While this may sound like drastic advice, it is well founded. Nitrite-free hot dogs and, to a lesser extent, bacon are now becoming available in some supermarkets; these products must be kept refrigerated. Their availability will increase if you firmly make your preferences known to your supermarket manager or grocer.

Avoid all food products containing petroleum-derived protein, either as a flavor enhancer or as a food ingredient. As far as is known, Amoco Foods Company, a subsidiary of Standard Oil of Indiana, is the exclusive U.S. manufacturer of petroleum protein.[18] Marketed under the trade name of Torutein, this is a high-protein yeast culture grown on "food grade" ethanol derived from hydrocarbons (usually ethylene), isolated from crude oil, which has been manufactured at the rate of about 15 million pounds per year since 1975. Torutein is now being sold to U.S. food processors for use in meat products, baked

---

freshwater fish which, depending on the purity of the water from where they are caught, may accumulate and concentrate these carcinogens.
* For instance, avoid coffee decaffeinated by the standard U.S. process which uses methylene chloride, currently under test in the NCI Bioassay Program. Coffex Ltd. of Switzerland now markets coffee (available through a few U.S. distributors including the White House Coffee Company in Long Island City, New York) which is decaffeinated by a more expensive pure water process which uses no chemical solvents.
† The USDA is now taking vigorous steps to reduce nitrosamine levels in bacon by ordering meat manufacturers to decrease amounts of nitrite that may be added to bacon.

foods, infant foods, and frozen and other prepared foods, particularly for the institutional food market — hotels, restaurants, and schools. Torutein is found in Prince's macaroni, French's croutons, Health Snacks Limited's breadsticks and cake mixes, La Choy food products, and Gerber baby foods. It is difficult, if not impossible, for the consumer to find out whether a particular product contains Torutein. Under current labeling laws, its presence as a flavor enhancer can be hidden in the catch-all term "natural flavorings." Its presence as a protein booster can be described by the term "torula yeast," without giving any indication as to whether this is natural torula yeast or petroleum-derived.

There are many unresolved questions about the safety of Torutein. The only data voluntarily submitted by Amoco to FDA are the negative finds of subacute rodent toxicity tests, on the basis of which FDA informally approved the use of Torutein in March, 1974. There are no data available on the nutritional value of Torutein (particularly with regard to its high, 10 percent content of nucleic acids), its chronic toxicity, reproductive or mutagenic effects, or carcinogenicity. While various foreign governments, including Japan, Great Britain, and Italy, have withheld approval of petroleum protein because of such questions on safety, there are no current restrictions in the United States, where its use is burgeoning.

There is a critical and overdue need for the regulation of the use of petroleum protein. In the meantime, to be on the safe side, avoid any food whose label bears any reference to torula yeast. You may express your concerns by writing directly to both the FDA and Amoco Foods Company to demand the immediate curtailment of this market until full toxicological and nutritional testing has been completed and independently evaluated.‡ Should Torutein be then found acceptable, its presence in food must be acknowledged by clear and explicit labeling.

Avoid organ meats, particularly liver (even though this is high in protein and vitamins and relatively low in calories), pancreas or sweetbreads, and kidney, as these concentrate residues of both accidental carcinogenic contaminants and carcinogenic feed additives. Avoid any food, oil, or beverage sold or stored in rigid PVC containers. Although banned, these are still on the market. Residues of carcinogenic and other chemicals from the plastic are dissolved in the contents.

4. *Water.* It is now common knowledge that drinking water in most cities, particularly downstream from chemical industries, contains a great variety of synthetic organic chemicals, of which more than 700 have so far been identified, including many known carcinogens.*[19] Demand from local EPA offices as much specific information as possible on the impurities of your drinking water. Do not accept unsubstantiated assurances of safety from water treatment engineers. Your personal options are limited, however. Boiling water will remove some volatile organics, but will actually concentrate others. Distilling is not particularly effective, since many organic chemicals, such as benzene, form "constant-boiling mixtures" with water and will be carried over with the distillate. De-

‡ The needs for such testing prior to the marketing of petroleum protein were in fact spelled out in detail at a tripartite meeting between the United States, Canada, and the United Kingdom at the FDA on December 16, 1974, whose recommendations were spelled out in a working document entitled "Single Cell Protein." The Protein Advisory Group of the United Nations made similar recommendations on February 7, 1972 (PAG Guideline No. 12, "Single Cell Protein"). According to the FDA, Torutein is a "likely candidate" for early consideration in their recently implemented cyclic review of GRAS food additives, with relation to its nutritional adequacy, besides carcinogenicity.

* The chemicals so far identified account for only a small fraction of total organic contaminants in water.

pending on source and purity, bottled water may be an improvement on your tap water, but there is no way of knowing, as bottled water labels give no information at all on levels of organic chemical pollutants.

Until polluting industries can be regulated and until municipal water treatment plants install appropriate water-purifying technologies, you have little option but to install carbon filtration or the more expensive and more efficient reverse osmosis units, preferably to your water mains supply.† Carbon units require regular and frequent replacement to reduce bacterial contamination and to prevent filter exhaustion. The efficiency of domestic carbon units in removing organic contaminants is under current study by EPA.

5. *Drugs.* A wide range of drugs are known to be carcinogenic, as shown by human experience and animal tests.[20] It is unfortunate, but true, that the most effective drugs used to treat cancer can also cause it. Considering the long latency period of most cancers, it may well be worthwhile taking the risk of being treated with carcinogenic drugs if you have cancer or some other equally serious disease. A possible example of such worthwhile risks is the case of kidney transplants. The recipient of a kidney transplant, for example, must be treated to suppress the immune response and to prevent rejection of the new kidney, and the drugs used for this purpose increase the risk of developing lymphomas up to thirty-five times. It is not, however, worthwhile taking carcinogenic drugs for relatively trivial conditions, such as Flagyl for tricho-

monal vaginal infections, griseofulvin for athlete's foot or for scalp infestation with ringworm, and Lindane shampoos for head lice. There are alternative noncarcinogenic treatments for all these conditions. Discuss this with your doctor if he appears to be well informed. If he is not, don't be lulled into false security or intimidated by reassurances such as "Those carcinogenicity data are just based on animal tests," or, "I've been using this drug for over twenty years and have never had any problems." Read the label and insert or stuffer in the packaged medicine bottle, and ask the pharmacist whether he has additional information. Check carefully for any reference to cancer.‡

If you are a menopausal woman, do not take estrogens unless your symptoms are really crippling, and if you do, take the lowest possible dose for the shortest possible time. Your risk of uterine cancer will be greatly increased by "estrogen replacement therapy" with Premarin. If you are a fertile woman who had unprotected intercourse last night, and you would rather not risk pregnancy, never take DES, as commonly prescribed in campus clinics, which apart from being highly carcinogenic may not be particularly effective.

After tranquillizers, the most commonly prescribed drug is "the Pill." Millions of women the world over are taking it for a substantial part of their lives. This is the largest carcinogenicity test in human experience, and the answers are not yet all in. Estrogens are carcinogenic in animals, Premarin induces uterine cancer in menopausal women, and the

---

† If you have even minimal mechanical skills, your best plan is to contact the Environmental Defense Fund Washington Office and ask for a copy of their pamphlet ($1.00 fee) on how to construct your own activated carbon unit.

‡ In May, 1979, the NCI announced that the following four widely used drugs were carcinogenic in the Bioassay Program: methapyrilene, an antihistamine used in most non-prescription sleeping

aids such as Nytol (Block Drug Co.), Excedrin (Bristol Myers), and Sominex (J. B. Williams Unit of Nabisco) and common nasal sprays and allergy medicines; reserpine (Ciba Geigy Co.), used for treatment of high blood pressure; selenium sulfide, an ingredient in antidandruff shampoos such as Selsun (Abbott Laboratories); and disulfiram, used as a fungicide and as the anti-alcoholic drug Antabuse.

synthetic DES induces vaginal cancer in adolescent girls whose mothers took it while they were pregnant. Epidemiological studies on users of birth control pills have so far been inconclusive, probably because most women have been taking them for too short a time for possible cancers to show up. The pill has, however, been associated with liver tumors, stroke, and other diseases. So consider other forms of contraception. And make up your own mind about this; your gynecologist or physician is likely to tell you not to worry.

6. *Cosmetics.* Under the authority of the 1938 Federal Food, Drug, and Cosmetic Act, the FDA has recently required the ingredients of all cosmetics to be listed on the label. Exemptions are granted to ingredients constituting less than 1 percent of the product, and to the names of specific flavors and fragrances. While the agency does not have the authority to require the industry to test their products for safety, it does require that if a product has not been tested, then the label must read: "Warning: The safety of this product has not been determined." Do not buy any

products carrying such a warning, nor products containing known carcinogens, such as 2,4-toluenediamine or 4-methoxy-mphenyl-enediamine, which are used in permanent (oxidative) hair dyes, particularly the darker colored ones. Nor should you allow your hairdresser to use these carcinogenic products on your hair.* The FDA still lacks the current statutory authority to ban the carcinogenic hair dyes, which are exempt from the requirements of the Federal Food, Drug, and Cosmetic Act. Recognizing this problem, the General Accounting Office in December, 1977, called for a legislative change to bring hair dyes under food, drug, and cosmetic regulations. This was followed in January, 1978, by the announcement of Congressman John Moss (D-Calif.) that his House subcommittee would hold hearings on whether to abolish the hair dye exemption. The dyes, however, could be regulated by OSHA, as about 400,000 workers, including hairdressers, cosmetologists, and furriers, are potentially exposed to them. Accordingly, on January 13, 1978, NIOSH urged that these dyes

---

* Several epidemiological studies have demonstrated an increased risk of lung, bladder, and thyroid cancer, and leukaemia in beauticians. However, none of these studies specifically incriminate any known carcinogens, such as 2,4-toluene-diamine or vinyl chloride propellants and nitrosamine contaminants in cosmetics and hair dyes. In February, 1979, R. E. Shore and a group of co-investigators from the New York University Institute of Environmental Medicine reported on preliminary case control studies on women using hair dyes. These studies, stimulated by the finding that the majority of oxidative hair dyes are mutagenic in the Ames system, and that several are also carcinogenic in animals, indicated that the incidence of breast cancer is increased in women who had used hair dyes for over ten years. The study controlled for other factors (such as family history of breast cancer, childbearing history, and socio-economic class) known to also influence the risk of breast cancer. A possible limitation in this study is that no relationship was

found between the color of the dye used and the degree of cancer risk, although dark dyes contain more chemical ingredients than blond dyes. While the number of women (129 breast cancer cases vs. 193 controls) involved in this study is too small and the risk estimates (1.4) too low to allow definitive conclusions, these findings add yet further information on the potential carcinogenic hazards of hair dyes. The industry, with its $300 million market involving 25 million consumers, has responded by insisting that no chemical in hair dyes is carcinogenic. Clairol and other manufacturers have, however, recently introduced new formulations devoid of known carcinogens. John Corbett, vice-president for technical development at Clairol, made it clear that the only reason for the industry action was because it would otherwise be required to carry a cancer warning on hair dye labels. "It's not good business to have to market a product with a cancer warning on it. We don't want our product used by worried women."

be handled as occupational carcinogens and proposed a 50 ppm standard. On December 12, 1977, the FDA banned further use of six color additives in drugs and cosmetics: Yellow #1, Blue #6, and Reds #10, 11, 12, and 13, the red colors mainly being used in lipsticks and soaps, but did not require these products to be removed from the market.

A small market based on cosmetics containing only natural ingredients and free from synthetic chemicals such as coal tar dyes, is now developing. You are encouraged to explore this to see if it meets your needs. If it doesn't, you may want to consider changing your needs.

7. *X-rays*. X-rays are carcinogenic. The more X-rays you submit to and the greater the dose, the greater is your risk of cancer.[21] Avoid unnecessary X-rays like the plague. Make your doctor or dentist spell out to you in detail the benefits you may get from exposure to X-rays. Are they given for "routine reasons," or for "defensive medical practice" to protect against possible malpractice suits, or because they are paid for by Medicaid and Medicare from which your physician may get a fee, or because critical choice of treatment in serious disease or injury is at stake?

You should raise these questions before you consider submitting to X-rays, even at the risk of offending "professional dignity." If you are convinced that X-rays are essential, only have them done in the office of a physician who is a specialist in radiology or in the radiology department of a hospital. Also, make sure that the technician is certified, not just "office trained," that modern equipment is used, that the smallest dose is given, and that your non-irradiated areas are protected with a lead shield.

Whatever you may be told, refuse routine mammograms to detect early breast cancer, especially if you are premenopausal. The X-rays may actually increase your chances of getting cancer.†[22] If you are older, and there are strong reasons to suspect that you may have breast cancer, the risks may be worthwhile. Very few circumstances, if any, should persuade you to have X-rays taken if you are pregnant. The future risks of leukaemia to your unborn child, not to mention birth defects, are just not worth it.

At issue here is not the occasional obvious necessity of X-rays, but their indiscriminate use. According to U.S. Public Health surveys, over 150 million Americans are given 210 million medical and general X-ray examinations annually.‡ The number of medical X-ray examinations per person has increased steadily from 50 per 100 population in 1964 to 56/100 in 1970, a 12 percent jump.[23] Medical uses of ionizing radiation now account for 90 percent of all uses. The number of dental X-rays per person increased from 27/100 in 1964 to 36/100 in 1970, a 29 percent jump. Not only is the number of exposures increasing, but the dosage is much larger than necessary. Many doctors and hospitals use old, outdated equipment, which is not properly controlled and has not been given needed annual inspections by a qualified health physicist.*

Dentists are also often guilty of overexposing their patients.[24] Some dentists require a full set of sixteen to eighteen films every time a patient comes in for a routine checkup. The additional diagnostic information furnished by such a series, over and above inspection aided by a dental pick, is difficult to imagine. The

---

† When first introduced in the 1960s, mammography exposed women to about 7 rads per examination, compared to the 0.02 rads of today's most up-to-date equipment, found only in a relatively few centers. Until very recently, the lowest amount of mammography exposure was about 2 rads.

‡ This excludes more than 2 million Americans

occupationally exposed to nuclear radiation in the last thirty years, including over 500,000 soldiers who were deliberately exposed to nuclear blasts.

* Federal expenditures on the health effects of ionizing radiation are trivial. The Department of Energy's annual budget for this purpose is about $12.6 million, of which nearly two thirds is allo-

American Dental Association advises that a full set need not be taken more often than every three to five years; and other authorities extend this to between six and ten years.

More than 20 million Americans consult chiropractors, instead of or in addition to physicians. Some chiropractors base entire treatments on extensive use of full body X-rays. Avoid such treatments and all chiropractors who offer them.

8. *Sex.*[25] Cancer of the cervix seems in some way related to sex. The earlier in life you start intercourse, the more your partners, marriages, and pregnancies, and the poorer your prenatal and postnatal care, the greater are your chances of cervix cancer. Intercourse during and immediately after menstruation is thought to increase risk, possibly accounting for the relative rarity of cervix cancer in orthodox Jewish women, who abstain during and immediately after menstruation. The relatively increased risk of this cancer in non-Jewish women has also been attributed to their sexual partners being uncircumcised. These sexual risk factors are further aggravated by poverty, possibly because of poor nutrition and limited opportunities for personal hygiene. The rate among lower socioeconomic groups, particularly low-income blacks, is double that for middle-class whites, and its incidence among other low-income ethnic groups, such as Mexican-Americans, is higher still. There is some evidence that a venereally transmitted Herpes virus is in some way responsible for this cancer.

Risks of breast cancer are increased in women who menstruated before the age of twelve, who have never had children or who had their first child after the age of thirty, who have had a history of benign cysts or breast tumors, and who have a familial predisposition.[†] If you fall into any of these high-risk categories, monthly breast self-examination is imperative.

If you are a Jewish male, your chance of getting cancer of the penis is virtually zero, as this is prevented by circumcision. If you are uncircumcised, make sure to retract your foreskin daily and wash away the secretions with soap and water.

There are also some suggestions, based on epidemiological studies, that promiscuity increases risk for prostate cancer, possibly due to a sexually transmitted virus. Rates of prostate cancer in black males are increasing at about twice those in whites.

9. *Sunlight.* This makes you feel and look good. But too much sun or exposure to ultraviolet lamps will age your skin and may give you skin cancer, especially if you have a light skin and blond complexion. You have much less to worry about if you are black. Besides avoiding too much sun, wear a good sunscreen ointment; those containing para-aminobenzoic acid are particularly effective. If you work outdoors, use sunblocking creams such as zinc oxide around your lips and nose.

The incidence of skin cancer and melanomas is greatest in farmers and fishermen, who spend a great deal of time outdoors.[‡] The incidence is also greater in southern latitudes, where sunlight is more intense. While most

---

cated to follow-up studies on Japanese atomic bomb survivors and on the Marshall Islanders, and the establishment of a radiation emergency assistance center and exposure data file. All other agency efforts total under $9 million. Responsive to these deficiencies, the Biomedical Research and Training Act (P.L. 95-622), introduced in November, 1973, by Congressman Paul Rogers (D-Fla.), makes provision for a new major coordinated federal research effort on the biological effects of ionizing radiation within HEW, as op-

posed to other agencies more concerned with promotion of nuclear energy uses.

† Other high risk factors include living in the vicinity of petrochemical plants, particularly those manufacturing, handling, or processing carcinogens, and prolonged use of hair dyes.

‡ The role of environmental factors other than sunlight is suggested by the striking recent increase in the incidence of melanomas in white males, from 2.6 per 100,000 in 1947 to 6.3 per 100,000 in 1975.

skin cancers are easily curable, melanomas are not, and account for approximately 9,600 new cases and 4,000 deaths a year in the United States.

10. *Where you live.* This influences your overall risks of cancer, and also the particular type you may get. For some, this advice may well be academic; but, you may nevertheless want to think about this if you are about to move or if you have the luxury of choosing where you live. If you can possibly avoid it, do not live close to a chemical plant, refinery, asbestos plant, or metal mining processing or smelting plant, or hazardous waste disposal site, even if claimed to be well managed. Also avoid living close to major highways and expressways.

From 1969 to 1971, the NCI conducted an intensive survey of new cancers in nine regions of the country and found wide geographic variations in the incidence of different types.[26] Many of these patterns paralleled those previously found in the twenty-year NCI cancer death rates study in each of the nation's counties. This study led to publication of the "cancer maps," which show that an excess of many cancers are clustered in regions of heavy industrialization and concentration of petrochemical plants. The excess incidence of cancers in the heavily industrialized counties includes women as well as men, and thus cannot be mainly due to occupational exposures. Rather, it is probably

also due to breathing and drinking carcinogens discharged into the air and water or dumped with chemical waste products into land disposal sites by the local petrochemical, metal mining, smelting, or asbestos plants. There is chemical monitoring information that confirms this for growing numbers of industrial carcinogens.

Among all states, for the survey period of 1950 to 1969, New Jersey leads in overall cancer mortality and in the variety of mortal cancers as well.[27] Every known major industrial chemical carcinogen is manufactured or otherwise handled in bulk in New Jersey[28] (Table 11.1). Nineteen of the twenty-one counties in the state have an incidence of bladder cancer in the top 10 percent of the nation. Salem County, New Jersey, has been singled out as having the highest national death rate from bladder cancer in both men and women, possibly related to the location there of a concentration of chemical industries, including a giant Du Pont organic chemical complex, and the fact that 25 percent of the male population in the county work in the chemical industry.* New Jersey is now attempting to control the discharge of carcinogens from industry into the environment of the surrounding community.†

New Jersey is not unique. In New Orleans, there is also an excess of overall cancer mortality, as well as of cancer of the bladder and large bowel. This is probably associated with

---

* Du Pont has acknowledged compensation of 330 workers who have so far contracted bladder cancer from working in its Chamber Works Plant, Deepwater, Salem, since 1919. Most of these cases occurred prior to 1955, when production of the carcinogen primarily responsible, 2-naphthylamine, was stopped. Some new cancer cases are still developing.

† Regulations effective by 1979 will require about half of all industries in New Jersey to install new anti-pollution devices designed to sharply curtail carcinogenic emissions from industry, though these regulations will initially apply to only eight known

carcinogens. Questionnaires are also being sent to 12,000 companies in the state to determine whether they use any of 188 known or suspect carcinogens in their operations. Additionally, New Jersey has established a computer terminal linked to an NCI data bank which will enable rapid studies on correlation of cancer mortality rates with geographical, ethnic, and other data. Industry has responded by the usual threats to move elsewhere. A September, 1978, interim report of the New Jersey Department of Health and Environmental Protection was "unable to confirm a specific cause for the outbreak of disease, despite exhaustive analysis

Table 11.1 Carcinogens Made or Handled at Major Facilities in New Jersey

Carcinogens	City
Aromatic Amines	Linden, Parsippany
Arsenic	Elizabeth
Asbestos	Manville, Paterson (closed)
Benzene	Wayne, Newark, Phillipsburg, Trenton, Garfield
Benzidine	Linden, Newark, Clifton, Carteret
Beryllium	Elizabeth, Parsippany
Cadmium	Elizabeth
Carbon black	Clifton
Chromium ore and oxides	Menlo Park, Teaneck, South Plainfield, Clifton
Coal-Tar Chemicals	Linden, Paterson, Cranford, Hackensack
Epichlorhydrin	Cranford
Nickel	Elizabeth
Pitch	Cranford
Radioisotopes	New Brunswick, Lawrenceville
Tetrachloroetbylene	Morristown, Clark, Cinnaminson, Monmouth Junction
Vinyl chloride	Middlesex, Lyndhurst, East Rutherford, Rahway, South Plainfield, East Orange, Moorestown
Vinylidene chloride	Haddonfield, West Orange

the heavy concentration of organic carcinogens in the drinking water, these being discharged from countless industries along the banks of the lower Mississippi. The increased incidence of birth defects, and possibly brain tumors, in certain Ohio counties where VC/

PVC plants are located has been associated with the discovery of VC leaking from the plants into the air of the nearby communities.

Petrochemical industries are by far the main, but not the only danger. Avoid, if possible, living in the vicinity of hazardous waste

of a wide variety of causes." However, it appears questionable whether this conclusion is justified by the restricted monitoring undertaken, particu-

larly as this has not yet been extended to an investigation of numerous local chemical industries for the carcinogens they manufacture, process, or emit.

disposal sites or the innumerable other sites where hazardous wastes have been improperly dumped. Love Canal, Niagara Falls, New York, is such an example. This is a sixteen-acre tract, housing about ninety families and a school which was used as a dump for disposal of hazardous wastes by Hooker Chemical Company from 1942 to 1952; the U.S. Army is also suspected of dumping during this time. In 1953, the site was sold to the board of education which built a school and sold the rest for residential construction. Since 1976, the site has been oozing chemical wastes and even containers into backyards and basements of homes. About 82 toxic chemicals including 11 carcinogens, such as benzene, chloroform, trichloroethylene, and perchloroethylene, have so far been identified in these wastes. An excess of miscarriages, birth defects including mental retardation, breast cancer, and leukaemia have been reported in the local population. On August 7, 1978, the U.S. Senate approved by voice vote a "sense of Congress" amendment, stating that a serious environmental disaster had occurred, and demanded that immediate Federal aid be made available. On the same day, President Carter approved emergency financial aid for the Love Canal area.

A further, though less dramatic, example is Wilsonville, a small county of about 700 residents in Macoupin County, central Illinois. Earthline Corporation operates a 130-acre disposal site, 90 acres of which is in the city limits and the main entrance to which is four blocks from downtown. The site is, in part, located on a disused mine, operated from 1918 to 1954 by Superior Coal Company, posing problems of surface cracking of the clay subsoil through mine subsidence, with the likelihood of waste leakage and contamination of water supplies, underground wells, and sewage systems of Macoupin County. In the spring of 1977, concerns were triggered by the discovery that Earthline had been dumping PCB wastes from Missouri and Indiana. Illinois EPA has refused to identify what hazardous wastes are being dumped at the landfill under a clause in the state Environmental Protection Act that exempts agency files constituting a "trade secret" from public disclosure requirements. Following a court order, (viewed as a national precedent) shutting down the Earthline disposal site at Wilsonville, Illinois, Attorney General William J. Scott filed suit in September, 1978, against the Federal EPA for having failed to issue regulations for hazardous waste disposal by April, 1978, as required to do so by the 1976 Natural Resources and Recovery Conservation Act. Scott cited the Wilsonville example and stated that the State of Illinois has become "the dumping ground" for the nation's hazardous wastes.‡

Avoid, if possible, living downtown in heavily air-polluted cities and live as far as you can from heavily traveled major expressways and highways. A recent Swiss study, based on a relatively small population sample, claims that there is a strong correlation between cancer incidence and proximity of residence to highways.[29] Quite apart from any possible excess cancer risks, levels of carbon monoxide, lead, and other automobile pollutants are also increased near major highways.

11. *Your home.* Your house or apartment can expose you to hidden carcinogenic hazards. These include asbestos insulation and lining of ventilation and heating ducts, and

---

‡ A further example of what is now becoming commonplace was the discovery by EPA in April, 1977, of 600 drums of highly toxic chemical wastes dumped by Donald E. Distler, President of Kentucky Liquid Recycling, Inc., New Albany, Indiana, in a field (owned by his family) flooded by the high waters of the Ohio River. Recent heavy rains caused the drums to scatter over a widespread area and to rupture. In December, 1978, in a landmark case, Distler was criminally convicted by a federal court for discharging pollutants into a federal waterway.

pesticides used for termite treatment and other purposes. Make sure that the apartment house manager is not allowed to disinfect with pesticides he "is sure are safe."

12. *Race.* You should recognize that race and color are factors that may be associated with excess risks of cancer. However, these excess risks are probably due to environmental factors rather than any intrinsic or genetic susceptibility. This is the only reason why questions of race have anything to do with ways and means by which you can possibly reduce your own cancer risks.

The overall cancer risks of black U.S. males are higher than those of white men and higher than those of blacks anywhere in the world.[30] The incidence of lung cancer in black males is particularly high, despite the fact that substantial underreporting is suspected. This is probably due to heavy cigarette smoking, particularly of unfiltered cigarettes, among blacks. The highest incidence of lung cancer in U.S. black males in ten major national areas recently surveyed is in Pittsburgh, Pennsylvania, and probably reflects their extensive employment in the most hazardous jobs in the steel industry.

Both black men and women are experiencing an increase in the incidence of esophageal cancer at a time when this is declining in whites. Cancer of the large bowel has increased sharply in blacks, compared to a slow increase in whites. Black women have more cervix cancers than whites.

Factors which have been incriminated in the excess incidence of cancer in blacks are varied. These include discriminatory employment of black males in high risk jobs; heavy smoking, particularly of unfiltered cigarettes; the high proportion of blacks in the populations of city centers, where air pollution is greatest and where there is likely to be heavy pesticide use; living in areas near high risk industries; and heavy consumption of dairy products and animal fats, rather than veg-

etables and fiber. Various surveys have shown that human fat residues of carcinogenic chlorinated hydrocarbon pesticides such as dieldrin and heptachlor epoxide are substantially higher in blacks than in whites.

Consumer Products

1. *Spray cans.* A wide range of consumer products — including insecticides, hair sprays, disinfectants, deodorants, furniture polishes, and cleaners — are marketed as aerosols. While vinyl chloride is no longer used as a propellant, existing stocks of VC-containing aerosols have not been recalled, nor has there been any clear brand identification of these stocks. Labeling may not necessarily help, for although the presence of propellants is stated their identities are not generally disclosed. The fluorocarbon Freons® are being phased out as propellants and are known to escape into the upper atmosphere and attack the ozone layer, which filters the sun's ultraviolet rays.* This will increase your chance — and everyone else's — of getting skin cancer.

Avoid all aerosols, no matter what their propellant. Every time you use one for any purpose, you will inhale high concentrations of its chemical contents, whatever they happen to be.

2. *Pesticides.* A number of common pesticides used in and around the home and garden are carcinogens. Among the more dangerous are chlordane and heptachlor, which are widely used as common garden insecticides, moth and termite proofing, and other purposes.

In the last decade, there have been major advances in the understanding of biological control of insects using integrated pest management systems. These are equally applicable for home, lawn, and garden infestations and other urban uses as for agriculture.

3. *Tris.* Until recently, children's sleepwear was treated with the flame retardant Tris.

* Since December, 1978, fluorocarbons may no longer be manufactured or packaged.

Don't buy such sleepwear. Tris is absorbed through the skin, persists in fabric even after repeated laundering, and has been recently shown to be both carcinogenic and mutagenic. Instead, try to use only inherently fire-resistant natural and semi-synthetic textiles.

4. *Cleaning agents and solvents.* Do not use *any* products containing carbon tetrachloride, trichloroethylene, perchloroethylene, or benzene, which are all carcinogenic. Use alternatives based on detergents. Be especially careful to avoid all products containing benzene, particularly paint and varnish removers, adhesives, and cements.

Work

1. *Industry.* Your choice of work can greatly affect your chances of getting cancer. Workers in petrochemical, asbestos, steel, smelting, and some mining industries are recognized "high risk" groups (See Table 5.1). While risks are clearly greatest in these manufacturing industries, they also extend to industries that subsequently fabricate products derived from these carcinogens.

The conditions you will experience in different industries vary from the totally uncontrolled, especially in smaller, non-unionized plants, to the partially controlled. One of the major problems, however, has been the chemical industry as a whole, through its politically powerful trade association, the Manufacturing Chemists Association, refusing to disclose the identity of most chemicals used in trade name products in the workplace on the grounds that these are "trade secrets." The likelihood is that you will not even know the names of many or most of the chemicals you work with. Instead you will find yourself handling and breathing chemical mixtures labeled something like AB-347. If you ask your foreman or plant manager what this is, the answer may be "We don't know, we buy it like this," from such a company as Monsanto or Du Pont, who in turn will not be eager to tell you what is in their product, again claiming trade secrecy. Alternatively, management may know what is in the mix, but will tell you that "it is none of your business."

Unless you are fully and completely prepared to take the consequences, you should not go to work in an uncontrolled, high-risk industry, especially one with a bad track record. If you are already working in one, you may only have very limited options, other than leaving, at the expense of loss of seniority and other rights, and trying to find other, safer work.† If you decide to stay, work with your union to make conditions safer.

If you do plan to seek work in one of the high-risk industries, try to choose a large, well-organized plant with reliable and informed union leadership, one in which carcinogens are handled in closed systems and the workplace is monitored with sensitive instrumentation. Also make sure the results of the monitoring are promptly made available to you. Avoid any non-organized industry, particularly one that refuses to give you complete information on the names of the chemicals you will be working with. Do not otherwise accept assurances of safety from the plant manager or even the company physician, who is employed by management and may not consider you his first loyalty. Finally, if you possibly can, try to find out from your union or some other independent source the record of this particular industry in the health and cancer area before you accept employment there. But be forewarned that your chances of getting such information are not good.

2. *Arts and crafts.* Arts and crafts are to some a full-time occupation, and to others a hobby. Whichever is the case, you should

---

† You have legal rights to refuse work you consider to be hazardous. Your options include suing the Department of Labor to force an injunction restraining employers from exposing employees to imminent hazards; rights under Sections 7 and 502 of the Labor Management Relations Act; and rights under Section III of the Occupational Safety and Health Act.

Table 11.2 Carcinogenic Materials Encountered in the Arts and Crafts

Material	Process	Type of Cancer
Arsenic and alloys	Textile prints, metal alloys	Skin and lung
Beryllium	Vapors in sculpture, dust in ceramics	Lung and liver
Cadmium	Silver soldering, brazing, welding	Lung and prostate
Chromium	Paints, lithographic dyes, mordants, printing	Lung
Nickel, oxides, and carbonyl	Welding, nickel alloys and carbonyl	Lung
Asbestos	Mold-making, foundry welding, soldering, spackling	Lung, pleura, and peritoneum
Wood	Carpentry and cabinet making	Nasal sinus
Arsene	Etching	Lung, skin
Benzene	Solvent for resins, glues, and rubber cement	Leukaemia and aplastic anemia
Carbon tetrachloride	General solvent, cleaner	Liver cancer
Trichloroethylene	Solvent for oils, resins, dry cleaning, scouring	Liver cancer
Tetrachloroethylene	Solvent for oils, resins, dry cleaning, scouring	Liver cancer
Formaldehyde	Preserving	Produces BCME, a lung carcinogen in acid solution

Source: Based on B. W. Carnow, "Health Hazards in the Arts and Crafts," University of Illinois, School of Public Health, April 19, 1974.

know as far as possible the composition of all your materials so that you can handle them with due care, and find substitutes for any which are carcinogenic (Table 11.2).

Some construction materials, such as plasterboard and spackle, contain asbestos. Many paints are based on carcinogenic pigments, including chromium, cadmium, nickel, and arsenic, and may also contain carcinogenic solvents, particularly benzene. Artists, especially, should take meticulous precautions when mixing dry pigments, since the dust generated is easily inhaled. Spray paints may still contain VC as propellants, even though its use for this purpose has been banned. Whether an occasional hobbyist or a serious artist, you should avoid handling carcinogenic materials. If you must handle them, do so either with complete ventilation and personal protection, such as a respirator, or with the process completely enclosed.

3. *Schools.* Schools may contain hidden and unexpected hazards, including the hazard of cancer, and children spend as much time there every day as does any workman in a factory or plant. Parents should check on the location of the school, to make sure that it is not near a chemical, mining, or smelting plant, or too close to busy highways and other sources of chemical emissions. The elementary school in Saugus, California, where VC levels of about 3 ppm were found in classrooms in the summer of 1977, is a good case in point. The construction of the school building should also be examined to avoid the now common experience of schools such as those in Howell Township, New Jersey, in which friable asbestos-sprayed surfaces, such as soundproof ceilings, were found in 1976 to be liberating large quantities of asbestos fibers into the air.

The cafeteria menu may also be of concern. Through your PTA, work for the ban of "junk" or convenience foods. Encourage the sale of nuts and fruit for snacking. The trailblazing example set by the West Virginia Board of Education should be followed on a national basis:

. . . Effective with the 1976-77 school year, the sale of the following non-nutritional foods or beverages is prohibited during the school day in all public schools of the state: candy, chewing gum, soft drinks, flavored ice bars.[31]

In November, 1977, the USDA, under an amendment to the Child Nutrition Act, regained the authority it had lost in 1972 to regulate what food items can be sold in vending machines on á la carte lunch lines or at snack stands at schools. USDA Secretary Bergland subsequently initiated action to restrict "competitive (junk) foods" in schools. However, under threats of legal action from "junk" food industries, including Hershey Candy Company, the USDA announced in December, 1978, that it would postpone such action for at least a further year in order to elicit public comments on the proposal.‡

Laboratory courses should not expose students to harmful chemicals.[32] Wood and metal shops should avoid the use of organic cleaning fluids and solvents containing benzene, carbon tetrachloride, trichloroethylene, or other carcinogens. Ventilation must be adequate. Chemistry laboratories and stockrooms should be completely cleared of all carcinogenic and other toxic chemicals, such as benzene. Some people question whether organic chemistry should be taught at all at the high school level. If it is, all chemicals used in classroom or laboratory work should be cleared by a knowledgeable independent authority. Finally, the unsupervised use of toxic

---

‡ In these negotiations, Hershey was represented by its attorney Peter Barton Hutt, formerly FDA General Counsel, supported by Ogden Johnson, Hershey's senior nutritionist and former Chief Nutritionist of the FDA. This is a not unusual example of the "revolving door" between agencies and industry which the Carter administration is attempting to limit.

and carcinogenic pesticides by janitorial staff should be completely stopped.

Early Detection and Treatment

Early detection is no substitute for preventing cancer, but it may result in a cure, or at any rate, increase your survival time. The prognosis of a wide range of cancers, particularly skin, breast, cervix, colon, and larynx, depends on how early they are picked up and treated effectively, in which case there is a good likelihood of a complete "cure."* Cancers which are localized to their organ of origin at the time of diagnosis and treatment are more curable than cancers that have spread to regional lymph nodes or beyond (Figure 11.1). Curability is usually expressed in terms of cases surviving without apparent recurrence of disease for over five years past initial treatment.

In view of the importance of early diagnosis, particularly for some of the more curable cancers, you should be on the lookout for any warning signs or symptoms and should check for these regularly. Additionally, you should make arrangements to have the following regular screening tests:

• Pap smears for cervix cancer.† Women over the age of twenty, especially sexually active ones, should have this test periodically. Black women should be more insistent on this, as their risk is higher than for white women.

• Pelvic examination for uterine cancer. Women over fifty years old should have this done periodically, especially if there is abnormal discharge or bleeding.

• Proctosigmoidoscopy for colon cancer. This unpleasant but lifesaving procedure is recommended routinely for men and women over forty, especially those with a family history of high-risk precancerous diseases, such as polyposis or ulcerative colitis.

• Self-examination of breasts. Every woman from adolescence on should learn and practice this procedure monthly.

• Laryngoscopy. This is recommended regularly for smokers and drinkers, particularly if there is a history of "laryngitis" or hoarseness.

Screening is even more important if you are already at a particular "high cancer risk," several categories of which are recognized:

1. *Familial predisposition.* Certain cancers tend to run in families, for poorly understood reasons.[33] These include cancer of the lung, large bowel, uterus, stomach, and breast, and childhood sarcomas and brain tumors. Your chances of contracting any of these particular cancers seem to be two to four times higher if a close relative has previously developed one of them. The excess risk is restricted to cancers of specific sites; a family history of lung cancer will not predispose to breast cancer.

Familial predisposition to breast cancer is particularly well established. Sisters or daughters of women who developed breast cancer before menopause are known to be about nine times more likely to get breast cancer than the general population. The risk is still further increased if the relative had cancer in both breasts. Risks for postmenopausal breast cancers are much lower.

* A specific example of the importance of early diagnosis is the mammography program of the Health Insurance Plan of New York sponsored by the NCI in the late 1960s and directed by Samuel Shapiro. This is the first and only completely controlled trial of early cancer diagnostic techniques, which proved that mammography in women over the age of 50 could lead to a reduction in mortality of breast cancer by 30 to 50 percent. (Mammography in younger women, however, is associated with increased risks of breast cancer, which may balance possible diagnostic advantages.)

† The value of the Pap test appears to have been exaggerated. The decline of cervix cancer deaths, commonly attributed to the Pap test, began before this test was widely introduced, and more probably reflects the high rate of unnecessary hysterectomies.

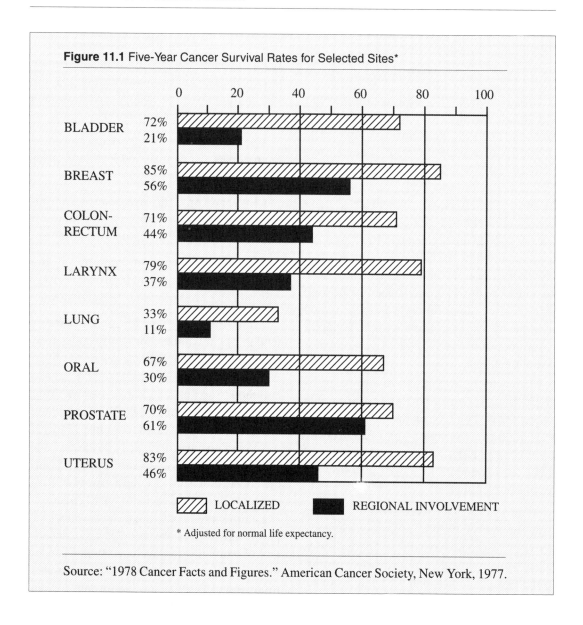

Figure 11.1 Five-Year Cancer Survival Rates for Selected Sites*

LOCALIZED   REGIONAL INVOLVEMENT

* Adjusted for normal life expectancy.

Source: "1978 Cancer Facts and Figures." American Cancer Society, New York, 1977.

2. *Genetic predisposition.* Certain rare cancers or predisposing conditions can be directly inherited. These include multiple polyposis of the colon, which predisposes to colon-rectal cancer, and xeroderma pigmentosum, which predisposes to skin cancer.

3. *History of occupational exposure to carcinogens.* The degree of excess risk will depend on the nature of the carcinogens you work with and the intensity and duration of exposure.

4. *History of treatment with carcinogenic drugs or X-rays.* As for occupational carcinogens, the excess risks depend on the degree and duration of exposure.

There are certain cancers, however, which are generally death sentences, regardless of how early they are diagnosed. Some of the claims which have been made for improved survival with early diagnosis probably reflect the extra time apparently gained before the cancer would have otherwise been diagnosed.

These poorly curable cancers include lung, brain, liver, pancreas, and stomach. Early treatment may, however, improve chances of survival and increase the quality of remaining life.‡

For Hodgkin's disease and some forms of leukaemia, particularly acute lymphocytic leukaemia of childhood, complete remissions, and prolonged survival are possible with early diagnosis and treatment, particularly in specialized centers. The importance of going to such a center for these and certain other cancers is critical. It may mean the difference between survival and death, or between prolonged and short survival. Find out what are the best centers in the country, and insist on going there if you possibly can.*

Recognizing the reality that one in four of us will sometime need cancer treatment, and that the costs will not be adequately covered by conventional policies, the ever-responsive insurance industry is now offering cancer policies which you may want to investigate. About 60 percent of these policies are writ- ten by the American Family Corporation, at a cost of about $75 a year for individual policies. Profits and a growth rate of 35 percent are expected by this industry in 1978.

Legal Remedies

If you have developed cancer and have reason to believe that this is due to the fault of industry or possibly even government, then there are some legal remedies available to you or your heirs. Your ability to succeed in these, apart from the inherent validity of the case, will depend on your persistence and on the expertise of your attorney. Any successful legal action you take against the industry responsible for your cancer may act as an incentive to prevent further such cancers.†

1. *Medical or drug-related suits.* More often than not, drug companies will settle out of court when faced with an obviously legitimate claim for damages in order not to implicate a particular drug or medicine as a precedent for other suits, which would inevitably follow. As for treatment-related cancer, such

---

‡ It is important to note that the "cancer surveillance programs" adopted by industry for lung or liver cancer most certainly do not offer prevention, but merely the earlier diagnosis of an inevitable death.

* There are three major guides to this: accreditation by the American College of Surgeons for cancer treatment; accreditation by the Joint Commission of the American Hospital Association; membership of the Comprehensive Cancer Centers, nineteen NCI-funded national centers for advanced cancer treatment. In addition, there are certain hospitals and centers that specialize in treatment of specific types of cancer and have the best survival rates. The importance of specialized treatment and specialized centers with their highly skilled and enthusiastic oncology teams has been recently emphasized in *Strike Back at Cancer* by Steven Rappaport (Englewood Cliffs, N.J.: Prentice Hall Inc., 1978), and in *The Conquering of Cancer* by Lucien Israël (New York: Random House, 1978). While Israël's optimism appears to reflect his humanity rather than documented over- all improvements in curability of the major cancer killers, the importance of "limited benefits" that can be achieved in the best modern centers, particularly the improvement in the quality of terminal life, must be clearly appreciated.

† Pressures from the insurance business may act as similar incentives. Robin Jackson, an executive of Merret Dixey Syndicates of London (a powerful force in the Lloyd's market) has warned:

As manufacturers move into new fields of product technology, so we in the insurance markets move into new areas of liability coverage that we can't fully understand yet. It's got to the point where a number of us in the underwriting market in London are starting to question whether we'll be able to provide coverage for certain products against cancer or similar diseases. (J. H. Miller, "Jackson's Leisure Study Reinforces Policy Fears," *Business Insurance,* February 14, 1979; see also S. S. Epstein, "Criticizes Insurers," *Business Insurance,* April 30, 1979.)

as that of the thyroid which developed following irradiation of children for "enlarged thymus glands," a malpractice suit may be difficult to prosecute. Not only has it been a problem to get doctors to testify against each other, but it has also been successfully argued that a given treatment was justified provided it was considered safe and effective at that time, even if it later turned out to be harmful and useless.

2. *Product liability suits.* If you or any member of your family develops cancer following the use of or exposure to a carcinogenic product, then you have the basis for a product liability suit. The burden to prove your case is less for a food or drug than for other types of products, such as pesticides or paint strippers. In cases involving food and drugs, the courts usually assume that the seller warrants his product as fit and safe for human consumption, and the plaintiff then usually only needs to show that damages were sustained and were caused by the product in question.

For a successful product liability suit, you must prove a "breach of duty of care"; that is, the manufacturer or supplier knew, or it was general knowledge among the industry, that the product was carcinogenic. This duty, when breached, constitutes negligence when the party affected is within the "ambit of risk," and could thus reasonably have been anticipated to be exposed to the product and consequently injured. The product in question must be the proximate or immediate cause of the disease, and the disease itself must be a genuine damage, such as cancer. When all these conditions can be established, grounds then exist for an award for negligence. Some states disqualify the plaintiff if the defense can prove that he somehow contributed to the negligence, while more liberal states, such as New York and Wisconsin, permit partial judgments based upon comparative negligence of both parties.

An alternative, but less well tested, legal approach is based on contract theory. The courts have often recognized that the purchaser of a product expects and receives an implied warranty from the manufacturer that the product is fit for use, or "merchantable." This warranty cannot be waived by mere labeling. The instances where this attack has failed, cigarette suits in particular, have usually involved jury trials, where the purchaser was found to have knowingly assumed a risk. Apart from this, chances of success in product liability suits are increased if the product label contained no indication or warning of its carcinogenicity.

3. *Tobacco cancer.* Suits against the tobacco industry for lung cancer have so far been unsuccessful. There is, however, some reason for guarded optimism based on as yet untested new legal strategies, which you or your heirs may wish to explore if you have developed lung cancer or other tobacco-induced diseases following smoking. Probably the single most effective measure for the prevention of cancer would be a series of large, successful lawsuits against the industry. This is a potential solution whose time is overdue.

4. *Occupational cancer.* Should you develop cancer after exposure to a known carcinogen, if you are both lucky and persistent, you may be awarded workman's compensation if you can legally prove that the exposure was work-related. This, however, is rarely sufficient to cover the total costs of your cancer, quite apart from deprivation of future earnings. It has also the added disadvantage that your acceptance of a settlement absolves the industry of all further liability from tort actions. An exception in theory may be made only if gross negligence can be proven, at best a difficult task for you when pitted against the resources of a giant industry or corporation.

State compensation systems have abjectly failed to deal with occupational health problems, particularly for diseases with long latency such as cancer.‡ Workman's compensation laws vary from state to state only in their degree of inequity. Theoretically, these laws are based on an implied trade-off in which workers surrender their rights to sue their employer in exchange for the guarantee of adequate compensation in a nonadversarial process. The courts have almost consistently upheld the legality of the denial of right to sue, but have generally failed to maintain the right to a noncontested adequate compensation. Impossibly heavy burdens are placed on workers or their heirs to unequivocally demonstrate causal and exclusive relationships between their cancers or other diseases and prior occupational exposures to carcinogenic and toxic agents.[34] Workers are obliged to hire a lawyer on a contingency basis (most lawyers are reluctant to accept such cases because of the poor chances of success and minimal nature of awards) to represent them before compensation boards which are often both unsympathetic and poorly informed. State compensation systems further make no provisions for identification and medical examination of retired or active workers previously exposed to carcinogens, but who are not yet clinically ill. Recent surveys by the Department of Labor have shown that the average length of time from onset of disability to the first disability payment is one year for a disease claim, compared to two months for an injury case; that less than 3 percent of compensation awards are for oc-

cupational diseases; that 60 percent of disease cases which were eventually compensated were contested, compared to 10 percent of injury awards; the probability of litigation approaches 90 percent for serious diseases; 55 percent of disease claims are settled by compromise and release agreements, compared with 16 percent of injury cases; the total compensation payment for permanent occupational disease is less than $10,000, compared to $23,400 for similar injury cases; compensation for death caused by occupational disease averages $3,500, compared to $57,500 for an injury case; foreign countries settle proportionately more disease claims than do the U.S. (in the case of Sweden the disparity is about twelve-fold); and the claims determination process in most foreign countries is in the hands of a disinterested party, in contrast with the U.S.

A more practical option, which may sometimes be available, is a third-party or product liability suit. You can bring one against the manufacturer supplying a carcinogenic product or process, especially in the absence of appropriate labels and warnings, to the industry in which you worked and contracted your cancer.

The principle of the third-party suit was expanded in 1972 in *Dole v. Dow Chemical et al.* (New York Court of Appeals, March 11, 1972) by the heirs of an employee of a small exterminating company who had died of exposure to methyl bromide, a pesticide

---

‡ An important recent development in attempts to reform the inequities of current workers state compensation systems has been the introduction of S.3060 by the Senate Human Resources subcommittee on labor. This bill is designed to provide comprehensive reform of compensation programs, and to mandate uniform national guidelines while allowing a reasonable degree of autonomy at the state level. Industry has reacted critically. The Alliance of American Insurers testified that the bill would impose "further liberalization of benefits without curtailing the abuses — [and that it would]

explode costs and create administrative chaos." John F. Burton, chairman of the 1972 National Commission on State Workers Compensation Laws, however, testified on behalf of the bill, expressing the view that "for the first time a workers' compensation bill had been introduced in Congress that deserves to be enacted." Other important proposed reforms include the Toxic Substances Pollution Victim Compensation Act of March, 1978 (H.R. 9616), which addresses problems of causality by establishing procedures of standards of proof and shifts the burden of proof of safety to industry.

widely used in fumigation. Unhappy with the trivial workman's compensation award, the heirs sued the third party, Dow Chemical, the manufacturer of the chemical. The grounds of the lawsuit were that the pesticide was not appropriately labeled, and that the worker had thus not been adequately warned of the hazard. Dow, while not explicitly accepting blame, sued the worker's employer for contributing to the negligence by failing to instruct him properly in the chemical's safe use. Dow thus won damages from the company, some of which it then paid the worker's family in its own settlement. The two major precedents set by this case were that liability for negligence could be shared between the defendant and a third party, and that a negligent employer could no longer hide behind workman's compensation to limit his liability for exposing workers to toxic chemicals or other hazards.

The third party principle was substantially strengthened, especially for carcinogens, when the government, late in 1977, settled a $20 million suit brought by families and former employees of a defunct asbestos plant in Tyler, Texas. The plant, which had been literally dismantled and buried because asbestos levels were so high that it could not be cleaned up, belonged to PPG Industries, which will pay $8 million, and before it, Union Asbestos and Rubber, which will pay $1 million. The government itself will pay the survivors $5 million, admitting that because of a secret agreement with the industry it had failed to warn workers of hazards of asbestos, even after several government inspections over a ten-year period turned up extremely high levels.

As the causal relationship between past exposure and delayed onset of cancer has become increasingly appreciated, the courts have more and more come to apply the doctrine of strict liability, and the prospects of success in third-party suits is now increasing. It seems likely that the recent disclosure of the asbestos "Pentagon Papers" will have a favorable impact on the multimillion dollar asbestos cases now before the courts. While large adverse judgments may act as an incentive to manufacturers to produce carcinogen-free products and to be more candid and explicit if they persist in manufacturing carcinogenic products, the financial impact of out-of-court settlements is blunted by current IRS law, allowing the carrying forward of such costs for tax purposes.

Another important option you have is suing your company doctor for medical malpractice if you can show that he failed to warn you of any findings that could have allowed you to limit further exposure or seek early treatment.* Such malpractice suits are likely to increase in the future. It is also likely that the scope of such actions will be extended to hold culpable other professionals in the workplace, such as industrial hygienists or chemists who fail to warn workers of exposure to carcinogenic or other toxic hazards.

Another possible avenue by which a diseased worker or his heirs may circumvent the legal barricade of the workman's compensation system is based on a fraud theory. Two Northern California courts have recently rendered conflicting decisions on whether a worker can sue his employer directly if he can prove that the company deliberately concealed or manipulated information on the hazards that ultimately led to the disease and

---

* Over ten lawsuits, totaling more than $50 million, have been filed against Kent Wise, the former physician of a Johns-Manville plant in Pittsburg, California, on the grounds that he deliberately withheld information from workers on X-ray evidence of asbestos-induced lung disease. Wise in turn is suing Johns-Manville for $100 million, claiming that in his original terms of employment he was "told not to have anything to do with X-rays," which would be read at the Trudeau Institute in Saranac Lake, New York. However, Wise also contends that he had no duty to report the results of the X-rays to the workers concerned but only to Johns-Manville.

claim. These suits are precedential and, if allowed to go forward, are likely to create a powerful deterrent to future suppression or manipulation of health and safety data by industry and its consultants. More salutary still would be the successful prosecution of guilty parties for criminal acts, including manslaughter.

5. *Community cancer suits.* Assume you are a middle-aged or elderly nonsmoking lady living in Salem County, New Jersey, who has developed bladder cancer. It should seem reasonable to take the position that there is a significant probability that your cancer was caused by discharge of aromatic amine carcinogens into your air and water from nearby plants known to be handling these carcinogens. The NCI cancer maps would be helpful in supporting your position, especially if these can be supported by evidence of the leakage of carcinogens from the industry to the outside air. This approach has not yet been tested in the courts, but when it eventually is, it will probably be done on a class action basis for high claims, because the expense is likely to be large and the case difficult to prove. The plaintiffs will also need to establish their case through arguments based on correlation in order to show proximate causes.

Finally, it must be realized that industry itself is not always legally passive. However, the recent failure of industry in the Galaxy v. Capurro case, besides the climate of current opinion, is likely to dampen any latent initiatives or ambitions in this direction.

The Goal of Public Action

The time has come to summarize the goals of the actions recommended in this book to reduce the national toll of cancer:

1. Cancer must be regarded as an essentially preventable disease.

2. The hidden political and economic factors which have blocked and continue to block attempts to prevent cancer must be recognized.

3. The ineffective past track record of government in cancer prevention must be recognized.

4. The critical roles in cancer prevention that public interest groups and informed labor leadership have exercised must be recognized and their further efforts fully encouraged and supported.

5. Congress must resolve the major inconsistencies in a wide range of legislation on environmental and occupational carcinogens.

6. Substantially higher federal priorities for the prevention of cancer must be developed.

7. Policies of the various federal agencies with responsibilities in cancer prevention must be effectively integrated and coordinated.

8. Top business management must recognize the essential similarities between their long-term interests and goals and those of society. Prevention of occupational cancer and cancer in the community-at-large is of primary importance to both.

9. The American Cancer Society must be influenced to balance its preoccupation with treatment with activist programs designed to prevent cancer.

10. The medical and scientific community must accept a higher degree of responsibility and involvement in the prevention of cancer by actions on both the professional and political levels.

11. Medical schools and schools of public health must be persuaded to massively reorient their educational and training programs from the diagnosis and treatment of disease and cancer to prevention.

12. Chemicals in consumer products and in the workplace must be clearly and simply identified and labeled.

13. Additional new approaches must be developed for obtaining and for retaining honest and scientifically reliable data on the carcinogenicity and toxicity of new chemicals, besides of untested or poorly tested chemicals already in commerce; such data must be made accessible to public scrutiny. Maximum legal penalties should be directed against all those responsible, directly and indirectly, for distortion or manipulation of toxicological and epidemiological data on the basis of which decisions on human safety and risk are based.

14. Apart from actions on a political level, we all have limited personal options. To some extent, it may be possible to reduce our own chances of developing cancer by making informed changes in lifestyle, use of consumer products, and work.

15. The major determinants of preventable cancer are political and economic, rather than scientific, and as such must be addressed in the open political arena. Cancer prevention must be made, at least, to rank with inflation on the next political ticket of your local and state representative, congressman, and President.

The vigorous implementation of policies based on these goals will reverse the growing epidemic of modern cancer and restore it to its rightful role of an uncommon disease.

Epilogue

Over the past few decades, there has been a progressive escalation of available information on the chemical causes of cancer. There has also been a parallel increase in our ability to test for carcinogenic effects of chemicals in animals and also to recognize such effects in humans. Not only is the level of this information in general adequate, but there are also ample laws, in spite of their occasional ambiguities and inconsistencies, to translate such information into regulatory action. The problem is thus not one of inadequate information or inadequate laws.

So then, what is the problem? As the case studies in this book make clear, there has been and continues to be a massive failure to utilize available knowledge and to implement the law. A combination of powerful and well-focused pressures by special industrial interests, together with public inattention and the indifference of the scientific community, has created a major imbalance in decision-making and public policies. In spite of efforts by organized labor and public interest groups, this imbalance has consistently and effectively thwarted, and still continues to thwart, meaningful attempts to prevent the carnage of chemical-cancer, a carnage whose unrecognized costs run each year into the tens of billion dollars.

It is not as if there is any necessary conflict between long-term industrial growth and the prevention of cancer. Many carcinogens are used for purposes that are trivial, or under conditions where they can be replaced by noncarcinogenic substitutes. In those special circumstances where carcinogens perform critically needed and irreplaceable functions, they can be used much more safely, provided industry invests in the appropriate engineering controls.

While much is known about the science of cancer, its prevention depends largely, if not exclusively, on political action. This then is the message of the book.

PART II

THE POLITICS OF CANCER, 1998

Cancer is a major cause of misery and death. Moreover, the distribution of hardship falls unevenly on those with least resources. Cancer cannot be explained away as something that just "happens" to people. Rather, we need to see many cancers as being caused by exposure to carcinogens in the workplace, in consumer products, and in the general environment. *These cancers are largely preventable* — if the real nature of their causes is understood and the fight against them becomes a political priority.

Foreword

Cancer remains one of the deadliest forces known to mankind, as it has been for centuries. Beyond the millions of people living with cancer, millions more live in fear of one day being diagnosed with the disease. Probably everyone in the country has known someone who has struggled to overcome cancer, or who has eventually succumbed to it. Although physicians and scientists continually try to improve diagnosis and treatment of this dreaded disease, over half a million Americans will die of cancer in this year alone.

The Federal government enjoined the medical crusade against cancer in 1927 with a funding allocation for cancer research, and in 1937 Congress established the National Cancer Institute which operated with modest funding for several decades. However, it wasn't until 1971 that President Nixon declared a national "War Against Cancer" and the National Cancer Act was passed. At that time, Congress was led to believe that an infusion of funding devoted to cancer research could produce a cure before the American Bicentennial in 1976.

When Dr. Epstein published *The Politics of Cancer* in 1978, Congress had increased the budget for the National Cancer Institute to $872 million, from $233 million in 1971, a cure was still nowhere in sight, and there was considerable debate as to how the war against cancer should be fought. Dr. Epstein and many of his colleagues in the public health community argued for a more aggressive assault on the preventable causes of cancer that people are unknowingly exposed to on a daily basis — at home, on the job, and in the environment — and often at low doses over a long period of time.

Today, the annual budget for the National Cancer Institute is over $2.5 billion, half a billion more than all of the combined budgets from the year it was founded to the year the war against cancer was declared. One thing that we have learned from this massive investment is that the hope for a simple cure was naive. The uncontrolled and destructive cell growth that can attack any part of the body is far more complex than was once thought. Although scientific knowledge about cancer has continued to expand, and significant progress has been made in new areas such as cancer genetics and improved techniques for detection, diagnosis, and treatments, the goal for a cure remains elusive and distant.

Despite NCI's growth, Dr. Epstein contends that cancer prevention is still greatly overlooked. In 1992, Dr. Epstein and a group of national experts and former federal officials in public health and cancer prevention held a press conference to engage the public on this imbalance. The group argued that the national cancer program should break from a focus on cancer treatment and do more to reduce the number of people getting cancer in the first place. Pointing to the continued onslaught of new cases of cancer, they urged that the NCI devote as many resources in research and outreach for cancer cause and prevention as for diagnosis and treatment. The NCI could then provide workers, consumers, Congress, and regulatory agencies vital information to reduce our exposure to carcinogens in air, water, food, and the workplace. The underlying goal of this change in policy is to reduce the rate of people getting cancer in each age group down to a level seen in the first half of the century.

In recent years, the National Cancer Institute has released some seemingly encouraging news. In 1997, the NCI reported the first sustained, significant decrease in cancer mortality rates since these statistics were collected in the 1930s. More recently, in March 1998, the NCI reported that the overall rate of new cancer cases being diagnosed, or the incidence rate, increased by 1.2 percent per year from 1973 to 1990, then declined by 0.7 percent per year through 1995. The reduction occurred in three of the most common cancers, including lung, colorectal and prostate cancer. Breast cancer rates have leveled, after increasing at 1.8 percent per year. Non-Hodgkin's lymphoma had been rising at the rate of 3.5 percent per year, and is now increasing at a rate of 0.8 percent per year. The NCI reported the rate of people dying from cancer declined overall by 0.5 percent per year.

These figures sound promising, and it is easy to interpret them as significant medical achievements, and as the precursor to the eventual eradication of this disease in our generation. I wish that they were. In this book, Dr. Epstein critiques the NCI statistics and provides a skeptic's view to help us understand these figures in a historical context. The fact remains that the overall incidence of cancer is much higher than it was twenty-five years ago, and survival rates for most common cancers remain unchanged.

The direction the Federal government takes in investing public resources in cancer research should be guided in the context of an open and vibrant debate among NCI, outside experts, and the public. The Institute of Medicine recently published a set of recommendations on setting priorities at the National Institutes of Health that emphasize a need to increase public participation in the agency's funding decisions. The recommendations confirm that the public's priorities should be included in the patchwork of factors used to decide how we invest finite research dollars to improve the nation's health.

As the National Cancer Institute continues its scientific investigations, with periodic announcements of achievements, discoveries, and hopes for the future (some recent studies suggest a reason for controlled optimism), *THE POLITICS OF CANCER Revisited* provides a highly critical review of the current state of our nation's struggle to reduce the incidence and mortality of cancer. Twenty years ago, the author's publication brought attention to the dangers of ignoring chemical hazards in our environment. I hope this new book will reinvigorate the debate on the direction of our cancer research and prevention efforts with the aim to optimize our nation's resources to spare as many lives as possible from this deadly disease.

Congressman David Obey
August 1998

Chapter Twelve

1987: Report to Congress

In 1987, Congressman Henry Waxman invited me to draft a position paper on the "War on Cancer." The paper was subsequently printed in the Congressional Record.* By way of introduction, Congressman Waxman stated:

"Mr. Speaker, just over 15 years ago, the country declared a war on cancer. Today, cancer is still the major killing disease in the industrialized world. With over 900,000 new cases and 450,000 U.S. deaths last year, cancer has now reached epidemic proportions.

"Last month, the Subcommittee on Health and the Environment received a very important statement from Dr. Samuel Epstein, professor of occupational and environmental medicine at the University of Illinois Medical Center. Dr. Epstein, one of our nation's leading cancer researchers, provides answers to who's responsible for the rising cancer rates and what we need to do about it. The statement follows."

Losing the War Against Cancer:
Who's to Blame and What to do About It

Increasing Cancer Rates

Cancer is now the only major killing disease in the industrialized world whose rates are sharply rising.† In contrast, there have been major reductions in deaths from cardiovascular disease, still the number one killer in the U.S., probably because of a recent decline in smoking and attention to diet and exercise.

With over 900,000 new cases and 450,000 U.S. deaths last year, cancer has now reached epidemic proportions with an incidence of one in three and a mortality of one in four.

Analysis of overall cancer rates, standardized for age, sex and ethnicity, has demonstrated steady increases since the 1930s, with more recent sharp annual increases in incidence rates by some 2% and in mortality rates by some 1%. Striking confirmation of these recent increases comes from estimates of the lifetime probability of getting cancer for people born at different times. For white males born in 1975 to 1985, for instance, the probability of developing cancer has risen from 30 to 36% and from 19 to 23% for dying from cancer. Such increases in overall can-

---

* Congressional Record. E3449-E3654, September 8, 1987.

† Just by way of quantitative contrast, mortality from AIDS (another eminently preventable disease) although highly alarming, if not catastrophic, is relatively low. About 33,000 cases, more than half already fatal, have been reported

since 1981 when the disease was first detected: additionally, it is estimated that 2-3 times as many Americans suffer from advanced symptoms of the AIDS-related complex which often progresses to frank AIDS. Rapidly increasing numbers of cases, totalling some 270,000, are projected by 1991.

cer rates are also reflected in increasing rates for cancers of organs including lung, breast, colon, prostate, testis, urinary bladder, kidney, and skin, malignant melanoma and lymphatic/hematopoietic malignances, including non-Hodgkin's lymphoma. (It should, however, be noted that there have been substantial decreases in rates for some stomach and cervix, and less so, for rectal cancer.) Lung cancer is responsible for about one-third of the overall recent increase in incidence rates. It should be stressed that some 75% of all cancer deaths occur in people over 55 years, and that recent increases are largely restricted to these ages.

Static Cure Rates

The overall cancer "cure rate," as measured by survival for over five years following diagnosis, is currently 50% for whites but only 38% for blacks. There is no evidence of substantial improvements in treatment over the last few decades, during which five-year survival and age-adjusted mortality rates for the major cancer killers, lung, breast and colon, besides for most other organs, have remained essentially unchanged. The only improvements have been for cancer of the cervix, and for relatively rare cancers, such as testicular seminomas, Hodgkin's disease, and childhood leukemias treated with radiation and/or chemotherapy. Apart from immediate toxicity, such treatment, while effective, can increase the subsequent risk of developing a second cancer by up to 100 times.

Increasing Carcinogenic Exposures

Cancer is an age-old and ubiquitous group of diseases. Its recognized causes and influ-

ences are multifactorial and include natural environmental carcinogens (such as aflatoxins and sunlight), lifestyle factors, genetic susceptibility, and more recently, industrial chemicals. Apart from modern lifestyle factors, particularly smoking, increasing cancer rates reflect exposure to industrial chemicals and runaway modern technologies whose explosive growth has clearly outpaced the ability of society to control them. In addition to pervasive changes in patterns of living and diet, these poorly controlled technologies have induced profound and poorly reversible environmental degradation, and have resulted in progressive contamination of air, water, food and work places with toxic and carcinogenic chemicals, with resulting involuntary exposures.

With the dawn of the petrochemical era in the early 1940s, when technologies including fractional distillation of petroleum, catalytic and thermal cracking and molecular splicing became commercially established, annual U.S. production of synthetic organic chemicals was about one billion pounds. By the 1950s, this had reached 30 billion pounds, and by the 1980s over 400 billion pounds annually. The overwhelming majority of these industrial chemicals have never been adequately, if at all, tested for chronic toxic, carcinogenic, mutagenic, and teratogenic effects, let alone for ecological effects, and much of the limitedly available industrial data is at best suspect.

Occupational exposure to industrial carcinogens has clearly emerged as a major risk factor for cancer.‡ The National Institute for Occupational Safety and Health (NIOSH) estimates that some 10 million workers are now

---

‡ In 1978, a blue ribbon governmental commission (under the auspices of then HEW Secretary Califano) estimated, on the basis of the only available exposure data, that up to 38% of all cancers in coming decades would reflect past and continuing exposures to just six high volume occupational carcinogens. In spite of the recognized limitations of these estimates, both in the direc-

tion of overestimating exposure to certain of the named carcinogens, particularly asbestos, and failure to reflect a wide range of other possibly more significant exposures, their magnitude was surprisingly confirmed by industry consultants, Stallones and Downs of the University of Texas School of Public Health, in a confidential report commissioned by the American Industrial Health

exposed to 11 high volume carcinogens. Five to 10-fold increases in cancer rates have been demonstrated in some occupations. Also persuasive are British data on cancer mortality by socio-economic class, largely defined by occupation, which show that the lowest class, particularly among males, has approximately twice the cancer mortality rate of the highest class.

Living near petrochemical and certain other industries in highly urbanized communities increases cancer risks, as evidenced by clustering of excess cancer rates; high levels of toxic and carcinogenic chemicals are deliberately discharged by a wide range of industries into the air of surrounding communities. Fallout from such toxic air pollutants is also an important source of contamination of surface waters, particularly the Great Lakes. While there still are no regulatory requirements for reporting and monitoring these emissions, unpublished government estimates indicate that they are in excess of 3 billion pounds annually.*

Another example of runaway technologies is the hazardous waste crisis. From the disposal of under one million tons of hazardous wastes in 1940 to well over 300 million tons annually in the 1980s, in excess of one ton per person per year, the industries involved — fossil fuel, metal mining and processing, nuclear, and petrochemical — have littered the entire land mass of the U.S. with some 50,000 toxic waste landfills, 20,000 of which are recognized as potentially hazardous, 170,000 industrial impoundments (ponds, pits, and lagoons), 7,000 underground injection wells, not to mention some 2.5 million

underground gasoline tanks, many of which are leaking. Not surprisingly, an increasing number of rural and urban communities have found themselves located on or near hazardous waste sites, or downstream, down-gradient, or downwind. Particularly alarming is growing evidence of contamination of ground water from such sites, contamination which poses grave and poorly reversible hazards for centuries to come.

Environmental contamination with highly potent carcinogenic pesticides has reached alarming and pervasive proportions. Apart from high level exposure of workers in manufacturing, formulating and applicating industries, contamination of ground and surface waters has become commonplace. Residues of ethylene dibromide in excess of 1,000 ppb in raw grains, cereals and citrus fruits have been well known to industry and the Environmental Protection Agency (EPA) as long as ten years after its very high carcinogenicity was first demonstrated; not until 1984 however, did EPA develop a 30 ppb tolerance, which was rejected by the Commonwealth of Massachusetts and the States of New York and Florida, and replaced by much lower and less hazardous levels. While the exact numbers are uncertain, it is probable that tens of millions of homes nationwide are contaminated with varying levels of chlordane/heptachlor, pesticides still registered by EPA for termite treatment. It should be noted that, on the basis of extensive hearings some 14 years earlier, the Agency concluded that exposure to such pesticides posed an "imminent hazard" due to cancer besides other chronic toxic effects, leading to a subsequent ban on their agricul-

---

Council.

* The Environmental Protection Agency has diverted attention away from its failure to regulate such toxic emissions, although so authorized by Sec. 112 of the 1970 Clean Air Act, by attempting to shift responsibility to local and state agencies, and by a barrage of poorly supportable claims that indoor air pollution, from pollutants

such as cigarette smoking, radon and pesticides, is a more important regulatory target than toxic air emissions. In spite of this near exclusionary emphasis on indoor air pollution, EPA still refuses to ban the continued use of carcinogenic pesticides, notably Chlordane and Aldrin used extensively for domestic termite treatment.

tural uses.

Much cancer today reflects events and exposures in the 1950s and 60s. Production, uses and disposal of synthetic organic and other industrial carcinogens were then minuscule compared to current levels, which will determine future cancer rates for younger populations now exposed. There is every reason to anticipate that even high current cancer rates will be exceeded in coming decades.

While most concern has understandably focused on increasing cancer rates, these substantially underestimate the extent and scope of the public health effects of environmental pollutants. Only a small proportion of the tens of thousands of petrochemicals in commerce, well under 500, are carcinogenic. However, many of these, together with other noncarcinogenic petrochemicals, can induce other chronic toxic effects, including neurological, respiratory, reproductive, hepatic, and probably immunological diseases, whose true causation is generally not suspected, let alone investigated.

Who's to Blame

Industry

Twentieth century industry has aggressively pursued short-term economic goals, uncaring or unmindful of harm to workers, local communities and the environment. So far, industry has shifted responsibility for such costs and harm to society-at-large. Belated governmental efforts to control polluting industries have generally been neutralized by well organized and financed opposition. Excepting special purpose legislation for drugs, food additives, and pesticides, there were no regulatory requirements for pretesting industrial chemicals until the 1976 Toxic Substance Control Act, legislation which the industry had stalled for

years, and which is now honored more in the breach than in the observance.

Apart from failure to pretest most chemicals, key in industry's anti-regulatory strategy has been the generation of self-serving and misleading data on toxicology and epidemiology, besides on regulatory costs and cost-benefit analysis. The track record of such unreliable and often fraudulent data is so extensive and well documented as to justify the presumption that much industry data must be treated as suspect until proven otherwise.

Attempts by the Carter Administration to develop comprehensive, "generic" regulation of occupational carcinogens, later reversed by the Reagan Administration, were attacked by the Manufacturing Chemists Association, which created the American Industrial Health Council to organize opposition. Such reactions generally reflect reflex ideology and short-sighted preoccupation with perceived self-interest rather than with efficiency and economy. The virtual uniformity of industry opposition to regulation is in marked contrast to the heterogeneity of size and interests of the industries involved. Regulation has, in fact, generally resulted in substantial improvements in industrial efficiency and economy, particularly in large industries, by forcing development of technologies for recovery and recycling of valuable resources. A deplorable result of regulation, however, has been and continues to be export of the restricted product or process to the so-called lesser developed countries.†

Apart from well documented evidence on control and manipulation of health and environmental information, industry has used various strategies to con the public into complacency and divert attention from their own recklessness and responsibility for the cancer epidemic. Key among these is the "blame-the-victim" theory of cancer causation, de-

---

† Information on such exports is being systematized by Consumer Interpol, a program of the International Organization of Consumers Union (IOCU) based in Penang, Malaysia, which promotes protection for the consumer from dangerous products. The participants in this network are consumer, environmental, health and other citizen groups concerned about unrestricted trade in

veloped by industry scientists and consultants and a group of conservative pro-industry academics, and tacitly supported by the "cancer establishment." This theory emphasizes faulty lifestyle — smoking, fatty diet, sun bathing, etc. — or genetic susceptibility as the major cause of preventable cancer, while trivializing the role of involuntary exposures to occupational and environmental carcinogens. Another misleading diversion is the claim that there is no evidence of recently increasing cancer rates other than lung cancer, for which smoking is given the exclusive credit. While the role of lifestyle is obviously important and cannot be ignored, the scientific and exclusionary basis of this theory is as unsound as it is self-serving. Certainly, smoking is a major, but not the only, cause of lung cancer. Evidence such as the following clearly incriminates the additional role of exposure to occupational carcinogens and carcinogenic community air pollutants: some 20% of lung cancers occur in nonsmokers; there have been major recent increases in lung cancer rates in nonsmokers; an increasing percentage of lung cancer is of a histological type (adenocarcinoma) not usually associated with smoking; high lung cancer rates are found with certain occupational exposures independent of smoking; and excess lung cancer rates are found in communities where certain major industries are located. The chemical industry clearly uses tobacco as a smoke screen to divert attention from the role of carcinogenic chemicals in inducing lung cancer besides other cancers.

When it comes to diet, the much touted role of high fat consumption, while clearly linked to heart disease, is based on tenuous and contradictory evidence with regard to breast and colon cancers (page 375). The evidence certainly does not justify the wild claims by lifestyle theorists that some 30 to 40% of all can-

cers are due to faulty diet (Chapter 14). For instance, a 1982 National Academy of Sciences report concluded that "in the only human studies in which the total fiber consumption was quantified, no association was found between total fiber consumption and colon cancer." Similarly, a large-scale 1987 study, based on the eating habits of nearly 90,000 nurses, concluded that ". . . there is no association between dietary fat and breast cancer."

Another illustration of grossly misleading strategies relates to the identification of chemical carcinogens. When a particular chemical or product is threatened with regulation on the basis of animal carcinogenicity tests, the industry invariably challenges the significance of these tests, while routinely using negative test results as proof of safety. At the same time industry insists on the need for long-term prospective epidemiological investigations to obtain definitive human evidence. To test this apparent reliance on direct human evidence, researchers at Mt. Sinai Hospital in New York compiled a list of some 100 chemicals accepted as carcinogenic on the basis of animal tests, but for which no epidemiological information is available, and sent this list to some 80 major chemical industries. Respondents were asked whether any of the listed carcinogens were in use and, if so, whether epidemiological studies had been conducted, whether they were being conducted, or whether it was intended to conduct them in the future, and if not, why not. The responses were revealing. The great majority of those industries using particular carcinogens replied that they had done no epidemiological studies, were not doing any, and didn't intend to do any for various reasons, including alleged difficulty, impracticality, expense, or because of their belief that these chemicals could not possibly be carcinogenic to humans. A perfect catch-22. Knock the animal tests and in-

---

hazardous substances. Besides the global dissemination of such hazards, the multinational corporations involved are also responsible for the loss of U.S. jobs and their replacement by cheap "expendable" foreign labor.

sist on human studies, but make sure that the human studies are never done.

Industry positions are vigorously advocated by trade associations, such as the Chemical Manufacturers Association; public relations firms, such as Hill and Knowlton; front organizations, such as the American Council on Science and Health (the contributions of whose director, Whelan, have been aptly characterized as "voodoo science"); and lay writers such as Efron (who charges that the American scientific community has been terrorized into submission by environmental "apocalyptics"). Disturbingly, another major source of support for anti-regulatory strategies is a stable of academic consultants who advance the industry position in arenas including the scientific literature, federal advisory committees, and regulatory and congressional hearings.‡

Government

Presidents play a powerful role in setting national public health priorities, not unnaturally reflecting their own political agendas. Reagan, however, is unique in having run for office on an ideological anti-regulatory platform, and in having then systematically used his office to implement this ideology, often in contravention to the spirit and letter of the law.

Reagan has thus neutralized legislative mandates on controls of toxic and carcinogenic exposure by frontal assaults on regulatory agencies.* Strategies employed include: staffing senior positions with unqualified, ideologically selected staff hostile to their agency mandates; budget cutting; insisting on formal cost-benefit analyses which focus on industry costs with little or biased consideration of costs of failure to regulate and which effectively stall the regulatory process; illegal, behind-closed-doors meetings with industry; and making regulation dependent on the Office of Management and Budget with its subservience to the White House. An informative example is the White House decision to block the $1.3 million 1984 request by the National Institute for Occupational Safety and Health (NIOSH) to notify some 200,000 workers of risks from previously undisclosed exposure to workplace carcinogens, as identified in some 60 government studies, in order to enable medical follow-up and early diagnosis of cancer. The reason for this refusal of modest funding seems to have been a desire to shield corporations from possible legal claims.† Such a track record justifies the conclusions of a 1984 Congressional Study Group report that "efforts to protect public health and the environment from the dangers of toxic pollution have ground to a

---

‡ These consultants include: MacMahon, a Harvard epidemiologist who has cleared his contracted studies with industry before submitting them for publication; Demoupoulos, a pathologist at NYU Medical Center who claims that asbestos and vinyl chloride are weak carcinogens and that the high cancer mortality rates in New Jersey are due to poor treatment by foreign-trained doctors in that state; Olson, a clinician at Pittsburgh University School of Medicine who has testified that benzene cannot be carcinogenic in humans because it does not induce tumors in animals; Hayes, ex-CDC and Vanderbilt University School of Medicine, a toxicologist repeatedly on record as rejecting the human significance of animal carcinogenicity data on organochlorine pesticides; and Harbison, a toxicologist from University of Ar-

kansas Medical School, who in 1980 testified as a governmental witness that rodents are "good predictors of human cancer risk," and who, as an industry expert, testified just the opposite in 1985.

* Such successes of the Reagan Administration at the regulatory level are, however, in striking contrast to its failure to make any impression on the scientific underpinning of public health and environmental regulations. For instance, a 1985 report by the Office of Science and Technology Policy of the White House clearly affirmed such critical tenets as the value of animal carcinogenicity data in extrapolating to human risk, and the inability to set "safe levels or thresholds" for exposure to carcinogens.

† On February 26, 1987, hearings were held before the Labor and Human Resources Committee

standstill under the Reagan Administration . . . [which was charged with being] a public health hazard."

The U.S. Congress has become sensitized to public health and environmental concerns, exemplified in a plethora of legislation in recent decades.‡ Such legislation has evolved fragmentarily, reflecting particular interests and priorities. New laws have focused on individual media, air, water, food, or the workplace, or on individual classes of products or contaminants, such as pesticides or air pollutants, with little or no consideration of needs for more comprehensive and integrated approaches. Furthermore, legislative language traditionally has been ambiguous, thus allowing maximal regulatory discretion to bureaucracies which, in some instances, have subsequently become closely associated with or even "captured" by the regulated industries. A noteworthy exception is the 1958 Delaney Amendment to the Federal Food Drug and Cosmetic Act, with its absolute prohibition against the deliberate introduction of any level of carcinogen into the food supply. Even so, the Reagan FDA is redefining the Delaney Amendment to allow carcinogenic food additives at levels alleged to be devoid of significant risk.

Congress has also tended to abdicate decision-making to scientific authority (or perceived authority), rather than questioning its basis in the open political arena. Of particular importance was passage of the 1971 Cancer Act in response to orchestrated pressures from the "cancer establishment" — the National Cancer Institute (NCI), American Cancer Society (ACS), and clinicians aggressively pushing chemotherapy as a primary cancer treatment. The cancer establishment misled Congress into the unfounded and simplistic view that the cure for cancer was just around the corner, *provided* that Congress made available massive funding for cancer treatment research. The Act did just this, while failing to emphasize needs for cancer prevention, and also gave the NCI virtual autonomy from the parent National Institutes of Health, while establishing a direct chain of command between the NCI and the White House. Some 16 years and billions of dollars later, Congress still has not yet appreciated that the poorly informed special interests of the cancer establishment have minimized the importance of and failed to adequately support critically needed cancer prevention efforts. Nor has Congress appreciated the long overdue need for oversight on the conduct and priorities of the NCI. Given the heterogeneity of congressional interests, the complexity of the problem involved, the heavy industry lobbying, the indifference of the general scientific community, and the well orchestrated pressures of the cancer establish-

---

on a bill sponsored by Senator Metzenbaum to require the Department of Health & Human Services to notify past or present workers known to be at risk of cancer and other occupational diseases. To the annoyance of Republican Committee members, NIOSH officials supported the bill, which was opposed by Administration spokesmen who claimed that it would duplicate existing efforts and generate "too much litigation." The senior dissenting officials received a subsequent "dressing down" from the Administration. However, unexpected support for the bill on March 27, 1987 came from the 3,000-member American Electronics Association, a trade group, and from IBM, the Digital Equipment Corporation, and the General Electric Company.

‡ Congress, however, has yet to recognize the need to consider certain industry practices from the perspective of white collar crime. White collar crime legislation has heretofore been exclusively directed to economically motivated crimes with economic consequences, such as antitrust violations. Efforts, such as the 1979 and 1984 bills by Cong. John Conyers (H.R. 4973 & 6350), to extend such legislation to economically motivated crimes with public health or environmental consequences, resulting from willful suppression or "non-disclosure" of risks from hazardous products and processes have not, yet may be, measured in countless cancer deaths.

ment, it is not surprising that Congress has still to recognize that we are losing the war against cancer.

Until recently, state governments have largely deferred to federal authority, exercising relatively minor roles in cancer prevention. Reagan's federal de-regulatory efforts have begun to reverse this relationship. Regulatory actions against carcinogens are now emerging at the state level, such as the banning of chlordane/heptachlor and aldrin/dieldrin for termite treatment by Massachusetts and New York, banning of daminozide (Alar) for apple ripening, and tough restrictions on ethylene dibromide food tolerances by Massachusetts, and by informative occupational labeling laws by various states, such as the "right-to-know" workplace legislation of New Jersey. Some such state initiatives have evoked federal preemption by restricted regulations, such as the 1983 Hazard Communication Standard of the Occupational Safety and Health Administration, in striking paradox to the Reagan ideology of the new federalism and getting big government off the backs of the people. In February 1987, a coalition of labor and citizen organizations asked the U.S. Court of Appeals to enforce its 18-month-old order directing OSHA to expand coverage of its communication standard from manufacturing to all workers. In an apparent about-face turn, the Chemical Manufacturers Association is supporting the expansion in conformity with regulations developed for various states.

The Cancer Establishment

The cancer establishment still continues to mislead the public and Congress into believing that "we are winning the war against cancer," with "victory" possible only given more time and money. The NCI and ACS also insist that there have been major advances in treatment and cure of cancer, and that there

has been no increase in cancer rates (with the exception of lung cancer which is exclusively attributed to smoking). Yet the facts show just the contrary.

The cancer establishment periodically beats the drum to announce the latest "cancer cure" and dramatic "breakthrough." These announcements reflect optimism and wishful thinking, rather than reality. The extravagant and counterproductive claims for interferon as the magic cancer bullet of the late 70s have been followed by the unpublicized recognition of its limited role in cancer treatment.* The latest NCI "breakthrough" claims for interleukin-2 as a cancer cure are grossly inflated and rest on questionable data (page 490). These claims fail to reflect the devastating toxicity and lethality of this drug, and gloss over the high treatment costs, which can run into six figures. Equally questionable are claims by the NCI and ACS that overall cancer survival rates have improved dramatically over recent years. These claims, based on "rubber numbers" according to one prominent critic, ignore factors such as "lead-time bias," earlier diagnosis of cancer resulting in apparently prolonged survival even in the absence of any treatment, and the "over-diagnosis" of essentially benign tumors, particularly of the prostate, breast and thyroid, as malignant. Defensively revealing is the recent finger-pointing by the director of the NCI, DeVita, at community physicians for using inadequate doses of chemotherapy drugs as the "real" reason why cancer cure rates are no better than they are.

The NCI misrepresentations are well reflected in budgetary priorities which are largely and disproportionately directed to cancer treatment research, to the neglect of cancer prevention. Even the very modest funding on cancer prevention is largely directed to endorsing industry's "blame-the-victim" concept of cancer causation. Thus, the NCI ex-

---

* Interferon is particularly effective, if not often curative for two rare neoplasms — hairy cell leukaemia and juvenile laryngeal papillomatosis.

aggerates the role of tobacco for a wide range of cancers besides lung, and treats as fact the slim and contradictory evidence relating diet to colon, breast, and other cancers. Apparently still oblivious to mounting criticisms, the NCI continues to vigorously propagate these misrepresentations. A 1986 NCI document on cancer control objectives, the executive summary of which fails to even mention environmental and occupational exposures to carcinogens and focuses on diet and tobacco as the major causes of cancer, rashly promises that annual cancer mortality rates could be reduced by 50% by the year 2000.

More disturbing than indifference to cancer prevention is evidence uncovered in September 1982 by Cong. Dave Obey that the NCI has pressured the International Agency for Research on Cancer (IARC), funded in part by the NCI, to downplay the carcinogenicity of benzene and also formaldehyde in IARC monographs which review and rank the carcinogenicity data on industrial and other chemicals. Such evidence is noteworthy since, contrary to the scientific literature and its own explicit guidelines, IARC has also downgraded the carcinogenicity of other carcinogenic industrial chemicals, such as the pesticides aldrin/dieldrin and chlordane/heptachlor, and the solvents trichloroethylene and perchloroethylene.†

Following nearly a decade of fruitless discussions with the ACS, at a February 7, 1987 press conference, a national coalition of major public interest and labor groups headed by the Center for Science in the Public Interest (and by the author of this position paper), and supported by some 24 independent scientists, charged that the ACS "is doing virtually nothing to help reduce the public exposure to cancer causing chemicals. . . . Despite its promises to the public to do everything to 'wipe out cancer in your lifetime,' the ACS fails to make its voice heard in Congress and the regulatory arena, where it could be a powerful influence to help reduce public exposure to carcinogens." More specific criticisms included the following:

• ACS fails to support, and at times has been hostile to, critical legislation that seeks to reduce or eliminate exposure to environmental and occupational carcinogens. For example, ACS refuses to join a coalition of major organizations, including the March of Dimes, American Heart Association, and American Lung Association, to support the Clean Air Act. ACS has rejected requests from Congressional subcommittees, unions, and environmental organizations to support their efforts to ban or regulate a wide range of occupational and environmental carcinogens. Giant corporations, which profit handsomely while they pollute the air, water and food with cancer causing chemicals, must be greatly comforted by the ACS's silence (Chapter 16).

• ACS's record on supporting efforts to ban carcinogens is dismal. Often ACS's statements are expressly or implicitly hostile to regulation.

• ACS's approach to cancer prevention largely reflects a "blame the victim" philosophy, which emphasizes faulty lifestyles, rather than workplace or environmental carcinogens. For instance, ACS blames the higher incidence of cancer among blacks primarily on their diet and smoking habits, which diverts attention from the fact that blacks work in the dirtiest, most hazardous jobs, and live in the most polluted communities.

A few days after the press conference, ACS announced a "new set of policies," passing resolutions for improved regulation of such chemicals as asbestos and benzene, and for cleanup of toxic waste sites. However, there has been no evidence of any real change of

---

† With the noted exceptions, the IARC monographs are unique and well-systematized compendia of information on chronic toxicity, carcinogenicity and use data of a wide range of industrial and other chemicals.

heart in the ACS since then.

The Lifestyle Apologists

The lifestyle academics are a group of conservative scientists including Doll, Warden and Director of the industry-financed Green College, Oxford,‡ his protégé Peto, a statistician also from Oxford, and more recently Ames, a California geneticist (Chapter 14). The puristic pretensions of the lifestyler apologists for critical objectivity are only exceeded by their apparent indifference to or rejection of a steadily accumulating body of information on permeation of the environment and workplace with industrial carcinogens, and the impact of such involuntary exposures on human cancer. Consciously or subconsciously, these academics have become the mouthpiece for industry interests, urging regulatory inaction and public complacency. Among the more noteworthy contributions of these academics is a series of publications claiming that smoking and fatty diet each is responsible for 30-40% of all cancers, that sunlight, drugs, and personal susceptibility account for another 10%, leaving only a few percent unaccounted for which, just for want of any other better reason, was then ascribed to occupation. According to the lifestylers, this then proves that occupation is an unimportant cause of cancer, which really does not warrant much regulatory concern (page 374). Apart from circularly referencing each other as authority for these wild guesses, the lifestylers have never attempted to develop any estimates of how many workers are exposed to defined levels of specific carcinogens. Without such estimates there is no way of attempting to determine just how much cancer is due to occupation.

The lifestyle theory was further advocated in a 1981 report dealing with causes of cancer in the USA by Doll and Peto where they denied evidence of increasing cancer rates other than for lung cancer, which was largely ascribed to tobacco without adequate consideration of the importance of carcinogenic community and occupational exposures (page 374).* To reach their misleading conclusions on static cancer rates, Doll and Peto excluded from analysis people over the age of 65 and blacks, those groups with the highest and increasing cancer mortality rates. Not content with such manipulation, they claimed that occupation was only responsible for some 4% of all cancers, without apparent consideration of a wide range of recent studies dealing with the carcinogenic effects of such exposures.† This wild 4% guess was matched by "guesstimates" that diet was determinant in some 35% of all cancers. To trivialize the significance of animal carcinogenicity data on industrial chemicals, Doll and Peto minimized the predictive value of these tests, while emphasizing epidemiological data as the basis of regulation.

Doll is prompt to side with industry in downplaying evidence on carcinogenicity of industrial chemicals. Illustratively, he recently lent enthusiastic support to the Australian Agent Orange Royal Commission in their dis-

---

‡ According to a founding fellow, Hermann, Green College was established in 1978 as a "special point of entry for industrial interests wishing to collaborate with university departments in research."

* This study was sponsored by the Office of Technology Assessment, whose contract officer Gough was apparently unable to find any U.S. experts with knowledge of cancer in the U.S., and so selected British lifestyle advocates for the project. (Gough is also subsequently on record in a book on Agent Orange as dismissing evidence on hazards of di-

oxin, including rejection of its carcinogenicity based on extensive animal data. Gough recently left OTA for a position in a chemical industry consulting firm.) Apparently responsive to criticisms of a draft report, The Office of Technology Assessment decided against its publication, which instead was independently published.

† Even if only 4% of cancers in the general population are occupational in origin, this implies that occupation is responsible for some 20% of all cancers in exposed workers.

missal of the experimental and epidemiological carcinogenicity data on the herbicides 2,4-D and 2,4,5-T (page 386).‡

Ames is a geneticist who, in the 1970s, developed bacterial assays for mutagenicity which he advocated as short-term tests for carcinogens. He then published a series of articles warning of increasing cancer rates and of the essential need for tough regulation of industrial carcinogens, such as the fire retardant Tris and the fumigant ethylene dibromide. By the 1980s, however, Ames did an unexplained 180-degree switch, now claiming just the opposite, that overall cancer rates are not increasing, that industrial carcinogens are unimportant causes of cancer which do not need regulating, and that the real causes of cancer are natural dietary carcinogens, largely because mutagens can be found in a variety of foods (page 422).*

What to Do About It

The cancer epidemic poses the nation with a grave and growing crisis of enormous cost to health, life and the economy. A 1979 book, *The Politics of Cancer,* concluded with the following specific recommendations designed to reduce the toll of preventable cancer.

- Cancer must be regarded as an essentially preventable disease.

- The hidden political and economic factors which have blocked and continue to block attempts to prevent cancer must be recognized.

- The ineffective past track record of government in cancer prevention must be recognized.

- The critical roles in cancer prevention that public interest groups and informed labor leadership have exercised must be recognized and their further efforts fully encouraged and supported.

- Congress must resolve the major inconsistencies in a wide range of legislation on environmental and occupational carcinogens.

- Substantially higher federal priorities for the prevention of cancer must be developed.

- Policies of the various federal agencies with responsibilities in cancer prevention must be effectively integrated and coordinated.

- Top business management must recognize the essential similarities between their long-term interest and goals and those of society. Prevention of occupational cancer and cancer in the community-at-large is of primary importance to both.

- The American Cancer Society must be influenced to balance its preoccupation with treatment with activist programs designed to prevent cancer.

- The medical and scientific community must accept a higher degree of responsibility and involvement in the prevention of cancer by actions on both the professional and political levels.

- Medical schools and schools of public health must be persuaded to massively reorient their educational and training programs from the diagnosis and treatment of cancer to prevention.

---

‡ The 2,4,5-T component of Agent Orange was contaminated with high concentrations of 2,3,7,8-tetrachlorodibenzodioxin which, according to the Carcinogen Assessment Group of EPA, is the most potent carcinogen it has ever evaluated, some sevenfold orders of magnitude greater than the potent carcinogen vinyl chloride.

* Ames fails to extend his logic by claiming that feces are carcinogenic, although they are a rich source of bacterial mutagens! Moreover, assuming that Ames' exclusionary emphasis on dietary carcinogens has scientific validity, the critical issue is not what carcinogens are "natural" and what are industrial (asbestos is an example of a carcinogen belonging to both categories), but what exposures are preventable or at least reducible.

- Chemicals in consumer products and in the workplace must be clearly and simply identified and labeled.

- Additional new approaches must be developed for obtaining and for retaining honest and scientifically reliable data on the carcinogenicity and toxicity of new chemicals, besides of untested or poorly tested chemicals already in commerce; such data must be made accessible to public scrutiny. Maximum legal penalties should be directed against all those responsible, directly and indirectly, for distortion or manipulation of toxicological and epidemiological data on the basis of which decisions on human safety and risk are based.

Apart from actions on a political level, we all have limited personal options. To some extent, it may be possible to reduce our own chances of developing cancer by making informed changes in lifestyle, use of consumer products, and work.

The major determinants of preventable cancer are political and economic, rather than scientific, and as such must be addressed in the open political arena. Cancer prevention must be made, at least, to rank with inflation on the next political ticket of your local and state representative, congressman, and President.

A decade later, these goals still stand as valid, but none have been achieved, while cancer rates have steadily risen. To prevent similar conclusions a decade from now the cancer prevention rhetoric must be translated into reality.

To compete with well financed propaganda of industry, tacitly supported by the cancer establishment and lifestyle academics, an educational offensive must be mounted to inform the public and develop grass roots pressures for a cancer prevention campaign. The cutting edge for such campaigns can be provided by the major public interest organizations, including the Natural Resources Defense Council, Sierra Club, Environmental Defense Fund, Health Research Group of Public Citizens, Environmental Action, Consumer Federation of America, National Campaign Against Misuse of Pesticides, the National Campaign Against Toxic Hazards, Greenpeace, the Rachel Carson Council, and the Center for Science in the Public Interest.† Equally critical will be involvement of the Industrial Union Department, AFL-CIO, and key unions, such as the United Steel Workers of America, United Rubber Workers, Linoleum and Plastic Workers of America, International Association of Machinists, Oil, Chemical, and Atomic Workers, Amalgamated Clothing and Textile Workers, and the United Auto Workers.‡ Many of these organizations have well informed professional staff, and some have played major roles in whatever limited legislative and regulatory successes have been achieved over the last two decades.

Active support at the local level is being provided by activist citizen and labor groups that have formed in response to community or regional concerns such as hazardous waste dumps, contaminated drinking water, or lawn care chemicals; the motto of such groups is "Think globally, act locally." Further support

---

† Support for the EDF should be qualified pending clarification of its recent ultra-conservative and poorly informed positions on public health hazards from environment pollutants.

‡ Left-wing liberal organizations and progressive labor, through effective research, writing, direct mail and public advertising, are now challenging the ability of conservative business to formulate the national agenda and shape the debate on basic social issues, such as worker rights, taxation and environmental concerns, and on foreign policy. Such organizations include the Center for National Policy, Citizens for Tax Justice, The Democracy Project headed by Mark Green, The Economic Policy Institute headed by Jeff Faux, and the Council for Economic Priorities.

can be provided by a small network of independent and government scientists, whose thinning ranks, however, have been recently boosted by the welcome involvement of professional organizations such as the American Public Health Association and the American Lung Association.

A potential source of cancer prevention funding is the multimillion dollar budget of the American Cancer Society (ACS) raised by voluntary public contributions. An economic boycott of the ACS is now well overdue. Funding inappropriately used by the Society should be diverted to public interest organizations and labor, who are more likely to achieve the goal of winning the war against cancer. Other potential funding sources include certification to participate by designation in the United Way and Combined Federal Campaign.

Public interest and labor organizations should develop coalitions with initially limited objectives, focused around specific areas of cancer prevention of local concern. These could be subsequently expanded into wider rainbow coalitions with more comprehensive goals. The 100th Congress, revitalized by the defeat of the Reagan revolution and by a democratic renaissance, is now more likely to be receptive to such initiatives. This receptivity should be directed into increasing priorities for governmental concerns on cancer prevention, besides restoring the fragmented regulatory apparatus of government. It is also likely that key Congressmen could be galvanized into making cancer prevention one of their major political priorities, and that presidential candidates could be interested in the potential grass roots appeal of a cancer prevention ticket.

Equally important are initiatives at the state level, whose recent track record offers encouraging precedents. These include the banning of chlordane and heptachlor for termite treatment by Massachusetts in 1985 and New York in 1986, largely at the impetus of a citizen group, People Against Chlordane (PAC), passage of a $1.5 billion hazardous waste cleanup bond by New York, the Environmental Quality Bond Act of 1986, and passage of Proposition 65, the Safe Drinking Water and Toxic Enforcement Act of 1986, by California. Proposition 65, masterminded by the Sierra Club and Environmental Defense Fund and supported by a rainbow coalition of California public interest citizen and labor groups, is a sophisticated referendum which imposes tough financial penalties on industries knowingly discharging carcinogens into the drinking water supplies, and which mandates full public disclosure of such discharges by industry and state officials. A vocal opponent of Proposition 65 was Ames, who failed to impress the California public with his lifestyle advocacy and his trivializing the significance of carcinogens in drinking water. Potential opposition by the major petrochemical industry was anticipated and muted by the earmarking of some 50% of revenues from fines for the state superfund budget. However, Governor Deukmejian, responsive to special interest lobbying, has recently neutralized the scope of the new legislation by restricting its scope only to epidemiologically confirmed carcinogens. This restriction is now under legal challenge. Irrespective of the outcome of this challenge, Proposition 65 has excited national interest and is being used as a model for similar regional initiatives, such as the 1987 Safe Drinking Water Act of New York which is currently being drafted.

Among early Congressional priorities should be enactment of comprehensive white collar crime legislation. This would impose tough sanctions on individual executives, managers and professionals of industries found guilty of willful "nondisclosure" of information on hazards to workers, local communities and the nation. White collar crime legislation should also be extended to U.S. and multinational corporations which export carcinogenic products or processes which have been banned or regulated in the U.S. to "lesser developed countries," especially in the absence of full disclosure of hazards directed to ultimate users and consumers. Attention should also be directed to developing comprehensive new "cradle-to-the-grave" and material balance legislative approaches to the regulation of toxic and carcinogenic chemicals. Such legislation can be designed to complement regulation by the judicious application of marketplace pressures, in the form of financial incentives and disincentives designed to wean industry from unsafe practices, and to insure that responsible industry is not penalized and subject to unfair competition. At present, other than the prospect of toxic tort litigation, there are virtually no incentives for industry to develop safer new products and processes. Legislation is needed to develop federal R&D funding to promote such benign technologies and also to ensure that they are closely coordinated with environmental, energy and resource policies.

A critical legislative priority is amendment of the National Cancer Act to give the highest possible priority to cancer prevention, to redress the historical unbalance existing in the NCI between cancer prevention and research, diagnosis, treatment and the basic sciences, and also to insulate the NCI from direct Presidential influence. In addition to replacing NCI's director DeVita who, in spite of his contrary protestations, has been indifferent if not hostile to cancer prevention efforts and who has played a major role in perpetuating the myth that we are winning the war against cancer, senior NCI staff should be restructured and boosted by a critical mass of professionals competent in environmental and occupational cancer and committed to cancer prevention. The National Cancer Advisory Board should be reconstituted with a balanced mix of independent cancer prevention professionals, representatives of public interest and labor organizations and concerned citizens, and should be subject to close Congressional oversight. Such oversight should insure that the institutional resources are largely directed to cancer prevention, that grants and contracts reflect this priority and that NCI staff play a key role in providing the supporting scientific basis for legislative and regulatory cancer prevention efforts at the national and state levels.

Cancer is essentially a preventable disease. Given high national priority, this goal will be achieved.

Postscript

NCI director Vincent DeVita submitted a response in attempted rebuttal of the criticism of the NCI in this position paper. His response, however, was considered to be unsubstantive and was not published in the Congressional Record.

Chapter Thirteen

1992-1993: Challenge to the Cancer Establishment

The Experts' Press Conference

The following statement was released at a press conference in Washington, D.C., on February 4, 1992. The statement was co-authored by former directors of federal agencies Drs. Eula Bingham, Anthony Robbins, and David Rall, by Dr. Irwin D. Bross and the author. It was also endorsed by 64 leading national experts in cancer prevention, public health, and preventive medicine.

Cancer now strikes one in three and kills one in four Americans, with over 500,000 deaths last year. Over the last decade, some 5 million Americans died of cancer and there is growing evidence that a substantial proportion of these deaths was avoidable.

We express grave concerns over the failure of the "war against cancer" since its inauguration by President Nixon and Congress on December 23, 1971. This failure is evidenced by the escalating incidence of cancer to epidemic proportions over recent decades. Paralleling and further compounding this failure is the absence of any significant improvement in the treatment and cure of the majority of all cancers. Notable exceptions are the successes with some relatively rare cancers, particularly those in children.

A recent report by the American Hospital Association predicts that cancer will become the leading cause of death by the year 2000 and the "dominant specialty" of American medicine. The costs in terms of suffering and death and the inflationary impact of cancer, now estimated at $110 billion annually (nearly 2% of the GNP), is massive. These costs are major factors in the current health care crisis, with per-case Medicare payments exceeding those of any other disease.

We express further concerns that the generously funded cancer establishment, the National Cancer Institute (NCI), the American Cancer Society (ACS) and some twenty comprehensive cancer centers, have misled and confused the public and Congress by repeated claims that we are winning the war against cancer. In fact, the cancer establishment has continually minimized the evidence for increasing cancer rates which it has largely attributed to smoking and dietary fat, while discounting or ignoring the causal role of avoidable exposures to industrial carcinogens in the air, food, water, and the workplace.

Furthermore, the cancer establishment and major pharmaceutical companies have repeatedly made extravagant and unfounded claims for dramatic advances in the treatment and "cure" of cancer. Such claims are generally based on an initial reduction in tumor size ("tumor response") rather than on prolongation of survival, let alone on the quality of life, which is often devastated by highly toxic treatments.

We propose the following reforms, not as a specific blueprint, but as general guidelines for redefining the mission and priorities of the NCI:

1. The NCI must give cancer cause and prevention at least equal emphasis, in terms of budgetary and personnel resources, as its other programs including diagnosis, treatment and basic research; NCI's current annual budget is $1.8 billion. This major shift in direction

should be initiated immediately and completed within the next few years. This shift will also require careful monitoring and oversight to prevent misleading retention of old unrelated programs under new guises of cancer cause and prevention.

2. A high priority for the cancer prevention program should be a large-scale and ongoing national campaign to inform and educate the media and the public, besides Congress, the administration and the industry, that much cancer is avoidable and due to past exposures to chemical and physical carcinogens in air, water, food and the workplace, as well as to lifestyle factors, particularly smoking. It should, however, be noted that a wide range of occupational exposures and urban air pollution have been incriminated as causes of lung cancer, besides smoking. Accordingly, the educational campaign should stress the critical importance of identifying and preventing carcinogenic exposures and reducing them to the very lowest levels attainable within the earliest practically possible time.

3. The NCI should develop systematic programs for the qualitative and quantitative characterization of carcinogens in air, water, food and the workplace, with particular emphasis on those that are avoidable. Such information should be made available to the general public, and particularly to sub-populations at high risk, by an explicit and ongoing "right-to-know" educational campaign, such as the specific labelling of food and consumer products with the identity and levels of all carcinogenic contaminants. While taking a lead in this program, the NCI should work cooperatively with federal and state regulatory and health agencies and authorities, industry, public health and other professional societies, labor, and community-based citizen groups.

4. The NCI should cooperate with the National Institute of Environmental Health Sciences (NIEHS), and other NIH institutes, in investigating and publicizing other chronic toxic effects induced by carcinogens, including reproductive, neurological, hematological and immunological diseases, besides cancer.

5. The NCI should cooperate with the National Institute for Occupational Safety and Health, and other agencies to develop large-scale programs for monitoring, surveillance and warning of occupational, ethnic, and other sub-population groups at high risk of cancer due to known past exposures to chemical or physical carcinogens.

6. In close cooperation with key regulatory agencies and industry, the NCI should initiate large-scale research programs to develop noncarcinogenic products and processes as alternatives to those currently based on chemical and physical carcinogens. This program should also include research on the development of economic incentives for the reduction or phase-out of the use of industrial carcinogens, coupled with economic disincentives for their continued use, especially when appropriate noncarcinogenic alternatives are available.

7. The NCI should provide scientific expertise to Congress, federal and state regulatory and health agencies and authorities, and industry on the fundamental scientific principles of carcinogenesis including: the validity of extrapolation to humans of data from valid animal carcinogenicity tests; the invalidity of using insensitive or otherwise questionable epidemiological data to negate the significance of valid animal carcinogenicity tests; and the scientific invalidity of efforts to set safe levels or thresholds for exposure to chemical and physical carcinogens. The NCI should stress that the key to cancer prevention is reducing or avoiding exposure to carcinogens, rather than accepting and attempting to "manage" such risk. Current administration policies are, however, based on questionable mathematical procedures of quantitative risk assessment applied to exposures to individual carcinogens, while concomitant

exposures to other carcinogens in air, water, food and the workplace are ignored or discounted.

8. The NCI should provide Congress and regulatory agencies with scientific expertise necessary to the development of legislation and regulation of carcinogens. Illustrative of such need is the administration's revocation in 1988 of the 1958 Delaney amendment to the Federal Food Drug and Cosmetic Act, banning the deliberate addition to foods of any level of carcinogen. This critical law was revoked in spite of the overwhelming endorsement of its scientific validity by a succession of expert committees over the past three decades. Neither the NCI nor others in the cancer establishment provided any scientific evidence challenging the validity of this revocation, including its likely impact on future cancer rates.

9. The limited programs on routine carcinogenicity testing, now under the authority of the National Toxicology Program (NTP), should be expanded and expedited with the more active and direct involvement of the NCI. (On a cautionary note, it should be emphasized that this program, which is clearly the direct responsibility of the NCI, was transferred to the NTP in 1978 because of mismanagement and disinterest of the NCI.) Underutilized federal resources, particularly national laboratories, should be involved in carcinogenicity testing programs. The cost of carcinogenicity testing of profitable, and potentially profitable, chemicals should be borne by the industries concerned, and not by NTP and the NCI and ultimately the taxpayer.

10. The NCI should undertake large-scale intramural and extramural research programs to characterize known carcinogenic exposures, both industrial and lifestyle, in terms of their estimated impact on cancer, and the practical feasibility of their avoidability or elimination within defined early periods.

11. The NCI should substantially expand its intramural and extramural programs on epidemiology research and develop large-scale programs on sensitive human monitoring techniques, including genetic and quantitative analysis of body burdens of carcinogens, and focus them specifically on cancer cause and prevention. The NCI should also take a key role in the design, conduct and interpretation of epidemiologic investigations of cancer by federal and state regulatory and health agencies and authorities.

12. The NCI should develop large-scale training programs for young scientists in all areas relating to cancer cause and prevention.

13. Continued funding by the NCI of its comprehensive cancer centers should be made contingent on their developing strong community outreach programs in cancer cause and prevention, as opposed to their present and almost exclusive preoccupation with diagnosis and treatment. Centers should also establish tumor registries focused on identifying environmental and occupational carcinogens, and on the surveillance of occupational and other populations at high risk of cancer.

14. With Congressional oversight and with advice from the NIH Office of Scientific Integrity, the NCI should take early action to disclose information on any interlocking financial interests between its Panel, Advisory Board, advisory committees, and others in the cancer establishment, and major pharmaceutical companies involved in cancer drugs and therapy, and other industries. The NCI should also take the necessary precautions to prevent any such future conflicts.

15. The NCI should be enjoined from making or endorsing claims for new "cancer cures" unless these are clearly validated by data on reduced mortality rates and unless they conform to standard FDA regulations on claims for therapeutic efficacy.

16. The NCI should be removed from direct Presidential authority, and reintegrated

within NIH, and thus made directly responsive to the scientific community at large and the advice and consent of Congress. Currently, the President appoints the Director of the NCI, who reports directly to the President, the twenty-three member executive National Cancer Advisory Board (NCAB), and three member National Cancer Advisory Panel (NCAP) which controls the policies and priorities of NCI. The NCAP should be replaced by an executive committee recruited from advisory committees conforming to standard requirements of the Federal Advisory Committee Act for openness and balanced representation. Half of all appointees to NCI advisory committees should be recruited from scientists with credentials and record of active involvement in cancer cause and prevention. Appointments should also be granted to representatives of citizens', ethnic, and women's groups concerned with cancer prevention.

There is no conceivable likelihood that such reforms will be implemented without legislative action. The National Cancer Act should be amended explicitly to re-orient the mission and priorities of the NCI to cancer cause and prevention. Compliance of the NCI should then be assured by detailed and ongoing Congressional oversight and, most critically, by House and Senate Appropriation committees. However, only strong support by the independent scientific and public health communities, together with concerned grassroots citizen groups, will convince Congress and Presidential candidates of the critical and immediate need for such drastic action.

Samuel S. Epstein, M.D.
 Professor of Occupational
  and Environmental Medicine
 School of Public Health
 University of Illinois
 Chicago, Illinois

Eula Bingham, Ph.D.
 (Former Assistant Secretary of Labor and
  Former Director of OSHA)
 Professor of Environmental Health
 University of Cincinnati Medical Center
 Cincinnati, Ohio

David Rall, M.D., Ph.D.
 (Former Assistant Surgeon General
  and Former Director NIEHS)
 Washington, D.C.

Irwin D. Bross, Ph.D.
 (Former Director Biostatistics, Roswell
  Park Memorial Institute)
 President, Biomedical Metatechnology
 Buffalo, New York

This statement also was endorsed by the signatories listed below:

Jerrold L. Abraham, M.D.
 Dept. of Pathology
 College of Medicine
 State University of New York
 Syracuse, New York

Dean Abrahamson, M.D., Ph.D.
 Professor of Public Affairs
 University of Minnesota
 Minneapolis, Minnesota

Nicholas A. Ashford, Ph.D., J.D.
 Professor of Technology and Policy
 Massachusetts Institute of Technology
 Cambridge, Massachusetts

Dr. Louis S. Beliczky
 United Rubber, Cork, Linoleum and
  Plastic Workers of America
 Akron, Ohio

Rosalie Bertell, Ph.D.
 International Institute of Concern for
  Public Health
 Toronto, Canada

Elizabeth A. Bourque, Ph.D.
  Boston, Massachusetts

Bryan O. Budholz, Ph.D.
  Dept. of Work Environment
  University of Lowell
  Lowell, Massachusetts

Walter Burnstein, D.O.
  President, Food & Water, Inc.
  New York, New York

Leopoldo E. Caltagirone, Ph.D.
  Chairman, Div. of Biological Control
  University of California
  Berkeley, California

Barry Castleman, Ph.D.
  Environmental Consultant
  Baltimore, Maryland

Richard Clapp, Ph.D.
  Director, JSI Center for
    Environmental Studies
  Boston, Massachusetts

Shirley Conibear, M.D.
  Carnow, Conibear & Assoc.
  Chicago, Illinois

Paul Connett, Ph.D.
  Professor of Chemistry
  St. Lawrence University
  Canton, New York

Donald L. Dahlsten
  Division Biological Control
  University of California
  Berkeley, California

Susan Daum, M.D.
  Consultant in Occupational Medicine
  Mt. Sinai Medical Center
  New York, New York

Brian Dolan, M.D., M.P.H.
  Consultant in Preventive and
    Occupational Medicine
  Santa Monica, California

Ellen A. Eisen, M.D.
  Professor of Work Environment
  University of Lowell
  Lowell, Massachusetts

Michael Ellenbecker, Ph.D.
  Professor of Work Environment
  University of Lowell
  Lowell, Massachusetts

Arthur L. Frank, M.D., Ph.D.
  Dept. of Preventive Medicine
  University of Kentucky
  College of Medicine
  Lexington, Kentucky

Richard Garcia, Ph.D.
  Professor of Entomology
  University of California at Berkeley
  Berkeley, California

Michael R. Gray, M.D., M.P.H.
  Chief of Staff, Benson Hospital
  Benson, Arizona

Ruth Hubbard, Ph.D.
  Harvard University
  Cambridge, Massachusetts

David Kriebel, Sc.D.
  Professor of Work Environment
  University of Lowell
  Lowell, Massachusetts

Marc Lappe, Ph.D.
  Professor of Health Policy and Ethics
  University of Illinois
  College of Medicine
  Urbana, Illinois

Marvin S. Legator, Ph.D.
   Professor of Preventive Medicine
   University of Texas
   Galveston, Texas

Stephen U. Lester, M.S., M.P.H.
   Church, Virginia

Charles Levenstein
   Professor of Work Environment
   University of Lowell
   Lowell, Massachusetts

Edward Lichter, M.D.
   Professor of Preventive Medicine
   University of Illinois
   College of Medicine
   Urbana, Illinois

Thomas Mancuso, MD.
   Emeritus Professor of
      Occupational Medicine
   University of Pittsburgh
   Pittsburgh, Pennsylvania

Sheldon Margen, M.D.
   Professor of Public Health
   University of California at Berkeley
   Berkeley, California

Anthony Mazzocchi
   Oil, Chemical, and Atomic
      Workers Union
   Denver, Colorado

Myron A. Mehlman, M.D.
   R.W. Johnson Medical School
   Piscataway, NJ

Franklin E. Mirer, Ph.D.
   Health and Safety Department
   International United Auto Workers
   Detroit, Michigan

Rafael Moure, Ph.D.
   Professor of Work Environment
   University of Lowell
   Lowell, Massachusetts

Vicente Navarro, M.D.
   Professor of Health Policy and
      Management
   Johns Hopkins University
   Baltimore, Maryland

Herbert Needleman, M.D.
   Professor of Psychiatry and Pediatrics
   University of Pittsburgh
   Pittsburgh, Pennsylvania

B. Paigen, Ph.D.
   Consultant Toxicologist
   The Jackson Laboratories
   Bar Harbor, Maine

Richard Piccioni, Ph.D.
   Senior Staff Scientist, Food & Water, Inc.
   Seattle, Washington

Michael J. Plewa, Ph.D.
   Institute for Environmental Studies
   University of Illinois
   Urbana, Illinois

Laura Punnett, Sc. D.
   Professor of Work Environment
   University of Lowell
   Lowell, Massachusetts

Melvin Reuber, M.D.
   Consultant in Carcinogenesis and
      Toxicology
   Baltimore, Maryland

Knut Ringen, M.D.
   Laborer's Health and Safety Fund of
      North America
   Washington, D.C.

Anthony Robbins, M.D.
   (Former Director National Institute for
      Occupational Safety and Health)
   Professor of Public Health
   Boston University School of Medicine
   Boston, Massachusetts

Kenneth Rosenman, M.D.
  Professor of Medicine
  Michigan State University
  East Lansing, Michigan

Ruth Shearer, Ph.D.
  Consultant Toxicologist
  Issaquah, Washington

Janette D. Sherman, M.D.
  Consultant in Internal Medicine and
    Toxicology
  Alexandria, Virginia

Victor W. Sidel, M.D.
  Professor of Epidemiology and Social
    Medicine
  Montefiore Medical Center
  New York, New York

Joseph H. Skom, M.D.
  Professor of Clinical Medicine
  Northwestern University Medical School
  Chicago, Illinois

Noel Sommer, Ph.D.
  Professor of Environmental Science
  University of California
  Davis, California

Theodore D. Sterling, Ph.D.
  Professor, School of Computing Science
  Simon Fraser University
  Burnaby, Canada

Alice Stewart, M.D.
  President, Childhood Cancer Research
  Boston, Massachusetts

Joel Swartz, Ph.D.
  Consultant in Epidemiology
  Emeryville, California

David Teitelbaum, M.D.
  Professor of Preventive Medicine
  University of Colorado
  Denver, Colorado

Vijayalaxmi, Ph.D.
  Research Geneticist
  Research Triangle Park
  North Carolina

George Wald, Ph.D.
  Nobel Laureate
  Harvard University
  Cambridge, Massachusetts

Bailus Walker, Ph.D.
  (Past Commissioner of Health,
  Commonwealth of Massachusetts)

  Dean, College of Public Health
  University of Oklahoma
  Oklahoma City, Oklahoma

David H. Wegman, M.D.
  Professor of Work Environment
  University of Lowell
  Lowell, Massachusetts

Susan Woskie, Ph.D.
  Professor of Work Environment
  University of Lowell
  Lowell, Massachusetts

Arthur C. Zahalsky
  Professor of Immunology
  Southern Illinois University
  Edwardsville, Illinois

Grace Ziem, M.D., Dr. P.H.
  Consultant in Occupational Medicine
  Baltimore, Maryland

Emanuel Farber, M.D.
  Chairman, Department of Pathology
  University of Toronto
  Toronto, Canada

D.J.R. Sarma, M.D.
  Department of Pathology
  University of Toronto
  Toronto, Canada

Additional signatures received after February 3, 1992:

Arnold Schecter, M.D.
 Professor of Preventive Medicine
 SUNY Health Science Center
 State University of New York
 Syracuse, New York

Charles F. Wurster, Ph.D.
 Professor Environmental Toxicology
 Marine Sciences Research Center
 State University of New York
 Stony Brook, New York

The following exchange — three press releases: from the NCI, the American College of Radiology (ACR), and the author — together with the text of the experts' press conference, was subsequently published in The International Journal of Health Services.*

NCI Reaffirms Commitment to Prevention

NCI Press Release
February 4, 1992

Allegations that the nation is "losing the war on cancer" because of a lack of prevention research were characterized by spokesmen for the National Cancer Institute (NCI) today as old charges, lacking any basis in fact.

NCI officials also disputed the claim by Dr. Samuel Epstein, professor of Occupational and Environmental Medicine at the University of Illinois, and 60 other scientists, that little or no progress has been made in treating cancer, and backed the continuing use of mammography as the best available, early detection tool for breast cancer.

---

* *International Journal of Health Services.* 22(3):1992.

"The NCI's efforts in research in cancer biology, cancer causation, cancer treatment, and cancer prevention and control are well balanced and peer reviewed," said Dr. Richard Adamson, director of the Division of Cancer Etiology, in a prepared statement. Moreover, he added, the Institute is "able to shift research into appropriate programs as science dictates" in order to reduce suffering and death from cancer.

In the coming year, the NCI will spend approximately one-third of its total budget on causation and prevention-related research, including the study of environmental agents in the workplace that may contribute to cancer risk. Over the past two years, NCI has also instituted new guidelines for intensified outreach and prevention programs at the nation's 57 NCI-designated cancer centers. These NCI-supported centers are engaged in all aspects of cancer research from basic research to clinical applications as well as prevention and control.

As part of its prevention efforts, NCI supports numerous studies of the total environment contributing to cancer causation, Adamson said, including studies on viruses, natural and synthetic chemicals, dietary and nutritional factors, fibers, ultraviolet radiation, ionizing radiation, and other factors.

"Unquestionably, however, lifestyle factors contribute to the toll of human cancer," Adamson stressed, "and the single most identifiable causes of cancer — and other diseases — in the United States is tobacco smoking." Numerous independent scientific studies now link tobacco use, particularly cigarette smoking, to lung cancer, as well as cancers of the larynx, oral cavity, pharynx, and esophagus. Tobacco use also has been implicated as a contributing factor in bladder, kidney, and pancreatic cancers.

In a separate statement, Dr. Edward Sondik, deputy director of NCI's Division of Cancer Prevention and Control, criticized Epstein's release of mortality data from the Canadian National Breast Cancer Screening Study, which has not yet been completely analyzed. The data purportedly show that women aged 40 to 49 who have annual mammograms have a 52 percent increase in breast cancer mortality over women who have physical exams only. "The dissemination of this [information] without any scientific basis is unethical," he said.

Although NCI does not view mammography as the ultimate technology for detecting early breast cancer, Sondik said, mammography, coupled with physical exam, has the potential to reduce mortality from breast cancer by at least 30 percent in women over 50. In addition, while studies in younger women have not been conclusive, he said, the evidence to date is that breast cancer screening is prudent for women between the ages of 40 and 49.

ACR Refutes Epstein's Comments on Mammography

ACR Press Release
February 4, 1992

Dr. Samuel Epstein's comments on mammography, which have been published in several major newspapers nationwide, are a mixture of partial truths and outdated data, according to the American College of Radiology (ACR). The ACR, which is a national medical specialty association, added that Dr. Epstein's comments could unfortunately discourage women from having regular screening mammograms — the only tests proven to detect breast cancer at an early enough stage to reduce mortality.

The increase in the number of women who develop breast cancer is indeed alarming. Contrary to Dr. Epstein's suggestion that the increased incidence is a recent phenomenon, in fact the increase has been progressive over the past 50 years — long before the routine use of mammography. Extensive research is being done to determine the reasons for the in-

crease. The most recent jump in incidence is primarily an artifact due to breast cancers being detected years earlier through the use of mammography. This produces an apparent increase in incidence. Another reason is that women are living longer and the older a woman, the greater the chance she has of developing the disease.

Dr. Epstein comments that there is no clear evidence that mammography benefits premenopausal women. There are, in fact, studies which show the benefit of screening women under 50. These include the Breast Cancer Detection Demonstration Project conducted by the National Cancer Institute and the American Cancer Society, and the Health Insurance Plan of New York study.

Dr. Epstein also raises the question of radiation risk. Studies of women exposed to high doses of radiation such as those women who survived the atomic bomb blasts in Japan show, along with other studies, that women 35 and older are at no demonstrable risk from radiation exposure to the breast, a fact which particularly applies to the very low doses which are used in modern mammography.

The Canadian study Dr. Epstein mentions is, unfortunately, seriously flawed because mammographic techniques and equipment varied throughout the trial. Quality control measures were not undertaken until late in the study. The researchers themselves noted that the quality of mammography was "poor" to "unacceptable" in the early years of the trial. Moreover, there is evidence that Canadian women with palpable cancers (usually later stage cancers) were encouraged to enroll in the screening trial. Many of these women died from their disease, leading Dr. Epstein to come to the erroneous conclusion that the increase in cancers and deaths was due to mammography screening.

The American College of Radiology has a peer review program which evaluates staff, equipment, and quality control procedures. Mammography facilities which meet the program's stringent requirements are accredited. This program also reviews exposure dose to ensure that mammography is performed at the lowest and safest dose possible while maintaining a high-quality test.

Researchers are constantly looking for other ways of detecting early breast cancer. Dr. Epstein mentions magnetic resonance imaging (MRI) and lightscanning. MRI is expensive and requires that contrast material be injected into the patient. It is one to two years away from the development of a prototype to exclusively evaluate the breast. Lightscanning has been shown to have absolutely no efficacy for detecting early breast cancers.

Investigations are underway to determine possible methods for preventing breast cancer. Numerous researchers are trying to determine its elusive causes. Until its causes are discovered or preventative measures devised, mammography screening provides the safest and best opportunity for detecting breast cancer at a stage at which curative treatment is possible.

Screening by mammography beginning at age 40 is widely accepted. It is recommended by the following organizations:

American Academy of Family Physicians

American Association of Women Radiologists

American Cancer Society

American College of Radiology

American Medical Association

American Osteopathic College of Radiology

American Society of Internal Medicine

American Society of Clinical Oncology

American Society for Therapeutic Radiology and Oncology

College of American Pathologists

National Cancer Institute

National Medical Association

Cancer Establishment Continues to Mislead Public

Press Release
By Samuel S. Epstein, M.D.
February 7, 1992

At a news conference Tuesday, February 4, a group of 60-plus prominent scientists and physicians released a statement condemning the National Cancer Institute (NCI) for ignoring or trivializing evidence of how carcinogens in air, food, water, and workplaces are major factors in the cancer epidemic in America. In addition, Dr. Samuel Epstein, professor at the University of Illinois School of Public Health presented data indicating significant cancer risks in mammograms and their lack of effectiveness for premenopausal women.

The NCI and the American College of Radiology (ACR) responded to these charges in separate statements. The following are Dr. Epstein's rebuttals, which show both groups selectively use scientific data to mislead the public about both the hazards of industrial carcinogens in our environment and of mammograms for younger women:

ACR Statement Reflects Ignorance, Self-Interest

Contrary to the ACR, the increase in breast cancer incidence since the 1970s has been steeper than in previous decades. Furthermore, these increases exclude effects of aging as they have been age-adjusted.

Also contrary to the ACR, a wide range of studies have failed to demonstrate any benefit from routine mammography in premenopausal women (as opposed to benefits in older women). These include the 1963 Health Insurance Plan of New York, and the 1975 Dutch and 1977 Swedish studies (Skrabanek, 1985; Bailar, 1988). The 1973-81 Breast Cancer Detection Demonstration Project studies, on which the ACR ineptly relies for alleged evidence of benefit, were "not designed for research purposes, were not carried out in accordance with rigorous research standards, and lack even an appropriate control group" (Bailar, 1988; also Eddy *et al.*, 1988).

The high cancer risk from mammography was well known before the National Cancer Institute and American Cancer Society, with active involvement of the ACR, initiated their large-scale routine screening of premenopausal women in the 1970s. The Biological Effects of Ionizing Radiation committee of the National Academy of Sciences, the world's leading authority on radiation, warned in 1972 of a "relative risk of about 0.8 percent increase in the spontaneous rate (of breast cancer) per rad" exposure. Thus, routine annual mammography over 10 years of premenopausal women with two rads per exposure (although much higher exposures were then commonplace) would lead to approximately a 20 percent increased cancer risk. Women were never warned of these risks while being falsely assured of benefits. Risks of routine mammography in premenopausal women still persist today, though at lower levels, at the best centers using designated equipment with lower exposures. However, women are still not warned of these risks or of the absence of any benefits (page 534).

The ACR has misrepresented the recent Canadian study which confirms mammography risks. This study reported a 52 percent increase in breast cancer mortality in young women given annual mammograms as opposed to unscreened controls. A 1991 editorial in *The Lancet* concluded that these findings could not be discounted by the criticisms on randomization and quality of mammography which ACR has resurrected. The editorial further pointed out that the Canadian findings are supported by similar results in several previous studies. *The Lancet* finally concluded that "there is no evidence to support introduction of service mammography for women under 50." It should be noted that this warning is endorsed by the American College of Physicians

and the Canadian Breast Cancer Task Force.

Finally, ACR seems unaware of evidence that transillumination with infrared light scanning is a safe and highly promising alternative to mammography.

Considerations of malpractice aside, the recalcitrance of the ACR reinforces a growing grass roots conviction that cancer is too important to be left to self-interested professionals.

NCI Release Reaffirms Its Denial that We're Losing the War on Cancer

As detailed in a statement by 60-plus distinguished national scientists at a Washington D.C. news conference on February 4: cancer rates are escalating; our ability to treat and cure cancer, apart from childhood and other rare cancers, has not improved for decades; and our environment, air, water, food and workplace have become permeated with industrial carcinogens.

Meanwhile, the NCI and the American Cancer Society (ACS) have trivialized the evidence for increasing cancer rates and their relation to avoidable exposure to industrial carcinogens. Instead, together with the chemical industry, they focus on dietary fat itself (ignoring its carcinogenic contaminants including pesticides), and smoking (ignoring increasing lung cancer rates in nonsmokers, and the important role of occupational exposures and urban air pollution) as the predominant causes of the cancer epidemic.

Furthermore, the NCI and ACS, with their fixations on diagnosis, treatment and basic research, are indifferent to cancer cause and prevention, which accounts for only five percent of the NCI $2 billion budget (see budget line item of $90 million for Cancer Prevention and Control), and not 33 percent as the NCI alleges. The position of the NCI and ACS on prevention is further illustrated by their recent silence while the administration rolls back regulations designed to reduce avoidable exposure to industrial carcinogens, including the 1958 Delaney law banning the deliberate addition of any level of carcinogens to food; overwhelming evidence supports the scientific validity of this law.

The NCI and ACS position on prevention is compounded by their exaggerated claims on ability to treat and cure cancer. As detailed by authorities including the General Accounting Office (1987), these claims reflect gross statistical manipulation, including the use of "relative survival" rather than mortality rates.

The statement by the 60-plus scientists calls for urgent reforms in federal cancer policies. These reforms must ensure that the NCI gives greater emphasis to cancer prevention, rather than to chasing the elusive but ever-promised cure for cancer, coupled with continuing oversight to ensure compliance. These reforms demand drastic legislative action and strong grassroots support.

The Debate Continues

Subsequent to the February 4 press conference, The Washington Post *printed a favorable report of the event by its medical correspondent, Dr. David Brown. In spite of this, the* Post *also, a few days later, published a letter from the American Cancer Society and the* Post's *own editorial, attacking the contents of the conference statement, and also vilifying the author personally. Many of the* Post's *so-called "facts" were incorrect, and the newspaper's ad hominem argument was unjustifiable. The three pieces are printed below, as is the author's response.*

Cancer Research Groups' Efforts Called Misdirected

Article by David Brown, M.D.
From *The Washington Post*
February 5, 1992

Two major institutions responsible for cancer research in the United States have paid little attention to environmental hazards, ex-

aggerated gains in cancer diagnosis and treatment, and in some cases endorsed controversial medical practices, a group of 64 physicians and scientists said yesterday.

In a wide-ranging indictment, the group called on the National Cancer Institute (NCI) and the American Cancer Society to redirect their attention to research and education on preventable causes of cancer in the home and workplace.

The cancer establishment has grossly confused and misled the public into thinking we are winning the war on cancer. "Nothing could be further from the truth," said group spokesman Samuel Epstein, a pathologist and toxicologist at the University of Illinois in Chicago.

"The cancer establishment is fixated on diagnosis and treatment, to the neglect of cause and prevention," and "has trivialized the risk of environmental causes," Epstein said at a news conference yesterday sponsored by Food & Water Inc., a nonprofit activist organization whose main campaign until now has been against irradiated food.

Among the allegations made yesterday by the group, which included occupational medicine and environmental health specialists from around the nation:

• Cancer researchers have under-emphasized the importance of pesticide and hormone residues in food and water, and have promoted the concept of "acceptable" levels of such chemicals. "The NCI," Epstein said, "should stress that the key to cancer prevention is reducing or avoiding exposure to carcinogens rather than accepting and attempting to 'manage' such risk."

• "NCI should be removed from direct presidential authority and re-integrated" into the National Institutes of Health, Epstein said. It would thus be made "directly responsive to the scientific community at large and to the advice and consent of Congress." At present, the president appoints the director of NCI — a legacy of President Nixon's 1971 "War on Cancer."

• Many physicians have promoted X-ray mammography to detect early breast cancer, even though some studies suggest the test may increase the risk of breast cancer.

NCI strongly contradicted Epstein's allegations, saying, among other things, that the research on environmental causes of cancer accounts for $270 million of nearly $600 million in the "causation, prevention and control" portion of its current budget.

John Laszlo, a medical oncologist and vice president of the American Cancer Society, said "there is a degree of paranoia to all of this. There is a claim that an establishment is conspiring to stifle promising leads for cancer prevention. . . . These charges are totally unfounded."

Cancer Cause and Prevention

Letter by Walter Lawrence, Jr., M.D.
President of the American Cancer Society
From *The Washington Post*
February 12, 1992

The American Cancer Society is greatly concerned about allegations of environmental medicine professor Samuel Epstein that the efforts of the society and the National Cancer Institute should be redirected away from research and education efforts we believe are designed to track down the best leads in cancer prevention, early detection and treatment.

Dr. Epstein insisted [news story, Feb. 5] that we are "losing the war on cancer," because we lack his singular focus on the possible effects of environmental pollution on cancer incidence. He further insisted that the American Cancer Society and the National Cancer Institute are "fixated on cancer diagnosis and treatment," while "trivializing the risk of environmental causes." Both asser-

tions are absurd.

Part of the mission of the American Cancer Society is to promote research and education that saves lives and diminishes suffering from cancer. A case in point is the emergence of mammography as our most important weapon in the fight against breast cancer. Dr. Epstein loosely referred to studies he said indicate that mammography may harm patients. He discussed screening procedures from the 1970s, when a radiation dose many times higher than is used today was used, which concerned some researchers. He further referred to a more recent study that he said indicates mammography might cause harm to premenopausal women even though scientists call the unpublished and incomplete study inconclusive and insist that it is unethical and invalid to disseminate such information.

The benefits of mammography in both pre- and postmenopausal women have been borne out in long-term studies. Even with the older technology of the '60s and '70s mammography has been shown to reduce breast cancer mortality in a substantial way.

As to the area of cancer prevention, the American Cancer Society has devoted huge amounts of its resources to research and programs on the carcinogenicity of substances.

On the other hand, despite points to the contrary by Dr. Epstein, there is no question that certain lifestyle factors are important to cancer cause and prevention. We know, for example, that the use of tobacco is responsible for 30 percent of all cancer deaths. Should we not pursue these productive leads?

Progress in the war on cancer has been significant but uneven. Most childhood cancers were universally fatal just a few decades ago. Now we're able to cure these children most of the time. Other cancers, such as that of the lung, continue to rise, but for a reason we know — smoking. The death rates from cancer of the bladder, ovary, stomach, lymphoma, cervix and others are falling. We believe death rates will also soon fall for breast cancer because of earlier diagnosis (mammography) and better treatment. Localized breast cancer is curable in more than 90 percent of those affected. Still, progress in other forms of cancer continues to elude us, and scientific research goes on.

The Cancer War and Its Critics

Editorial
From *The Washington Post*
February 16, 1992

One of the continuing intramural conflicts in the government's "war on cancer" made an appearance last week when Samuel Epstein, a professor of environmental medicine from the University of Illinois, held a press conference to denounce the priorities of what he calls the "cancer establishment." Dr. Epstein, a longtime gadfly, accuses the major research groups and their funders of being "fixated on diagnosis and treatment" to the disadvantage of "preventive" research on environmental causes, like toxins. It's an argument based partly on a false distinction — obviously, "basic" research figuring out the mechanism by which cancer is triggered in an individual would mean great strides for both cure and prevention. The argument is fueled by the frustration of people watching the rates of many cancers actually go up. Breast cancer, the main example and the most mysterious, has risen 57 percent since 1950, and lung, pancreas, and some kidney cancers are also higher. Nobody knows why.

Scientists from both the National Cancer Institute, which the federal government funds, and the private American Cancer Society sharply dispute Dr. Epstein's charges. Many call him a menace. They say that his demands for "preventive" research go at the matter backward — you can't work on "preventive" for a disease whose causes you don't know — and that he assumes a relationship with environmental toxins that they have in fact been unable to find. An added complicating

factor is that tracing something like contaminants in body fat is a lot more difficult than looking at airborne factors, and a fistful of studies can be waved for almost every conceivable link. These same cancer groups have been a major force in raising public awareness of the environmental factors that *have* been shown to be cancer-related — cigarettes, asbestos, and radon.

The "establishment" Dr. Epstein attacks is, of course, responsible for myriad advances over two decades, not only in cancer research but in spin-off discoveries in genetics, immunology and the mechanism of other diseases — including current AIDS research. At least some of the apparent rise in incidence (how much is in dispute) is due to the improved detection methods they have developed. Dr. Epstein goes further than mere scientific criticism in some cases, alleging collusion with drug companies and hospital boards. On the level of purely scientific disagreement, it's not such a bad thing for scientific bureaucracies to field criticism, whether it likes the source or not. But given these organizations' proven record of advances, it seems ridiculous to accuse them of conspiracy or bad faith.

The Cancer Establishment

Opinion Piece by Samuel S. Epstein, M.D.
From *The Washington Post*
March 10, 1992

"The Cancer War and Its Critics" (editorial, Feb. 16) is a welcome expression of the overdue debate on federal cancer policies. However, the editorial misattributes criticisms of the cancer establishment, the National Cancer Institute (NCI) and American Cancer Society (ACS), exclusively to me — as well as seriously misrepresenting such criticisms.

These criticisms were based on a statement released on Feb. 4 by 65 prominent authorities in cancer research, public health and preventive medicine, including former senior government scientists.

We expressed grave concerns about the failure of the war against cancer, evidenced over the past four decades by escalating cancer rates (now striking one in three and killing one in four), paralleled by absence of significant improvement in treatment except for relatively uncommon cancers. We expressed further concern that the lavishly funded establishment has "misled and confused the public and Congress by repeated claims that we are winning the war on cancer."

As recently as 1986, the NCI promised annual cancer mortality rates would be halved by the year 2000. The establishment now belatedly admits that cancer rates are increasing sharply. However, with the enthusiastic support of the chemical industry, these are ascribed exclusively to smoking, dietary fat itself (ignoring the tenuous evidence relating this to colon, breast and other cancers) and "mysterious" causes. Meanwhile, it discounts substantial evidence incriminating a wide range of chemical and radioactive carcinogens permeating the environment, air, water, food, and the workplace. Examples include occupational carcinogens causing lung cancer in nonsmoking workers; parental exposure to occupational carcinogens (implicated in more than 20 studies as causes of cancer, which increased by 28 percent between 1950 and 1987) and carcinogenic pesticides in food, which are estimated to cause tens of thousands of excess cancers annually.

Non-mysterious causes of breast cancer, which the establishment ignores, let alone investigates, include carcinogenic contaminants in dietary fat, particularly pesticides; PCBs; and estrogen (with extensive and unregulated use as growth promoting animal feed additives).

Mammography, claimed as a diagnostic triumph, is an important and ominous cause. The high sensitivity of the breast, especially in younger women, to radiation-induced cancer was known by 1970. Nevertheless, the estab-

lishment then screened some 300,000 women with X-ray dosages so high as to increase breast cancer risk by up to 20 percent in women aged 40 to 50 who were mammogramed annually. Women were given no warning whatever. How many subsequently developed breast cancer remains uninvestigated.

Mammography risks persist with lower X-ray doses at modern centers. This is evidenced by excess breast cancer mortality in younger women noted in a Canadian study, besides four other published studies, reported in a June 1991 editorial of *The Lancet*. Strangely, the NCI and ACS castigate my reference to this public information as "unethical and invalid." Moreover, there is no known benefit from screening of younger, as opposed to postmenopausal, women — a warning endorsed by the American College of Physicians and Canadian Breast Cancer Task Force. Additionally, the establishment ignores safe and effective alternatives to mammography, particularly transillumination with infrared scanning.

While explaining away soaring cancer rates, the establishment, abetted by cheerleading science journalists, grossly exaggerates treatment successes. Periodic announcements of dramatic advances are based on initial reduction in tumor size rather than on prolonged survival. For most cancers, survival has not changed for decades. Contrary claims are based on rubber numbers.

Furthermore, the establishment is financially interlocked with giant pharmaceutical companies (grossing $1 billion annually in cancer drug sales), with inherent conflicts of interest.

The establishment devotes minimal resources to research and education on cancer cause and prevention — only 5 percent of the $1.9 billion NCI budget. Furthermore, the establishment provides no scientific support for legislation and regulation to reduce avoidable exposures to industrial carcinogens.

As emphasized by critics of the cancer establishment, drastic reforms are needed.

The "700-to-1 Debate"

Subsequent to the February 4 press conference,[1,2,3] the cancer establishment — the NCI and ACS — responded with a media campaign of personal attack akin to scientific McCarthyism. Furthermore, the NCI and ACS misrepresented the February 4 statement as exclusively the author's,[4,5] rather than that of a group of over 60 leading national experts in cancer prevention and public health. Reacting to the author's responses[6] and the ensuing adverse publicity and congressional concerns, the NCI invited the author to present an "Evaluation of the National Cancer Program" at the 82nd National Cancer Advisory Board Meeting, on May 5, 1992. Present at the meeting, chaired by Dr. Paul Calabresi, were the members of the President's Cancer Board and the entire NCI scientific and administrative staff. This meeting became known as the "700-to-1 Debate."

Articles on the author's presentation and the discussion which followed were published in The Lancet, Science and Government Report, Environmental Health Letter, The Blue Sheet, *and* The Cancer Letter. *Perhaps the most succinct summaries were those from* The Lancet *and* The Cancer Letter. *Both are reprinted below.*

Washington Perspective: The Two-by-Four Factor in Cancer Politics

By Daniel S. Greenberg
From *The Lancet**
May 30, 1992

"The first time we got your attention is when you were, with due respect, hit over

* *The Lancet.* 339:1343-1344, 1992. © by The Lancet Ltd.

the head by a two-by-four," said Prof. Samuel Epstein, resolute antagonist of the reigning priorities in the disheartening war on cancer. His audience, the high command of the Government's $2-billion-a-year cancer research program, listened intently, as though confronted by an apparition.

Epstein, professor of occupational and environmental medicine at the University of Illinois School of Public Health, scoffs at the search for cures and pleads for a commitment to prevention. Long ignored by the cancer establishment as a bothersome crank and tunnel-visioned zealot, Epstein charges that he has been a target of its "vilification." He feels he has been classed with the charlatans and eccentrics who deprecate orthodox science and medicine. But there he was, after being disregarded for two decades by the managers and strategists of the National Cancer Institute, delivering an invited address on May 5 before NCI's elite, senior body of counselors, the 17-member National Cancer Advisory Board. In attendance, too, were the senior executives of NCI and the three-member President's Cancer Panel, created in that long-ago declaration of war to link NCI directly to the White House.

At times, the session turned into a rhetorical duel, with Epstein and several of his listeners exchanging accusations of "scientific McCarthyism." Nonetheless, after Epstein spoke, the NCI Director Dr. Samuel Broder asked the audience, "Can we learn from this dialog?" "I think the answer is yes," he said, adding that the issues of environmental carcinogenesis and prevention "are important enough, and they are complicated enough, that they will require full attention on a scientific and scholarly basis."

A week later, NCI sent a letter of thanks and commentary to Epstein, including an assurance that "We are very committed to the principle that a scholarly discussion informed by facts is the only way to address important issues." Moreover, said the letter, from NCI's Deputy Director, Dr. Daniel Ihde, "the National Cancer Institute must always stand ready to hear divergent views and will become a better agency by having its ideas tested and probed through a process of constructive criticism and disputation."

How could it be otherwise, the naive might wonder. But, in fact, Epstein's invitation to address the board was preceded by a splashy public-relations gambit in which he and an assemblage of allies came to Washington, expressed scorn about the cancer program, and reaped a good deal of press notice. In the high councils of this intensely politicized disease, that's the equivalent of a two-by-four timber over the head.

The build-up to Epstein's NCI address occurred on Feb. 4 at a well-advertised and well-attended Washington press conference built around a paper, "Losing the 'War Against Cancer;' A Need for Public Policy Reforms," published in the *International Journal of Health Services* (vol. 22, no. 3, 1992). The co-authors were Epstein; David Rall, retired director of the National Institute of Environmental Health Sciences, a sister institute of NCI; Eula Bingham, professor of environmental health, University of Cincinnati, a former director of the federal Occupational Safety and Health Administration; and Irwin Bross, former director of biostatistics, Roswell Park Memorial Institute. Some 65 researchers, physicians, and others involved in cancer research and treatment endorsed the paper.

The gist of the paper, presented by Epstein, was that cancer is on the rise, despite victory claims by NCI and the American Cancer Society; that the "cancer establishment" focuses on the tobacco menace, serious as it is, to the neglect of "avoidable carcinogens" in air, water, food, and the workplace; that NCI's alarms against dietary fat are scientifically baseless and a diversion from avoidable carcinogens that accumulate in fat; and finally, that NCI neglects preventive research in favor of a futile quest for

cures. The allegations received wide attention in the press, and shortly afterwards, at the suggestion of NCI Director Broder, Epstein was invited to address the next session of the Advisory Board.

Meeting with the Board on the NIH campus, Epstein essentially put on a rerun of his press conference statement, but with the addition of ideological accusations — namely, that the cancer program is under the sinister influence of industrial polluters and pharmaceutical firms that, in tandem, he contended, steer policy and priorities toward cures rather than prevention. The late Armand Hammer, the oil tycoon who chaired the President's Cancer Panel during the Reagan administration, was "one of the nation's leading polluters with carcinogenic chemicals," Epstein said. Hammer's predecessor in that post, Benno Schmidt, a New York financier and philanthropist, was assailed for "deep and close ties with drug companies." And, turning to one of the nation's premier cancer centers, Memorial Sloan-Kettering, in New York, Epstein charged that its board members and its endowment are heavily invested in cancer-causing industries.

These influences, he continued, have skewed NCI's policies, so that a mere $19 million of its $2 billion budget is assigned to research on occupational sources of cancer. Scoffing at NCI's insistence that $335 million is currently devoted to all forms of research on primary prevention of cancer, Epstein denounced the claim as a "shell game," asserting that the overall prevention budget is "well under $100 million."

In his finale, Epstein veered to another issue, declaring: "I see no reason why scientific McCarthyism should be the response to well-based concerns, which I can assure you, ladies and gentlemen, are reaching a significant level in the general population."

While Director Broder was conciliatory in his remarks, two senior NCI executives responsible for the program criticized by Epstein fired back at him. Dr. Richard Adamson, director of the cancer etiology division, credited NCI with "a comprehensive and balanced program of experimental, epidemiologic, clinical, and prevention research that gives us credibility and capability at both a national and international level." He accused Epstein of disregarding what he described as substantial research activities focused on environmental carcinogens. Dr. Peter Greenwald, director of the Cancer Prevention and Control Division, said that all cancer research is under budget pressure but that prevention is not disproportionately affected.

Several board members then had a go at Epstein. "I think the tone of some of these comments is highly adversarial," said Dr. Frederick M. Becker, Vice President for Research at the Tumor Institute, M.D. Anderson Cancer Center, Houston. Becker added, "I agree with you 100 percent that we should not, and I will use your term, recede to scientific McCarthyism. But I think you come perilously close to it yourself," Becker said, as several other board members indicated agreement. Epstein responded: "I have never attacked a person or any individual in the NCI in any statement that I have made. The *ad hominem* attacks have come from NCI, being called a menace, being called a gadfly, being called unethical. That is what I call scientific McCarthyism, and you are repeating that now by suggesting that the attacks come from me." The meeting, prolonged 40 minutes beyond the one hour originally scheduled, then ended.

What is the meaning of this extraordinary confrontation? Does it signal a serious rethinking of cancer-research strategy? Was it merely a sop to a pesky critic? Will NCI Director Broder, in office since December, 1988, reorient resources in the direction that Epstein advocates? The answer may be known by the leaders of NCI, but elsewhere there's only speculation. To be noted, however, is a potent factor in the affairs of NCI

and all of the National Institutes of Health — an acute sensitivity to public and Congressional pressure. That was the origin of the ill-conceived war on cancer, and, with skillful manipulation, it could again become a force in this tumultuous branch of biomedical politics.

Epstein Alleges Conflict Of Interest Of Former Panel Chairmen And Sloan-Kettering Directors

From *The Cancer Letter*
May 15, 1992

Invited to the inner sanctum of what he calls "the cancer establishment," Samuel Epstein intensified his offensive by alleging conflict of interest on the part of two former chairmen of the President's Cancer Panel speaking before the National Cancer Advisory Board last week, Epstein said Benno Schmidt, the first Panel chairman, "has deep and close personal ties with drug industries." The late Armand Hammer, Epstein said, "was chairman of Occidental Petroleum, one of the nation's leading producers of carcinogenic chemicals."

Further, Epstein said, the Board of Overseers of one of the nation's leading cancer centers, Memorial Sloan-Kettering, is dominated by representatives of the pharmaceutical and chemical industries. MSK directors also serve as directors of drug, oil, steel, automotive, and other companies and the center owns stock in several drug companies, Epstein said.

This is an important concept because the Sloan-Kettering clearly represents a very substantial segment of the scientific community which constitutes a powerful national lobbying and pressure group," Epstein said. "The Memorial Sloan-Kettering is an excellent example of how the major decision making body in the prototype national cancer center is dominated by industrial and drug company interests.

Schmidt, who chaired the committee whose recommendations led to the National Cancer Act of 1971, was traveling and unavailable for comment early this week.

"We will decline the opportunity to comment," a spokesman for Memorial Sloan-Kettering told *The Cancer Letter*.

A Two-By-Four

"For the last 20 years, I have been attempting, and others have been attempting, to influence NCI more and more in the direction of primary cancer prevention," said Epstein at the May 5 presentation. "The first time we got your attention was when you were hit over the head with a two-by-four. And I'm delighted we have your attention now."

The proverbial piece of lumber Epstein was referring to was the publicity he received as a result of a Feb. 4 press conference in Washington, paid for by Food & Water Inc., an environmental group that has received funding from a tobacco family foundation. The publicity figured heavily into the decision to invite Epstein to the NCAB, NCI sources said.

Epstein, professor of occupational and environmental medicine at Illinois Univ., repeated the arguments he made in a statement signed by more than 60 supporters: NCI has misled the public and Congress by overstating gains in treatment of cancer while ignoring the role of industrial carcinogens. The statement was inserted in the April 2 "Congressional Record" by Rep. John Conyers (D-MI), chairman of the House Government Operations Committee.

"Let me assure you that we welcome criticism and any discussion on a high scientific plane." NCAB Chairman Paul Calabresi said to Epstein.

Basic Research Not Relevant?

Much of Epstein's presentation echoed the claims he made at the February press conference and in newspaper opinion pieces (*The Cancer Letter*, Feb. 14 and May 1). New allegations included:

• Basic research, particularly molecular biology, is not relevant to cancer "in general." Epstein quoted a remark attributed to David Baltimore to that effect, and called research on mechanisms "a game."

• Cancer survival rates are "near static" and treatment results are based mainly on tumor response, Epstein quoted, among others, NCI Div. of Cancer Treatment Director Bruce Chabner.

• Epstein said NCI's estimates on lifestyle risk factors are based on an "obsolete analysis" by Richard Doll and Richard Peto. NCI calculates that 35% of cancer is related to diet, 30% tobacco, 7% reproductive/sexual behavior, 4% occupational, 3% alcohol, 3% geophysical factors, 2% pollution, 1% industrial products, and 1% medicine and medical procedures.

• NCI's definition of primary cancer prevention is too broad. "Chemoprevention is important but irrelevant to primary prevention," Epstein said.

• NCI's response to his criticism amounted to "scientific McCarthyism," he said.

He recommended that NCI conduct a national campaign to inform the public "that much cancer is avoidable and due to past exposures to chemical and physical carcinogens" and "provide scientific expertise to Congress on primary cancer prevention."

In particular, Epstein said, NCI should tell Congress about, "the validity of extrapolation to humans of data from valid animal carcinogenicity tests; the invalidity of using insensitive or otherwise questionable epidemiological data to negate the significance of validity of efforts to set safe levels or thresholds for exposure to chemical and physical carcinogens. NCI should stress that the key to cancer prevention is reducing or avoiding exposure to carcinogens, rather than accepting and attempting to manage such risk."

Further, Epstein called for the expansion of the NCI program for occupational and environmental cancer studies.

"Do You Have Any Data?"

"I think the bottom line is, are we a perfect institute? No. Do we try to do what is right? I think we do. Can we learn from dialogue? I think the answer is yes," NCI Director Samuel Broder said.

"There are important issues related to environmental carcinogenesis and prevention, and they are important enough, and they are complicated enough that they will require our full-time attention on a scholarly basis," Broder said. "I would hope that one need not invoke on either side of the debate some additional nonscientific agenda or some issue related to motivation or conflicts."

President's Cancer Panel member Geza Jako, who has been critical of NCI in the past, asked Epstein about the NCI estimate of 4% incidence of occupational cancers: "Do you have any scientific data that would show that it is greatly different than 4%?"

"There is no evidence whatsoever to support this 4%," Epstein said. "These estimates of Doll and Peto are based on data from 1933 to 1977, times at which occupational exposures were very low. Doll, Peto and (former NCI staff member Marvin) Schneiderman, who examined these issues in great detail, have agreed that the estimates would account for up to 20-40%, as opposed to 4%."

The latter statement was resourceful. Doll and Peto, in a 1981 paper published in the *Journal of the National Cancer Institute* and later published as a book, *The Causes of Cancer*, disparaged the 20-40% estimate as politically motivated and the method used to reach it "defective." However, as Epstein said, Doll and Peto agreed that the (erroneous) method would account for the (erroneous) estimate.

Schneiderman was a contributor to the

1978 paper that proposed the 20-40% estimate of occupational cancer incidence, along with former NIEHS director David Rail, who some consider the key force behind the estimate. The paper listed 10 "contributors," but no one has been publicly identified as the author, and the paper was never published in a scientific journal. It was filed by the Occupational Safety & Health Administration in a post-hearing record, and became known as "the OSHA paper."

HEW Secretary Joseph Califano first used the estimate in a speech to the AFL-CIO.

Over the next few years, Epstein and others used it to pressure for funding for occupational studies, while other scientists criticized NCI for producing an inaccurate estimate. NCI was in a difficult position unable to issue a correction for an unpublished study.

The Congressional Office of Technology Assessment commissioned Doll and Peto to analyze the estimate. They wrote:

"It seems likely that whoever wrote the OSHA paper did so for political rather than scientific purposes, and it will undoubtedly continue in the future as in the past to be used for political purposes by those who wish to emphasize the importance occupational factors. . . . we would suggest that the OSHA paper should not lie regarded as a serious contribution to scientific thought and should not be cited or used as if it were. (Furthermore, any suggestions which derive directly or indirectly from it that 20, 23, 38 or 40% of cancer deaths are, or will be, due to occupational factors should be dismissed.)"

"Ad Hominem Attacks from NCI"

In his response to Jako's question, Epstein also said a New York group studied occupational cancer deaths in that state and made "a conservative estimate of minimally 10 percent of cancer deaths in New York are occupational."

"My question, which you didn't answer, was whether your institution has any scientific data or statistics that would greatly change this estimate," Jako said. "This is what Dr. Broder was referring to — let's leave this discussion on a scientific basis."

"I think the terminology you use is highly controversial and adversarial," NCAB member Fred Becker told Epstein. "I don't know if those were the terms used in that [New York] article. What would have been given in an accurate scientific article was the actual percentage estimated and then the statistical variation."

"I agree with you 100% that we should not recede to scientific McCarthyism," Becker said. "But I think you come perilously close to it yourself. You referred repeatedly to the 'cancer establishment' as if there were some vast conspiracy — and perhaps you feel there is — of the hundreds and thousands of people who work tirelessly. . . . I know many of the workers at Sloan-Kettering are dedicated scientists and not driven by what the board thinks.

"I think we would do better not to use a term that was last popularized by the defenders of laetrile when they talked about the 'cancer establishment,'" Becker continued. "If we go to Congress, let's plead for more money to be given equally to all of the disciplines, because I assure you those of us who work in cancer institutes could not ignore the people who are suffering from cancer today. So I plead with you to join in with what Sam [Broder] said, avoid these terms and these suggestions of accusation and really keep this on the basis where, by providing the data, you can identify the proper target. And we would certainly support you on that basis."

"Dr. Becker, this approach was a carefully considered document based on the input of 65 scientists who have been frustrated over the last two decades," Epstein said. "The ad hominem attacks have come from NCI — being called a menace, being called a gadfly, being called unethical, that's what I call scientific McCarthyism."

In Defense of Treatment, Chemoprevention

"I agree there are different approaches to prevention," Board member Sydney Salmon told Epstein, "but I think you've lost sight of the fact that the mission of the National Cancer Institute is to overcome cancer as a problem and do it as quickly and effectively as we can, whether it be with treatment, or with prevention. And if it's prevention, whether primary or secondary, if we can prevent it, treat and cure it, those are the goals."

Salmon said the Breast Cancer Prevention Trial, the largest chemoprevention trial to date, "may make a major reduction in breast cancer incidence, and that could give a far quicker result than the longer term approaches to primary prevention."

In addition, Salmon said he objected to Epstein's statement that treatment results are based on tumor shrinkage: "I have to point out that the Food and Drug Administration does not approve anticancer drugs on the basis of tumor shrinkage. Complete remission, disappearance of all evidence of cancer, is accepted as an intermediate marker for improved survival."

Epstein replied: "As far as treatment is concerned, I simply quoted from the General Accounting Office, from Rifkin, from Chabner, saying we haven't achieved any significant advance in our to ability to treat and cure cancer with the exception of childhood cancers. That's all there is to it."

"You've misquoted me!" Chabner interrupted. "You've used my name twice!"

"Hold on a second. I have a direct quote from you which I put on a slide," Epstein went on.

The Chabner quote on the slide read: "In patients with disseminated forms of the common epithelial tumors, both complete remissions and cures continue to elude us."

(NAGAM, 1992)

"Yes, one sentence out of a whole article. You neglected the rest of it," Chabner said.

"As far as the tamoxifen study, the fact is this, tamoxifen is a potent carcinogen," Epstein continued. "Whether or not one should give tamoxifen to a significant number of women without warning is a matter which I haven't discussed now."

"You, Sir, are Unfamiliar with the Literature"

After the presentation Epstein faced a small group that gathered around the lectern.

"I cannot believe that basic research and basic researchers are playing a game and that the advances that have been made as part of that game will not be of significance," said Becker to Epstein.

Epstein: I've probably done as much basic research in cancer as you or many other people in this room. I believe in basic research. I believe, however, that the overwhelming budget on basic research, particularly oncogenes and molecular biology is irrelevant, because, number one, I don't think mechanisms is relevant to prevention. Number two, this work should be more appropriately undertaken in [the National Institute of] General Medical Sciences. This is the view of a growing body in Congress that we're starving other institutes.

Becker: You think it's irrelevant unless it's done in General Medical Sciences.

Epstein: I think that what we're talking about is basic molecular biology —

Becker: And it's not going to be relevant.

Epstein: — which is basic to the whole field of interest in the whole field of biology. It so happens that it's easier to get money for cancer research, and this is the point of the quotes I gave.

Becker: You really believe that if you got Dave Baltimore here today in front of us, he would say that his discoveries are not relevant to cancer?

Epstein: Now, look, Dave is an old friend of mine. I can't answer what he would say. I have quoted to you what he stated —

Becker: You also quoted a conversation about a study done in New York and gave it as if it were data.

Epstein: Yes.

Becker: The data said 10% minimal —

Epstein: That trivializes it —

Becker: "Trivializes" is a word you have used 36 times today.

Yodaiken: I think you've done something that's lovely. I've sat on this board for nine years and there's never been any discussion of pesticides, and this is the first time we've discussed them.

Epstein (to Becker): Oh Fred, listen to this a second, will you please?

Becker: No.

Epstein: He just said he's sat on this board for nine years and there's never been a discussion of pesticides. It's the first time the subject has come up.

Becker: My grant on chlordane proving that it was a carcinogen came from NCI.

Jako (to Epstein): Do you subscribe to *The Cancer Letter*?

Epstein: I'm afraid not, no.

Jako: Because that gives you a general overview of what goes on at the Board. Now, when you refer to the cancer establishment —

Yodaiken: It's not enough to say the exposures in the 1933 to 1977 series were less. There might have been fewer exposures or fewer substances.

Epstein: No, no, you see, essentially, the point was, in the early '30s and '40s, the studies on occupational were very few and far between. Now what we've seen is a plethora of studies. This is the whole point. . . . So, Ralph, what are you doing these days?

Yodaiken: I'm a senior advisor to the Dept. of Labor, and I went to Sam Broder previously and said, why don't you get somebody up here to talk about occupational cancer. And he dismissed it like that.

Epstein: They've been impossible to persuade. The only reason NCI invited me is because of the publicity. However, I hope it's going to be a constructive dialogue.

Jako: You always refer to the cancer establishment.

Epstein: Yes, not only I. The group of 65 refer to it.

Jako: I served on the NCAB and do you think the Board action is to approve everything which the director says?

Epstein: No, not at all.

Jako: There is quite a bit of discussion, and quite a bit of controversy.

Epstein: I've read the transcripts for many years.

Jako: There are different views.

Epstein: The representation of those interested in primary prevention is minimal. Minimal to nonexistent. This is my point.

Jako: Because the government deals with those areas in the Agriculture Department, in —

Epstein: Oh, come on. There are innumerable mechanisms where NCI could provide scientific expertise and guidance. I'm not talking about regulation.

Jako: But, you see —

Epstein: I'm talking about providing scientific expertise to Congress, when Congress —

Jako: But we need your scientific expertise backed up with scientific data.

Epstein: The scientific data are there.

Jako: No, there isn't.

Epstein: You're unfamiliar with the literature.

Jako: I asked you, provide the Cancer Institute with scientific data —

Epstein: Oh, come on. You're unfamiliar with the literature, the literature on pesticides are overwhelming. The literature on occupational cancer are overwhelming. You, sir, are unfamiliar with the literature!

Exeunt.

Evaluation of the National Cancer Program and Proposed Reforms

The International Journal of Health Services *subsequently published* an article based on the author's invited verbal presentation to the NCI, with full documentation and references.*

A statement by 68 prominent national experts in cancer prevention, carcinogenesis, epidemiology, and public health, released at a February 4, 1992, press conference in Washington, D.C., charged that the National Cancer Institute (NCI) has misled and confused the public by repeated claims of winning the war against cancer. In fact, age-standardized incidence rates have escalated to epidemic proportions over recent decades, while the ability to treat and cure most cancers has not materially improved. Furthermore, the NCI has minimized evidence for increasing cancer rates, which are largely attributed to smoking, trivializing the importance of occupational carcinogens as nonsmoking attributable causes of lung and other cancers, and to diet per se, in spite of tenuous and inconsistent evidence and ignoring the important role of carcinogenic dietary contaminants. Reflecting this near exclusionary blame-the-victim theory of cancer causation, with lockstep support from the American Cancer Society and industry, the NCI discounts the role of avoidable involuntary exposures to industrial carcinogens in air, water, food, the home, and the workplace. The NCI has also failed to provide any scientific guidance to Congress and regulatory agencies on fundamental principles of carcinogenesis and epidemiology, and on the critical needs to reduce avoidable exposures to environmental and occupational

---

* *International Journal of Health Services.* 23(1):15-44, 1993. Basically the same article was published in *The American Journal of Industrial Medicine.* 24:109-133, 1993.

carcinogens. Analysis of the $2 billion NCI budget, in spite of fiscal and semantic manipulation, reveals minimal allocations for research on primary cancer prevention, and for occupational cancer, which receives only $19 million annually, 1 percent of NCI's total budget. Problems of professional mindsets in the NCI leadership, fixation on diagnosis, treatment, and basic research, much of questionable relevance, and the neglect of cancer prevention, are exemplified by the composition of the National Cancer Advisory Board. Contrary to the explicit mandate of the National Cancer Act, the Board is devoid of members authoritative in occupational and environmental carcinogenesis. These problems are further compounded by institutionalized conflicts of interest reflected in the composition of past executive President's Cancer Panels, and of the current Board of Overseers of the Sloan-Kettering Memorial Cancer Center, the NCI's prototype comprehensive cancer center, with their closely interlocking financial interests with the cancer drug and other industries. Drastic reforms of NCI policies and the priorities are long overdue. Implementation of such reforms is, however, unlikely in the absence of further support from industrial medicine professionals, besides action by Congress and concerned citizen groups.

Discrepant NCI Objectives

The National Cancer Institute launched the cancer prevention awareness program in 1984 as part of the NCI's overall effort to reduce the rate of cancer mortality to one-half of the 1980 rate (from 168/100,000 to 84/100,000) by the year 2000.[9]

Within the next few years, however, the NCI made the poorly publicized and startling admission that its objective of reducing cancer mortality was totally unrealistic. The NCI now actually anticipates further increases, and not decreases, in cancer mortality rates, from 171/100,000 in 1984 to 175/100,000 by the

year 2000.[10] This is a remarkable admission of the NCI's failure to even hold the line against increasing cancer mortality rates and the nation's second leading cause of death.

Incidence and Mortality Trends in the General U.S. Population

Cancer now strikes one in three and kills one in four, up from an incidence of one in four and a mortality of one in five in the 1950s. Age-standardized incidence rates in the overall U.S. population have increased sharply by 43.5 percent from 1950 to 1988.[11] Rates for some common cancers have increased more sharply: lung by 263 percent, prostate by 100 percent; and male colon and female breast by about 60 percent. Rates for some less common cancers have also increased more sharply: malignant melanoma, multiple myeloma, and non-Hodgkin's lymphoma by well over 100 percent, and testis and male kidney by about 100 percent. The only major declines have been for stomach and cervix cancers (Table 13.1).

Increasing incidence rates have been accompanied by less sharply increasing mortality rates. From 1975 to 1984, overall age-standardized mortality rates increased by 5.5 percent from 162/100,000 to 171/100,000, while rates for those over 75 years increased by 9.0 percent from 1,212/100,000 to 1,351/100,000.[12] Americans 65 and over are now at a ten-fold higher risk of developing cancer than younger age groups.[11] The discrepancy between incidence and mortality trends probably reflects the overdiagnosis of benign as malignant neoplasms, especially for the breast and prostate.[13,14]

Contrary to their own data, both the NCI and ACS have insisted until very recently that cancer incidence and mortality rates, other than those due to tobacco, are not increasing: "We are not certainly experiencing an overall epidemic of cancer, except for that attributable to cigarette smoking."[15] Support for such unfounded assertions, however, persists from

Table 13.1 Summary of changes in cancer incidence, United States, 1950-1988*

Primary site	No. of new cases, all races, 1988†	Percent incidence changes in whites, 1950-1988
Stomach	24,800	-72.9
Colon/Rectum	147,000	10.6
Larynx	12,200	58.7
Lung and bronchus	152,000	262.8
Males	100,000	222.5
Females	52,000	511.7
Melanoma of skin	27,300	303.3
Breast (females)	135,000	56.9
Cervix uteri	12,900	-77.7
Corpus uteri	34,000	-5.2
Ovary	19,000	2.9
Prostate gland	99,000	100.3
Testis	5,600	96.1
Urinary bladder	46,400	54.5
Kidney and renal pelvis	22,500	102.1
Hodgkin's disease	7,400	20.6
Non-Hodgkin's lymphoma	31,700	154.1
Leukemia	26,900	4.0
Childhood cancers	6,600	21.3
All sites, excluding lung	833,000	29.1
All sites	985,000	43.5

* Source: reference 11.
† Excluding basal and squamous skin cancers and all in situ cancers.

sources still relied on by the NCI as authoritative: "The increase in mortality from cancer can be accounted for in all industrialized countries by the spread of cigarette smoking."[16] Overwhelming contrary data have recently been summarized:[17]

In the USA and United Kingdom, mortality rates for lung cancer . . . have actually begun to decline in men, due in large part to reductions in smoking.[18, 19] Moreover, despite these reductions in lung cancer, incidence and mortality for many other types of cancer increased from 1969 to 1986 in 15 industrial countries, especially in persons over age 65.[20] The causes of these recent increases in cancer cannot simply be explained by smoking, but appear to reflect other exposures to changing factors in the environment.

Furthermore, even assuming incorrectly that all lung cancer is due to smoking (page 373), about 75 percent of the increased cancer incidence since 1950 is due to cancers at sites other than the lung (Table 13.1).

Near Static Survival Rates
for Common Cancers

Over the last two decades, the NCI and ACS leadership, with support of the cancer drug industry, have made overly optimistic and poorly founded claims for success with the latest anticancer drugs, based sequentially on cytotoxic chemotherapy, interferons, and recent biotechnology products including tumor necrosis factor, monoclonal antibodies, and interleukins. Responding to criticisms of such claims,[21] the NCI asserted: "There is clear and striking evidence for improvements in cancer treatment, not only for the less common diseases in younger age groups, but also for the common tumors that affect older age groups."[15]

The NCI's position is poorly supportable. The overall five-year survival rates for all cancers have not materially improved, with the notable exception of pediatric and other uncommon cancers, even in more recent years. From 1974 to 1987, survival rates increased marginally from 49.1 to 51.1 percent for all ages and races, and decreased from 38.6 to 38.4 percent for blacks.[11]

The NCI and ACS claims for advances in ability to treat and cure cancer are meeting increasing skepticism:[14,22]

> For the majority of the cancers we examined, the actual improvements [in survival] have been small or have been overestimated by the published rates. . . . NCI does not systematically alert readers of its annual statistics reviews to potential sources of bias that affect changes in survival rates. . . . It is difficult to find that there has been much progress. . . . [For breast cancer], there was a slight improvement . . . [which] is considerably less than reported.
>
> The real survival rates [for the common cancers] have hardly changed since the sixties and seventies.

Based on a recent comprehensive review of the clinical oncology literature and a questionnaire survey of over 350 oncologists and research units worldwide (page 475), a leading German biometrician concluded:

> At least 80% of cancer deaths in Western industrial countries are due to advanced epithelial malignancies. Apart from lung cancer, particularly small-cell lung cancer, there is no direct evidence that chemotherapy prolongs survival in patients with advanced epithelial malignancies.
>
> The majority of publications equate the effect of chemotherapy with [tumor] response, irrespective of survival. Many oncologists take it for granted that response to therapy prolongs survival, an opinion which is based on a fallacy and which is not supported by clinical studies. To date there is no clear evidence that the treated patients, as a whole, benefit from chemotherapy as to their quality of life.
>
> With few exceptions, there is very little scientific basis for the application of chemotherapy in symptom-free patients with advanced epithelial malignancy. Although this is the opinion of a good number of well-known oncologists, the ongoing studies do not take this fact into account.[23]

The NCI's current claims for cancer cures are now more muted: "In patients with disseminated forms of the common epithelial tumors, both complete remissions and cures continue to elude us."[24]

Professional Mindsets in the NCI

The key problem in the leadership of the cancer establishment is a professional mindset fixated on diagnosis, treatment, and research, coupled with relative indifference to and ignorance of cancer cause and prevention. Critically, the current 18-member National Cancer Advisory Board (Table 13.2) "almost totally lacks expertise in occupational and environmental carcinogenesis."[25] This is clearly in violation of Section 407(a)(1)(B) of the National Cancer Act, which requires that no less than five members "shall be individuals knowledgeable in environmental carcinogenesis." Similarly lacking in such expertise is the three-member executive President's Cancer Panel.

Conflicts of Interest in the NCI

Problems of professional mindsets in the NCI leadership appear further compounded

Table 13.2 Members of the National Cancer Advisory Board, 1992*

Member	Date term ends	Scientific/Public		Expertise
Zora K. Brown	3/09/92		X	Public service, health policy
John R. Durant	3/09/92	X		Medical oncology, cytogenetics, immunology, university administration
Bernard Fisher	3/09/92	X		Surgery, surgical oncology
Phillip Frost	3/09/92		X	Civic leader, public service
Irene S. Pollin	3/09/92		X	Social work, counseling
Erwin P. Bettinghaus	3/09/94		X	Health education, communications
David G. Bragg	3/09/94	X		Radiology, radiologic technology, diagnostic oncology
Walter Lawrence	3/09/94	X		Surgery, oncologic surgery, cancer center administration, oncologic education
Howard M. Temin	3/09/94	X		Virology, oncology, carcinogenesis
Samuel A. Wells	3/09/94	X		Surgery, immunology, microbiology
Brenda L. Johnson	3/09/94		X	Public service, management
Frederick F. Becker	3/09/96	X		Carcinogenesis, pathology, tumor biology
Paul Calabresi (Chair)	3/09/96	X		Cancer research
Kenneth Chan	3/09/96	X		Drug metabolism, pharmacokinetics, pre-clinical and clinical pharmacology of anticancer drugs
Marlene A. Malek	3/09/96		X	Nursing, community programs
Deborah K. Mayer	3/09/96	X		Oncology nursing, public and professional education, public policy, clinical trials
Sidney Salmon	3/09/96	X		Medical oncology, immunology, hematology

* Source: National Cancer Institute, March 12, 1992.

by poorly recognized institutionalized conflicts of interest[26-28] (page 494). For decades, the war on cancer has been dominated by powerful groups of interlocking professional and financial interests, with the highly profitable drug development system at its hub — and a background that helps explain why "treatment," not prevention, has been and still is the overwhelming priority, as indeed it is for most physicians. The members of the generously funded cancer establishment include the NCI, ACS, the comprehensive cancer centers such as New York's prototypical Memorial Sloan-Kettering, whose annual budget exceeds $350 million, NCI and ACS contractees and grantees at universities, and major pharmaceutical companies. Cancer care is big business, with annual cancer drug sales of ap-

Table 13.3 Potential conflicts of interest at the Memorial Sloan-Kettering Comprehensive Cancer Center (MSKCC)*

Ownership of cancer drug company securities by MSKCC, 1987

Security description	Shares	Market value (12/31/87)	Cancer drugs
American Home Products	1,800	$ 130,950	Cerubine
Bristol-Myers	13,500	561,938	Blenoxane, Cytoxan, etc.
IC Industries	10,000	329,877	Bolvadex
Eli Lilly	14,600	1,138,000	Oncovin, Velban. etc.
Merck & Co.	8,700	1,378,950	Cosmagen. Mustargen, etc.
Schering Plough Corp.	8,700	408,900	Intron A
Squibb	12,500	762,500	Hydrea, Teslac

Drug company ties of MSKCC overseers, 1988

Frederick R. Adler	Bio Technology General, Life Technologies, Inc., Scitex Corp., etc., director
Richard M. Furlaud	Squibb, president; Pharmaceutical Manufacturers Association, director
Richard L. Gelb	Bristol-Myers, chairman of the board
Louis V. Gerstner, Jr.	Squibb, director
Paul A. Marks, M.D.	Pfizer, director
John K. McKinley	Merck & Co., director
James D. Robinson, III	Bristol-Myers, director

Industrial ties of MSKCC overseers, 1988

Peter O. Crisp	Rockefeller Family & Associates
Richard M. Furlaud	Olin, director
Clifton C. Garvin, Jr.	Exxon, president
Louis V. Gerstner, Jr.	RJR Nabisco, Inc., chairman of the (tobacco company) board
Albert H. Gordon	Allen Group, Inc., director (automotive parts, etc.)
Elizabeth J. McCormack, Ph.D.	Philip Morris, director
John K. McKinley	Texaco, chairman of the board (ret.): Martin Marietta Corp., director
W. Earle McLaughlin	Algoma Steel, director
Thomas A. Murphy	General Motors, chairman of the board (ret.)
Ellmore C. Patterson	Bethlehem Steel Corp., director
John S. Reed	Philip Morris, United Technologies, director
Laurance S. Rockefeller	Exxon, Mobil, Standard Oil of Indiana, Standard Oil of California, etc., major shareholder
Robert V. Roosa	Owens-Corning Fiberglas, Texaco, director
Benno C. Schmidt	Freeport-McMoRan, Inc. (gas, oil, uranium oxide, etc. production), chairman of the executive committee
Fayez Z. Serafim	Pennzoil, etc., major investor
Frederick Seitz, Ph.D.	Ogden Corporation (waste incineration, aviation fueling, etc.), director
Virgil H. Sherrill	Reliance Electric Co., chairman

proximately $10 billion.

The connections between the cancer establishment and the drug development industrial complex, chemical, pharmaceutical, and biotechnology companies, include Bristol-Myers Squibb, the nation's largest chemotherapy drug producer, which also controls key positions on Sloan-Kettering's board. Other board members have close affiliations with oil, steel, and various large corporations (Table 13.3); of particular additional interest is the interlocking relationship of Sloan-Kettering's board with the media giants. Another major component of the cancer drug industry is Sandoz Pharma Ltd., a huge pharmaceutical company, which recently signed a $100 million cancer drug development deal with Boston's Dana Farber Cancer Institute. Furthermore, a "revolving door" operates among the NCI, the major cancer centers, and the drug companies. For example, Stephen Carter, head of drug research and development at Bristol-Myers Squibb, is a former director of NCI's Division of Cancer Treatment. Based on these concerns, I have requested the National Institutes of Health (NIH) Office of Scientific Integrity to investigate the NCI for possible conflicts of interest, with a view to minimizing any such future problems.[29]

A more obvious conflict of interest has related to the three-member Presidentially appointed Cancer Panel that controls NCI priorities and policies. The most long-standing past chairman of the panel was Benno C. Schmidt, an investment banker, senior drug company executive, and member of the Board of Overseers of the Memorial Sloan-Kettering Comprehensive Cancer Center. He was followed by the late Armand Hammer, Chairman of Occidental Petroleum, a major polluting industry and manufacturer of carcinogenic chemicals. Congress has recently warned against such conflicts of interest in the Public Health Service:[30] "The Secretary shall by regulation establish criteria for preventing, and for responding to the existence of, any financial interest . . . that (a) will create a bias in favor of obtaining results . . . that are consistent with financial interest; or (b) may be reasonably expected to create such a bias."[30]

Questionable Relevance of Some Major Basic Research Programs in the NCI to Cancer in General and to Cancer Prevention in Particular

The NCI has traditionally maintained that basic research is one of its highest priorities to which major resources are allocated: "NCI has had a long-standing commitment to basic research."[31] The relevance of such research to the NCI's overall mission is, at best, questionable. There is no apparent evidence, or any basis for belief, for its relevance to cancer prevention. The views of some of the nation's leading molecular biologists and recipients of substantial

NCI funding (including Dr. Harold Varmus, now NIH director) are illuminating:[32-34]

> I have no idea when we'll know enough to develop anything that's clinically applicable, and I don't know who's going to do it. . . It's not a high priority in my thinking. I'm happy to work on the model systems we're working on. . . . [Responding to questions on the relevance of oncogene research, he replied,] I think all of us would say honestly that it's the normal processes of the cell that are our real concern.
>
> If you're giving me money, I'll talk about cures. Since you're not, I won't. Talking about cures is absolutely offensive to me. In our work, we never think about such things even for a second.
>
> You can't do experiments to see what causes cancer. It's not an accessible problem, and it's not the sort of thing scientists can afford to do. You've got to live, and you've got to eat, you've got to keep your postdocs happy. Everything you do can't be risky.

Congressional skepticism on the NCI's high priority for basic research appears fully justified:[35]

Research is serendipitous . . . and many of the important discoveries that enable us to fight cancer today originate at an institute other than the NCI. A number of them originated at [the National Institute of] General Medical Sciences, which devotes almost all of its budget to basic medical research, . . .[which] we starved [of funds]. . . . There will be a tremendous pressure on researchers who want to get dollars for their research grants to find some way to claim that they have a cancer angle in their research. . . . The fact is that from 1988 through this year, the NCI budget went up by 35%. Meanwhile heart-lung-blood [Institute's] budget went up 24%. Almost twice as many people die of those diseases as die of cancer. . . . [Yet] we would be funding 48% [of competitive grants] . . . at

NCI, but we will be funding only half that research at heart-lung-blood.

The NCI Budget for Cancer Prevention

Of an approximate $2 billion budget for 1992, the NCI allocates about $645 million, or 30 percent, to "cancer prevention," of which the Division of Cancer Etiology (DCE) receives about 82 percent and the Division of Cancer Prevention and Control (DCPC) the remainder (Table 13.4). Included in the "cancer prevention" budget is an allocation of some $335 million, 17 percent of the total budget, for "primary cancer prevention," defined as "those research activities designed to yield results that are directly applicable to the identification of risk and to interventions to prevent disease or the progression of detectable but asymptomatic disease."[31]

It should, however, be emphasized that the NCI has apparently never initiated any scientific or other "interventions" in legislative, regulatory, or public arenas (by a wide range of available mechanisms) designed to prevent or reduce avoidable exposures to any carcinogens other than tobacco.

The entire budget of DCPC is included in that of "primary cancer prevention," nearly half of which is allocated to investigator-initiated grants, with the remainder allocated to contracts and intramural research (Table 13.5). Included also is $19 million for research on occupational cancer — about 6 percent of the "primary prevention" budget and about 1 percent of the total NCI budget. Also included are pass-through funds of $500,000 to the National Institutes of Occupational Safety and Health (NIOSH), only 10 percent of the $3 million 1977 allocation (adjusting for inflation). Review of the 1991 line item grant and contract obligations for "primary prevention" and for in-house DCPC programs (Appendix VI) reveals a predominant emphasis on smoking and nutrition. Also included are well-funded and highly questionable, if not hazardous, chemoprevention trials, particu-

Table 13.4 1992 NCI budget on cancer prevention, in thousands of dollars

Total appropriation		$1,951,541
Cancer prevention (including primary prevention)		645,185
Division of Cancer Etiology (DCE)	$531,575	
Division of Cancer Prevention and Control (DCPC)	113,610	
As percent of total appropriations	30%	
"Primary cancer prevention"		334,693*
As percent of cancer prevention	52%	
As percent of total appropriations	17%	
Occupational cancer		19,000†
As percent of cancer prevention	3%	
As percent of total appropriations	1%	
NIOSH pass-through funds		500
As percent of 1977 allocation (adjusted for inflation)	10%	

* Includes the total DCPC allocation of $113,610.
† Included in the "Primary Cancer Prevention" allocation.

larly tamoxifen chemoprevention of breast cancer in healthy women, and studies on secondary cancers following treatment. With the exception of widely ranging antismoking programs, only minimal funding, $50 million at most, appears to be obligated for research on avoidable carcinogens in air, water, food, home, and the workplace. Furthermore, there is no evidence of any funding for interventions directed to reducing such avoidable exposures. Not surprising is the Congressional reaction: "A number of scientists have suggested that cancer prevention receives an even smaller percentage of the budget than what NCI considers primary prevention."[3]

The NCI leadership has misled and confused Congress as to its allocations for "cancer prevention" in general, and "primary cancer prevention" in particular, by a combination of budgetary manipulation and semantics. Illustrative is the following statement in the 1991 Congressional report on NCI authorization and appropriations, which relied on and quoted from NCI representations in its 1991 and 1992 budget estimates:[30]

NCI Director Samuel Broder has written,

Table 13.5 1992 NCI budget on "Primary Cancer Prevention," in thousands of dollars

Grants	$147,053
Contracts	45,660
Intramural research	28,370
Cancer prevention and control (DCPC)	113,610
Total	334,693

Source: National Cancer Institute. Letter to S. S. Epstein, June 2, 1992.

"Prevention is the most cost-effective way to deal with any disease or set of diseases; cancer is not an exception. Ultimately, the real gains in reducing cancer incidence and mortality will come from prevention." The prevention and control agenda outlined by the NCI in its proposed FY 1992 budget is comprehensive, scientifically valid and, most important, achievable. By increasing the percentage of the budget allocated to prevention from approximately 5 percent to 10 percent over two fiscal years, the Committee believes the real gains to which Dr. Broder referred can be achieved. . . . The cancer prevention and control program of NCI provides "the bridge between knowledge derived from basic and clinical research programs and its application in clinical and public health settings. . . . The primary focus of the Cancer Prevention Research Program is to develop and evaluate strategies for the prevention of cancer." The primary goal of cancer control "is to change personal behavior and patterns of practice to maximize the impact of cancer prevention and control regimens on cancer morbidity and mortality." For this reason, cancer prevention and control activities hold the greatest promise of achieving the goal of significantly reducing cancer incidence and mortality by the year 2000.

Particularly noteworthy is the NCI's equation of cancer prevention with "blame-the-victim" concepts of cancer causation, to the virtual exclusion of avoidable and unknowing exposures to industrial carcinogens in air, water, food, the home, and the workplace. This misrepresentation is further confounded by the NCI's failure to admit to Congress that it has totally abandoned its unrealistic objective of "significantly reducing cancer incidence and mortality by the year 2000."

It is furthermore clear that the NCI has no intention of making any substantial changes in its current policies and priorities. The NCI fiscal year 1993 "bypass" budget, which is presented directly to the President, circumventing the NIH and Department of Health and Human Services bureaucracy, calls for an allocation of $2.7 billion. The bypass budget itemizes a total of $205 million for DCPC for the expansion of itemized current prevention programs, with no reference whatsoever to research and interventions relating to occupational cancer and other avoidable exposures to environmental carcinogens.[36] The same reservations relate to the 1993 NIH reauthorization bill, which earmarks $325 million for research on breast cancer, besides $75 and $72 million for research on ovarian and prostate cancers, respectively.

NCI Estimates on the Contribution of Lifestyle and Environmental Factors to Cancer Mortality

Current NCI estimates on the causes of cancer (Table 13.6) are largely based on an obsolete analysis of trends in cancer mortality from 1933 to 1977 reported a decade ago.[37] However, such estimates reflect a lack of recognition of the multiple causes of some, if not most, cancers. Thus, the true sum total of all "causes" should well exceed 100 percent. It is of further interest to note that the Doll and Peto[37] report concluded that "there is no evidence of any generalized increase [in cancer mortality] other than that due to tobacco." (Chapter 14.) This conclusion, however, was reached by excluding consideration of blacks and of all people over the age of 65, just those groups in which more than half of all cancer deaths have been reported, and by incorrectly ascribing lung cancer almost exclusively to smoking. It should also be emphasized that the 1981 Doll and Peto estimates are devoid of any cited quantitative scientific data, apart from tobacco, for which the confounding variable of occupational exposures was ignored.

The basis of Doll's and Peto's estimates is as follows: they assumed that diet causes 35 percent (even up to 70 percent) of cancers and that smoking causes 30 percent and that these

Table 13.6 NCI estimates on the contribution of "lifestyle and environmental factors" to cancer mortality*

Diet	35%
Tobacco	30%
Reproductive/sexual behavior	7%
Occupation	4%
Alcohol	3%
Geophysical factors	3%
Pollution	2%
Industrial products	1%
Medicine and medical procedures	1%
Total	86%

* Source: reference 10.

together with other causes, such as alcohol and sunlight, total 96 percent. This leaves a balance of 4 percent. To bring these figures neatly up to 100 percent, Doll and Peto conveniently ascribed 4 percent to occupational causes. They attempted to dignify this tenuous hypothesis by circular references to other blame-the-victim advocates, including Higginson, Armstrong, and Wynder, who in turn cited earlier publications of Doll and Peto as their authority.[37] Doll's continuing insistence on his obsolete blame-the-victim hypothesis, which trivializes the role of environmental and occupational exposure to industrial carcinogens,[16] is scientifically unsupported.[25] Doll's position is also consistent with his industrial interests, as illustrated by his position until recently as Warden and Director of the industry-financed Green College, Oxford. Green College was established in 1978 as a "special point of entry for industrial interests wishing to collaborate with University departments in research."[38]

The NCI Trivializes Causes of Lung Cancer Other Than Smoking

Smoking is indisputably a leading cause of disease and death from cardiovascular disease and lung cancer, and cancers at other sites generally to a much lesser extent.* However, the NCI leadership has trivialized the substantial evidence for a major role of occupational and urban causes of lung cancer. This evidence includes the following:

1. The incidence of lung cancer in nonsmokers has more than doubled over recent decades.[39]

2. Lung cancer rates in black men are some 40 percent higher and have been increasing more rapidly than in whites over the last few decades. While more black men identify themselves as current smokers, they have in fact smoked less and started smoking later in life than white men.[40-42]

* From 1973-1991, annual lung cancer mortality rates in females increased nine time faster than in males, 4.6% compared with 0.5%, and lung cancer is up to three times more likely to develop in females than in males with comparable smoking habits. Based on such trends, more women, especially teenaged, than men will be smoking by the millennium. In contrast, lung cancer mortality rates in men are declining significantly due to reductions in smoking.

3. The incidence of adenocarcinoma of the lung, which is less clearly related to smoking than are squamous and oat cell carcinoma,[43] has increased sharply over recent decades.[44] The most recent data (1983-1987) for the percentage of all lung cancer that is due to adenocarcinomas are 26.5 and 32.4 percent in whites and blacks, respectively.[11]

4. The role of occupation as a major confounding variable was ignored in nearly all of the 30 or so retrospective studies associating lung cancer with smoking.[45]

5. There are strong positive associations, largely independent of smoking habits, between lung cancer and occupational exposure to a wide range of carcinogenic products, such as arsenic, chrome, nickel, and BCME, and carcinogenic processes, such as copper smelting, uranium, zinc, and lead mining, spray painting, and tanning.[17]

6. The high lung cancer rates in workers in casting areas of iron foundries are related to their daily inhalation of levels of polycyclic aromatic hydrocarbon carcinogens equivalent to 10 to 20 packs of cigarettes;[46] these estimates ignore the incremental role of silica.

7. On the basis of studies linking urban air pollution and lung cancer,[47] the 1970 "National Panel of Consultants on the Conquest of Cancer" concluded that "lung cancer [is] undoubtedly attributable to the air pollution in certain environments."[48] Subsequent studies, including those on diesel exhaust, have also incriminated air pollution as a significant cause of lung cancer.[49-52] Other studies have demonstrated excess lung cancer rates in communities residing near large petrochemical plants.[53] Of clear relevance is evidence that U.S. industries in 1991 discharged into the environment some 3.6 billion pounds of chemicals, including a wide range of carcinogens.[54]

8. Age-adjusted lung cancer death rates not attributable to smoking have recently been commuted from published data on the proportion of active smokers, the proportion of former smokers, and the amounts smoked.[55] Nonsmoking attributable causes of lung cancer were found to range from 13 percent in white men to 28 percent in black women, and to be 67 percent higher in black than in white men and 16 percent higher in black than in white women (Table 13.7). "These residual rates place nonsmoking attributable lung cancers among the three or four most common cancers [in terms of mortality] in the U.S."[42]

Finally, it should be noted that until very recently, the NCI and ACS have tried to explain away increasing cancer incidence rates by ascribing them almost exclusively to smoking.[e.g., 15]

The NCI Trivializes Occupational Cancer as a Major Cause of Cancer Mortality

The NCI's current estimate that occupational cancer is responsible for only 4 percent of total cancer mortality[10] is largely based on obsolete analyses of cancer trends from 1933 to 1977.[37] Contrary evidence includes the following:

1. Over the last decade, a plethora of new studies have identified a wide range of additional carcinogenic products and processes inducing cancers in a wide range of organs, particularly lung, brain, bladder, and kidney tumors and multiple myeloma.[e.g., 17, 56-58]

2. Based on exposure data, NIOSH[59] has estimated that approximately 11 million workers are exposed to occupational carcinogens. Surveillance of these workers by the NCI and NIOSH is minimal, at best.

3. In the same year that Doll and Peto published their 4 percent estimate, which the

Table 13.7 Smoking and nonsmoking attributable causes of lung cancer*

	Age-adjusted lung cancer mortality rates, per 100,000, 1984			
	Male		Female	
	White	Black	White	Black
Rate	71.8	101.0	25.2	24.1
Smoking attributed	62.5	85.5	19.4	17.3
Nonsmoking attributed	9.3	15.5	5.8	6.8
Percent nonsmoking attributed	13.0%	15.4%	23.0%	28.2%

* Source: reference 51.

NCI leadership regularly cites, Peto also admitted to divergent estimates of up to an order of magnitude greater:[60]

> Occupational factors are likely to account for . . . a "large" percentage (e.g., 20-40%) of all U.S. cancer. . . . [Even low estimates] represent large enough absolute numbers of deaths to justify both intensive research and political action. . . . A mere 2.5% of all U.S. cancer deaths would represent some 10,000 deaths per year.

4. Of 37,000 total cancer deaths each year in New York State, 10 percent (3,700) are estimated to be due to occupational exposures.[61] Since the exposure patterns of the New York and national work forces have been shown to be similar, the annual U.S. mortality from occupational cancer would thus be approximately 50,000, or about 10 percent of all cancer deaths.

5. The relative risks for cancers induced in a wide range of organs following exposures to occupational carcinogens, such as aromatic amines, benzene, and BCME, are orders of magnitude greater than the risks for the general population.

6. Asbestos, clearly the single most important *known* occupational carcinogen, is es-

timated to cause some 300,000 cancer and other deaths by 2030, including 60,000 nonsmoking related mesotheliomas.[62] As recently emphasized,[20] such evidence negates continuing assertions by Doll — on whom the NCI still heavily relies for its low 4 percent estimate of occupational causes of total cancer mortality — that asbestos is only responsible for a "few cases of mesothelioma."[16]

7. Some 20 U.S. and international studies have incriminated parental exposures to occupational carcinogens as major causes of childhood cancer,[63] whose incidence has increased by 21 percent since 1950.

8. Based on a recent analysis of cancer mortality trends in 15 industrialized countries from 1969 to 1986, it was concluded that "we have identified changes in the incidence and mortality rates for cancers at other sites [than those related to smoking]. . . in the middle and older age groups throughout the industrialized world."[19]

The NCI Accepts Tenuous Evidence for the Role of a High-Fat Diet Itself as a Major "Cause" of Breast and other Cancers

A high intake of fat has been associated with

cancer of the breast, colon, rectum, and prostate, and possibly pancreas, uterus and ovary. Dietary factors are estimated to account for approximately 35% of cancers.[10]

This "high-fat" hypothesis, however, is largely based on Doll and Peto[37] and related reports by other "blame-the-victim" advocates, which provide only weak and inconsistent supporting evidence. It should further be noted that Peto subsequently retracted this 35 percent estimate: "[Recommendations for reducing dietary fat] should chiefly be because they *will* help avoid heart disease, rather than because they *may well* avoid cancer. . . . the evidence in this respect is less secure." [64] "We'd like to have definitive evidence [on diet and cancer], but we don't have it. There is nothing in the league with smoking, which is a big and definite risk factor." [65]

Furthermore, with reference to the role of dietary fat as a major cause of breast cancer, which NCI policy-makers explicitly accept, a recent review concluded: "The results of case-control and cohort studies[e.g.,66] have produced at best inconsistent results."[67]

The NCI Fails to Recognize Preventable Causes of Breast Cancer (page 477)

Despite expenditures of over $1 billion on breast cancer over the last two decades,[68] "we must conclude that there has been no progress in preventing the disease."[69] NCI programs on breast cancer prevention reflect myopia and questionable science, as illustrated by emphasis on a high-fat diet by itself as the major cause (Table 17.6). This is further compounded by neglect and by an apparent unfamiliarity with evidence incriminating a wide range of carcinogenic pesticides and other xenobiotic dietary contaminants. None of the NCI's past heavily funded nutritional studies claiming associations between dietary fat and breast cancer, besides colon and other cancers, have investigated or apparently even considered the confounding variable of carcinogenic contaminants. Less understandable

is the NCI's failure to consider investigation of the role of dietary contaminants in its proposed multimillion dollar studies on the relation of diet and breast cancer. Evidence for the role of these contaminants includes the following:[70]

1. Carcinogenic pesticides, such as DDT, chlordane, and dieldrin, which concentrate in animal fats, induce breast cancer in rodents.[71,72] This creates a strong presumption for a causal role of such dietary contaminants and breast cancer in women, particularly as the sites of tumor induction are generally similar in experimental animals and humans.[73]

2. Promotion by DDT of mammary tumors induced in rodents by the potent carcinogen acetamidophenanthrene "might be considered possible contributors to the high incidence of breast cancers."[74]

3. DDT and PCBs concentrate in human breast cancer itself in contrast to adjacent non-neoplastic tissue,[75] and in breasts with cancer in contrast to those with fibrocystic disease.[76]

4. Breast cancer mortality in premenopausal Israeli women declined by 30 percent following regulations reducing levels of DDT and other carcinogenic pesticides in dietary fat, in spite of increasing fat consumption and decreasing parity.[77]

5. In view of the known carcinogenicity of exogenous estrogens, lifelong exposure to estrogenic contaminants in animal fat, due to their unregulated use as growth-promoting feed additives, is clearly a risk factor for breast cancer. Warnings of such breast cancer risks, including by the NCI's former leading expert in endocrinology, have gone unheeded by the cancer establishment.[78]

6. Exogenous estrogens are synergists for the carcinogenicity of irradiation in the rodent breast.[79, 80] Estrogens are also synergists in the induction of mammary cancer

in rats by polynuclear hydrocarbon carcinogens.[81]

Apart from ignoring the role of avoidable carcinogenic dietary contaminants, the NCI and ACS have also failed to investigate the carcinogenic hazards of mammography, particularly the relation between increasing breast cancer rates and the high-dose mammograms administered without warning to some 300,000 women in the 1970s Breast Cancer Detection and Demonstration Program (BCDDP). Based on a wide range of previously published epidemiological data, an authoritative international expert group in 1972 estimated incremental breast cancer risks of approximately 1 percent per rad of exposure.[82] Thus, a premenopausal woman given one mammogram annually, for 10 years, with a conservative estimated dose of two rads per exposure, would be at a 20 percent excess risk. A confidential memo by a senior NCI physician in charge of the screening program[83] may explain why, in spite of warnings by the National Academy of Sciences in 1972 and by the NCI's own key scientific staff,[84] women were not warned of this risk. The memo may also account for the cancer establishment's enthusiasm for the BCDDP program: "Both the [ACS] and NCI will gain a great deal of favorable publicity because they are bringing research findings to the public and applying them. This will assist in obtaining more research funds for basic research and clinical research which is sorely needed."[83]

It may be further noted that the NCI has also failed to adequately explore safe alternatives to mammography, particularly transillumination with infrared light scanning.[85,86] This is all the more serious in view of recent reports of excess breast cancer mortality in premenopausal women following mammography, together with accumulating evidence of its diagnostic ineffectiveness in younger women,[87] including the recent large-scale Canadian study of Cornelia Baines and Anthony Miller: "There is no evidence to support introduction of service mammography for women under 50, and some may argue that there should be a moratorium on all mammography for symptom-free women in this age group outside randomized control trials."[88]

The NCI still ignores carcinogenic dietary contaminants and high-dose mammography in the 1970s as preventable causes of breast cancer.[70] Meanwhile, the NCI designates its tamoxifen chemoprevention trial as "primary cancer prevention" (page 485). In May 1992, the NCI initiated this trial on 16,000 healthy women at increased risk of breast cancer, for familial and more questionable reasons, including age over 60 years.[89] The tamoxifen trial is a prospective experiment in human carcinogenesis whose scientific invalidity is compounded by a misleading patient consent form, trivializing risks and exaggerating benefits;[90,91] participating oncologists and institutions clearly risk future malpractice claims.

Tamoxifen, which is structurally related to DES, induces covalent DNA adducts in rodents, thus making "this drug a poor choice for the chronic preventive treatment of breast cancer."[92] Tamoxifen induced 15 percent of liver tumors in rats at doses equivalent to the daily 20mg low dose in human adjuvant therapy, and 71 percent at the higher 40mg dose;[93,94] these tumors were highly malignant.[95] This experimental evidence of potent carcinogenicity is confirmed by two case reports of liver cancer among 931 women receiving 40mg tamoxifen doses in the Stockholm adjuvant therapy trials,[96] and more strikingly by several reports of endometrial cancer, particularly in the Stockholm trial documenting a 6.4 relative risk of endometrial cancer.[97] It should further be emphasized that the median follow-up for all the seven reported tamoxifen trials was only 80 months;[94] very few healthy women have taken the drug for more than five years.[95] Thus, tamoxifen may well be a much more potent human carcinogen than is currently recognized.

The NCI Trivializes Environmental Pollutants as Causes of Avoidable Cancer

According to the NCI, "pollution" and "industrial products" are together responsible for only 3 percent of cancer deaths (Table 13.6). Estimates such as these fail to reflect an extensive body of evidence. This includes the exponential production and manufacture of a wide range of synthetic organic chemicals, particularly industrial carcinogens,[26] from one billion pounds per annum in the 1940 dawn of the petrochemical era to over 400 billion pounds annually by the 1980s.[40] Only some 10 percent of these new industrial chemicals have been adequately tested for carcinogenicity.[98] More critically, of some 120 carcinogens identified in experimental animals over the last two decades, less than 10 percent have yet been subjected to epidemiological study by the NCI or by industry.[99]

The role of environmental pollution as a substantial cause of increasing cancer rates is illustrated by reference to just one class of industrial chemicals, carcinogenic pesticides:

1. Some 53 carcinogenic pesticides are registered for use on major crops, such as apples, tomatoes, and potatoes, which become contaminated with detectable residues. Consumption of common foods with residues of 28 of these pesticides has been associated with some 20,000 excess annual cancer deaths.[100] It was further estimated that if then-current exposure levels were to continue, 6,000 preschool children would develop cancer from exposure to residues of carcinogenic pesticides in fruits and vegetables.[101] Environmental Protection Agency (EPA) policies now allow residues of a single carcinogenic pesticide on a single food item at levels posing a "negligible cancer risk" of 1/100,000 excess cancers, equivalent to some 35 excess annual cancer deaths. However, based on EPA estimates, aggregate risks from consumption of about 30 food items contaminated by residues of 30 carcinogenic pesticides would thus result in about 30,000 excess cancers each year, assuming conservatively that risks are no more than additive.[102,103] It should be further stressed that the NCI has failed to undertake epidemiological studies on the great majority of pesticides known, in some instances for decades, to induce cancer in experimental animals and which are common dietary contaminants.

2. Some 34 pesticides are commonly used for professional lawn care treatment at application rates up to fivefold in excess of agricultural. Ten of these pesticides (29 percent) are known to induce cancer in rodents;[104] this evidence has been confirmed for one of these pesticides, 2,4-D, in occupational studies by NCI epidemiologists.[105,106] Recent studies have also demonstrated major excesses of lymphomas in dogs living in homes with gardens that receive regular lawn care treatment.[107] Infants and children are also clearly at major excess risk from such exposures. Of relevance in this connection is the EPA's recent report that the theoretical maximum levels of some dietary pesticide residues, including carcinogens, may exceed published standards by a factor of more than 10,000.[108]

3. Over the last three decades, tens of millions of U.S. homes have been treated for termites by subterranean application of the slowly degradable carcinogenic pesticides chlordane and heptachlor.[109] These pesticides are a complex mix of some 150 components, including undisclosed potent carcinogenic contaminants, termed "inert" by the EPA and industry.[110] The agricultural use of these pesticides was phased out after 1975 EPA suspension/cancellation hearings concluded that their food residues posed an "imminent hazard" of cancer.[109]

It was subsequently determined that routine termite treatment could result in persistent air contamination with exposure levels greater than those that the EPA had determined to pose an imminent cancer hazard on food, and which posed risks in the order of 300 to 3,000 excess annual cancer deaths. Commonplace misapplication of these pesticides resulted in higher air contaminant levels and still higher cancer risks. No epidemiological studies have ever been conducted on the very large number of people living in contaminated homes, in spite of repeated recommendations.[111-113] While NCI scientists agreed, in principle, to conduct an epidemiological feasibility study on people living in chlordane-contaminated homes,[114] this has not yet been undertaken.

Reforming the NCI

Obstacles. Drastic reforms of NCI policies, with their minimal priorities on "primary cancer prevention," are long overdue. However, a complex of powerful constraints limits the practical feasibility of implementing such reforms, particularly in the near future. These include: direct control of the NCI, uniquely and in contrast to all other National Health Institutes, by the President, who appoints the NCI's Director, executive Cancer Panel, and advisory National Cancer Board; the nearly total lack of expertise in environmental and occupational carcinogenesis in the NCI leadership, particularly the Cancer Panel, and in the Advisory Board, in violation of Section 407 of the National Cancer Act; professional mindsets of past and present directors and senior staff who are fixated on diagnosis, treatment, and basic research; powerful self-interested support for NCI priorities by a national network of cancer clinicians, basic researchers, and academic and clinical institutions; powerful support from the ACS, whose policies lockstep with the NCI; indifference to and poor comprehension of primary prevention, which is restrictedly focused on simplistic and obsolete blame-the-victim theories and chemoprevention; failure to recognize the relation between escalating cancer rates and avoidable exposure to carcinogens in air, water, food, the home, and the workplace; support from giant cancer drug pharmaceutical industries, with interlocking financial and personal interests; pressures from chemical industries in support of exclusionary blame-the-victim theories of cancer causation; an apparent conscious or subconscious duplicity of the NCI leadership in attempting to persuade the public and Congress that we are winning the war against cancer, the NCI's semantic and budgetary manipulations or fundamental misunderstanding, designating a wide range of unrelated and marginal programs as "primary prevention" programs in order to justify grossly inflated claims for primary prevention allocations; and the historic lack of effective scientific, Congressional, grassroots, and labor constituencies for primary cancer prevention.

Proposed Reforms. The group of 68 experts, signatories to the statement "Losing the War against Cancer," proposed a series of reforms, not as a specific blueprint but as general guidelines for redefining the mission and priorities of the NCI (pages 341-344).

Recognizing the powerful complex of interlocking obstacles to their proposed reforms, the group of 68 experts concluded:[2, p.344]

There is no conceivable likelihood that such reforms will be implemented without legislative action. The National Cancer Act should be amended explicitly to reorient the mission and priorities of the NCI to cancer cause and prevention. Compliance of the NCI should then be assured by detailed and ongoing Congressional oversight and, most critically, by House and Senate Authorization and Appropriation committees. However, only strong support by the independent scientific and public health communities, together with concerned grass roots citizen groups, will convince Congress and Presidential candidates of the critical and immediate need for such drastic action.

The emergence of the group of 68 experts poses a unique challenge to the current policies and priorities of the NCI, and a unique opportunity for developing appropriate drastic reforms. Of critical importance is the need for additional industrial medicine professionals to join this group, endorse its objectives, and actively participate in the planning and implementation of future strategies. Endorsement should also be solicited from other scientific and public health professionals. Tens of thousands of avoidable cancer deaths each year should prove an adequate stimulus to abandon customary scientific reticence and proceed instead with aggressive action programs, including media campaigns and the enrollment of support from organized labor and from nationwide grass roots citizen groups.

Equally critical is the need for active support for Congress, particularly members of NCI appropriations and authorization committees who have demonstrated concern for setting high priorities for primary cancer prevention. They should be encouraged to develop initiatives, including the following: encouraging the NCI to accept a realistic definition of primary cancer prevention (excluding both important but irrelevant programs on chemoprevention and scientifically questionable programs, such as nutrition per se), based on research and interventions for reducing or eliminating exposure to avoidable carcinogens in air, water, food, the home, and the workplace; requiring the NCI to submit a detailed annual report on all primary prevention programs, with abstracts and line item budget allocation for each; developing appropriate mechanisms for the scientific evaluation of NCI primary prevention programs by qualified independent experts; developing progressive "set-aside" appropriations, such as 10 percent of the total budget each year, for primary prevention, until they reach parity with all other NCI programs combined, ideally within a five-year period; complying with the National Cancer Act requirement that at least five members of the NCI's Advisory Board should be scientists with recognized authority in environmental and occupational carcinogenesis; requiring NCI scientists to provide expertise to Congress, Federal and regulatory agencies, and local authorities concerned with legislation and regulation of avoidable exposures to environmental and occupational carcinogens; and amending the National Cancer Act as follows:[2, p.344]

> The NCI should be removed from direct Presidential authority, and reintegrated within NIH, and thus made directly responsive to the scientific community at large and the advice and consent of Congress.

For the fiscal analysis of NCI In-House Prevention Programs, see Appendix VI.

Chapter Fourteen

The Academic Apologists Rebutted

Efforts have been made to trivialize escalating cancer rates and to minimize the role of environmental and occupational carcinogens by a small but influential group of academic cancer establishment apologists who have become leading spokesmen for regulatory inaction and industry interests. Notable among them are Great Britain's epidemiologist Sir Richard Doll, his statistician Richard Peto, and California geneticist Bruce Ames.

Doll and Peto have vigorously espoused the lifestyle or "blame-the-victim" theory of cancer causation, with its virtually exclusionary emphasis on the role of smoking, fatty diet, and sunlight exposure. Ames embraces the lifestyle theory and expands it with the creative claim for a major role for "natural carcinogens" in food.

Doll and Peto:
The "Lifestyle" Theorists

Martin Walker wrote the following article for the British Journal The Ecologist. *The article exposes Doll's self-interested bias and shows him to be a spokesman for the petrochemical and other industries.*

Sir Richard Doll:
Discredited Pillar of the
British Cancer Establishment

By Martin Walker*
From *The Ecologist*
March/April 1998

The Imperial Cancer Research Fund writes in its current publication, *Preventing and Curing:* "One of the biggest myths in recent years is that there is a cancer epidemic caused by exposure to radiation, pollution, pesticides and food additives. The truth is that these factors have very little to do with the majority of cancers in this country. In fact, food additives may have a protective effect — particularly against stomach cancer." One would presume that the Imperial Cancer Research Fund would only dare make a statement of this sort, which runs counter to endless serious studies on the subject, after exhaustive research over many decades on the possible carcinogenic effects of exposure to these environmental factors. However, unbelievable as it may seem, this august institution fully admits that it has never carried out any such research! How then can it conceivably make such a statement? The answer is that it is entirely based on the pronouncements of Sir Richard Doll, seen to be the greatest living expert on the subject, and whose every word is gospel among the members of Britain's cancer establishment. Let us look carefully at the career of Sir Richard Doll in order to trace the origin and development of this most questionable pillar.

On October 17, 1997, the news programs and the newspapers made frequent mention of new evidence from three studies supervised by Sir Richard Doll, and originally published in the *British Medical Journal,* which pur-

---

* **Martin J. Walker, M.A.,** is the author of six books. He is a writer, investigator, and lecturer, who since the publication of his last book *Dirty Medicine* has been writing mainly about the social history of environmental health. At the pres-ent time, he is researching organophosphate pesticides, factory farming, and the history of alternative cancer therapies in Britain. This article is reprinted with permission from *The Ecologist,* March/April 1998.

ported to show that "passive smoking" caused lung cancer.[1]

That same day, in London's High Court, Mrs. Justice Smith handed down her judgement in the case of John Hill, who had taken a civil action against the owners of a farm upon which he had worked. He claimed that exposure to organophosphate (OP) insecticide at work had adversely affected his health. Mrs. Justice Smith ruled that his ill health was partly at least "attributable to psychological factors." With the exception of Britain's most subversive 6 am radio program, *Farming Today,* little publicity was given to the court hearing.[2,3]

Curious Double Standards

These separate sets of circumstances, occurring as they did on the same day, give voice to a number of issues relating to the way we perceive health and the environment. The first and most obvious is that thirty years after Richard Doll and Bradford Hill published their first epidemiological study on the high rates of lung cancer amongst GPs who smoked,[4] the public are still in thrall to the idea that cigarette smoking is the single most important public health problem we face in Britain.

Secondly, the judgement in the OP case demonstrates something which is difficult to understand within the context of truthful scientific research. It has been recognized for hundreds of years that agricultural and industrial chemicals, especially those of which we have had no evolutionary experience (xenobiotic chemicals), can have serious adverse effects upon humans, but, unlike the public issue of cigarette-induced lung cancer, the history of both academic judgements and plaintiff actions with respect to chemicals is almost a secret history.

Research by the Medical Research Council into the use of organophosphorus compounds predates the work of Doll and Bradford Hill on cigarette smoking.[5] Initial scientific conclusions in the late 1940s and 1950s were not

in the least reassuring. There are presently hundreds of OP cases waiting to come before the courts, including over 100 Gulf War syndrome cases. The great majority of complaints involving OPs have been made by farmers who were pressed, by law, between 1975 and 1993 to dip sheep and treat cattle with washes of OP as a deterrent to warble fly. Almost all the cases which have so far reached court have, like cases brought by others suffering from Multiple Chemical Sensitivities (MCS), floundered on two medical, legal, and scientific arguments. First, that it cannot be "proved" that exposure to apparently toxic chemicals can cause long-term and ongoing systemic damage to health. Secondly, that any damage caused by chemicals is relative, dependent first upon their method and duration of use, and second upon the susceptibility of the injured party. In this way the chemical company is defended and the sufferer blamed for having a weak constitution.

One question raised by these issues is why the medical research establishment and the State have allowed a confused, unscientific and sometimes almost mystical appraisal of the risk of cigarette smoking to entirely shape the public policy debate over cancer? Why have so many research scientists in developed societies, and particularly in Britain, refused to investigate the chemical causes of cancer, despite their increasingly telling effect upon the epidemiological picture of cancer, ill-health and the quality of life?

In comparing the responses of scientists, doctors and the media to both cigarette smoking, chemicals and cancer, the career and philosophy of Sir Richard Doll emerges as a convincing guide and marker to changing perceptions and modalities.

The Career of Sir Richard Doll

Sir Richard Doll has been considered England's most influential epidemiologist for the last thirty years. Doll first did work on mortality in asbestos workers in the 1950s, producing a paper in 1955.[6] His conclusions came down decidedly on the side of asbestos workers, whose health he said was being put in jeopardy.

In his first Rock Carling Fellowship Lecture in June 1967, Richard Doll stated clearly that prevention of cancer was a better strategy than cure.[7] He considered that an "immense" number of substances were known to cause cancer. In 1954, for instance, he stated, along with Bradford Hill, that besides cigarette smoking, exposure to nickel, asbestos, tarry products in gas production, and radioactivity, were major causes of cancer.[8] He believed that cancer rates varied with environment, geography and class, and he argued that poor, working class people, able to afford only a poor diet, were more likely to get cancer of the stomach. In the late sixties, Richard Doll could have been considered a radical.

Following the announcement of a 1968 study, which suggested that more women than was previously realized might suffer complications from the Pill, Doll found himself in a head-on confrontation with both the pharmaceutical companies and the moral hegemony of his profession. The "medical authorities" chose to interpret his report in such a way as to justify the conclusion that "the new assessment need cause no alarm among the million British women now believed to be using the pill."[9]

In common with other "public health" scientists of the pre-war and immediately post-war periods, Richard Doll considered that workers faced the greatest and most consistent threat to their health in the workplace. In October 1977 Doll spoke out against the research carried out by the National Radiological Protection Board (NRPB) and British Nuclear Fuels (BNFL) into the health risks of the nuclear industry; his message was unequivocal. Research by these organizations, he said, "had not been carried out in a way that would satisfy even an ordinary university department. They did not do what was recognized as necessary in

epidemiological studies — analyze all the available data."[10]

Again, in 1977, Doll came into conflict with the medical establishment, when he was outspoken about the yellow card scheme, a scheme used by doctors to report adverse drug reactions to the Committee on the Safety of Medicines. In that year it had become apparent that there were adverse effects to the use of Practolol (Eraldin), a heart drug which was withdrawn after five years, when it became apparent that it caused various illnesses in patients.

The importance of Doll's earlier work in shaping public health policy is beyond dispute. As he has grown older, however, his frequent public appearances on the world stage, like those of an aging rock star, have increasingly articulated an industry-accommodating view of public health risks.

The Two Paradigms

In the contemporary world, two paradigms vie for ideological power over public health, especially in the area of cancer diagnosis and treatment. The two paradigms do not present whole or homogeneous conceptual worlds; there are conflicts between them and on occasions they confoundingly dissolve into each other. Within the first paradigm, which has for some time been referred to, by detractors, as the "lifestyle" paradigm,[11] it is held primarily that lifestyles by themselves, and without reference to the environmental conditions in which they are conducted, determine the individual's susceptibility to cancer and other chronic illnesses. For Sir Richard Doll, the leading exponent of this view, the cancer rate is not increasing — nor indeed could it increase, because lifestyles are becoming healthier. In fact, he assures us, in the most important areas cancer cases are now falling and will continue to fall. Indeed, in 1985[12] Doll was of the opinion that cancer could be largely eradicated within the next few decades, which meant, in his opinion, that there was clearly no need for any further corporate or political regulation. (See also Peto, page 401.)

In reality there is a rising level of certain specific cancers, such as male testicular cancer, myeloma, cancer of the bone marrow, female breast cancer, male cancer of the mouth (which has doubled over 30 years), and deaths from cancer of the pancreas, which have increased considerably in women while staying level in men. There have been increases in cancer of the cervix and melanoma in the 20-44 age group and a rising death rate among men suffering from prostate cancer. In 1990, Sir Richard, discussing these figures, was still sure that *on the whole* "there is, to my mind, good evidence we have been winning the fight in Britain."[13] He reiterated this same message in 1992, when the *Independent* reported his views under the title of "Doctors gaining ground in war against cancer."

Nevertheless, Doll favors more cancer research and he is personally very much involved with the Imperial Cancer Research Fund (ICRF). However, like other lifestyle proponents, he insists that the focus should be largely on research into the minutest details of cell biology in order to determine the exact mechanism of carcinogenesis. Doll has stated that major cancer charities like the ICRF should not become involved in education or preventive work. The ICRF, he said, "as its name implies, is there to do research."[14] Needless to say, this does not include research into the effects of environmental carcinogens, which the ICRF generally refuses to consider.

The second paradigm, which we might call the "dissident" paradigm, represents a more socially holistic view of disease. Dissidents argue that many forms of cancer are rising alarmingly. Research as to the exact mechanism of carcinogenesis is a waste of energy and money, for chemical toxicity is partially or even largely to, blame for many, if not most, cancers, as well as for the fall in the general level of public health. Dissidents argue that policy makers have got to act now to

phase out the production of all reasonably well-established carcinogens.

Though Doll started off as a dissident, one who was clearly concerned with the health of the people he was serving, as his career developed his views gradually changed and he became one of the most powerful and influential promoters of entrenched industrial and political interests.

The Controversies

Smoking and Lung Cancer. Sir Richard first began publishing on smoking and lung cancer with Professor Bradford Hill in 1950. His two most effective early papers, published in 1954 and in 1956[15] recorded the results of a longitudinal epidemiological study based upon 40,000 postal interviews sent out to general practitioners in 1951. The first results analyzed the deaths of 789 of the doctors aged 35 and over who had died during the three years of the study. Thirty-six of them had died of lung cancer.

The conclusion, as has been continually reflected in the media, was, and has continued to be, that smoking is responsible for the huge increase in deaths from cancer of the lung. However, some responsible health care workers have asked whether or not smoking was perhaps not the sole cause, but one of a number of factors which might be "weakening the system in a way which makes it susceptible to cancer."[16] Major concerns along these lines have been raised by research carried out in China where the peasant population smokes heavily and where there appears to be little difference in the rates of lung cancer between smokers and nonsmokers.

Nevertheless, Sir Richard Doll's first major study has been bolstered by further studies that have come out with the same answer — lung cancer is almost entirely attributable to smoking. The political, social and economic effects of this singular message are still reverberating, despite the fact that today, lung cancer mortality rates for *nonsmokers* are rising.[17] To a degree, the success of this first work has become a screen behind which Sir Richard has dodged with increasing frequency, to avoid awkward but substantial issues about other man-made carcinogens.

Medical professionals, politicians, and health educationalists, reached a very speedy consensus on this issue, and other lines of investigation were consequently quickly abandoned.

By 1986 when *The Big Kill*, a 15-volume series, was published by the Health Education Authority[18] with consultative advice from Doll, an exact figure of individuals killed by smoking in England and Wales was given as 77,774, even though these deaths included those in which heart disease, bronchitis, and emphysema clearly also played an important role. In 1993 when Sir Richard was interviewed,[19] he cited a figure of 150,000 individuals who died prematurely as a consequence of smoking.

Questions have also been raised about the recorded incidence of death from lung cancer, said to be caused from smoking in the elderly. In the deaths of those over 65 it is exceptionally difficult to assess cause and even more difficult to establish what brought it on. These figures are not even addressed in *The Big Kill*, because as the Royal College of Physicians makes clear, ". . . this could not be done with much confidence, partly because certification of the cause of death in older people, who may suffer from a variety of disabilities, is less accurate than in younger people . . . no attempt has been made to estimate the number of deaths due to cigarette smoking in older people".[20]

This is a very weak excuse for excluding the elderly from the study — precisely those people who are most susceptible to cancer, and until recently those who constituted the major statistical group for the disease.

In the USA, Doll's thesis has always been rejected by Professor Samuel Epstein, Professor of Environmental Medicine at the University of Illinois, and founder of the Cancer Prevention Coalition, who for decades has fought a lonely battle against the medical establishment on this issue, though today at least sixty other scientists working in the field have now endorsed his position. In Great Britain, opposition to Doll's views came from Professor Simon Wolff, a toxicologist who was, before his premature death in 1995, the most committed of a new generation of scientists. Professor Wolff was particularly concerned about the effects of diesel and petrol exhaust pollution, which he saw as major factors in the development of lung cancer. He said:

There is no doubt that cigarette smoking causes lung cancer, but there is also no doubt that air pollution, particularly from diesel, is a contributory factor, so important that perhaps without air pollution we would see a much lower rate of lung cancer than we have. For example, in rural China, where people tend to smoke very heavily and where air pollution is much less, the differences in lung cancer rates between smokers and nonsmokers is very small, and lung cancer rates are about one tenth of the lung cancer rates in industrialized countries.[21]

Cancer and Diet. Doll does not accept that air pollution of any kind may be regarded as a cause of lung cancer or of any other diseases of the respiratory tract. These can only be attributed to smoking, which he sees as accounting for 30 percent of cancer deaths. Nevertheless, he does incriminate various natural — as opposed to man-made carcinogens. In a study commissioned by the American Academy of Sciences, which Doll conducted with his colleague Richard Peto in 1981,[22] he identified various natural contaminants of raw food as natural carcinogens produced during cooking. He sees these, together with obesity and the consumption of unspecified refined foods, as responsible for 35 percent of cancer deaths. In this report pollution and exposure to industrial products are seen to account for no more than 3 percent of cancer deaths.

Another "natural carcinogen" — alcohol — was incriminated in a report to the ICRF in 1982,[23] as both a cause of cancer of the respiratory tract and of the digestive tract. By 1983, the accent had shifted to the consumption of fats as a dietary factor in the induction of cancer.

Doll has advised people to consume more fresh fruit and vegetables, though, needless to say, he does not distinguish between fruits and vegetables produced organically and those produced by means of chemical agriculture, which contains all sorts of pesticide residues. Nor does he see the large number of food additives in the average modern diet as playing any role in the development of cancer. On the contrary, he has denied this over and over again, notwithstanding the fact that an ever increasing number of these chemicals have been classified by such organizations as the World Health Organization (WHO) and the Environmental Protection Agency (EPA) as proven or suspected carcinogens. This attitude very much colored his 1992 keynote address entitled "The Lessons of Life" at the Nutrition and Cancer Conference in Great Britain.

Agent Orange. Doll's refusal to accept that any man-made chemicals can cause cancer and other serious health problems could not have been better reflected than in the testimony he gave against the Australian veterans of the Vietnam war whose health had been devastated by exposure to "Agent Orange." Agent Orange was a mixture of the two well-established carcinogenic herbicides 2,4,5-T and 2,4-D (the former having since been taken out of production in every country in the Western world). Produced by the Monsanto Corporation, Agent Orange was used as a defoliant by the U.S. forces, and it was in the interest of that company that Doll acted.

2,4,5-T is generally contaminated with an impurity known as dioxin, one of the most toxic substances known. The smallest amounts of this substance can produce a total degeneration of the liver, and it has been found to be 70,000 times more deadly than cyanide. This did not prevent the American forces from using 2,4,5-T to defoliate Vietnam — to strip away the tree cover, so important for their Vietcong opponents. Great swatches of jungle were destroyed and as much as one tenth of South Vietnam's rural countryside was devastated. Monsanto did very well out of it, as production of 2,4,5-T rocketed from 5.8 million pounds in 1958 to 13 million pounds in 1964, and to 42 million pounds in 1968.[24]

In 1964, the National Cancer Institute commissioned a report to test the carcinogenicity of 2,4,5-T and it was found to cause birth defects, cleft palate and malformation of the kidneys in the animals tested. The report was kept secret.

In the meantime a large number of Australian veterans, whose health had been seriously affected while serving in Vietnam, campaigned for an inquiry into its effects.

A Royal Commission was eventually set up. Its focus was on soft-tissue sarcoma, the incidence of which had been linked in Sweden with the use of 2,4,5-T by two Swedish researchers, Olar Axelson and Lennart Hardell, at the University of Umea.[25] The Commission went out of its way to discredit the evidence provided by these researchers and ended up by giving 2,4,5-T a clean bill of health. Axelson and Hardell, however, refused to give in. Supported by other scientists, they accused the Royal Commission report of being "a most questionable document" and of being "full of misquotations, distortions of information, and even falsification of facts." In a later paper they accused the Royal Commission of "lying in order to be able to disregard apparently inconvenient results."[26] Going even further, they showed that *almost all the conclusions* of the report had been taken word for word from the evidence of Monsanto's Australia Ltd.

Sir Richard Doll wrote a personal letter to the judge who headed the Royal Commission, in which he gave the Commission's report his seal of approval, validated the defence evidence of Monsanto, and defended Agent Orange, while also attempting to destroy Hardell's scientific reputation.

"Hardell's conclusions," Doll wrote, "cannot be sustained, and in my opinion his work should no longer be cited as scientific evidence. It is clear, too, from your review of the published evidence relating to 2,4-D and 2,4,5-T (the phenoxy herbicides in question) that there is no reason to suppose that they are carcinogenic in laboratory animals and that even TCDD (Dioxin), which has been postulated to be a dangerous contaminant of the herbicides, is at the most, only weakly and inconsistently carcinogenic in animal experiments."[27]

This letter, the contents of which are irreconcilable with all the serious evidence on the subject, coming as it did from one of the most prestigious scientists in the field, had an electrifying effect. It could not have done more for Monsanto had he taken out a full-page advertisement in the world's biggest circulation newspapers.

Low-level Radiation. Establishment scientists, politicians, medical researchers, and doctors, have almost always argued that exposure to low levels of radiation has a negligible effect on human health. If the opposite could be proved to be true, the consequences for the nuclear weapons and the nuclear power industries would be intolerable.

William H. Taft, U.S. State Department attorney, in 1981 stated himself that "the mistaken impression (that low-level radiation is hazardous) has the potential to be seriously damaging to every aspect of the Department of Defence's nuclear weapons and nuclear propulsion programs. . . . It could adversely affect our relationship with our nuclear allies."[28]

Of course this view has not been endorsed by serious and objective scientists. Professor Linus Pauling, the double Nobel Laureate in the U.S., and Professor Andrei Sakharov in the USSR, calculated in the 1950s that millions of people would die prematurely from the ingestion of fission products resulting from fallout from atmospheric bomb tests,[29] and many others have said likewise.

Inevitably, Sir Richard Doll has been heavily involved in this field. In the 1950s, he was asked by the Government to look at the possible carcinogenic effects of strontium-90, a radionuclide generated by nuclear installations that mimics calcium and is taken up in the bones of growing children.

Doll was also engaged by the Medical Research Council (MRC) at that time to review all the research conducted on the Hiroshima survivors. In his report on this issue Doll accepted that those who had been directly exposed to the bomb when it exploded would have a higher risk of leukaemia and other cancers; not so, however, those who had been exposed only indirectly to the bomb. For them there was little risk of cancer or other health damage, and hence no evidence that low-level radiation in the form of fallout could do any damage.

In 1957 Doll had been engaged by the Government to assess the quantitative relationships between exposure to radiation and the development of cancer. He had carried out two epidemiological studies, the results of which suggested that there could be a quantitative relationship between radiation and leukaemia. At that time he still had an open mind on the subject.[30] However, by 1992 his tune had totally changed and he stated quite explicitly that "the effects of low-level radiation are so small as to be virtually zero." This has been the view he has expressed ever since, in spite of the mounting evidence to the contrary.

In 1987 Doll presented the findings of a study on "Cancer near nuclear installations" in *Nature,*[31] which looked at the cancer rate in the vicinity of all Britain's 15 nuclear power stations (made up of 36 nuclear reactors). Predictably it concluded that there was "no increase in childhood leukaemia near any nuclear power station." However, very shortly afterwards reports clearly demonstrating the existence of leukaemia clusters around nuclear installations began to appear. In August 1987, for instance, a government advisory group tried to establish the causes of the alleged increases in child leukaemia at Aldermaston, where atom bombs are produced, Harwell, the nuclear research centre south of Oxford, and Burghfield. The fact that leukaemia clusters existed in these areas was no longer denied, but the government advisory group still reported, very predictably, that they could not possibly be attributed to the activities of these three nuclear installations.

Even more embarrassing to Sir Richard Doll was the report, published in the *British Medical Journal* in October 1987.[32] The report contained the results of two studies of childhood leukaemia in Seascale, the village which borders on the Sellafield nuclear reprocessing plant. The first study looked at one group of 1,068 children born near Sellafield between 1950 and 1984, and another a group of 1,546 children born outside the area but attending local schools. The leukaemia and cancer cases occurred only in those children born in Seascale. This fitted in well with the findings of a report by Sir Douglas Black, former chief scientific adviser to the Department of Health, in 1985.[33] Both studies were conducted by Dr. Martin Gardner, Professor of medical statistics at Southampton General Hospital, and Dr. John Terrell, District Medical Officer of Health at West Cumberland Hospital, Whitehaven.

Gardner and Terrell concluded that the children with leukaemia and other cancers were those whose parents had worked at the Sellafield processing plant. These results endorsed the campaigning views of CORE (Cumbrians Opposed to a Radioactive Environment), the key environmental group in that area, who believed that "the damage is from radioactive particles first inhaled by prospective mothers from the atmosphere. In pregnancy the radioactivity is transferred to the fetus where it collects in concentrations up to a thousand times the level in the mother." Needless to say BNFL could not accept these findings. Their spokesman, Jake Kelley insisted that the retreatment plant was not to blame, and that "leukaemia in children can be caused by many things." It was predictably Sir Richard Doll who was engaged to give scientific weight to this denial.

In March 1989 Doll was engaged by the MRC and the ICRF to conduct yet another research program to assess cancer risks (lymphoid leukaemia) in under-25-year-olds in the population living within ten miles of a nuclear installation. The results of the study were again embarrassing.[34] The death rates were found to be 21 percent higher than the national average, yet this still did not persuade Sir Richard that there was a connection between radiation and leukaemia. In an interview with the *Daily Mail* he admitted that "until we find some other cause, we cannot say that it (radioactivity) is not responsible." Clearly though, he was very keen to find another cause, and hit on the idea of a leukaemia virus, which could easily have been introduced by newly arrived workers coming to work at the Sellafield installations. The novel theory was also advanced that the over-clean homes of nuclear workers rendered their children more susceptible to leukaemia viruses.[35] Shamefully, this speculative viral infection, for which there is not a shred of evidence, remains the official explanation spouted by the nuclear industry and the Government alike.

That same year the conference organized by the United Kingdom Atomic Energy Authority (UKAEA) advised the Government not to reduce the maximum annual dose for radiation workers, as had been proposed the year before by the National Radiation Protection Board (NRPB) and also by the United Nations Scientific Committee on the effects of low-level radiation, in the face of mounting evidence of the carcinogenicity of even extremely low levels of radioactivity. Clearly industry interests had to come first. Indeed, the new safety levels proposed from (50 to 15 millisievers a year) would have led the nuclear industry to incur extra costs which it would have had difficulty in meeting.[36]

In March 1992, the U.K. Co-ordinating Committee on Cancer Research, which consists of the major cancer charities, announced a £6 million study to test the various hypotheses that have been put forward to explain childhood cancer around nuclear installations. Doll, predictably, expressed his firm belief in the viral hypothesis. A colleague of Doll's, Professor Mel Greaves, tried to rationalize an embarrassingly unconvincing thesis on the grounds that homes had become much cleaner and that the risk of leukaemia increases with rising living standards. In this way cleaner homes, which made us vulnerable to persistent viruses, rather than the much more chemicalized environment of our more affluent society were conveniently incriminated.[37]

The Bomb Test Service Men. In the same way that Doll offered evidence against the Australian Vietnam war veterans, whose health had been devastated by exposure to Agent Orange, so was he engaged to demolish the case brought by Mr. Ken McGinley, Chairman of a group of 1,500 members of the Nuclear Test Veterans Association, who in the 1950s were used as guinea pigs in test trials and whose health was seriously affected by radiation.

The case was first investigated by the Ministry of Defence. The study was then funded by the NRPB and the ICRF, who, in spite of the fact that not one of the servicemen had been examined clinically, decided that there was no evidence to prove that any of them had suffered from higher than normal radiation exposure. The testimony given by Doll and Darby, based on a statistical study that revealed a high incidence of deaths from leukaemia and multiple myeloma (attributed, Doll said, to a "statistical quirk") among those servicemen who had been exposed to radiation, confirmed the conclusion of the study.[38]

A further study in 1993 on this same issue, by Doll and Darby, further confirmed their previous position, with minor reservations.

Significantly, though Doll has always refused to accept the connection between man-made radioactivity and cancer, he has always seen, for reasons best known to himself, *natural* background radiation as a major cause of leukaemia and other cancers.

Quite early on the NRPB had estimated that at least 2,500 people who lived in areas where there is a lot of granite, as in Cornwall, and were exposed to high levels of radon gas in their homes died of lung cancer every year in Britain. In 1990 however, Doll and Darby published a report for the ICRF in *Nature* which suggested that the figure may be as high as 5,000 cases a year.[39] Why, we might ask, if man-made radioactivity is so totally harmless, is natural radioactivity on the contrary so incredibly dangerous?

Doll's estimates of natural low-level radiation from radon were based on an assessment of the levels of lung cancer among uranium miners exposed to high levels of radon gas. They came only months after Doll and Darby had yet again denied cancers at sites of nuclear installations. They showed that a decreasing exposure to radiation, instead of leading to a lower risk of cancer, actually increased the risk of cancer — in other words, that very low levels of exposure to this natural radioactivity were particularly harmful. Given these conclusions, why have Doll and his colleagues always insisted that only very high levels of *man-made radioactivity* were harmful?

It is easy to demonstrate that in every field in which Doll has been involved he has systematically defended the interests of industry and the State, even when these are in total conflict with those of people in general, and are irreconcilable with all the established knowledge on the subject.

Asbestos and Cancer. In 1955 Doll had carried out a study of mortality in asbestos workers. His report[40] was considered a landmark publication showing that workers in the asbestos industry had a high risk of cancer.

By 1983 he was singing a different tune. His career as a defender of corporate interests was now well under way. A new report done by him and his assistant Richard Peto came to a totally different conclusion.[41]

The Society for the Prevention of Asbestosis and Industrial Diseases (SPAID) criticized the methodology used by Sir Richard in a letter to the *Sunday Times* on the 26th April 1985: "Sir Richard Doll," SPAID insisted, has "used so many estimates, adjustments, approximations, and hypothetical figures in order to assure us that only one person in 100,000 working in an office containing undamaged asbestos risks death, that SPAID is not reassured."[42]

Nor, for that matter, one must assume, were the 30,000 people in the USA whose health had been devastated by exposure to asbestos and who were seeking compensation from their insurance companies — not to mention the 500 new ones who were deciding to do likewise every month.

Anesthetics. There is some evidence that substances used as anesthetics have a damaging effect on health.[43] The results of a study carried out on the subject were published in the April 1979 issue of the *British Medical Journal*.[44] The study was based on a survey of the health of 10 percent of all the anesthetists in England and Wales — and it suggested that working with anesthetics had a generally adverse affect on their health status. In particular it noted that there were excess spontaneous abortions in the families of anesthetists, a lower fertility rate, a greater incidence

of cancer, and a greater likelihood that children of anesthetists would be born with congenital defects. The Medical Research Council predictably qualified the paper as "a one-sided review,"[45] and Sir Richard Doll, one of its leading lights, did not waste any time in stating his complete rejection of the study's findings.

Fluoridation of Drinking Water. Sir Richard Doll's role in the debate on the fluoridation of water supplies was equally predictable. It has been known for a long time that fluoride is a poison. In October 1944 the *Journal of the American Medical Association* published an editorial stating "that the use of drinking water containing as little as 1.2 to 3 parts per million of fluoride will cause such developmental disturbances in bones as osteosclerosis, spondylosis, and osteopetrosis, as well as goitre."[46]

In 1990 the American National Toxicology Program announced that it had established a clear link between fluoride and a type of bone cancer called osteosarcoma. It also indicated that fluoride might be responsible for a particular type of cancer of the mouth. However, it was in the interest of many powerful bodies that fluoride be added to our drinking supplies. This included the sugar industry and the aluminum industry, which was desperate to get rid of the vast amount of fluoride waste that its activities had generated.

Industrial interests were sufficient to influence the Royal College of Physicians' 18-member committee, which included Doll, to recommend the addition of fluoride to drinking water in January 1976.[47] The widespread criticism was raised that to impose this medication on the population at large without its prior informed consent, would be a breach of medical ethics.

Sir Richard Doll fully backed the report's conclusions, going even further than they did in declaring that, if anything, it was "unethical *not* to add fluoride to drinking water."[48]

Lead in Petrol. The role played by Sir Richard Doll in the long controversy over the effects of exposure to lead in petrol on the health of children was equally predictable. Lead was originally added to petrol in the form of the organic lead compounds: tetramethyl and tetraethyl, both of which are absorbed through the skin and are extremely neurotoxic.[49] In the 1960s and 1970s, it became increasingly clear that children absorbed this lead into their blood through their lungs and by eating contaminated fruit and vegetables. Clear evidence of health damage from organic lead in petrol began to appear in the late 1970s. However, in Britain and America, the petrochemical companies ran a continuous campaign in favor of maintaining lead in petrol and generally denying its deleterious health effects.

In May 1980 the Department of Health and Social Security (DHSS) published the report of a study carried out by the MRC entitled *Lead and Health,* written by the Lawther Working Party set up by the Department of the Environment (DOE).[50] The Working Party concluded that there was no evidence for clinical lead poisoning, which fitted in perfectly with the propaganda of the petrochemical companies. It even went further, claiming that the removal of lead from petrol would lead to increased cancer-causing hydrocarbon emissions.

A study carried out by two members of the Lawther Working Party, Dr. Yule and Dr. Lansdown,[51] drew conclusions that totally contradicted those of the Lawther Working Party.

Vehicle Exhaust: Lisbon, Portugal. They found that, in almost every case, among a group of schoolchildren whom they examined, body-lead levels correlated with IQ and school performance, more strongly than did the social class of the children. The *British Medical Journal* (BMJ) declined to publish this paper.

In 1983 Professor Derek Bryce-Smith and Dr. Robert Stephens refuted the DHSS report, accusing the MRC team of being hypercritical of all the studies which showed evidence of a relationship between levels of lead in petrol and mental function.[52] They also showed that the blood lead safety levels set by the DHSS report were without "real scientific or medical basis."[53]

However, in 1983 Sir Richard Doll was still arguing the case of the petrochemical companies. He insisted that there was not enough lead in the air to damage children's brains. Any adverse health effects caused by lead, he also insisted, were due to drinking water that had passed through lead piping. Lead in petrol could not be incriminated.[54]

From a Friend of the People to a Friend of the Powerful

What lessons can be drawn from the career of Sir Richard Doll? How can we explain, in particular, his and other research scientists' failure to appraise seriously the subject of cancer and the environment?

Today nearly all the major institutions of scientific research which study the effect of chemicals and other toxins on health are financed, managed, supported, or aided by chemical and pharmaceutical companies. As a result it is increasingly difficult to find independent scientists within the area of environmental health. Those academics who fight the corner for sufferers of chemically induced illnesses are an eclectic grouping of medical clinicians, social scientists, philanthropists and community activists. They have, however, one thing in common: they lack funding and have on the whole been prised away from real power.

The first British Labor government which came to power in 1945, was open to the idea that science and government could work *for* the people. In 1947, the Medical Research Council, which had been created before the war, set up a toxicology research unit.[55] Its aim was to monitor the growing use of chemicals, including insecticides, fungicides, and organic solvents, and their effects on human health.

In the early fifties, the MRC Toxicology Unit did indeed research pesticides, and especially the effect of organophosphate insecticides on human health. By the mid-fifties, however, the unit was moving slowly away from its original brief, pushing chemicals to one side and liberally extending the research to cover more esoteric subjects. Significantly, in 1956, one of the Unit's nine research subjects was the "toxic properties of certain plants used as herbal remedies in primitive societies."[56] The accent was already on *natural* rather than *man-made* poisons.

Over the next thirty years, the MRC, while preserving its Toxicology Unit, gradually dropped its research into toxic chemicals. During the 1970s and 1980s, as the drug companies increasingly offered funding, support, and partnership projects, the focus of research turned towards cell-biology, pharmaceuticals, and genetics. The emphasis was on the *good* rather than the *harm* that chemicals and industrial scientific processes could do. In the mid-1980's the Wellcome Foundation used the MRC as a vehicle for providing the scientific justification for the production of the first AIDS drug, AZT.[57] This was possible because by then the Council of the MRC was already dominated by individuals with vested interests in the chemical and pharmaceutical industry.[58] The very companies whose products should have been critically investigated by the MRC were, in one form or another, represented on the Council of Britain's most prestigious medical research body. It is no coincidence that Sir Richard Doll has held office in that august institution for most of his professional career. Nor is it a coincidence that its present Chairman, Sir David Plastow, instead of being someone with a lifetime professional preoccupation with the health of the British people, is a man whose interests have

been with the motor industry, whose polluting activities are a major source of lung disease, including lung cancer.

What is true of the MRC is also true of the main cancer charities. Decades ago they were relatively independent from industry, arguing the case for "the people." Now they are all but departments of large pharmaceutical companies. The Imperial Cancer Research Fund, for which Doll worked for a large part of his career, is a case in point. While most lay people imagine that it is simply a worthy charity collecting money to research cancer, few will understand that it is itself a multi-million pound corporation which hardly makes a move independently of professional science, or its industrial pharmaceutical patrons and backers.

Through its council and its benefactors, the ICRF is run by, and mainly for, the profit of the pharmaceutical companies, the very corporations whose products would have to be investigated in any wide-ranging investigation of cancer and the environment. The sort of cancer research that is supported by the ICRF and other cancer charities is that which seeks to find "cures" for specific forms of the disease.

The dissident position is of course that most of the money should go into searching for the environmental causes of cancer and then into wide-ranging preventive campaigns to eliminate the environmental factors involved. This emphasis, however, would bring cancer research into head-on conflict with its industrial backers.

In the introduction to his book *Wings of Death,* Dr. Chris Busby notes how ". . . the control of research and publication in the area of radiation-dose and effect, has been assumed by the nuclear and military establishment, a powerful international lobby which grew out of the need for secrecy relating to defense uses of nuclear fission, and the realization of the opportunities that there were for making immense amounts of money in this area."[59]

Thus, much of the research undertaken by the Great Britain Co-ordinating Committee on Cancer Research (CCR) on leukaemia and radiation, from the early 1990s onwards, has been funded by British Nuclear Fuels, the very company that operates the Sellafield nuclear retreatment plant right next to Seascale, where the biggest child leukaemia cluster in Great Britain has been found. BNFL and other nuclear industry groups gave Great Britain's CCR between £3 million and £6 million. The research undertaken was headed by none other than Sir Richard Doll.[60]

From 1979 to the end of his career, Sir Richard also received a very substantial yearly reward for research into cancer from General Motors.[61] This is of course hardly surprising given the wide range of problems which are increasingly associated with motor vehicle exhaust emissions, from global warming to cancer and various respiratory diseases.

Sir Richard has never hidden the source of this funding and has not even bothered to defend it. He does not feel there is any need to. In 1993, Doll wrote to Cumbrians Opposed to a Radioactive Environment (CORE), that had brought up the matter of Great Britain's CCR BNFL grant: "To imply that Great Britain's CCR was in some way under the influence of the nuclear industry . . . this is certainly untrue."[62]

The answer to that, of course, is that industry is not in the habit of funding research for the publication of studies which demonstrate the carcinogenicity of their products. On the contrary, all the evidence shows that it goes out of its way to suppress any such information which may occasionally surface.[63,64]

In 1996, researchers from the Center for Public Integrity (CPI), an American non-profit investigative research organization, set out to discover "how chemical companies manufacture controversial products, year in and year out, in the face of government regulatory efforts, civil litigation by citizens who feel victimized, and investigative news stories."[65]

They found that time and again Congress and regulatory agencies put the interests of the chemical industry before those of the public; that scientific studies financed by the chemical industry tended to find that suspected carcinogens, such as atrazine, formaldehyde and perchloroethylene, were "innocent," while scientific studies by non-industry sources tended to find them dangerous to human health.[66]

The CPI also uncovered an extensive PR machine operated by the chemical industry, often with the complicity of the regulatory agencies, as well as a million-dollar service industry organized by chemical companies and associated organizations, to provide courtesy trips for regulatory officials.[67]

"Today in Europe and America, wherever chemicals are likely to become the subject of criticism, the companies move in, balancing, propagandizing, controlling, mediating protests, funding pseudo-scientific research, buying people off, and funding social ventures to enhance their reputation."[68]

The dissident who questions the chemical companies, the industrial food companies, and inevitably the State, is branded as irrational, anti-science, and anti-technology, and hence as a subversive standing in the way of progress.

In his 1983 Harveian Oration, Sir Richard Doll warned against environmentalists, who might "whip up irrational prejudice, unfounded in science."[69]

Again, in 1992, writing in the *Daily Mail* at the time of the Rio Summit, Doll warned that we may be seeing "a new attitude emerge; an irrational ideology opposed to science, to industry, and to progress."[70] That attitude, he told us, exists already.

"There is, for example, a large and powerful lobby against pesticides, which they say leave cancer-causing residues in our food. Yet scientific research has shown that those residues are some 1,800 times less than the amount of cancer-causing agents naturally present in the plants. The lobby does not seem to object to natural carcinogens; only to the infinitesimally small amounts introduced by man."[71]

If this is the level of intellectual reasoning of Britain's greatest epidemiological scientist, then we should all pray for British science. Which edible plants have carcinogens in them 1,800 times more powerful than *which* pesticides? This, of course, he doesn't tell us. Nor could he, because these and similar statements routinely made by Doll and his sponsors, are pure fabrications.

The unbridled alliance of science and industry is transparent in Doll's *Daily Mail* article.[72] He defended industry on six different occasions in the short article and asked us, not without a dash of desperation, to trust industry and industrialists, science and scientists. These, he said, are the people with the key to the future. He ended the article with a warning that we must stop environmentalists whom he describes as the "anti-science Mafia," from "hijacking" the Rio summit.[73]

Sir Richard Doll believes strongly that whatever criticisms might be "laid at the door of industry and science," only "industry and science" can solve the problems of the modern world.[74]

He tells us too, against all the evidence, that the continual, unregulated, and untested introduction of chemicals into our food, can do the land, the farmers, and ultimately the consumers, nothing but good.

Fortunately Sir Richard and his colleagues are fighting a losing battle. It is becoming increasingly clear to the people that all this is not only false but the very opposite to the truth — mere propaganda for the chemical and nuclear industries that are, like the tobacco industry also, responsible for the present cancer pandemic. How many people today really believe that the leukaemia clusters found around just about all nuclear installations in Great Britain and elsewhere are caused by *viruses* introduced by outsiders? Who will believe that the main environmental carcinogens are natural ones like blue cheese, mushrooms, and radon gas? How many people really believe that asbestos, lead in petrol, and organophosphate pesticides are harmless? Fewer and fewer, as the serious, independent evidence inexorably accumulates.

The following two articles appeared in the March 27, 1980 and January 15, 1981 issues of Nature, *respectively. The first is a critical review of the first edition of* The Politics of Cancer *by Richard Peto, statistician to British cancer establishment spokesman Sir Richard Doll. The second is a response by the author and Joel B. Swartz.*

Peto's position is largely a defense of Doll's highly questionable "lifestyle" theory of cancer causation, which excludes any significant role for involuntary exposure to environmental and occupational carcinogens. Not surprisingly, this is attractive to industrial and governmental interests opposed to regulation of these carcinogens. But the response to Peto makes clear that the lifestyle theory is rebutted by a substantial body of scientific evidence. It may be further noted that Peto's review was triggered by the public discrediting of the British cancer establishment at a Labor (Trades Union Congress) Conference in Great Britain in June, 1979 (Chapter 15).

Distorting the Epidemiology of Cancer: The Need for a More Balanced Overview

By Richard Peto
From *Nature*†
March 27, 1980

There exist, both in the general environment and in certain occupations, chemical or physical agents which increase the likelihood of human cancer. Our political response to this would, in an ideal world where sufficient

---

† *Nature* 284:297-300, 1980.

knowledge was available, depend on the direct and indirect costs of the various possible measures of control, and on how many cancers each such measure would prevent. In the real world, estimates of the direct financial costs of the control of particular agents can easily differ by one or two orders of magnitude, the indirect costs may be grossly exaggerated, or some major indirect costs may be completely overlooked. Worst of all, we have in general no remotely reliable estimates of the numbers of cancers which particular legislative controls would prevent. Consequently, there is wide scope for pressure groups to have considerable influence on public policy.

Historically, the most powerful pressure groups in U.S. society have been the large financial interests, which have almost always put financial advantage before human health. Over the past few years the major tobacco companies have launched massive sales drives in the third world, which if successful will kill millions of people. (About one in four regular cigarette smokers is killed prematurely by smoking.) In the USA, where cigarettes cause well over 100,000 deaths every year from lung cancer or chronic obstructive lung disease, the tobacco industry refuses to accept in public that cigarettes cause either disease, let alone to collaborate in serious public information, and no epithet can suitably describe the collective efforts of their advertisers.

No other industry kills people on anything like the scale that the tobacco industry does, but where other industries have been found to cause cancer (or dust-induced lung disease) in their workers or in the consumers of their products, their immediate response has usually been to delay acceptance of the findings, to minimize their relevance to current practice, and in general to delay or obstruct any hygienic measures which will cost money. Even when human danger has been unequivocally demonstrated, industrial consortia may actively lobby for controls so weak that (as with the new British government regulations

limiting inhaled asbestos to 1 fiber/ml from 1981) they leave no reasonable safety margin. Large amounts of money are available to mount press or TV publicity campaigns about the homely apple-pie virtues of asbestos, journals financed by the tobacco industry run populist articles which misrepresent research results to lay readers, and some American television journalists are explicitly told always to censor all reference to the dangers of smoking.

Even the scientific literature is not immune from distortion by financial interests. The decades-long argument that "threshold" dose levels of carcinogens must exist below which the general population is absolutely safe has not been entirely motivated by the scientific plausibility of the hypothesis. With increasing understanding of the derivation of tumors from single cells acted on by mutagenic carcinogens, industry is slowly abandoning "threshold" arguments in favor of arguments[1,2] (where the biological fallacies[3,4] are somewhat better concealed by the mathematics) that thousandfold reductions in dose can conveniently be "statistically guaranteed" to produce a million-fold or some other enormous reduction in risk.

Even if the scientists who propounded such models are disinterested, industrial endorsement of them is not. Much excellent toxicology may be done by industry, and many industrial scientists and managers may be directly and honestly concerned with the prevention of hazards. But so many examples of financially-motivated bias exist that the motives and work of industrial scientists and consultants are inevitably distrusted.

Over the past quarter century, the "environmentalist" camp in North American society has pressed for (and achieved) stricter control of particular carcinogens in the workplace, the general environment, and the diet. Usually, their efforts have been directly resisted by the relevant financial interests. Inevitably, in view of the scantiness of reliable quantitative knowledge about the cancer risks to man of nearly all carcinogens, the argument has polarized. In the politics of cancer, each side takes a very extreme position. Industry usually argues for the irrelevance to man of animal or *in vitro* cancer tests, or minimizes the quantitative hazards and exaggerates the costs of control. The environmentalists usually exaggerate the likely hazards and are largely indifferent to the costs of control. The vacuum of reliable scientific knowledge is such that each side can find scientists who will maintain in courts, in public hearings or in the scientific literature whatever is politically convenient, and it is important to recognize that scientists on both sides of this debate now have career interests at stake in it.

A particularly good example of the biased writings of politically active environmentalists is Samuel Epstein's *The Politics of Cancer* (Sierra Club Books, 1978, revised in Anchor Press, 1979). Epstein outlines, for university-educated but not necessarily science-educated readers, his view of our present state of knowledge about prevention of death from cancer. He concludes that the cure rates for the major cancers have not been improving much over recent years, but that we do know enough now about the causes of cancer for the testing and regulation of environmental contaminants to prevent the majority of American cancer deaths, and that the main obstacles to our doing so are political rather than scientific. He therefore reviews the scientific and political circumstances surrounding a dozen or so disputed consumer products or occupational hazards, providing much fascinating political detail, and then describes at length the internal politics of the various agencies which research, regulate and litigate in Washington.

Epstein's book has been written to inflame political passions against environmental carcinogens, and parts of it are well worth reading. However, the political punch is often achieved at the expense of scientific accuracy

and balance. Despite this, the book has already gained wide and apparently uncritical acceptance even among scientists. For that reason, it is worth considering some of the misrepresentations of scientific evidence which it contains, and some of the more general defects in the environmentalist perspective on cancer.

First, a few details. Epstein's book is very useful as a source of reference to original papers, but it is not in itself a reliable secondary reference because the material presented is so often distorted. Sometimes this distortion is due to the effects of Epstein's vigorous campaigning style on his scientific judgement and is, perhaps, forgivable; at other times it appears to be deliberate, which cannot so easily be forgiven.

For example, consider the (by now generally agreed) finding that incorporation of about 5 percent by weight of saccharin into rat diets gives a few rats bladder cancer, but has no generally accepted effects on any other type of cancer. By human standards, 5 percent represents a vast saccharin intake (and so, of course, the industrial "Calorie Control Council" has tried to shrug off these findings). To refute the common reaction that "anything given in large enough doses will cause cancer in animals," Epstein's chief argument is to report that 0.01 percent saccharin has also been shown to be carcinogenic. In support of this extraordinary claim, he presents in tabular form the control and 0.01 percent data for selected cancers from certain multi-group feeding experiments, leaving out the observations from those same experiments which would have refuted it (Table 14.1). This appears to be a deliberate attempt to deceive the reader. It is not a casual slip in a 600-page book, as Epstein devotes twenty pages and two full-page tables to saccharin. His entire table 6.4, entitled "Tumors other than the bladder in rodents fed saccharin," appears to be so subject to artifacts of selection that it provides no evi-

Table 14.1 Data from OTA report[5] on the tumor sites selected for presentation in Epstein's book to substantiate the claim that 0.01 percent saccharin is carcinogenic. Groups selectively omitted in Epstein's book are marked with an asterisk. These omissions substantially alter the implications of the original data.

Saccharin dose (% in rat diet; these doses have no material effect on longevity)	Male or female lymphosarcomas (FDA, 1948)	Female breast (FDA, 1973)	Male breast (FDA, 1973)
0 (control)	0/20† (0 %)	6/26 (23%)	6/29 (21%)
0.01	8/14 (57%)	14/30 (47%)	14/25 (56%)
0.1	5/16 (31%)*	13/34 (38%)*	9/27 (33%)*
0.5	2/15 (13%)*	—	—
1	1/18 (6%)*	12/30 (40%)*	8/27 (30%)*
5	10/17 (59%)	12/27 (44%)*	7/25 (28%)*

* Omitted in Epstein's book.

† In addition to these 20, since some other sweeteners were being tested concurrently, 34 other control animals were studied in the same experiment, and the 1977 OTA review of these data, considering all the control animals to be equivalent, cited 9/54 control lymphosarcomas. (0/10 saccharin controls of each sex were studied, not 0/20 as Epstein inadvertently indicated.)

dence that saccharin does cause any rodent tumors other than in the rat bladder.‡

Saccharin is not an isolated example of bias; indeed, I found that in many places where he discussed data with which I was familiar, inaccuracies were present, almost always in the direction of accentuating the need for battle with the devils of industry.

Turning to more important matters, Epstein asserts that any benefits from the "less dangerous" cigarettes which the tobacco industry has developed will be outweighed by people increasing their consumption to get more nicotine, and he is therefore in many places particularly scathing about (or even downright opposed to) research into changed cigarette composition. This is a distorted perspective on one of the more promising immediate means

of preventing fatal cancers, a quarter of which in America are currently due to smoking.

Smokers of "less dangerous" cigarettes have already been found in various epidemiological studies to have disease rates which are materially lower than smokers of other cigarettes;[6,7] at autopsy they have far fewer "premalignant" histological changes in their bronchi and, perhaps due to the changes in cigarette composition 10 or 20 years ago male lung cancer death rates in early middle age are now decreasing in North America, in Britain and in Finland.[9]

After lung, the next commonest fatal cancers in the USA are those of the breast and the large intestine, for which the most striking epidemiological finding to date is a 90 percent correlation between fat consumption in different countries and their breast or colon cancer rates (see Figure 14.1; similar correlations exist for colon cancer).[10] Epstein suggests that dietary fat may merely be act-

‡ This accusation is totally without merit, and was fully rebutted in the author's letter to the editor of *Nature* (p. 411).

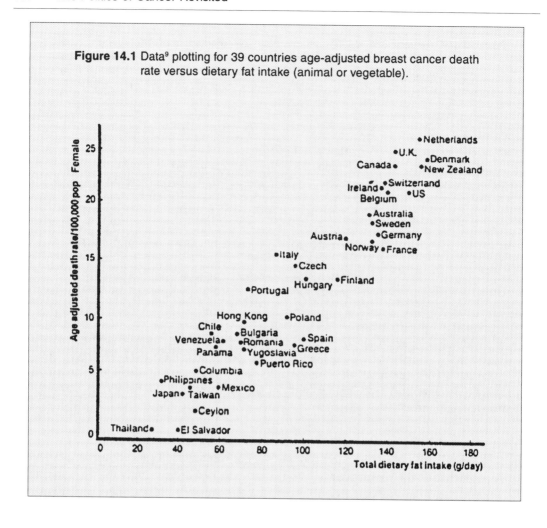

Figure 14.1 Data[9] plotting for 39 countries age-adjusted breast cancer death rate versus dietary fat intake (animal or vegetable).

ing as a vehicle for fat-soluble pesticides and industrial chemicals, which predictably emerge as his villains yet again. However, his suggestion is implausible: countries with high levels of contamination do not stand out from the general cancer/fat relationship, colorectal and breast cancer were common long before the widespread use of pesticides, and in experimental animals high-fat or low-fat diets can greatly enhance or reduce the risk of cancer.*[11] Something more interesting is waiting to be discovered in our diet than simple contamination by carcinogens.

The fat-associated and smoking-derived cancers collectively account for more than half of all cancer deaths, and people concerned with cancer politics should try to understand them considerably more accurately than Epstein appears to. One can list many other instances where Epstein's content or style are misleading or unbalanced. For example:

• The discussion of alcoholism and cancer is entirely erroneous because of failure to standardize properly for age.

• One of Epstein's chapters ends: "Eisen-

---

* By 1987, Peto had totally reversed his position on fat. At that stage, he recommended that the role of fats (particularly the absence of saturated fat from land animal products) was chiefly "be-

cause [it] *may well* avoid heart disease rather than because [it] *may well* avoid cancer." (*Science* 235, 1501, 1987.)

hower warned against the growing national threat of the military-industrial complex. The medical-industrial complex now appears to be as serious a threat."

• There is idealization of the value of long-term animal tests with concomitant denigration of the value of the Ames test and other short-term tests. This is one of Epstein's most inexplicable errors of scientific judgement, unless he wants cancer tests to be difficult and expensive for industry.

• He is irritatingly puritanical, sneering at "the plastic age which symbolizes how the value of our lifestyle has been degraded."

• He seeks by stylistic tricks to attribute to oral contraceptives some of the established hazards of hormone replacement therapy and of diethylstilbestrol.

• He claims that cancer costs the American economy over $25 billion per year. (In fact, cancer must be prevented for humane, not for economic reasons; without cancer, there would be three or four million more retired North Americans to support, costing over $25 billion per year).

And so on. He seems so certain about everything — how can anybody be justified in being so certain about so many details? Sometimes I know he's wrong, but more often (especially in the many places where inconclusive scientific results are presented as established fact) I know that nobody knows for sure. Lewis Thomas once wrote, in another context:

> The sceptics in medicine have a hard time of it. It is much more difficult to be convincing about ignorance concerning disease mechanisms than it is to make claims for full comprehension, especially when the comprehension leads, logically or not, to some sort of action. When it comes to serious illness, the public tends, understandably, to be more sceptical about the

sceptics, more willing to believe the true believers.

Epstein (like many others) is unjustifiably definite about three major issues. He seems certain that even after the effects of cigarettes have been allowed for, Americans live in an era of rapidly increasing cancer rates. But trends in recorded cancer death rates (and, perhaps more so, recorded incidence rates) over the past quarter century are biased upwards (since the cure rates for the major cancers have not materially improved) by improvements in medical care and cancer counting. These improvements have affected all sectors of U.S. society, but most particularly old people and previously poor people, especially blacks. Epstein, along with most other American commentators, does not allow for these biases even to the limited extent of restricting his attention to trends in age-specific mortality rates among middle-aged whites, where they might be expected to be least prominent.

Among middle-aged whites during the past quarter century, cancer cure rates have not materially improved, but some U.S. cancer mortality trends seem to be genuinely down (stomach, cervix) while some seem to be genuinely up (pancreas, melanoma, and certain lymphomas). I can discern no net pattern other than that due to the massive effects of smoking on lung cancer, although no extension to 1978 yet exists of the excellent 1950-67 trend analyses in NCI monograph 33. In Britain, the same is true[12] as long as we examine mortality in middle age. (Interestingly, although Epstein emphasizes that bladder cancer death rates among whites in the industrial northeastern USA are high, this may not be chiefly due to any current industrial hazard, for they have been decreasing both relatively and absolutely for a quarter of a century.)[13]

Epstein also seems certain that the majority of human cancer is caused by chemical and physical agents in the environment and could be prevented by their testing and regulation. There is no sound scientific basis for this certainty. Since the cancers (lung, breast, large intestine) which are commonest in the USA are rare in certain other countries, and *vice versa*, they probably really are preventable, but (Figure 14.1) not necessarily by regulation of any environmental pollutants or food additives. Indeed, one of the most intriguing animal findings is the effect in many studies of gross aspects of diet on cancer; for example, mice randomized between 5g of food once daily and *ad lib* consumption averaging 6g/day of the same food, had respectively 8 percent and 64 percent spontaneous mammary tumors,[14] and the role of dietary fat[11] has already been discussed.

Thirdly, Epstein seems certain that at least a quarter of all cancer deaths are attributable to occupational exposure to carcinogens. There is as yet no good evidence for hazards of anything like this magnitude, and there is clear evidence that many of his particular claims are exaggerated. For example, he says that asbestos has led to approximately 50,000 deaths per year in the USA from cancer and related disease (referencing a paper by Selikoff[15] which actually neither makes nor implies any such claim). This is sheer nonsense; of 50,000 asbestos deaths, several thousand should be certified as being due to pleural mesothelioma, yet only several hundred per year are thus certified.

Likewise, Epstein cites with approval (indeed, he describes it as being of "epochal significance") Health, Education, and Welfare Secretary Califano's absurd 1978 estimate, in a speech to labor union leaders, that as many as half of the 8-11 million workers who have been exposed to asbestos could develop serious diseases such as cancer or asbestosis. In his second edition, Epstein draws extensively on Califano's source, a curious but extremely influential document which has been circulating privately for the past year or more. This

unpublished typescript, with no listed authors, was prepared by a working group of nine well-known scientists including Arthur Upton and David Rall, the National Cancer Institute and National Institute of Environmental Health Sciences directors, both of whom still seem more ready to defend than to repudiate it.

Entitled "Estimates of the fraction of cancer in the U.S. related to occupational factors," it shows how a group of reasonable men can collectively generate an unreasonable report. The group multiplied the 12 million workers exposed in any way in 1972-4 to any of asbestos, As, Ni, Cr, benzene or petrochemicals by the very large risk factors (e.g. fivefold lung cancer excesses) typical of much more extensively exposed industrial populations, finally multiplying again by "4-5" to allow for the additional cancers that will be caused by these six agents among workers exposed to them at times other than 1972-4. (In casual disregard of dosimetry, this whole process is very like predicting 100,000 occupational lung cancer deaths per year among nonsmokers due to their exposure to other people's cigarette smoke at work, "since 20 percent of heavy smokers get lung cancer.")

These assumptions "predict" over 200,000 extra respiratory tract cancers per year in the near future due to the above six agents alone (and are the sole source of the currently widespread prediction of "20-30 percent" of cancers being due to occupation). But, in reality, fewer than 90,000 males/year get respiratory tract cancer in the U.S. (and most of these are due to cigarettes and not to occupation at all) and moreover the USA male rates in the first 25 years of working life are currently decreasing! A prediction of 100,000-200,000 extras due to the above six agents is clearly very unrealistic.

The unreality of the whole method is further highlighted by the fact that the assumptions "predict" 7,300 X 4.5 nickel-oxide induced occupational lung cancers/year. Since nickel refining causes a lot of nasal as well as lung cancer, we would presumably then also soon "expect" something like 13,000 nasal cancer death certificates per year among nickel workers. Nickel has already been widely used for decades, so many thousands of these should presumably already be evident. In reality, each year in the American population there are only 300-odd male and 200-odd female nasal cancer death certificates. The majority of these are not ex-nickel workers and no marked trends are evident. This demonstrates the unsoundness of the NCI-NIEHS methodology.

Unfortunately, such exaggerated estimates are so much what many people want to believe of modern society that they have now achieved a life of their own, and although they are utterly without foundation they are quoted widely, repeatedly and reputably both in the lay and scientific press. In Geneva the International Labor Organization reportedly endorsed them, as did the Toxic Substances Strategy Committee in their recent draft report to the American president,[16] and they have been used in OSHA to emphasize the need for stricter laws. Most recently, the British trade union the Association of Scientific, Technical and Managerial Staffs (ASTMS) released a policy document which appears to have been strongly influenced by Epstein's book, and which is notable for its prominent but erroneous assertion, derived solely from the foregoing unpublished American typescript, that 20-40 percent of current British cancer deaths are caused by occupational carcinogens.

Epstein now claims that these exaggerated estimates seriously underestimate the impact of industrial carcinogens. There is obviously a valid political need to exaggerate the importance of the preventive measures we can already implement, but in the long run we do also still need to discover the main preventable causes of cancer other than smoking. Bearing both these needs in mind, there are limits beyond which it is not even politically wise to distort the science of cancer, and some of today's exaggerations may well transgress those limits. Reliable reviews of the known and suspected causes[17-19] of human cancer and of trends in British death rates[12] should be more widely known.

My criticisms of Epstein's science, however, must be viewed in the light of the continued resistance of many industries to reasonable controls. One has only to read some of his descriptions of industrial behavior to see where his passion comes from, and a suitably sceptical reader could derive much important information from the dozen or so detailed case-histories of particular carcinogens that make up the bulk of this book. But, although I cannot prove it, I suspect that environmentalists as a whole (including Epstein and those U.S. and British trade unions which have already modelled their public statements closely on his book) would be better respected and could therefore press more effectively for controls in particular instances if their overview of cancer was more balanced in the following ways:

• if they accepted that present-day cancer rates and trends are probably not dominated by occupational carcinogens or environmental pollutants (especially since they could still warn that future rates might perhaps be so dominated unless present-day exposures are regulated);[20]

• if their chief concern was with the identification and control of the few major determinants of human cancer (or, in an industrial context, the few major industrial carcinogens) rather than the large multitude of sins which Epstein denounces;

• if they discussed the costs and benefits of research into the control of toxic substances in the context of other possible ways of improving longevity (bad diet and tobacco in rich countries, malnutrition and infective and parasitic diseases elsewhere);

• if they took the costs of imposing restrictions on society more seriously. Epstein's general assertion is that the total direct and indirect costs of failing to regulate usually exceed the real costs of the testing and regulation, but I suspect that this is a slogan to avoid political embarrassment rather than a carefully researched conclusion;

• if they accepted that for most toxic chemicals we have both qualitative and vast quantitative uncertainty about the health benefits of restriction.

Particularly, even if the sort of grossly biased interpretation which Epstein applied to the animal saccharin data is avoided, the results of animal experiments simply are not an uncomplicated key to human hazard identification. First, moderate alteration of gross aspects of the diet of animals greatly modifies their spontaneous tumor onset rates:[12] (so, for example, increasing the sugar content of rat diets may increase their cancer rates more than the equivalent amount of dietary saccharin would have done).[11] Also any chemical which causes proliferation or necrosis in any organ that is subject to spontaneous cancers is likely to modify the onset rate of tumors in that organ, and since the aim of most animal experiments is to study a dose which is nearly, but not quite, sufficient to cause significant weight loss or mortality within three months, it is not surprising that so many chemicals at such doses can cause cancer in animals.

However, it may be that where adversary politics operate one needs views at both extremes in order to get a balanced outcome. And there is a possibility that overemphasis on the avoidance of scientific error would emasculate the environmentalist passions and merely lead to my own rather inactive conservatism. (After all, no scruples about scientific certainty of safety usually precede the widespread introduction of new chemicals, so should the imposition of prudent restrictions require absolute proof?)

Environmentalists with biased judgements and a quasi-religious certainty of right will fight more battles than any reasonable sceptic would do, and even if their victories confer 10 or 100 times less benefit on humanity than they imagine, they will in the long run probably do more good than harm — unless they materially reduce food production, distort research priorities, or direct attention away from the smoking problem in the process. Epstein justly quotes, from the 1st century AD, the Plutarch chronicles: "He who in time of faction takes neither side shall be disenfranchised." So, I feel, should both environmentalists and industrialists who suppress or deliberately misinterpret data, but they probably won't be. For the moment, the "politics of cancer" is dominated on both sides by exaggeration.

Rebuttal
Fallacies of Lifestyle Cancer Theories

By Samuel S. Epstein and Joel B. Swartz
From *Nature*†
January 1981

Peto's article,[1] purporting to be a review of the book *The Politics of Cancer*,[2] is largely a restatement of the lifestyle theory of cancer causation. This theory postulates that if you get cancer it is essentially your own fault, and that the causal role of past involuntary exposure to environmental and occupational carcinogens is trivial. Not surprisingly, the lifestyle theory has emerged as the major professed basis of the chemical industry's objections to the regulation of its carcinogenic products and processes.[3] As an enthusiastic proponent of this theory, Peto asserts that smoking-derived and fat-associated cancers "collectively account for more than half of all cancer deaths." As a corollary, of Peto's emphasis on lifestyle factors, he denigrates the role of occupational and environmental carcinogens and the need for their effective regulation, claiming that

† *Nature* 289(5794):127-130, 1981.

Table 14.2 Age-adjusted cancer mortality rates per 100,000 U.S. population for selected sites by sex and year 1969-76, and average percent change[15]

Site	Sex*	Mortality rate per 100,000		Average % change 1969-76	
		1969	1976	Annual	7-Year
All sites	WM	195.0	210.2	0.9	7.8
	WF	129.0	133.8	0.5	3.7
Stomach	WM	10.6	8.7	-2.9	-17.4
	WF	5.3	4.1	-3.6	-22.6
Colon	WM	18.7	20.7	1.3	10.7
	WF	16.2	16.5	0.0	1.9
Rectal	WM	6.9	5.6	-3.0	-18.8
	WF	3.9	3.2	-3.1	-17.9
Pancreas	WM	11.0	11.0	0.0	0.0
	WF	6.6	6.8	0.3	3.0
Lung	WM	55.0	66.7	2.6	21.3
	WF	10.2	17.8	7.6	74.5
Melanoma	WM	2.0	2.6	4.0	30.0
	WF	1.4	1.6	0.8	14.3
Breast	WF	26.2	27.2	0.3	3.8
Cervix	WF	5.5	3.9	-4.9	-29.1
Uterus	WF	4.6	4.2	-1.7	10.5
Prostate	WM	19.0	21.0	1.2	8.7
Bladder	WM	7.1	7.5	0.6	5.6
	WF	2.1	2.0	-1.4	-4.8
Kidney	WM	4.3	4.5	0.6	4.7
	WF	2.0	2.1	0.7	5.0
Leukaemia	WM	9.4	9.2	-0.4	-2.1
	WF	5.7	5.2	-1.7	-8.8

For age adjustment the 1970 United States population was used as standard.
* WM, white male; WF, white female.

there has been no recent increase in cancer mortality rates other than that due to smoking. We shall demonstrate that there is scant scientific basis for the lifestyle theory, and that it is in fact contradicted by a substantial body of published evidence.

Cancer Rate Trends

Peto justifies his emphasis on lifestyle factors by dismissing evidence for recently increasing cancer rates, apart from "that due to the massive effects of smoking on lung cancer." However, there is substantial evidence to the contrary. Standardized cancer death rates, adjusted to the 1940 age structure of the total United States population, show a progressive overall increase of about 7% from 1935 to 1970[4] despite marked reductions of stomach cancer rates for unexplained reasons and of cervix cancer rates for reasons including the frequency of elective hysterectomy for non-malignant disease and the success of

Table 14.3 Crude cancer mortality rates per 100,000 population for selected sites by sex and year, England and Wales 1971-77, and average percent change[16]

Site	Sex	Mortality rate per 100,000		Average % change 1971-77	
		1971	1977	Annual	6-Year
All sites	M	265	283	1.1	6.8
	F	215	233	1.3	8.4
Stomach	M	30	28	-1.2	-6.7
	F	21	19	-1.7	-9.5
Large intestine	M	30	32	1.1	6.7
and rectum	F	34	35	0.4	2.9
Respiratory	M	106	112	0.9	5.7
	F	22	29	5.3	31.8
Breast	F	45	47	0.7	4.4
Uterus	F	15	16	1.1	6.7
Prostate	M	17	19	1.9	11.8
Bladder	M	12	12	0.0	0.0
	F	4.1	5.1	3.7	24.4
Leukaemia	M	7.0	7.2	0.4	2.9
	F	5.5	6.0	1.5	9.1

screening programs. These trends are consistent with standardized mortality data for the United States (Table 14.2),[5] where they are even more marked in black males, and with crude mortality data for Great Britain. (Table 14.3).[6] The overall rate of increase in U.S. cancer mortality in the 7-year period from 1969 to 1976 (5.5%), adjusted to the 1970 age structure, is substantial and comparable with that for the preceding 35 years, 1935 to 1970 (7%). The overall increase in incidence rates is even more marked than mortality rates in the past decade, involving a wide range of organs besides the lung (Table 14.4).[5] Moreover, the increase in incidence for all sites is comparable with that when lung cancer is excluded (Table 14.5).[7, 8]

Reliance on overall age-adjusted incidence or mortality rates alone is simplistic, as such rates can mask steep increases in organ-specific cancers in high risk population sub-groups, such as asbestos insulation workers or menopausal women treated with estrogen replacement therapy. The overall probability, at today's death rates, of a person born now getting cancer by the age of 85 is 27% for both men and women; this is increased from the 19% for men and 22% for women born in 1950.[9] Furthermore, recent cancer rate trends reflect exposures and events beginning some 20 or 30 years ago, when the production of synthetic organic chemicals was relatively trivial compared with the present levels. The production of synthetic organic compounds in the United States in 1935, 1950 and 1975 was about 1, 30 and 300 billion pounds per annum, respectively;[16] sharp increases have also been observed for a wide range of derived industrial products such as chlorinated hydrocarbon solvents, plastics and resin materials, and of industrial carcinogens, such as vinyl chloride and acrylonitrile. It is reason-

Table 14.4 Age-adjusted cancer incidence rates per 100,000 U.S. population (whites) for selected sites by sex and year, 1969-76, and average percent change[15]

Site	Sex	Incidence rate per 100,000		Average % change 1969-76	
		1969	1976	Annual	7-Year
All sites	M	346.6	374.0	1.3	7.9
	F	271.5	301.2	2.0	10.9
Stomach	M	15.4	12.6	-2.3	-18.2
	F	7.1	5.6	-3.7	-21.1
Colon	M	34.5	36.9	1.5	7.0
	F	30.6	31.4	0.7	2.6
Rectal	M	17.5	19.4	1.3	10.9
	F	11.1	11.4	1.2	2.7
Pancreas	M	12.1	11.5	-0.5	-5.0
	F	7.5	8.0	0.9	6.7
Lung	M	70.6	77.8	1.4	10.2
	F	13.3	23.7	8.6	78.2
Melanoma	M	4.4	6.8	6.8	54.5
	F	4.1	6.1	6.2	48.8
Breast	F	73.9	83.5	1.8	13.0
Cervical	F	16.0	10.6	-5.9	-33.8
Uterine	F	22.6	31.2	5.9	38.1
Ovarian	F	14.9	13.6	-0.4	8.7
Prostate	M	59.0	68.6	2.3	16.3
Bladder	M	23.8	26.4	2.3	10.9
	F	6.3	7.3	2.5	15.9
Kidney	M	9.0	9.6	1.2	6.7
	F	4.3	4.8	1.3	11.6
Leukaemia	M	13.2	13.1	-0.2	-0.8
	F	8.0	7.1	-1.0	-11.3

The 1970 population was used as standard for age-adjustment.

able to anticipate that greater production has been paralleled by increased exposure of increasing numbers of both the work force and the general public, which is likely further to accentuate increasing trends in cancer rates. It must also be recognized that before the 1976 Toxic Substances Act, which the chemical industry so effectively stalled for so long,[11] there were no requirements for testing chemicals before their introduction into commerce (with the exception of special-purpose legislation for drugs, pesticides, and food additives). Thus, the overwhelming majority of industrial chemicals now in use have never been tested for chronic toxic and carcinogenic effects, let alone for ecological effects.

Role of Smoking

As emphasized in *The Politics of Cancer*, (p. 104), "Smoking is the single most important cause of lung cancer, as well as of cancer at other sites, chronic bronchitis and em-

Table 14.5 Changes in U.S. cancer incidence rates from 1970 to 1975[17, 18]

| | Average % increase in incidence rate, 1970-75 | | | |
| | Cancers of all sites | | Cancers of all sites except lung | |
Groups	Annual	5-Year	Annual	5-Year
White male	0.9	4.7	0.9	4.6
Non-white male	2.3	11.9	2.7	14.3
White female	2.2	11.6	1.8	10.2
Non-white female	6.1	34.6	5.7	32.2

physema, and cardiovascular diseases." Less well appreciated by lifestyle advocates is that overemphasis on smoking is widely used to divert attention from occupational causes of lung and other cancers. Of the approximately 100,000 annual lung cancer deaths in the United States, at least 20% occur in nonsmokers. It is relevant that lung cancer death rates in nonsmokers approximately doubled[12] from 1958 to 1969, an increase maintained since. Furthermore, the role of occupational exposure to carcinogens was not recognized in most of the classic epidemiological studies which linked lung cancer with smoking. This led to overestimation of the contribution of smoking compared with occupational risks or to their possible interactions.

Thus, "we are unable to say how much of the risks attributed to cigarettes is a 'pure' cigarette risk and how much is cigarette times another, possibly on the job hazard."[8] Moreover, smoking and occupation are confounded variables, smoking among men being more prevalent in "blue-collar" workers than in professional and managerial classes.[13] Occupational causes of lung cancer include asbestos, radon daughters, nickel ores, chromium, arsenic, beryllium, mustard gas, vinyl chloride, and bischloromethyl ether, apart from incompletely identified carcinogens in

a wide range of industries such as rubber curing, tanning, steel (coke ovens), foundries, automobile, and petrochemicals. Thus, lung cancer rates in asbestos insulation and topside coke oven workers are as much as 10 times greater than general population rates.

Underestimation of the role of such occupational carcinogens has been assisted by the fact that lung cancer mortality rates, based on the International Classification of Diseases, fail to distinguish pleural mesotheliomas from lung cancers; there is evidence of substantial under-reporting of mesotheliomas (by about 75%) in high risk groups,[14] and even more so in occupations, such as automobile mechanics, where asbestos exposure has not been well recognized. There is a further lack of distinction between lung cancers of different histological types, some of which, such as adenocarcinomas, are less likely to be due to smoking than to occupational carcinogens.[15, 16] "In several instances where the risk of bronchogenic carcinoma has been shown to be increased among occupationally exposed groups, there has been an accompanying shift in the distribution of histologic types of tumors," away from the small-cell undifferentiated and squamous cell carcinoma of the lung, the principal types whose frequency is increased by smoking, in the direction of other types, particularly adenocarcinoma.[16] "This (shift) has been noted among metal miners, uranium miners, copper smelter workers, vinyl chloride polymerization workers, chloromethyl methyl ether production workers, and mustard gas manufacturers."[16]

Possible variations of smoking patterns fail to account for the marked excess in U.S. lung cancer rates identified in specific occupational exposures, particularly among ethnic minorities and migrants from southern states.[17] A further challenge to the dominant role ascribed to smoking seems to be provided by observations that the risk of lung cancer in certain occupational groups, such as American Indian uranium miners,[18] Swedish zinc-lead miners,[19] mustard gas workers,[20] copper smelters exposed to arsenic,[21] and chloromethyl methyl ether workers,[22] is about as high among nonsmokers as smokers, although the latency period is reduced in smokers, suggesting a possible promotional effect of smoking. It appears that the relative risks of lung cancer for smokers as against risks for nonsmokers may have been overestimated, particularly in less-than-lifetime studies.[23] Variations in smoking do not account for geographic excesses in lung cancer rates in U.S. males and females, which overall reflect proximity of residence to petrochemical and certain other industries;[23, 24] there are also data showing associations between levels of atmospheric carcinogens and lung cancer mortality rates.[25] It may be noted that a report[26] from Peto's own institution demonstrates that the correlation coefficient between lung cancer and smoking internationally explains only one-third as much of the variation as does the correlation between lung cancer and solid fuel consumption (0.4 versus 0.7; $r^2 = 0.16$ versus 0.49).

Overemphasis on the carcinogenic effects of smoking, and ignoring or discounting the role of occupational and other exposures, is extended by Peto and others to cancers of the bladder and pancreas which are variously characterized as related to or caused by smoking.[27,28] However, the relative risks for these cancers are several times less in smokers compared with nonsmokers than is the case for lung cancer. Excess bladder cancer rates have been identified in several occupational categories, including rubber, paint manufacturing and textile dyeing workers,[29] and among residents in highly industrialized countries,[30] particularly those with large chemical industry complexes.[31] Excess pancreatic cancer rates have also been reported in various occupations including steel and metal workers[32] and organic chemists.

Recognition of the important role of occupational exposures in lung cancers previously ascribed, exclusively or largely, to smoking in no way detracts from the recognition, emphasized in *The Politics of Cancer*, that the impact of smoking constitutes a "national disaster." There is no basis for regarding the smoking/lifestyle and occupational theories as mutually exclusive, particularly as these exposures may operate interactively. Furthermore, lifestyle is a somewhat misleading rubric for smoking as it restrictively implies voluntary personal choice. Placing responsibility for personal choice of an addictive lethal habit on young teenagers, the fastest growing group of new smokers, seems inappropriate. Failure to control smoking reflects a wide range of political and economic constraints, including massive press advertising by the industry which omits the word "death" from the guarded small print warning of danger, massive revenues to federal, state and local government from tobacco taxes, federal subsidies to the industry and unwillingness of governments to increase tobacco taxation or to develop incentives to tobacco farmers to diversify. It is also important that the industry has moved to open up massive new markets with high-tar cigarettes in less developed countries, where the population is poorly informed on the hazards

Table 14.6 International correlations between breast, colon and liver cancers and possible etiological variables[28]

	Correlation coefficients			
	Consumption of fat	Consumption of animal protein	Gross National Product	Total energy production
Breast cancer				
Incidence	0.79	0.77	0.83	0.70
Mortality	0.89	0.83	0.72	0.60
Colon cancer (M)				
Incidence	0.74	0.74	0.81	0.68
Mortality	0.05	0.86	0.77	0.69
Colon cancer (F)				
Incidence	0.78	0.80	0.82	0.67
Mortality	0.81	0.84	0.69	0.62
Liver cancer (M)				
Incidence	-0.49	-0.59	-0.42	-0.25*
Liver cancer (F)				
Incidence	-0.59	-0.67	-0.53	-0.31*

* "Liquid energy"

of smoking.

Role of Diet

Lifestyle proponents are on less sure ground when they bracket diet, excess fat and over-nutrition with smoking as the causes of the majority of cancer deaths. This claim is based largely on international correlations between consumption of total fat and rates for cancer of the breast and colon;[26] however, such correlations by themselves are not proof of causality. Similar correlations were found, in the same study from Peto's institution, between breast and colon cancers and other variables, such as Gross National Product and consumption of animal protein, which also appear to reflect industrialization[16] (Table 14.6). Furthermore, "epidemiologically, the case against fat is weak because there are populations that have a high fat intake and little bowel cancer."[33] Of two case control studies on the as-sociation between diet and breast cancer, one found no effect[34] and the other found trivial effects of fat and caloric intake, concluding that ". . . recommendations of major dietary modification as a possible preventive measure for breast cancer are clearly premature."[35]

Equally unconvincing are the studies, cited by Peto as corroborative evidence on the experimental effects of diet, which were largely concerned with the influence of fat on the incidence of tumors induced by chemical carcinogens and ionizing radiation, and the influence of caloric intake on the incidence of spontaneous and induced tumors. Not only were different variables defined in the animal and human studies — percent fat in the diet and total dietary fat, respectively — but increasing fat levels in the animal experiments were associated with increased incidence of skin, liver and breast cancers, whereas the reported correlations between fat consumption and liver cancer mortality are negative for both men and women (Table 14.6). Moreover, these experiments often failed to differentiate between variations of total dietary fat and caloric intake in test animals and to adjust caloric intake in controls to reflect dietary fat variations in test animals; the magnitude of the variations in fat and caloric intake required substantially to influence the incidence of induced and spontaneous tumors in experimental animals is generally far in excess of the dietary differences observed among the various human populations studied.[33] These experiments invariably failed to adjust the intake in controls of fat soluble carcinogens, present in fat as accidental environmental contaminants, to reflect variations of fat intake of test animals.

Peto's claim for the causal role of dietary fat in human cancer overstates the conclusions of those cited as the basis for his claims. Armstrong and Doll,[26] for instance, merely suggest that dietary fat levels may influence the incidence of colon and breast cancers, without asserting causality. Doll considers that diet may act by modifying the incidence of tumors induced by carcinogens or by acting as a vehicle for exogenous carcinogens[36] — a suggestion also made in *The Politics of Cancer* which Peto dismisses as "implausible." Carrol concludes that "although caloric intake may be a factor in human carcinogenesis, it does not appear to offer a practical approach to the problem."[37] As recognized by current concepts on the multifactorial etiology of cancer, there is a substantial probability that a wide range of influences, diet and other lifestyle factors included, modify individual responses to carcinogenic agents. To ascribe causality to any particular modifying factor requires a degree of scientific evidence that has not yet been presented for dietary fat.

Role of Occupation

Peto associates himself with the insistence by the chemical industry[2] and other lifestyle proponents that occupational exposures account for about 5%[2 (refs 38-40)] or "a very small proportion"[41] of all cancers. This view is based on ascribing given percentages to known or alleged lifestyle factors, including smoking, fatty diet and sunlight, leaving a small unaccounted-for residue to which occupational factors are arbitrarily assigned by exclusion. The authors of this simplistic hypothesis compensate for its tenuous basis by reliance on "educated estimates" and by making circular references to each other, often by "personal communication," as the responsible authority.

However, there are problems with such "guesstimates." First, they fail to consider the multifactorial etiology of cancer and the role of multiple causal agents, such as asbestos and smoking;[42] thus, the summation of known causes of cancer should properly exceed 100%. As one of the lifestyle authors recently stressed,[36] "there is now strong evidence to suggest that the risk of cancer is commonly increased by interaction of two or more factors." Second, current cancer rates reflect exposures 20 to 30 years ago, when production levels of occupational carcinogens were a small fraction of the present; such estimates should thus now be adjusted to reflect increasing numbers of workers exposed. Third, the authors of these guesstimates failed to consider the very limited nature of the data base on exposure to occupational carcinogens. Nor have they at any stage protested or even commented on the persistent refusal of the chemical industry to make such critical data available. In the absence of exposure data, it is even less clear how the "lifestylers" confidently arrive at their estimate of less than 5%.

Rather than addressing himself to such problems, Peto dismisses recent estimates of the importance of occupational carcinogens in a report by the U.S. Public Health Service[43] as exaggerated, unsound, and unreasonable. This report, prepared by nine named and internationally recognized experts in cancer epidemiology, statistics and carcinogenesis from three federal research agencies, is based on a National Occupational Hazard Survey which between 1972 and 1974 surveyed nearly 5,000 workplaces chosen to provide a cross-section of industry in the United States. The report estimated the total number of workers exposed to asbestos, nickel ores, chromium, arsenic, benzene and petroleum fractions, including aromatics. The excess cancers attributable to each of these carcinogens were derived by multiplying the number of exposed workers by known risk ratios and subtracting the "normal incidence" of the cancer.

The report concluded that "as much as 20% or more" of cancers in the near term and future may reflect past exposure to the six carcinogens considered. The uncertainties and limitations in these conclusions, including the possibility that exposures and risk ratios may have been overestimated in some instances, were clearly stated in the report, as were other considerations including the multifactorial etiology of cancer, and the role of lifestyle factors and their possible interactions with occupational exposures.

The possibility that this government report underestimates rather than overestimates the role of occupational exposures, for several reasons some of which are recognized in the report, has not been considered by its denigrators, including Peto. First, the calculations in the report ignore the role of radiation and of some ten epidemiologically recognized occupational carcinogens, other than the six considered. Second, the risk ratios considered may be artificially low as they were largely derived from less-than-lifetime epidemiological studies, which may thus underestimate the true risk in view of the long latencies commonly involved. Third, the report does not consider the many statistical and methodological constraints common to most occupational epidemiological studies[44] such as relatively small numbers of workers in many locations, changes in exposure patterns over

time due to employee turnover, plant shutdown, process and production changes and changes in management, all of which lead to fragmentation of health and exposure records, access to which is often restricted by industry. Fourth, the estimates fail to take account of the many chemicals recognized as carcinogenic in animals for which there are no exposure or epidemiological data. Thus, of 442 chemicals and industrial processes recently evaluated by the International Agency for Research on Cancer (IARC), epidemiological data are available for only 60 (14%), although evidence of experimental carcinogenicity was considered to be sufficient for 143 (32%).[45] Fifth, the estimates exclude high risk occupations with incompletely defined carcinogens, such as the steel, rubber and tanning industries. Sixth, the estimates do not adequately reflect conditions in small business where exposure levels are likely to be higher than in major chemical companies. Seventh, the report does not reflect major increases in the production of the occupational carcinogens it considered such as benzene, with the likelihood of recently increasing exposures. Eighth, the study examined only a limited number of sites, excluding cancers such as skin and bladder which are known to be occupationally related. Finally, the estimates neglect the possible role of fugitive point-source emissions of industrial carcinogens as causes for the excess of overall and organ-specific cancers, including lung, bladder, colon, pancreas and breast, in residents of certain highly industrialized counties.

This government report has received extensive support from various expert bodies, such as the Toxic Substances Strategy Committee, whose position has been endorsed by 17 federal agencies, and international groups, such as the International Labor Organization, and the U.S. and British trades union. The report has also received additional support in the critique of two consultants to the chemical industry's American Industrial Health

Council which concluded that "... the full range (of total cancer attributable to occupational exposure) using multiple classifications may be from 10 to 33% or perhaps higher if we had better information on some other potentially carcinogenic substances ... The annual number of cancer deaths attributable to asbestos is in the range from 29,700 to 54,000, which corresponds to a percentage range of the total cancer of 7 to 14%. ... Any argument over these numbers cannot detract from the fact that asbestos exposure was, as the authors (of the Government report) state, a major public health disaster. ... We also believe that reduction of exposure to carcinogens in the course of employment can certainly be expected to affect major reductions in the frequencies of occurrence of cancer and is one of the most promising applications of preventive medicine."[47] The American Industrial Health Council failed to release this critique until the record of the recent Occupational Safety and Health Administration hearings on regulation of occupational carcinogens closed.

Finally, there is no basis whatsoever for recent unsubstantiated allegations by Peto and others that all or most authors of the government report have disowned or rejected it or its conclusions (K. Bridbord, M. Schneiderman, and A. Upton, personal communication). It should be further emphasized that this 50-page report was prepared as a government document specifically for inclusion in public hearing records, and not for submission to a scientific journal.

Conclusions

Cancer is a disease of multifactorial etiology to which occupational exposure and smoking can contribute importantly, sometimes interactively. There have been substantial recent increases in cancer rates which cannot be accounted for by smoking alone. Smoking is the major lifestyle factor of importance in cancer, and evidence for the causal role of other lifestyle factors, particularly diet, is slender. The role of lifestyle factors has been exaggerated by those with an economic or intellectual investment in this theory, by largely excluding involuntary exposures to carcinogens and minimizing the role of occupational carcinogens. These considerations further illustrate the primary thesis of *The Politics of Cancer:* cancer is essentially a preventable disease which requires intervention and regulation at several levels, particularly the occupational and smoking. Failure to prevent cancer reflects major political and economic constraints which have hitherto been largely unrecognized or discounted.

Peto's Misrepresentations

The following letter was written by the author and published in Nature, *January 15, 1981.‡ It is a rebuttal of Peto's libellous charge (page 397) "a deliberate attempt to deceive the reader" with regard to the carcinogenicity of saccharin.*

Sir:

In reviewing my book *The Politics of Cancer,*[1] Peto[2] charged that one table (Table 6.4) selectively and deliberately omitted data that would otherwise have questioned the conclusion that low dietary doses of saccharin (0.01 percent) are carcinogenic in rats. This statement is incorrectly based on comparison of Table 6.4 with data in an appendix to the report of the office of Technology Assessment.[3] However, the caption of Table 6.4 clearly states that it is based on another table, prepared by Melvin Reuber for use in the congressional testimony on saccharin by the Health Research Group on 21 March 1977.[4] Peto persisted in publishing this serious allegation in spite of two warnings.

Peto also appears unfamiliar with the content of the Office of Technology Assessment's

---

‡ *Nature.* 289:115-116 (1981).

report, which he cites as the basis for his charges on saccharin. This report explicitly discusses Reuber's low-dose data and his conclusion that "the increased incidence of lymphosarcoma of the thorax in rats at the 0.01 percent . . . are highly significant in the saccharin study."[5] Reuber also emphasizes that the carcinogenic effects of saccharin in various studies were not always dose-related.

Contrary to Peto's impressions, inversions in dose-response data are not uncommon in both experimental and epidemiological carcinogenicity studies. Reasons for such inversions include competing risks, heterogeneity in tested populations, and statistical fluctuation, particularly when dose-response curves are shallow. Peto, also fails to recognize that saccharin has produced tumors in experimental animals at low as well as at relatively high doses.

Contrary to Peto's impression that "it is not surprising that so many chemicals (such as saccharin) at such (high) doses can cause cancer in animals," there is an overwhelming consensus in the qualified, independent scientific community that high-dose testing does not produce false positive results, and that this is necessary to reduce the insensitivity of carcinogenicity tests, reflecting the small number of animals tested, compared with large human populations at presumptive risk.[6] It is also well recognized that carcinogenicity testing in excess of maximally tolerated doses (MTD) can produce false negatives due to competing toxicity.

Peto's charge of selective omission of the saccharin data is not his only misrepresentation. After his circulation of drafts of his review to various U.S. experts in the autumn of 1979, Schneiderman, then Associate Director for Science Policy of the National Cancer Institute (NCI) and co-author of the government report on the importance of occupational carcinogens,[7] explained in a letter to Peto that breast cancer correlates as well with Gross National Product as fat, that occupation had

been ignored in studies exclusively associating lung cancer with smoking, that there have been major recent increases in lung cancer among nonsmokers and that there have been "big and frightening" recent increase in cancer incidence which cannot be accounted for by smoking or other lifestyle factors.

Similarly, Upton, then-director of NCI and a co-author of the report,[7] challenged the erroneous charge that a "4-5" multiplication factor was used to inflate the 1978 government estimates of cancer anticipated from occupational exposures. ". . . This simply is not true . . ."

Repeatedly, Peto dismisses as personal views statements in *The Politics of Cancer* to which he takes exception, rather than recognizing that they are based on fully referenced primary sources and without attempting to challenge these sources directly. For instance, he disparages the conclusion "that the cure rates for major cancers have not been improving much over recent years" without noting that this reflects cited NCI data. Peto refers to the "claims that cancer costs the U.S. economy over $25 billion per year" without recognizing that such figures are derived from NCI sources. Similarly, Peto criticizes as "misleading or unbalanced" references to the term "medical-industrial complex" without attribution to its source, referenced and identified in the text (page 52), as the caption of an editorial in *The Lancet*.[8]

Peto charges that the book denigrates the value of short-term carcinogenicity tests, which he asserts is a "most inexplicable error of scientific judgement." While problems of such tests, particularly the limited associations between carcinogenicity and Ames test data for compounds from a wide range of structural classes[9,10] are recognized, the book concludes (page 48) that there is a "range of useful applications" for these tests, particularly when incorporated into battery protocols.

Peto accepts that industries "delay or obstruct any hygienic measures which will cost money. . . . (and) that the scientific literature is not immune from distortion by financial interests." Peto apparently also accepts the wide range of case studies in *The Politics of Cancer*, which document a common pattern of constraints, including manipulation, distortion and destruction, in health, safety and economic data generated or interpreted by industry and its consultants. Yet he seems willing to accept studies sponsored or endorsed by industry as authority for the nearly exclusive lifestyle theory of cancer causation. Moreover, he is opposed to further regulatory controls on grounds of costs, professed "inactive conservatism," and because "for most toxic chemicals, we now have both qualitative and quantitative uncertainty about the health benefits of restriction." This seems a questionable basis for prudent public health policy.

Ames:
The "Natural Carcinogen" Proponent

The following four articles were published in Science *between September 1983 and May 1988. Geneticist Bruce Ames has characterized the importance of natural dietary toxins as cancer-causing agents and trivialized the importance of synthetic petrochemicals as carcinogens.*

Dietary Carcinogens and Anti-Carcinogens

By Bruce N. Ames
From *Science*, 1983*

Summary: "Comparison of data from different countries," writes Ames, "reveals wide differences in the rates of many types of cancer. This leads to hope that each major type of cancer may be largely avoidable, as is the case for cancers due to tobacco, which constitute 30 percent of the cancer deaths in the United States and Great Britain. Despite numerous suggestions to the contrary, there is no convincing evidence of any generalized increase in U.S. (or British) cancer rates other than what could plausibly be ascribed to the delayed effects of previous increases in tobacco usage. Thus, whether or not any recent changes in lifestyle or pollution in industrialized countries will substantially affect future cancer risks, some important determinants of current risks remain to be discovered among long-established aspects of our way of life.

"Epidemiologic studies have indicated that dietary practices are the most promising area to explore. These studies suggest that a general increase in consumption of fiber-rich cereals, vegetables, and fruits and decrease in consumption of fat-rich products and excessive alcohol would be prudent. There is still a lack of definitive evidence about the dietary components that are critical for humans and about their mechanisms of action. Laboratory studies of natural foodstuffs and cooked food are beginning to uncover an extraordinary variety of mutagens and possible carcinogens and anticarcinogens."

Professor Ames discussed certain possibilities — namely that 1) many of these mutagens and carcinogens may act through the generation of oxygen radicals; 2) oxygen radicals may play a major role as endogenous initiators of degenerative processes, such as DNA damage and mutation (and promotion), that may be related to cancer, heart disease, and aging; 3) dietary intake of natural antioxidants could be an important aspect of the body's defense mechanism against these agents; 4) many antioxidants are being identified as anticarcinogens; and 5) characterizing and optimizing such defense systems may be an

---

* *Science*. 221:1256-1264, 1983.

important part of a strategy of minimizing cancer and other age-related diseases.

Rebuttal

By Samuel S. Epstein and Joel B. Swartz, and co-signed by 16 leading experts in carcinogenesis and epidemiology.[†]
From *Science*, 1984[‡]

We commend Ames for his review of natural dietary toxins, but not for concluding that, rather than reducing exposure to environmental and occupational carcinogens, "dietary practices are the most promising area to explore" for reducing cancer risks. Ames' article, moreover, is flawed by substantial errors, omission of relevant data and reliance on tenuous hypotheses. These limitations are more significant in view of the major public health implications of Ames' article and the accompanying editorial by Abelson, press release, and publicity in the mass media.

Ames' position that there is no evidence for generalized recent increases in U.S. or British cancer rates, other than for cancers attributed to tobacco, is based on epidemiological analyses that, with tenuous justification, exclude people over the age of 65 and also blacks of all ages and attribute a near exclusive tobacco etiology to cancers of various organs in addition to the lung.[1] In fact, overall cancer rates have increased sharply since 1970.[2] Incidence and mortality rates in the United States, age standardized to 1970, have risen sharply since the late 1960s par-

ticularly for persons over 60, blacks of all ages, and a wide range of occupational subgroups.[2-4] From 1969 to 1976, mortality rates increased for white and black males by 8 percent and 17 percent, respectively, and for white and black females by 4 percent and 6 percent, respectively. While this increase was pronounced for lung cancer — 21 percent and 32 percent for white and black males, respectively, and 74 percent and 56 percent for white and black females, respectively — increases also occurred in other organs, including, for whites, the prostate (11 percent), male and female kidney (5 percent), and female breast (4 percent); sharper increases were noted for less common cancers, including those of brain, liver, esophagus, and multiple myeloma. Incidence rates rose more rapidly than mortality on an overall basis and for cancers of various organs, such as the colon, bladder, kidney, skin (melanoma), uterus, female breast, and prostate, besides lung;[2] for whites, cancers of sites other than the lung accounted for approximately 70 percent of the increase. The most recent data show persistence of these trends through 1980.[5] These trends are consistent with the theory that past exposure to industrial carcinogens, whose production have increased exponentially since the 1940s, are responsible for recently increasing cancer burdens.[3,4]

The assertion that smoking is responsible for essentially all lung cancer, and thus accounts for almost all recent increases in cancer rates, is negated by substantial evidence,[3] including (i) the more than doubling of lung cancer

[†] Eula Bingham, University of Cincinnati Medical School; Donald Dahlsten, University of California, Berkeley; Susan Daum, Albert Einstein College of Medicine, New York; John Gofman, University of California, Berkeley; Robert Harris, Princeton University; Joseph Highland, Princeton University; Ruth Hubbard, Harvard University; Marvin Legator, University of Texas Medical Branch, Galveston; Kenneth Miller, Oil, Chemical, and Atomic Workers, Washington, D.C.; Rafael Moure and Michael Silverstein, International Union, United Auto Workers, Detroit, Michigan; Glenn Paulson, National Audubon Society, New York; Marvin Schneiderman, Bethesda, Maryland; Joseph Wagoner, Springfield, Virginia; George Wald, Harvard University; and Bailus Walker, Commonwealth of Massachusetts.
[‡] *Science* 224:660-667, 1984.

rates among nonsmokers over the last two decades, with the proportion of these cancers in nonsmokers approaching 20 percent;[3,6] (ii) the sharply increasing incidence of adeno-carcinoma of the lung, which is less closely related to smoking than are squamous and oat cell carcinomas;[7] (iii) over the last three decades,[8] the decline in the proportion of smoking males and the tar content of ciga-rettes, while lung cancer mortality increased at a rate that cannot be accounted for by co-hort effects; (iv) the strong positive associa-tions, largely independent of smoking hab-its, between lung cancer and exposure to a wide range of occupational carcinogens, in-cluding vinyl chloride, mustard gas and chlo-romethylmethylether, and carcinogenic pro-cesses, such as copper smelting and uranium, zinc, and lead mining;[3,4] (v) lung cancer rates in black men that are now about 40 percent higher and have been increasing more rap-idly than in whites over the last 30 years, al-though blacks smoke less and start smoking later in life;[4,9] (vi) lung cancer rates that are almost equal in white and black women, al-though the proportion of whites smoking more than one pack a day is twice that of blacks;[9] (vii) a threefold increase in lung can-cer rates among women between 1950 and 1975, a steeper increase than could be ac-counted for by the modest rise in their smok-ing prevalence;[8] (viii) the major geographic variations in mortality rates due to cancers of the lung (besides other organs) that have been associated with workplace and commu-nity air pollution[10] and are not explainable by differences in smoking patterns; (ix) the shift of the highest lung cancer rates from northeastern to southeastern and south-cen-tral states after World War II industrializa-tion of the South; and (x) the divergent trends and directions observed between cancers of the lung, on the one hand, and, on the other hand, of other organs, including the esopha-gus, buccal cavity, and pharynx,[4] which have also been strongly associated with cigarette smoking.[1] These considerations in no way de-tract from the critical importance of tobacco as a major cause of preventable disease and death.

In his statement that high-dose exposure to occupational carcinogens "*might* also turn out to be important for particular groups of people" [emphasis added], Ames does not acknowledge the substantial literature on oc-cupational cancer. According to a 1978 fed-eral estimate, occupational exposure just to asbestos and five other carcinogens could, on a worst case basis, account for 18 to 38 percent of all male cancers in coming de-cades.[11] Even outspoken critics of these esti-mates, whose analyses Ames cites, concede that "the minimum proportion of all current cancer deaths attributable to occupation can hardly be less than 2% or 3%,"[1] 4000 to 6000 male deaths per annum. Asbestos and coke plant workers both have lung cancer rates five to ten times those of appropriate controls.[11] Some 10 million workers are now potentially exposed to 11 "high volume human carcino-gens and there are major excesses of cancers throughout a wide range of occupational groups, including oil refinery and petrochemi-cal workers, rubber and tire workers, weld-ers and metal-trades workers,[4] and atomic plant workers.[12] These studies are all the more important as two- to fivefold excesses in can-cer rates have generally been necessary be-fore they could be detected by standard epi-demiological techniques.[13]

Contrary to Ames, substantive studies have documented the carcinogenic effects of ur-ban air pollution or some related urban fac-tor. Accordingly, the World Health Organi-zation concluded that "it is probable that some urban atmospheric factor is involved [in the etiology of lung cancer], resulting from the air pollution from car exhausts, fumes from heating systems and industrial fumes;"[14] au-tomobile exhaust contains a wide range of car-cinogens, many common to tobacco smoke. In addition, many epidemiological studies have documented large geographical variations in standardized cancer mortality rates, on an overall and organ-specific basis, with higher rates in communities located near smelters, petrochemical plants and facilities producing nuclear weapons, and in communities with high levels of atmospheric pollution;[10, 15] definitive epidemiological evidence of carcinogenic and reproductive hazards from proximity of residence to hazardous waste landfills or industrial impoundments is not yet available, although preliminary data from sites such as Woburn, Massachusetts, are highly suggestive.[16]

Ames dismisses the possibility that carcinogenic synthetic pesticides, marketed since the 1940s, may contribute substantially to cancer rates, as their dietary intake is claimed to be 10,000 times lower than that of age-old "nature's pesticides." There is, however, much evidence to the contrary. For example, a number of widely used chlorinated hydrocarbon pesticides have accumulated by many orders of magnitude in certain foods to levels comparable to those inducing cancer in small groups of experimental animals.[17] Chub and trout in Lake Michigan have been found with aldrin and dieldrin residues above 0.3 part per million, and similar residues of chlordane and heptachlor have been found in the Great Lakes and in Long Island and New York City lakes: in 1983 Montana health officials warned against eating game contaminated with concentrations of heptachlor epoxide more than 100 times the Environmental Protection Agency's (EPA's) "acceptable intake level." Aldrin and dieldrin were found to be carcinogenic at dietary concentrations of between 0.1 and 20 parts per million in five separate rodent bioassays, and residues of chlordane and heptachlor have been found in concentrations in human fat similar to those found in rats in whom carcinogenic effects had been induced by these pesticides.[18] By all principles of extrapolation, such exposures would be expected to result in a significant excess of human can-

cers. The widespread use of chlordane and heptachlor for termite treatment represents additional major carcinogenic exposures. Indoor chlordane concentrations greater than an arbitrary interim guideline of 5 micrograms per cubic meter have led to the evacuation of more than 1500 contaminated homes at Air Force bases across the country[19] and to the petition by a New York State citizens' group, after the finding in April 1983 that 63 percent of 443 treated homes were contaminated, to ban the use of chlordane for termite treatment. Exposure to 5 micrograms per cubic meter of chlordane, approximately 50 micrograms per day for an average adult, according to EPA extrapolations that considerably underestimate risk for several reasons, including neglect of high-dose fattening, would be expected to increase lifetime cancer risks by as much as 0.1 to 0.5 percent.[20]

Ames' position on the significance of dietary burdens of carcinogenic synthetic pesticides is not supported by recent data on ethylene dibromide (EDB) residues, with concentrations up to 5000 parts per billion in flour and citrus pulp. EPA estimated, again using procedures that minimize risk, that lifetime exposures to "realistic worst case" dietary concentrations of 31 parts per billion of EDB would result in cancer risks of from 10^{-4} to 10^{-3},[21] about 300 to 3000 deaths per year: occupational risks were estimated to be as high as 40 percent. Ames has also objected to the regulation of EDB, saying that the "trace of the carcinogen EDB now allowed in food is insignificant;"[21] this in spite of the fact that available noncarcinogenic alternatives include aluminum phosphide for grains and cold storage for fruits and vegetables.

The minimal references by Ames to problems of poorly regulated exposures to a wide range of environmental and occupational carcinogens are in contrast to his exaggerated emphasis of the roles of high-fat and low-fiber diets and of charred foods as "major risk factors," although evidence for such risks, where not negative, is generally inconclusive. A recent report concludes that "in the only human studies in which the total fiber consumption was quantified, no association was found between total fiber consumption and colon cancer."[23] The position that high fat consumption is a major cause of breast and colon cancer is based on experimental and epidemiological studies.[1, 24] However, this evidence is weak and inconsistent.[3, 25] There appear to be no data on the correlation between the proportion of fat in the diet, the critical variable examined in the animal experiments, and rates of colon and breast cancers on a nation-by-nation basis; while those rates are strongly correlated with absolute fat consumption, this correlation is equally good with other measures of industrialization, such as per capita energy production.[3] Moreover, up to 20-fold increases in dietary fat were generally necessary to increase tumor yields in rodents after the administration of carcinogens, whereas between-country differences in total fat consumption are generally less than a factor of 2.[3] Finally, no evidence was found in two major case control studies of an association between fat consumption and breast cancer rates.[26] These considerations do not denigrate the importance of a prudent diet in the promotion of health nor the need for research in this area which could lead to future cancer prevention strategies; a low-fat and high-fiber diet not only decreases intake of fat-soluble synthetic carcinogenic contaminants but also reduces risks of cardiovascular disease and diverticulitis.

Evidence on the qualitative and quantitative significance in generalized diets of Ames' examples of "nature's pesticides" and on their carcinogenicity is unimpressive. For instance, conclusions about the carcinogenicity of pepper are based on the results of a single questionable study,[27] and the inference that mushrooms are carcinogenic is based on the identification in certain mushroom extracts of un-

stable diazonium compounds that are carcinogenic in mice only after artificial *in vitro* stabilization.

The implicit identification of mutagens with carcinogens, the implication of an identity in their underlying mechanisms, the blurring of the distinction between different types of mutagens, the identification of quantitative mutagenicity with the results of Ames' bacterial assay, and the derivation of carcinogenic potency from quantitative mutagenicity data are all of questionable validity.[28] Many mutagens are inactive in carcinogenesis tests, and many carcinogens are inactive in short-term tests for mutagenicity;[29] glutathione is positive in the Ames test,[30] although Ames recognizes it as an anti-carcinogen and an anti-mutagen. Furthermore, recent evidence has suggested that gross mutagenic events, such as chromosome translocations, are more likely to be crucial in carcinogenesis than are the point mutations or deletions detected in the Ames assay.[28] Moreover, while somatic mutations are likely to be involved in carcinogenesis, epigenetic events also appear critical.

Ames' discussion of free radicals and the potential anti-carcinogenic effects of antioxidants is speculative and of dubious relevance. Even one of the authors cited in support of the thesis that carotenoid antioxidants are protective in smokers has admitted that various studies revealed only "a slightly lower than average incidence of cancer among people with above average intake of B-carotene" and that even this slim association may be artifactual.[31] A recent large-scale case control study[32] produced no evidence "relating intake or serum levels of antioxidant vitamins to a reduced cancer risk."

Evidence for major carcinogenic effects of trace natural components of U.S. diets is speculative. Strategies based on this hypothesis offer little hope for cancer prevention, and the hypothesis affords no basis for Ames' trivializing the importance of reducing exposure to occupational and other environmental carcinogens. Understandably, such strategies are applauded by corporations resisting regulation of their carcinogenic products and processes and seeking, with others, to explain away cancer causation largely in terms of diet and faulty lifestyle.[1] Strangely, Ames' current proposals appear at variance with his strongly argued recent positions.[33] These include warnings that EDB is "a potent carcinogen whose presence as an impurity in tris-BP [tris (2.3-dibromopropyl) phosphate] is one of the reasons why this flame retardant "should not be used"; that there are "enormous possible [carcinogenic] risks" from inadequately tested industrial chemicals, such as flame retardants; that a "steep increase in the human cancer rate from [industrial] chemicals may soon occur . . . as the 20- to 30-year lag time for chemical carcinogenesis in humans is almost over;" that "tens of thousands of man-made chemicals have been introduced into the environment in the last few decades — with widespread human exposure to low but disturbing doses of these carcinogens" and that such chemicals should be tested for mutagenicity and carcinogenicity; and that priorities must be established to "minimize human exposure to these chemicals."[33] Clearly there is substantial evidence that, besides smoking, involuntary exposures to occupational and industrial environmental carcinogens are major and generally avoidable contributors to the burgeoning national cancer burden and to a wide range of other chronic diseases. Vigorous public health measures are essential to reduce such exposures.

Ranking Possible Carcinogenic Hazards

By Bruce N. Ames, *et al.*
From *Science**
1987

Summary: This review discusses reasons why animal cancer tests cannot be used to predict absolute human risks. Such tests, however, may be used to indicate that some chemicals might be of greater concern than others. Possible hazards to humans from a variety of rodent carcinogens are ranked by an index that relates the potency of each carcinogen in rodents to the exposure in humans. This ranking suggests that carcinogenic hazards from current levels of pesticide residues or water pollution are likely to be of minimal concern relative to the background levels of natural substances, though one cannot say whether these natural exposures are likely to be of major or minor importance.

Rebuttal:
Carcinogenic Risk Estimation

By Samuel S. Epstein and Joel B. Swartz and co-signed by 15 leading experts in carcinogenesis and epidemiology†
From *Science*‡
1988

In their widely publicized and popularized article "Ranking Possible Carcinogenic Hazards," Bruce N. Ames *et al.* (17 Apr. 1987, p. 271) conclude that "analysis on the levels of

---

* *Science.* 236:271-280 (1987).
† John Bailar, McGill University, Montreal; Eula Bingham, University of Cincinatti Medical School; Donald L. Dahlsten, University of California, Berkeley; Peter Infante, Washington, D.C.; Philip Landrigan and William Nicholson, Mount Sinai School of Medicine, New York; Marc Lappe and Michael Moreno, University of Illinois Medical Center; Marvin Legatot, University of Texas Medical Branch, Galveston; Franklin Mirer, Rafael Moure and Michael Silverstein, United Auto Workers, Detroit; David Ozonoff, Boston University Medical School; Beverly Paigen, Oakland Children's Hospital, Oakland, CA.; and Jacqueline Warren, Natural Resources Defense Council, New York.
‡ *Science.* 240:1043-1045 (1988).

synthetic pollutants in drinking water and of synthetic pesticide residues in foods suggests that this pollution is likely to be a minimal carcinogenic hazard relative to the background of natural carcinogens" and thus that the "high costs of regulation" of such environmental carcinogens are unwarranted. These conclusions reflect both flawed science and public policy.

Although Ames *et al.* challenge the validity of animal carcinogenicity data for quantitative estimation of human risk, they nevertheless use such extrapolations, based on the percentage Human Exposure dose/Rodent Potency dose (HERP), for ranking carcinogenic hazards. Apart from the fact that HERP rankings are based on average population exposures excluding sensitive subgroups, such as pregnant women, the derived potencies of Ames *et al.*, doses inducing tumors in half the tumor-free animals, are misleading. Potencies for "synthetic pollutants," such as trichloroethylene, are derived from bioassays in which lowest doses are large fractions of the maximally tolerated dose (MTD), whereas potencies for more extensively studied "natural carcinogens," such as aflatoxins, are generally derived from titrated doses, orders of magnitude below the MTD. Since dose-response curves are usually flattened near the MTD,[1] potencies derived from high-dose testing yield artificially low risk estimates; HERPs for "synthetic" carcinogens are thus substantially underestimated compared with many "natural carcinogens."

Compounding this misconception, Ames *et al.* maintain that carcinogenic dose-response curves rise more steeply than linear curves and that tumor incidences increase more rapidly than proportional to dose. At high doses, dose-response curves are usually less steep than linear curves,[1] as also recognized elsewhere by Ames and his colleagues.[2] Thus at MTD doses, large further dose increases may induce only small increases in tumor incidence, perhaps reflecting compe-

tition between transformation and cytotoxicity;[3] linear extrapolations from high-dose tests thus underestimate low-dose risks.

For Ames *et al.*, the term "carcinogen" heterogeneously includes direct and indirect influences, including promoting and modifying factors and mutagens. Caloric intake is considered "the most striking rodent carcinogen." However, no correlations have been established between food intake and tumor incidence among animals eating ad libitum, despite wide variations in caloric intake and body weight,[4] nor have correlations been established between obesity and most human cancers. In the statement by Ames *et al.*, "at the MTD a high percentage of all chemicals might be classified as 'carcinogens'," toxicity and carcinogenicity are confused. However, among some 150 industrial chemicals selected as likely carcinogens and tested neonatally at MTD levels, fewer than 10 percent were carcinogenic.[5] Many highly toxic chemicals are noncarcinogenic, and carcinogen doses in excess of the MTD often inhibit tumor yields. While Ames *et al.* revive the discredited theory that chronic irritation causes cancer, most irritants are noncarcinogenic, and there is no correlation between nonspecific cell injury and carcinogenic potency.[6]

Ames *et al.* classify ethanol as carcinogenic, "[one of the two] largest identified causes of neoplastic death in the United States" along with tobacco; their HERP indices for a daily glass of wine and "average" occupational exposure to formaldehyde are similar. In four rodent tests cited by Ames *et al.*, alcohol was noncarcinogenic; in the fifth, an experiment with alcohol of undefined purity, carcinogenicity was "extremely low." While epidemiologic studies have incriminated alcohol — particularly in promoting or synergizing tobacco smoke, in upper digestive tract cancers, and also in inducing cirrhosis, a risk factor for liver cancer[7] — there is no evidence incriminating alcohol per se as a potent carcinogen for the general population, particularly nonsmokers. Although two cohort studies not cited by Ames *et al.* demonstrate weak associations between breast cancer and alcohol consumption,[8] their significance is limited by minimal dose-response relationships, several contrary studies, and the contamination of alcoholic beverages with carcinogens including urethane, methylglyoxal, nitrosamines, and pesticide residues.

While diffusely defining carcinogens, Ames *et al.* artificially categorize them as "natural" or "industrial," saying that the former hazards should somehow limit concerns on the latter. However, dietary levels of "natural carcinogens" such as aflatoxins and dimethylnitrosamine are influenced by harvesting and storage technologies and nitrite additives, respectively. Moreover, predominant exposure to other "natural carcinogens" results from industrial activity; examples include asbestos, heavy metals, uranium, and formaldehyde. While emphasizing "natural carcinogens" and "nature's pesticides" in food as major carcinogenic exposures, Ames *et al.* ignore natural dietary anticarcinogens and antimutagens, such as porphyrins, phenolics and retinoids.[9] Although risks from aflatoxin and alcohol, described as two most important and potent carcinogens, depend on synergism with hepatitis B virus and tobacco smoke, respectively, risk estimates for most synthetic carcinogens are based on single-agent exposures only. While "natural carcinogens" have long played a role in human cancer, concerns must also focus on recent incremental effects of increased production of and exposure to nonsynthetic carcinogens, such as asbestos and heavy metals, and on the novel and escalating production and exposure to "synthetic carcinogens."[10] Although some petrochemicals have been proved to be carcinogenic, most have not been tested; moreover, much industrial data is at best suspect or unavailable.[11]

The National Institute for Occupational Safety and Health estimates that 11 million workers are exposed to ten high volume industrial carcinogens.[12] Up to tenfold increases in organ-specific cancer rates are reported among those who work with asbestos, uranium and arsenic and in coke plants and among those exposed to specific petrochemicals and to some 20 less well-defined processes, such as dry cleaning, spray painting, and plumbing;[12] excess childhood leukemia is also associated with parental occupational exposures to organic solvents and related chemicals.[13] Just one of the few well-studied occupational carcinogens, asbestos, responsible for up to 10,000 annual cancer deaths,[14] is second only to tobacco of all known causes of human cancer.

Growing evidence demonstrates that pervasive contamination of air, water, soil, and food with a wide range of industrial carcinogens, generally without public knowledge and consent, is important in causation of modern preventable cancer. Even if hazards posed by any industrial carcinogen are small, their cumulative, possibly synergistic, effects are likely substantial. Eating food contaminated with residues at maximum legal tolerances of only 28 of 53 known carcinogenic pesticides, excluding numerous other carcinogenic pesticides and incremental exposure in drinking water, is estimated to be potentially responsible for 1.5 million excess lifetime U.S. cancers.[15] Trichloroethylene is a common contaminant of drinking water, generally resulting from improper disposal of industrial wastes; lifetime consumption levels of 250 parts per billion found in contaminated wells in Woburn, Massachusetts, together with other related carcinogens not considered by Ames *et al.*, is associated with excess risks of cancer,[16] childhood leukemia, perinatal deaths, and birth defects.[17] Some 20 retrospective and case control studies have associated trihalomethane-contaminated water with gastrointestinal and urinary tract cancers.[18] As only a few organic drinking water contaminants are characterized,[19] and as inhalation and cutaneous exposures may be as important as ingestion,[20] risk estimates, excluding possible interactive effects, are likely to be misleadingly low. Nevertheless, Ames *et al.* ignore these limitations and also the substantive epidemiologic data and assert that "the animal evidence provides no good reason to expect that chlorination of water or current levels of man-made pollution of water pose significant carcinogenic hazards," and that the risk from contaminated Woburn water is 1/10,000 that of a glass of wine.

Community air pollution from industrial emissions, and thus proximity of residence to certain industries, is a recognized cancer risk factor. Numerous studies, controlled or stratified for smoking, demonstrate associations between excess lung cancer rates and heavy metal and aromatic hydrocarbon emissions;[20] exposure to benzo[a]pyrene, a conventional combustion index, increased lung cancer mortality by 5 percent per nanogram per cubic meter of air.[21] Others estimate that "the proportion of lung cancer deaths in which air pollution is a factor is 21 percent."[22] Concerns have recently focused on defined industrial emissions, including arsenicals, benzene, chloroform, vinyl chloride, and acrylonitrile, which in both sexes are associated with excess overall and organ-specific, standardized community cancer rates; carcinogenic trace metals and volatile organic community air pollutants, have been incriminated in some 0.6 to 2.3 per 1,000 excess lifetime cancers.[23] Ames *et al.*, however, trivialize risks from "general outdoor air pollution."

Ames *et al.* state that cancer mortality rates "have mostly been steady for 50 years" apart from "lung cancer due to tobacco and melanoma due to ultraviolet light." This is based on analyses that exclude people over 65 and blacks of all ages[24] and which ignore the following: effects on mortality rates of the approximately 70 percent reduction in gastric and cervical cancer mortality since the 1940s which have been masked by increasing mortality from cancers at other sites; probability estimates that have projected marked increases in mortality rates for a wide range of malignancies for those born in 1985 compared with those born in 1975;[25] very recent increases in premenopausal breast cancer mortality;[26] the role of nonsolar causes of melanoma;[26] and the role of other major causes of lung cancer besides smoking.[27] While smoking is a major cause of lung cancer, the importance of other causes is evidenced by increasing rates in highly urbanized and highly industrialized communities; disproportionately increasing rates for black males not attributable to smoking pattern differences; increasing rates in nonsmokers while rates for other tobacco-related cancers, such as those of the buccal cavity and pharynx, are declining; increasing rates in some groups of nonsmoking workers; increasing rates in women, greater than can be accounted for by increased smoking; and, increasing proportions of lung cancers that are adenocarcinomas, which are less closely associated with tobacco smoking.[12, 27] Incidence rates, not considered by Ames *et al.* and which can "reveal changes in cancer occurrence that are not apparent in the mortality data,"[26] from 1950 through 1985 increased overall by 37 percent; by 20 percent or over for pancreas cancer; by 51 percent for urinary bladder cancers; by over 100 percent for non-Hodgkin's lymphoma, multiple myeloma, and malignant melanoma in both sexes; by 31 percent for female breast cancer; by 92 percent for testis cancer; by 67 percent for prostate cancer; and by 63 percent for colorectal and 142 percent for kidney cancers in males.[26, 28]

Apart from fundamental problems inherent in Ames's views on carcinogenesis and his dismissal of concerns about industrial carcinogens as "chemophobia," positions editorially endorsed,[29] his current views and recommendations contrast strikingly with those previously and strenuously propounded.[30]

Besides proper concerns about naturally

occurring carcinogens and tobacco, prudent policy must reflect overwhelming data on incremental exposure to industrial carcinogens and their association with increasing cancer rates, besides reproductive, neurotoxic, and other toxic effects.[31] The existence of natural hazards clearly does not absolve industry and government from the responsibility for controlling industrial hazards. From public health, ethical, and policy perspectives, the important distinction is not between "natural" and "synthetic" carcinogens, but between preventable and non-preventable cancers.

Note:

With the advent of the Reagan Administration, and the abrupt shift in federal policies and research funding away from indus-

---

Figure 14.7 Ames's flip-flop

In the 1970s:

In 1977, Ames demands urgent steps to "minimize human exposure to (synthetic) chemicals," pointing to "enormous possible (carcinogenic) risks" from inadequately tested industrial chemicals and predicted that a "steep increase in the human cancer rate from these suspect . . . chemicals may soon occur . . . as the 20-30 year lag time of chemical carcinogenesis in humans is almost over."

In 1977, Ames warned that the pesticide ethylene dibromide (EDB) is a potent carcinogen whose structural similarity to Tris is one of the reasons why EDB "should not be used."

In 1977, Ames emphasizes need for high-dose testing in an effort to compensate for the "inherent statistical limitation in animal cancer tests" and expresses concern about "the effects of the large-scale human exposure to the halogenated carcinogens [including] vinyl chloride, strobane-toxaphene, aldrin-dieldrin, DDT, trichloroethylene and chlordane/heptachlor." Ames urges the need to establish "priorities for trying to minimize human exposure to these synthetic chemicals."

In 1979, Ames shows that cancer dose-response curves usually rise less steeply than linear curves and criticizes the view that many carcinogens have activity only at very high doses.

In the 1980's:

In 1983, Ames claims cancer rates are not rising, that synthetic carcinogens pose only trivial risks and that the real culprits are natural carcinogens, faulty lifestyles, tobacco, and high-fat diets." Ames later (1987) further revised his thoughts on the role of high-fat diets as merely "a possible risk factor in colon cancer."

In 1986, Ames argues that before EDB was banned, it was present in 'trivial' amounts in food and that "the average daily intake was about 1/10 the possible carcinogenic hazard of aflatoxin in the average peanut butter sandwich, a trivial risk itself."

In 1987, Ames challenges the validity of using animal tests to estimate human carcinogenic risks claiming "there is little sound scientific basis for this type of extrapolation." Ames calls for the "need for more balance in animal cancer testing to emphasize . . . natural carcinogens as well as synthetic chemicals."

In 1987, Ames maintains that cancer dose-response curves rise more steeply than linear curves and that tumor incidence increases more rapidly than proportional to dose.

trially generated hazards in the direction of generous allocations to research on lifestyle and the blame-the-victim theories of cancer causation, without apparent embarrassment, Ames developed positions diametrically opposed to those he had enthusiastically advocated only a few years previously (Figure 14.7). By 1984 (*Science.* 221:1256-1264), Ames was trivializing the role for industrial carcinogens, concluding that "natural carcinogens and mutagens" represented a much greater public health hazard. The wide range of errors of omission and commission reflected in the Ames *volte face* were subsequently detailed in a rebuttal letter in *Science* (S. S. Epstein and J. Swartz. 224:660-667, 1984).

Chapter Fifteen

The British Parallel

Labor Protests Against the Cancer Establishment

The following two articles from British journals reported on a seminar given by the author in London on June 20, 1979, which dealt primarily with cancer in the workplace. These articles illustrate the striking similarities between the politics of cancer in the U.S. and Great Britain.

Scientists Reticent

By Lawrence McGinty
From *New Scientist* (Great Britain)
June 28, 1979

When the General and Municipal Workers Union (GMWU) decided to organize a series of seminars on cancer in the workplace — a thoroughly commendable idea — it tried hard to find British scientists to address the three meetings it planned. The GMWU is one of the few British trade unions to have a safety officer, and there are clear signs that it intends to campaign vigorously for stricter control of carcinogens in the workplace. Such a campaign is much overdue — too long have trade unions been content merely to win compensation for their members disabled or debilitated by exposure to chemicals at work, leaving the more political problem of controlling carcinogens to "the experts." This abdication of responsibility left the Health and Safety Executive (HSE), which has responsibility for controlling carcinogens at work, at the mercy of the chemical industry.

Scientists unconnected with the chemical industry might therefore be expected to leap at the opportunity to help the GMWU to develop its campaign. But *the union could not find a single British scientist of stature willing and able to give any of the three seminars it was organizing.* Instead, it invited Bruce Ames from California to talk about short-term testing for carcinogens and last week it paid for Sam Epstein to fly from Illinois to the second of its seminars (held jointly with the Association of Scientific Technical and Managerial Staffs). Epstein is a leading member of a group of scientists in the U.S. which, in the past five years or so, has put its expertise at the service of trade unions and public interest groups campaigning for tighter control of carcinogens (and other dangerous chemicals).

Could it be that scientists in Britain are not happy to be linked — financially and otherwise — to the chemical industry, an industry which, as Epstein has detailed in his book *The Politics of Cancer,* has deliberately destroyed, distorted, and suppressed inconvenient research findings? Outspoken criticism on environmental issues has certainly cost some scientists advancement and recognition in their fields. The platform and political protection that campaigns such as the GMWU's provide for scientists may not be ideal — trade unions are not above criticism. But at least it is a platform.

The Politics of Cancer

From *Medical World* (Great Britain)
June/July 1979

A searchlight was swept over the problem

Press Release General and Municipal Workers' Union (Essex, England)

The Politics of Cancer
June 20, 1979

Dr. Sam Epstein, Professor of Occupational and Environmental Medicine at the University of Illinois, has been invited to the country to give the second in a series of seminars on the evidence for carcinogenicity which the GMWU began last year. We have asked him to give a seminar tomorrow on the use and limitations of animal testing and a lecture in the afternoon on how carcinogens are identified and controlled in the USA.

The main points that Dr. Epstein makes in his recent book *The Politics of Cancer* are:

1. Cancer is reaching epidemic proportions and is likely to increase with the rise in consumption of chemicals;

2. The cost of not controlling cancer is enormous. Apart from incalculable human costs the community in the USA pays $25 billion a year for its cancer problem — the equivalent of about £3,000 million for Great Britain's population;

3. Most cancer resources go to treatment and basic research, with little effect on the survival rate or incidence of cancer;

4. Most cancer is preventable if we reduce or eliminate exposure to carcinogenic agents;

5. There is sufficient knowledge of carcinogenicity and of the laws needed to prevent exposures to carcinogenic agents. However, the short-term needs of industry predominate over the medium- and long-term needs of the community so that effective control of carcinogens is not achieved;

6. Industry has produced inadequate and distorted data in the past and cannot be relied on. Independent testing and quality control of industry testing are needed;

7. There is only a very limited role that individuals can play by changing their lifestyle;

8. Only concerted political action by trade unions and public interest groups can force Governments to recognize and legislate for cancer prevention;

9. Dr. Epstein's points are illustrated with case studies from the Workplace (asbestos, vinyl chloride, Bischloromethylether, Benzene) from Consumer Products (Tobacco, Red Dyes 2 and 40, Saccharin, Acrylonitrile, Female Sex Hormones) and from the General Environment (Pesticides, Aldrin/Dieldrin, Chlordane/ Heptachlor, and Nitrosamines.

Dr. Epstein's book has helped the GMWU to reach the following conclusions:

(a) A British version of his book could not be written because there is little published evidence available about either the testing; the views of scientists and industry; the costs of controlling and not controlling cancer, etc. Our closed and confidential system of controlling carcinogens and other toxic substances does not lead to the publication of the type of information which makes *The Politics of Cancer* so illuminating. The U.S. Freedom of Information Act, the use of open hearings to determine control limits, and the use of the courts are some of the ways in which U.S. society opens up the debate for public participation. We need something similar in Great Britain.

(b) The trade unions need to establish close links with sympathetic scientific expertise to assist them in developing their own policies on particular substances and issues.

(c) The Government, trade unions and public interest groups need to have access to independent testing and research institutions so that we are not reliant on industry data.

(d) The urgency of the situation requires immediate action. We have therefore produced a preliminary Cancer Prevention Program which we hope will speed up the process of cancer control in Great Britain.

of the cancer epidemic now afflicting the wealthy nations when ASTMS held a joint seminar with the General and Municipal Workers at the TUC Centenary Institute in London on June 20.

The main speaker was Dr. Sam Epstein, Professor of Occupational and Environmental Medicine at the University of Illinois, who has recently published in America a book entitled *The Politics of Cancer.*

Dr. Epstein's thesis is that cancer has reached epidemic proportions and is likely to increase with the rising consumption of chemicals. It is enormously costly to the community, both in human and money terms.

Yet most cancers can be prevented if the exposure to carcinogenic agents is reduced. The necessary controls are not being achieved because the short-term needs of industry are taking precedence over the long-term needs of the community. Industry has produced inadequate and distorted data that cannot be relied on. Prof. Epstein condemns as "white collar crime" this suppression and even destruction of data about carcinogens.

He makes a powerful call for independent testing, regulation within industries and concerted action by trade unions and public interest groups to force governments to legislate for cancer prevention. Among the many substances with which he is concerned are:

- In the workplace: asbestos, vinyl chloride, and Benzene.

- In consumer products: tobacco, Red Dyes 2 and 40, Saccharin, Acrylonitrile, and female sex hormones.

- In the environment: pesticides, Aldrin/Dieldrin, Nitrosamines, and Chlordane/Heptachlor

Addressing the afternoon session of the Seminar, which was chaired by Professor J. Corbett McDonald, director of the TUC Centenary Institute of Occupational Health, Prof. Epstein said his major thesis was that cancer was a disease, the major determinants of which were economic and political, not scientific.

It was the only major disease on the increase, affecting one in every four and killing one in every five. Between 1933 and 1970, there had been an overall basic increase in cancer mortality rates of 11 percent. But between 1970 and 1976 the overall increase had been 2 percent per annum.

"Cancer is not a disease of the elderly exclusively," he said. "It affects all ages. It is a major cause of child disease and death. Cancer is not a disease of degeneration but a consequence of exposure to carcinogens."

Contrary to optimistic assurances, our ability to cure cancer had not materially increased over decades. The increased rates of survival for five years from one in every four people affected to one in every three, reflected, not an improved ability to cure and treat, but advances in antibiotics, surgical skills and blood transfusion. "Progress has been abysmal," he said.

"But the information we have developed over the last few decades on the influence of cancer in the environment — in food, water and workplace — has accumulated. How is it that such information has not been implemented in regulating practice so as to reduce the incidence of cancer?" The reasons lay in political and economic constraints.

Of the 400,000 cancer deaths per annum in the U.S., some 100,000 were due to lung cancer — and of these 100,000 victims, 80,000 smoked. Did this mean smoking caused 80,000 cancer deaths a year? Criticizing the assumption of such an exclusive relationship between tobacco and lung cancer, he said that of 25 retrospective epidemiological studies, all had omitted taking into account the occupational history and the possible interaction between tobacco and industrial carcinogens such as asbestos. "Automatically, the authorities blame the victim for smoking as the cause of his lung cancer, irrespective of whether he has been exposed to occupational carcinogens."

Dealing with environmental hazards, he said there were areas in the U.S. where people living in proximity to the chemical industry — women as well as men — suffered an excess of cancer mortality. "The closer you live to petrochemical industries, the greater your chances of getting cancer."

In the U.S. when the government had attempted to ban certain chemicals or institute certain work practices, they were faced with two- or three-year court battles during which industry still had the right to maintain production and exposure of people to the suspect materials.

In 1940, in the U.S., they were manufacturing and liberating into the atmosphere one billion pounds per annum of synthetic organic chemicals. By 1976, it was 300 billion pounds per annum. In 1976, the Toxic Substances Regulations gave the government agency the authority to require testing of materials before production.

Five Factors

He listed five factors supporting evidence for the environmental and occupational causes of cancer:

1. An absolute increase in cancer, over and above increases reflected in increased longevity.

2. Greater still increases in high risk groups.

3. Major variations in incidence from area to area. These cannot be ascribed to genetic factors since when people migrate from a high risk area to a low risk area, the cancer incidence decreases.

4. The results of a wide range of studies of carcinogenic effects in animals.

5. The massive increase in exposure to synthetic organic chemicals.

In the U.S., every major piece of regulation against environmental and occupational carcinogens had stemmed from labor or public interest groups. None had emerged from the so-called independent scientific community. None had emerged from government and, of course, none had emerged from industry. But these regulatory authorities were pitifully small, he said.

Prof. Epstein dealt in scathing and satirical terms with the response of medical authorities to this 20th century epidemic. Some $200 billion dollars were spent on health care in the U.S. "Medical expenditure is a leading growth industry. Short of some catastrophe, such as National Health Insurance, it will give you an excellent return on your dollar," he said. He contrasted this with the total amount spent on cancer prevention from all federal agencies — $200 million dollars.

He examined the strategies used by the chemical industry to block regulatory efforts to limit the exposure of public and workers to carcinogens:

1. Blame the victim. The victim was told: "It is your own fault. You smoke too much, drink too much" or "you are highly susceptible."

2. Whenever evidence of hazards develops, industry says it is just animal, not human data.

3. Exaggeration of the utility of the product and of the difficulty of regulation. There were numerous chemical agents to which public and workers were exposed, the value of which to society was problematic or absent. The only possible benefits went to shareholders.

4. Exhaust the agencies. When an agency attempts to regulate, appeals in the courts made by industry go on for two or three years and the regulatory process grinds to a halt.

5. Flight of the multi-nationals. If you have to restrict or regulate the materials, export them to yellow and black peoples. There

has been a massive flight of materials to Mexico and the East, to countries ignorant of the crop of diseases which will await them 10 to 20 years from now.

6. Propagandizing. Millions are spent on advertising which says chemicals are safe unless mishandled.

7. Control of information. Data is developed by in-house scientists eager for promotion or by commercial testers eager for next year's contract with the industry. In both instances there are unspoken pressures to produce information consistent with the short-term interests of industry.

Prof. Epstein gave examples of the "white collar crime" committed under these pressures.

Experiments were designed to prove what industry wanted. Data was suppressed or destroyed. Records were manipulated and reports made on non-existent experiments. There was also manipulation of the economics.

"The Asbestos Papers"

Prof. Epstein referred to documents which he called the "Asbestos Pentagon Papers," which show that the asbestos industry in the 1930s had overwhelming evidence of the hazards and conspired to suppress it. He gave the example of a Canadian plant where workers were not told of X-ray evidence of asbestosis.

"As long as the man is not disabled, it is felt he should not be told of his condition so that he can live and work in peace and the company can benefit by his many years of experience," said a report from the firm's medical director.

Prof. Epstein called for a "national constituency of labor, public interest, and consumer groups." It could also include the churches, who were trying to find a mission in modern society, and old-age pensioners who were strongly affected by failure to regulate.

"Every society has its own political tools and it would be presumptuous of me to offer

blueprints," he said. It would probably be more difficult in Britain than in America because of the draconian Official Secrets Act and crippling libel laws.

In the discussion which followed, Jean Robinson, on behalf of the Cancer Prevention Society, said her field was cancer in women where there was blame of the victim. In cancer of the cervix, the victim's sexual behavior was blamed, whereas it was known, for example, that there was more risk to a woman with a miner husband. A high breast cancer rate was associated with the clothing trade. Yet in the last occupation and mortality study, there had been no analysis of female cancer. "Even experts in this country are not looking at causes," she said. "Some of us lowly amateurs are trying hard, but by God it is a battle."

Prof. Epstein said he sympathized with her problems of access to information and that he was ignorant of the excess of breast cancer and cancer of the cervix in people with husbands in certain occupations. "In the U.S. there is a major excess of breast cancer in women living in the vicinity of certain industries. You have raised very important issues, well deserved of the highest priority and attention," he said.

Prof. Bob Williamson of ASTMS, who is a member of the Genetic Manipulation Advisory Group (GMAG), said that in relation to genetic engineering, there was statutory provision for workers in industry, universities and research institutions, under the Health and Safety at Work Act.

"Safety committees are a statutory right and must have trade union representation," he said. The trade unions on GMAG had delegated significant powers to local safety committees and through these an enormous amount had been achieved.

"Our attitude has been that it is the worker in the factory who is at immediate risk from any hazard and will have most concern in operating safety procedures," he said. The multinationals, he added, were fleeing to the U.S. from Britain in order to manipulate under no control.

Prof. Epstein commented, "I wish we could persuade our academic colleagues in the U.S. to be unionized. On genetic engineering we are doing badly because of professional self-interest of distinguished geneticists." He was puzzled by the implication that because of unionization of the professions in Great Britain, the trade unions here had access to a body of professional expertise. "I have yet to see such expertise being actively harnessed in this area of occupational hazard," he said.

Sheila McKechnie, ASTMS Health and Safety Officer, said the union's membership in the scientific field had taken a low profile stand on carcinogens. "Some scientists have been very useful to me on a person-to-person basis, but far more are not prepared to stick their necks out in the work situation," she said. "The real crunch from genetic manipulation control has yet to come."

Prof. J. W. Jeffery, ASTMS, of Birkbeck College, gave the example of plutonium of which particles might cause cancer in man. But experiments were not designed to test this theory directly and did not go on long enough to establish whether cancer would develop. They had got to the stage where lesions had developed which might be pre-cancerous. Yet no action had been taken either in this country or the U.S. "Apparently it is believed that unless the case is proved, we need do nothing about it," he said.

Prof. Epstein who said he shared Prof. Jeffery's concern, declared that the whole question of where the burden of proof lies should be more aggressively put. The burden of proof should rest on those who initiated the risk and profited from it.

A speaker from Aston University called for a "deeper analysis of why chemicals are being introduced into society as a whole." There should be a test of utility before chemicals were allowed on the market. "But testing for needs is complicated," he said.

Prof. Epstein agreed that testing for utility was very important. About 700 new chemicals were introduced into commerce every year. The cost of carcinogen testing on one new chemical was 200,000 dollars and so to test them all would cost 140 million dollars — not an inflationary figure. Scientists now unemployed in the U.S. could do this work, but the cost should be borne by industry, not by the taxpayers.

Animal Testing

At the morning session, which was chaired by Sheila McKechnie, ASTMS Health and Safety Officer, Prof. Epstein spoke on testing for carcinogenicity. He has 12 major criticisms of such tests as performed by U.S. industry in support of its petitions to the regulatory agencies:

1. Too few animals used.

2. Exposures in excess of the maximally tolerated doses result in premature animal deaths before the possible onset of cancer.

3. Doses too low for the size of the animal test group failed to obtain a statistically significant incidence of tumors.

4. Deliberate premature sacrifice of animals for other "studies" during the course of the main test depletes the number of animals remaining alive and at risk for cancer.

5. Premature termination of the test before sufficient time has elapsed for the animals to develop tumors.

6. Poor housing, diet and care cause infection, sickness, and premature death.

7. Failure to ensure that each test and control group receive appropriate prescribed treatments as originally intended.

8. Failure to inspect cages regularly so that dead animals become decomposed, results

in the possibility that tumors may be missed at autopsy.

9. Inadequate autopsies.

10. Failure to examine appropriate tissues and organs for histological study.

11. Poor record-keeping.

12. Alteration, falsification, and even destruction of records.

Addressing the seminar, Prof. Epstein said it was now regarded as appropriate in the U.S. that consumer products should be tested in animals prior to their introduction into commerce, but there was no such presumption about industrial chemicals and chemicals in the workplace.

"The presumption is — we will use the material and if we have evidence of hazard on a retrospective basis, we will develop regulatory concern," he said.

So there was a wide range of testing for consumer products, but until recently, there had been no such requirement for the testing of industrial chemicals — an amazing dichotomy of approach.

He described at some length the various methods of testing in animals — mice and rats — discussing the numbers used, the nature of control groups, feeding methods, dosages, and threshold problems.

A "mythology" of the subject which served the interests of the chemical industry, had been aided by professionals some of whom held august positions in academia. One myth was the distinction between tumors and carcinoma. Tumor, it was said, just induced a little lump and was nothing to get excited about. When a member of the audience commented that not all tumors were carcinogenic, Professor Epstein replied: "I am unaware of any chemically-induced tumor which, if followed up, does not behave in a malignant fashion."

Another myth was that there are two kinds of carcinogens: one which induced cancer in

animals and the other which induced the disease in humans.

In this whole field, he said, there was a "massive distortion of the democratic decision-making process by special interests. . . . If the trade unions are not capable of dealing with this problem, who the hell is?" he asked.

He was delighted, he said, by the emergence of people like Health and Safety Officers Sheila McKechnie of ASTMS and David Gee of the General and Municipal Workers Union, who were unwilling to be bamboozled by scientific jargon.

"I know the enormous pressures on the scientists. I know what happens to the guy who steps out of the old boy network," he said. It was also difficult for the decent government agency official who, with political protection, could be more helpful.

The unions, he said, should acquaint themselves with the jargon, understand the mythologies and create a cadre of scientists they could trust.

The Science and Politics of Cancer in Britain

The following section is comprised of the first three chapters from Cancer in Britain, *a book co-authored with Lesley Doyal, and published in 1983 by Pluto Press in London. The section surveys the history and scope of the cancer problem in Britain. It also rebuts the misleading and self-interested policies of the British cancer establishment. Clearly, the situation in Britain mirrors that in the U.S., with minimal progress in regard to cancer prevention in both nations.*

Cancer is increasingly regarded as a preventable disease; accordingly, there has been growing criticism of the curative emphasis that dominates most research. It is generally accepted that most cancers are caused by the way we live and work, and that changes are an essential first step towards prevention.

However, there is considerable disagreement about what these changes should be and how they could be brought about.

Why has there been a swing towards prevention in the case of cancer in particular? The most immediate reason is probably the sheer size of the problem. The disease now kills one in five of all people dying in Britain. Furthermore, cancer is now the disease that people fear most. Just as tuberculosis appeared to symbolize the wretched conditions of nineteenth-century towns, so cancer has come to be seen as an epidemic that is somehow characteristic of the "affluent society" of the post-war period.[1] This fear is exacerbated by the fact that western medicine has so far proved remarkably ineffective in helping cancer patients — survival rates for most of the common cancers have improved very little over the past 30 years. Indeed, there is a growing belief that, far from providing a cure, cancer treatment often serves merely to reduce the quality of the patient's remaining life-span.

This growing emphasis on prevention has been reinforced by the recognition that, like the other "diseases of affluence," cancer is usually both environmental and multi-causal in origin. That is to say, there is not usually a simple relationship between the onset of cancer and exposure to a particular carcinogen. Rather, most cases are related to several different elements in a victim's physical, social, and economic environment which interact with his/her own genetic make-up to produce a cancer. The fact that the majority of cancers are largely environmental in origin is evidenced by the marked differences found in cancer rates between different social groups. ("Environmental" is used here in the widest sense, encompassing all those external influences impinging on an individual organism.) This applies to the variations in incidence between different countries but especially to the marked differences between social classes in the *same* country. In Britain, for example, most of the major cancers are more common among semi-skilled and unskilled workers than among their more affluent compatriots. Lung and stomach cancers in particular show a very marked social class differential of this kind. These class differences are important, not just because they illustrate yet another of the burdens disproportionately borne by the underprivileged in our society, but because they demonstrate that cancer cannot be explained simply in natural or genetic terms. Instead, it has to be understood as one outcome of the material differences that exist between the lives of people in different social groups.

Two Approaches to Cancer Prevention

From a public health perspective, the central tasks in any prevention campaign would therefore be the removal or transformation of those aspects of people's lives that render them more likely than others to develop cancer. However, as soon as we move into the formulation of practical strategies for achieving such a goal, political concerns immediately become apparent. Contrary to popular mythology, issues of this kind are never resolved by reference to purely scientific considerations, as we can see if we look at the current debate about cancer prevention in Britain. Two distinct positions are clearly identifiable. Each has its own view about the relative importance of the different causes of cancer, its own recommendations about how the disease could be prevented, and, underlying both of these, its own political philosophy. At the risk of oversimplification, we will call these the "establishment" and the "radical" approaches, though there is inevitably some degree of overlap between the two.

If we look first at the "establishment" approach, it is clear that the most vociferous proponents of this view are industrial interests — the Chemical Industries Association (CIA) in particular. However it is also to be found in many official government publications where the emphasis is on individuals looking after their own health, rather than expecting the state to do it for them. The "establishment" approach rests on two major assumptions. First, it is argued that industrial products and processes play very little part in causing cancer. Thus, occupational factors are said to cause less than 5 percent of all cancers and pollution some 2 percent. Instead, the major causes of cancer are said to be smoking (causing some 30 percent of all cancers) and diet (about 35 percent). Additional factors often mentioned are alcohol, food additives, sunshine, and "sexual habits." According to this view, the most significant causes of cancer are things to which individuals willingly expose themselves, so that social class differences are explained by the assumption that working-class people *voluntarily* lead less healthy lives than their more enlightened fellows. Whether this is because of moral weakness, intellectual inferiority, lack of education, or sheer laziness is never made clear. In any case, the main hope for prevention is seen to lie in more health education — in trying to persuade people to "look after themselves."

In order to back up their analysis, exponents of the "establishment" approach tend to draw heavily on the work of Richard Doll and Richard Peto (Chapter 14). Doll and Peto are influential cancer epidemiologists; their volume *The Causes of Cancer* (1982) has been extremely important in supporting industry's position. It is necessary, therefore, to look carefully at the social implications of their approach and at the uses to which their work has been put. In particular, we need to look at the ways in which their ideas have been used to reinforce the "victim-blaming" approach that has been prominent in recent discussions of ill-health in general and cancer in particular. Of course, the technical arguments used to support the "establishment" position are always put forward in apparently neutral and value-free terms and Doll and Peto have gone to considerable trouble to assert their own impartiality.[2] However, their ideas have been eagerly seized upon by industry and widely disseminated by the CIA in their attempts to resist further regulation.

The alternative approach to cancer — which we have called the "radical" view — is taken by trade unions, environmental groups and others concerned to expose the role of industry in the creation of ill-health. According to this view, industrial processes and hazardous chemicals play a far more significant part in the causation of cancer than the "establishment" position would admit. It recognizes the importance of smoking, diet, and other factors individuals could perhaps control, but it places more emphasis on industrial exposures over which the individual has little or no say.

Supporters of this approach have drawn particularly on the work of Samuel Epstein, Professor of Occupational and Environmental Medicine at the University of Illinois and an international authority on the toxic and carcinogenic hazards of chemicals. Epstein supports the 20-40 percent minimal estimates calculated by a group of American federal experts for the proportion of cancers that are work-related.[3] He also stresses industrial pollution and the chemicals used in consumer products as significant causes of cancer. Furthermore, he demonstrates that the contribution of smoking, while clearly major, has been overestimated because it is often seen as the *only* cause of a cancer which in fact often has an occupational component. Diet he sees as having little proven relationship with cancer except in the very specific case of deliberate or accidental carcinogenic food additives.

According to this view then, the answer to the cancer problem lies not merely in health education — in the moral persuasion of individuals — but in the identification and regulation of hazardous industrial chemicals, whether in the workplace, in consumer products, or in the wider environment. Moreover, there is a clear realization that this greater control will not be achieved by individuals acting alone, and that neither industry nor government can be left to their own devices on the assumption that they will act in the public interest. Thus, it is assumed that the social and economic changes required for any real progress in cancer prevention can only be achieved through collective political action.

In the same way that the CIA have used the Doll-Peto analysis to bolster their case against further regulation of industry, so trade unions have used the analysis of Epstein (and others) in their fight for better health and safety measures at work. Three unions in particular — the Association of Scientific, Technical, and Managerial Staffs (ASTMS), the General and Municipal Workers' Union (GMWU), and the National Graphical Association (NGA) have all produced their own documents exposing the possible carcinogenic hazards facing their workers."[4] In addition the National Union of Agricultural and Allied Workers (NUAAW) has drawn on this analysis in their campaign against 2,4,5-T.

In Britain there is, therefore, a continuing debate between what we have called the "establishment" and the "radical" positions, with skirmishes ranging from debates in the scientific literature[5] to more overtly political battles of words between the CIA and the unions.[6] These debates have been summarized by Peto and Epstein.

So who is right? This remains a matter of considerable dispute and certainly more information is required before we can come to definitive conclusions about the relative importance of different causes of cancer. However, there are good reasons for suggesting that the CIA calculation of 4-5 percent of cancers being work-related is a considerable underestimate. The main problem with figures of this kind is that they are based on a supposedly unaccountable residue of cancers when all the causes of the major lifestyle cancers are added up. Additionally, they ignore consideration of at least 130 substances recognized as animal carcinogens by the International Agency for Cancer Research (IARC) as well as a growing number of potentially hazardous substances in daily use that have not yet been adequately tested.[7] Furthermore, it is becoming increasingly clear that many of the carcinogens found in the workplace may spread or be discharged into the air and water of local communities and also may be transmitted directly to others — especially the worker's family. Evidence of this has been found among the families of asbestos workers, and there is also growing concern that some proportion of cervical cancer may be caused by the male worker exposing his partner to carcinogens during intercourse.[8] Thus figures reflecting only direct (usually male) exposure are inevitably too low. Finally, it is clear that we still know far too little about the environmental pollution caused by industrial production in Britain, so that it is impossible to make an accurate estimate of its effects on the incidence of cancer.

It seems likely then, that the proponents of the "radical" view are right in claiming that the industrial-occupational causes of cancer are far more significant than industry cares to admit. A campaign for the identification and control of these substances is therefore of paramount importance if avoidable cancers are to be prevented. Indeed, it is worth pointing out that Doll and Peto themselves (if not their corporate supporters) have recognized that even if "only" about 4 or 5 percent of cancers (i.e. 6,000-7,000 per year) are work-related, then the detection of such hazards should have a greater priority in any program of cancer research. Once they are identified, it is usually practicable to remove such hazards — or at least to reduce them quite markedly — and, given the multi-causality of most cancers, this would be likely to reduce the incidence not just of known occupational cancers but also of some not usually seen as directly occupational in origin.

It is important to emphasize, however, that any cancer prevention campaign that restricted itself to the control of industrial carcinogens would inevitably be limited in its effectiveness. Even if we achieve a greater degree of control over industrial chemicals, we would still be left with significant causes of cancer untouched — smoking in particular. While continuing to campaign for the removal of carcinogenic hazards, we also need to treat smoking, unhealthy diets,* and possibly other "lifestyle" factors as serious problems that necessitate the development of an appropriate political response.

If we take the example of smoking, for instance, we must accept that cigarettes are probably the single most important cause of preventable cancer and that they kill proportionately more semiskilled and unskilled workers. It is also clear that not only is smoking a major cause of illness among smokers themselves but what is called "passive smoking" may also pose a serious threat to those around them. It is essential, therefore, that we develop a clearer understanding of why people smoke cigarettes (or eat unhealthy food) and particularly why such activities should be class-related. Whilst not ignoring the question of personal responsibility entirely, we do need to challenge the simplistic "victim-blaming" approach of industry. We need to highlight the activities of the tobacco industry in persuading people to smoke, and to show how conditions at work and at home may push people to seek solace in cigarettes. Thus, a progressive approach to cancer prevention needs to identify both the industrial causes of cancer and also the social and economic pressures that may lead individuals to act in ways that damage their health. It is only on this basis that an effective strategy for the prevention of cancer can be formulated.[9]

The Cancer Problem in Britain

During the twentieth century there has been a dramatic increase in the number of people suffering and dying from cancer in Britain. In 1901, infectious diseases were the major killers — influenza, pneumonia, and bronchitis caused 16 percent of all deaths, while dysentery and diarrhoea accounted for another 7 percent.[1] Tuberculosis alone killed twice as many people as cancer, which was responsible for only 4.5 percent of all deaths. By contrast, at least 20 percent of people now alive in Britain can expect to die from cancer, and the so-called "diseases of affluence" — cancer and heart disease — now account for about 50 percent of all deaths.[2] In the following pages, we examine the main features of the cancer problem in Britain. We show that a considerable proportion of the cancer burden arises from past exposure to carcinogenic substances in the general environment, at home, and at work, and that much of this exposure results from the pursuit of corporate profit in a situation where public controls are weak.

The Overall Impact

Over 130,000 men and women died of cancer in England and Wales in 1980 and the disease was the cause of about 22 in every 100 deaths. Cancer is a major cause of death among men and women of all ages. It is the most common cause of death for people aged 35-54 and the second most common cause (after heart disease) for those aged 55-74. Moreover, contrary to popular belief, cancer is not only a disease of middle or old age, but is second only to accidents as a cause of death in those aged 5-34 (Figure 15.1).

In 1979, cancer of the lung claimed most male cancer victims (39 percent), cancers of the intestine (11 percent) and stomach (9 percent) being the other major killing sites (Table 15.1). In the same year, most cancer deaths among women were due to breast cancer (21 percent), followed by cancers of the intestine (16 percent), and lung (14 percent).

---

* In particular, with reference to the relation between high fat diet and cardiovascular disease and the intake of fat-soluble carcinogens.

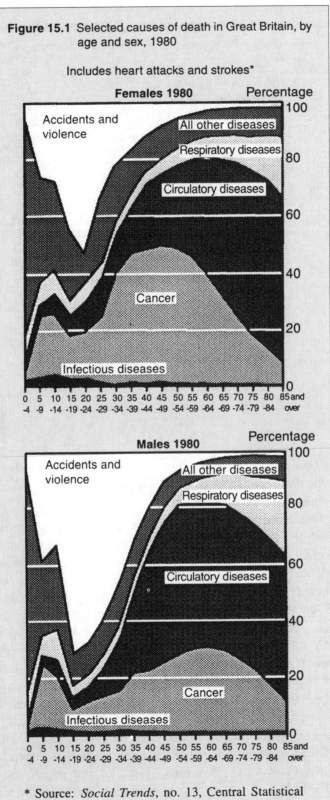

Figure 15.1 Selected causes of death in Great Britain, by age and sex, 1980

Includes heart attacks and strokes*

Females 1980   Percentage

Accidents and violence

All other diseases

Respiratory diseases

Circulatory diseases

Cancer

Infectious diseases

Males 1980   Percentage

Accidents and violence

All other diseases

Respiratory diseases

Circulatory diseases

Cancer

Infectious diseases

* Source: *Social Trends*, no. 13, Central Statistical Office, 1982.

Table 15.1 Male and female deaths from cancer in England and Wales, 1979

	Male			Female		
Site	Number of deaths (thousands)	As % of all cancer deaths		Site	Number of deaths (thousands)	As % of all cancer deaths
Lung, bronchus, trachea	26.8	39		Breast	12	21
Intestine, rectum	7.8	11		Intestine, rectum	8.9	16
Stomach	6.5	9		Lung, bronchus, trachea	7.9	14
Prostate	4.8	7		Stomach	4.7	8
Bladder	2.9	4		Ovary	3.7	6
Pancreas	3.0	4		Cervix	2.1	6
Other	18.4	26		Pancreas	2.8	5
				Uterus	3.6	2
				Other	13.0	22
Total	67.7	100			58.7	100

Source: *Mortality Statistics*, 1979, series DH I no. 8, OPCS, 1982

So far we have been talking about the numbers of people who die from cancer (cancer mortality rates) rather than the number who contract it (cancer incidence rates). In the case of an illness which has a high rate of cure, mortality figures of this kind would obviously provide an inaccurate picture of the real extent of the problem. However, in Britain, as in the USA, the "curability" of most major cancers, particularly of the lung, breast, and colon, has improved only slightly over the past three decades.[3] Hence, on an overall basis, and for most major sites, mortality rates closely reflect incidence rates. In the case of lung cancer, for instance, only about 7 patients out of every 100 remain alive 5 years after diagnosis. Even for the more "curable" breast cancer, just over half of its victims survive 5 years (Table 15.2).

Evidence of Recent Increase in Cancer Rates

Cancer is therefore a major cause of death in Britain and its contribution to the total mortality rate is increasing. There has been a steady rise in crude cancer death rates during this century, and, between 1951 and 1975, rates among British males increased by about 1 percent per year.[4] Cancer death rates among women fell by some 7 percent between 1943 and 1963; since that period, they have been on the increase and, like male rates, rose by about 1 percent per year during the 1970s.[5] Obviously the "epidemic" of lung cancer during the post-war period has been the major factor in this rise, but in men, there have also been increases in deaths from leukaemia and bladder and pancreatic cancers, while in women there has been a marked increase in

Table 15.2 Number of male and female patients surviving 5 years or more out of every 100 diagnosed with cancer*

		Year of diagnosis		
		1959	1964-6	1971-3
Stomach	M	5.5	5.8	7.3
	F	5.7	5.6	7.2
Large intestine	M	23.6	26.2	29.6
	F	23.4	26.3	29.3
Pancreas	M	1.8	1.8	3.78
	F	1.7	2.0	3.12
Lung	M	4.3	6.0	7.8
	F	4.6	5.0	7.0
Breast	M	54.5	51.6	59.5
	F	42.4	51.4	56.8
Cervix	F	39.1	62.0	54.4

* Corrected survival rates.
Source: *Cancer Statistics: Survival, 1971-73 Registration*, series MBI no. 3, OPCS, 1980

breast cancer since 1961 and steady increases in cancers of the ovary and pancreas. Rates for stomach and intestinal cancer declined among both sexes between 1951 and 1971, but mortality rates from intestinal cancer are now beginning to rise again among men. In fact, stomach and cervical cancers are the only major cancers to have shown a consistent decline during the post-war period.[6]

It is often suggested that this increase in cancer mortality is merely an artifact of the statistics, reflecting the increasing number of older people in the population. Thus, it is argued, the increase would disappear if we adjusted for these demographic changes. However, when the crude mortality figures are adjusted to take into account the proportion of the population in different age groups, the adjusted death rate from cancer has still risen — though not quite so steeply as the crude death rate.[7] It is clear, therefore, that we are dealing with a real and absolute rather than an apparent and relative increase in cancer deaths.

How are we to explain these real increases in cancer mortality? The most obvious explanation might be that the figures simply reflect improvements in diagnosis — that more cancer deaths are now recognized for what they are and recorded as such. There is no doubt that this has played some part in the increase, but the overall effect is likely to be small, particularly in recent decades. An alternative and widely held assumption is that the increase in the number of people dying from cancer, if not an artifact of the statistics, is nevertheless a "natural" and inevitable consequence of an aging population. "You've got to die of something," is a comment frequently heard. Thus it is claimed that with the decline in infectious diseases and an overall improvement in standards of living, people live longer and an increase in cancer is unavoidable — that cancer is simply a "degenerative" disease which is part of the ageing process itself. But there are certain problems with this argument, the most important being that there has been a real rise in cancer rates in *all* age groups, and a theory which attributes cancer only to "degeneration" cannot account for this excess mortality at all ages. Given this fact, a more plausible explanation is that an individual's chance of contracting cancer *increases* with greater exposure to carcinogenic substances whose production has in general been much increased in recent decades. For most people, the longer they live the greater that exposure is likely to be and the greater is the opportunity for cancers to develop, following exposure earlier in life. This provides an important additional element in explaining the link between cancer and longevity. Viewed in this way, historical trends in cancer incidence point to the role of environmental factors in producing many types of cancer — an interpretation which is borne out both by comparative evidence of cancer rates in different societies and also, very importantly, by the marked differences that exist in cancer rates for different groups in the *same* society.

Social Class Differences in Cancer Rates

In the United States, evidence concerning different cancer rates among blacks and whites has been used to demonstrate the importance of environmental influences.[8] In Britain, we know very little about such racial differences, but the very obvious and dramatic *class* differences in cancer mortality provide powerful evidence of the impact of environmental factors.[9] An examination of standardized mortality ratios (SMRs)[10] shows that there is a marked difference in death rates from cancer among different social classes, so that people belonging to social classes IV and V[11] are considerably more likely to die from cancer *at any age* than their counterparts in social classes I and II (Figure 15.2). Moreover, this social class gradient is steeper among men than among women — a fact which probably reflects in part their greater exposure to occupational carcinogens.

There are also important variations in the social class gradients for different *types* of cancer (Figure 15.3). Social class gradients are most pronounced for lung and stomach cancers which together accounted for more than half the total number of male cancer deaths in 1970-72; the gradient is much shallower for bladder, esophageal and rectal cancers. Only two forms of cancer — intestinal and pancreatic — are apparently class "impartial;" while brain cancer has a *negative* social class gradient — i.e. is commonest among those in higher social classes. Thus, among men, cancer at five of the major sites shows a positive social class gradient. Comparable tables are not available for female cancers, and most mortality data classifies married women according to their husbands' occupation, thus obscuring possibly important relationships between women's own work and their cancer risk. However, class differentials are observable in female cancer rates (Figure 15.2). Cervical cancer in particular is much more common among women of social classes IV and V. However, it is important to note that breast cancer, the commonest cancer among women, is more frequent in *higher* social classes.

It is clear then that there are very significant class differences in overall cancer rates in Britain, as well as in the rates of cancer at different sites. It is unlikely that variations of this kind are merely random, or the result of genetic differences between social groups. We therefore need to examine the lives of people in different social classes in order to assess why men and woman in social classes IV and V are more likely to die prematurely of some form of cancer than those who are more affluent.

Most epidemiologists argue that there are two sets of factors primarily responsible for producing these class differences in cancer rates: occupational hazards and the so-called "lifestyle" factors.[12] As we have seen, there is still considerable controversy about how many cancers are directly work-related, but we can reasonably assume that a significant, though not precisely quantifiable proportion of cancer can be explained in this way. Leav-

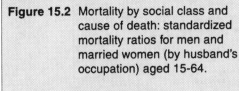

Figure 15.2 Mortality by social class and cause of death: standardized mortality ratios for men and married women (by husband's occupation) aged 15-64.

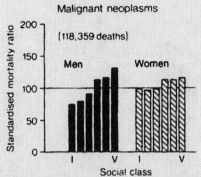

Malignant neoplasms

Note: This figure includes six bars for five social classes as a result of changes in classification made in 1970. Class III is now divided into two subgroups: IIIN (non-manual skilled occupations) and IIIM (manual skilled occupations).

Source: *Occupational Mortality: Registrar General's Decennial Supplement*, 1970-72, series DS no. 1, OPCS, 1978

ing these aside, we are then left with the so-called lifestyle factors commonly used to explain all those cancers that are either unrelated to, or not explicable in terms of occupational exposure alone. Explanations of this kind usually imply that the risks associated with these habits are easily avoidable (compared with the "unavoidable" ones at work), and result primarily from the moral weakness of the victim. But how useful is "lifestyle" as an explanation of class differentials in cancer rates?

As we have seen, the most important problem with this approach is that the way people live is not simply a matter of individual choice — not even in the case of smoking or drinking — but is structured in a multitude of ways by their wider social and economic environment.[13] Moreover the resulting differences in degrees of exposure to carcinogens are not random, but affect those in lower social classes

more acutely. People who are most exposed to carcinogens at work are *also* more likely to live in industrially polluted areas, and to smoke heavily; it is this concentration which is largely responsible for such marked class differences in cancer rates. Moreover, it is this very combination of exposures which makes the problem of the relationship between smoking and, say, occupational factors so difficult to disentangle. (In epidemiological terms, smoking and occupation are confounding variables.) Since very few of the studies — other than recent ones — relating smoking to lung cancer have even considered occupation as a relevant variable, there are good grounds for concluding that the relationship between smoking *alone* and lung cancer may well have been overestimated. Indeed such a conclusion is borne out by recent data showing a marked rise in lung cancer rates among nonsmokers.[14] "Lifestyle" arguments which ignore these facts and offer entirely individualistic explanations are therefore of little value in understanding the real causes of cancer — but of considerable value in covering them up.

We now go on to illustrate these points in more detail by looking at the three most important sources of exposure to carcinogens — the workplace, consumer products, and the environment.

1. Carcinogens in the workplace

Ever since Percival Pott first pointed out the relationship between scrotal cancer and employment in the chimney-sweeping trade in eighteenth-century Britain, there has been a growing acceptance that certain occupations involve an excess risk of contracting cancer. Indeed, some of these relationships are now so well established that certain cancers are designated as "prescribed diseases," entitling the victim to possible compensation. Occupational cancers granted this status in Britain include skin cancer caused by exposure to soot, tar, and mineral oil (prescribed in 1921); lung cancer caused by exposure to gaseous

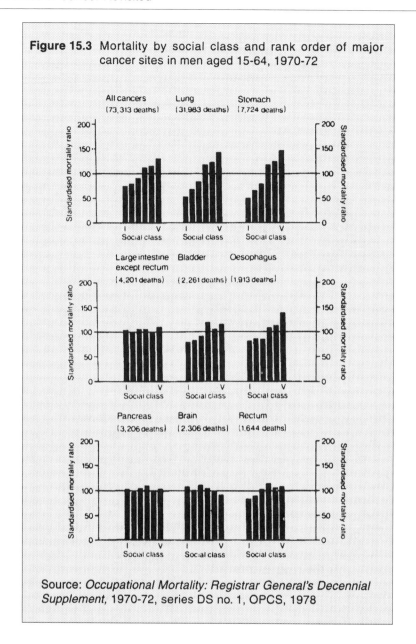

Figure 15.3 Mortality by social class and rank order of major cancer sites in men aged 15-64, 1970-72

Source: *Occupational Mortality: Registrar General's Decennial Supplement,* 1970-72, series DS no. 1, OPCS, 1978

nickel compounds (1949); bladder cancer caused by aromatic amines in chemical dye-stuffs and in rubber production (1953); meso-theliomas caused by exposure to asbestos (1969); adenocarcinoma of the nose caused by exposure to wood dust (1969); angiosar-coma of the liver resulting from exposure to vinyl chloride monomer (1976); and finally, cancer of the nasal cavity contracted in the manufacture and repair of footwear (1979). Thus, for some workers who contract cancer,

their disease is recognized as being *possibly* due to occupational exposure and they (or their family) *may* be "compensated."

However, only some of the relatively rare cancers are "prescribed" in this way, and not all workers contracting even these are accepted as victims of occupational exposure. Out of the 4,300 people who died of bladder cancer in Britain in 1976, only five were officially recognized as being entitled to industrial-death benefit.[15] Similarly, we have already seen that

Table 15.3 Occupational cancer in men, 1966-69

Cancer site and sufferer's occupation	Cancer registrations in men aged 15-74	Expected registrations	Excess registrations due to occupational exposure	Excess cancer risk factor*
Lip				
Agricultural laborers	68	15	53	5.0
Farmers	66	22	34	2.5
Construction workers	88	43	45	2.0
Laborers	203	116	87	1.8
Salivary gland				
Armed forces	34	13	21	2.6
Esophagus				
Agricultural laborers	69	42	27	1.6
Textile workers	53	35	18	1.5
Stomach				
Miners and quarrymen	1,014	709	305	1.4
Glass and ceramic workers	90	65	25	1.4
General metal workers and jewellers	192	136	56	1.4
Boiler firemen	138	104	34	1.3
Rectum				
Miners and quarrymen	462	362	100	1.3
Liver				
Carpenters and joiners	31	20	11	1.3
Pancreas				
Coal miners	33	13	20	2.5
Tailors	23	12	11	2.0
Nose				
Woodworkers	29	15	14	2.0
Larynx				
Machine tool operators	80	58	22	1.4
Lung, trachea, bronchus				
Ceramic formers	71	48	23	1.4
Foundry molders and coremakers	306	214	92	1.4
Fettlers and metal dressers	114	81	33	1.4
Metal plate workers and riveters	372	281	99	1.3
Plumbers, lead burners	491	387	104	1.3
Bricklayers and tile setters	845	668	177	1.3

continued on next page

continued from previous page

Cancer site and sufferer's occupation	Cancer registrations in men aged 15-74	Expected registrations	Excess registrations due to occupational exposure	Excess cancer risk factor*
Plasterers	238	184	52	1.3
Charmen, window cleaners and Chimney sweeps	260	198	62	1.3
Skin				
Farmworkers, foresters and fishermen	1,148	890	258	1.3
Prostate				
Farmworkers, foresters and fishermen	667	496	171	1.3
Bladder				
Clothing workers	103	83	20	1.2
Rubber workers	42	26	16	1.5
Brain				
Farmers and market gardeners	114	78	36	1.5
Hodgkin's disease				
Machine tool operators	66	50	16	1.3

* Elevated risk factors do not necessarily imply causal relationships, but should be considered as leads for further epidemiological investigation.

Source: Tables 5G and 5Q in *Occupational Mortality, Registrar General's Decennial Supplement,* 1970-72, series DS no. 1, OPCS, 1978

even the most minimal estimates recognize that 1-5 percent of cancers are work related. In the British context, this would give a figure of between 1,200 and 6,000 occupational cancer victims each year. However, in a typical year the Department of Health and Social Security (DHSS) agrees to pay occupational disease-related death benefit to only around a hundred cancer victims.[16] It would seem obvious, then, that even according to the lowest industry estimates, the bulk of occupational cancer still remains uncompensated and even unrecorded. If we look in more detail at the example of asbestos, official statistics acknowledge that 600 people die each year of asbestos-related cancers. Richard Peto suggests that this figure should be 1,000 (with a twofold uncertainty) while Dave Gee, health and safety officer of the General and Municipal Workers Union, has argued that 2,000 deaths would be more accurate.[17]

But we also need to go beyond the *known* — usually unacknowledged — carcinogenic hazards in the workplace, and consider those that have not, as yet, been investigated. Strong hints of where we might look can be found in the *Registrar General's Decennial Supplement,* as the ASTMS document *The Prevention of Cancer* emphasizes (Table 15.3 and Appendix I).

The information in Table 15.3 is based on the number of cancer registrations from 1966 to 1969 for men in different occupations. These figures are then compared with the number of cancer registrations that would be expected in the general population, making it possible to make some estimate of the number of cancer cases that might be related to particular kinds of industrial exposure. Thus, we find that coal miners, for instance, are two-and-a-half times more likely to get cancer of the pancreas than the rest of the population, while woodworkers are twice as likely to get nasal cancer. With data of this kind, it is obviously difficult to isolate specific causal relationships but as the ASTMS document points out: "These tables reveal a multitude of links that cannot be ascribed to any substance in particular — but are nonetheless real and deadly."[18]

Although we cannot yet explain many of these apparent associations, there are others where the cause — or at least a major contributory factor — is only too obvious. Thus, lung and stomach cancer are strongly associated with work which involves exposure to dusts of various kinds, and exposure to certain metal dusts and fumes is clearly related to an excess risk of lung cancer. Furthermore, it has recently been suggested that we are getting only a very partial view of the carcinogenic effects of such industries by looking at male mortality rates. An examination of the incidence of cervical cancer among married women shows a remarkable association between increased rates of the disease and marriage to men in specific occupations — "dirty jobs" involving the use of mineral oils, for example.[19]

2. Carcinogens in consumer products

Cigarette smoking is well recognized as a major cause of lung and other cancers, as well as of other major diseases. There may be synergistic or multiplicative interactions between smoking and certain types of occupational exposure — especially asbestos — in producing an increased risk of lung cancer. Nevertheless, the tobacco industry continues to manufacture and strongly promote cigarettes — a fact which is reflected particularly dramatically in the rising rates of lung cancer among women who are now both smoking more heavily[20] and also becoming increasingly exposed to occupational hazards. Cigarette smoking is, of course, different from most other forms of exposure to carcinogens since it does involve a much greater degree of volition than, say, occupational or environmental exposure. However, as we have already seen, this apparent "choice" can only be understood in a broader context, since the pressures on people to continue smoking often make it difficult for them to "choose" to stop — whatever the consequences for their health.

The second potentially carcinogenic consumer product we will be considering is food — a very different sort of commodity from cigarettes. We "need" food in a way we do not "need" cigarettes, and yet, like tobacco, some foods may be dangerous to health.[21] Firm evidence has yet to be found, but it seems clear that we need to consider the impact of general dietary composition on cancer incidence. We also need to look particularly carefully at the growing consumption of clearly carcinogenic additives which are either deliberately added to food as coloring agents, preservatives or flavorings, or find their way indirectly into our diet through their use in plastic containers or food wrappings, in cattle feed or as pesticides. Contamination of food with these direct and indirect additives is becoming increasingly common in Britain, yet they are difficult to avoid, since information about their effects is hard to obtain and there are no adequate rules governing the labelling of foods.

Doctors supply us with another important class of consumer product. In Britain, as in the USA, oral contraceptives are now widely used, and injectable contraceptives, such as Depo Provera (banned in the USA), appear to be growing in popularity. Hormone-replacement therapy, too, is being prescribed

Table 15.4 County and London boroughs with the greatest excess mortality from cancer of trachea, bronchus, and lung, 1969-73

Males		Females	
Borough	SMR	Borough	SMR
Bootle	172	Camden	193
Islington	159	Hammersmith	176
Gateshead	152	Westminster	172
Liverpool	152	Southwark	170
Kingston-upon-Hull	152	Lambeth	167
Manchester	151	Islington	162
Salford	151	Salford	158
Newcastle-upon-Tyne	148	Newcastle-upon-Tyne	157
Hammersmith	147	Lewisham	156
Southwark	146	Liverpool	155

Source: *Area Mortality, 1971*, OPCS, 1980

frequently for postmenopausal women.[22] All these drugs have been implicated as causes of some reproductive tract cancers and they do represent a growing — yet largely preventable — cause of cancer among women.

3. Carcinogens in the general environment

Finally, the general environment is another major potential source of carcinogens. Thus, people may be at risk not only from their jobs and the commodities they consume, but also from the air they must breathe and the water they must drink. The differences between urban and rural cancer rates are very marked in the USA and the same pattern is evident in Britain (Tables 15.4 and 15.5). Thus, it is the industrialized inner-city areas such as Bootle, Islington, Gateshead, Hartlepool, and Stoke-on-Trent which show very high rates of lung and stomach cancer.

It is frequently assumed that these high rates can be explained simply in terms of differences in smoking habits and job patterns, and in the general deprivation found in inner-city areas. However, we do know that the benzpyrene found in soot is a carcinogen, and this gives us good reason to assume that generalized atmo-

Table 15.5 Mortality from stomach cancer in selected county boroughs in England and Wales, 1969-73

	SMR	
	Males	Females
Bootle	163	119
Hartlepool	162	147
Stoke-on-Trent	159	138
Oldham	155	133
Salford	151	134
West Bromwich	148	139
Newport	143	122
Sunderland	138	160
Swansea	133	153
Teesside	132	132
St Helens	127	157
Bolton	125	139
Bury	125	140
Bradford	124	123
Wolverhampton	121	136
Walsall	114	145
Birmingham	113	109
Wigan	111	158
Barrow-in-Furness	104	170

Source: *Area Mortality, 1971*, OPCS, 1980

spheric pollution also plays a significant part.[23] It is also becoming clear that living close to certain industries and to hazardous waste disposal sites is associated with an increased risk of contracting cancer.[24] So far, we have no cancer maps of the kind that have proved so informative in the USA — indeed, it is only now that British researchers are beginning to look at the relationship between industrial pollution and local patterns of cancer mortality. However, a study carried out in one Scottish town between 1968 and 1974 has revealed a significant excess of deaths from respiratory cancer in those parts of the town exposed to pollution from a steel foundry.[25] This is clearly in line with American findings of increased cancer mortality rates in men and women in communities exposed to industrial pollution — particularly from local petrochemical plants — and we can expect more such data to appear in the near future. Interesting evidence is also emerging from a team in Southampton, about the geographical concentration of occupationally related cancers — an excess of mesothelioma in the dock area of Portsmouth, for instance, and of nasal cancer around High

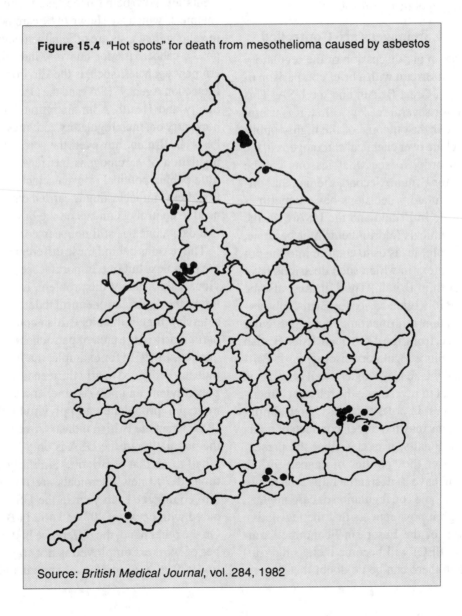

Figure 15.4 "Hot spots" for death from mesothelioma caused by asbestos

Source: *British Medical Journal*, vol. 284, 1982

Wycombe where there is a concentration of furniture production (Figure 15.4).[26]

Cancer is a major cause of misery and death in Britain. Moreover, the distribution of hardship falls unevenly on those with least resources. Cancer cannot be explained away as something that just "happens" to people. Rather, we need to see many cancers as being caused by exposure to carcinogens in the workplace, in consumer products, and in the general environment. These cancers are largely preventable — if the real nature of their causes is understood and the fight against them becomes a political priority.

How Carcinogens are Controlled

We begin our discussion of the regulatory process in Britain with a brief comparison of policies in Great Britain and the USA. This is done for several reasons. First, it is useful to consider the outcome of the highly publicized debate over chemical carcinogens in the USA in order to see what lessons can be learned for Britain. Second, the fact that different regulatory decisions have sometimes been made in Britain and the USA over the *same* chemicals (aldrin/dieldrin or benzene, for example) leads us to enquire into the political context in which such decisions have been taken in Britain. Third, it must also be said that it is often easier for British observers to obtain information about a particular substance from the USA than from British sources. Since regulatory discussions in Britain usually take place under a veil of secrecy, it is useful to investigate the relevant American debates, in order to "guess" how similar discussions may have been conducted in this country. Finally, it is clear that the present debate over the "politics of cancer" in the USA will have a substantial impact on future British policies on regulation of carcinogens. Although it now appears that the legislative activities of the European Economic Community (EEC) will become increasingly influential, there can be no doubt that American developments will continue to have important international repercussions.

The Regulatory Process in Britain and the United States: A Comparison

There are striking differences between the British and American systems for the regulation of carcinogenic substances. In the USA, far greater progress has been made in identifying such chemicals and stricter standards have been set for their control. An increasing number of carefully designed animal experiments are now being undertaken, and those chemicals which are shown to be carcinogenic in valid animal tests are officially presumed to pose a cancer risk for humans. Indeed, government agencies, such as the Environmental Protection Agency (EPA) and the Occupational Safety and Health Administration (OSHA), now carry out their regulatory activities on this basis. In Britain, however, the screening and regulation of carcinogens has received very little public, political or even scientific attention. Less animal testing is carried out and the need to control chemicals on the basis of animal data alone has still not been conceded.

The reasons behind these different policies are complex, but one important factor is obviously the scale of the problem. In absolute terms, the American chemical industry is considerably bigger than its British counterpart, particularly in the area of petrochemical production. In 1979, for example, the American industry produced nearly thirteen times more polyethylene and polystyrene, and six times more polypropylene and polyvinyl chloride (PVC) than the British industry, even though the population of the USA is only four-and-a-half times that of Britain.[1] Similarly, an estimated 700 new chemicals are introduced into commerce each year in the USA, compared with between 200 and 400 in Britain.[2] On the other hand, the difference in the number of workers employed is not so great — in 1979, the American chemical industry employed some 1,100,000 compared with 440,000 in Britain. Thus, we cannot explain the greater degree of progress made in controlling carcinogenic chemicals in the USA simply in terms of the larger size of their problem. There are, in addition, a number of social and political differences between the USA and Britain which have been, and still are, especially significant in their effects on carcinogenic regulation policies.

Public Participation in the Regulatory Process

During the post-war period, there has been a growing awareness in the USA of the dangers of many chemicals — both new substances and also those already in use — and this has led to demands for greater public involvement in the relevant decision-making bodies. American environmental and consumer lobbies are larger and more broadly based than they are in Britain. In association with the trade unions, they have been able to use their power to achieve some degree of success in pressing specific arguments related to cancer prevention. In particular, they have monitored the relationship between government regulatory officials and representatives of industry, so as to bring out into the open any collaboration that might develop between the two groups.

By contrast, there are very few organizations in Britain which can claim to represent the broader "public interest" — certainly none on the scale of the movement in the USA.[3] So far, only the trade unions have managed to exert any degree of pressure on the regulatory process, and even they have varied very considerably in the resources they have chosen to allocate to campaigns over health and safety issues.

The growth of public interest groups in the USA is closely linked to the more open style of regulation and decision-making which has traditionally existed there. An important aspect of this is the Freedom of Information Act which has allowed individuals and groups outside government and industry considerable access to relevant technical reports as well as to statements of intended policy. In addition, federal agencies are required to hold public meetings so as to allow open debate on regulatory questions and on other important public issues. Congress also has a network of subcommittees, whose duties include overseeing the activities of various governmental bodies and scrutinizing the general direction of their policies. These subcommittees have the power to call government officials as witnesses before hearings which are usually open to the public; a written record is kept of all transactions. Taken together, these aspects of the American system allow interested parties at least to be aware of the policy alternatives under discussion and to make an independent assessment of the case being made both by the "regulators" and the "regulated." Without such basic information, no effective participation by "outside" groups can take place. Thus, although existing American procedures could certainly be improved, they do at least provide for the possibility of citizen participation and offer the opportunity to influence policymaking at various stages. It must, however, be noted that the American regulatory system is now under attack as a consequence of the changed political climate in that country since Ronald Reagan became president. It is now clear that Reagan's rhetoric of deregulation — freeing business from "unnecessary restraints" — has substantially weakened the operation of carcinogen controls.

The style of British regulatory activity differs very considerably from that in the USA. Since 1974, the control of workplace hazards has been supervised by the "tripartite" structure of the Health and Safety Commission (HSC), which includes representatives from industry, local government and trade unions. However, this structure is by no means typical of the rest of the regulatory system, which consists mainly of advisory committees working behind closed doors and in close cooperation with civil servants. Confidentiality appears to be a dominant concern. Consequently, the minutes and proceedings of these committees are never published, the criteria by which they operate are rarely made public, and few detailed reports of their findings and decisions are made available. The committees consist predominantly of supposedly independent experts and virtually no provision is made for public interest groups to be involved in the decision-making process. In addition, committee members are not usually required to disclose any conflicting interest they may have in general or on a particular issue. Unlike the adversarial situation in the USA, the British regulatory system is geared towards the achievement of a consensus between regulators and the regulated. In this way controversy can be avoided and existing assumptions about carcinogenic risks, and how they should be calculated, can survive without "outside" challenge.

The Use of the Legal System

In the USA, citizen participation is also facilitated by the structure of the legal system. Claims for workers' compensation and product liability are relatively frequent and high levels of damages from a few cases of the latter have been awarded in recent years. In part, this easier access to the courts stems from the fact that lawyers are generally paid by results on a contingency basis (that is to say, they take a proportion of any damages awarded, up to 33 percent, but do not charge an unsuccessful claimant), and this provides a major incentive for lawyers to involve themselves. Thus, the judicial system provides one way in which the effectiveness of regulation can be monitored and — where necessary — effectively challenged. In addition, pressure groups have been able to use the courts to petition regulatory

activity by the various agencies. Indeed, legal action by "public interest" groups has been behind many of the regulatory decisions made in the USA in recent years. The Oil, Chemical, and Atomic Workers' Union (OCAW), for example, with the assistance of various health pressure groups, helped to push OSHA into issuing its first carcinogen list (of 14 chemicals) in 1974. On the other hand, the legal system can of course be used by industry to obstruct regulatory action. An illustration of this is provided by industry's successful petition in the American courts against OSHA's proposal to lower benzene standards.

In Britain, the legal system is far less accessible to groups or individuals wishing to influence policymaking. No direct equivalent to product liability exists, and the use of common law is typically cumbersome, slow and extremely expensive. In addition, there is no provision for a "group" or "class" action, so that financial responsibility for legal proceedings has to be assumed by an individual victim. Finally, the rights of groups and individuals in Britain to use the courts to force action by regulatory bodies are virtually nonexistent. Generally, then, the British courts have not proved useful as a way of influencing political action over the control of hazardous chemicals.

The Collection and Dissemination of Safety Data

The USA is now the major country in the world for toxicological and epidemiological research on the hazards of industrial products and processes. Both state and industrial expenditure on research have increased to cope with recent and anticipated schemes for the regulation of new chemicals. Thus, the American chemical industry has been forced to conduct increasingly stringent toxicological testing before putting new products on the market. Similarly, the federal government has allocated more resources to this area of research. In 1972, total federal government expenditure on environmental health research was in the region of $215 million of which $24 million (some 11 percent) was spent on research into chemical carcinogens.[4] By 1976, these figures had grown to $485 million and $76 million (15.8 percent) respectively.[5] When these figures are added to the $500 million spent by industry in the same year[6] it becomes clear that toxicology, and to a lesser extent epidemiology, have become big business in the USA.

In Britain, the volume of similar research is minute by comparison. In 1977, total government expenditure on toxicological research and training amounted to only about £2 million.[7] Moreover, British toxicology is even more massively dominated by industry than its American counterpart. Industry spending on toxicology amounted to some £50 million in 1977[8] and the vast majority of toxicologists are both trained by industry and work in industry. Many academic toxicologists either receive research funds from industry or are employed as industry consultants. Not surprisingly, therefore, they tend to exhibit a uniformity of approach towards the problem of cancer causation, and this approach often reflects industrial interests. Thus, most British toxicologists take an extremely conservative approach to the identification of carcinogens. They tend to pay little attention to data on animal carcinogenicity and emphasize instead the need to wait for evidence of cancer in *human* subjects before "proof" can be established — a policy which has been aptly described by several trade unions as "counting the bodies."

A serious problem is posed by this lack of British toxicologists who are truly independent of direct or indirect economic links with industry, and who, in other circumstances, could be used by trade unions and other public interest groups to intervene in the regulatory process. In the USA by contrast, a group of toxicologists and epidemiologists who are free of any dependence on industry have been able to challenge industry data and have also been willing to become involved in debates over public policy. The ensuing technical and regulatory controversies have served both to make areas of disagreement overt and also to encourage public education, participation and debate. Indeed, the fostering of this critical stance on questions of carcinogenicity control played a major part in ensuring the ultimate acceptance of the "generic" approach to carcinogen control adopted by the EPA and other regulatory agencies.

In the rest of this chapter we examine the strengths and weaknesses of the British approach to regulating carcinogens in the workplace, in consumer products, and in the general environment. If our account appears complicated at times, this reflects both the complexity of the regulatory process itself and also the very low level of public knowledge about what is an extremely important, but almost invisible, area of government activity.

The Regulation of Carcinogens in the Workplace

1. The history of regulation before 1974

The history of factory legislation extends back to the early nineteenth century when the Factory Acts were introduced to deal with the crisis conditions engendered by the Industrial Revolution.[9] Since then, legislation has been characterized by its partial and fragmentary nature. The 1953 Mule Spinning Regulations, for example, finally prohibited the use of carcinogenic mineral oils only when the industry itself had virtually ceased to exist and some 78 years after the first recorded death of a mule spinner from scrotal cancer. Moreover, no other industries using carcinogenic mineral oils were regulated, even though scrotal cancer was notifiable from the early 1920s and prescribed as a compensatable industrial disease. This illustrates the fact that the British control system has typically been more concerned with compensating the worker than with controlling the original hazards. However, this emphasis should not be taken to mean that Britain actually has an adequate compensation system. The medical panels which assess whether victims of industrial disease are eligible for benefit from the Department of Health and Social Security have come under repeated criticism for their ultra-cautious approach. The pneumoconiosis medical panels are known to reject about 50 percent of all applications, and the Society for the Prevention of Asbestosis and Industrial Diseases (SPAID) has criticized these panels for their excessively secretive mode of operation.

Cancers induced by nickel, arsenic, wood and leather dusts, and benzene are also prescribed industrial diseases (under the National Insurance Industrial Injuries Act) yet the industrial processes using these various carcinogens are not themselves extensively regulated. Thus, by offering compensation, the state recognizes the risk to workers. However, it also accepts the continuation of the risk at its existing level and as a result it is the British worker who bears the burden of proof. Such flagrant discrepancies are not due to lack of information, but reflect the influence of industry on the regulatory process and a lack of commitment by government bodies to the removal of unnecessary cancer hazards from the workplace.

The regulations introduced between 1900 and 1974 to control certain categories of a few carcinogens were very limited in their scope. Only four classes of carcinogens were covered over these years — asbestos, aromatic amines, polycyclic hydrocarbons and chromates — and the final two were controlled only in certain sectors of industry. Thus, the Carcinogenic Substances Regulations of 1967 despite the comprehensiveness implied in the title — dealt only with certain aromatic amines known to cause bladder cancer and used in the dye-stuffs, rubber, and other industries. The regu-

lations prohibit the manufacture and use in factories of beta-naphthylamine, benzidine, 4-aminodiphenyl, 4-nitrodiphenyl, and their salts, *except* when any of these is present in some other material, as a by-product of a chemical reaction in a total concentration not exceeding 1 percent. Nevertheless, the industrial use of benzidine-based dyes imported from France and Poland has been the subject of a recent trade union campaign in Britain. It is estimated that, despite the regulations, some ten thousand workers continue to handle such dyes each year, and pressure for a total ban on their use has come from the National Union of Dyers, Bleachers, and Textile Workers, the TUC General Council, ASTMS, and the Cancer Prevention Society.[10]

2. The Health and Safety at Work Act 1974

This act deals with all industrial hazards — not just carcinogens — and provides a framework for gradually reforming all previous legislation relating to health and safety at work. For the first time all workers were covered by a single law and certain provisions were also made for people living near a workplace who might be affected by emissions from it. The Act imposes the general requirement on employers to provide a safe and healthy working environment — but only "so far as is reasonably practicable." It also obliges manufacturers, importers, suppliers and designers to ensure that their products are safe by carrying out the necessary testing. They must also supply "adequate information" relating to the use of the product and to any particular safety precautions which must be adopted. In practice, however, the important phrase "so far as is reasonably practicable" qualifies all these duties and permits a broad range of compromises between the safety of workers and the expense of safer procedures and processes.

A most important section of the Act allows trade unionists to select shop-floor safety representatives. These representatives can then act for the work force on health and safety issues and they have the right to request information from their employers on existing and future hazards. Whilst the strength of safety representatives obviously varies between workplaces, the system does at least provide the opportunity for greater trade union influence over the enforcement of safety standards.

The major administrative change enacted by the Health and Safety at Work Act was to bring the various existing inspectorates (i.e. factory, mines and quarries, alkali and clean air, nuclear installations, explosives, agricultural, and the Employment Medical Advisory Service) together into one agency — the Health and Safety Executive (HSE). Policy was then delegated to another new body the Health and Safety Commission (HSC). The HSC is built on a tripartite principle with equal representation from the trade union movement, employers, and local authorities, but its secretariat is drawn from the HSE — i.e. from civil servants. This tripartism also applies to the advisory committees which operate within the HSC for the establishment of safety standards and codes of practice, the most important being the Advisory Committee on Toxic Substances (ACTS). The advisory committees prepare recommendations for the HSC itself (usually after an advisory committee working party has been formed), and these recommendations are often published as consultative documents and criticism and comment invited. The HSC then carries out further consultation with interested parties before returning the matter to the relevant advisory committee. However, at each stage in the regulatory procedure, every attempt is made by HSC and HSE officials to achieve some kind of consensus and to iron out major disagreements *before* a consultative document appears. Thus, in sharp contrast to the explicitly adversarial and open nature of the American system, this ensures that at least an appearance of unanimity continues to be maintained. However, its weakness is that an intransigent party can block attempts to reach any decision at all, thereby seriously delaying the whole regulatory process.

3. The control of carcinogens and other toxic hazards since 1974

The British HSC/E have as yet no official policy for the regulation of carcinogens. Indeed, the HSE insists that control of carcinogens should be subsumed under the general control of toxic chemicals. The HSE used to point to one of its publications, *Toxic Substances: A Precautionary Policy* (1977) as its major statement of intent. This four-page document argues the case for an overall plan for the control of the potential carcinogens only in the most general terms:

> When a substance is known to cause cancer in humans, rigorous control measures, including prohibition where appropriate, are essential and their implementation is enforced at all times. When a substance is suspected of being carcinogenic, increasingly strict control measures are taken concomitant with the available evidence of carcinogenicity.[11]

However, the document gave no detailed guidance as to precisely what such control measures might involve. So far, the HSE has itself set only four carcinogen control standards — for vinyl chloride (VC), acrylonitrile, benzene, and asbestos.

It has recently become clear that there is some difference of opinion within the occupational health and safety authorities (or rather between the HSC and the HSE) over the creation of a specific policy for occupational carcinogens. The Advisory Committee on Toxic Substances set up the Carcinogens Working Party, in 1978, which drafted proposals for separate regulations for the control of carcinogens — but these proposals have never been published. In 1982, however, the HSE published a so-called technical report *(Carcinogens in the Workplace),*[12] written by H. J. Dunster, Deputy Director General of the HSE, in which he expressed the view that the HSE "hopes to move towards a *single comprehensive* set of regulations dealing in fairly general terms with the control of substances hazardous to health" (emphasis added). Carcinogens would simply be

> subject to the more stringent requirements of the regulations . . . the more certain it appears that a substance is or will be a human carcinogen and the more potent a carcinogen it appears to be, the more stringent will be the control requirements, but the process of identification as a carcinogen will not take the substance out of one control regime into another.

This report, and the philosophy underlying it were strongly criticized by several trade unions since it appeared to be a firm statement that carcinogens would not be treated differently from other toxic substances; yet no such policy had been agreed upon by the tripartite HSC which is supposedly responsible for broad policy matters of this kind. The HSC promptly dissociated itself from the report, claiming (in March 1982) that "policy for control of all substances hazardous to health (including carcinogens) for use at work is under consideration by the Commission who expect to issue a consultation document in due course."[13]

It would seem, then, that there is some degree of confusion and disagreement within the state regulatory authority over how potential carcinogens should be controlled. But however these disputes are resolved, it is also clear that there is a further obstacle to setting new and more adequate safety standards. This stems from the lack of accurate information about the carcinogenic effects of many industrial materials on either animals *or* humans. As Edward Langley of the Hazardous Substances Division of the HSE pointed out in 1978, "the testing of industrial and commer-

cial chemicals in the past has been rudimentary and directed primarily toward the acute effect rather than the chronic."[14] Similarly, industry has usually carried out systematic testing only when there is a legal requirement — in the case of food additives or drugs, for instance — but not for industrial chemicals. In recent years, however, experiences with VC in particular have led to serious concern about the safety of many of the chemical industry's most widely used products. They have also demonstrated the crucial importance of testing materials on animals rather than insisting on the delaying and often impracticable tactic of investigating these problems exclusively on humans. This has posed two separate but interconnected problems for the HSE. First, what should be done about carcinogenic or untested materials already in use, and, second, how should the safety of new chemicals be assessed?

4. The assessment of chemicals already in use

So far there has been no systematic attempt to review the hazards of the 20,000-30,000 chemicals already in commercial or industrial use in Britain. HSE policy is that industry has the legal duty to test these materials under section 6 of the Health and Safety at Work Act, and that firms will notify them of any toxic hazards that are discovered. However, it is open to some doubt whether firms will do this without explicit legislation. It was recently revealed, for instance, that Coalite Chemical Products Ltd. had misrepresented the results of a survey into the effects of the highly toxic and carcinogenic dioxin (TCDD) on the workers in their 2,4,5-T plant.[15] In addition, sections of the report (commissioned by the firm in the aftermath of the Seveso explosion) were not made available to either the HSE or the trade unions concerned.

Neither the HSE nor the various state-supported research institutions in Britain are involved in systematic animal research to explore the carcinogenic and other effects of materials in widespread use. This is in contrast to the activities of the National Cancer Institute (NCI) and National Toxicology Program (NTP) in the USA, which have been carrying out a "bioassay program" of animal cancer tests on major industrial chemicals. This independent testing has had a significant effect in re-evaluating the hazards of certain materials that had previously been considered "safe" on the basis of either chemical industry testing or even mere assumption. The American NIOSH (National Institute for Occupational Safety and Health), although a separate research agency, in part acts as the research wing of the enforcing agency OSHA. In 1980, it spent about one-fifth of its $50 million budget on research into carcinogens. It has produced over eighty criteria documents reviewing the scientific evidence on hazards of particular chemicals and industrial processes, and recommending precautions and control standards as a basis for regulation. In addition to epidemiological surveys, NIOSH has also carried out a national occupational hazard survey, for 1972-74, which covers 5,000 plants employing over a million workers; it is embarking on a second survey of this type. The British HSE, by contrast, has no developed research wing equivalent to NIOSH. Work is contracted out to the Medical Research Council, but on a much smaller scale, and the only current systematic research program is attempting to validate short-term cancer screening tests. The HSE does not have — and does not seem to want — the resources to perform the kind of research work in which NCI, NTP and NIOSH have been engaged.

5. The regulation of new substances

Like most industrialized countries, Britain has at last begun to draw up schemes for pre-market testing of industrial chemicals. In the USA, comprehensive legislation of this sort has already been enacted (the 1976 Toxic Substances Control Act (TOSCA)), although

it has not yet been adequately implemented. In the EEC such "notification" procedures have been adopted in the form of the "sixth amendment" to the 1967 EEC directive on the classification, packaging, and labelling of dangerous substances, and this scheme has now been adopted for implementation in Britain. The HSC, in 1981, proposed a stronger scheme than that derived from the sixth amendment but, after strong industry opposition, was obliged to abandon it.

In brief, the sixth amendment requires that companies wishing to market new chemicals within the EEC must supply the following information at least 45 days before sales commence:

- a technical dossier containing evaluations of the hazardous potential of the chemical concerned;

- a declaration of its "unfavorable effects;"

- proposals for classification and labelling;

- recommended precautions for safe use.[16]

The technical dossier must give various chemical details — such as formula and purity — as well as estimates of quantities to be produced, proposed uses and storing and handling procedures. It must also include the results of some short-term animal tests — acute toxicity (LD_{50}), skin and eye irritation, and a sub-acute 28-day exposure study. Also required are the results of two short-term tests for the substance's carcinogenic potential (one using bacteria and one using some other such system).

The details of the scheme were the subject of much negotiation, and British officials had considerable success in getting their "flexible" approach to pre-market testing adopted. This was in marked opposition to the Dutch who wanted a stricter scheme similar to the American TOSCA.[17] Obviously, any scheme for notification is an improvement on the present situation and therefore welcome, but the EEC scheme has serious inadequacies.

These can be seen most clearly if it is compared with TOSCA.

(1) TOSCA's requirements on testing are much stricter than those of the EEC scheme. All notifiable chemicals (that is, those to be produced in quantities greater than 1 ton per year) have to be subjected to full animal testing, including long-term tests for carcinogenic effects. Under the EEC scheme, requirements for such long-term testing are, in effect, at the discretion of the regulatory authority (in Britain, the HSE). Such discretion is only likely to be exercised if the chemical is to be produced in very large quantities (over 1,000 tons per year).

(2) TOSCA requires the publication of information on chemicals provided by the manufacturer to the enforcing agency — in this case, the EPA — so that the information can then be subject to public scrutiny. However, under the EEC scheme, publication of the technical dossiers is at the discretion of the regulatory agency. This discretion was strongly supported by the HSE on the grounds of preserving "commercial secrecy," though as ASTMS rightly pointed out:

> The chemical companies have no secrets from one another; each can analyze the products of its rivals within hours in an analytical laboratory. The real object of "commercial secrecy" is to keep information out of the hands of the unions.[18]

(3) Manufacturers have to notify the EPA 90 days in advance of marketing the chemical, giving the EPA plenty of time to require further tests. The EEC scheme allows 45 days (and indeed the HSE argued for only 30 days).

(4) TOSCA gives the EPA the power to ban a hazardous chemical outright. There are no such powers under the EEC scheme, though they may be included in a future set of EEC regulations on the control of toxic substances.

TOSCA was only enacted in the USA after a bitter six-year struggle against the opposi-tion of American manufacturers who eventually succeeded in modifying the thrust of some of its requirements. However, the EEC scheme is even more acceptable to European chemical companies than a TOSCA-style one would be. Indeed the HSE, reflecting the views of the British chemical industry, are of the opinion that too vigorous pre-market testing requirements would actually impede innovation. Their 1977 discussion document on the subject of notification alleges (without supporting evidence) that the £12,000-20,000 (in 1977 prices) cost of carrying out the minimum toxicity tests (i.e. *excluding* tests for carcinogenicity and mutagenicity) "would cause the abandonment of many projects — perhaps 30-50 percent of the total."[19] It might well be asked whether products which do not justify the spending of such relatively small sums of money on basic testing are worth developing at all.

Early in 1981, the HSC, in response to the requirements of the sixth amendment to the EEC directive, published a revised and more extensive scheme *(Notification of New Substances,* consultative document),[20] which included the basics of the EEC scheme with two principal additions. First, chemicals produced during a production process which are not themselves the final product, but to which workers might be exposed (so-called "intermediates") would also be included in the notification regulations. Toxic intermediates would therefore have to be notified to the HSE and full assessments of their toxicity might have to be produced. Second, included for notification in addition to obvious industrial chemicals would be pharmaceuticals, food additives, pesticides and tobacco substitutes. Although these substances were already regulated by other committees, the HSE might require further information on them for the purpose of assessing their toxicity to *workers* rather than just to consumers.

Industry, particularly the pharmaceutical

industry and those firms represented by the CIA, was vehemently opposed to these additions, arguing that they would lead to higher costs and would put the British chemical industry at a disadvantage compared to its European rivals. The refusal of industry representatives to agree to the HSC's proposed scheme led the HSC to abandon it in late 1981 (though a "working party" was set up to examine particularly contentious issues). The weaker EEC scheme was therefore adopted instead.

It is important to stress one major consequence of the comparative laxity of British (and European) testing requirements. American firms will be attracted overseas — where pre-marketing requirements are much less stringent — for the initial marketing of new chemicals. Thus, if control procedures in this country are not brought up to American standards, there is a danger of Britain becoming a testing ground for "dirty" chemicals.

The overall conclusion must therefore be that, inasmuch as they necessitate some pre-market testing for new chemicals, the EEC notification schemes do represent an advance on the existing situation. However, they can only be a tiny step in the political struggle to reduce public exposure to carcinogens.

The Regulation of Carcinogens in Consumer Products

The Department of Trade is responsible for the safety of all consumer products used in and around the home which are not the specific concern of other government departments. The main products falling outside their jurisdiction are pharmaceuticals, which are regulated by the Department of Health and Social Security (DHSS), and food products and pesticides, which are both under the supervision of the Ministry of Agriculture, Fisheries, and Food (MAFF). Under the Consumer Safety Act of 1978, the Secretary of State has, for the first time, the power to pro-

hibit the supply of any dangerous goods which appear on the market, and also to insist that hazardous consumer products which are already available should be the subject of published warnings. Within the department itself, the Minister of State for Consumer Affairs takes special responsibility for consumer protection and information and also for product liability. So far, two prohibition orders which relate to carcinogenic substances have been made under the 1978 Act. These concern children's nightwear treated with the flame-retardant chemical Tris and balloon-making compounds containing benzene.[21]

The most striking features of the British system for the control of known or suspected carcinogens in consumer products are the diversity of the regulatory authorities concerned and the lack of public participation in the process. These can be illustrated most effectively by reference to three types of product: food additives, medicines, and pesticides.

1. Food additives

Under the Food and Drugs Act of 1955, it is illegal to sell food which is either "unsound" or "injurious to health." A special section of the Act (part V) covers regulations dealing with food additives and contaminants. These regulations list permitted additives according to their function (e.g. preservatives, artificial sweeteners, and coloring agents), and specify the permitted levels for each substance. The devising and amending of the permitted lists are the responsibility of MAFF, which acts on the recommendations of the Food Additives and Contaminants Committee (FACC). FACC is a committee of experts and does not include formal representation from interested parties — either the food industry or the general public. However, it should be noted that many of the experts serving on FACC are, or were until recently, employed by companies concerned with food manufacturing, such as Smedley-HP, ICI, Unilever, and Reckitt and Colman.

When an additive is considered by FACC, recommendations are made on the basis of two explicit criteria — need and safety. The judgement of "need" may be based on a range of factors including either supposed "consumer demand" or the potential of the relevant chemical for solving technical problems faced by the food industry. The onus is on the manufacturers themselves to submit evidence of both need and safety. In principle, strictly economic criteria are excluded from the discussion of need, but, in practice, it appears inevitable that the economic interests of companies are paramount in their decision to introduce a new additive. Moreover, because FACC basically functions "behind closed doors," a full and open discussion of various assessments of "need" is impossible. In such circumstances, there is a distinct danger of a close and friendly relationship developing between the regulators and the regulated industries. This means that industrial claims about the potential social utility of a product can continue without external challenge.

2. Medicinal products

The thalidomide tragedy of the early 1960s suddenly brought to public attention the lack of any systematic procedure in Britain for the testing and clearance of drugs. The 1968 Medicines Act was designed to remedy this situation by establishing a system within the Department of Health and Social Security (DHSS) for the granting of clinical trial certificates, product licences and permission to market new medicines. The day-to-day operation of the Medicines Act is carried out by the medicines division of the DHSS and by a series of advisory committees. The most important of these are the Committee on the Safety of Medicines (CSM), which gives advice on applications for licences of new drugs, and the Committee on the Review of Medicines (CRM), which considers those products which are already on the market. Both committees are composed of independent experts and do not include any wider public representation.

Broadly speaking, British controls over the safety of medicines are more systematic and stringent than those for any other type of consumer product. The DHSS has produced a series of *"Notes for Guidance on Carcinogenicity Testing on Medicinal Products,"* which specify those occasions when such testing should be conducted and lay out broad principles for the form that toxicological studies should take. However, the Association of the British Pharmaceutical Industry (ABPI) has been involved in lengthy negotiation with the DHSS and its relevant expert committee over these guidelines. While the original notes for discussion (published by the DHSS in September 1977) stated that carcinogenicity testing should be carried out where a substance would be administered to humans for any period greater than six months, the ABPI argued that this period should be extended to twelve months. After protracted negotiations this longer period was eventually accepted by the DHSS. There has also been an important debate between the pharmaceutical industry and the DHSS over the number of species to be included in carcinogenicity testing. The ABPI claims that one species alone is sufficient, while the DHSS have argued that two species must be involved.

These negotiations over carcinogenicity testing illustrate the fact that although such decisions may appear to be purely technical, they are in fact taken within a wider political and economic context which cannot be ignored. Clearly, the pharmaceutical companies have a strong interest in maintaining their profits, and therefore will be likely to oppose any regulatory policy which they see as expensive to themselves. We have already seen, for instance, that they opposed pharmaceuticals being included under the HSC's proposed scheme for pre-market assessment of chemicals to which *workers* are exposed. However, as in the case of food additives, the relevant advisory committees and decision-making bodies are structured in such a way that the results of testing are not made public and economic and political arguments of this kind cannot be explicitly debated. Rather, they operate on the basis of an assumed — but mythical — consensus between government regulators, the regulated industry and consumers, a situation which can lead to a disregard for the wider public interest.

3. Pesticides

The efficacy and safety of pesticides is under the control of MAFF. Efficacy is assessed by the Agricultural Chemicals Approval Scheme and a list of approved products is published each year. However, there is no legal restriction on the sale of unapproved products. Safety is regulated under the Pesticides Safety Precautions Scheme (PSPS) which was created in 1957. It functions through the Advisory Committee on Pesticides (ACP), consisting of ten academics and civil servants, with a scientific subcommittee of technically qualified civil servants and academics, who review all pesticide applications. Four grades of clearance are available for pesticides, from limited trials to full commercial clearance — all based on chemical, toxicological and usage data supplied by companies. An impressive list of toxicological requirements is given in an appendix to the PSPS handbook, but in practice companies only carry out tests as they see fit.

PSPS is voluntary, inasmuch as no individual firm is forced to join it. However, once the decision to join has been made, the firm is then obliged to be bound by government decisions. The scheme has been reinforced by the British Agrochemicals Supply Industry Scheme (BASIS), under which agricultural merchants undertake to sell only those products cleared by PSPS. In turn, members of the British Agrochemicals Association (which initiates the manufacture of about 95 percent of the active ingredients of all pesticides marketed in Britain) have agreed to supply only those companies that are members of BASIS. In practice, however, the voluntary nature of the scheme, and the lack of worker or consumer representation on the appropriate committees has led to widespread criticism of the pesticide regulatory scheme.

The Regulation of Carcinogens in the General Environment

Mechanisms for regulating environmental pollution and carcinogens in Great Britain are similar in character to those we have already examined in relation to consumer goods. That is to say, they are complex and fragmented and provide little or no opportunity for independent experts or concerned citizens to participate in the regulatory process. Indeed, both these criticisms probably apply even more in the area of environmental carcinogens than elsewhere.

To begin with, there are at least six separate pieces of legislation which form the basis for this area of regulatory activity.

(1) Alkali, etc., Works Regulation Act, 1906. This consolidated existing legislation on environmental pollution. However, it specifies actual emission limits for only three processes;[22] for all others, the idea of "best practicable means" is used as a basis for regulation, although operating guidelines and "presumptive standards" do exist.

(2) Health and Safety at Work Act, 1974. This imposes a general duty on manufacturers to use the best practicable means to prevent fugitive emissions from a workplace into the environment of local communities.

(3) Public Health Acts, 1936 and 1961; Public Health (Recurring Nuisances) Act, 1969; Public Health (Scotland) Act, 1897. These lay out the responsibility of local authorities for pollution control.

(4) Clean Air Acts, 1956 and 1968. These acts extend the provisions of the Public Health Acts in regard to smoke nuisances. However they relate only to those processes which are outside the jurisdiction of the Alkali Inspectorate.

(5) Control of Pollution Act, 1974. This allows local authorities to obtain full information about emissions from industrial premises.

(6) Road Traffic Acts, 1972 and 1978. These acts regulate the constitution of fuels used in motor vehicles and are supervised by the Department of Transport.

The above breakdown of legislative provisions illustrates the extremely confusing and fragmented nature of the British framework for pollution control. Moreover, these laws govern a wide range of different kinds of environmental contaminants (e.g. air, freshwater, marine, noise, and solid wastes), and the responsibility for implementing them is divided between a large number of government departments and regulatory bodies. Government agencies involved in the control of environmental pollution include the following:[23]

• Cabinet Office — interdepartmental decisions
• Department of Transport — vehicle emissions
• Department of the Environment — general co-ordinating functions and responsibility for policy in a number of areas
• Ministry of Agriculture, Fisheries, and Food (MAFF) — protection of fisheries and responsibility for Pesticides Safety Precautions Scheme (PSPS)
• Department of Trade (DOT) — marine pollution
• Department of Industry (DOI) — industrial and economic aspects of pollution
• Department of Health and Social Security (DHSS) — provides medical advice, especially through its Committee on Carcinogenicity of Chemicals in Food, Consumer Products and the Environment
• Department of Energy — advises on nuclear installations
• Department of Employment — responsibility for health, safety and welfare of persons at work
• Health and Safety Commission (HSC) — responsibilities under the Health and Safety at Work Act, 1974
• Department of Education and Science (DES) — funds basic science through its research councils
• Foreign and Commonwealth Office — international implications of environmental policies
• Ministry of Defence — supports various types of relevant research
• Scottish Office and Welsh Office — various environmental responsibilities in their respective countries
• Royal Commission on Environment Pollution (RCEP) — advises on national and international matters concerning the pollution of the environment

This division of responsibilities is further complicated by the lack of clarity concerning the functions undertaken by each agency. Thus, in the case of research for example, the Department of Industry has three relevant research establishments (Warren Springs Laboratory, the Laboratory of the Government Chemist, and the National Physical Laboratory), while the Department of Education and Science also funds environmental analysis through its research councils (particularly the National Environment Research Council). Other agencies may also sponsor research related to a specific environmental problem. So far as policymaking is concerned, initiatives may come from almost any of the above agencies — although the Royal Commission on Environmental Pollution and the Department of

the Environment play an especially significant role. Similarly, advice for future policy
may come from any of the listed agencies.
Overall, then, it is very difficult if not impossible to characterize the specific function of
each institution — each operates on a flexible basis and each is able to play a role in
research and policymaking according to the
particular circumstances.

The complexity of the system is further
exacerbated by the fact that *regulatory* duties are not concentrated in any one body and
even the responsibility for one specific type
of pollution can often be divided between
various departments — as we show below
with reference to air pollution. The fragmented and even chaotic nature of the British regulatory system is best illustrated by
comparing it with the American situation,
where the EPA combines most of the responsibilities listed above in a single authority.
Such a model is undoubtedly more efficient,
allowing for the creation of a general policy
rather than a piecemeal and incremental approach to the problem of controlling environmental carcinogens.

An additional feature of the British system
is that it frequently grants an individual department the conflicting responsibilities both
for regulating an industry and also for promoting its growth. The Department of Trade,
for example, in addition to stimulating British export sales and promoting general economic growth is also responsible for controlling oil pollution at sea. This creates an obvious danger that the development of a close
working relationship between government
officials and industry representatives will discourage the establishment of stricter environmental standards. Thus, MAFF has been criticized for being concerned more with the prof-
itability of farms than with the health and
safety of agricultural workers. In the USA,
public interest groups have paid particular
attention to situations of this kind, where there
is conflict of interest and the possibility of an

agency being captured by industrial interests.
In Britain, however, such problems have received little or no attention.

The Alkali Inspectorate: A Case Study

As an example of the British control system in practice, we now look at the regulation of air pollution by the Alkali and Clean
Air Inspectorate (AI).

The AI was originally created under the
1906 Alkali, etc. Works Regulation Act. Since
its transfer from the Department of the Environment in 1974, the AI has been located
within the HSE. It has responsibility for airborne emissions from some two thousand registered works,[24] other emissions being largely
the responsibility of local authority Environmental Health Departments (EHDs). The division of responsibility between the AI and
the EHDs is made partly according to mere
tradition and partly on the principle that the
AI should deal with the more complex and
problematic types of emission control. Fundamental to the AI is its special relationship
with the industries which it regulates. As a recent Royal Commission Report commented:

> The essence of their approach lies not in
> standing back from the industry but, on the
> contrary, in being intimately involved in it.
> The Inspectorate collaborate closely with the
> industry in seeking solutions to pollution
> problems.[25]

Central to this approach is the use of the
important concept "best practicable means."
That is to say, national air quality standards
have been rejected in favor of a case-by-case
strategy as outlined by a former chief alkali
inspector:

> There must be a compromise between: (1)
> the natural desire of the public to enjoy
> clean air; (2) the legitimate desire of the
> manufacturers to meet competition by pro-
> ducing their goods cheaply and therefore

to avoid unremunerative expenses; and (3) the overriding national interest.[26]

The operation of "best practicable means" has been succinctly described as being rather like "a good system of contract bridge played with a cooperative partner."[27] This regulatory approach is geared towards the achievement of a compromise between factory owners and the local inspectorate. Although general guidelines are provided by "presumptive limits," the system is highly flexible and the emission controls imposed on any individual workplace are the result of a process of negotiation. The economic effects of regulation on a factory are therefore taken into account by the alkali inspectors although explicit cost-benefit analyses are rarely carried out. Quite obviously, the alkali inspectors are given large discretionary powers under this system. Unfortunately, however, these powers are not balanced by any degree of accountability to local communities. Although there are provisions under the 1974 Control of Pollution Act for local authorities to obtain accurate information on pollution, and to make this available in a public register, such information has rarely been provided. Moreover, the AI has not tended to be helpful to individuals in search of details about specific emissions. Indeed one chief alkali inspector has recently referred to media coverage of pollution issues in the following terms: "Mischievous and exaggerated publicity . . . can cause fears in the public and introduce gulfs. It can also lead to social problems, unrest, and militancy."[28]

In the light of comments of this kind, it is perhaps not surprising that the AI's attitude to the public was itself criticized as follows in a recent Royal Commission Report:

To the public whose interests they serve they sometimes appear remote and autocratic. There has been some clumsiness and insensitivity in the Inspectorate's public pronouncements and an air of irritation with those who presume to question the

rightness of their decision.[29]

Thus, in contrast to the situation in the USA, public knowledge about environmental pollution is sparse, and it is very difficult to discover even what standards are being used to regulate carcinogens. Following the recent EEC directive, regulations are now being developed which will provide the public with information on the hazards of new substances about which the manufacturers will be required to notify relevant authorities such as the Department of Environment. However, notification of this kind is likely to be of little value if it merely states that the authorities consider a substance to have certain hazards without giving details of the reasons for that conclusion or specific proposals for control. Meanwhile, the secrecy of the British system has encouraged various public interest groups to demand a greater degree of public participation in the control of environmental pollutants. While the "contract bridge" approach may be acceptable to the two partners concerned, it is inevitably unsatisfactory for those outside who may well suffer the consequences of any decisions that are made and therefore not unreasonably wish to be included in the decision-making process itself.

Conclusion

We have seen that, in contrast to the USA, the procedures for the regulation of carcinogenic substances in Britain are generally fragmented and conducted in private. They operate on the basis of consensus between government-appointed experts rather than the more adversarial, open and participative approach which has developed in the USA. The only exception to this is the regulation of workplace hazards where, after a long history of piecemeal reform, the Health and Safety Commission and its advisory committees now operate on a tripartite basis. This system has given one public interest group at least — trade unions — a right both to be heard and, equally importantly, to hear and challenge the views of government officials, industry representatives, and medical and scientific experts. However, this system is far from perfect in practice. Although the HSC has held public hearings (when it was collecting views regarding the control of asbestos in the late 1970s), most of its decision-making processes are not open to public scrutiny.

Finally, it is important to emphasize that there is a clear distinction between the process by which standards for exposure to toxic and carcinogenic substances are set and the mechanisms by which these standards are then implemented and enforced. Despite its various deficiencies, the American standard-setting system is superior to the British equivalent. However, in the area of the enforcement of those few standards which exist, the British system appears more effective — at least so far as the workplace is concerned. Thus, the number of inspectors per workplace and their legal powers are greater in Britain, particularly since the 1974 Health and Safety at Work Act. The USA therefore has more satisfactory standards, but less effective means of enforcing them, whilst Great Britain has less adequate standards, but more effective enforcement — though the British Factory Inspectorate is currently experiencing financial cut-backs.

This situation illustrates the serious defects of the policies being practiced in *both* countries and the critical need for sweeping reform. It is particularly important that the *relatively* greater effectiveness of the enforcement procedures in Britain should not be used as a justification either for not improving the regulatory system itself — which has serious faults — or for leaving standards at their present unsatisfactory level.

Call for Accountability

On May 15, 1998, Lord Baldwin of Bewd-

ley wrote to the London *Times* with a "call for accountability from the scientists and doctors who work in the important field of cancer research." Lord Baldwin also expressed concern on the high cancer mortality rate in Great Britain, and called for an evaluation of alternative or complementary cancer treatment.[1]

The response to Lord Baldwin came from Dr. Gordon McVie, Director General of Britain's Cancer Research Campaign, in a letter to the *London Sunday Times* —

Sir:

Lord Baldwin of Bewdley [in his letter of May 15] calls for accountability from the scientists and doctors who work in the important field of cancer research.[2]

Let me reassure him. Twenty-five years ago, all children with leukaemia died: now, over 70 percent survive. Twenty years ago, all young men with advanced testicular cancer died: now, thanks to a drug discovered by the Cancer Research Campaign, 90 percent survive.

Deaths from all adult cancers, excluding those due to tobacco, have been 1 to 2 percent fewer, year on year, for a decade. Simultaneously, and most pertinent to Lord Baldwin's criticism, mortality from breast cancer has fallen by over 12 percent in England and Wales. All of these are the fruits of cancer research.

Our "qualified failure" has been in the fight against the tobacco industry which has successfully targeted young children, particularly girls. This has led to a sorry state of affairs in Scotland and the North of England, where more women now die of lung cancer than breast cancer.

Lord Baldwin wishes complementary medicine to be given a hearing. So it should, but it requires the same strict evaluation as conventional medicine. The Cancer Research Campaign and others have just agreed on funding for the first-ever randomized trial of aromatherapy and relaxation therapy in cancer.

We are always receptive to innovative ideas, and totally accountable to the thousands of people who support our work and who place their faith in our pioneering research.

Yours faithfully,
J. Gordon McVie
Director General
Cancer Research Campaign
May 19, 1998

McVie Misses the Point

It should be noted that, in his letter, Dr. McVie studiously avoided any reference to the "call for accountability," a call more than justified by the dominant role in national cancer policies of the indentured Richard Doll. Doll has trivialized the critical need for research and outreach on the avoidable causes of cancer (other than smoking), and has attempted to explain away the escalating incidence of cancer. McVie also made no reference to the failure, or minimal success, of conventional toxic chemotherapy to have improved survival rates for the overwhelming majority of common cancers over the last few decades. McVie's call for strict evaluation of alternative therapies would disqualify most conventional cancer therapy concerning which he is, to say the least, uncritical. Furthermore, his claim for reduction in cancer mortality is misleading, as it largely reflects improved access to health care and reduction in lung cancer from smoking in men, rather than improved survival rates. McVie also appears unaware that the incidence of cancer, including breast cancer and various nonsmoking cancers, is still steadily increasing.

McVie's claim to be "always receptive to innovative ideas" is in sharp contrast to his subsequent speech recommending that the government should actively regulate grant making by cancer charities to prevent funding of research "that is redundant or scientifically deficient" as small charities can find it difficult to obtain high quality advice from external experts.[8] McVie clearly implied that CRC, which awarded about £49 million in research grants in 1997, second only to the Imperial Cancer Research Fund's £56 million, should have a virtually exclusive monopoly on cancer research in Great Britain, research that focuses on damage control — treatment and diagnosis — to the virtual exclusion of prevention. Typical of the response to McVie's revealing mindset was a comment that his recommended oversight "gets into the field of big brother knowing what is best all the time."[1]

Chapter Sixteen

American Cancer Society: The World's Wealthiest "Nonprofit" Institution

The ACS is accumulating great wealth in its role as a "charity." According to James Bennett, professor of economics at George Mason University and recognized authority on charitable organizations, the ACS held a fund balance of over $400 million with about $69 million of holdings in land, buildings, and equipment in 1988.[1] Of that money, the ACS spent only $90 million — 26 percent of its budget — on medical research and programs. The rest covered "operating expenses," including about 60 percent for generous salaries, pensions, executive benefits, and overhead. By 1989, the cash reserves of the ACS were worth more than $700 million.[2] In 1991, Americans, believing they were contributing to fighting cancer, gave nearly $350 million to the ACS, 6 percent more than the previous year. Most of this money comes from public donations averaging $3,500, and high-profile fund-raising campaigns such as the springtime daffodil sale and the May relay races. However, over the last two decades, an increasing proportion of the ACS budget comes from large corporations, including the pharmaceutical, cancer drug, telecommunications, and entertainment industries.

In 1992, the American Cancer Society Foundation was created to allow the ACS to actively solicit contributions of more than $100,000. However, a close look at the heavy-hitters on the Foundation's board will give an idea of which interests are at play and where the Foundation expects its big contributions to come from.

The Foundation's board of trustees included corporate executives from the pharmaceutical, investment, banking, and media industries. Among them:

• David R. Bethune, president of Lederle Laboratories, a multinational pharmaceutical company and a division of American Cyanamid Company. Bethune is also vice president of American Cyanamid, which makes chemical fertilizers and herbicides while transforming itself into a full-fledged pharmaceutical company. In 1988, American Cyanamid introduced Novatrone, an anti-cancer drug. And in 1992, it announced that it would buy a majority of shares of Immunex, a cancer drug maker.

• Multimillionaire Irwin Beck, whose father, William Henry Beck, founded the nation's largest family-owned retail chain, Beck Stores, which analysts estimate brought in revenues of $1.7 billion in 1993.

• Gordon Binder, CEO of Amgen, the world's foremost biotechnology company, with over $1 billion in product sales in 1992. Amgen's success rests almost exclusively on one product, Neupogen, which is administered to chemotherapy patients to stimulate their production of white blood cells. As the cancer epidemic grows, sales for Neupogen continue to skyrocket.

• Diane Disney Miller, daughter of the conservative multi-millionaire Walt Disney, who died of lung cancer in 1966, and wife of Ron Miller, former president of the Walt Disney Company from 1980-84.

• George Dessert, famous in media circles for his former role as censor on the subject of "family values" during the 70s and 80s as CEO of CBS, and now Chairman of the ACS board.

• Alan Gevertzen, chairman of the board of Boeing, the world's number one commercial aircraft maker with net sales of $30 billion in 1992.

• Sumner M. Redstone, chairman of the board, Viacom Inc. and Viacom International Inc., a broadcasting, telecommunications, entertainment, and cable television corporation.

The results of this board's efforts have been very successful. A million here, a million there — much of it coming from the very industries instrumental in shaping ACS policy, or profiting from it.

By 1992, *The Chronicle of Philanthropy* reported that the ACS was "more interested in accumulating wealth than in saving lives." Fund-raising appeals routinely stated that the ACS needed more funds to support their cancer programs, all the while holding more than $750 million in cash and real estate assets.[3]

A 1992 article in the *Wall Street Journal*, by Thomas DiLorenzo, professor of economics at Loyola College and veteran investigator of nonprofit organizations, revealed that the Texas affiliate of the ACS owned more than $11 million worth of assets in land and real estate, as well as more than fifty-six vehicles, including eleven Ford Crown Victorias for senior executives and forty-five other cars assigned to staff members. Arizona's ACS chapter spent less than 10 percent of its funds on direct community cancer services. In California, the figure was 11 percent, and under 9 percent in Missouri:[4]

Thus for every $1 spent on direct service, approximately $6.40 is spent on compen-

sation and overhead. In all ten states, salaries and fringe benefits are by far the largest single budget items, a surprising fact in light of the characterization of the appeals, which stress an urgent and critical need for donations to provide cancer services.

Nationally, only 16 percent or less of all money raised is spent on direct services to cancer victims, like driving cancer patients from the hospital after chemotherapy, and providing pain medication.

Most of the funds raised by ACS go to pay overhead, salaries, fringe benefits, and travel expenses of its national executives in Atlanta. They also go to pay Chief Executive Officers, who earn six-figure salaries in several states, and the hundreds of other employees who work out of some 3,000 regional offices nationwide. The typical ACS affiliate, which helps raise the money for the national office, spends more than 52 percent of its budget on salaries, pensions, fringe benefits, and overhead for its own employees.

Salaries and overhead for most ACS affiliates also exceeded 50 percent, although most direct community services are handled by unpaid volunteers. DiLorenzo summed up his findings by emphasizing the hoarding of funds by the ACS:[4]

If current needs are not being met because of insufficient funds, as fund-raising appeals suggest, why is so much cash being hoarded? Most contributors believe their donations are being used to fight cancer, not to accumulate financial reserves. More progress in the war against cancer would be made if they would divest some of their real estate holdings and use the proceeds — as well as a portion of their cash reserves — to provide more cancer services.

Aside from high salaries and overhead, most of what is left of the ACS budget goes to basic research and research into profitable patented cancer drugs.

The current budget of the ACS is $380 million and its cash reserves approach one billion dollars. Yet its aggressive fund-raising campaign continues to plead poverty and lament the lack of available money for cancer research, while ignoring efforts to prevent cancer by phasing out avoidable exposures to environmental and occupational carcinogens. Meanwhile, the ACS is silent about its intricate relationships with the wealthy cancer drug, chemical, and other industries.

A March 30, 1998 Associated Press Release has just shed unexpected light on questionable ACS expenditures on lobbying.[5] National Vice President for federal and state governmental relations Linda Hay Crawford admitted that the ACS was spending "less than $1 million a year on direct lobbying." She also admitted that over the last year, the society used 10 of its own employees to lobby. "For legal and other help, it hired the lobbying firm of Hogan & Hartson, whose roster includes former House Minority Leader Robert H. Michel (R-IL)." The ACS lobbying also included $30,000 donations to Democratic and Republican governor's associations. "We wanted to look like players and be players," explained Crawford. This practice, however, has been sharply challenged. The AP release quotes the national Charities Information Bureau as stating that it "does not know of any other charity that makes contributions to political parties."

Tax experts have warned that these contributions may be illegal, as charities are not allowed to make political donations. Marcus Owens, director of the IRS Exempt Organization Division also warned that: "The bottom line is campaign contributions will jeopardize a charity's exempt status."

Track Record on Prevention

Marching in lockstep with the NCI in its "war" on cancer is its "ministry of information," the ACS. With powerful media control and public relations resources, the ACS is the tail that wags the dog of the policies and priorities of the NCI.[7,8] In addition, the approach of the ACS to cancer prevention reflects a virtually exclusive "blame-the-victim" philosophy. It emphasizes faulty lifestyles rather than unknowing and avoidable exposure to workplace or environmental carcinogens. Giant corporations, which profit handsomely while they pollute the air, water, and food with a wide range of carcinogens, are greatly comforted by the silence of the ACS. This silence reflects a complex of mindsets fixated on diagnosis, treatment, and basic genetic research together with ignorance, indifference, and even hostility to prevention, coupled with conflicts of interest.

Indeed, despite promises to the public to do everything to "wipe out cancer in your lifetime," the ACS fails to make its voice heard in Congress and the regulatory arena. Instead, the ACS repeatedly rejects or ignores opportunities and requests from congressional committees, regulatory agencies, unions, and environmental organizations to provide scientific testimony critical to efforts to legislate and regulate a wide range of occupational and environmental carcinogens. This history of ACS unresponsiveness is a long and damning one, as shown by the following examples:[6]

• In 1971, when studies unequivocally proved that diethylstilbestrol (DES) caused vaginal cancers in teenaged daughters of women administered the drug during pregnancy, the ACS refused an invitation to testify at congressional hearings to require the FDA to ban its use as an animal feed additive. It gave no reason for its refusal.

• In 1977 and 1978, the ACS opposed regulations proposed for hair coloring products that contained dyes known to cause breast and liver cancer in rodents in spite of the clear evidence of human risk.

• In 1977, the ACS called for a congressional moratorium on the FDA's proposed ban on saccharin and even advocated its use by nursing mothers and babies in "moderation" despite clear-cut evidence of its carcinogenicity in rodents. This reflects the consistent rejection by the ACS of the importance of animal evidence as predictive of human cancer risk.

• In 1977 and 1978, the ACS opposed regulations proposed for hair coloring products that contained dyes known to cause breast cancer. In so doing, the ACS ignored virtually every tenet of responsible public health as these chemicals were clear-cut liver and breast carcinogens.

° In 1978, Tony Mazzocchi, then senior representative of the Oil, Chemical, and Atomic Workers International Union, stated at a Washington, D.C., roundtable between public interest groups and high-ranking ACS officials: "Occupational safety standards have received no support from the ACS."

• In 1978, Congressman Paul Rogers censured the ACS for doing "too little, too late" in failing to support the Clean Air Act.

• In 1982, the ACS adopted a highly restrictive cancer policy that insisted on unequivocal human evidence of carcinogenicity before taking any position on public health hazards (pages 484-490). Accordingly, the ACS still trivializes or rejects evidence of carcinogenicity in experimental animals, and has actively campaigned against laws (the 1958 Delaney Law, for instance) that ban deliberate addition to food of any amount of any additive shown to cause cancer in either animals or humans. The ACS still persists in an anti-Delaney policy, in spite of the overwhelming support for the Delaney Law by the independent scientific community (Appendix VII).

• In 1983, the ACS refused to join a coalition of the March of Dimes, American Heart Association, and the American Lung Association to support the Clean Air Act.

• In 1992, the ACS issued a joint statement with the Chlorine Institute in support of the continued global use of organochlorine pesticides — despite clear evidence that some were known to cause breast cancer. In this statement, Society Vice President Clark Heath, M.D., dismissed evidence of this risk as "preliminary and mostly based on weak and indirect association." Heath then went on to explain away the blame for increasing breast cancer rates as due to better detection: "Speculation that such exposures account for observed geographic differences in breast cancer incidence or for recent rises in breast cancer occurrence should be received with caution; more likely, much of the recent rise in incidence in the United States . . . reflects increased utilization of mammography over the past decade."

• In 1992, in conjunction with the NCI, the ACS aggressively launched a "chemoprevention" program aimed at recruiting 16,000 healthy women at supposedly "high risk" of breast cancer into a 5-year clinical trial with a highly profitable drug called tamoxifen. This drug is manufactured by one of the world's most powerful cancer drug industries, Zeneca, an offshoot of the Imperial Chemical Industries (page 487). The women were told that the drug was essentially harmless, and that it could reduce their risk of breast cancer. What the women were not told was that tamoxifen had already been shown to be a highly potent liver carcinogen in rodent tests, and also that it was well-known to induce human uterine cancer.[9]

• In 1993, just before PBS *Frontline* aired the special entitled, "In Our Children's Food," the ACS came out in support of the pesticide industry. In a damage-control memorandum sent to some forty-eight regional divisions, the ACS trivialized pesticides as a cause of childhood cancer, and reassured the public that carcinogenic pesticide residues in food are safe, even for babies. When the media and concerned citizens called local ACS chapters, they received reassurances from an ACS memorandum by its Vice President for Public Relations: "The primary health hazards of pesticides are from direct contact with the chemicals at potentially high doses, for example, farm workers who apply the chemicals and work in the fields after the pesticides have been applied, and people living near aerially sprayed fields. . . . The American Cancer Society believes that the benefits of a balanced diet rich in fruits and vegetables far outweigh the largely theoretical risks posed by occasional, very low pesticide residue levels in foods."[10]

• In September 1996, the ACS together with a diverse group of patient and physician organizations, filed a "citizen's petition" to pressure FDA to ease restrictions on access to silicone gel breast implants. What the ACS did not disclose was that the gel in these implants had clearly been shown to induce cancer in several industry rodent studies, and that these implants were also contaminated with other potent carcinogens such as ethylene oxide and crystalline silica (pages 540-542).

This abysmal track record on prevention has been the subject of periodic protests by both independent scientists and public interest groups. A well publicized example was a New York City January 23, 1994 press conference, sponsored by the author and the Center for Science in the Public Interest. The press release stated:

A group of 24 scientists charged that the ACS was doing little to protect the public from cancer-causing chemicals in the environment and workplace. The scientists urged ACS to revamp its policies and to emphasize prevention in its lobbying and educational campaigns.

The scientists, who included Matthew Meselson and Nobel laureate George Wald, both of Harvard University; former OSHA director Eula Bingham; Samuel Epstein, author of *The Politics of Cancer*; and Anthony Robbins, past president of the American Public Health Association, criticized the ACS for insisting on unequivocal human proof that a substance is carcinogenic before it will recommend its regulation.

This public criticism by a broad representation of highly credible scientists reflects the growing conviction that a substantial proportion of cancer deaths are caused by exposure to chemical carcinogens in the air, water, food supply, and workplace, and thus can be prevented by legislative and regulatory action.

Calling the ACS guidelines an "unrealistically high-action threshold," a letter to ACS executive Vice President Lane Adams states that "we would like to express our hope that ACS will take strong public positions and become a more active force to protect the public and the work force from exposure to carcinogens."

ACS's policy is retrogressive and contrary to authoritative and scientific tenets established by international and national scientific committees, and is in conflict with long established policies of federal regulatory agencies.

Speakers at the conference warned that unless ACS became more supportive of cancer prevention, it would face the risk of an economic boycott. Reacting promptly, ACS issued a statement claiming that cancer prevention would become a major priority. However, ACS policies have remained unchanged. More recently, the author has issued this warning again, a warning echoed by activist women's breast cancer groups.

In "Cancer Facts & Figures, 1998," the latest annual ACS publication designed to provide the public and medical profession with "Basic Facts" on cancer — other than information on incidence, mortality, signs and symptoms, and treatment — there is little or no mention of prevention.[11] Examples include: no mention of dusting the genital area with talc as a known cause of ovarian cancer; no mention of parental exposure to occupational carcinogens as a major cause of childhood cancer; and no mention of prolonged use of oral contraceptives and hormone replacement therapy as major causes of breast cancer. For breast cancer, ACS states: "Since women may not be able to alter their personal risk factors, the best opportunity for reducing mortality is through early detection." In other words, breast cancer is not preventable in spite of clear evidence that its incidence has escalated over recent decades, and in spite of an overwhelming literature on avoidable causes of this cancer.[12]

In the section on "Nutrition and Diet," no mention at all is made of the heavy contamination of animal and dairy fats and produce with a wide range of carcinogenic pesticide residues, and on the need to switch to safer organic foods.

Conflicts of Interest

Of the members of the ACS board, about half are clinicians, oncologists, surgeons, radiologists, and basic molecular scientists — and most are closely tied in with the NCI (page 494). Many board members and their institutional colleagues apply for and obtain funding from both the ACS and the NCI. Substantial NCI funds go to ACS directors who sit on key NCI committees. Although the ACS asks board members to leave the room when the rest of the board discusses their funding proposals, this is just a token formality. In this private club, easy access to funding is one of the "perks," and the board routinely rubber-stamps approvals. A significant amount of ACS research funding goes to this

extended membership. Such conflicts of interest are evident in many ACS priorities, including their policy on mammography and their National Breast Cancer Awareness campaign.[13]

Mammography. The ACS has close connections to the mammography industry. Five radiologists have served as ACS presidents, and in its every move, the ACS reflects the interests of the major manufacturers of mammogram machines and film, including Siemens, DuPont, General Electric, Eastman Kodak, and Piker. In fact, if every woman were to follow ACS and NCI mammography guidelines, the annual revenue to health care facilities would be a staggering $5 billion, including at least $2.5 billion for premenopausal women.

Promotions of the ACS continue to lure women of all ages into mammography centers, leading them to believe that mammography is their best hope against breast cancer. A leading Massachusetts newspaper featured a photograph of two women in their twenties in an ACS advertisement that promised early detection results in a cure "nearly 100 percent of the time." An ACS communications director, questioned by journalist Kate Dempsey, responded in an article published by the Massachusetts Women's Community's journal *Cancer*:

> The ad isn't based on a study. When you make an advertisement, you just say what you can to get women in the door. You exaggerate a point. . . . Mammography today is a lucrative (and) highly competitive business.

In addition, the mammography industry conducts research for the ACS and its grantees, serves on advisory boards, and donates considerable funds. DuPont also is a substantial backer of the ACS Breast Health Awareness Program; sponsors television shows and other media productions touting mammography; produces advertising, promotional, and information literature for hospitals, clinics, medical organizations, and doctors; produces educational films; and, of course, lobbies Congress for legislation promoting availability of mammography services. In virtually all of its important actions, the ACS has been strongly linked with the mammography industry, ignoring the development of viable alternatives to mammography.

The ACS exposes premenopausal women to radiation hazards from mammography with little or no evidence of benefits. The ACS also fails to tell them that their breasts will change so much over time that the "baseline" images have little or no future relevance. This is truly an American Cancer Society crusade. But against whom, or rather for whom?

National Breast Cancer Awareness Month. The highly publicized "National Breast Cancer Awareness Month" campaign further illustrates these institutionalized conflicts of interest. ACS and NCI representatives help sponsor promotional events, hold interviews, and stress the need for mammography every October. The flagship of this month-long series of events is National Mammography Day on October 17 in 1997.

Conspicuously absent from the public relations campaign of the National Breast Cancer Awareness Month is any information on environmental and other avoidable causes of breast cancer. This is no accident. Zeneca Pharmaceuticals — a spin-off of Imperial Chemical Industries, one of the world's largest manufacturers of chlorinated and other industrial chemicals, including those incriminated as causes of breast cancer — has been the sole multimillion-dollar funder of National Breast Cancer Awareness Month since its inception in 1984. Zeneca is also the sole manufacturer of tamoxifen, the world's top-selling anticancer and breast cancer "prevention" drug, with $400 million in annual sales. Furthermore, Zeneca recently assumed direct management of eleven cancer centers in

United States hospitals. Zeneca owns a 50 percent stake in these centers known collectively as Salick Health Care.

The link between the ACS and NCI and Zeneca is especially strong when it comes to tamoxifen. The ACS and NCI continue aggressively to promote the tamoxifen trial, which is the cornerstone of its minimal prevention program (page 485). On March 7, 1997, the NCI Press Office released a four-page "For Response to Inquiries on Breast Cancer." The brief section on prevention reads:

> Researchers are looking for a way to prevent breast cancer in women at high risk. . . . A large study (is underway) to see if the drug tamoxifen will reduce cancer risk in women age 60 or older and in women 35 to 59 who have a pattern of risk factors for breast cancer. This study is also a model for future studies of cancer prevention. Studies of diet and nutrition could also lead to preventive strategies.

Since Zeneca influences every leaflet, poster, publication, and commercial produced by National Breast Cancer Awareness Month, it is no wonder these publications make no mention of carcinogenic industrial chemicals and their relation to breast cancer. Imperial Chemical Industries, Zeneca's parent company, profits by manufacturing breast-cancer-causing chemicals. Zeneca profits from treatment of breast cancer, and hopes to profit still more from the prospects of large-scale national use of tamoxifen for breast cancer prevention. National Breast Cancer Awareness Month is a masterful public relations coup for Zeneca, providing the company with valuable, if ill-placed, good will from millions of American women.

The Pesticide Industry. Just how inbred the relations between the ACS and the chemical industry are became clear in the spring of 1993 to Marty Koughan, a public television producer. Koughan was about to broadcast a documentary on the dangers of pesticides to children for the Public Broadcasting Service's hour-long show, "Frontline." Koughan's investigation relied heavily on an embargoed, ground-breaking report issued by the National Academy of Sciences in June of 1993 entitled "Pesticides in the Diet of Children." This report declared the nation's food supply "inadequately protected" from cancer-causing pesticides and a significant threat to the health of children.

An earlier report, issued by the Natural Resources Defense Council in 1989, "Intolerable Risk: Pesticides in our Children's Food," had also given pesticide manufacturers failing marks. The report was released in high profile testimony to Congress by movie actress Meryl Streep. A mother of young children, Streep explained to a packed House chamber the report's findings, namely, that children were most at risk from cancer-causing pesticides on our food because they consume a disproportionate amount of fruits, fruit juices, and vegetables relative to their size, and because their bodies are still forming.

Shortly before Koughan's program was due to air, a draft of the script was mysteriously leaked to Porter-Novelli, a powerful public relations firm for produce growers and the agrichemical industry. In true Washington fashion, Porter-Novelli plays both sides of the fence, representing both government agencies and the industries they regulate. Its client list in 1993 included Ciba-Geigy, DuPont, Monsanto, Burroughs Wellcome, American Petroleum Institute, Bristol-Meyers-Squibb, Hoffman-LaRoche, Hoechst Celanese, Hoechst Roussel Pharmaceutical, Janssen Pharmaceutical, Johnson & Johnson, the Center for Produce Quality, as well as the USDA, the NCI, plus other National Institutes of Health.

Porter-Novelli first crafted a rebuttal to help the manufacturers quell public fears about pesticide-contaminated food. Next, Porter-Novelli called up another client, the American Cancer Society, for whom Porter-Novelli had done pro bono work for years. The rebuttal that Porter-Novelli had just sent off to its industry clients was faxed to ACS Atlanta headquarters. It was then circulated by e-mail on March 22, 1993, internally — virtually verbatim from the memo Porter-Novelli had crafted for a backgrounder for 3,000 regional ACS offices to have in hand to help field calls from the public after the show aired.

"The program makes unfounded suggestions . . . that pesticide residue in food may be at hazardous levels," the ACS memo read. "Its use of a 'cancer cluster' leukemia case reports and non-specific community illnesses as alleged evidence of pesticide effects in people is unfortunate. We know of no community cancer clusters which have been shown to be anything other than chance grouping of cases and none in which pesticide use was confirmed as the cause."

This bold, unabashed defense of the pesticide industry, crafted by Porter-Novelli, was then rehashed a third time, this time by the right-wing group, Accuracy in Media. AIM's newsletter gleefully published quotes from the ACS memo in an article with the banner headline: "Junk Science on PBS." The article opened with "Can we afford the Public Broadcasting Service?" and went on to disparage Koughan's documentary on pesticides and children. "In Our Children's Food . . . exemplified what the media have done to produce these 'popular panics' and the enormously costly waste (at PBS) cited by the *New York Times.*"

When Koughan saw the AIM article he was initially outraged that the ACS was being used to defend the pesticide industry. "At first, I assumed complete ignorance on the part of the ACS," said Koughan. But after repeatedly trying, without success, to get the national office to rebut the AIM article, Koughan began to see what was really going on. "When I realized Porter-Novelli represented five agrichemical companies, and that the ACS had been a client for years, it became obvious that the ACS had not been fooled at all," said Koughan. "They were willing partners in the deception, and were in fact doing a favor for a friend — by flakking for the agrichemical industry."

Charles Benbrook, former director of the National Academy of Sciences Board of Agriculture, worked on the pesticide report by the Academy of Sciences that the PBS special would preview. He charged that the role of the ACS as a source of information for the media representing the pesticide and product industry was "unconscionable."[14] Investigative reporter Sheila Kaplan, in a 1993 *Legal Times* article, went further: "What they did was clearly and unequivocally over the line, and constitutes a major conflict of interest."[15]

Cancer Drug Industry. The intimate association between the ACS and cancer drug industry, with current annual sales of about $12 billion, is further illustrated by the unbridled aggression which the Society has directed at potential competitors of the industry.[16]

Just as Senator Joseph McCarthy had his "black list" of suspected communists and Richard Nixon his environmental activist "enemies list," so too, the ACS maintains a "Committee on Unproven Methods of Cancer Management" which periodically "reviews" unorthodox or alternative therapies. This Committee is comprised of "volunteer health care professionals," carefully selected proponents of orthodox, expensive, and usually toxic drugs patented by major pharmaceutical companies, and opponents of alternative or "unproven" therapies which are generally cheap, non-patentable, and minimally toxic.[16]

Periodically, the Committee updates its statements on "unproven methods," which are then widely disseminated to clinicians, cheerleader science writers, and the public. Once a clinician or oncologist becomes associated with "unproven methods," he or she is blackballed by the cancer establishment. Funding for the accused "quack" becomes inaccessible, followed by systematic harassment.

The highly biased ACS witch-hunts against alternative practitioners is in striking contrast to its extravagant and uncritical endorsement of conventional toxic chemotherapy. This in spite of the absence of any objective evidence of improved survival rates or reduced mortality following chemotherapy for all but some relatively rare cancers.

In response to pressure from People Against Cancer, a grassroots group of cancer patients disillusioned with conventional cancer therapy, in 1986 some 40 members of Congress requested the Office of Technology Assessment (OTA), a Congressional think tank, to evaluate available information on alternative innovative therapies. While initially resistant, OTA eventually published a September 1990 report that identified some 200 promising studies on alternative therapies. OTA concluded that NCI had "a mandated responsibility to pursue this information and facilitate examination of widely used 'unconventional cancer treatments' for therapeutic potential."[17]

Yet the ACS and NCI remain resistant, if not frankly hostile, to OTA's recommendations. In the January 1991 issue of its *Cancer Journal for Clinicians* ACS referred to the Hoxsey therapy, a nontoxic combination of herb extracts developed in the 1940s by populist Harry Hoxsey, as a "worthless tonic for cancer." However, a detailed critique of Hoxsey's treatment by Dr. Patricia Spain Ward, a leading contributor to the OTA report, concluded just the opposite: "More recent literature leaves no doubt that Hoxsey's formula does indeed contain many plant substances of marked therapeutic activity."[16]

Nor is this the first time that the Society's claims of quackery have been called into question or discredited. A growing number of other innovative therapies originally attacked by the ACS have recently found less disfavor and even acceptance. These include hyperthemia, Tumor Necrosis Factor, (originally called Coley's Toxin), hydrazine sulfate, and Burzynski's antineoplastons. Well over 100 promising alternative non-patented and nontoxic therapies have already been identified.[18] Clearly, such treatments merit clinical testing and evaluation by the NCI using similar statistical techniques and criteria as established for conventional chemotherapy. However, while FDA has approved approximately 40 patented drugs for cancer treatment, it has still not approved a single non-patented alternative drug (Appendix VIII).

Subsequent events have further isolated the ACS in its fixation on orthodox treatments. Bypassing the ACS and NCI, the National Institutes of Health in June 1992 opened a new Office of Alternative Medicine for the investigation of unconventional treatment of cancer and other diseases. Leading proponents of conventional therapy were invited to participate. ACS refused and still refuses. NCI grudgingly and nominally participates while actively attacking alternative therapy with its widely circulated Cancer Information Services. Meanwhile, NCI's police partner, the FDA uses its enforcement authority against distributors and practitioners of innovative and nontoxic therapies (Appendix VIII).

In an interesting recent development, the Center for Mind-Body Medicine in Washington, D.C. held a two day conference on "Comprehensive Cancer Care: Integrating Complementary and Alternative Medicine." According to Dr. James Gordon, President of the Center and Chair of the Program Advisory Council of the NIH Office of Alternative Medicine, the object of the conference was to bring together practitioners of mainstream and alternative medicine, together with cancer patients and high ranking officials of the ACS and NCI. Dr. Gordon warned alternative practitioners that "they're going to need to get more rigorous with their work — to be accepted by the mainstream community."[19] However, no such warning was directed at the highly questionable claims by NCI and ACS for the efficacy of conventional cancer chemotherapy. As significantly, criticism of the establishment's minimalistic priority for cancer prevention was effectively discouraged.

The Role of ACS in the War Against Cancer

The launching of the 1971 War Against Cancer provided the ACS with a well-exploited opportunity to pursue it own myopic and self-interested agenda. Its strategies remain based on two myths — that there has been dramatic progress in the treatment and cure of cancer, and that any increase in the incidence and mortality of cancer is due to aging of the population and smoking while denying any significant role for involuntary exposures to industrial carcinogens in air, water, consumer products and the workplace.

As the world's largest non-religious "charity," with powerful allies in the private and public sectors, ACS policies and priorities remain unchanged. In spite of periodic protests, threats of boycotts, and questions on its finances, the Society leadership responds with powerful PR campaigns reflecting denial and manipulated information, and pillorying its opponents with scientific McCarthyism.

The verdict is unassailable. The ACS bears a major responsibility for losing the winnable war against cancer.

Chapter Seventeen

1994-1998: NCI Track Record

The policies and priorities of the National Cancer Institute have remained virtually unchanged since the 1992 Experts' Press Conference and subsequent "700-to-1 Debate" (Chapter 13). If anything, these events have triggered a series of damage-control initiatives and aggressive public relations campaigns claiming commitment to cancer prevention, reversal of escalating cancer rates, more effective methods of cancer treatment, and success in chemoprevention of breast cancer.

Apart from the merits or otherwise of these claims, NCI's recent campaigns have been primarily directed to creating a groundswell of public and Congressional support for substantial increases in budgetary appropriations and also to deflecting criticism of NCI's minimal prevention priorities. These concerns were detailed in the author's March 20, 1998 testimony to the House Committee on Appropriations, on which this chapter is largely based.[1] This testimony prompted key Committee member Cong. David Obey (D-WI) to seek further clarification by directing a series of questions to NCI director Klausner. This exchange, together with the author's comments, are included in this chapter.

Turning the Tide Against Cancer?

Incidence, Mortality, and Survival Rates

The incidence of cancer continues to escalate. From 1950 to 1994, based on the latest published NCI data, the overall percentage in whites increased by 54%, an increase of approximately 1% per annum, while overall rates increased more sharply, by 23% from 1973 to 1994.[2] These increases are real, and persist after adjusting for a slowly aging population and for smoking. Nevertheless, NCI persists in its claims that cancer is a declining public health threat.

On December 16, 1996, defensively anticipating the twenty-fifth anniversary of the National Cancer Act which launched the "War Against Cancer," in a highly publicized press release, NCI claimed that we have "turned the tide against cancer."[3] As evidence, the NCI pointed to a "nearly 3% reduction" in cancer mortality from 1991 to 1995. NCI admitted, however, that this is mostly due to a decline in lung cancer deaths from smoking in men, and to improved access to health care, particularly among African Americans.

More importantly, however, the number of Americans getting cancer has been and still is on a steady increase. The "tide against cancer" has not only *not been turned back*, but now strikes one in two men and one in three women, up from an incidence of less than one in four a few decades ago. Cancer incidence is not only increasing overall, but also in a broad range of cancers at all ages, including: childhood leukemia and brain cancer; testicular cancer; non-Hodgkin's lymphoma and melanoma among young and middle-aged adults; and prostate and breast cancer in older age groups. Cancer incidence — the total number of people getting cancer as opposed to the smaller numbers developing fatal cancers — is a more significant measure of cancer trends than is mortality. However, incidence rates may overestimate true increases for certain cancers, particularly breast and prostate, due to the over-diagnosis of pre-invasive or pro-liferative lesions.[4] On the other hand, mortality rates are insensitive, if not misleading, for those cancers with high cure or survival rates.

Further, the picture on mortality, when examined closely, is much less rosy than the NCI would have us believe. Since 1991, cancer mortality rates for Americans over the age of 65 has continued its four-decades-old climb. Also, there has been a sharp increase in mortality from nonsmoking related cancers, including multiple myeloma, non-Hodgkin's lymphoma, chronic leukemia, and pancreatic cancer. Similar mortality trends have also been reported in major industrial nations.[5,6]

The recent 3% decline in mortality rates claimed by NCI is statistically suspect, as this is based on age-adjustment to the 1970 U.S. population. As emphasized by leading former NCI epidemiologist Dr. John Bailar in a May 1997 publication[7] and subsequent testimony before the Senate Subcommittee on Labor, Health, and Human Services,[8] the decline is only 1% when rates are more appropriately adjusted to the 1990 population. Bailar further testified that this minimal decline is more likely due to early detection and improved access to health care than to improved treat-ment, and that the decades-old claim "that 'the cure is just round the corner' is old now. We are not questioning the value of treatment; treatments are curing half of all patients. This is not a dispute over whether the glass is half full or half empty. The problem is that it is the same half full now as it was several decades ago."[7] Bailar thus agreed with the February 4, 1992 experts' report and recommended reforms (Chapter 13): "I'm convinced that a major emphasis in cancer research should be shifted from cancer treatment to cancer prevention. The war against cancer could be judged as a qualified failure."[7]

Furthermore, despite NCI's continued hype about major advances in cancer cures, overall 5-year survival rates from 1974 to 1990 have improved only minimally, from 49 to 54% for all races, from 50 to 55% for whites, and from 39 to 40% for African Americans.[7] Improvements in organ-specific survival rates are also generally small (Table 17.1). Moreover, in most cases they are accounted for by earlier diagnosis, or "lead-time bias," and diagnostic overkill and bias, particularly for pre-invasive breast cancer (ductal carcinoma in situ) and pre-invasive prostate cancer. In fact, the evidence for advances in treatment and survival

Table 17.1 Mortality and survival rates for the ten most lethal cancers

Cancer	Deaths, 1998*	% Five Year Survival Rates† 1981-87	1989-94
Lung/Bronchu	160,000	13.4	14.1
Colon/Rectum	56,000	57.0	62.1
Breast (Female)	43,900	78.2	85.3
Prostate	39,200	75.6	93.4
Pancreas	28,900	3.1	3.9
Non-Hodgkin's Lymphoma	24,900	51.4	51.4
Leukemias	21,600	36.3	42.8
Ovary	14,500	38.7	49.9
Stomach	13,700	16.0	20.8
Brain/Nervous System	13,300	25.0	30.3

* Estimated
† SEER Cancer Statistical Reviews

rates over recent decades for most common cancers is highly questionable. An extensive and rigorous statistical analysis by Dr. Ulrich Abel of the Institute of Epidemiology and Biometry of the University of Heidelberg, Germany (page 366) concluded that for most patients chemotherapy is at best, nothing more than a placebo.

After decades of intensive clinical research and development of cytotoxic drugs, there is no evidence for the vast majority of cancers that chemotherapy exerts any positive influence on survival or quality of life in patients with advanced disease. To say the least, reports of therapeutic progress commonly made public are misleading . . . They are usually based on false conclusions from inappropriate data.[9]

In spite of such compelling evidence, the cancer establishment persists in extravagant and misleading claims of high cure rates. A recent flagrant example of such claims is contained in the January 26, 1998 annual fundraising appeal from the University of Texas, MD Anderson Comprehensive Cancer Center, one of the largest in the country. The appeal states:

The fact is that well over 50% of people with cancer who are cared for at the University of Texas MD Anderson Cancer Center return home cured. That's great news for you and every Texan.

This claim is now under legal challenge on the grounds that the "outright unqualified claim of a cancer cure rate of 50% [is] a false statement . . . which violates the prohibition against mail fraud" (Appendix IX).

At a highly publicized March 12, 1998 Washington, D.C. press briefing, the NCI and ACS, together with the Centers for Disease Control and Prevention, released a "Report Card" announcing a recent reversal of "an almost 20-year trend of increasing cancer causes and deaths,"[10] as detailed in a simul-

taneously released publication.[11] "These numbers are the first proof that we are on the right track," enthused NCI director Klausner. Media coverage was extensive and uncritical. A *New York Times* headline reported "A sharp reversal of the incidence (of cancer and that) the nation may have reached a turning point" in the war against cancer.[12] The journal *Science* commented: "The news could not have come at a better time for cancer researchers. Just as Congress began working on the 1999 biomedical budget, a group of experts announced . . . that the U.S. has 'turned the corner' in the war on cancer."[13]

NCI's March 12 claims were based on a comparison between data from its 1973 to 1990 Surveillance, Epidemiology and End Results (SEER) report[14] and the most recent SEER data for 1973 to 1995.[15] However, according to its senior editor, the latest SEER report will not be published for a few months as "we are still analyzing the data."[16] Apart from these concerns, critical review of the publication on which NCI's claims were based[10] is hardly reassuring. The "reversal" in the overall mortality rates is not only minimal but exaggerated, and more likely due to improved access to health care rather than to advances in treatment and survival and to a reduction in lung cancer deaths from smoking in men. Additionally, as Bailar emphasized,[7] the true decline would have been much less if rates were more appropriately standardized to the 1990 population rather than to the 1970 rate used in the latest SEER report."[15]

The claimed reversal in the incidence of cancers of "all sites" is statistically insignificant, as are similar claims for leukemia and cancer of the prostate. Even the minimal reduction for prostate cancer was admittedly questionable. "The decreased incidence rates (of prostate cancer) may be the result of decreased utilization of PSA screening tests . . . during the early 1990s."[11] While there were significant reductions in the incidence of lung, colon/rectum and bladder cancers, there were significant increases in uterine cancer, melanoma, and non-Hodgkin's lymphoma. Moreover, there was no decline in breast cancer rates, which remain unchanged at their current high level. Curiously, no reference at all was made to testicular or to childhood cancer, whose rates have dramatically increased in recent decades. Clearly the "Report Card" merits a failing grade.[17] Report Card apart, there are disturbing questions on the overall reliability of NCI incidence data. This is well illustrated by the wild variations in the incidence of childhood cancer reported by NCI (Table 17.2).

Indifference to Cancer Prevention

Faulty Science

Complementing NCI's fixation on treatment, diagnosis, and basic genetic research is its ignorance, trivialization, or manipulation of the burgeoning and well-documented scientific evidence on avoidable and involuntary causes of cancer. Fundamental to this is NCI's continued reliance on 1981 "guesstimates" that "occupation, pollution, and industrial products" are responsible for only 7% of cancer deaths.[18] Apart from the fact that these myths have been fully rebutted in a peer reviewed scientific publication,[19] there is substantive evidence of extreme bias of the principle "guesstimate" author — Sir Richard Doll — in his gross exaggeration of the "blame-the-victim" causation of cancer, apart from his indentured relationship with industry (Chapter 14).

Among the more egregious examples of NCI's faulty or manipulative science are the following:

• Explaining away escalating cancer incidence rates as due to diagnostic advances such as CAT scans, to aging of the population, although such rates are age-adjusted, and to smoking, while ignoring the fact that lung cancer mortality rates for males in the U.S. and Great Britain are declining. Also

Table 17.2 Reported changes in the incidence of childhood cancer, 1973-1994

SEER Reports	% Incidence
1973-1980	+21.3
1973-1989	+9.8
1973-1990	+1.3
1973-1991	-8.0
1973-1994	+31.1

ignored is the 100% or greater increase in the incidence over recent decades of a wide range of nonsmoking cancers including multiple myeloma, non-Hodgkin's lymphoma, and testicular cancer, and the 40% increase in brain and nervous system childhood cancers.

• The virtual equation of lung cancer with smoking, ignoring the strong evidence incriminating a wide range of occupational causes included among "nonsmoking-attributable" cancers, particularly in women, accounting for 23% and 28% in whites and blacks, respectively. Nonsmoking attributable lung cancers are now among the three or four most common causes of cancer deaths.[19]

• Continued insistence on the role of fat per se as a major cause of many cancers, in the absence of documented evidence, while ignoring unarguable evidence of the role of a wide range of industrial carcinogenic contaminants in fat.

• In common with the position of the American Cancer Society (ACS), NCI maintains that breast cancer is "simply not a preventable disease."[20] In fact, there is a well-documented wide range of avoidable risk factors and measures which women can take to reduce such risks (Table 17.3).

More egregious than its manipulative trivialization of involuntary and avoidable cancer risks is NCI's minimalistic research on

Table 17.3 Unpublicized common breast cancer risk factors[20]

Medical Risks

- Oral contraceptives, with early and prolonged use.
- Estrogen replacement therapy, with high doses and prolonged use.
- Premenopausal mammography, with early and repeated exposures.
- Nonhormonal prescription drugs, such as some anti-hypertensives.
- Silicone gel breast implants, especially those wrapped in polyurethane foam.

Environmental and Occupational Risks

- Diets high in animal and dairy fats contaminated with carcinogenic and estrogenic environmental pollutants.
- Exposure to carcinogenic household products or pollutants from neighboring chemical plants or hazardous waste sites.
- Workplace exposure to a wide range of carcinogens.

Lifestyle Risks

- Alcohol, with early and excessive use.
- Tobacco, with early and excessive use.
- Inactivity and sedentary lifestyle.
- Dark hair dyes, with early and prolonged use.

such cancer prevention. This includes failure to have undertaken comprehensive epidemiological studies on population groups exposed to carcinogens identified in rodent tests, such as consumer products and common prescription drugs. Most seriously, NCI has failed to undertake systematic research on risk factors of every cancer whose incidence has increased over the last few decades, and which must have reflected avoidable carcinogenic exposures. In short, rather than undertaking research on cancer prevention, NCI's priorities remain dedicated to research on damage control treatment efforts.

Silence on Avoidable Cancer

In spite of the massive resources at its disposal, and in sharp contrast to the prodigious stream of information, press releases, and data bases dedicated to cancer drugs and treatment, NCI has made no effort to warn the public of involuntary exposures to a wide range of avoidable carcinogens in air, water, consumer products, and the workplace, nor of avoidable cancer risks from common prescription drugs and medical procedures such as premenopausal mammography. Nor has NCI attempted to develop systematic reader-friendly registries on all such avoidable carcinogenic exposures.

Apart from the absence of public outreach, NCI has never initiated any formal or informal intervention in Federal or State legislative and regulatory arenas designed to provide government with well-documented scientific information on involuntary carcinogenic risks. Nor has NCI made even passing reference to them in the programmatic basis of requests to Congress to increase its $2.5 billion 1998 budget to $5 billion by 2003. All this is in striking contrast to NCI's highly publicized, but questionable, claims of striking success with chemoprevention and new cancer drugs, and its plethora of publications and educational materials, including the comprehensive Public Cancer Database System, dealing with information on cancer diagnosis, treatment and clinical research. NCI remains silent or even dismissive of risks from unknowing or involuntary exposure to a wide range of environmental and occupational carcinogens as major causes of avoidable cancer while insisting that this is the exclusive responsibility of Federal regulatory agencies. However, these agencies are charged with a wide range of other responsibilities and lack the authority and wealth of scientific and educational resources specifically directed to cancer which are invested in NCI. This longstanding abnegation of responsibility and myopic professional mindset has made NCI, besides the ACS, actively complicit in losing the otherwise winnable war against cancer.

The impact of NCI's silence is well illustrated by consideration of a complex of avoidable risk factors involving the entire U.S. population. A survey of over 3,000 consumer products, published in the 1995 *Safe Shopper's Bible,*[21] revealed that many common brand name products contain a wide range of unlabeled and avoidable carcinogenic, and otherwise toxic, ingredients and contaminants (Table 17.4). The scientific basis of this information, which is presented in reader-friendly charts and text, is fully documented. As importantly, information on readily available safer alternatives are identified.

A wealth of evidence on carcinogens in consumer products — food, cosmetics and toiletries, and household products including home and garden pesticides — remains buried in government and industry files and in scattered scientific literature, and is virtually inaccessible to the general public but not to NCI. The Federal agencies involved, the Food and Drug Administration (FDA), Consumer Product Safety Commission, and Environmental Protection Agency (EPA), have taken minimal if any regulatory action to ban unsafe products or to require explicit labelling of carcinogenic ingredients and contaminants with warnings of their risks. A good recent example is diethanolamine (DEA), a very common ingredient in cosmetics and toiletries, which is readily absorbed through skin and recently been shown to be carcinogenic (see facing page). DEA has also been known for decades to interact with nitrites yielding carcinogenic nitrosamines in various consumer products, particularly preserved meat and hot dogs and cosmetics and toiletries (pages 575-584). A single and notable exception is FDA's requirement for labelling diet foods containing saccharin with warning of evidence on its carcinogenicity in rodents (Chapter 6). This warning has been recently strongly opposed by the Calorie Control Coun-

cil. Of related interest is FDA's failure to require such warnings in saccharin-containing tooth paste, posing particular hazards to children.

The pervasiveness of this problem is illustrated by the multiplicity of carcinogens listed in the examples of 12 brand name products — the "Dirty Dozen" — listed in Table 17.4. In addition to experimental evidence of carcinogenicity, there is epidemiological confirmation for some of the listed ingredients and products.[21] Examples include statistically significant associations between: consumption of nitrite dyed or preserved meat, such as hot dogs, and childhood brain and nervous system cancer and leukemia (page 575); frequent application of cosmetic talc to the genital area and ovarian cancer (page 569); long-term use of black or dark brown permanent or semi-permanent hair dyes and non-Hodgkin's lymphoma, multiple myeloma, leukemia, and breast cancer; exposure to crystalline silica and lung cancer; and exposure to 2,4-D herbicides and non-Hodgkin's lymphoma, soft tissue sarcoma, and other cancers.[21]

There is also substantial evidence associating breast and other reproductive cancers with consumption of meat in view of its high residues of estrogen and other sex hormones used to fatten cattle in feed lots prior to slaughter (Appendix XI), and also associating breast, prostate, colon, and other cancers with drinking milk from cows treated with bovine growth hormone (rBGH) to increase their milk production (Appendix XII).

Another major class of poorly recognized, and often avoidable cancer risks, includes prescription drugs. Last year, more than 2.4 billion prescriptions, were written in the United States, about nine for every man, woman and child.[22] Of the estimated 3,200 drugs on the U.S. market, 50 (1.5%) are so-called "Top Sellers,"[23] which account for nearly 30% of all prescriptions written annually, almost three per person. By retirement age, about 80 percent of the population are taking prescription

Major Cosmetic and Toiletry Ingredient
Poses Avoidable Cancer Risks

Press release by Samuel S. Epstein, M.D.
February 22, 1998

As reported on CBS Morning News today, the National Toxicology Program (NTP) recently found that repeated skin application to mouse skin of diethanolamine (DEA), or its fatty acid derivative cocamide-DEA, induced liver and kidney cancer. Besides this "clear evidence of carcinogenicity," NTP also emphasized that DEA is readily absorbed through the skin and accumulates in organs, such as the brain, where it induces chronic toxic effects.

High concentrations of DEA-based detergents are commonly used in a wide range of cosmetics and toiletries, including shampoos, hair dyes and conditioners, lotions, creams and bubble baths, besides liquid dishwashing and laundry soaps. Lifelong use of these products thus clearly poses major avoidable cancer risks to the great majority of U.S. consumers, particularly infants and young children.

Further increasing these cancer risks is long-standing evidence that DEA readily interacts with nitrite preservatives or contaminants in cosmetics or toiletries to form nitrosodiethanolamine (NDELA), another carcinogen as well recognized by Federal agencies and institutions and the World Health Organization, which, like DEA, is also rapidly absorbed through the skin. In 1979, FDA warned that over 40% of all cosmetic products were contaminated with NDELA and called for industry "to take immediate action to eliminate this carcinogen from cosmetic products." In two 1991 surveys, 27 out of 29 products were found to be contaminated with high concentrations of this carcinogen, results which were subsequently confirmed by the FDA. Based on this information, the European Union and European industry have both taken strong action to reduce or eliminate DEA and NDELA from cosmetics and toiletries. In sharp contrast, the FDA has taken no such action, nor has it responded to a 1996 petition from the Cancer Prevention Coalition to phase out the use of DEA or to label DEA-containing products with an explicit cancer warning. The mainstream U.S. industry has been similarly unresponsive, even to the extent of ignoring an explicit warning by the Cosmetics, Toiletries and Fragrance Association to discontinue uses of DEA. Such reckless intransigence is in strong contrast to the responsiveness of the growing safe cosmetic industry.

Tom Mower, CEO of Neways Inc., a major distributor of carcinogen-free cosmetics, emphasizes: "I see no reason at all to use DEA, as there are safe and cost-effective alternatives which we have been using in a wide range of our cosmetics and toiletries for the last decade."

Faced with escalating cancer rates, now striking more than one in three Americans, FDA should take immediate action to prevent further exposure to the avoidable carcinogens DEA and NDELA in cosmetics, toiletries and liquid soaps. Safe and effective alternatives to DEA are readily available.

Table 17.4 Avoidable causes of cancer from consumer products: **The Dirty Dozen**

FOOD

Beef Frankfurters — (e.g. Oscar Mayer Foods Corporation)
Unlabeled Toxic Ingredients — *Benzene Hexachloride,* Carcinogenic; *Dacthal,* Carcinogenic (Can be contaminated with dioxin); *Dieldrin,* Carcinogenic; *DDT,* Carcinogenic; *Heptachlor,* Carcinogenic; *Hexachlorobenzene,* Carcinogenic; *Lindane,* Carcinogenic; *Hormones,* Carcinogenic and feminizing; *Antibiotics,* Some are carcinogenic, e.g. Sulfamethazine.
Labeled Toxic Ingredient — *Nitrite,* Interacts with meat amines to form carcinogenic nitrosamines.
Note: Substantive evidence of causal relation to childhood cancer.
Whole Milk — (e.g. Borden or Lucerne)
Unlabeled Toxic Ingredients — *DDT,* Carcinogenic; *Dieldrin,* Carcinogenic; *Heptachlor,* Carcinogenic; *Hexachloro-Benzene,* Carcinogenic; *Antibiotics,* Some are carcinogenic; *Recombinant Bovine Growth Hormone* and *IGF-1*: Evidence of breast and colon cancer promotion.

COSMETICS and TOILETRIES

Talcum Powder — Johnson & Johnson, Inc.
Labeled Toxic Ingredient — *Talc,* Carcinogenic.
Note: Substantive evidence of causal relation to ovarian cancer.
Cover Girl Replenishing Natural Finish Make-Up (Foundation) — Procter & Gamble, Inc.
Labeled Toxic Ingredients — *BHA,* Carcinogenic; *Talc,* Carcinogenic; *Titanium Dioxide,* Carcinogenic; *Triethanolamine (TEA),* Interacts with nitrites to form carcinogenic nitrosamines; *Lanolin,* Often contaminated with DDT and other carcinogenic pesticides.
Crest Tartar Control Toothpaste — Procter & Gamble, Inc.
Labeled Toxic Ingredients — *FD&C Blue #1,* Carcinogenic; *Saccharin,* Carcinogenic; *Fluoride,* Possible carcinogen.
Alberto VO5 Conditioner (Essence of Neutral Henna) — Alberto-Culver USA, Inc.
Labeled Toxic Ingredients — *Formaldehyde,* Carcinogenic; *Polysorbate 80,* Can be contaminated with the carcinogen 1,4-dioxane; *FD&C Red #4,* Carcinogenic.
Clairol Nice 'n Easy (Permanent Haircolor) — Clairol, Inc.
Labeled Toxic Ingredients — *Quaternium-15,* Formaldehyde releaser, Carcinogenic; *Diethanolamine (DEA),* Interacts with nitrites to form a carcinogenic nitrosamine; *Phenylene-Diamines,* Includes carcinogens and other ingredients inadequately tested for carcinogenicity.
Note: Substantive evidence of causal relation to lymphoma, multiple myeloma, and other cancers.

HOUSEHOLD PRODUCTS

Ajax Cleanser — Colgate-Palmolive, Inc.
Unlabeled Toxic Ingredient — *Crystalline Silica,* Carcinogenic.
Zud Heavy Duty Cleanser — Reckitt & Colman, Inc.
Unlabeled Toxic Ingredient — *Crystalline Silica,* Carcinogenic.
Lysol Disinfectant Spray — Reckitt & Colman, Inc.
Labeled or Unlabeled Toxic Ingredient — *Orthophenylphenol (OPP),* Carcinogenic.
Zodiac Cat & Dog Flea Collar — Sandoz Agro, Inc.
Labeled Toxic Ingredient — *Propoxur,* Carcinogenic.
Ortho Weed-B-Gon Lawn Weed Killer — Monsanto Co.
Labeled Toxic Ingredient — *Sodium 2,4-Dichlorophenoxyacetic acid (2,4-D),* Carcinogenic.
Note: Substantive evidence of causal relation to lymphoma, soft tissue sarcoma, and other cancers.

drugs and each filling about 19 prescriptions per year. On a lifetime basis, this works out to 684 prescriptions per person at current rates of drug use.[24]

Since 1994, information on carcinogenicity testing has been available in the Physicians' Desk Reference (PDR) for only 241 relatively new drugs. An industry survey revealed that, in tests designed by the pharmaceutical industry to prove their safety, 101 (42%) of these drugs induce cancer in either mice or rats, 39 of which also induce cancer in both species.[25] Additionally, another 27 hormonal and cancer drugs are also recognized as carcinogenic in humans. Thus, nearly half of the 241 drugs surveyed pose potential cancer risks. The authors of the survey emphasized its limited nature: "Unfortunately, much of the data on carcinogenicity testing . . . remains unpublished in the files of the pharmaceutical companies."

Among the 50 top sellers there is epidemiological evidence of cancer risks for four hormonal drugs, such as the Pill.[22, 25] Another 12 drugs, including Mevacor, Dilantin and Prilosec, have also clearly been shown to be carcinogenic in rodent tests. A further 19 have apparently not been tested for cancer risk[26] or, if they have, the industry has failed to disclose this information. Thus, approximately one-third (16/50) of these drugs pose long-term cancer risks to the entire U.S. population.

Disturbingly, many carcinogenic drugs have been identified at test dosages near or at the therapeutic. For instance, the calcium channel blocker Plendil and the epilepsy drug Depokene induce cancer in rodents at levels as low as three times and at levels lower than the therapeutic, respectively.[22] The aggressively advertised new anti-osteoporosis drug Evista induces ovarian cancers at one-third of the recommended human dose (pages 534-5). This contrasts sharply with evidence on the carcinogenicity of pesticides and most other industrial carcinogens which

is based on tests at maximally tolerated doses (MTD), and MTD/4. Thus, based on comparative dose or exposure levels, prescription drugs as a class may pose higher cancer risks than most other recognized carcinogens.[22] These risks are compounded by the fact that many carcinogenic drugs are administered individually and in various combinations to tens of millions of patients, often for decades and sometimes starting in childhood. It would appear that prescription drugs may pose the single most important class of unrecognized and avoidable cancer risks for the entire U.S. population.[22]

To argue that such risks are more than justified by very real benefits is to posit a false dilemma. The risk-benefit equation is based on the premise that patients are affirmatively and explicitly informed of the cancer, and other risks, besides benefits of any drug, and also of the availability of safer and effective alternatives. However, this is not the case for most widely used drugs. Examples include very common non-hormonal prescription drugs, particularly anti-hypertensives and tranquilizers, known to induce breast cancer[20 Ch. 8] and drugs prescribed to many millions of children annually, such as Lindane shampoos for lice or scabies (page 572) and Ritalin for over-prescribed "attention deficit disorders."[27]

Attempts have been made to compare the carcinogenic effects of prescription drugs with smoking.[22] Estrogen-based drugs, one of the most clear-cut class of prescription drugs with long-standing evidence of carcinogenicity in a wide range of experimental animals and also with unarguable evidence of human cancer risks, induce uterine cancer in 1 of 200 women annually after 5 years of estrogen replacement therapy unopposed by progesterone, and in one of 100 women after 10 years. This is a very considerable risk, and comparable to the 1 in 250 annual incidence of lung cancer in heavy smokers.[22] Clearly, comparisons of this kind are even more difficult for most other prescription drugs known to be carcinogenic in humans and still more difficult for drugs inducing cancer in animals within human dose ranges.

Clearly, all such data should raise challenging questions for NCI which merit critical consideration, intensive research and scientific guidance to the FDA. However, not only has NCI ignored these concerns, it has gone even further by joining with ACS (Chapter 16) and industry in trivializing the significance of experimental evidence, on the basis of which the identification of carcinogenic prescription drugs, besides other chemicals, is largely based. Illustrative of this recklessness is a statement by Dr. Richard Adamson, past director of NCI's Division of Cancer Etiology, trivializing the risks of food contaminated with pesticides, such as Alar, found carcinogenic in rodent tests.[28] More recently, Dr. Leslie Ford, the senior NCI scientist in charge of chemoprevention trials to investigate whether tamoxifen can reduce risks of breast cancer in healthy women, has dismissed risks of its very high carcinogenic potency in rats, incorrectly alleging that they were only induced at high test doses.[29] Apart from the fact that the doses were equivalent to the human, based on blood levels, Ford's misleading logic would absolve virtually every carcinogen identified by rodent tests posing human risks, even though such data has preceded, in some instances by decades, epidemiological evidence on the approximately 28 recognized human carcinogens. Besides prescription drugs, medical procedures (notably premenopausal mammography and breast implants) and chemoprevention trials pose undisclosed risks of cancer (pages 535-544).

Some 11 million men and 4 million women are currently exposed, often at relatively high levels, to occupational carcinogens. As a result, occupation is the single most important source of involuntary carcinogenic exposures responsible for a wide range of avoidable can-

---

Table 17.5 Carcinogens incriminated as causes of breast cancer[19]

Carcinogen	Occupation	Approximate Numbers Exposed
Benzene	Solvents; petrochemical synthesis; electrical equipment industries; printing; hand painting, coating, and decorating	143,000
Ethylene oxide	Manufacture of products including detergents, glycol ethers, polyester fibers, and textile chemicals; past major use as hospital sterilant	121,000
Methylene chloride	Solvents; petrochemicals manufacturing; electrical equipment; molding and casting machine operators; metal plating; printing; textile; and photography	353,000
Phenylene-diamine dyes	Manufacture and formulation of dyes; cosmetologists	200,000

cers. These include breast cancer, as one million women are exposed to chemicals or processes which have been incriminated in rodent tests or epidemiological studies. The most important of these carcinogens are listed in Table 17.5.

Minimal Budgets for Prevention

Since the "War Against Cancer" was launched by President Nixon in 1971, the NCI budget has increased by over 10-fold from $223 million to an estimated $2.6 billion in 1998 (Table 17.6). This rate of increase, dwarfing escalating cancer incidence rates, has been steepest in recent years and is almost certain to increase even more steeply in the near future.

In a February 1997 budget breakdown, NCI claimed that funding for cancer prevention in its Division of Cancer Prevention and Control (DCPC) increased from $115 million in 1992 to $249 million in 1997.[30] However, in March 1998, NCI director Klausner informed Congress that "funding for primary prevention in 1997 was over $480 million" (page 498). Irrespective of this apparent gross inconsistency, past review of line item grant and contract obligations and intramural programs for "primary cancer prevention" reveals almost exclusive emphasis on smoking, nutrition, excluding carcinogenic contaminants in food, and chemoprevention. Otherwise only nominal funding, $50 million at most, is allocated to research on avoidable carcinogens in air, water, consumer products — food, cosmetics, and household products — and the workplace. Illustrative is NCI's minimal commitment to occupation — the single most avoidable involuntary exposure to carcinogens involving some 12 million male and 4 million female U.S. workers. As further illustration of its budgetary shell games, NCI's current allocation of $19.4 million to occupational cancer, representing less than 1% of its total budget, has remained virtually unchanged over the last six years. At the request

Table 17.6 NCI budgets 1992-1999

Year	NCI Budget (billions)
1992	1.8
1993	2.0
1994	2.1
1995	2.1
1996	2.3
1997	2.4
1998	2.6
1999	3.2 (requested)

of the House Committee on Government Reform and oversight, NCI submitted its latest budgetary estimates for prevention in July, 1998.

Defensive Strategies

With belated sensitivity to growing concerns on its minimal priorities for cancer prevention, NCI has developed a series of highly publicized damage-control initiatives. However, these reflect cosmetic obfuscation at worst or ignorance of the principles of primary cancer prevention at best.

In 1984, NCI launched a "Cancer Prevention Awareness Program" as part of NCI's claims that it would reduce the rate of cancer growth to one-half of the 1980 mortality rate — from 160/100,000 to 84/100,000 — by the year of 2000.[31] In spite of this assurance, mortality rates have actually increased to the current rate of 172/100,000. In a creative initiative floated in 1994, while finally admitting that it had lost the war against cancer, NCI blamed, not its own misdirected priorities, but lack of funding, Congressional support, and direct representation at the cabinet level.[32] A subsequent initiative was the April 1996 creation of a "Cancer Prevention Program Review Group" of 19 non-governmental scientists.[33] Their 70-page report, submitted to NCI in June 1997, focused on five alleged major approaches to cancer prevention:

1. *modifiable risk factors* — largely tobacco avoidance and the role of dietary macro- and micro-nutrients;

2. *animal models* — for investigating new chemopreventive agents and for studying markers of exposure to carcinogens;

3. *chemoprevention trials*;

4. *genetic predispositions to cancer*; and

5. *behavioral research.*

Avoidable exposure to occupational or environmental carcinogens received short shrift, about half a page. While stating that chronic exposure to these carcinogens "probably contributes 5 to 10% of the deaths due to cancer," it was claimed that this was a problem for regulatory agencies, and not for the NCI.

A more recent initiative was the convening of a "Cancer Control Program Review Group." Its report, submitted to NCI in September, 1997, virtually equated cancer prevention with behavioral modification.[34] The report emphasized tobacco avoidance, 5-a-day fruit and vegetable diets, and avoidance of excessive sun exposure. It also called for expansion of programs directed to this myopic and exclusionary "blame-the-victim" concept of cancer prevention. No reference whatsoever was made to avoidable exposures to environmental and occupational carcinogens.

A later initiative has been the appointment of the "First Director's Consumer Liaison Group," announced in NCI's November 6, 1997 press release.[34] The mandate of this 15-member advisory group, largely composed of cancer survivors, was to create a forum of exchange between the scientific community and cancer advocacy groups, and to develop "a mechanism by which NCI can obtain advice and feedback from the consumer community on a broad range of issues," focused on high-quality treatment, rehabilitation, and psychosocial support. Not surprisingly, these issues included no reference to cancer prevention. A most revealing defensive initiative, in response

to Congressional concerns and questions, has been a series of budgetary shell games with regard to alleged expenditures on prevention. Highlights include claimed increases from $115 million in 1992, to $249 million in 1997, to "over $480 million" in May 1998, and to approximately $1 billion in July 1998.

At the request of the House Committee on Government Reform and Oversight, NCI submitted its latest budgetary estimates for prevention in July, 1998.[35]

By including a grab bag of clearly unrelated programs, such as "Community Clinical Oncology," "Early Detection Activities," and "Immunology"; other broad and loosely defined programs such as "Physical, Chemical, and Biological Carcinogenesis," which largely deal with basic mechanism studies unrelated to prevention; and "Diet and Nutrition," which includes nutritional support for cancer patients, NCI has upped its estimated "prevention" expenditures to about $1 billion (Table 17.7). These rubber numbers reflect defensiveness at best and obfuscation at worst.

Chemoprevention of Breast Cancer

Tamoxifen

On April 6, 1998, NCI distributed a sensational press release. Headlined "The First Prevention Trial in the World to Show That a Drug Can Reduce the Incidence of Breast Cancer," it lauded a drug trial in which the incidence of breast cancer had been reduced by about half in tamoxifen-treated women. It further stated that, in view of these results, NCI had decided to terminate the trial 14 months ahead of schedule. This announcement was highly unusual in two particulars: (1) it was not accompanied by any scientific publication, and (2) none of the details of the so-called "Breast Cancer Prevention Trial" would be available for at least six months.

A leading tamoxifen researcher and pro-

Table 17.7 NCI 1998 budget estimates for "Total Prevention Research"

Program	$ (in thousands)
Chemoprevention Activities	32,393
Community Clinical Oncology Program (CCOP)	41,200
Diet and Nutrition	57,710
Early Detection Activities	31,036
Epidemiology	192,304
Immunology	6,470
Information Dissemination and Outreach	55,627
Physical, Chemical, and Biological Carcinogenesis	495,622
Smoking Prevention and Cessation Program	49,878
Special Studies in the Surveillance Program	19,058
Management and Support Costs Associated with the Prevention Program	18,870
Total NCI Prevention Research	$1,000,166

ponent of the short-term trial, Dr. Craig Jordan, was typically extravagant in his claims: "Within the next two years, it will be routine to prevent breast cancer in postmenopausal women" with tamoxifen.[36] Dr. Bernard Fisher, scientific director of the National Surgical Adjuvant Breast and Bowel Project that conducted the Breast Cancer Prevention Trial, proclaimed: "This the first time in history that we have evidence that breast cancer cannot only be treated but also prevented."[37] Dr. H. Varmus, NIH director and uncritical supporter of the cancer drug industry (page 493), whose disinterest in mission-oriented research is a matter of record (page 369), enthused about "a big deal."[38] After an initial outburst of uncritical enthusiasm, the media generally became more cautious, with warnings of side effects of the drug and also with headlines such as "British Scientists Criticize U.S. for Ending Trial of Cancer Drug — acting prematurely and perhaps raising false hopes."[39]

Involving 300 cancer centers in the U.S. and Canada, NCI, and ACS launched the $60 million trial in April 1992 (page 542). Some 16,000 healthy women at "high risk of breast cancer" were to be recruited, equal numbers of whom were to be randomly assigned to either a tamoxifen or placebo test group. Enrollment was closed in September 1997 and the trial was terminated in April 1998. Criteria for "high risk" included: the absence of parity and/or delayed parity; first degree relatives with breast cancer; the number of breast biopsies, especially if they revealed atypical hyperplasia; and age over 60. Based on these criteria, it has been estimated that about 29 million U.S. women would qualify as candidates for chemoprevention if the trials proved successful.

A summary report accompanying NCI's press release revealed a mixed pattern of benefits and risks for the 13,388 healthy participants, 6,681 in the tamoxifen group and 6,707 in the placebo group. In each group, 40% of the women were under the age of 50, and 60% were over the age of 50 (Table 17.8).

While short-term reduction in invasive breast cancer was seen in all age groups, serious and sometimes fatal complications

Table 17.8 Results of the tamoxifen trial

Risks	Tamoxifen Group	Placebo Group
Invasive Breast Cancer	85	154
Breast Cancer Deaths	3	5
Non-Invasive Breast Cancer	31	59
Bone Fractures	47	71
Pulmonary Embolism	17 (2 deaths)	6
Deep Vein Thrombosis	30	19
Uterine Cancer	33	14
Cataracts	"slight increase"	

were seen only in postmenopausal women. For women in this age group who had not had a hysterectomy, tamoxifen reduced the incidence of invasive breast cancer by 1.7% while resulting in a 2.2% increased incidence of serious complications.

What the Results Mean

These results make it clear that, at the very best, chemoprevention with tamoxifen is an *exercise in disease substitution rather than disease prevention,* and that the rationale for its use in healthy women is thus highly questionable. [20,40] Moreover, these results raise two basic and unanswered questions. First, does tamoxifen prevent breast cancer or does it merely delay its onset, by treating small undetected cancers, as queried by British critics. [41] Second, does the short duration of this, and other planned trials, preclude recognition of serious delayed, long-term health risks. In this connection, it may be noted that while calcium channel blockers are effective in reducing high blood pressure in the short-term, they subsequently increase the risk of cardiac death. Similarly, AZT has been shown to delay AIDS-related symptoms in asymptomatic patients, but has no effect on long-term survival. Of major concern in this connection is the unequivocal evidence of the high hepatocarcinogenic potency of tamoxifen in rats, [37]

as confirmed in February, 1996 by the International Agency for Research on Cancer, apart from the unusual production of stable DNA adducts in liver cells. [41] It should further be noted that liver cancer may take up to twenty years to develop and that only relatively few women have taken tamoxifen in breast cancer treatment trials for over five years. Astoundingly, while these risks were dismissed by senior NCI staffer and spokesperson Dr. Leslie Ford as just based on experimental data, NCI was sufficiently impressed by the experimental evidence of tamoxifen's teratogenicity to exclude pregnant women from this trial. Further compounding risks of liver cancer, apart from other reported risks including hepatitis, liver failure, and ocular toxicity, [41] are serious legal, ethical, and scientific considerations. These reflect the fact that the healthy women enrolled in these trials were given no information on such risks in spite of explicit warnings six years ago:

"The 'consent forms' waiver of compensation for illness and injury which participants must sign is unlikely to protect the NCI or its investigators and hundreds of U.S. and Canadian centers and institutions involved in the trial from a future flood of malpractice and punitive claims for cancer and other complications. The doctrine of informed consent is legally protective only when all facts relevant to benefits and risks are fully and affirmatively disclosed."[41]

On July 11, 1998, two articles in *The Lancet* effectively discredited NCI's claims, based on a press release rather than a scientific publication, that tamoxifen prevented breast cancer in short-term trials.[42] A six-year study by the Royal Marsden Hospital in London, based on some 2,500 women with a family history of breast cancer and a similar four-year study by the European Institute of Oncology in Milan, based on 5,400 women, found no difference in the incidence of breast cancer in women treated with tamoxifen or placebo.[43] Dr. Trevor Powles, leader of the British study, concluded: "I have grave concerns about the widespread use of [the drug] in healthy women."[42] Particularly in view of this most recent evidence on the ineffectiveness of tamoxifen for breast cancer prevention, besides its recognized short-term life-threatening complications and the strong likelihood of further delayed fatal complications, NCI's proposed new tamoxifen trial represents medical malpractice, verging on the criminal. The trial should have been embargoed pending urgent independent review. NCI, however, has made it clear that, irrespective of these considerations, it intends to proceed with the trial.

One other element of the tamoxifen chemoprevention trial merits comment; that is the role of Zeneca Pharmaceuticals,* the manufacturer of tamoxifen. Zeneca supplied all of the tamoxifen for the trials free of charge. Since 1984, Zeneca has also sponsored and financed the annual October National Breast Cancer Awareness Month, urging women to have regular mammograms (page 538). Conspicuously absent from Zeneca's aggressive promotion is any reference to prevention of breast cancer by reducing exposure to a wide range of avoidable environmental, occupa-

tional, lifestyle, and medical risk factors, including the well-documented evidence of risks from premenopausal mammography.[20]

Zeneca Moves for Fast-Track Approval

In August 1998, the Food and Drug Administration announced that it would review a New Drug Application (NDA) from Zeneca for the routine use of tamoxifen to prevent breast cancer in healthy women at "high risk." The FDA Advisory Committee hearing was set for September 2, 1998. In response, the author submitted the following critique for the hearing record:

Zeneca's Nolvadex NDA [tamoxifen] for preventing breast cancer in healthy women "at high risk of cancer," including all women over 60 years old, is primarily based on NCI's April 6, 1998 summary report, "Breast Cancer Prevention Trial (BCPT) Shows Major Benefits, Some Risks."[52] This report was unsupported by a peer reviewed scientific publication and was qualified by the admission that "Further analyses of the data are under way;" no further data have yet been released nor has the report yet been published. Additional evidence is derived from tamoxifen's partial protective effects in rats and mice against the induction of breast cancer by 7,12-dimethylbenzanthracene (DMBA), besides other carcinogens.[51] However, those DMBA-induced cancers which were not suppressed were hormone independent and highly aggressive.[44]

Evidence for Chemoprevention. NCI's report announced that the BCPT had been terminated prematurely on March 24 in view of "clear evidence that tamoxifen reduced breast cancer risks."[52] As indicated in the Table [17.8], based on data cited on

---

* Zeneca is a spin-off of Imperial Chemical Industries, one of the world's largest manufacturers

of carcinogenic pesticides and industrial chemicals.

the report, tamoxifen reduced the incidence of both invasive and non-invasive breast cancer in women of all ages. However, the short-term duration of the trial precludes determination as to whether the drug prevented cancer or merely delayed its onset by treating small undetected tumors.

On July 11, 1998, two publications in *The Lancet* reported no evidence for the efficacy of tamoxifen in preventing breast cancer. A six year trial by the Royal Marsden Hospital, London oncologic team, based on some 2,500 women with a family history of breast cancer,[53] and a similar four year study by the European Institute of Oncology in Milan, based on 5,400 women,[57] reported no difference in the incidence of breast cancer in women treated with tamoxifen or a placebo. An accompanying editorial warned:[54]

> The failure of these trials to confirm the results of the U.S. study, however, casts doubt on the wisdom of the rush, at least in some places, to prescribe tamoxifen widely for prevention. Longer follow-up of completed and current trials is clearly required, to clarify the relative preventive benefits and risks in different populations, and to confirm the BCPT findings. Most importantly, none of these trials provides reliable data on mortality, which should be the ultimate endpoint.

These concerns have been summarily dismissed by NCI. ". . . the chance that our results occurred by chance was 1 in 10,000."[50] However, *The Lancet* editorial did not challenge the results themselves, but their interpretation and significance.[54]

Evidence For Risks. Serious short-term complications in the BCPT, uterine cancer, pulmonary embolism, and deep vein thrombosis, were increased 2-3 fold in the tamoxifen group (Table 17.8); these complications were only seen in postmeno-

pausal women. Among non-hysterectomized women in this age group, the incidence of these serious complications was 2.2% in contrast to a 1.7% reduction in the incidence of breast cancer.

It must be recognized that the short-term duration of the BCPT, apart from the absence of any long-term follow-up, precludes recognition of possible further increases in the incidence of already recognized short-term life-threatening and other serious complications, and also of other, not yet reported, long-term or delayed complications. Of concern in this connection is the fact that tamoxifen induces ovarian necrosis[49] and ovulation in a manner similar to clomiphene, a recognized risk factor for ovarian cancer.[58] More serious still is the high hepatocarcinogenic potency of tamoxifen in the rat, as confirmed in February 1996 by the International Agency For Research On Cancer, at low doses and blood levels equivalent to those in the BCPT;[47, 56] tamoxifen also binds tightly to estrogen receptors in the human liver,[56] and induces highly stable DNA adducts in two rodent species.[48] Risks of liver cancer are not precluded by the absence of such reported complications among breast cancer patients treated with tamoxifen, as relatively few such women have taken the drug for over five years and [none have been] followed up for a further twenty years before which [time] the induction of liver cancer would be unlikely.

It should be noted that senior NCI staffer Dr. Leslie Ford dismissed risks of liver cancer on the grounds that no cases were reported in the short-term BCPT and also on the incorrect grounds that carcinogenic effects in rats were only seen at high doses;[45] Ford's logic, however, would exculpate virtually all recognized human carcinogens. Furthermore, NCI's denigration of the human relevance of the experimental carcinogenicity data on tamoxifen and its failure to warn BCPT participants of this grave risk is in striking contrast to its reliance on rodent teratogenicity data as the basis for warning against the administration of tamoxifen to pregnant women.[52] It is of further interest to note that while some 25 cases of liver toxicity in tamoxifen-treated breast cancer patients, acute hepatitis, liver failure and deaths, and hepatobiliary complications, had been reported in Great Britain by 1992, with similar evidence obtained from the FDA,[46] no such adverse effects were noted in the short-term BCPT.

Conclusions. NCI's preliminary April 6 report on the prevention of breast cancer by tamoxifen has still not yet been finalized and published in a scientific journal. The Advisory Committee should consider the propriety of Zeneca's NDA submission as it is based, in part, on data which have not been made fully available to the public although the underlying (NCI) research was funded by the public. Furthermore, the claimed evidence for chemoprevention has been rebutted by two subsequent scientific publications. Of as great concern is the well-documented evidence of short-term life-threatening complications, and also risks of delayed fatal complications evidence for which has been trivialized and suppressed by NCI. Based on these scientific and ethical considerations, the Advisory Committee is urged to deny approval of Zeneca's NDA.*

Raloxifene (Evista)

On April 20, 1998, summaries of two new unpublished studies involving less than 50 women treated with raloxifene (Evista), manufactured by Eli Lilly, were released by the American Society of Clinical Oncology.[59] Raloxifene is a second generation of a group of drugs known as "selective estrogen receptor modulators" (SERMs), of which tamoxifen was the first generation progenitor. Unlike tamoxifen, raloxifene does not pose risks of uterine cancer and was approved by FDA on December 10, 1997 for the prevention of osteoporosis. Based on one of two short-term clinical trials with small numbers of women, it was claimed that raloxifene reduced risks of breast cancer by about 50%. With knee-jerk alacrity, NCI director Klausner reacted to this minimal information by announcing "head to head" clinical trials this fall comparing the alleged ability of raloxifene to prevent breast cancer with that of tamoxifen.

Of particular concern is the fact that in experiments designed by Lilly to prove the drug's safety, raloxifene was shown to induce ovarian cancer in rats, and in mice at doses well below the therapeutic. However, Lilly suppressed this critical information in its full-page ads for Evista in major national and regional newspapers and in its prescription warnings (page 534).† NCI's reckless indifference to the grave risks of raloxifene gave a clear go-ahead to Lilly. Lilly began aggressively promoting and advertising Evista even before the onset of the clinical trials. As a result, Evista appears to be well on its way to becoming a household word, and is receiving comments from the popular press that range between tacit approval and outright blessing. In the September 1, 1998 issue of

---

* It may be noted that Chicago's Northwestern Memorial Hospital's Fall 1998 issue of "Lifetime of Health," widely circulated in early August, outlines guidelines for tamoxifen chemoprevention by Drs. Craig Jordan and Monica Morrow, and misleadingly assures women that the use of tamoxifen for breast cancer prevention has been "recently approved by the FDA."

† Lilly also reacted to the author's public disclosure of such risks by attempting to dismiss the human relevance of the experiments, and by protesting to the Provost of the University of Illinois, Chicago — where the author is Professor of Environmental Medicine — which is in receipt of funding from the company.

Family Circle magazine, the Medical News department reported:

> A widely used drug for the prevention of osteoporosis, raloxifene (Evista), may also protect against breast cancer. . . . In recent months researchers found that women taking raloxifene had a more than 50 percent reduction in their risk of developing breast cancer, and preliminary findings show it may not increase endometrial cancer like other anti-breast-cancer drugs.

There Are Alternatives

More fundamental is the fact that there are alternative methods for reducing risks of breast cancer which are not only effective but also safer (Table 17.3). A 1996 study showed that women taking aspirin three times weekly for five years reduced their breast cancer risk by as much as 30%;[60] there is similar protective evidence for other nonsteroidal anti-inflammatory drugs (NSAIDS) such as ibuprofen. These findings are confirmed by five earlier studies published in peer reviewed journals.[20]

Although gastrointestinal complications of NSAIDS may limit their role in chemoprevention, it is revealing to note that NCI has failed to mount clinical trials on this inexpensive and non-patentable non-prescription drug. More recent studies have shown that aspirin may have anti-angiogenic effects by inhibiting an enzyme, cyclooxygenase-2 (COX-2), that promotes growth of blood vessels into tumors.[61] Several COX-2 inhibitors have been developed which seem to be devoid of gastrointestinal toxicity and which induced prolonged regression in rodent tumors.

Additionally, lifestyle factors, particularly exercise, avoidance of obesity, low animal fat diets, and low alcohol intakes have also been shown to be effective protectants. In one recent study, such factors were reported to reduce risks of breast cancer by 30%.[62]

Cancer Drugs

The history of cancer chemotherapy over the last three decades is littered with a highly touted array of cancer drugs, such as tumor necrosis factor, alpha interferon, interleukin-2, and monoclonal antibodies, whose initial high promise of success was each greeted with a flurry of breathless headlines announcing the latest magic bullet or miracle cancer cure. With subsequent recognition of their high toxicity, drug resistance following temporary tumor responses, and failure to improve survival rates, initial enthusiasm was followed by sober reality and disillusion.[9, 63] This cyclical process was ironically described in a *Washington Post* article by Daniel Greenberg. See "Progress Reports," on the facing page.

Randomized Controlled Clinical Trials

The "gold standard" for determining the acceptability of new cancer drugs is the so-called *randomized controlled clinical trial.* Two groups of patients are randomly assigned either to treatment with the new drug, or to "controls" — generally drugs with assumed or established benefits or, less frequently, to a placebo. The impetus for the now-routine use of these trials came from the 1962 Kefauver-Harris amendments to the Federal Food, Drug, and Cosmetic Act requiring "substantial evidence" to prove the effectiveness of any new drugs. While the FDA has interpreted this law to require evidence from minimally two trials, it should be emphasized that a wide range of drugs, such as penicillin, insulin, and aspirin, are unquestionably accepted as highly effective without ever having been subjected to these trials.

The NCI and major oncology centers nationwide currently urge cancer patients to enroll in these clinical trials. Each year, NCI sponsors hundreds of trials, currently involving about 300,000 patients, with costs approaching $100 million, in a tangled web of

"Progress Reports"
An Exercise in Irony by Daniel S. Greenberg
From *The Washington Post*, June 8,1998

Professor: Class will come to order. Today we will discuss reporting news of medical progress. Why is this type of news popular and important?

Student: People are afraid of being sick and want good news.

Professor: Correct, but it's not only ordinary people who like good news about medical progress. Who else?

Students: (In unison) Investors.

Professor: Of course. But what I had in mind was that scientists and doctors like good news too. It shows they're helping people. That's why they let us know whenever they make progress. But new cures are actually very rare. Sometimes doctors and scientists go for years without finding a new cure for disease. For long stretches, there are no cures to report. So what do you do? (Silence).

Professor: Think hard. What do you do?

Student: Make up that there's a cure?

Professor: No. For the hundredth time. You'll get caught if you make it up, and you might lose your job. What do you do? (Silence).

Professor: You write about a step that might possibly lead to a cure. A step. There are few cures, but in the medical journals, there are many reports of steps.

Student: But if it's only a step, you can't be sure that it's leading to a cure. It could end up as nothing.

Professor: Right. And that happens lots of the time. That's why you don't report that it's leading to a cure. That would be unethical, because you don't know. You report progress.

Student: So, what do you write?

Professor: You write that there's a promising development and that researchers and doctors are excited. That clues people into knowing that something important is going on. Otherwise, the researchers and doctors wouldn't be excited. Also, that doctors are besieged by desperate patients and their families pleading for the new treatment. You might even call it an unprecedented clamor.

Student: For the cure?

Professor: That's what the patients want. But you have to point out that there is no cure, no treatment, no drug. There's nothing. Just a promising development in mice or maybe some bugs. That's all. As a medical communicator, it's your responsibility to make that clear.

Student: How do you do that?

Professor: With absolute honesty. You write that there's a development and that researchers are excited about it. You find a researcher who will give you a meaningful quote, along the lines of: "In 86 years of working on this problem, I've never seen anything like this." You should also point out that the new step was published in a peer-reviewed journal. Most people have no idea what that means, but it's a plus. But having set the stage, you now need to guard yourself and your readers.

Student: Against what?

Professor: Against undue optimism that a cure is coming.

Student: How do you do that?

Professor: You write that on many previous occasions, reports of promising developments have not panned out, and that it may be years before a drug is available just for human testing — if ever. Also that drugs sometimes work in rats but have no effect on people, or maybe even harmful effects. Look for a researcher in the field who will give you a skeptical quote, something like, "This development, if it stands up to verification, is interesting, but a great deal of work remains to be done to determine what, if anything, it means."

Student: So, it's not so hard to write about medical progress that can lead to cure even if it doesn't.

Professor: Not at all. It happens all the time.

The writer is a visiting scholar in the history of science, medicine and technology at John Hopkins University.

government, academia, and the now globalized pharmaceutical industry. The NCI proposes to expand these trials to enroll a five-fold increase in the number of participants over the next five years. However, many trials are marred by serious problems of bias, design, and interpretation.[63] Additionally, as patients are randomly and without their knowledge assigned to test or control groups, some may get only a placebo.

While entering a clinical trial may well sound attractive, particularly to patients with advanced cancer, the chances of any benefits are remote. Only about 1% of patients develop complete remissions, and only 5% get any "tumor response."[63] However, tumor response is by no means a cure. As defined by NCI and FDA, it is a shrinkage in the size of a measurable tumor by 50% lasting for a month or more, even if the tumor resumes its previous size and then grows rapidly. In fact, there is generally no relation at all between shrinkage of a tumor and any prolongation of survival. Worse still is the poorly predictable toxicity of the new drug — sometimes leading to marked deterioration in the quality of life, devastating toxicity, and earlier death than in untreated patients.[9] In one trial involving a three-drug regimen, called "ICE," the oncologists involved concluded, with revealing insensitivity, that the regimen was "well tolerated with acceptable side-effects," although 8% of the patients were killed by the treatment. In another clinical trial on patients with a leukemia-type syndrome, 42% of patients were killed by the treatment (Appendix VIII). Clearly, the ethical and legal doctrine of fully informed consent for patients enrolling in clinical trials is honored more in the breach than the observance. Similar charges have been leveled against the conduct of clinical trials in Great Britain.[64]

No wonder that resistance of patients, and also many oncologists, to controlled trials with cancer drugs is now sharply increasing. "In fact, only 10 percent of all oncologists enroll 80% of patients in clinical trials. In New York, oncologists have given these patients small doses of standard chemotherapy to make them ineligible for useless clinical trials."[63]

A recent draft report from the Inspector General of the Department of Health and Human Services warned that patients entering these trials were "often exposed to unsafe and unethical practices because no one policed the research to protect their interest."[65] The report further charged that "doctors and drug companies often recruited people for their research with misleading advertisements in buses and subways (and that) review boards in hospitals and medical schools . . . were riddled with potential conflicts of interest . . . (as they) were expected to be responsive to the financial pressures facing their parent institutions and/or sponsors."

Of all medical procedures, NCI's randomized trials with cancer drugs pose the greatest risks to patients with highly questionable, if any, potential benefits. Enrollment in these trials, as currently conducted is at best an exercise in Russian roulette.

The New Generation of Cancer Drugs

A new generation of biotechnology drugs is now emerging. These are based on naturally-occurring proteins or genetic materials which are more specific and focused in their action and have less than or minimal toxicity than conventional chemotherapy. These biotherapies include: anticancer vaccines; antisense and gene therapy; matrix metallo-proteinase inhibitors; more specific monoclonal antibodies; and angiogenesis inhibitors. Over 30 such drugs are now in the final phase of clinical trials, and a few have shown early signs of promise, either alone or in combination with conventional chemotherapy. Notable examples are the monoclonal antibodies Herceptin, used for treatment of breast cancer, and Rituxan, for non-Hodgkin's lymphoma.[66] However, in the absence of evidence on improved survival rates, which will take several years to develop, most oncologists and the media are reacting with cautious optimism and with talk of advances in treatment, rather than cures. A notable exception is the extravagant recent hype on angiogenesis inhibitors.

A Sunday (May 3, 1998) *New York Times* front-page article by Gina Kolata, followed by a flurry of other newspaper and television reports, proclaimed dramatic and ostensibly *new* news on experimental studies in mice with two angiogenesis inhibitors, endostatin and angiostatin. With awe-inspiring hyperbole, Kolata reported that a combination of endostatin, derived from collagen, and angiostatin, derived from plasminogen, eradicated tumors in mice without inducing resistance. Curiously, however, there was nothing new in Kolata's news. In November 1997, veteran *New York Times* science editor Nicholas Wade reported the identical information which had just been published in the journal *Nature*, accompanied by a cautious editorial warning that there had been equally impressive results in mice with many other drugs with subsequently disappointing results.[67] Lost also in Kolata's brouhaha was the fact that about 20 angiogenesis inhibitors are already being tested in humans, three of which are in Phase III trials.[68]

Even Folkman — a meticulous and modest researcher who has been working on angiogenesis inhibitors for nearly three decades — constantly faced with skepticism and a complete lack of support from the cancer establishment — was taken aback by Kolata's story: "I am puzzled by the response, because this is six months old." The answer to this puzzle seems based on a two-million dollar book deal that Kolata was negotiating the same day that her article appeared. Faced with challenges to her credibility and questions on conflict of interest, Kolata was obliged to withdraw her proposed book deal.[69] This challenge to Kolata's credibility was hardly surprising in view of her track record of extreme

anti-environmental and pro-corporate bias.[70]

Unquestionably, Folkman's research on angiogenesis inhibitors is of great interest. More than 30 pharmaceutical industries are now researching and manufacturing a wide range of angiogenesis inhibitors. While they appear to be nontoxic, complications from their effects on normal angiogenesis involved in wound healing, ovulation, menstruation, and fetal development may be anticipated. It must also be recognized that testing cancer drugs on mouse tumors has proved such an unreliable indicator of human responses that NCI abandoned their use several years ago in favor of screening with tissue culture systems. The reasons for this disparity between mice and humans include the greater genetic heterogenicity and sensitivity to drug toxicity of humans compared with highly inbred mice, and immunological differences between the two species. Additionally, small-scale clinical trials with one of Folkman's earliest angiogenesis inhibitors, the fungal derivative TNP-470, have met with only limited success. It is of further interest to note that the use of shark cartilage extracts, a highly potent source of endostatin, for treatment of patients with advanced or terminal cancer has reportedly yielded promising results.[63, 71, 72]

In spite of encouraging developments with the new generation of biotherapy drugs, cautious optimism is warranted until they can be evaluated in terms of improved survival rates. Meanwhile, the critical comments of veteran epidemiologist and NCI critic John Bailar seem justified: "We've had 40 years of hype about wonderful cancer cures that are just around the corner, down the road, hang on, we'll be there soon. I do not see anything that says the present situation is any different."[73]

Escalating Budgets

In November, 1997, Dr. Klausner sent Congress a blueprint request for $3.2 billion 1999 budget. In an urgent appeal for more money,

Klausner placed almost exclusive emphasis on the need for expanding research on genetics, cancer diagnosis, and treatment. "Knowledge about the fundamental nature of cancer is exploding." Noteworthy was the virtual absence of any reference to cancer prevention.

Powerful support for NCI's requests for further funding has been spearheaded by a well-orchestrated campaign to lobby Congress and persuade the public to accept the groundless and decades-old myth that further research — that is, research on treatment but not on prevention — is the only answer to the cancer epidemic. In January 1995, the National Coalition for Cancer Research, sponsored by the American Cancer Society and the cancer drug industry, launched an industry-funded "Research Cures Cancer" campaign, focused exclusively on finding newer and better cancer drugs without any reference whatsoever to prevention (Appendix XIII). An Op-Ed article entitled "Cancer: So Close to Success" appeared in *The Washington Post* on June 29, 1997. Authored by noted oncologist, Dr. Marc Lippman, and beginning with an urgent plea for still more spending on cancer research and treatment, the piece illustrates the powerful and self-serving support for the research cures cancer campaign among cancer clinicians and researchers in the nationwide network of some 60 National Cancer Centers funded by the cancer establishment.

A subsequent initiative, launched in October 1997, is "The March." This encompasses hundreds of events nationwide, culminating in a "Historic March on Washington, D.C. on September 26, 1998 — to encourage government to increase the woefully inadequate funding for research" to cure cancer. Like the National Coalition for Cancer Research, "The March" is sponsored and heavily financed by the cancer drug industry, with support from cancer survivor groups. Not surprisingly, the White House was warmly responsive to this PR onslaught. President Clinton announced his initiative to increase funding for cancer research at the National Institutes of Health (NIH) by 65% over the next 5 years. This is the largest increase in cancer-related spending in the history of NIH. Approximately 90% of the funds would go to the NCI, bringing its budget up from $2.5 billion this year to about $4.3 billion by 2003. At a February 1998 House Appropriation committee hearing, Dr. Klausner went still further in requesting a $5 billion budget for 2003 (page 500). As a first step, the President requested Congressional approval for a $2.8 billion budget for 1999. Strong public and Congressional support for these proposals has been encouraged by very recent uncritical media coverage of successes with chemoprevention of breast cancer, new "miracle cancer drugs," and randomized controlled clinical trials.

Conflicts of Interest‡

Clearly NCI, leadership is and has been fixated on diagnosis, treatment, and basic genetic research with relative indifference to cancer prevention. These problems of professional mind-sets are compounded by basic institutionalized conflicts of interest. For decades, powerful groups of interlocking financial interests, with the highly profitable cancer drug industry at their hub, have dominated the war on cancer. By linking their priorities with those of major pharmaceutical companies, the NCI has directed its own priorities away from prevention.[19, 20]

The NCI's prototype Comprehensive Cancer Center, New York's Memorial Sloan-Kettering Hospital, represents just one example of how deeply entrenched is this conflict of interest. Jointly funded by the NCI and ACS, the Sloan-Kettering annual budget exceeds $350 million — the equivalent of the com-

---

‡ This section is largely based on material from Chapter 13 of *The Breast Cancer Prevention Program,* 1998,[20] reprinted with permission.

bined total budgets of the nation's ten largest environmental organizations. Bristol-Myers Squibb, the world's largest manufacturer of cancer drugs and past manufacturer of carcinogenic breast implants, along with other major pharmaceutical companies, controls key positions on Memorial Sloan-Kettering board (368-9). Other board members have close affiliations with oil, petrochemicals, and other industries, and the media (pages 463-4). Further examples of this basic conflict of interest show up in employment and funding practices.[19]

A revolving door of employment between the cancer establishment and drug industry raises disturbing questions about conflict of interest among senior executives.[20] Dr. Stephen Carter, now head of drug research and development at Bristol-Myers Squibb, for instance, previously served as director of NCI's Division of Cancer Treatment. He was followed in August 1994 by Dr. Richard Adamson, former Director of the Division of Cancer Etiology, who later left NCI to head the Washington office of the National Soft Drinks Association, an organization that vigorously promotes the use of artificial sweeteners, including the carcinogenic saccharin. After six years as NCI Director, Samuel Broder, M.D., resigned in April 1995 to become Vice President and Chief scientific officer of IVAX Co. of Miami, a major manufacturer of cancer drugs. Broder was recruited to this new job by Dr. Phillip Frost, CEO of IVAX and key member of the National Cancer Advisory Board (page 367).[74]

This pattern is not new. The late Dr. Frank Rauscher, who was appointed NCI Director by President Nixon to spearhead his "War On Cancer," resigned in 1976 to become Senior Vice President for research of the ACS and moved from there in 1988 to become Executive Director of the Thermal Insulation Manufacturers Association, which promotes the use of carcinogenic fiberglass and fights against its regulation.[75] The late oil magnate Armand Hammer, chairman of Occidental Petroleum,

a major manufacturer of carcinogenic industrial chemicals and pesticides, chaired the President's Executive Cancer Panel of NCI in the 1980s. The previous chairman, for over a decade, was Benno C. Schmidt, an investment banker, senior drug company executive, and member of the Board of Overseers of the Memorial Sloan-Kettering Comprehensive Cancer Center. Not surprisingly, both Schmidt and Hammer showed little interest in cancer prevention research and programs, and virtually exclusionary interest in highly profitable drug development and marketing.

Illustratively, using taxpayers' money, NCI paid for the research and development of Taxol, an anticancer drug now manufactured by Bristol-Myers Squibb. Following completion of clinical trials — an extremely expensive process in itself — the public paid further for developing the drug's manufacturing process. Once completed, NCI officials gave Bristol-Myers Squibb the exclusive right to sell Taxol at an inflationary price. As investigative journalist, Joel Bleifuss, wrote in a 1995 *In These Times* article, "Bristol-Myers Squibb sells Taxol to the public for $4.87 per milligram, which is more than 20 times what it costs to produce."[76] Taxol has been a blockbuster for Bristol-Myers, posting sales of about $3 billion since its approval in 1992, and accounting for about 40 percent of the company's sales.[77]

Taxol is not the only drug involved in such murky funding practices. Bristol-Myers Squibb now sells nearly one-third of the approximately thirty-five cancer drugs currently available, often with highly inflated profits, and often developed with taxpayer funds. In 1995, NIH director Harold Varmus, a past major recipient of the NCI funds for basic genetic research (Chapter 13), decided that "reasonable pricing" clauses, which protect against pharmaceutical industry exorbitant profiteering from drugs developed with taxpayer dollars, were driving away private industry. So he struck these from agreements between industry and the NCI. Now, no controls on prices for cancer drugs made at taxpayers' expense exist. James P. Love of Ralph Nader's Center for Study of Responsive Law has extensively investigated conflicts of interest between the NIH, the NCI, and the cancer drug industry. In testimony before the Subcommittee on Regulation of Business Opportunity and Technology of the Committee on Small Business of the United States House of Representatives, Love protested:[78]

It is just one more example of NIH's efforts to accommodate the pharmaceutical industry's interest in a wide range of matters. ... NIH sees itself as a partner with industry, and it has become highly sympathetic to the industry views on issues such as drug pricing and reporting requirements. Why is it that the U.S. government does not collect data on drug prices, does not routinely collect data on drug development costs, even for drugs developed with government funding, and does not express the slightest interest in these matters? There are ... less benign reasons. NIH officials often seek employment in the private sector after their government service, or anticipate lucrative consulting arrangements with the private sector if they obtain a university appointment. What's good for the industry may eventually be good for them too. Indeed, as Dr. Robert Wittes has shown in the case of Taxol, one can work on a research project for NIH, then leave the government to help a drug company commercialize the discovery, and then return to the same government agency and begin a new research project.

Taxol is not an isolated example. Taxpayers have funded NCI's research and development for over two-thirds of all cancer drugs now on the market. In a surprisingly frank admission, Samuel Broder, who directed NCI from 1989 to 1995, stated the obvious: *"The NCI has become what amounts to a government pharmaceutical company."*[77] In this con-

nection, it is of interest to note that the U.S. spends about five times more on chemoprevention per patient than Great Britain, although this is not matched by any difference in survival rates.[79]

Imbalanced Priorities

The current status of non-Hodgkin's lymphoma (NHL) offers a paradigm of NCI's imbalanced policies and priorities with regard to research on cancer treatment and related genetics, in contrast to research and outreach on prevention.

The age-adjusted incidence of NHL has escalated dramatically by 187%, from 1950 to 1994.[2] From 1973 to 1994, its incidence increased by 91% for men and 67% for women — 1.8% annually for both sexes. Decades of research on the chemotherapy and genetics of NHL have met with limited therapeutic success, although recent developments with Rituxan therapy appear promising. Yet a substantial body of well-documented data since the 1970s, including those from NCI's minimally funded Occupational Studies Section, have provided substantial evidence incriminating occupational exposure to pesticides and the cosmetic use of hair dyes as major avoidable causes. Illustrative are studies showing up to a seven-fold increased risk in farmers exposed to 2,4-D herbicides for over three weeks a year,[80] and high risks for farmers exposed to several groups of pesticides and individual insecticides.[81] Also illustrative is evidence that use of black and dark brown permanent and semi-permanent hair dyes accounts for 30% of NHL cases in exposed women and 20% in all women, apart from additional risks of multiple myeloma and leukemia.[82]

Yet in spite of substantial evidence that the recent epidemic of NHL is largely avoidable, NCI has failed to conduct further research on its risk factors and failed to provide Congress and the FDA with such scientific information in order to enable the development of appropriate legislative and regulatory responses. As importantly, NCI has failed to warn the public and labor of these avoidable risks through its well-developed and well-funded outreach program. Instead, NCI still focuses on attempts to treat, rather than prevent, this avoidable cancer.

A similar scenario relates to most other cancers involved in the current cancer epidemic. There is, or should be, no conflict between priorities for treatment and basic research and for prevention. Both merit high priority, if not purity. But surely, preventing avoidable cancer is more effective and more humane than damage control, just attempting its treatment.

NCI Responses to Congressional Questioning

Following the author's March 20, 1998 testimony to the U.S. House of Representatives Committee on Appropriations, key Committee member Cong. David Obey (D-WI) directed a series of questions to NCI director Klausner. Selected questions and his May 1 responses are summarized below, followed by the author's comments and conclusions.

Question: Explain the basis of NCI's request for a $3.2 billion budget as opposed to the $2.8 billion proposed by President Clinton.

Answer: The extra $.4 billion is needed for further funding of NCI's "Extraordinary Opportunities (and) Challenge" in four major areas: cancer genetics; pro-clinical models of cancer; diagnostic imaging techniques; and defining distinctive "signature" molecules in blood of cancer patients for purposes of early diagnosis and selection of treatment methods.

In order to meet this "Challenge," NCI has developed a plan with "seven critical elements." These include the National Clinical Trials program on new cancer drugs, currently involving 300,000 patients, which NCI proposes to increase by five-fold, and expansion of the Cancer Centers' Program.

Comment: Apart from a single parenthetic reference in relation to cancer genetics, NCI's proposed plan makes no reference whatsoever to prevention. Moreover, the track record of NCI's clinical chemotherapy trials leaves little basis for optimism. Despite massive investment of resources in these trials over the last three decades, there is little if any objective evidence of therapeutic efficacy of chemotherapy for most common cancers as evidenced by prolongation of survival, in contrast to the current misleading criterion of a "tumor response" based on temporary tumor shrinkage. As importantly, many new drugs tested are highly toxic, sometimes resulting in impairment of the quality of life, devastating complications, and a high incidence of treatment deaths. Apart from problems of design and biased interpretation of these trials, there are serious ethical and legal questions with regard to the adequacy of informed patient consent. For these reasons, a growing number of patients and oncologists are becoming increasingly reluctant to participate in NCI's clinical trials. Also of concern is NCI's refusal to undertake systematic clinical trials on alternative, non-patented, and minimally toxic complementary treatments — in spite of the strong recommendations in a 1990 Office of Technology Assessment report on "Unconventional Cancer Treatments" and by the National Institutes of Health Office of Alternative Medicine.

In August 1997, the Office of Alternative Medicine (OAM), based on recommendations by over 100 conventional and alternative practitioners, proposed a mechanism — "Practice Outcomes Monitoring and Evaluation Systems" (POMES) — for NCI's evaluation of alternative therapies. NCI director Klausner has yet to respond, while professing to be "open-minded" on the problem. Klausner has gone still further in highly prejudicial and misleading attacks on alternative therapies through NCI's widely disseminated Cancer Information Service (Appendix VIII).

Responding belatedly to a growing groundswell of protests, from patient advocacy groups and their congressional supporters, against NCI's frank hostility to alternative cancer therapy, Klausner suddenly reversed his position. In July 31, 1998 written testimony before the House Government Reform and Oversight Committee, Klausner stated: "The NCI is moving very quickly in important directions to develop CAM (complementary alternative medicine) information and expand research opportunities for CAM investigation — including strengthening our relationship with the Office of Alternative Medicine." In the same testimony, Klausner reiterated NCI's misleading claims for declining cancer incidence and mortality and for "real progress against cancer" without any reference to prevention.

Moreover, the programs of the National Cancer Centers are dedicated to diagnosis, treatment, and basic molecular research, and they play no educational or interventional role relating to cancer prevention.

Question: "Provide a breakdown of cancer causes as a percentage of total cancer cases."

Answer: While NCI has not developed such estimates, it relies on those published by Doll and Peto which ascribe 35% to dietary factors, 30% to tobacco, and the balance to causes including 4% to occupation and 2% to pollution.[18]

Comment: There are serious scientific flaws in these estimates, based on an obsolete analysis of cancer trends from 1933 to 1997, which have been fully rebutted in peer-reviewed publications.[19] These include trivializing the role of occupation as major causes of lung and other cancers, ignoring

the role of parental occupational exposures as important causes of childhood cancer, and ignoring the wealth of scientific publications on cancer risks from involuntary exposures to industrial carcinogens in air, water, food, and other consumer products. As disturbingly, there is persuasive evidence of Doll's indentured relationship to industry (Chapter 14).

Question: "Provide a breakdown of NCI's cancer prevention funding by categories . . . where prevention is the primary purpose of the grant."

Answer: Funding for primary prevention in 1997 was over $480 million "almost 50% (of which) was directed towards environmental exposures, 19% was directed towards nutrition research, 14% involved smoking, and 2% was related to occupational exposures. . . . Opportunities in cancer prevention are emerging and we anticipate fully to take advantage of these opportunities."

Comment: The claim for expenditures of $480 million on primary cancer prevention, approximately 20% of the 1997 budget, is misleading. Curiously, this claim is flagrantly inconsistent with NCI's February 1997 budget for "research dollars by various cancers" listing an allocation of $249 million for "cancer prevention and control." Furthermore, no information at all is provided on the alleged 50% expenditure on "environmental exposures." The 19% for nutrition research is allocated to chemoprevention, in attempts to protect against avoidable exposures to environmental and occupational carcinogens, and to the protective effects of low-fat and high-fruit and vegetable diets. However, this research ignores substantial and long-standing evidence on the important role of dietary contamination with carcinogenic pesticides and other industrial chemicals. As disturbing is the less than 2% allocated to occupation, the single most important cause of involuntary and avoidable carcinogenic exposures. Even Doll and Peto, on whose 1981 publication NCI still explicitly relies,[18] ascribe 4% of all cancer mortality to occupation. This is about 20,000 deaths a year. Moreover, there is clear evidence that 4% is a substantial underestimate of occupational cancer mortality.[19] Interestingly, the balance of 15% of the NCI's alleged $480 million expenditures on primary prevention is unaccounted for in NCI's response. Still further straining credulity as to NCI's May 1, 1998 prevention estimate of $480 million, in response to a later request for information from the House Committee on Government Reform and Oversight, Klausner responded by doubling this figure to about $1 billion (Table 17.7).

According to the author's estimates,* expenditures on primary cancer prevention were under 3% — 50 million of its $2 billion budget — rather than 30% as claimed.[19] The only way for Congress to obtain reliable information on primary prevention funding is to request a General Accounting Office audit of the title, summary, abstract, and cost of every grant and contract claimed to have been specifically designed for primary prevention, and also similar information for all such intramural programs.

NCI's claim to take advantage of emerging opportunities in cancer prevention is difficult to take seriously. Such opportunities have been available for decades and NCI still fails to recognize and take advantage of them.

Question: "Other than tobacco and exposure to sunlight, do you think that the general public has been adequately informed about avoidable causes of cancer?"
Answer: The NCI and a number of other or-

ganizations including the American Cancer Society . . . have worked for years to inform the public about lifestyle choices that could increase or decrease the risks of cancer . . . through NCI's Cancer Information Services . . . and through distribution of millions of publications. . . . In addition, when testing shows that chemicals cause cancer, NCI and other agencies including the National Toxicology Program (NTP) and the International Agency for Research on Cancer (IARC) publicize the test results."
Comment: This revealing response illustrates NCI's persistent fixation on personal responsibility for cancer prevention. NCI still takes no responsibility for public dissemination of well documented scientific information on avoidable risks from involuntary exposure to a wide range of carcinogenic chemicals, including those identified and systematized by IARC in its monographs for over two decades and, more recently on a limited basis, by the NTP. Moreover, senior NCI scientists are on recent record as denigrating the human relevance of evidence of carcinogenicity from animal tests. It should further be emphasized that NCI has rarely if ever testified before Congress on the scientific validity of information on avoidable carcinogenic exposures nor has it provided such information and expertise to Federal regulatory agencies, notably FDA, EPA, and OSHA. This represents a virtual abnegation of responsibility for informing the nation of practical methods for reducing escalating cancer rates.

Question: "Should the NCI develop a registry of avoidable carcinogens and make this information widely available to the public?"
Answer: Such information is already available from NCI's Cancer Information Ser-

---

* Estimates which went unchallenged in the debate following my May 5, 1992 invited presenta-

tion to NCI's entire staff and advisory committee.

vice, which last year took nearly 50,000 calls about a variety of carcinogens, and also from IARC and the NTP.

Comment: IARC and the NTP have not developed such registries nor is it their mission to do so. This is clearly an integral scientific and outreach responsibility of NCI and should be one of its major priorities.

Question: "During the hearing, you stated the NCI could effectively spend $5 billion by 2003. Provide a budget mechanism table that shows how you would allocate this level of spending in 2003 compared to 1998.

Also provide the following for 1998 and 2003 —

a) The number of competing, continuation and total grants.

b) The average success rate.

c) The average grant size and length of the award.

d) The number of research centers and average center award.

e) Any other quantitative or budgetary comparisons that indicate how the additional $2.5 billion would be spent compared to existing resource levels."

Answer: "NCI envisions a three-pronged approach:

1. Sustain at full measure the proved research programs that have enabled us to come this far.

2. Seize extraordinary opportunities to further progress brought about by our previous successes. . . . Our goals in these areas are: Cancer genetics; pre-clinical models of cancer; imaging technologies defining the signatures of cancer cells.

3. Create and sustain mechanisms that will enable us to rapidly translate our findings from the laboratory into practical applications that will benefit everyone."

Comment: The five-page response is as broad in generalizations as sparse in detail. Furthermore, it is unresponsive to the specific questions posed, nor does it provide the requested "budget mechanism table."

Conclusions: Dr. Klausner's response to Cong. Obey's questions make it clear that NCI persists in its intransigent and long-standing indifference to primary cancer prevention. As disturbing is the deceptive and misleading nature of NCI responses to current and past expressions of Congressional concerns. NCI is a runaway institution fixated on its own myopic and self-interested agenda and unresponsive to national concerns on the losing war against cancer.

Recognizing these realities, the February 1992 statement by over 60 leading national experts in cancer prevention and public health urged the following legislative initiative (Chapter 13):

"The NCI must give cancer cause and prevention at least equal emphasis, in terms of budgetary and personnel resources, as its other programs including diagnosis, treatment and basic research. . . . This major shift in direction should be initiated immediately and completed within the next few years. This shift will also require careful monitoring and legislative oversight to prevent misleading retention of old unrelated programs under new guises of cancer cause and prevention."

The only possible legislative response to NCI's minimal priorities for cancer prevention, and the annual cancer toll of 1.2 million Americans, is for Congress to hold its appropriations hostage to such reforms and, more immediately, to block NCI's request for a further increase in its 1999 budget.

Chapter Eighteen

How to Win the
Losing "War Against Cancer"

This book has made it clear that the cancer establishment, with its overwhelming medical, educational, media and financial resources, has failed to direct even minimal priorities to research on primary cancer prevention. This failure is compounded by the virtual absence of outreach to Congress, regulatory agencies, and the public-at-large with regard to information on involuntary exposures to avoidable environmental, occupational, and other carcinogens. The establishment's highly restrictive blame-the-victim policies on prevention are in striking contrast to its disproportionate and myopic fixation on research on basic genetics, and on damage control, diagnosis and treatment, and related outreach programs. These misguided and imbalanced priorities have been the single most important disincentive to the development of corrective legislative and regulatory action, and to industrial initiatives to phase out the manufacture, use, and disposal of carcinogenic products and processes in favor of safer alternatives. In no small measure, these policies have also been responsible for escalating cancer rates over recent decades, culminating in the current cancer epidemic.

Faced with these realities, is it in any way possible for individual citizens to fight the losing cancer war? The answer to this question, posed and answered two decades ago (Chapter 11), is a resounding yes. This answer is based on two complementary strategies. The first — personal action which effectively bypasses the cancer establishment — is to prevent or reduce avoidable exposures to carcinogens, particularly for consumer products, prescription drugs, and the workplace. The second — involvement in political action, locally, regionally, and nationally — is to achieve similar and even broader objectives. The right-to-know is the key and common link to empowerment on both personal and political levels.

Personal Action

A recent reader-friendly book, *The Safe Shopper's Bible*, provides well-documented information on avoidable cancer risks from numerous brand name consumer products — foods, cosmetics and toiletries, and household products — which carry no warning label, risks which the cancer establishment has known but ignored (Appendix XIV).[1, 2]

Government offers little guidance. Indeed, while many local, state, and federal government agencies are entrusted with protection of the public health, most have failed to assure consumers they are being adequately protected, or that they are being provided with full, if any, label disclosures of carcinogenic (i.e., cancer-causing), neurotoxic (i.e., causing damage to the nervous system), and reproductive effects, including teratogenic (i.e., birth defect-causing) chemicals in their foods and household products.

Armed with such information on undisclosed carcinogenic ingredients and contaminants, you can boycott these products and instead shop for safer, in many instances organic, alternatives which are becoming increasingly available. Apart from protecting yourself and your family, such marketplace pressures punish reckless mainstream industries and reward those which are responsible. As increasing numbers of citizens vote for safety with their shopping dollars, the greater will be the economic incentive for industry to phase out the manufacture, use, and disposal of carcinogenic products and processes. There are several other reader-friendly books dealing with a wide range of environmental carcinogens and toxics, and with self-protection.[3-5]

When it comes to carcinogenic prescription drugs, no such sources of information are readily available (Chapter 17). However, there is one exception: the "Drug Disclosure Label" or "Patient Package Insert" which your pharmacist is legally required to provide on request. Similar information is also provided in the *Physicians' Desk Reference* (PDR), the "Bible" on drugs which is or should be on every M.D.'s bookshelf, and possibly even on your own bookshelf. Each label generally has ten or more sections, four of which are the most important from the standpoint of cancer risk: Warnings or Caution; Indication and Usage, Contraindications; and Precautions. Explicit warnings of cancer risk are infrequent, found only in the Warnings and/or Indications and Usage sections, rarely in boldface black type, and even then restricted to those few drugs with strong and well-recognized evidence of risks, such as those for the association between Premarin and uterine cancer. The great majority of carcinogenicity test data is summarized in a Precaution subsection entitled "Carcinogenesis, Mutagenesis, and Impairment of Fertility." The language of this subsection is highly technical and virtually deliberately unintelligible except to professional toxicologists. Nevertheless, the essential points can be grasped by any reader. Any reference to an increased incidence of tumors or cancers in mice or rats dosed with the drug (tumors or cancers especially when they are induced in both species) is a clear warning signal. Drugs so identified should be avoided —

especially if, following discussion with your physician, safe and effective alternatives can be identified. The same position should also be taken for drugs for which no carcinogenicity data are presented in the PDR. This process can be reasonably achieved by developing a productive relationship with your physician, making it clear that you want to be involved in medical decisions about your treatment. A good formula could be "I would like to discuss my patient preferences for avoiding any medication that is identified in the PDR as causing cancer in humans or rodents, or for which there is no evidence that it has been tested for cancer risk, except for urgent life-threatening conditions, especially when safe and effective alternatives are available."[6]

Although workers are generally provided with access to some information on the toxic and carcinogenic risks of products and processes to which they are exposed (Material Safety Data Sheets), this information is often inadequate if not frankly misleading. An alarming example of such inadequacy relates to the exposure of about one million women to known occupational carcinogens which have been incriminated as risk factors for breast cancer, in the absence of any warning to this effect (Chapter 17). Another more glaring example is the strong body of published evidence incriminating maternal and paternal exposures to occupational carcinogens as major causes of childhood cancers whose rates have dramatically escalated over recent decades (Chapter 13). Such information, once it became widely known, would be likely to galvanize strong legislative, regulatory, and public support for safer workplace conditions, including the phasing out of a wide range of occupational carcinogens and their replacement with safer alternatives.

Political Action

Right-to-Know Initiatives

The right-to-know is the most practical potential strategy in the war against cancer. It is a strategy whose political potency is unquestionable. As Cong. Henry Waxman (D-CA), the leading Congressional advocate of strict environmental standards, has recognized: "I think the public's right-to-know is a new flank in the environmentalist movement."[7] Only a foolhardy politician, regulatory agency, or administration would openly resist a well-orchestrated grass roots campaign demanding explicit labeling of carcinogenic ingredients or contaminants in consumer products, especially since this information on ingredients remains buried in government and industry files or is relatively inaccessible in the scientific literature — and, further, since safe alternatives are generally available.

There is, in fact, ample precedent for such a national initiative, thanks to California's 1996 Proposition 65 which requires public disclosure of carcinogenic and toxic reproductive chemicals in consumer products and the workplace. In this connection, a March 1993 poll, commissioned by Public Voice for Food and Health Policy, found that 86 percent of the public "strongly agreed" that Americans have an absolute right-to-know about the chemicals used on the foods they buy in their supermarket. Furthermore, 79 percent of those polled emphasized that they "strongly favor tough laws requiring clear labelling of chemicals and pesticides used to grow a food product." The meteoric growth of the organic food industry over recent years further attests to the impact of these concerns.

These initiatives should be extended to all other involuntary and avoidable carcinogenic exposures. Every municipality nationwide should be required to provide analytic data on carcinogenic contaminants, and their concentrations, in water, together with their annual bills. Such a proposal has been drafted by Cong. Waxman, with bipartisan support, requiring that consumers be presented each year with a complete list of contaminants in their drinking water, together with a simply-worded explanation of their risks. The EPA should also provide communities with information from its 1995 Toxic Release Inventory on atmospheric emission of carcinogens from local industries. Communities should demand that industries disclose the carcinogenic products or processes they use or manufacture, and what amounts of pollutants are released into surrounding air and water. No industry should be allowed to operate unless it provides ongoing quantitative information on smokestack and other atmospheric emissions of carcinogens in the air of its perimeter and in the local community.

Fortunately, progress is being made in the area of consumer's right-to-know legislation. Since publication of the first edition of *The Safe Shopper's Bible*, in 1995, Congressman Waxman has introduced a child's Right-to-Know bill into Congress. This bill, known as the Children's Environmental Protection and Right-to-Know Act of 1997, or H.R. 1636, would require manufacturers and importers of products with toxic ingredients to report the identity and concentration of these ingredients to the consumers Product Safety Commission, and to provide information regarding how these products would meet existing requirements of the Hazardous Substance Act. Although the act would initially apply to children's products, after three years it would cover all consumer products. Currently, the bill has 144 mainly Democratic co-sponsors in Congress.

Spurred on by the success of *The Safe Shopper's Bible* and the work of many public interest groups, the Consumer Labeling Initiative (CLI) got underway in early 1996. The CLI is a voluntary partnership between the Environmental Protection Agency, other government agencies, companies that make and distribute household cleaners, insecticides, and pesticides, and consumer groups. The goal of the CLI is to put consumers' needs first — helping them to find, read, and understand labeling information so they can compare household products and use these products safely and effectively. Presently, the CLI is investigating what information about ingredients consumers want and need on labels for pesticides and various household cleaning products.

State consumer right-to-know bills, based on the Proposition 65 law passed by California voters in 1996, have simultaneously been introduced in Massachusetts, New Jersey, and Connecticut, and soon will be in Hawaii.

The Massachusetts Citizen's Right-to-Know Act, introduced in the state Senate by state Senator Lois Pines, would mandate strict warnings on all consumer products containing toxic chemicals and is designed to guarantee the right of consumers "to know about toxic chemicals in commonly used consumer goods."

Each of these bills would require producers or packagers to label all consumer products containing known carcinogens and other toxic materials, and also provide an exemption if the packager or producer can demonstrate that the product poses no significant risk of cancer or other toxic effects.

On a worldwide scale, in July, 1996 the *International Green Network Conference* in England unanimously endorsed a consumer bill of rights (drafted by the author), which is firmly girded in the individual's fundamental right-to-know. The international resolution was presented to the United Nation's Food and Agriculture Organization at the Global Food Summit in Rome in November, 1996. As our diverse planet becomes ever more closely linked, such international resolutions are certain to have a huge impact worldwide. The consumer right-to-know movement, crystalized by the International Greens, heralds the clearest, most clarion call yet to address the fundamental rights of consumers in a free market worldwide. The Greens' resolution urges consumers to demand label information on the health hazards of ingredients and contaminants in consumer products and

further "urges governments worldwide to enact laws to require labeling of hazardous chemicals in consumer products and food." Soon, legislatures of the world will recognize this truth: labeling for ingredients in consumer products is fundamental to the free market. Indeed, if the European Union demands it — and the Greens are pushing hard for it — then the United States and other industrialized nations will have to follow suit.

Right-to-know initiatives have been facilitated by the very recent development of special Internet web sites, easy to use on home computers. An Environmental Defense Fund web site enables citizens to call up the following information on community industrial pollution: who are the polluters in any community; how serious is the pollution; what are the carcinogenic and other health effects of these pollutants; and what regulations govern these pollutants.[8] This site integrates information from over 150 data bases and provides detailed information on 2,000 counties, 5,000 zip codes, and 17,000 individual chemical plants based on information from EPA's Toxic Release Inventory. Two other new web sites deal with information on avoidable causes of cancer and the National Cancer Program.[9, 10]

In short, the greatest incentive for phasing out the manufacture, use, and disposal of industrial carcinogens — and their replacement by safe alternatives — is public knowledge of these avoidable exposures. Political pressure at the local, regional and national levels by citizen and public interest groups, individually or in concert (Appendix XV) would be politically difficult to resist. This strategy effectively empowers the public to self-protect against involuntary and avoidable carcinogenic exposures in addition to sending a resounding vote of no confidence to the cancer establishment. The effectiveness of industry sensitivity to public disclosure on avoidable carcinogenic exposures is illustrated by reference to the "Dirty Dozen" carcinogenic consumer products (Table 17.4). Since their

Resolution: Consumer Right-To-Know

Whereas,   The International Green Network Conference advocates the public's right-to-know about human health risks posed by industrial chemicals; and

Whereas,   The global environment is becoming increasingly permeated with industrial chemical contaminants; and

Whereas,   Substantial evidence has incriminated exposures to industrial carcinogens in escalating cancer rates in industrialized countries; and

Whereas,   There is also evidence that incriminates industrial chemicals as causes of endocrine disruption and other toxic effects; and

Whereas,   Consumers have an inalienable right-to-know about the human health risks from toxic ingredients and contaminants in food and other consumer products; and

Whereas,   Unlabeled toxic ingredients and contaminants in food, cosmetics, and household products pose avoidable health risks; and

Whereas,   Consumers are demanding safer and healthier products from the manufacturers of food, cosmetics, and household products; and

Whereas,   Government agencies have refused to require labeling of food and other consumer products with known toxic and carcinogenic ingredients and contaminants; and

Whereas,   Labeling of food and other consumer products will maintain consumer confidence in these products; therefore be it

Resolved,   The International Green Network Conference urges consumers to demand labeled information on the health hazards of ingredients and contaminants in consumer products; and be it further

Resolved,   The International Green Network Conference urges governments world-wide to enact laws to require labeling of hazardous chemicals in consumer products and food.

public disclosure in 1995,[1] several major companies have reformulated their products which are now carcinogen-free.[2]

Toxics Use Reduction Initiatives

A striking example of the successful political impact of well-organized environmental groups, in close collaboration with the University of Massachusetts Toxics Use Reduction Institute, has been the enactment of the 1989 Toxics Use Reduction Act, passed unanimously by the Commonwealth of Massachusetts legislature. In reporting on the impact of the act, Trudy Coxe, Secretary of Environmental Affairs recently stated:

> This law established the Commonwealth as a leader in environmental and public health policy by declaring that our first priority would be to prevent pollution at the source. Over the past six years, hundreds of industry professionals, and scores of government and university staff have worked to implement this innovative program and meet its legislated goals.[11]

The achievements of this Act include:

• Reducing the generation of toxic wastes from 1989 to 1997 by 50%, by reducing toxic use by 20%.

• Establishing toxic use reduction as the preferred means for achieving compliance with federal and state environmental statutes.

• Promoting reduction in the production and use of toxic chemicals.

• Enhancing and strengthening the enforcement of existing environmental laws.

• Promoting coordination between state agencies administering toxics-related programs.

• Sustaining and promoting the competitiveness of Massachusetts industry.

The Act is a specific form of pollution prevention that focuses on reducing the use of toxic chemicals and the generation of hazardous waste by improving and redesigning industrial products and processes. The Toxics Use Reduction Institute of the University of Massachusetts, Lowell has played a critical role by providing education and training, research on new materials and processes, a technical library and information source, and special laboratories for testing surface cleaning technologies.[12]

This Act, which should serve as a model for Federal legislature, has made a greater contribution to cancer prevention than all the combined activities of the NCI and ACS, since their inception decades ago.

In fact, this Act, has implemented one of the very specific following recommendations made by the coalition of experts at their February 1992 press conference, all of which have been ignored by NCI (Chapter 13):

> In close cooperation with key regulatory agencies and industry, the NCI should initiate large-scale research programs to develop noncarcinogenic products and processes as alternatives to those currently based on chemical and physical carcinogens. This program should also include research on the development of economic incentives for the reduction or phaseout of the use of industrial carcinogens, coupled with economic disincentives for their continued use, especially when appropriate noncarcinogenic alternatives are available.

Reforming the Cancer Establishment

Most difficult of all is political action directed to challenging and reforming the cancer establishment and the National Cancer Program. The first major public initiative in this direction came from a coalition of leading independent experts in cancer prevention and public health (Chapter 13). In the February 4, 1992, Washington, D.C. press conference, the coalition proposed a comprehensive set of reforms as guidelines for redefining the mission and priorities of the NCI. Their opening recommendations stated:

> The NCI must give cancer cause and prevention at least equal emphasis, in terms of budgetary and personnel resources, as its other program including diagnosis, treatment and basic research. This major shift in direction should be initiated immediately and completed within the next few years. This shift will also require careful monitoring and oversight to prevent misleading retention of old unrelated programs under new guises of cancer cause and prevention.
>
> A high priority for the cancer prevention program should be a large-scale and ongoing national campaign to inform and educate the media and the public, besides Congress, the administration and industry, that much cancer is avoidable and due to past exposures to chemical and physical carcinogens in air, water, food and the workplace, as well as to lifestyle factors, particularly smoking.... Accordingly, the educational campaign should stress the critical importance of identifying and preventing (involuntary and avoidable) carcinogenic exposures and reducing them to the very lowest levels attainable within the earliest practically possible time.

Although NCI and ACS attempted to discredit the coalition's critique by personal vilification, public and Congressional concerns forced the NCI to agree to the "700-to-1" debate in May, 1992, when its policies and faulty science were subjected to more detailed analysis and scrutiny (Chapter 13). However, apart from some immediate cosmetic responses, NCI's indifference to cancer prevention has continued unchanged, and its misleading claims that the cancer war is being won have further intensified.

The failure of the 1992 initiative by leading national professionals stimulated further interest and involvement of activist public interest groups in political efforts to reform NCI policies. A January 25, 1995 Cancer Prevention Coalition (CPC) Press Advisory, made the following explicit recommendations (Appendix XIII):

- The NCI must be held accountable for its failed policies and for over $30 billion taxpayer support for the "war against cancer."

- The NCI must undergo radical reforms in its programs, priorities and leadership.

- Cancer prevention must receive greater emphasis in NCI policies, achieving parity with all other programs combined over a five-year period.

- The NCI budget must be held hostage to such reforms under the terms of the 1998 Government Performance and Results Act, HR 2883, which requires Federal Agencies to define their goals, develop appropriate strategies and be accountable to taxpayers.[13]

The Cancer Prevention Coalition has taken further action to inform the public of a wide range of involuntary exposures to avoidable carcinogens, documenting the cancer establishment's indifference to cancer prevention coupled with conflicts of interest, rebutting misleading claims for "reversing the tide against cancer" and for "miracle cancer drugs," and acting as a watchdog with regard to critical developments in public policy on cancer. These outreach activities include publishing newsletters and "Cancer Alerts," press briefings and conferences, petitioning regulatory agencies, and developing resolutions on critical consumer and related issues for international ratification (Appendix XVI). A wide range of other activist groups have also played important roles in educating the public and in urging corrective legislative action (Appendix XV). Noteworthy among these are increasingly militant cancer patient advocacy and survivor groups, particularly People Against Cancer and The Cancer Control Society.

The most urgently needed legislative action is amendment of the 1971 National Cancer Act, as urged by the 1992 experts coalition (Chapter 13):

There is no conceivable likelihood that such reforms will be implemented without legislative action. The National Cancer Act should be amended explicitly to reorient the mission and priorities of the NCI to cancer cause and prevention. Compliance of the NCI should then be assured by detailed and ongoing Congressional oversight and, most critically, by House and Senate Appropriation committees. However, only strong support by the independent scientific and public health communities, together with concerned grass roots citizen groups, will convince Congress and Presidential candidates of the critical and immediate need for such drastic action.

The Act should be amended to redefine NCI's mission by specifically directing a parity of resources and allocations for primary prevention and for all other programs combined, diagnosis of treatment and basic genetic research. Such parity would help enforce the development of large-scale prevention research and outreach programs.

Prevention research programs should primarily focus on those cancers whose incidence and mortality rates have escalated since 1950. By definition, these increases clearly reflect recent avoidable carcinogenic exposures. All available experimental and epidemiological data, of varying degrees of strength, for such cancers should be reviewed, systematized and published. Examples of such data, largely unrecognized by Congress, regulatory agencies, and the public, include relationship between: parental occupational exposure and childhood cancers; use of black and dark brown permanent hair and semi-permanent hair dyes and non-Hodgkin's lymphoma, multiple myeloma, leukemia and breast cancer; occupational exposures and breast cancer; psychoactive and antihypertensive drugs and breast cancer; consumption of hormonal milk with elevated levels of IGF-1 and breast, prostate, colon, and other cancers; and consumption of meat contaminated with high residues of sex hormones and breast, prostate, testis and other reproductive cancers. Emphasis should also be directed to research on important data gaps, such as epidemiological studies on a wide range of prescription drugs and for a wide range of ingredients and contaminants in consumer products for which there is strong experimental evidence of carcinogenicity.

In parallel with prevention research, large-scale outreach programs should be developed to inform Congress, regulatory agencies, and the public of all available strong or suggestive experimental and epidemiological evidence on cancer risks from all known environmental and occupational carcinogenic exposures. Media for this outreach should include: testimony to Congress; liaison with Federal and state regulatory agencies; communications to industry; press releases; and public cancer information services, including computerized data bases.

This same recommendation was made in *The Politics of Cancer,* 1979 (see page 219):

Relation of NCI and regulatory agencies. NCI should preserve its primary function as a research agency, with emphasis on problem-solving, and should not become directly involved in regulatory specifics. NCI should, however, develop special formalized large-scale resources for providing guidance and counsel to regulatory agencies on all scientific matters relating to chemical carcinogens in the general environment and workplace.

A critical resource which NCI should develop is a documentation and analysis center, to collate and systematize available carcinogenicity data from sources including the Bioassay Program with particular reference to potential environmental and occupational exposure. Such a center should be directed by a scientist with recognition in chemical carcinogenesis and with experience and sensitivity to the needs of regulatory agencies, and should be adequately staffed with biometricians, statisticians, and epidemiologists so that it can also be capable of performing risk estimates. Finally, the center should be capable of analyzing the impact of failure to regulate a particular carcinogen in terms of total costs from induced or associated cancers and other diseases.

The current failure of NCI to have developed such a resource was critically noted in a recent United Nations document (*International Register of Potentially Toxic Chemicals Bulletin* June 1, 1978, p. 4): "The National Cancer Institute of the National Institutes of Health, U.S. Department of Health, Education, and Welfare, has certain program elements that relate directly or indirectly to concerns about exposure to specific agents that are environmental carcinogens. However, there is currently no identifiable program that assesses, on a holistic basis, the potential hazard from the carcinogenic insult of air and water pollutants, diet contaminants, and other composite stresses."

The development of such research and outreach programs would be greatly facilitated by restructuring the National Cancer Advisory Board, as required by the National Cancer Act, to ensure that at least one-third of its members have expertise and interest in environmental and occupational carcinogenesis. The current composition of the Board is in violation of such a requirement.

NCI's escalating claims for cancer prevention funding, from $115 million in 1992 to $1 billion in 1998 could, not unreasonably, be dismissed as a deceptive shell game. More constructively, it could be viewed as belated recognition of the Institute's long track record of indifference to prevention coupled with its difficulty in conceptualizing and implement-

ing large-scale comprehensive research and outreach prevention programs. The latest $1 billion claim should then be taken at face value as an expression of a new and highly welcome commitment to prevention. The effectiveness of such a commitment, however, would depend on Congressional and advocacy input and ongoing oversight.

Of interest in this connection is a July 8, 1998 report from a blue-ribbon panel of the National Academy of Sciences' Institute of Medicine.[14] The report urged that: the National Institutes of Health (NIH), including NCI, should define their priorities more clearly; each Institute should establish a "council of public representatives;" members of advocacy groups should sit on NIH committees that decide how Federal money is spent; and that ordinary citizens should have "more opportunities to present their views regarding research needs." However, the basic problem is not lack of public input and outreach, which is usually orchestrated by lobbyists and press releases, but lack of scientific productivity and accountability. "Contrary to the complaints of biomedical researchers, the problem is an excess of public money pumped into an aged institution . . . infested with scientific conservatives."[15]

Representative of such advocacy and citizens' input is a previous statement of concern in a January 25, 1995 Cancer Prevention Coalition press release endorsed by 15 major national organizations representing over 5 million citizens (Appendix XIII):

The reason for the failed war against cancer is not a shortage of funds but their gross misallocation. NCI has directed a minimal priority to cancer prevention. Furthermore, NCI has failed to inform Congress and the public of a wide range of avoidable carcinogens in the air, water, food, consumer products, and the workplace. Research on such exposures receives a minuscule 5% of NCI's annual budget. Reduction of exposures to carcinogens in the workplace and the environment are likely to reverse the current epidemic.

The ACS is even more indifferent, if not hostile, to prevention other than the role of lifestyle risk factors. The ACS is also more directly in conflict of interest with the cancer drug and other industries than is the NCI (Chapter 16). Reforming the ACS is, in principle, relatively easy and directly achievable.

Boycott the ACS.

Instead, give your charitable contributions to public interest and environmental groups involved in cancer prevention. Such a boycott is well overdue, and will send the only message this "charity" can no longer ignore. The Cancer Prevention Coalition and some breast cancer activist groups have already taken steps in this direction.[16, (Chapter 13)]

Epilogue

Over recent decades, the incidence of cancer has escalated to epidemic proportions while our ability to treat and cure most cancers remains virtually unchanged. Apart from the important role of tobacco, there is substantial and long-standing evidence relating this epidemic to involuntary and avoidable exposures to industrial carcinogens in air, water, the workplace, and consumer products. Nevertheless, the priorities of the cancer establishment, the NCI and ACS, remain narrowly fixated on damage control — diagnosis and treatment — and on basic molecular research, with relative indifference to, if not always benign neglect of, prevention. Concerns over this imbalance are further compounded by serious questions of conflicts of interest, particularly with the multibillion-dollar cancer drug industry.

In spite of overwhelming resources at its disposal, the cancer establishment has failed to allocate minimal priorities to research on cancer prevention. It has also failed to provide Congress and the Executive with well-documented scientific evidence on avoidable causes of cancer that would enable development of corrective legislative and regulatory action. Nor have U.S. citizens been advised of such information, which remains buried in confidential government and industry files or is relatively inaccessible in the scientific literature, to enable them to protect themselves. Even more seriously, both government and the public have been misled by repeated claims that we are "winning the war against cancer" and that we have "turned the tide against cancer." These claims are based on extravagant and unfounded announcements of dramatic advances in conventional treatment, coupled with highly prejudicial and unfounded attacks on alternative therapies. With this background, there has been little if any pressure on industry or incentive to phase out the manufacture, use, and disposal of carcinogenic chemicals and products and to replace them with safer alternatives.

In short, the NCI and ACS bear major responsibility for losing the winnable war against cancer. This failure is belatedly forcing realization that right-to-know citizen initiatives, on both personal and political levels, are the basis for the most practical and effective strategies for winning the losing cancer war. In addition to these initiatives, the National Cancer Act should be explicitly amended to reorient the mission and priorities of the NCI to cancer cause and prevention. ACS policies will remain impervious to reform absent well-orchestrated threats of economic boycott.

In view of the powerful influence of the U.S. cancer establishment over the policies of most major industrialized nations, the message of this book is truly global, rather than just national.

| Appendix I |

Chemicals Known to Induce Cancer in Humans

		Humans	
Chemicals or industrial process	Main type of exposure	Target Organ	Main route of Exposure*
1. Aflatoxins	Environmental, occupational	Liver	p.o., inhalation
2. 4-Aminobi-phenyl	Occupational	Bladder	Inhalation, skin, p.o
3. Arsenic compounds	Occupational, medicinal, and environmental	Skin, lung, liver	Inhalation, p.o., skin
4. Asbestos	Occupational	Lung, pleural cavity, gastrointestinal tract	Inhalation, . p.o.
5. Auramine (manufac-ture of)	Occupational	Bladder	Inhalation, skin, p.o.
6. Benzene	Occupational	Hemopoietic. system	Inhalation, skin
7. Benzidine	Occupational	Bladder	Inhalation, skin, p.o.

Animals		
Animal	Target Organ	Route of Exposure*
Rat	Liver, stomach, colon, kidney	p.o.
Fish, duck, marmoset, tree shrew, monkey,	Liver	p.o.
Rat	Liver, trachea	i.t.
	Liver	i.p.
Mouse, rat	Local	s.c. injection
Mouse	Lung	i.p.
Mouse, rabbit, dog	Bladder	p.o.
Newborn mouse	Liver	s.c. injection
Rat	Mammary gland, intestine	s.c. injection
Mouse, rat, dog	Inadequate, negative	p.o.
Mouse	Inadequate, negative	Topical, i.v.
Mouse, rat, hamster, rabbit	Lung, pleura	Inhalation or i.t.
Rat, hamster	Local	Intrapleutral
Rat	Local	i.p., s.c. injection
	Various sites	p.o.
Mouse, rat	Liver	p.o.
Rabbit, dog	Negative	p.o.
Rat	Local, liver, intestine	s.c. injection
Mouse	Inadequate	Topical, s.c. injection
Mouse	Liver	s.c. injection
Rat	Liver	p.o.
	Zymbal gland, liver, colon	s.c. injection
Hamster	Liver	p.o.
Dog	Bladder	p.o.

Humans			
Chemicals or industrial process	Main type of exposure	Target Organ	Main route of Exposure*
8. Bischloro-methylether	Occupational	Lung	Inhalation
9. Cadmium-using industries (possibly cadmium oxide)	Occupational	Prostate, lung	Inhalation, p.o.
10. Chloram-phenicol	Medicinal	Hemopoietic system	p.o., injection
11. Chloromethyl-methylether (possibly associated with bischloro-methylether	Occupational	Lung	Inhalation
12. Chromium (chromate-producing industries)	Occupational	Lung, nasal cavities	Inhalation
13. Cyclophos-phamide	Medicinal	Bladder	p.o., injection
14. Diethylstil-bestrol	Medicinal	Uterus, vagina	p.o.

Animals		
Animal	Target Organ	Route of Exposure*
Mouse, rat	Lung, nasal cavity	Inhalation
Mouse	Skin	Topical
	Local, lung	s.c. injection
Rat	Local	s.c. injection
Rat	Local, testis	s.c. or i.m. injection
	No adequate tests	
Mouse	Initiator	Skin
	Lung	Inhalation
	Local, lung	s.c. injection
Rat	Local	s.c. injection
Mouse, rat	Local	s.c., i.m. injection
Rat	Lung	Intrabroncial implantation
Mouse	Hemopoietic system, lung	i.p., s.c. injection
	Various sites	p.o.
Rat	Bladder	i.p.
	Mammary gland	i.p.
	Various sites	i.v.
Mouse	Mammary	p.o.
Mouse	Mammary, lympho-reticular, testis	s.c. injection, s.c. implantation
	Vagina	Local
Rat	Mammary, hypo-physis, bladder	s.c. implantation
Hamster	Kidney	s.c. injection, s.c. implantation
Squirrel monkey	Uterine serosa	s.c. implantation

	Humans		
Chemicals or industrial process	Main type of exposure	Target Organ	Main Route of Exposure*
15. Hematite mining (?radon)	Occupational	Lung	Inhalation
16. Isopropyl oils	Occupational	Nasal cavity, larynx	Inhalation
17. Melphalan	Medicinal	Hemopoietic system	p.o., injection
18. Mustard gas	Occupational	Lung, larynx	Inhalation
19. 2-Naphthyl-amine	Occupational	Bladder	Inhalation, skin, p.o.
20. Nickel (nickel refining)	Occupational	Nasal cavity, lung	Inhalation
21. *N,N*-Bis(2-chloroethyl) - 2-naphthyl-amine	Medicinal	Bladder	p.o.
22. Oxymetholone	Medicinal	Liver	p.o.
23. Phenacetin	Medicinal	Kidney	p.o.
24. Phenytoin	Medicinal	Lymphoreticular tissues	p.o., injection
25. Soot, tars, and oils	Occupational, environmental	Lung, skin (scrotum)	Inhalation, skin
26. Vinyl chloride	Occupational	Liver, brain, lung	Inhalation, skin

Source: L. Tomatis et al., "Evaluation of the Carcinogenicity of Chemicals: A Review of the Monograph Program of the International Agency for Research on Cancer," *Cancer Research* 38 (1978): 877–85.

Animals		
Animal	Target Organ	Route of Exposure*
Mouse, hamster, guinea pig	Negative	Inhalation, i.t.
Rat	Negative	s.c. injection
	No adequate tests	
Mouse	Initiator	Skin
	Lung, lympho-sarcomas	i.p.
Rat	Local	i.p.
Mouse	Lung	Inhalation, i.v.
	Local, mammary	s.c. injection
Hamster, dog monkey	Bladder	p.o.
Mouse	Liver, lung	s.c. injection
Rat, rabbit	Inadequate	p.o.
Rat	Lung	Inhalation
Mouse, rat hamster	Local	s.c., i.m. injection
Mouse, rat	Local	i.m. implantation
Mouse	Lung	i.p.
Rat	Local	s.c. injection
	No adequate tests	
	No adequate tests	
Mouse	Lymphorecticular tissues	p.o., i.p.
Mouse, rabbit	Skin	Topical
Mouse, rat	Lung, liver, blood vessels, mammary, Zymbal gland, kidney	Inhalation

* p.o.=per os or oral; s.c.=subcutaneous; i.m.=intramuscular; i.t.=intratracheal; i.v.=intravenous.

Evaluation of Environmental Carcinogens*

Report to the Surgeon General, USPHS
April 22, 1970

Ad Hoc Committee on the Evaluation
of Low Levels of Environmental
Chemical Carcinogens

*Members of the Ad Hoc Committee
on the Evaluation of Low Levels of
Environmental Chemical Carcinogens*

*National Cancer Institute
Bethesda, Maryland*

Umberto Saffiotti, Chairman, Associate Scientific Director for Carcinogenesis, Etiology, National Cancer Institute, Building 37, Room 3A21, Bethesda, Maryland.

Hans L. Falk, Associate Director for Laboratory Research, National Institute of Environmental Health Sciences, Research Triangle Park, North Carolina.

Paul Kotin, Director, National Institute of Environmental Health Sciences, Research Triangle Park, North Carolina.

William Lijinsky, Professor of Biochemistry, The Eppley Institute for Research on Cancer, University of Nebraska College of Medicine, Omaha, Nebraska.

Marvin Schneiderman, Associate Chief, Biometry Branch, National Cancer Institute, Wiscon Building, Room 5C10, Bethesda, Maryland.

Philippe Shubik, Director, The Eppley Institute for Research on Cancer, University of Nebraska, College of Medicine, Omaha, Nebraska.

Sidney Weinhouse, Director, Fels Research Institute, Temple University School of Medicine, Philadelphia, Pennsylvania.

Gerald Wogan, Professor of Food Toxicology, Massachusetts Institute of Technology, 77 Massachusetts Avenue, Cambridge, Massachusetts.

Staff Members: John A. Cooper, Executive Secretary, Richard R. Bates, James A. Peters, Howard R. Rosenberg, Elizabeth K. Weisburger, John H. Weisburger.

Introduction

Establishment of this Ad Hoc Committee was requested on October 24, 1969, by the Deputy Assistant Secretary for Health and Scientific Affairs. The task of the Committee is to review the problems relating to the evaluation of low levels of environmental chemical carcinogens, to consider the scientific bases on which such evaluations can be made, and to advise the Department of HEW on the implications of such evaluations. The Committee, in addressing itself to the problems of environmental exposures to chemical agents from all sources, has considered the

---

* This report was introduced as an exhibit and published in full in both the following Senate hearings: "Chemicals and the Future of Man," hearings before the Subcommittee on Executive Reorganization and Government Research of the Committee on Government Operations: United States Senate, April 6 and 7, 1971; and the "Federal Environmental Pesticide Control Act," hearings before the Subcommittee on Agricultural Research and General Legislation of the Committee on Agriculture and Forestry, United States Senate, March 23-26, 1971.

scientific criteria for evaluation of carcinogenic hazards. Many previous recommendations on the criteria to be used for evaluating environmental chemical carcinogenic hazards have been made for specific sources of exposure or for specific groups of substances (e.g., food additives, pesticides, certain occupational carcinogens). In some cases this approach has led to an uneven approach to preventive measures.

The task of this Committee covers a broader area and includes an appraisal of the scientific criteria for evaluation of chemical carcinogenesis hazards in the total environment.

I. Recommendations

In full consideration of the past and present states of carcinogenesis investigation this Committee offers the following recommendations:

1. a. Any substance which is shown conclusively to cause tumors in animals should be considered carcinogenic and therefore a potential cancer hazard for man. Exceptions should be considered only where the carcinogenic effect is clearly shown to result from physical, rather than chemical, induction, or where the route of administration is shown to be grossly inappropriate in terms of conceivable human exposure.

b. Data on carcinogenic effects in man are only acceptable when they represent critically evaluated results of adequately conducted epidemiologic studies.

2. No level of exposure to a chemical carcinogen should be considered toxicologically insignificant for man. For carcinogenic agents a "safe level for man" cannot be established by application of our present knowledge. The concept of "socially acceptable risk" represents a more realistic notion.

3. The statement made in 1969 by the Food Protection Committee, National Research Council, that natural or synthetic substances can be considered safe without undergoing biological assay should be recognized as scientifically unacceptable.

4. No chemical substance should be assumed safe for human consumption without proper negative lifetime biological assays of adequate size. The minimum requirements for carcinogenesis bioassays should provide for: adequate numbers of animals of at least two species and both sexes with adequate controls, subjected for their lifetime to the administration of a suitable dose range, including the highest tolerated dose, of the test material by routes of administration that include those by which man is exposed. Adequate documentation of the test conditions and pathologic standards employed are essential.

5. Evidence of negative results, under the conditions of the test used, should be considered superseded by positive findings in other tests. Evidence of positive results should remain definitive, unless and until new evidence conclusively proves that the prior results were not causally related to the exposure.

6. The implication of potential carcinogenicity should be drawn both from tests resulting in the induction of benign tumors and those resulting in tumors which are more obviously malignant.

7. The principle of a zero tolerance for carcinogenic exposures should be retained in all areas of legislation presently covered by it and should be extended to cover other exposures as well. Only in the cases where contamination of an environmental source by a carcinogen has been proven to be unavoidable should exception be made to the principle of zero tolerance. Exceptions should be made only after the most extraordinary justification, including extensive documentation of chemical and biological analyses, and a specific statement of the estimated risk for man are presented. All efforts should be made to reduce the level of contamination to the minimum. Periodic review of the degree of

contamination and the estimated risk should be made mandatory.

8. A basic distinction should be made between intentional and unintentional exposures.

    a. No substance developed primarily for uses involving exposure to man should be allowed for widespread human intake without having been properly tested for carcinogenicity and found negative.

    b. Any substance developed for use not primarily involving exposure in man but nevertheless resulting in such exposure, if found to be carcinogenic, should be either prevented from entering the environment or, if it already exists in the environment, progressively eliminated.

9. A system should be established for ensuring that bioassay operations providing data upon which regulatory decisions are made be monitored so that their results are obtained in accordance with scientifically acceptable standards.

10. A unified approach to the assessment and prevention of carcinogenesis risks should be developed in the federal legislation; it should deal with all sources of human exposure to carcinogenic hazards.

11. Clear channels should be identified for the regulatory function of different government departments and agencies in the field of cancer prevention. Establishment of a surveillance and information program would alert all concerned government agencies to the extent and development of information on formation on carcinogenic hazards.

12. An ad hoc committee of experts should be charged with the task of recommending methods for extrapolating dose-response bioassay data to the low response region ($1/10000\%$ to $1/10000000\%$). The low doses corresponding to the responses in this range are the ones which have direct relevance to the human situation.

II. Background

Knowledge of cancer causation by chemicals originates from clinical observations, going back as far as 1775 with Pott's discovery of soot as the causative agent in chimney sweeps' cancer. Several major classes of carcinogenic agents were first discovered by their effects on man. Experimental animal models for the determination of the potential carcinogenic activity of chemicals were only developed in the last 50 years, and most of them have been studied only in the last 20 years.

The effects of carcinogens on tissues appear irreversible. Exposure to small doses of a carcinogen over a period of time results in a summation or potentiation of effects. The fundamental characteristic which distinguishes the carcinogenic effect from other toxic effects is that the tissues affected do not seem to return to their normal condition. This summation of effects in time and the long interval (latent period) which passes after tumor induction before the tumor becomes clinically manifest demonstrate that cancer can develop in man and in animals long after the causative agent has been in contact and disappeared.

It is, therefore, important to realize that incidences of cancer in man today reflect exposure of 15 or more years ago; similarly, any increase of carcinogenic contaminants in man's environment today will reveal its carcinogenic effect some 15 or more years from now. For this reason it is urgent that every effort be made to detect and control sources of carcinogenic contamination of the environment well before damaging effects become evident in man. Similar concepts may apply to the needs for evaluation of other chronic toxicity hazards. Environmental cancer remains one of the major disease problems of modern man.

An agent which is causally related to the occurrence of cancer in man or animals is defined as a carcinogen or oncogen. The number of known carcinogenic agents includes several groups of viruses, various physical factors, and hundreds of chemicals.

Viruses of different types are known to induce cancer in animals; none has yet been proven to evoke cancer in man. If specific viruses are proven to be causally related to cancer induction in man, the frequency of certain human tumors might be reduced in the future by immunization procedures.

Physical factors are known to cause cancers in man and animals. For example, ultraviolet radiation causes skin cancer, and ionizing radiation cancer of various organs (e.g., leukaemias, lung cancer, bone sarcomas, skin cancer). Exposure to a "background level" has been widely considered as unavoidable and, in the case of ultraviolet light, even necessary as an integral part of our natural environment. Strong epidemiologic and experimental evidence indicates the existence of a direct dose-response relationship between exposure to radiation and carcinogenic effects. Tolerance levels have been suggested for various forms of radiation and health benefits have been realized from their application. Evaluation of radiation hazards has been approached through measurement of the total cumulative dose of radiation exposure. Some carcinogenic radiation hazards, such as certain occupational exposures (e.g., radiation in uranium mines), are still not effectively controlled.

Chemicals of many classes produce cancer in a large number of organ sites in animals. Cancers in man are known to be caused by several individual chemicals and by materials composed of mixtures of chemicals. Chemical carcinogens have been shown to act by surface contact with skin or mucosae, by inhalation, by ingestion, and occasionally by injection or implantation (medical or accidental). Chemicals may induce cancer at the site of initial contact (e.g., skin cancer from polynuclear hydrocarbons), the site of selective localization (e.g., bone cancer radionuclides), the site of metabolism and detoxification (e.g., liver or kidney cancer from aflatoxin or nitrosamines), or the site of excretion (e.g., urinary bladder cancer from aromatic amines). A complex and often uneven approach to the problem of preventing exposure to chemical carcinogens has developed over the years. It has become increasingly obvious that the hazard from a single chemical carcinogen cannot be evaluated out of context of the total environmental exposure.[1] Estimation of the "cumulative carcinogenic dose" resulting from all possible chemical carcinogens or even from all sources of a single type or class of chemical carcinogens is presently impossible.

Prevention of exposure to known carcinogenic chemicals depends largely on man's ability to control their entry into the environment. Certain chemical carcinogens are natural products (e.g., metabolities of the amino acid tryptophan) or naturally occurring contaminants (e.g., mycotoxins). Others are formed in the processing of natural products. Many, such as polynuclear hydrocarbons (e.g., benzo[a]pyrene), occur almost ubiquitously in our modern industrialized environment. They derive from most sources of organic combustion. A class of very potent carcinogens discovered only in recent years, the N-nitrosamines, include compounds that may be formed in the environment from nitrites and secondary amines. Many other known chemical carcinogens have been introduced as synthetic materials or by-products into man's present environment through a wide range of newly developed industrial processes. Some of these, such as food additives, medicinal products, cosmetics, and certain household products or pesticides, were developed for human use. Several carcinogens derive from products such as tobacco smoke, developed exclusively for human use. In other cases chemical carcinogens not intended primarily for human exposure are introduced into the general environment and eventually come in contact with its inhabitants; many substances (certain polynuclear hydrocarbons, pesticides, metals, dusts, and fumes, etc.) gain widespread environmental distribution, thereby becoming pollutants of the air, soil, water, and food. Prevention of exposure to this broad spectrum of chemical carcinogens must take a variety of forms.

The production of chemicals recognized as carcinogens for uses involving intentional human exposure can be identified and effectively eliminated. Exceptions to this approach should be made for substances that involve a well-defined health benefit (e.g., certain chemotherapeutic drugs). Use of such substances should be accepted on the basis of extraordinary evidence that their health benefit outweighs their risk.

The production of specific carcinogenic chemicals for uses that do not primarily involve an intentional exposure of man, but which result in such environmental contamination that extensive human exposure becomes inevitable, must also be controlled. The most effective prevention of exposure in man is the elimination of carcinogen production, or control of entry into the environment.

A large group of chemical carcinogens (e.g., combustion products, mycotoxins, and other natural products) is widely disseminated in the environment from sources that can only be partly controlled. For these contaminants, as well as for products which have been widely spread in the environment before their carcinogenicity was recognized, the only possible approach to exposure reduction is to monitor their environmental distribution and subsequently minimize their contact with humans.

Modifying factors are known to condition the development of neoplasia in man and animals. They can act intrinsically or extrinsically (e.g., hormonal imbalances, metabolic characteristics or abnormalities, caloric intake, dietary factors). Understanding of their specific effects in man, however, is still not adequate to serve as a reliable basis for preventive action.

Interactions among multiple factors have received limited attention to date. There are well-documented instances in animal studies of strong synergistic effects produced by chemicals in combination with radiation, viruses, or other chemicals. The epidemiological patterns of certain human cancers implicate combined effects of multiple agents (e.g., inhalation of radon and radon daughters in uranium mines and cigarette smoking).

The types of cancer in man that are due, directly or indirectly, to extrinsic factors are thought to account for a large percentage of the total cancer incidence.[2] These include tumors of the skin, the respiratory, gastrointestinal and urinary tracts, hormone-dependent organs (such as the breast, thyroid, and uterus), and the hemopoietic system. During the past decade considerable progress has been made in the detection of carcinogenic agents and the analysis of their biological effects. New approaches to the interpretation of quantitative relationships between exposures and carcinogenic effects in man and animals are being developed. It is estimated, therefore, that the majority of human cancers are potentially preventable.[3]

III. Animal Bioassay Results and Evaluation of Risks in Man

In order to evaluate the hazard of a chemical for man, one must extrapolate from the animal evidence. It is essential to recognize that no level of exposure to a carcinogenic substance, however low it may be, can be established to be a "safe level" for man. This concept, put forward in the 1950s, remains true in 1970. The current legislation in the field of food additives, with its "anticancer clause," is based on this principle (Federal Food, Drug and Cosmetic Act, as amended,

Sect. 409 (c) (3) (A)).

The reasons for retaining this "anticancer clause" were effectively summarized in 1960 by Secretary of Health, Education and Welfare Arthur S. Flemming in testimony to Congress[3] on the subject of extending the clause to cover the use of food colors, with the following statement.

The rallying point against the anticancer provision is the catch phrase that it takes away the scientist's right to exercise judgment. The issue thus made is a false one, because the clause allows the exercise of all the judgment that can safely be exercised on the basis of our present knowledge. The clause is grounded on the scientific fact of life that no one, at this time, can tell us how to establish for man a safe tolerance for a cancer-producing agent.

Until cancer research makes a breakthrough at this point, there simply is no specific basis on which judgment or discretion could be exercised in tolerating a small amount of a known carcinogenic color or food additive.

As I pointed out in my original testimony, the opposition to inclusion of an anticancer clause arises largely out of a misunderstanding of how this provision works. It allows the Department and its scientific people full discretion and judgment in deciding whether a substance has been shown to produce cancer when added to the diet of test animals. But once this decision is made, the limits of judgment have been reached and there is no reliable basis on which discretion could be exercised in determining a safe threshold dose for the established carcinogen.

So long as the outstanding experts in the National Cancer Institute and the Food and Drug Administration tell us that they do not know how to establish with any assurance at all a safe dose in man's food for a cancer-producing substance, the principle

in the anticancer clause is sound.

I want to emphasize the statement I made on January 26 that the Food, Drug, and Cosmetic Act, as it now stands, will be enforced to prohibit the addition of cancer-producing substances to food unless a law should be passed directing us to follow another course of action.

Even though we have this authority in the law, we urge the Congress to join with the executive branch to give added assurance to the consuming public by directing the anticancer clause in the proposed additives amendment.

Again, we say, however, that we believe the issue is so important that the elected Representatives of the people should have the opportunity of examining the evidence and determining whether or not the authority should be granted.

The scientific basis on which the government's position was established in 1960 remains valid. The progress of knowledge in carcinogenesis in the last decades has only strengthened the points made in Secretary Flemming's testimony.

IV. Detection of Low Levels of Carcinogens in the Environment

To establish the presence of "low levels of carcinogen in the environment" requires that (1) the presence of the material in question be recognized in the environment and (2) the material be recognized as carcinogenic. To evaluate the impact of a chemical in the human environment, it is useful to prepare an "environmental profile" to reflect the distribution of this material in time and space. Failure to detect the presence of a compound implies only that the compound is present, if at all, in concentrations below the detectable limit of the analytical method used. These "sub-detection levels" cannot be differentiated from "zero." From the distribution profile and additional information on the conditions of uptake in man the approximate level and extent of exposure for population segments can be estimated.

In recognizing a chemical as a carcinogen, the limiting factor is the sensitivity and specificity of the bioassay system used. A bioassay system designed to detect tumor induction only at or above a given level under the conditions of the test (e.g., a 25 percent incidence of a specific tumor type) will fail to reveal carcinogenicity below that level. Compounds whose carcinogenic effects fall below specific bioassay detection limits must not be considered innocuous. Such materials must be characterized as presenting a carcinogenic risk no greater than that defined by this lower limit.

Methodology for the determination of chemical contamination in the environment and of biological activity of carcinogens are discussed in the following sections.

A. Chemical Detection Methods

Methods for detection of low levels of carcinogens in the environment have increased in accuracy and reliability over the past several years. The lower limits of detection for different types of known carcinogenic substances are extremely variable, extending over several orders of magnitude from very sensitive methods (e.g., 1 part per billion of benzo[a]pyrene or aflatoxin) to rather insensitive ones (e.g., for aromatic amines). In principle, analytical methods should be capable of detecting carcinogenic materials at any level or in any condition which has relevance to human exposure. For this reason, increasingly sensitive analytical techniques are needed, and indeed many have been developed over the last 10 years. Much of the improvement in methodology is attributable to the application of gas-liquid chromatographic techniques. Within the next few years sizable additional improvements in the sensitivity of analytical methods are likely to be achieved.

It is important to consider how widely the new analytical methods can be applied for the detection of a given carcinogenic contaminant in different materials. While highly sensitive analytical methods can be devised to detect a chemical in specific materials, these same methods might be powerless in the analysis of the same chemical from other source materials (e.g., dimethylnitrosamine can be detected in the alcoholic beverages at 1 ppb, but in foods only at 10-100 ppb). An uneven evaluation of the sources of environmental contamination may result. Development of widely applicable procedures will provide a more balanced evaluation of environmental contamination.

B. Biological Detection Methods

The carcinogenic activity of materials can only be detected by long-term biological tests. At the present time the chemical structure or physico-chemical properties of a compound do not provide a reliable basis for prediction of freedom from carcinogenic activity. Several structure, activity correlations are valuable indicators of the possible carcinogenicity of a compound, but none can be used to classify the compound as noncarcinogenic. Short-term bioassays that determine the effect of certain chemicals on selected biologic targets have not been reliable for prediction of carcinogenic activity.

The present state of the art requires long-term bioassays in mammalian species for the experimental identification of carcinogenic activity. United States law requires that food additives and various other materials be tested in animals by the intended route of human exposure. Similar tests have not been required for some materials to which humans are exposed by other than the oral route. The expanding production and use of chemicals in household products results in extensive human exposure (via the skin and respiratory tract) to dusts and aerosols; little information is available on the chronic toxicity of these materials by these routes of administration. It would not be wise to wait for the results of these "experiments in man" before instituting animal experimentation.

Bioassays are always performed on a number of animals which is extremely small when compared with the millions of humans exposed to most environmental carcinogens. Such studies can only detect carcinogenic effects resulting in fairly high incidences. For example, an observed outcome of no tumors in a test group of 100 animals, as well as in 100 negative controls, only provides assurance, at the 99 percent probability level, that the true tumor risk is under 4.5 percent. The maximum probable risk is 0.46 percent if groups of 1,000 animals are used. It would require tumor-free results in 450 animals to establish with like probability that the risk is under 1 percent.[4]

The assessment of the carcinogenic activity of a chemical depends on a variety of parameters. These include not only the total number of tumors induced but also their multiplicity, latent period, morphologic type, and degree of malignancy. The induction of tumors diagnosed as benign as a result of treatments has been interpreted by certain groups in the past as not sufficient to demonstrate a "carcinogenic" effect. This is a dangerous position since few, if any, substances are known to have produced only benign tumors and no malignant ones when properly and repeatedly tested. This has been pointed out in the Report of the Subcommittee on Carcinogenesis of the FDA Committee on Protocols for Safety Evaluation.[5]

The important scientific problem of defining the sensitivity of a bioassay system used for testing materials of unknown activity has received insufficient attention. The interpretation of both positive and negative findings is strictly dependent on such definition as well as on the results obtained in negative, vehicle, positive and colony control animals. A bioassay result is meaningful only when accompanied by a statement of the sensitivity and specificity of the bioassay design used. An observed incidence of a given tumor type in a test group has no meaning without adequate information on the appropriate controls. Far too little work has been done using adequate positive controls. Lack of tumor response in a given experimental system cannot be interpreted as negative evidence if positive controls also yield negative results or if no positive controls have been included to show that the experimental system used is appropriate.

A body of knowledge has developed over the years on the response of experimental animals to chemical carcinogens. Several committees of experts in the field of carcinogenesis convened by national and international bodies over the past 15 years have formulated general principles for performance and evaluation on carcinogenesis studies in animals. The recommendations put forth by these committees have shown remarkable unanimity[2,5-10] and are widely accepted in principle by the scientific community.[11-15] General requirements for testing procedures, which have been outlined by these groups, include specification of criteria for the following.

1. Selection of materials to be tested
2. Chemical and physical characterization of the test materials
3. Selection of appropriate animal species and group size
4. Choice of appropriate routes and levels of administration

In addition, recommendations concerning the lifetime maintenance and pathological examination of experimental animals have been outlined.

Two principles are recognized as fundamental to the evaluation of carcinogenesis bioassays.

1. The minimum requirements for carcinogenesis bioassay should include adequate numbers of animals of at least

two species and both sexes with adequate positive and negative controls, subjected for their lifetime to the administration by appropriate routes of a suitable dose range of the test material, including doses considerably higher than those anticipated for human exposure.

2. Any substance which is shown conclusively to produce tumors in animals, when tested under these conditions, should be considered potentially carcinogenic for man.

V. Quantitative Relationships

The major new argument presented today against the "anticancer clause" is that the marked increase in sensitivity of many analytical methods makes it possible to detect low levels of carcinogens in a broader segment of the environment and that, therefore, the immediate enforcement of regulations requiring a zero tolerance becomes more difficult, in some instances impossible.

New and very potent classes of chemical carcinogens, such as aflatoxin and nitrosamines, have been detected in the environment. Striking examples of potentiation in cancer induction have been reported in experimental animal tests and in epidemiologic observations. Bioassays have revealed the carcinogenicity of such widespread environmental chemicals as DDT and cyclamate, to which a large majority of the American population has been exposed.

In contrast to the analytical methods, bioassay methods have remained tools of low sensitivity, capable only of detecting the highest peaks of carcinogenic activity. The factor which limits bioassay sensitivity is usually the small number of test animals used. If the bioassay design has a low probability of detecting carcinogenic effects produced by hazards at levels comparable to those present in environmental samples, then tests at such levels are wastes of time, effort and money. The need to test levels higher than those found in the environment is thus founded. Some substances, on the other hand, are potent carcinogens in animal test systems at levels not currently detectable in the environment. An example is provided by the recent evidence on aflatoxin. Its lowest analytically detectable level is 1 ppb. One hundred percent tumor incidence was produced in rats by a dose as low as 15 ppb in the diet. Experiments now under way suggest that aflatoxin, when fed to rats at the lowest detectable level (1 ppb), is still carcinogenic.[16] It has already been demonstrated to be carcinogenic at 1 ppb in the trout. These data indicate that aflatoxin may be present in food at undetectable levels and still be capable of producing cancer incidences so high as to be detectable in tests involving relatively small numbers of experimental animals.

It is impossible to establish any absolutely safe level of exposure to a carcinogen for man. The concept of "toxicologically insignificant" levels (as advanced by the Food Protection Committee of the NAS/NRC in 1969), of dubious merit in any life science, has absolutely no validity in the field of carcinogenesis. Society must be willing to accept some finite risk as the price of using any carcinogenic material in whatever quantity. The best that science can do is to estimate the upper probable limit of that risk. For this reason, the concept of "safe level for man," as applied to carcinogenic agents, should be replaced by that of a "socially acceptable level of risk."

While science can provide quantitative information regarding maximum risk levels, the task of ultimately selecting socially acceptable levels of human risk rests with society and its political leaders. The evaluation of the balance of benefits and risks, required for such a decision by society, should not be the result of uninformed guesswork but should be reached on the basis of complete and pertinent data, social as well as scientific. It is necessary, therefore, to define the extent in the processes of interpreting animal response data and subsequently extrapolating them to man. The principle of zero tolerance should be applied in all but the most extraordinary of cases.

VI. Conclusion

Modern society has been extremely fortunate — given the technical limits on detection of carcinogenic effects — that at least some environmental carcinogens have been identified. So-called negative data, obtained in bioassays often incapable of detecting effects below the 10 percent level, are grossly inadequate to give assurance of safety for man. Information on about 2,500 compounds tested for carcinogenic activity up through 1960 has been compiled and published.[17] Most of these materials, however, are of no environmental significance. Data on tests reported since 1960 will be published shortly. It is estimated that data on 3,500 previously unevaluated chemicals will be included in the forthcoming volume. It is seen, then, that about 6,000 chemicals are documented as having undergone carcinogenesis bioassay to date. Many of the referenced tests, however, were inadequate according to presently recommended standards.

If this nation wishes to identify a large segment of existing and potential carcinogenic hazards, it must institute a comprehensive program involving a concert of activities. Scientific and technical plans for the development of methodological standards should be provided by experienced agencies in collaboration with qualified advisors. It is essential that the objectivity of these advisors not be damaged by any conflicting interests.

Resources needed for the extensive bioassay screening of environmental chemicals will be considerable. In addition to the myriad of substances presently in the environment, several thousand new compounds are introduced each year. Up to 20,000 materials should be tested for carcinogenicity as a first screening of the environment. Testing 20,000 compounds by bioassay would cost about $1 billion. This estimate would increase accordingly for the more extensive testing required in less superficial evaluation. Yet even were such funds available today, they could not nearly be spent effectively. Bioassay laboratory and professional resources are just not available in quantities capable of supporting a huge testing program. A great deal of "tooling up" is prerequisite to any such expanded level of effort.

Because the latent period in human carcinogenesis is so long, epidemiologic evidence develops only over periods of 15 to 20 years. Timely decisions to exclude materials from uses involving exposure to man, therefore, must be based solely on adequately conducted animal bioassays. Retrospective human evidence of risk must not be allowed to show itself before controlling action is taken. Chemicals should be subjected to scientific scrutiny rather than given individual "rights"; they must be considered potentially guilty unless and until proven innocent. Valid evidence must come from biological assays; every bioassay report should include a statement of its limits of sensitivity. Experimental design should provide for reproducibility of test results. Since the bioassay plays such a key role in a total carcinogen control scheme, more effort must be devoted to setting standards for both the performance of tests and the interpretation of results. Only given good bioassay data can science possibly provide sound information to those who are charged with making social decisions regarding the acceptability of carcinogenesis risk levels.

An effective program to protect man from the mass of environmental cancer hazards is within reach. No more time should be allowed to pass before the recommendations set forth in this report are applied to reality.

References

1. Shubik P. Clayson DB. Terracini B: The Quantification of Environmental Carcinogens. UICC Technical Report Series, Volume 4. Geneve, Switzerland, Braillard E., 1970, p. 33

2. Report of a WHO Expert Committee: Prevention of cancer. Wld Hlth Org Techn Rep Ser 276: pp. 1-53, 1964.

3. Flemming AS: Statement of Arthur S. Flemming, Secretary, DHEW, In Hearings before a Subcommittee on the Committee on Interstate and Foreign Commerce of the House of Representatives Regarding Color Additives; 86th Congress, 2nd Session. Washington DC, U.S. Govt Print Office, 1960, pp. 499-501.

4. Mantel N. Bryan WR: "Safety" testing of carcinogenic agents. J Nat Cancer Inst 27: pp. 455-470, 1961.

5. FDA Advisory Committee on Protocol for Safety Evaluation: Panel on Carcinogenesis: Report on cancer testing and the safety evaluation of food additives and pesticides. Toxicol Appl Pharmacol: (in press), 1970.

6. Committee on Causative Factors of Cancer and Committee on Cancer Prevention: Report of symposium on potential cancer hazards from chemical additives and contaminants to foodstuffs. Acta Un Int Cancer 13: pp. 179-193, 1957.

7. Fifth Report of the Joint FAO/WHO Expert Committee on Food Additives: Evaluation of carcinogenic hazards of food additives. Wld Hlth Org Techn Rep Ser 220: pp. 1-32, 1961.

8. Food Protection Committee, Food and Nutrition Board: Problems in the Evaluation of Carcinogenic Hazard from Use of Food Additives. Washington DC, National Academy of Sciences–National Research Council Publ No 749, 1960, 44 p: Cancer Res 21: pp. 429-456, 1961.

9. Berenblum 1: Carcinogenicity Testing, UICC Technical Report Series, Volume 2, Geneve, Switzerland, de Bursen G, 1969, 56 p.

10. Technical Panel on Carcinogenesis: Carcinogenicity of pesticides. In Report of the Secretary's Commission on Pesticides and Their Relationship to Environmental Health. Washington DC, U.S. Govt Print Office, 1969, pp. 459–506.

11. Shubik P, Sice J: Chemical carcinogenesis as a chronic toxicity test: A Review, Cancer Res 16: pp. 728-742, 1956.

12. Clayson DB: Chemical Carcinogenesis. Boston, Massachusetts, Little Brown and Company, 1962, 467 p.

13. Hueper WC, Conway WD: Chemical Carcinogenesis and Cancers. Springfield, Illinois, Thomas CC, 1964, 744 p.

14. Weisburger, JH, Weisburger EK: Tests for chemical carcinogens. In Methods in Cancer Research, Volume I (Busch H, ed.). New York, New York, Academic Press Inc, 1967, pp. 307-387.

15. Arcos JG, Argus MG, Wolf G: Testing procedures. In Chemical Induction of Cancer, Volume I (Arcos JG, Argus MG, Wolf G. eds.). New York, New York, Academic Press Inc. 1968, pp. 340-463.

16. Wogan GN: Personal communication.

17. Hartwell JL: Survey of Compounds Which Have Been Tested for Carcinogenic Activity, 2nd ed., Public Health Serv Publ No. 149, Washington DC.

Substances Regulated as Recognized Carcinogens

1. Workplace Standards under § 6, Occupational Safety and Health Act

SUBSTANCE	DATE OF FINAL ACTION
Asbestos	June 7, 1972 (37 Fed. Reg. 11318)
14 Carcinogens 2-Acetylaminofluorene Alpha-naphthylamine 4-Aminobiphenyl Benzidine Beta-naphthylamine Beta-propiolactone Bischloromethylether 3,3´-Dichlorobenzidine 4-Dimethylaminoazobenzene Ethyleneimine Chloromethylmethylether 4,4´-Methylene bis(2-chloroaniline) (MOCA) (deleted) 4-Nitrobiphenyl N-Nitrosodimethylamine	Jan. 29, 1974 (39 Fed. Reg. 3756)
Vinyl chloride	Oct. 4, 1974 (39 Fed. Reg. 35890)
Coke oven emissions	Oct. 22, 1976 (41 Fed. Reg. 46741)

2. Hazardous Air Pollutants under §12, Clean Air Act

SUBSTANCE	DATE OF FINAL ACTION
Asbestos	April 6, 1973 (38 Fed. Reg. 8820) May 3, 1974 (39 Fed. Reg. 15396) Oct. 14, 1975 (40 Fed. Reg. 48302)
Vinyl chloride	Oct. 21, 1976 (41 Fed. Reg. 46559)

3. Toxic Pollutants Effluent Standards Under §307, Federal Water Pollution Control Act

SUBSTANCE	DATE OF FINAL ACTION
DDT (and DDE, DDD)	Jan. 12, 1977 (42 Fed. Reg. 2587)
Aldrin/dieldrin	Jan. 29, 1974 (42 Fed. Reg. 2587)
Benzidine	Jan. 12, 1977 (42 Fed. Reg. 2587)
PCBs	Feb. 2, 1977

4. Food, Color, and Cosmetic Products Banned Under Federal Food, Drug, and Cosmetic Act

SUBSTANCE	DATE OF FINAL ACTION
Dulcin, P-400	15 Fed. Reg. 321 (1950)
Coumarin	19 Fed. Reg. 1239 (1954)
Safrole, oil of sassafras, dihydrosafrole, iso-safrole	25 Fed. Reg. 12412 (1960)
DES (for use in poultry)	21 CFR 510.120 (1960)
Flectol H (1-2, Dihydro-2,2,4-trimethquinoline, polymerized)	32 Fed. Reg. 5675 (1967)
Oil of calamus	33 Fed. Reg. 6967 (1968)
Cyclamates	34 Fed. Reg. 17063 (1969)
MOCA (4,4´-methylenebis- (2-chloroaniline))	34 Fed. Reg. 19073 (1969)
DEPC (diethylpyrocarbonate)	37 Fed. Reg. 15426 (1972)
Mercaptoimidazoline	38 Fed. Reg. 33072 (1973)
FD&C Violet #1	38 Fed. Reg. 9077 (1973)
Vinyl chloride	39 Fed. Reg. 26842 (1976)
FD&C Red #2	41 Fed. Reg. 5823 (1976)
Chloroform	41 Fed. Reg. 26842 (1976)
FD&C Red #4	41 Fed. Reg. 41852 (1976)
Carbon black	41 Fed. Reg. 41857 (1976)
Acrylonitrile	42 Fed. Reg. 13546 (1977)
Nitrofurans	42 Fed. Reg. 17526, 18611, 18619, 18660 (1977)
Graphite	42 Fed. Reg. 60734 (1977)
D&C Red # 10-13	42 Fed. Reg. 62475 (1977)
D&C Yellow # 1	42 Fed. Reg. 62482 (1977)

5. Consumer Products Under Consumer Product Safety Act/Federal Hazardous Substances Act

SUBSTANCE	DATE OF FINAL ACTION
Vinyl chloride	39 Fed. Reg. 30114 (1974)
Tris	42 Fed. Reg. 18856, 61621, (1977)
Asbestos products	42 Fed. Reg. 63354 (1977)

6. Pesticides Under Federal Insecticide, Fungicide, and Rodenticide Act

SUBSTANCE	DATE OF FINAL ACTION
DDT	37 Fed. Reg. 13369 (1972)
Vinyl chloride	39 Fed. Reg. 14753 (1974)
Aldrin/dieldrin	39 Fed. Reg. 37265 (1974)
Heptachlor/chlordane	41 Fed. Reg. 7552 (1976)
Kepone	41 Fed. Reg. 24624 (1976)
Mirex	41 Fed. Reg. 56694 (1976)
DBCP (dibromochloropropane)	42 Fed. Reg. 57543 (1977)

Source: Marion F. Suter and Warren R. Muir. "Federal Programs in Cancer Research," unpublished report.

Appendix IV

Human Cancers Following Drug Treatment

DRUGS	RELATED CANCER
Radioisotopes	
Phosphorus (P^{32})	Acute leukaemia
Radium, mesothorium	Osteosarcoma and cancer of nasal sinuses
Thorotrast	Liver angiosarcoma
Immunosuppressive drugs (for renal transplantation)	
Antilymphocyte serum	Reticulum cell sarcoma
Antimetabolites	Soft tissue sarcoma, other cancers (skin, liver)
Cytotoxic drugs	
Chlornaphazine	Bladder cancer
Melphalan, cyclophosphamide	Acute leukaemia
Hormones	
Synthetic estrogens	
Prenatal	Cancer of the vagina and cervix
Postnatal	Cancer of the uterus
Androgenic-anabolic steroids (for treatment of aplastic anemia)	Liver cancer
Others	
Arsenic	Skin cancer
Phenacetin-containing drugs	Kidney cancer
Coal tar ointments	Skin cancer
Diphenylhydantoin?	Lymphoma
Chloramphenicol?	Leukaemia
Amphetamines?	Hodgkin's disease
Reserpine?	Breast cancer

Source: Based on R. Hoover and J. F. Fraumeni, Jr., "Drugs," ch. 12, in J. F. Fraumeni, Jr., ed., *Persons at High Risk of Cancer* (New York: Academic Press, 1975).

Women Beware:
Cancer Risks from Prescription Drugs,
Medical Procedures, and Clinical Trials

The following editorials and press releases deal with particular threats to women's health. These writings seek to provide the general public with cautionary research information that has been available to the medical, industrial, and scientific communities for as much as 35 years.

Prescription Drugs

Failure to Fully Document Risks of Osteoporosis Drug is "Reckless"

By Samuel Epstein, M.D. and Pat Cody
From *The Chicago Tribune*
April 19, 1998

Eli Lilly recently began running full-page color ads for Evista, a synthetic hormone with both estrogenic and anti-estrogenic effects, in major national and regional newspapers. The ads claim that Evista offers "a new way to prevent osteoporosis," but at the same time admit that "its effect on fractures is not yet known." The ads also claim that "women taking Evista had no increased risks of breast and uterine cancers," in contrast to conventional hormone replacement therapy, and that it reduces LDL, or bad cholesterol, blood levels. This should be welcome news to women worldwide, particularly as osteoporosis has now reached epidemic proportions, affecting 15 million to 20 million American women each year; osteoporosis causes more than a million fractures, including 250,000 hip fractures, and kills some 50,000 elderly women, from complications as

a result of their fractures.

While warning of some possible side effects, such as blood clots or hot flashes, Lilly fails to warn of the more serious risks of ovarian cancer. A company-sponsored article in the Dec. 4, 1997 issue of the *New England Journal of Medicine* also ignores this risk. Lilly's pre-market clearance study, however, clearly shows that Evista induces ovarian cancer in both mice and rats. Furthermore, carcinogenic effects were noted at dosages well below the recommended therapeutic level. However, the study concluded: "The clinical relevance of these tumor findings is not known." Lilly reached this conclusion despite the strong scientific consensus that the induction of cancer in well-designed tests in two rodent species creates the strong presumption of human risk. Nevertheless, Lilly fails to disclose this critical information in its ads and in its "warning" to patients.

Responding to such criticisms by one of us (Samuel Epstein) during a broadcast of the "Jim Lehrer Newshour" earlier this year (Jan. 12), a Lilly spokesman claimed that the carcinogenic effects of Evista in the ovaries of sexually mature rodents are irrelevant to such risk in postmenopausal women, as their ovaries are inactive, and therefore, no warning is necessary. Apart from the fact that the rodent studies were specifically designed to evaluate Evista's safety, ovarian cancer is a scientifically documented complication of long-term estrogen replacement therapy in post-menopausal women. Also disturbing is the claim that Evista poses no risks of breast and uterine cancers, based on clinical trials over only some 40 months, a period totally inadequate to possibly measure any such risks.

Ovarian cancer strikes about 24,000 women in the United States every year, accounting for 4 percent of all female cancers. About 15,000 women die annually from ovarian cancer, making it the most lethal of all female reproductive cancers. Lilly's suppression of its own evidence of ovarian cancer risks from Evista is reckless and threatening to women's health and lives. Equally reckless is the Food and Drug Administration's December 1997 marketing clearance, especially in the absence of any requirement for warning. Such conduct clearly merits urgent congressional investigation. Evista should be withdrawn from the world market immediately. As importantly, a "cancer alert" should be sent to the more than 12,000 women who have participated in U.S. and international clinical trials, in the absence of fully informed consent. The doctrine of informed consent is ethically and legally protective only when all facts relevant to benefits and risks are affirmatively disclosed. This is clearly not the case with women who have been involved in the Evista trials. These women should be offered semi-annual lifelong surveillance for the early detection of ovarian cancer at Eli Lilly's expense.

Medical Procedures: Mammography

Perspective on Women's Health: Mammography Radiates Doubts

By Samuel S. Epstein, M.D.
From *The Los Angeles Times*
January 28, 1992

It has been widely (and with reason) charged that the makers and marketers of silicone breast implants, and self-interested plastic surgeons, made women their guinea pigs. But what of that other, and greater, scourge of women, breast cancer? There is reason to believe that women are equally ill-served by the cancer establishment, especially in its unrelenting promotion of mammography.

Breast cancer now strikes one in nine women, a dramatic increase from the one in 20 measured in 1950. This year, 180,000 new cases and 46,000 deaths are expected. Hearings scheduled Feb. 5 in Washington by the Breast Cancer Coalition, an advocacy group loosely modeled on AIDS activists, could not seem more timely.

The coalition wants more federal funding for the National Cancer Institute (NCI) to increase its research into the causes and treatment of breast cancer, and to improve delivery of breast health care — including diagnostic screening. In pursuing these goals, the coalition has been co-opted into supporting the policies of the cancer establishment — NCI and the American Cancer Society — which is fixated on basic research, diagnosis, and treatment. Cancer prevention receives only an estimated 5% of the annual $1.8 billion NCI budget.

Breast cancer is not the only cancer on the rise. While its incidence has increased 57% since 1950, overall cancer has increased 44%, now striking one in three people and killing one in four. Male colon cancer is up 60%, testis, prostate, and kidney cancer up 100%, and other cancers, such as malignant melanoma and multiple myeloma, more than 100%. The cancer establishment trivializes evidence linking these increasing rates with avoidable exposure to cancer-causing industrial chemicals and radiation that permeate our environment — food, water, air, and workplace.

The cancer establishment maintains, on tenuous evidence, that a fatty diet itself is a major cause of breast cancer, while ignoring contaminants in fat. Carcinogenic pesticides, such as the highly persistent chlordane and dieldrin, which concentrate in animal fats, are known to cause breast cancer in rodents. Elevated levels of DDT and PCBs are found in human breast cancers. An Israeli study found that breast cancer deaths in younger women recently dropped by 30%, despite a substantial increase in consumption of animal fat. This drop followed, and seems linked to, regulations that reduced previously high levels of DDT and related pesticides in dairy products. These pesticides act by mimicking the action of estrogens or by increasing estrogen production in the body, which in turn increases the risk of breast cancer. A related concern is lifelong exposure of all women to estrogenic contaminants in animal fat, because of their unregulated use as growth-promoting additives in cattle feed.

In 1977, NCI's director of endocrinology, Dr. Roy Hertz, warned, without effect, of breast cancer risks from these contaminants.

More ominous is the enthusiastic endorsement by the cancer establishment of massive nationwide expansion of X-ray mammography, including routine annual screening. While there is a general consensus that mammography improves early cancer detection and survival in postmenopausal women, no such benefit is demonstrable for younger women.

Furthermore, there is clear evidence that the breast, particularly in premenopausal women, is highly sensitive to radiation, with estimates of increased risk of breast cancer of up to 1% for every rad (radiation absorbed dose) unit of X-ray exposure. This projects up to a 20% increased cancer risk for a woman who, in the 1970s, received 10 annual mammograms of an average two rads each. In spite of this, up to 40% of women over 40 have had mammograms since the mid-1960s, some annually and some with exposures of 5 to 10 rads in a single screening from older, high-dose equipment.

Significant studies on radiation risks to the breast have been well known since the late 1960s, including evidence that mammography, especially in younger women, was likely to cause more cancers than could be detected. A confidential memo by Dr. Nathaniel Berlin, a senior NCI physician in charge of large-scale mammography screening in 1973, may explain why women were not warned of this risk; "Both the [American Cancer Society] and NCI will gain a great deal of favorable publicity [from screening, and] . . . this will assist in obtaining more research funds for basic and clinical research, which is sorely needed."

Thus, once again, suspect technology was applied to women on a large scale, in spite of clear warning signals and with insufficient knowledge of the likely consequences. (On a smaller scale, but even more ethically appalling, was the use until last April of industrial polyurethane foam to coat silicone breast inserts, despite clear evidence that its manufacturing contaminants and breakdown products were carcinogenic. As with mammography, no serious studies have been launched to find out what happened to women in whom the foam was implanted, or indeed to women carrying any type of silicone implant.)

The risks of mammography, especially for premenopausal women, persist with the lower radiation doses (about one-half rad per screening) found in modern facilities with dedicated equipment and licensed operators. A large Canadian study conducted from 1980 to 1988 found a 52% increase in early breast cancer deaths in women aged 40 to 50 who had 10 annual mammograms, compared to women given just physical examinations. More recent concern comes from evidence that 1% of women carry a gene that increases their breast cancer risk from radiation fourfold.

The coalition should insist that the NCI and American Cancer Society initiate an immediate, large-scale, well-publicized study to further investigate the role of past mammography in increasing breast cancer rates, and to investigate future cancer risk from mammography as currently conducted under widely varying conditions. Women should also be informed of their X-ray exposure and individual and cumulative risks each time they undergo mammography. The coalition should demand an immediate ban on obsolete high-dose X-ray equipment, and the abandonment of routine mammograms on premenopausal women.

The coalition should also encourage a crash program to develop and make available safe alternatives to mammography, apart from physical examination. Two that show the most promise are magnetic resonance imaging and transillumination with infrared light. The expansion of mammography should be put on hold, especially in view of the 1991 conclusion of the General Accounting Office that "there are more than enough machines to meet the screening needs of American women."

The Breast Cancer Coalition represents a welcome trend toward active grass roots involvement in public health. However, its current goals are too narrowly defined within the context of existing perspectives and institutional policies. The coalition needs broader and more radical strategies if it is to reverse the modern epidemic of breast cancer.

National Mammography Day

Press Release
From the Cancer Prevention Coalition
October 18, 1995

Chicago — Commenting on tomorrow's National Mammography Day, Dr. Samuel Epstein, Chairman of the Cancer Prevention Coalition (CPC), charged that "this is a recklessly misleading and self-interested promotional event more aptly named NATIONAL MAMMOSCAM DAY."

National Mammography Day, October 19, is the flagship of October's National Breast Cancer Awareness Month (NBCAM). NBCAM was conceived and funded in 1984 by Imperial Chemical Industries (ICI) and its U.S. subsidiary and spin-off Zeneca Pharmaceuticals. NBCAM is a National Cancer multi-million dollar deal with the cancer establishment, the National Cancer Institute (NCI) and American Cancer Society (ACS) and its multiple corporate sponsors, and the American College of Radiology.

ICI is one of the largest manufacturers of petrochemical and organochlorines. And Zeneca is the sole manufacturer of tamoxifen, the world's top-selling cancer drug, widely used for breast cancer. Zeneca/ICI's financial sponsorship gives them control over every leaflet, poster, publication, and commercial produced by NBCAM.

ICI supports the NBCAM blame-the-victim theory of cancer causation, which attributes escalating rates of breast (and other) cancers to heredity and faulty lifestyle. This theory diverts attention away from avoidable exposures to carcinogenic industrial contaminants of air, water, food, the workplace, and consumer products — the same products which ICI has manufactured for decades. NBCAM also ignores other avoidable causes including prolonged use of oral contraceptives and prolonged use of hormone replacement therapy. Ignoring prevention of breast cancer, NBCAM promotes "early" detection by mammography.

There is a wide range of serious problems with mammography, particularly with premenopausal women:

- There is no evidence of the effectiveness or benefit of mammography in premenopausal women.
- By the time breast cancers can be detected by mammography, they are up to 8 years old. By then, some will have spread to local lymph nodes or to distant organs, especially in younger women.
- Missed cancers (false negatives) are commonplace among women, as their dense breast tissue limits penetration by x-rays.

- About 1 in every 4 "tumors" identified by mammography in premenopausal women turns out not to be cancer following biopsy (false positive). Apart from needless anxiety, repeated surgery can result in scarring and delayed identification of early cancer that may subsequently develop.
- Regular mammography of younger women increases their cancer risks. Analysis of controlled trials over the last decade has shown consistent increases in breast cancer mortality within a few years of commencing screening. This confirms evidence of the high sensitivity of the premenopausal breast, and on cumulative carcinogenic effects of radiation.
- Premenopausal women carrying the A-T gene, about 1.5 percent of women, are more radiation sensitive and at higher cancer risk from mammography. It has been estimated that up to 10,000 breast cancer cases each year are due to mammography of A-T carriers.
- Radiation, particularly from repeated premenopausal mammography, is likely to interact additively or synergistically with other avoidable causes of breast cancer, particularly estrogens (natural; medical; contaminants of meat from cattle feed additives; and estrogenic pesticides).
- Forceful compression of the breast during mammography, particularly in younger women, may cause the spread of small undetected cancers.

Pressured by this evidence on the ineffectiveness and risks of premenopausal mammography, NCI recently withdrew recommendations for such screening. This evidence is still ignored by NBCAM, supported by radiologists and giant mammography machine and film corporations, which have specifically targeted premenopausal women with high-pressure advertisements.

CPC urges the immediate phaseout of premenopausal mammography. Postmenopausal mammography should be restricted to major centers and exposure reduced to a minimum. Women should be provided with actual dose measurements, rather than estimates. NCI and ACS should develop large-scale use of safe screening alternatives, including imaging techniques, and blood or urine tumor markers or immunologic tests.

Dr. Epstein urges that a medical alert be sent to women subjected to the Breast Cancer Detection Demonstration Project high-dose radiation experiments commencing in 1972. These experiments were conducted in spite of explicit prior warnings by a National Academy of Science's committee. Finally, Dr. Epstein calls for an "immediate investigation of the cancer establishment's reckless conduct by the President's Committee on Human Radiation Experiments."

Awareness Month Keeps Women Perilously Unaware

By Samuel S. Epstein
From *The Chicago Tribune*
October 27, 1997

This October marks the 13th anniversary of the National Breast Cancer Awareness Month (NBCAM), with its flagship Oct. 17 National Mammography Day. Enthusiastically promoted by the cancer establishment — the American Cancer Society and the National Cancer Institute, the American College of Radiology, and mainstream women's groups — NBCAM is dedicated to reducing breast cancer mortality through early detection by mammography screening. With an estimated 180,000 new cases and 44,000 deaths in 1997, breast cancer is second only to lung cancer as the leading cause of cancer death in women — what could be a more worthy objective?

Unfortunately, the primary focus of NBCAM reveals profoundly misguided priorities and a disturbing lack of commitment to prevention. NBCAM is based on the insistence, exemplified by the American Cancer Society's statement in its "Cancer, Facts and Figures — 1997," that there are no "practical ways to prevent breast cancer. . . . Since women may not be able to alter their personal risk factors, the best opportunity for reducing mortality is through early detection" by mammography. Similarly, the National Cancer Institute's 1995 Special Presidential Commission on Breast Cancer maintained that breast cancer is "simply not a preventable disease," while requesting more funding for research on detection and treatment.

In fact the benefits of annual screening to women age 40 to 50, who are now being aggressively recruited, are at best controversial. In this age group, one in four cancers is missed at each mammography. Over a decade of premenopausal screening, as many as three in 10 women will be mistakenly diagnosed with breast cancer. Moreover, international studies have shown that routine premenopausal mammography is associated with increased breast cancer death rates at older ages. Factors involved include: the high sensitivity of the premenopausal breast to the cumulative carcinogenic effects of mammographic X-radiation; the still higher sensitivity to radiation of women who carry the A-T gene; and the danger that forceful and often painful compression of the breast during mammography may rupture small blood vessels and encourage distant spread of undetected cancers.

Apart from the dangers and questionable value of premenopausal screening is its apparently unrecognized and prohibitive cost of $2.5 billion annually — based on an average of $125 per mammogram for approximately 20 million U.S. women age 40-50 — which is more than the budgets of the National Cancer Institute and American Cancer Society combined.

While the benefits of postmenopausal screening are less controversial, there is little evidence that the usual U.S. overkill of taking four or more mammograms per breast

annually is any more effective than the more restrained European practice of a single view every two to three years. Furthermore, there is no evidence that screening at any age is more effective than monthly breast self-examination, especially by women trained in this procedure, combined with an annual clinical examination whose costs are minimal.

Underlying this indifference to prevention are interlocking conflicts of interest between the cancer establishment and the cancer drug industry, and between the American Cancer Society and American College of Radiology and the powerful mammography machine and film industries. More significantly, NBCAM was conceived and funded in 1984 by Imperial Chemical Industries, one of the world's largest petrochemical manufacturers, and its U.S. subsidiary and spin-off Zeneca Pharmaceuticals.

Zeneca is the sole manufacturer of tamoxifen, the world's top-selling cancer drug, widely used for treating breast cancer and also for ill-advised trials to see whether it can prevent the disease in healthy women even though it is itself strongly carcinogenic. Of further concern, Zeneca has recently acquired 11 major cancer centers from Salick Health Care, posing disturbing and precedent-setting conflicts of interest between drug manufacture and prescription. Financial sponsorship by Zeneca gives it editorial control over every leaflet, poster, publication and commercial produced by NBCAM. As such, NBCAM is a masterful public relations coup for Zeneca.

With this background, it is hardly surprising that NBCAM fails to inform women how they can reduce their risks of breast cancer. In fact we know a great deal about its avoidable causes, which include:

• Prolonged use of oral contraceptives and estrogen replacement therapy.
• High-fat animal and dairy product diets that are heavily contaminated with chlo-

rinated pesticides that are estrogenic and carcinogenic to the breast, and meat contaminated with potent sex hormones following their use to fatten cattle in feed lots prior to slaughter.

- Exposure to petrochemical carcinogens in the workplace that put about 1 million U.S. women at increased risk.
- Exposure to carcinogenic chemicals from hazardous waste sites and petrochemical plants that pollute soil, air and water.
- Exposure to indoor air pollutants, including carcinogenic pesticides and solvents.
- Prolonged use of black and dark brown permanent or semi-permanent hair dyes.
- Heavy smoking and drinking commencing in adolescence.
- Inactivity and obesity.

Making women aware of these avoidable risks rather than fixating just on early detection should be the goal of a truly effective National Breast Cancer Awareness Month.

Medical Procedures: Breast Implants

Women at Risk Are Still in the Dark

By Samuel S. Epstein, M.D.
From *The Los Angeles Times*
September 9, 1994

Last week's establishment of a $4.25 billion settlement fund seems to add finality to the breast-implant controversy, even though the judge in the case believes that the amount, contributed by manufacturers, will be insufficient for current claims. The settlement also is insufficient because it ignores the risk of breast cancers developing decades later.

The Food and Drug Administration has consistently down-played any cancer risk from silicone gel implants. But the agency's sanguine position is contradicted by substantial research, including its own. Why is no

one sounding an alarm? Why is no one informing women of their risk and offering all women with breast implants the option of removal?

Studies by manufacturer Dow Corning, discovered in 1987 FDA inspections, showed that silicone-gel injection induced malignant tumors in rats. Internal memoranda by FDA scientists concluded that "while there is no direct proof that silicone causes cancer in humans, there is considerable reason to suspect that it can do so" and urged that "a medical alert be issued to warn the public of the possibility of malignancy following long-term implant[ation]." The FDA's response was to reassign the report's writers. Another report, in the July, 1994 *Journal of the National Cancer Institute*, confirmed that silicone gel is carcinogenic in mice as well.

Supporting this experimental evidence, a 1989 FDA internal report stated: "A survey of the literature indicates numerous case reports of cancer" long after implantation and warned of the "possibility of worsened diagnosis" and prognosis when implanted women developed breast cancer. The report stressed that population studies claimed as proof of safety by industry and surgeons were too short-term and flawed to "negate the potential risk of cancer."

At known higher risk of breast cancer are 350,000 women with foam-wrapped implants. These consist of a silicone pouch wrapped in industrial polyurethane foam made from the carcinogenic synthetic petrochemical toluene diisocyanate (TDI). The foam is unstable in the body and breaks down into TDI and another carcinogen, TDA, which was removed from hair dyes in 1971 for that reason.

The foam-wrapped implants were developed to reduce scar-like hardening in some women following silicone implantation. However, their use beginning in the early 1980s ignored unequivocal evidence published two decades previously. Beginning in 1960, Wilhelm Hueper, the National Cancer

Institute's leading carcinogenesis authority showed that foam degraded and induced malignant tumors in rats following injection and warned: "Since the polyurethane plastics have been used in cosmetic surgery . . . these observations are of practical importance . . . [and] should caution against indiscriminate use." He also noted that carcinogenic effects "might require an induction period of some 30 years or more," as with other carcinogens, notably asbestos. Hueper's finding have since been fully confirmed and extended by other independent studies.

Polyurethane-wrapped implants are thus carcinogen-impregnated sponges. These gradually disintegrate, releasing carcinogens to which the breast cells of premenopausal women are particularly sensitive.

Scientific publications apart, there is extensive documentation on industry's secret knowledge of cancer risks from implants, which were nevertheless aggressively marketed with assurances of safety. Dow Corning's carcinogenicity information on silicone implants is two decades old. Shortly after foam implants were first manufactured, the industry admitted that carcinogenicity data were significant in those applications ". . . for use inside the body." In 1985, Medical Engineering Corp., a Bristol-Myers Squibb subsidiary, admitted that "degradation products of polyurethane are toxic and in some cases carcinogenic. . . . Whether they are released in such low levels as to be no threat, only time will tell. . . . The breakdown products of the fuzzy implant material may well be carcinogenic. How would anyone defend himself in a malpractice suit if a patient developed a breast malignancy?" At industry-sponsored meetings in 1985, leading plastic surgeons cautioned that "foam could be a time bomb . . . [in view of its] carcinogenic potential. Surgeons should not go on implanting."

Without mentioning cancer risk, in April, 1992 the FDA banned all silicone implants except for controlled trials. This action was aggressively challenged by the American Society of Plastic and Reconstructive Surgery, the American College of Radiology, and the American Medical Association.

Responsibility for undisclosed cancer risks in 2 million implanted women, most seriously in the 350,000 with foam implants, is broadly shared among: the industry, for egregious conduct; plastic surgeons, for self-interested complicity; the FDA, for reckless unresponsiveness; the American Cancer Society, for silence; and the media, for minimal coverage of long-standing evidence. An immediate medical alert should be sent to all implanted women, with priority for those with foam implants. This should be followed by long-term surveillance with offers to remove the implants of any concerned women, at industry's but not taxpayers' expense. And all of this should be thoroughly apart from the inadequate $4.25 billion settlement.

New Study Warns Implants Pose Risk of Breast Cancer

Press Release
From the Cancer Prevention Coalition
November 9, 1995

Chicago — In the first comprehensive review of the scientific literature, internationally-recognized cancer expert Samuel Epstein, M.D. concludes that implants pose significant risks of breast cancer. The study will appear in the November issue of the peer-reviewed *International Journal of Occupational Medicine and Toxicology*.

The review presents a detailed analysis of the scientific literature, and confidential industry and government documents on the carcinogenicity of silicone and polyurethane breast implants.

"Risks of breast cancer have been ignored in the current controversy over implants," stated Dr. Epstein, Chair of the Cancer Prevention Coalition and pathology expert at the School of Public Health, University of Illinois at Chicago. "Evidence on the carcinogenicity of implants, particularly polyurethane, is strong. Recent epidemiological studies claimed as proof of safety are grossly flawed. Such studies would have even given a clean bill of health to asbestos."

Dr. Epstein continued, "Both industry and the Food and Drug Administration (FDA) have suppressed evidence on the cancer risk of silicone breast implants. FDA has still failed to act on the recommendation by their leading scientists to send Medical Alerts to women with silicone implants warning them of their cancer risks."

Based on his report, Dr. Epstein renews the call for a medical alert. He also urges the development of a long-term surveillance program, at industry's expense, with priority for women with polyurethane implants.

Clinical Trials

Perspectives on Medicine: A Travesty, at Women's Expense

By Samuel S. Epstein, M.D. and Susan Rennie
From *The Los Angeles Times*
June 22, 1992

The government's National Cancer Institute this spring launched a large-scale breast cancer prevention trial, recruiting thousands of healthy women at increased risk of breast cancer — including those with close relatives with the disease, and also anyone over 60. Half are to be treated with tamoxifen, a potent chemotherapy drug; the remainder will get a placebo. NCI believes tamoxifen can reduce breast cancers by 30%, while also reducing heart attacks and preventing osteoporosis.

With one in nine women expected to develop breast cancer over a lifetime, the trial would seem worthy of unqualified support.

However, the evidence that tamoxifen can prevent breast cancer is largely wishful thinking. To make matters worse, the risks to healthy women of a wide range of serious complications, including uterine cancer, fatal liver cancer, liver failure, life-threatening blood clots, and crippling menopausal symptoms are unacceptable. This trial must be halted in its tracks.

The NCI's rationale is that tamoxifen, which is modestly successful in treating breast cancer, appears to reduce the risk of new cancers of the other breast. This benefit has only been seen in some patients in about half of the studies that have been done. The protection also appears largely restricted to postmenopausal women. However, the NCI ignores this and misleadingly offers healthy younger women the hope of prevention.

In addition, Swedish studies suggest that tamoxifen increases mortality in postmenopausal women who do develop cancer in the other breast during treatment, these cancers being highly aggressive and treatment-resistant. This evidence appears confirmed by studies showing that while tamoxifen reduces breast cancer in rats, cancers that do develop are highly malignant. There are also questions concerning whether heart benefits actually exist, and to what extent.

If tamoxifen's effectiveness were the only question, our alarm would not be so great. But the drug is implicated in a range of serious and sometimes life-threatening complications, although the NCI dismisses these as "infrequently severe."

Tamoxifen triples the risk of uterine cancer, even in patients followed for relatively short periods. Reaching a new low in medical sexism, statistician Richard Peto, a leading British supporter of the trial, dismisses the risk as "no big deal," since uterine cancer is curable by hysterectomy.

Tamoxifen is also a "rip-roaring liver carcinogen," according to Gary Williams, medical director of the American Health Foundation, inducing aggressive cancers in 100% of rats at high doses, and 20% at lower doses equivalent to those being used in the prevention trial. This is acknowledged by the drug's manufacturer, ICI Americas, Inc. The prestigious British Medical Research Council warns of the absence of any safety margin at the trial dose. Yet the NCI misleadingly trivializes evidence of liver cancer to rats and ignores reports of two liver cancers in women on just double the dose used in the trials. Tamoxifen also promotes liver cancer in rats previously exposed to low doses of other carcinogens.

Moreover, as the British council emphasized, "Few women have received tamoxifen for longer than five to seven years, whereas the maximum incidence of liver tumors induced by known carcinogens occurs at eight to 10 years." Indeed, it is probable that a significant number of healthy women receiving tamoxifen may die from liver cancer after a decade or so.

Recent Swedish data suggest a more-than-50% increase in new cancers, including gastrointestinal, among breast cancer patients treated with tamoxifen.

Shortly before the NCI started its trial, the blue-ribbon British Committee on Safety of Medicines reported five cases of liver failure with four fatalities, five hepatitis with one fatality, and 11 other liver complications in breast-cancer patients treated with tamoxifen. Previously-undisclosed similar evidence has just been obtained from the U.S. Food and Drug Administration.

The NCI recognizes a six-fold risk of often-fatal blood-clotting problems with tamoxifen, but the trial's coordinator suggests, with no supporting evidence, that this is due not to tamoxifen itself, but to "the interactive effect of [other] chemotherapy." Sometimes severe menopausal symptoms, including hot flashes and vaginal discharge, are other recognized complications that the NCI seeks to downplay.

Incredibly, the NCI claims that theirs is "one of the most comprehensive informed-consents

we've ever seen." The consent form exaggerates tamoxifen's possible and questionable benefits and trivializes probable and high risks. These concerns have stimulated a congressional inquiry led by Rep. Ted Weiss (D-NY). The consent form's waiver of compensation for illness and injury, which participants must sign, is unlikely to protect the NCI or its investigators and hundreds of U.S. and Canadian centers and institutions involved in the trial from a future flood of malpractice and punitive claims for cancer and other complications. The doctrine of informed consent is legally protective only when all facts relevant to benefits and risks are fully and affirmatively disclosed.

The use of women as guinea pigs is familiar. There is revealing consistency between the tamoxifen trial and the 1970s trial by the NCI and American Cancer Society involving high-dose mammography of some 300,000 women. Not only is there little evidence of effectiveness of mammography in premenopausal women, despite NCI's assurances no warnings were given of the known high risks of breast cancer from the excessive X-ray doses then used. There has been no investigation of the incidence of breast cancer in these high-risk women. Of related concern is the NCI's continuing insistence on premenopausal mammography, in spite of contrary warnings by the American College of Physicians and the Canadian Breast Cancer Task Force and in spite of persisting questions about hazards even at current low-dose exposures. These problems are compounded by the NCI's failure to explore safe alternatives, especially transillumination with infrared light scanning.

Meanwhile, the NCI ignores other preventable causes of breast cancer, particularly fat contamination with pesticides and other carcinogens. It recently canceled a proposed $100-million study on dietary fat in favor of the tamoxifen trial.

The tamoxifen project is a travesty of science and a parody of cancer prevention. It also strikingly illustrates fundamental problems with federal cancer policies. The NCI suffers from a mindset myopically fixated on diagnosis, treatment and basic research, with relative indifference to cancer prevention.

Drastic reforms of NCI priorities and policies are essential to curbing the cancer epidemic, including escalating breast cancer rates. Only congressional action and strong support by women's and other concerned citizen groups can make this come about.

NCI In-House Programs

Fiscal Year 1991 Obligations
for Primary Prevention

DCPC In-House

The Division of Cancer Prevention and Control (DCPC) of the National Cancer Institute (NCI) has as its mandate the conduct of research on cancer prevention, cancer control, and the surveillance and monitoring of the incidence, mortality, and morbidity of cancer. Priorities include research to develop and evaluate cancer prevention regimens, research on special populations, and research to effect the full translation of research into applications. The Division is comprised of four Programs and includes the Cancer Prevention Research Program, the Cancer Control Science Program, the Early Detection and Community Oncology Program, and the Surveillance Program. The overall goal of these efforts is to achieve significant reductions in cancer incidence, mortality, and morbidity with a concomitant increase in cancer survival.

The Office of the Director (OD) is responsible for the coordination and direction of DCPC's programs. Total in-house costs for the OD in Cancer Control were $2,209,000.

The research in the Cancer Prevention Research Program (CPRP) is divided into two broad categories — chemoprevention, and diet and nutrition — that are pursued through both extramural and intramural mechanisms. The aim of chemoprevention research is to identify specific chemical substances that demonstrate anti-cancer activity in humans. Ultimately, these specific substances may be prescribed for high-risk individuals through dietary supplementation. A wide variety of

pharmacological and chemical substances are being investigated, for example, tamoxifen, ibuprofen, and calcium. The goals of the diet and nutrition program are to conduct research in nutritional and molecular regulation, prevention-related epidemiology, clinical trials and nutrition studies; identify and validate cancer-preventive dietary patterns; and — through NCI's information dissemination channels — encourage and change the dietary patterns of the public. Total in-house costs for Cancer Control in the CPRP were $3,429,000.

The Cancer Control Science Program (CCSP) is designed to identify the most effective strategies for bringing cancer prevention and control methods to the public and to the nation's health care providers. The Program identifies and develops strategies to surmount the barriers limiting the full transfer of new scientific results to practice. It also fosters cancer control research across the country and works with state and local health organizations/agencies on developing cancer control plans for their regions and making maximal use of existing data on cancer. Total in-house costs for Cancer Control in the CCSP were $3,997,000.

The Early Detection and Community Oncology Program is responsible for the identification and evaluation of technologies for early detection, biomarker research, rehabilitation for cancer patients, and community-based clinical trials in prevention, control, and treatment. The goal of early detection research is to increase the effectiveness of early detection practices that could lead to a reduction in cancer morbidity and mortality. Emphasis is also placed on the application of early cancer detection in medical practice. Research initiatives on new methods and approaches in early detection are undertaken with the goal of extending this research to comparative trials in high-risk groups, and in other defined populations.

In addition, research is aimed at finding intermediate endpoints of cancer prevention that can be used as markers of cancer risk or as early detection tests prior to the development of cancer. Such markers would also be validated in clinical trials so that they can be used to measure the success of prevention strategies.

Another mission of the Program is to train the next generation of scientists and practitioners in order to provide the field with qualified people to advance all facets of cancer prevention and control. Total in-house costs for EDCOP in Cancer Control were $5,515,000.

The Surveillance Program monitors the cancer burden on the population of the United States through the measurement of cancer incidence, mortality, and survival and the assessment of individual and societal factors that mediate these cancer measures both directly and indirectly. The ultimate purpose of cancer surveillance is to guide future programmatic and resource allocation decisions of the National Cancer Program.

The surveillance effort includes the development of information and statistical analysis systems, such as population-based registries and national probability surveys, and conduct of a broad series of studies focused on specific cancer control indicators. Programmatically and operationally, cancer surveillance requires a strong interface between methodologic techniques and cancer control initiatives in prevention, early detection, and treatment. Total in-house costs for Cancer Control in the SP were $1,670,000.

The research program in epidemiology spans a variety of areas and includes second-

ary data analysis from the cancer control supplement of the National Health Interview Survey as well as the Surveillance, Epidemiology and End Results (SEER) program. Total in-house costs for Epidemiology were $2,720,000.

The Physical and Chemical research categories include support to NCI's Smoking, Tobacco and Cancer Program, the evaluation of the "Working Well," a worksite-based cancer prevention and control program, and support related to research on oncologic pain. Total in-house costs were $73,000.

The Nutrition research category includes support for activities related to the retinoid skin cancer trial as well as a beta-carotene skin cancer trial in albinos, a computer-based dietary intervention program for worksites, and general support for nutrition-related activities. Total in-house costs were $292,000.

DCE In-House

The Division of Cancer Etiology (DCE) of the National Cancer Institute (NCI) is responsible for planning and directing a national program of basic research including laboratory, epidemiologic, and biometric research on the cause and natural history of cancer and means for preventing cancer. The DCE evaluates mechanisms of cancer induction and promotion by chemicals, viruses, and environmental agents and serves as the focal point for the federal government on the synthesis of clinical, epidemiological, and experimental data relating to cancer causation. Division staff participate in the evaluation of program-related aspects of other basic research activities as they relate to cancer cause and prevention. The DCE is comprised of three research program organizations: the Epidemiology and Biostatistics Program; the Chemical and Physical Carcinogenesis Program; and the Biological Carcinogenesis Program.

The Epidemiology and Biostatistics Program plans, directs, manages, and evaluates a program of epidemiologic, demographic, statistical, and mathematical research activities, and provides statistical and relevant automatic data processing services to support the research programs throughout the NCI. The Program is comprised of four intramural branches and one extramural branch: Clinical Epidemiology Branch; Environmental Epidemiology Branch; Radiation Epidemiology Branch; Biostatistic Branch; and the Extramural Programs Branch. The total in-house costs for prevention activities in FY 1991 were $13,243,000.

The Chemical and Physical Carcinogenesis Program (CPCP) plans, develops, directs, and evaluates a national program of basic and applied research in which agents known or suspected to have carcinogenic and/or tumor-promoting activity are evaluated from the standpoint of mechanism of action, metabolism, interactions with biologically important macromolecules, and related areas. The Program also supports basic research involving the development of effective agents to prevent or reverse the process of carcinogenesis. A significant portion of the activities of the CPCP intramural laboratories listed below involves primary prevention and nutrition studies.

The Laboratory of Chemoprevention plans, develops, and implements a research program on the use of pharmacological agents for the prevention of cancer; studies molecular mechanisms of action of chemopreventive agents such as retinoids; studies polypeptide growth factors, including their isolation, characterization, and mechanism of action; and develops new methods to control the activity of peptide growth factors, utilizing techniques of molecular genetics and immunology. Total in-house prevention expenditures in FY 1991 were $1,535,000.

The Laboratory of Human Carcinogenesis plans, develops, and conducts a research program assessing mechanisms of carcinogenesis in epithelial cells from humans and experimental animals; experimental approaches in biological systems for the extrapolation of carcinogenesis data and mechanisms from experimental animals to the human situation; and host factors that determine differences in carcinogenic susceptibility among individuals. The total in-house prevention expenditures in FY 1991 were $2,733,000.

The Laboratory of Cellular Carcinogenesis and Tumor Promotion plans, develops, and implements a comprehensive research program to determine the molecular and biological changes that occur at the cellular and tissue level during the process of carcinogenesis. For FY 1991, the total in-house prevention expenditures for physical and chemical carcinogenesis were $1,250,000 and for nutrition research, $400,000.

The Laboratory of Comparative Carcinogenesis plans, develops, and conducts a research program to compare effects of chemical carcinogens in rodents and non-human primates; identifies determinants of susceptibility and of resistance to carcinogenesis; identifies, describes, and investigates mechanisms of interspecies differences and of cell and organ specificity in carcinogenesis; investigates the perinatal age period and pregnancy in modifying susceptibility to chemical carcinogens; and conducts biologic and morphologic studies on the pathogenesis of naturally occurring and induced tumors in experimental animals. The total in-house prevention expenditures in FY 1991 were $1,783,000.

The Laboratory of Experimental Carcinogenesis plans, develops, and implements a research program aimed at elucidating mechanisms of malignant transformation in human and animal cells by chemical carcinogens and other cancer-causing agents; to determine critical cellular and genetic factors involved in initiation, promotion, and progression of these transformed cells; and to apply, whenever possible, the knowledge obtained from these studies towards effective prevention of cancer in humans. For FY 1991, the total in-house prevention expenditures for physical and chemical carcinogenesis were $1,250,000 and for nutrition, $610,000.

The Laboratory of Molecular Carcinogenesis plans, develops, and conducts a research program designed to clarify the molecular biology of carcinogenesis; elucidate the fundamental nature of the interactions of carcinogenic agents, especially chemical, with biological systems in the induction of cancer; define those environmental and endogenous factors that relate to and modify the carcinogenic process; and clarify the metabolic regulatory processes that are related to carcinogenesis. The total in-house prevention expenditures in FY 1991 were $770,000.

The Laboratory of Biology plans, develops, and conducts in vitro and in vivo investigations aimed at elucidating the role of chemical, physical, and biological agents in the modulation of carcinogenesis. Coordinated biochemical and biological studies utilizing human and animal cell models are used to characterize the cellular alterations associated with carcinogenesis. These include assessment of the effect of physiologic host mediating factors; determination of CCU surface changes; and evaluation of the relationships between differentiation, chromosome alterations, and carcinogenesis. The total in-house prevention expenditures in FY 1991 were $260,000.

The Laboratory of Experimental Pathology plans, develops, and implements research on the experimental pathology of carcinogenesis, especially concerned with the induction of neoplasia by chemical and physical factors in epithelial tissues, the total in-house prevention expenditures in FY 1991 were $100,000.

Statement on Administration Policies
on "Acceptable" Risks of Cancer
March 26, 1990

We express grave concerns at October 1988 EPA regulations (55FR 411030) allowing the intentional addition of carcinogenic pesticides to processed foods at levels allegedly posing "acceptable" risks of cancer. In October 1989, the Bush Administration proposed a Food Safety Plan which formally ratifies this new regulation. These new policies contravene the 1958 Delaney Amendment to the Federal Food, Drug and Cosmetic Act banning the intentional addition to food of any level of chemical carcinogen. Congress is now considering legislation ratifying the principle of "acceptable" risk.

The validity of the Delaney law, that there is no scientific way to determine safe levels or tolerances for chemical carcinogens, has been repeatedly examined and unequivocally endorsed over the last three decades by a succession of independent expert committees. The remarkable advances over the last three decades in our understanding of the molecular mechanisms of carcinogenesis are fully consistent with the scientific basis of the Delaney law, with our inability to meaningfully define carcinogenic risk quantitatively, and with recognition of the importance of environmental and occupational carcinogens as major causes of cancer. The Delaney law thus provides a valid scientific basis for regulatory policies designed to *prevent* avoidable exposures to carcinogenic contaminants in food. In contrast, the "negligible" or "de minimis" policies of EPA and FDA, respectively, are based on attempts to *manage* risks at "acceptable" levels of 1/100,000 to 1/1

million excess lifetime cancers as estimated by quantitative risk assessment: in instances of alleged economic necessity, risks even in excess of 1/100,000 are allowed. However, quantitative risk assessment is based on mathematical models and questionable assumptions. The uncertainty and flexibility of these models allow their misapplication to reflect pre-determined nonscientific considerations and special interest pressures. Furthermore, these estimates are restrictedly based on residues of a single carcinogenic pesticide or food additive on a single food item; based on this simplistic assumption, EPA estimates that a 1/100,000 risk would result in some 2,500 excess lifetime cancers or 35 annual cancers in the U.S. However, EPA has admitted that it does not attempt to estimate aggregate cancer risks in a total diet; most fruit and vegetables contain residues of as many as 25 carcinogenic pesticides. Thus, based on EPA's risk estimates for a single carcinogenic pesticide, it becomes clear that residues of 25 carcinogenic pesticides on 25 food items eaten daily would result in some 22,000 excess annual cancers. Furthermore, these estimates are minimal as they ignore the following incremental exposures: undisclosed inert carcinogenic pesticide ingredients; other carcinogens in food, notably color additives and residues of animal feed additive; and other chemical and radioactive carcinogens in air, water, and the workplace. EPA estimates also ignore unpredictable synergistic interactions from these multiple exposures. Additional flaws in EPA and FDA estimates include:

their basis on extrapolation from high-dose carcinogenicity tests in animals, thus underestimating low-dose response effects; their basis on lifetime carcinogenicity tests, thus underestimating responses from exposures of shorter duration; differences in risks posed by early and late stage carcinogens; ignoring the increased sensitivity of the fetus and infant; and ignoring other important toxic effects of carcinogenic food contaminants, particularly genetic, reproductive and behavioral.

The new policy for regulation of carcinogenic pesticides in food, based on risk management rather than risk prevention, is likely to reverse major current trends on reduction in the manufacture and use of agricultural pesticides in general and carcinogenic pesticides in particular. More seriously, this new policy creates dangerous precedents for opening the floodgates to "acceptable" risks from innumerable carcinogens, in air, water and food, regulation of which is totally ceded to the discretionary authority of highly politicized federal agencies. Very recently, following a court enforced ban on the food color Red No. 3, DHHS Secretary Sullivan announced that he would request Congress to repeal the Delaney law on which the ban was based in view of recent scientific advances which have allegedly made this law obsolete. Still more ominously, OMB economists have attempted to enforce on OSHA's scientists new definitions of chemical carcinogens, which would restrictively exclude from regulation the majority of chemicals found to be carcinogenic in valid animal tests, and which would impose requirements for epidemiological confirmation of animal carcinogenicity data.

We urge staunch opposition to Administration policies and proposed Congressional legislation allowing and legitimizing avoidable residues of carcinogenic pesticides in food. Instead, the Delaney law must be strengthened and enforced, and uniformly applied to all avoidable carcinogens in food — pesticides, food and feed additives. The principles of the Delaney law should also be extended to the regulation of avoidable exposures to carcinogens in air and water.

Samuel S. Epstein, M.D.
   Professor of Occupational and
      Environmental Medicine
   School of Public Health
   University of Illinois Medical Center
   Chicago, IL

Marvin Legator, Ph.D.
   Professor and Director
   Division Environmental Toxicology
   University of Texas Medical Branch
   Galveston, TX

William Lijinsky, Ph.D.
   Cancer Researcher
   Maryland

Scientist Co-Signers

Dean Abrahamson, M.D.
   University of Minnesota
   Minneapolis, Minnesota

Nicholas Ashford, Ph.D., J.D.
   Center for Policy Alternatives

Elizabeth Bourque, Ph.D.
   Environmental Toxicologist
   Massachusetts

Barry Castleman, Sc.D.
   Environmental and Occupational
   Consultant
   Baltimore, MD

Richard Clapp, Ph.D.
   John Snow Institute
   Boston, MA

Barry Commoner, Ph.D.
   Center for Biology of Natural Systems
   Queens College
   Queens, NY

Donald Dahlsten, Ph.D.
   University of California
   Berkeley, CA

Susan Daum, M.D.
  Occupational Physician
  New Jersey

Roger Detels, M.D.
  School of Public Health
  University of California
  Los Angeles, CA

Brian Dolan, M.D., Ph.D.
  Occupational Physician
  Santa Monica, CA

Vincent Esposito, M.D.
  St. Joseph Hospital
  Patterson, NJ

Emanuel Farber, M.D.
  Department of Pathology
  University of Toronto
  Toronto, Canada

Richard Garcia, M.D.
  University of California
  Berkeley, CA

Jack Geiger, M.D.
  CUNY Medical School
  New York, NY

John Gofman, M.D.
  Professor Emeritus of Medical Physics
  University of California
  Berkeley, CA

Allen Goldman, M.D.
  University of Illinois Medical Center
  Chicago, IL

Andrew Gutierrez, Ph.D.
  University of California
  Berkeley, CA

Marc Lappe, M.D.
  University of Illinois Medical Center
  Chicago, IL

Stephen Lester, Ph.D.
  Citizen's Clearinghouse for
    Hazardous Wastes, Inc.
  Arlington, VA

Alan Levine, M.D.
  San Francisco, CA

Edward Lichter, M.D.
  University of Illinois Medical Center
  Chicago, IL

Thomas Mancuso, M.D.
  Professor of Occupational Health
  University of Pittsburgh
  Pittsburgh, PA

Laurie Martinelli, J.D., M.P.H.
  Massachusetts Audubon Society
  Lincoln, MA

Michael McCann, Ph.D.
  Center for Occupational Hazards
  New York

Peter Orris, M.D.
  Director of Occupational Medicine
  Cook County Hospital
  Chicago, IL

Melvin Reuber, M.D.
  Pathologist
  Columbia, MD

Anthony Robbins, M.D.
  School of Public Health
  Boston University
  Boston, MA

Ken Rosenman, M.D.
  Michigan State University

Ruth Shearer, Ph.D.
  Genetic Toxicologist
  Washington

Jannette Sherman, M.D.
  Alexandria, VA

Allen Silverstone, M.D.
  State University of New York
  Syracuse, NY

Joel Swartz, Ph.D.
  University of Minnesota
  Minneapolis, Minnesota

David Teitelbaum, M.D.
University of Colorado
Boulder, CO

Arthur Zahalsky, Ph.D.
University of Southern California

Grace Ziem, M.D.
Occupational Physician
Baltimore, MD

Additional Co-Signers, Non-Scientific

Louis Beliczky
United Rubber, Cork, Linoleum
Plastic Workers of America
Akron, OH

Jay Feldman
National Coalition Against the
Misuse of Pesticides
Washington, D.C.

Rick Hind
U.S. Public Interest Research Group
Washington, D.C.

Ralph Lightstone
California Rural Legal Assistance
Sacramento, CA

Anthony Mazzocchi
Oil, Chemical, Atomic Workers Union
Denver, CO

Esther Peterson
Washington, D.C.

Michael Picker
National Toxics Campaign
Sacramento, CA

Local community-based organizations from across the country (too numerous to list here).

Appendix VIII

Ralph W. Moss:
Congressional Testimony on Clinical Trials and Alternative Treatments

Testimony before the House Committee
on Government Reform and Oversight
February 4, 1998

Mr. Chairman and Members
of the Committee,

Congress was deceived when the war on cancer was launched in 1971. Experts swore under oath that they would deliver a cure for cancer in time for the Bicentennial (1976). That is ancient history. But Congress continues to be fooled by a new generation of "experts" who testify that the war on cancer is being won, and that all we need to do is trust them to conquer this terrible disease.

Recently, Dr. Richard Klausner, M.D., director of the National Cancer Institute (NCI), appeared before this Congress and claimed that we have turned the corner in the fight against cancer. He promised that advances in genetics were ushering in a golden age of research. However, I believe that the rosy picture he paints is misleading.

Back in 1962, 278,000 Americans died of cancer. Last year, cancer deaths were over 560,000, double the figure of 35 years ago. Certainly, part of this increase is due to the growth and aging of the population. But even when one adjusts for these factors, the overall U.S. mortality rate from cancer increased over 10 percent from 1950 to 1991. And the incidence rate during that time increased nearly 50 percent.

There has been a leveling off in recent years.

But we have still witnessed a tremendous worsening of the cancer situation throughout this century. In particular, the rates of lung cancer have risen astronomically, more than 500 percent among women. There has been a tripling in the incidence of melanoma, and nearly a doubling of cases of prostate cancer and multiple myeloma.[1]

Breast Cancer Statistics

Many of us are understandably alarmed at the prevalence of breast cancer in America today. When Pres. Nixon launched the war on cancer in 1971, a woman's lifetime risk for contracting breast cancer was one in fourteen. Today, it is one in eight. Between 1973 and 1992, the incidence of breast cancer rapidly increased by 34 percent, and among black women by 47 percent. And the chances of being cured have not improved very much. Since 1960, nearly one million American women have died of breast cancer. Dr. Klausner has made much of the recent leveling off or even downturns in some of the cancer statistics. These are encouraging.

However, a slight downturn in mortality does not make up for millions of personal tragedies.

When the Diagnosis Is Cancer

Let us consider what happens to a person who is diagnosed with cancer.

First of all, there are the so-called "proven"

methods, surgery, radiation therapy, and chemotherapy. Sometimes these are brutal methods, that involve the loss or damage of body parts and functions. Surgery is an ancient approach, known to the Egyptians, Greeks and Romans. It is a sad commentary that this is still the mainstay of therapy. New ideas are urgently needed in the treatment of even so-called "curable" cancers.

But what about those patients whose tumors are inoperable or widespread at the time they are discovered? Similarly, what about the patients whose tumors have returned after being "successfully" treated with "curative" therapies?

Such cancers are, by and large, incurable with today's conventional methods. The best that conventional medicine has to offer is palliation. And despite the war on cancer about half of all cancer patients will eventually find themselves in this deplorable position.

What are they supposed to do?

The Pitfalls of Clinical Trials

If you read the statements of the NCI, they urgently appeal to cancer patients to join their clinical trials. This message is picked up and amplified by all the beneficiaries of the war on cancer. You can even see it on billboards in airports. A "clinical trial" is made to sound very attractive to cancer patients. However, as the President's Commission for the Study of Ethical Problems in Medicine stated (in 1983), "Patients who are asked to participate in tests of new anticancer drugs" should "not be misled about the likelihood (or remoteness) of any therapeutic benefit they might derive."

In fact, there is little chance of therapeutic benefit to patients in such trials. Studies in both the United States and Japan have shown that only about one percent of patients in Phase I clinical trials have a complete response to the treatment, and only about 5 percent have any response at all.[2]

You may think that five percent is not bad odds when you are in a desperate situation. But here you have to understand some of the peculiar terminology of the field. For a "response" is not a "cure." Far from it. The FDA defines a response as the *shrinkage* of 50 percent or more, of the measurable tumors for a period of one month or more.

It is a change in size of a mass. This *might* be important, if the tumor is painfully pressing on a nerve or another vital structure. But usually such shrinkages are absolutely meaningless to the patient. It is essentially a numbers game played among oncologists — who can shrink tumors the most. In the majority of cases, these temporary shrinkages do not correlate with an increase in median overall survival, which is the most meaningful measurement of patient benefit in such trials.

Sometimes, in fact, a high response rate actually correlates with a lower period of survival. It may do more harm than good.

"Treatment Deaths"

I want to call your attention to the fact that these trials can be very dangerous for patients. The drugs approved by the FDA for treating cancer are all toxic. Some of them have astonishing toxicity, especially when given in combination. In one clinical trial of drugs on patients with the leukemia-like myelodysplastic syndrome, 42 percent of participants were killed by the treatment itself.

In another study, of a three-drug regimen called "ICE," 13 patients (8 percent of the total) died as a consequence of the treatment itself, so-called "treatment deaths." But the scientists in charge had the nerve to conclude that this regimen was "well tolerated, with acceptable . . . side effects and predictable organ toxicity."[3]

Acceptable to whom? Not the patients who died after contracting raging bacterial infections, capillary leak syndrome, bleeding inside the brain, and irreversible kidney failure — all caused by these drugs. And certainly not their families.

This is the "scientific" approach of the NCI. Not surprisingly, there is tremendous resistance among patients and doctors to such trials. Only three to five percent of cancer patients go into them. Many oncologists want nothing to do with them. In fact, just 10 percent of all oncologists enroll 80 percent of the patients in clinical trials.[4] In New York, oncologists have given their patients small doses of standard chemotherapy to make them ineligible for useless clinical trials.

Looking for Alternatives

Drugs that don't work — clinical trials that measure meaningless shrinkages — doctors who think that horrible side effects are perfectly acceptable . . . no wonder cancer patients today are desperately looking for alternatives. They are exploring the realm of unapproved, complementary, nontoxic treatments in record numbers.

You can be sure that one of the reasons the NCI and FDA so hate these alternative treatments is that they siphon away "adventurous" patients who might otherwise go into clinical trials.

Historically, all of the agencies involved in the war on cancer have lied about the nature of these alternatives. They have painted a distorted picture of them as quackery. They have prejudged them, refusing to carry out the most basic tests that could evaluate their efficacy. Tests were only performed under duress (often because the Congress insisted) and these tests were at best ill-conceived and at worst marked by outright fraud.

Yet, the history of medicine tells us that many treatments and techniques once considered "alternative" or "fraudulent" later became an established part of the mainstream. Radiation and chemotherapy themselves started out on the fringe. Acupuncture was derided as "quackupuncture" for decades. But a recent Consensus Conference of the National Institutes of Health endorsed its use for such conditions as pain and nausea related to cancer.

The Office of Alternative Medicine (OAM) was established by Congress at the National Institutes of Health precisely because of the historic failure of the NCI to fulfill its mission and examine all possible options in the fight against cancer. But little progress has been made because of the intransigent attitudes of the cancer establishment.

Are there frauds among the alternatives? Certainly. How can we separate the wheat from the chaff? We need good research, with open-minded attitudes and adequate funding, to carry out studies of these alternatives. The OAM is ready to perform these studies. But the NCI stands in the way. Along with its police partner, the FDA, it is the great roadblock to the examination of promising new ways of treating cancer.

Great Promise

Dr. Klausner is betting on the genetic revolution to produce a cure for cancer. Even some geneticists warn that cancer breakthroughs, if they do come from this field, may be decades away. I believe there is enormous potential in the various alternative and complementary approaches to cancer.

In my book, *Cancer Therapy* (1992), I discuss over 100 such methods. One could add another hundred or so of promise. These include vitamin and mineral regimens, herbal formulas, unusual drugs from land and sea, immunological techniques, electromagnetic treatments, and utilization of the mind-body connection.

On a recent trip to Germany I was astonished to see the scope and freedom with which many progressive oncologists treat cancer. They use a combination of the conventional approaches with such things as tumor vaccines; mistletoe therapy; local, regional, and whole-body hyperthermia; thymus and other organ extracts; fever therapy; orthomolecular and antioxidant therapies; psychoneuroimmunology; music and art therapy; sports and physical therapy; and many, many others. Their government not only allows such approaches, but encourages and pays for them as well.

It is astonishing that the average American oncologist knows little or nothing about any of these approaches. The FDA has done everything in its power to block their development over here. The NCI has not seriously examined a single one of these. Our war on cancer has fallen woefully behind developments in other parts of the world, not just Germany but Japan, China, and many other countries as well.

The approach of the war on cancer has been relentlessly that of chemotherapy. Reliable estimates put the sales of cancer therapeutics at over $12.3 billion this year.[5] Most of that is controlled by American firms. And so it has been a big business success story, with double-digit growth rates every year for over a decade. But it has done little for the cancer patient.

The FDA has approved approximately 40 drugs for the treatment of cancer. *But it has never approved a nontoxic agent or one that was not patented by a major pharmaceutical company.* The approved drugs are all toxic and many of them cause second cancers in those who are lucky enough to survive the treatment. And the NCI, FDA, and comprehensive cancer centers are tied by a thousand strings to the multi-billion dollar pharmaceutical industry. Recently, a top FDA official went to work for Elan Pharmaceuticals. But this is nothing new. Two past directors of the FDA became drug company officials, as did Dr. Klausner's predecessor at the NCI. It is a time-honored tradition, the "revolving door."

Meanwhile, the FDA spends a good deal of its resources hunting down and harassing those who use innovative methods in treating cancer.

They have carried out a vendetta against Dr. Stanislaw R. Burzynski, MD, PhD, a Texas physician who has used nontoxic peptides in the treatment of brain cancer and other kinds of malignancy. They have repeatedly raided his clinic, seized his records, harassed his patients. In 1995, they instigated charges that would have put him in federal prison for life. Luckily, the jury saw otherwise and Dr. Burzynski is a free man. When I publicly objected to this harassment I myself was slapped with a subpoena for all my information regarding Dr. Burzynski. When I pointed out the illegality of this request, and indicated my willingness to fight the FDA, the subpoena was just as suddenly quashed by the U.S. Attorney.

FDA has also impeded the work of Dr. George Springer of the Finch Medical School, who has developed a promising vaccine for breast cancer. It has hindered the work of Arnold Eggers, M.D., of Downstate Medical School, who has a promising treatment based on concepts first proposed by William B. Coley a century ago. And it has used its resources to attack the distributors of nontoxic medications. The most recent victim was a distributor of the nontoxic drug hydrazine sulfate, who was raided by FDA enforcement agents on January 16, 1998.

The approach of the NCI and FDA is overwhelmingly in support of toxic chemotherapy. They have abrogated their duties as the defenders and protectors of the cancer patients. They function today on behalf of the industry they were supposed to challenge and oversee. They are the drug testing and law enforcement arms of a vast $100 billion a year business, the cancer industry.

CIS Fiasco

The promotion of toxic treatments and the venomous hatred of alternatives is not restricted to court battles. Both FDA and NCI are active in the court of public opinion, trying to destroy confidence in any nontoxic or less-toxic treatment.

Their main vehicle in this regard is the Cancer Information Service of the NCI. Their reckless attacks on alternative and complementary treatments are disseminated at taxpayer's expense via print, fax, and especially the Internet.

Their statements are filled with prejudice, errors and innuendo. Each one contains an "advertisement" for NCI's clinical trials. When I was an advisor to the Office of Alternative Medicine, I tried to find out exactly who wrote these erroneous statements and what sort of "peer review" they possibly could have undergone before being released. I never could find out. It is clear that no bona fide experts were involved in their creation, and that the proponents of such methods were not consulted or even interviewed before these statements were drawn up and released.

These harmful, hateful statements have become an integral part of the "war on cancer" which, quite frankly, more often looks like a "war on alternative practitioners" than a war on any disease. Treatment approaches that threaten the hegemony of the drug industry are prone to vicious attack.

The NCI's statements on alternative and complementary cancer treatments should be immediately withdrawn. New statements that are factual and unbiased should be drawn up for release by the Cancer Information Service.

The statements that have already been prepared by Dr. Mary Ann Richardson and her group at the University of Texas School of Public Health could provide a good starting point for these new statements.

Reform of FDA

In addition, the FDA should be reformed so that it no longer exerts a stranglehold on innovators in cancer treatment and diagnosis. That is why I strongly support passage of the Access to Medical Treatment Act and urge you all to co-sponsor this important legislation.

The FDA does little to protect citizens from the ravages of chemotherapy, which is overwhelmingly given without any proof of patient benefit. In the past, FDA at least paid lip service to the idea that anticancer drugs should extend life or improve quality of life. But in 1996, they caved in and agreed that new drugs could be approved based on partial remissions in clinical trials. Such partial remissions are nothing but the shrinkages of tumors. As we have shown, such temporary and partial shrinkages do not necessarily lead to improvements in survival or quality of life.[6]

POMES

Finally, Mr. Chairman and members of the committee, I have an urgent request.

In August, 1997, the Office of Alternative Medicine (OAM) in conjunction with the National Cancer Institute (NCI) convened a meeting in Bethesda, MD to consider how they could evaluate the practices of doctors who use unconventional methods to treat cancer. The name of this meeting was "POMES," which stands for "Practice Outcomes Monitoring and Evaluation Systems." Over 100 leaders of the cancer field attended, including not just alternative researchers and practitioners, but the director of the Comprehensive Cancer Center of the University of Wisconsin, the president of the American Health Foundation, two department chairs from Memorial Sloan-Kettering Cancer Center, representatives from major food companies, and many others.

There were great hopes for this meeting, since we were told that it was funded by Dr. Klausner's office at the NCI. Perhaps this signaled a change in attitude at NCI, the change we have all been waiting for. But not only was Dr. Klausner unable to attend, but his key deputy, Robert Wittes, M.D., Director of the Division of Cancer Treatment, Diagnosis and Centers, also failed to put in an anticipated appearance. The FDA and NCI scientists who did appear lacked decision-making power in this area.

After several days of heated discussion, the participants finally hammered out statements that could lay the basis for future evaluations of alternative cancer treatments. It felt like history in the making. These guidelines called for the creation of an Oversight Board, a body of experienced people who could guarantee a "level playing field" in the evaluation of alternative practices. No longer would NCI have complete power to serve as lawyer, judge, and jury in every case.

Most of the participants left that meeting excited by the prospects before us. Then, silence. Since August, we have not received a single official communication regarding POMES. Has POMES died a natural death . . . or did someone kill it?

I know for a fact that the problem does not lie with the Office of Alternative Medicine, whose leaders remain enthusiastic about the prospect of fairly evaluating such treatments. I can only conclude, therefore, that the roadblock is the top leadership of the NCI and possibly the NIH as well.

You have to ask yourself why these high-placed medical leaders so fear an impartial test of unconventional approaches to cancer? Why do they hate the idea of an impartial Oversight Board, which could detect fraud or malfeasance on either side of the cancer controversy?

Perhaps they are afraid of the competitive threat such nontoxic and less-toxic methods might pose to the cancer industry? Do they fear the ridicule of prejudiced colleagues? Or perhaps they fear the repercussions in Congress, if it turns out that an effective treatment for cancer was overlooked — or even suppressed — by NCI and FDA?

Mr. Chairman, I urgently appeal to you to help revive POMES.

I am sure you agree that patients and their caregivers need reliable information about the safety and potential effectiveness of alternative and complementary cancer treatments.

Many American citizens are impatient with the foot-dragging at NCI and the obstructionism of the FDA. Yet we as individual citizens have no way to force these agencies and individuals to act properly or fairly. It is up to you, our elected representatives, to do that. There is no time to waste. Since August, another 270,000 Americans have died of cancer. Many of them were desperately seeking reliable scientific information on alternatives at the time they died.

The Congress created the OAM to bring about the fair evaluation of alternative methods. We appreciate the fact that you have increased OAM's funding to $20 million this year. It is a heartening vote of confidence in the future of this field. And, in some respects, under the leadership of Wayne Jonas, M.D., it has done a brilliant job. But OAM by itself does not have the political clout to force the testing of alternative cancer treatments. That is the main reason that OAM has not carried out a single evaluation of a controversial cancer treatment. It has not and it will not, because at every turn, the NCI has been there, insisting on a major role. It now turns out that the role NCI wanted was to block and obstruct such trials from taking place.

Block NCI's Appropriations!

Just one month ago, Dr. Klausner appeared before the Appropriations Committee and requested $2.2 billion for his agency for fiscal year 1998. This is an increase of $61 million over last year. I am here to ask you to do everything in your power to block that appropriation until NCI changes its attitude towards alternative and complementary treatments. As a first step they should actively implement the POMES process.

In his speech to Congress, Dr. Klausner stated that "there is no one intervention or even one type of intervention that will successfully conquer the many diseases we call cancer. Our approach must be open and broad-based."

Fine words! But it happens to be the *exact opposite* of the course that NCI is actually pursuing. It is only an aroused Congress that can make Drs. Klausner and Wittes open the doors of NCI to alternative treatments. They must not be allowed to serve as a branch of the pharmaceutical industry, but must be convinced to test a wide variety of treatments, as they are currently practiced around the world.

If these individuals will not comply, they should be replaced by open-minded scientists who will.

Mr. Chairman, for the 1.2 million Americans and the 9 million people worldwide who will develop cancer this year, such reforms cannot come a moment too soon.

References

1. L. A. G. Ries *et al.* "SEER Cancer Statistics Review, 1973-1991: Tables and Graphs," NCI, Bethesda, 1994.
2. *J. Clin. Oncol.* 14:287, 1996.
3. *J. Clin. Oncol.* 13:323, 1995.
4. *J. Clin. Oncol.* 12:1796 1994.
5. Frost & Sullivan. *World cancer therapeutics markets* (executive summary), Frost & Sullivan, Mountain View, CA, 1993. Cited in Moss, *Questioning Chemotherapy*, p.75.
6. H. Stout and L. McGinley. "Cancer drugs to get speedier FDA review," *The Wall Street Journal*, March 29, 1996.

Appendix IX

Legal Challenge
to High Cure Rate Claims

The Claims

THE UNIVERSITY OF TEXAS
MD ANDERSON
CANCER CENTER

1997·1998
ANNUALFUND

January 26, 1998

Mr. Henry J. Novak
P.O. Box 26162
Austin, TX 78755-0162

Dear Mr. Novak:

When it comes to cancer, the odds are in your favor!

The fact is that well over 50% of people with cancer who are cared for at The University of Texas M. D. Anderson Cancer Center return home cured.

That's great news for you and every Texan.

Today, M.D. Anderson is known throughout the world for its innovations in the treatment and prevention of cancer. Here, dedicated physicians and scientists have found ways to cure and treat many forms of once-deadly cancers.

That translates into hope for more than 52,000 patients who come to us every year for help.

But it's not all good news . . . because the sad truth is that the number of new cancer cases continues to grow and many cancers are not yet curable. Through research, we must investigate every possible way to cure cancer . . . and we need your help to accomplish this goal.

Your gift to our Annual Fund will help conquer cancer and help your fellow Texans have an even better chance of beating this disease.

Please, join other Texans who share our vision of a day when cancer is eliminated as a major health threat to us all. Make a gift to M. D. Anderson's Annual Fund today.

Sincerely,

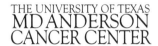

John Mendelsohn, M.D.
President

P.S. We urgently need your help to maintain our cutting-edge research and patient-care programs. Please send your gift by March 16. Thank you.

1515 HOLCOMBE BOULEVARD·135 · HOUSTON, TEXAS 77030 · (713) 792-3450

Enclosure with the Claims

Here's How Your Gift Saves Lives

Thanks to the help of good people like you, we now have hope against cancer — in fact, well over 50% of the cancer patients who come to us for help are cured! Here's how your gift works today — to safeguard lives tomorrow . . .

• Support research into the exact roles played by cancer-causing genes . . . so one day we can actually prevent cancer before it strikes.
• Funds research into marshaling the body's defense systems against cancer.
• Funds our unique in-hospital center where patients and their families can learn about cancer and caring for themselves.
• Helps us develop new conservative surgery techniques and much, much more!

Your neighbors have helped put us on the cutting edge of research and treatment. Please help us continue this fight against cancer. Send what you can today.

Attorney Novak's Challenge to the Claims

LAW OFFICES

HENRY J. NOVAK

A PROFESSIONAL CORPORATION
SUITE 402, SPICEWOOD BUSINESS CENTER
4412 SPICEWOOD SPRINGS ROAD
P. O. BOX 26162
AUSTIN, TEXAS 78755-0162

March 5, 1998

<u>CERTIFIED MAIL RETURN RECEIPT REQUESTED NO. Z 110 876 752</u>
John Mendelsohn, M.D., President
The University of Texas M D Anderson Cancer Center
1515 Holcombe Boulevard - 135
Houston, Texas 77030

<u>Re: M. D. Anderson Cancer Center Annual Fund Solicitation Letter. 1998</u>

Dear Dr. Mendelsohn,

The M. D. Anderson Cancer Center's Annual Fund letter, dated January 26, 1998, which solicits contributions from members of the general public (a copy of which is enclosed), makes the following representation:

> The fact is that well over 50% of people with cancer who are cared for
> at . . . M. D. Anderson Cancer Center return home cured.

And, again, on the back of the contribution card

> . . . in fact, well over 50% of the cancer patients who come to us for
> help are cured.

It is the opinion of this office, and the opinion of numerous observers of the results being obtained by the medical profession in its efforts to solve the problem of cancer in the United States, that an outright, unqualified claim of a cancer cure rate of 50% is a false statement. If it is in fact false, then Title 18 of the United States Code, §1341 applies to your conduct and to the M. D. Anderson Cancer Center in authoring and causing the 1998 Annual Fund solicitation letter to be distributed through the United States Postal Service. Section 1341 provides in pertinent part as follows:

> §1341. Frauds and swindles. Whoever . . . for obtaining money . . . by means of
> false . . . representations . . . places in any post office of authorized depository
> for mail matter, any matter or thing whatever to be sent or delivered by the
> Postal Service . . shall be fined under this title or imprisoned not more than five
> years, or both.

(continued on next page)

John Mendelsohn, M.D.
March 5, 1998
Page 2

Because of the politics of the cancer industry, it is unlikely that federal or state prosecutors would entertain imposing criminal sanctions on the M. D. Anderson Cancer Center even if your representation is in fact, false or substantially misleading.

The responsibility of protecting the public from the deceptive consequences of such a claim, if it is false, therefore falls upon private citizens who are willing to call your institution to account for such conduct. This letter seeks such an accounting.

Please provide this office, within 30 days of your receipt of this letter, copies of all statistics, studies, calculations, and source materials upon which the above-quoted representation is based. Please ensure that your response contains (i) a clear, layman's explanation of the meaning and significance of the data constituting the evidentiary basis for the cancer care representation, (ii) articulate statements of exactly what the M. D. Anderson Cancer Center means by its use of the words "cancer," "cancer patients," "cared for," "return home," and "cured" in the January 26, 1998 Annual Fund letter; and, if the M. D. Anderson Cancer Center is selective in the species of cancer which it admits for treatment, then (iii) a statement of those kinds of cancers which it treats and those which it does not treat and the reasons for the discrimination.

Should you fail to provide the foregoing information, or should the information you do provide fail to materially substantiate the cancer cure rate representation, a class action lawsuit will be filed against the M. D. Anderson Cancer Center in a court of appropriate jurisdiction, without further notice, alleging that the mailing of the January 26, 1998 Annual Fund letter violates the prohibition against mail fraud contained in U.S.C. §1341. The lawsuit will ask the court to issue an injunction against the M. D. Anderson Cancer Center compelling it (1) to cease and desist from any further publications, utterances, or mailings of the 50% cancer cure rate representation which are accompanied by any solicitation for money; (2) to issue a retraction of the cancer cure claim made in the January 26, 1998 Annual Fund letter; and (3) to offer to refund to any contributor the monies it contributed to the M. D. Anderson Cancer Center in response to the January 26, 1998 Annual Fund letter.

Very truly yours,

Henry J. Novak

Enclosure: (as stated)

The MD Anderson Response

THE UNIVERSITY OF TEXAS
MD ANDERSON
CANCER CENTER

April 1, 1998

Office of the Chief Legal Officer
Telephone: (713) 794-4000
Fax: (713) 799-8801
Box: 537

Henry J. Novak
Suite 402, Spicewood Business Center
4412 Spicewood Springs Road
P.O. Box 26126
Austin, Texas 78755-0162

Dear Mr. Novak:

Your letter of March 5, 1998, addressed to Dr. John Mendelsohn, President of The University of Texas M. D. Anderson Cancer Center, has been forwarded to this office for response.

Please be advised that M. D. Anderson stands by any and all statements made in its annual fund letter of January 26, 1998. Your suggestion that the 1997-1998 annual fund letter is somehow a false statement covered by Title 18 of the United State Code §1341, and that §1341 provides any type of private cause of action against this institution, is insupportable under any theory of law.

The University of Texas M. D. Anderson Cancer Center is a component of The University of Texas System and therefore, is a state agency entitled to Eleventh Amendment immunity.

The Eleventh Amendment of the United States Constitution bars suits by a citizen against the citizen's own state, as well as suits by citizens of another state. *Hans v. Louisiana,* 134 U.S. 1, 10 S. Ct. 504 (1890). Eleventh Amendment immunity extends not only to states, but also to state agencies and individuals sued in their official capacities. *United Carolina Bank v. Bd. Of Regents of Stephen F. Austin State Univ.,* 665 F. 2d553, 561 (5th Cir. 1982) (state agencies); *Will v. Michigan Dept. of State Police,* 491 U.S. 58, 109 S. Ct. 2304 (1989) (individuals sued in their official capacities). Because The University of Texas M. D. Anderson Cancer Center is a component institution of The University of Texas System, it is a state agency; and therefore it is entitled to Eleventh Amendment immunity.

The U.S. Supreme Court's interpretation of the Eleventh Amendment has two parts: "first, that each State is a sovereign entity in our federal system;" and second, that "it is inherent in the nature of sovereignty not to be amendable to the suit of an individual

TEXAS MEDICAL CENTER
1515 HOLCOMBE BOULEVARD · HOUSTON, TEXAS 77030 · (713) 792-2121
A Comprehensive Cancer Center Designated by the National Cancer Institute

(continued on next page)

without its consent." *Seminole Tribe of Florida v. Florida,* U.S. 44, 116 S. Ct. 1114, 1122 (1996).

Congress may abrogate a state's sovereign immunity if it has: (1) " unequivocally expressed its intent to abrogate the immunity," and (2) acted "pursuant to a valid exercise of power." *Seminole Tribe of Florida v. Florida,* U.S. 44, 116 S. Ct. 1114, 1123 (1996). Not only has the Supreme Court held that Congress' intent to abrogate a state's immunity from suit must be obvious from a clear legislative statement: but also that the Fourteenth Amendment is the only valid means by which Congress can abrogate state sovereign immunity.

Only in the event that the U.S. Congress, or the legislature of the State of Texas, has provided for a waiver of sovereign immunity may a claim be brought against this institution, as any general claim against the institution is prohibited by the Eleventh Amendment of the United States Constitution.

The Supreme Court of Texas has long recognized that sovereign immunity, unless waived, protects the State of Texas, its agencies and its officials from being subjected to suit or damages in its own courts. *Federal Sign v. Texas Southern University,* 951 S. W.2d 401, 405 (Tex. 1997). Sovereign immunity has two components — immunity from suit and immunity from liability. Sovereign immunity bars suits against units of state government unless express consent has been given. A party suing a governmental entity protected by sovereign immunity may allege consent to suit either by reference to statute or express legislative permission.

There is nothing in the Texas Revised Civil Statutes indicating that the Texas Legislature has waived sovereign immunity for a claim such as the one that you suggest you will make. Specifically, no cause of action arises under the Texas Tort Claims Act for the sort of claim that you allege nor do you have legislative permission to bring such a claim. Furthermore, even in the event that 1x U.S.C. §1341 was being violated by the institution, which it is not, that statute, as you admit in your correspondence, does not offer any private cause of action, nor injunctive relief, nor damages to an individual. Accordingly, your position is completely and wholly without legal basis.

Your position is so completely without merit that I find it appropriate to advise you of the Texas Disciplinary Rules of Professional Conduct should you choose to pursue this matter. As I am sure you are aware, the Texas Disciplinary Rules of Professional Conduct, Rule 3.01, Meritorious Claims and Contentions, provides:

> A lawyer shall not bring or defend a proceeding, or assert or controvert an issue therein, unless the lawyer reasonably believes that there is a basis for doing so that is not frivolous.

A pleading filed with a court is frivolous if the lawyer is unable to make a good faith argument that the action is consistent with existing law or that it may be supported by a

(continued on next page)

good faith argument for an extension, modification, or reversal of existing law. (Texas Disciplinary Rules of Professional Conduct. Rule 3.01, Comment 3).

Your insinuation that there is a cause of action against this agency for its annual fund letter has no basis in fact, and more importantly, is completely without support in the law. It therefore can hardly be argued that you have any reasonable belief that there is any legal basis for your claim, as the slightest degree of research would have indicated that no such legal basis exists.

Accordingly, please be advised that not only will The University of Texas M. D. Anderson Cancer Center not provide you with the information requested in your correspondence, but it is also the Cancer Center's position that any effort on your part to institute a class action suit on the basis stated in your correspondence is completely without legal basis. Since the Cancer Center, through this office, has advised you of its position, in the event that you were to bring a claim as stated in your correspondence, and the Cancer Center appropriately sought and obtained a summary judgment against such a claim, this matter would be reported to the Travis County Bar Association for whatever disciplinary action is deemed appropriate.

If I can be of any further assistance in this matter, please do not hesitate to call.

Sincerely,

Dan Fontaine
Chief Legal Officer

DF:mf

cc (w/encl.): John Mendelsohn, M. D.
              Ray Farabee
              Kevin Wardell
              Leon Leach
              Andrew von Eschenbach, M. D.
              Steve Stuyck
              Pat Mulvey

NOTE: In view of the unresponsiveness of Fontaine's letter, Attorney Novak filed the lawsuit against MD Anderson Cancer Center on August 10, 1998.

The Request for Substantiation of the Claims

DIANNA LOPER
18314 OAKHAMPTON DRIVE
HOUSTON, TEXAS 77084

June 19, 1998

<u>CERTIFIED MAIL NUMBER:</u>

Mr. Dan Fontaine
Legal Services Department
Box 537, M.D. Anderson Hospital
1515 Holcombe Blvd.
Houston, Texas 77030

Dear Mr. Fontaine:

Pursuant to Chapter 552 of the Texas Government Code, I request that you send me copies of the following public information maintained by or in the possession of the M.D. Anderson Cancer Center:

a. A listing of all cancer cases admitted for treatment to M.D. Anderson from 1980 through 1993, classified (identified) by (i) date of entry for treatment, (ii) the site of the cancer, (iii) the type(s) of treatment administered, and (iv) whether the patient is now alive and, if not, the date of death;

b. A listing of the foregoing cases grouped by cancer sites;

c. Compilation of Ratios and/or percentages derived from the information identified in paragraph a.;

d. Guidelines, policies, or directives that establish or identify the kind of cancers that M.D. Anderson admits for treatment and/or those which it declines to admit or treat;

e. All written and electronic correspondence between officers, agents, and employees of M.D. Anderson and any third party or parties which discuss directly or indirectly statistics, percentages, or ratios derived from the information identified in paragraphs a. and b.; and

f. An index of all material that are provided to me in response to this request.

Please provide me within 10 days of your receipt of this letter with an estimate of the costs of reproduction and advise whether a prepayment for costs will be required.

Thank you for your cooperation.

Sincerely yours,

Dianna Loper

The MD Anderson Response

(The response from M.D. Anderson appears to be a frank admission that they do not have any systematized data on 5-year survival rates, and that they have no statistical basis for their highly misleading, if not fraudulent, March 5, 1998 claim for an overall 50% cancer cure rate.)

THE UNIVERSITY OF TEXAS
MD ANDERSON
CANCER CENTER

June 29, 1998

Associate Vice President
for Business Affairs
Telephone: (713) 792-7550
Fax: (713) 794-4566
Box: 194

Dianna Loper
18314 Oakhampton Drive
Houston, Texas 77084

Dear Ms. Loper:

Your recent Public Information Request has been forwarded to me for resolution. I have reviewed your recent request and need to discuss it with you. I have left two messages on your recorder to call me.

For your information the Public Information Act provides access to many records maintained at The University of Texas M.D. Anderson Cancer Center. However, the Act only applies to information already in existence and it does not require a governmental body to prepare new information in response to a request. The Act does not require a governmental body to prepare answers to questions or to perform general research to prepare the response. Items a, b, c, and f, in your request are not in existence and would take time and effort to prepare this information from underlying data elements. Such an effort would result in substantial interference with ongoing operations to prepare this information as you have requested it. Item e is a derivative of items a and b and, thus, would not exist. I do not believe that I will find any documentation in item d as we are a comprehensive cancer center. I know of no guideline, policy, or directive that establishes admittance criteria based on the type of cancer.

Documents that identify medical patients, including medical records, are confidential by law and are protected from disclosure.

Please call me so we may discuss your request. If you wish to revise, limit or clarify your request, it would be helpful to receive a written letter modifying your request at this time.

Sincerely,

Michael J. Best
Associate Vice President
for Business Affairs

TEXAS MEDICAL CENTER
1515 HOLCOMBE BOULEVARD · HOUSTON, TEXAS 77030 · (713) 792-2121
A Comprehensive Cancer Center Designated by the National Cancer Institute

Appendix X

Citizen Petitions to the FDA

on Avoidable Cancer Risks

Citizen Petition Seeking Carcinogenic Labeling on all Cosmetic Talc Products

17 November 1994

David A. Kessler, M.D.
Commissioner
Food and Drug Administration, Room 1-23
12420 Parklawn Drive
Rockville, MD 20857

The undersigned submits on behalf of the Cancer Prevention Coalition, Inc. (CPC), Samuel S. Epstein, M.D., Chair and National Advisor of the Ovarian Cancer Early Detection and Prevention Foundation (OCEDPF), Nancy Nehls Nelson, member of the Ovarian Cancer Early Detection and Prevention Foundation, Peter Orris, M.D. and Quentin Young, M.D. This citizen petition is based on scientific papers dating back to the 1960s which warn of increased cancer rates resulting from frequent exposure to cosmetic grade talc.

The undersigned submits this petition under 21 U.S.C. 321 (n), 361, 362, and 371 (a); and 21 CFR 740.1, 740.2 of 21 CFR 10.30 of the Federal Food, Drug, and Cosmetic Act to request the Commissioner of Food and Drugs to require that all cosmetic talc products bear labels with a warning such as "Talcum powder causes cancer in laboratory animals. Frequent talc application in the female genital area increases the risk of ovarian cancer."

A. Agency Action Requested

This petition requests that FDA take the following action:

1. Immediately require cosmetic talcum powder products to bear labels with a warning such as "Talcum powder causes cancer in laboratory animals. Frequent talc application in the female genital area increases the risk of ovarian cancer."

2. Pursuant to 21 CFR 10.30 (h) (2), a hearing at which time we can present our scientific evidence.

B. Statement of Grounds

Ovarian cancer is the fourth deadliest women's cancer in the U.S., striking approximately 23,000 and killing approximately 14,000 women this year. Ovarian cancer is very difficult to detect at the early stages of the disease, making the survival rate very low. Only three percent of ovarian cancer cases can be attributed to family history.[1] One of the avoidable risk factors for ovarian cancer is the daily use of talcum powder in the genital area.[2]

Research done as early as 1961 has shown that particles, similar to talc and asbestos particles, can translocate from the exterior genital area to the ovaries in women.[3, 4, 5] These findings provide support to the unexpected high rate of mortality from ovarian cancer in female asbestos workers.[6, 7, 8] Minute particles such as talc are able to translocate through the female reproductive tract and cause foreign body reactions in the ovary.

There is a large body of scientific evidence, dating back thirty years, on the toxicity and mineralogy of cosmetic talc products. As early as 1968, Cralley et. al. concluded:

All of the 22 talcum products analyzed have a . . . fiber content . . . averaging 19%. The fibrous material was predominantly talc but probably contained minor amounts of tremolite anthophyllite, and chrysotile (asbestos-like fiber) as these are often present in fibrous talc mineral deposits . . . Unknown significant amounts of such materials in products that may be used without precautions may create an unsuspected problem.[9]

As a follow-up to previous findings, Rohl, *et al.*, examined 21 samples of consumer talcums and powders, including baby powders, body powders, facial powders and pharmaceutical powders between 1971 to 1975. (See Addendum.) The study concluded:

. . . cosmetic grade talc was not used exclusively. The presence in these products of asbestiform anthophyllite and tremolite, chrysotile, and quartz indicates the need for a regulatory standard for cosmetic talc . . . we also recommend that evaluation be made to determine the possible health hazards associated with the use of these products."[10]

Talc is a carcinogen, with or without the presence of asbestos-like fibers. In 1993, the National Toxicology Program published a study on the toxicity of non-asbestiform talc and found clear evidence of carcinogenic activity.[11]

Recent cancer research in the United States has found conclusively that frequent talcum powder application in the genital area increases a woman's risk of developing ovarian cancer.[12, 13, 14, 15] Cramer, *et al.*, suggested that talc application directly to the genital area around the time of ovulation might lead to talc particles becoming deeply imbedded in the substance of the ovary and perhaps causing foreign body reaction (granulomas) capable of causing growth of epithelial ovarian tissue.[16, 17]

Harlow, *et al.*, found that frequent talc use directly on the genital area during ovulation increased a woman's risk threefold.

That study also found:

The most frequent method of talc exposure was use as a dusting powder directly to the perineum (genitals) . . . Brand or generic "baby powder" was used most frequently and was the category associated with a statistically significant risk for ovarian cancer.

In Harlow's report, arguably the most comprehensive study of talc use and ovarian cancer to date, 235 ovarian cancer cases were identified and compared to 239 controls, women with no sign of ovarian cancer or related health problems. Through personal interviews, Harlow, *et al.*, found that 16.7% of the control group reported frequent talc application to the perineum.[18] This percentage is useful in estimating the number of women in the general population exposed to cosmetic talc in the genital area on a regular basis. Harlow, *et al.*, concludes:

. . . given the poor prognosis for ovarian cancer, any potentially harmful exposures should be avoided, particularly those with limited benefits. For this reason, we discourage the use of talc in genital hygiene, particularly as a daily habit.

Clearly, large numbers of women — an estimated 17% — are using cosmetic talc in the genital area and may not be adequately warned of the risk of ovarian cancer from daily use.

C. Claim for Categorical Exclusion

A claim for categorical exclusion is asserted pursuant to 21 CFR 25.24 (a) (11) .

D. Certification

The undersigned certifies, that, to the best knowledge and belief of the undersigned, this petition includes all information and views on which the petition relies, and that it includes representative data and information known to the petitioner which are unfavorable to the petition.

This petition is submitted by:

Samuel S. Epstein, M.D.
Cancer Prevention Coalition
520 North Michigan Avenue, Suite 410
Chicago, Illinois 60611
Phone 312-467-0600
Fax 312-467-0599

Council to the Cancer Prevention Coalition:
Center for Constitutional Rights
Michael E. Deutsch, Legal Director
666 Broadway
New York, NY 10012
212-614-6427

Addendum: Results from an informal survey of talc products in Chicago drug stores.

Baby Powders:

Johnson & Johnson Baby Powder (Johnson & Johnson, Skillman, NJ)
Contains: TALC, fragrance

Osco Brand Baby Powder (Osco Drug, Oak Brook, IL)
Contains: TALC, fragrance

Body Powders:

Jean Naté Perfumed Talc (Revlon, New York, NY)
Contains: TALC, kaolin, magnesium carbonate, fragrance.

Shower to Shower (Johnson & Johnson, Skillman, NJ)
Contains: TALC, cornstarch, sodium bicarbonate, fragrance, polysaccharides.

Osco Brand Body Powder (Osco Drug, Oak Brook, IL)
Contains: TALC, cornstarch, sodium bicarbonate, fragrance, polysaccharides.

Ammens Medicated Powder (Bristol-Myers Squibb, New York, NY)
Contains: Zinc oxide, cornstarch, fragrance, isostearic acid, PPG-20, methyl glucose ether, TALC.

Cashmere Bouquet Perfumed Powder (Colgate, New York, NY)
Contains: TALC, magnesium carbonate, zinc stearate, fragrance

Gold Bond Medicated Powder (Martin Himmel, Hypoluxo, FL)
Contains: Menthol, Zinc oxide, boric acid, eucalyptol, methyl salicylate, salicyclic acid, TALC, thymol, zinc stearate.

Feminine products:

Vagisil Feminine Powder (COMBE, Inc., White Plains, NY)
Contains: Cornstarch, aloe, mineral oil, magnesium stearate, silica, benzethonium chloride, fragrance.

Vaginex Feminine Powder (Schmid Laboratories, Sarasota, FL)
Contains: Zinc oxide, cornstarch, fragrance, 6-hydoxquinole, 8-hydroxquinole sulfate, isostearic acid, PPG-20, methyl glucose ether, TALC.

Summer's Eve Feminine Powder (CB Fleet Co., Lynchburg, VA)
Contains: Cornstarch, tricalcium phosphate, oxoxynol-9, benzethonium chloride, fragrance.

FDS Feminine Deodorant Spray (Alberto Culver, Melrose Park, IL)
Contains: isobutane, isopropyl myristate, cornstarch, mineral oil, fragrance, lanolin alcohol, hydrated silica, magnesium stearate, benzyl alcohol.

References

1. SEER. *Cancer Statistics*, 1973-1990.
2. B.L. Harlow, D.W. Cramer, D.A. Bell, W.R. Welch. "Perineal Exposure to Talc and Ovarian Cancer Risk," *Obstet.*

Gynecol. 80: 19-26, 1992.

3. G.E. Egli and M. Newton. "The transport of carbon particles in the human female reproductive tract," *Fertility Sterility,* 12:151-155, 1961.

4. P.F. Venter and M. Iturralde. "Migration of particulate radioactive tracer from the vagina to the peritoneal cavity and ovaries," *S. African Med. J.* 55: 917-919, 1979.

5. W.J. Henderson, T.C. Hamilton, M.S. Baylis, C.G. Pierrepoint, K. Griffiths. "The demonstration of migration of talc from the vagina and posterior uterus to the ovary in the rat," *Environ. Research*, 40: 247-250, 1986.

6. M.L. Newhouse, G. Berry, J.C. Wagner, M.E. Turok. "A study of the mortality of female asbestos workers," *Brit. J. Indust. Med.* 29: 134-141, 1972.

7. B.K. Wignall, A.J. Fox. "Mortality of female gas mask assemblers," *Brit. J. Industrial Med.* 39: 34-38, 1982.

8. E.D. Acheson, M.J. Gardner, E. Pippard, and L.P. Grime. "Mortality of two groups of women who manufactured gas masks from chrysotile and crocidolite asbestos: a 40-year follow-up," *Brit. J. Industrial Med.* 39: 344-348, 1982.

9. L.J. Cralley, M.M. Key, O.H. Groth, W.S. Lainhart, and R.M. Ligo. "Fibrous and mineral content of cosmetic talcum products," *Am. Industrial Hygiene Assoc. J.* 29: 350-354, 1968.

10. A.N. Rohl, A.M. Langer, I.J. Selikoff, A. Tordini, R. Klimentidis, D.R. Bowes, and D.L. Skinner. "Consumer talcums and powders: mineral and chemical characterization," *Technical Report* Series N: 421, September 1993.

11. National Toxicology Program. "Toxicology and carcinogenesis studies of talc (CAS N 14807-96-6) in F344/N rats and B6C3F, mice (Inhalation studies)," *Technical Report* Series N:421, September 1993.

12. P. Hartge, R. Hoover, L.P. Lasher, L. McGowan. "Talc and ovarian cancer" letter, *JAMA* 250:1844, 1983.

13. K.A. Rosenblast, M. Szklo, N.B. Rosenshein. "Mineral fiber exposure and the development of ovarian cancer,"

Gynecol. Oncol. 45: 20-25, 1992.

14. A.S. Whittemore, M.L. Wu, R.S. Paffembarger, D.L. Sarles, J.B. Kampert, S. Grosser, D.L. Jung, S. Balloon, and M. Hendrickson. "Personal and environmental characteristics related to epithelial ovarian cancer, II. Exposures to talcum powder, tobacco, alcohol, and coffee," *Am. J. Epidemiol.* 1128:228-1240, 1988.

15. Harlow, 1992.

16. Ibid.

17. D.W. Cramer, W.R. Welch, R.E. Scully, and C.A. Wojciechowski. "Ovarian cancer and talc: a case control study," *Cancer* 50:372-376, 1982.

18. Harlow, 1992.

Citizen Petition Seeking to Ban the Use of Lindane (gamma-hexachlorocyclohexane) as Treatment for Lice and Scabies

17 January 1995

David A. Kessler, M. D.
Commissioner
Food and Drug Administration, Room 1-23
12420 Parklawn Drive
Rockville, MD 20857

The undersigned submits on behalf of the Cancer Prevention Coalition, Inc. (CPC), Samuel S. Epstein, M.D., Chair, Quentin Young, M.D., and Peter Orris, M.D, and on behalf of the Center for Constitutional Rights, Michael Deutsch, Esq. This citizen petition is based on recent scientific information on risks of brain cancer in children resulting from the use of lindane shampoo, other evidence of carcinogenicity, and evidence of hematotoxicity and neurotoxicity.

The undersigned submits this petition under 21 U.S.C. 321 (n), 361, 362, and 371 (a); and 21 CFR 740.1, 740.2 of 21 CFR 10.30 of the Federal Food, Drug, and Cosmetic Act to request the Commissioner of the Food and

Drug Administration (FDA) to immediately ban the use of lindane as a treatment for lice and scabies.

A. Agency Action Requested

This petition requests that FDA take the following action:

(1) Immediately ban the use of lindane as a treatment for lice and scabies.

(2) Pursuant to 21 CFR 10.30 (h) (2), a hearing at which time we can present our scientific evidence.

B. Statement of Grounds

Lice and scabies are endemic among the population. An estimated six million Americans, mainly children, are infested with lice each year. Most children are treated with pesticide-containing products marketed as shampoos. Lindane (gamma-hexachlorocyclohexane) is one of the most widely prescribed treatments for lice and scabies.

In a recent case-control study, Davis *et al.* reported a statistically significant increase of brain cancer in children following treatment with lindane shampoo:

> . . . use of Kwell® [lindane] was significantly associated with childhood brain cancer in comparison to friend controls (OR-4.6; 95% CI -1.0-21.3).[1]

These findings are of particular significance in relation to the striking increase, 38%, in the incidence of brain and nervous system cancers in children from 1973 to 1991.[2]

Further evidence on carcinogenicity is provided by two epidemiological studies by the National Cancer Institute.[3,4] Statistically significant increases, up to six-fold, in the incidence of non-Hodgkin's lymphoma were reported in farmers exposed to lindane.

In addition to these epidemioloical data, a series of case reports on blood disorders, including aplastic anemia, with case fatality rates of some 50%, and leukemia have appeared in the literature over the last three decades. [5,6] Of related interest is recent evidence on the high toxicity of lindane to human red blood stem cells.[7]

These epidemiological data are further supported by experimental evidence on the carcinogenicity of lindane. Lindane is classified as Group 2B by the International Agency for Research on Cancer,[8] and as 2B/C by the Environmental Protection Agency. The EPA has restricted lindane's use as an agricultural pesticide.[9] Agricultural and other uses of lindane and other isomers of hexachlorocyclohexane have been severely restricted or banned by other countries.[10]

The neurotoxic effects of lindane are well known. A 1976 FDA alert was issued to warn physicians of such risks.[11] Numerous case reports have documented seizures and brain damage following lindane exposure.[12] Recent studies have emphasized that recommended dosages of lindane may cause seizures:

> Therefore, given the extremely narrow range of safety of this drug and the risk imposed by the kindling effect, which potentiates convulsive seizures, and that this potentiation may be carried on for a considerable period of time, there is no good reason to use lindane in children or adults when other perfectly effective, safer pediculides are available.[13]

Lindane is readily absorbed through the skin.[14] After topical application to the adult skin without washing for 24 hours, almost 10% can be recovered from urine.[15] Absorption is further increased when lindane is administered in warm water or followed by oil-based hair care preparations.

C. Claim for Categorical Exclusion

A claim for categorical exclusion is asserted pursuant to 21 CFR 25.24 (a) (11).

D. Certification

The undersigned certifies, that, to the best knowledge and belief of the undersigned, this petition includes all information and views on which the petition relies, and that it includes representative data and information known to the petitioner which are unfavorable to the petition.

This petition is submitted by:

Samuel S. Epstein, M.D.
Cancer Prevention Coalition
520 North Michigan Avenue, Suite 410
Chicago, Illinois 60611
Phone: 312-467-0600
Fax: 312-467-0599

Council to the Cancer Prevention Coalition:

Michael E. Deutsch, Esq.
Legal Director
Center for Constitutional Rights
666 Broadway
New York, NY 10012
212-614-6427

References:

1. J.R. Davis, R.C. Brownson, R. Garcia, B.J. Beniz, and A. Turner. "Family Pesticide Use and Childhood Brain Cancer," *Arch. Environ. Contam. Toxicol.* 24:87-92, 1993.

2. L.A.G. Reis, B.A. Miller, B.F. Hankey, C.L. Kosary, A. Harras, B.K. Edwards, Eds. *SEER Cancer Statistics Review, 1973-1991: Tables and Graphs*, National Cancer Institute, NIH Pub. No. 94-2789:428, Bethesda, MD, 1994.

3. K.P. Cantor, A. Blair, G. Everett, R. Gibson, L.F. Burmeister, L.M. Brown, L. Schuman, and F.R. Dick. "Pesticides and other agricultural risk factors for non-Hodgkin's lymphoma among men in Iowa and Minnesota," *Cancer Res.* 52: 2447-2455, 1992.

4. A. Blair, O. Axelson, C. Franklin, O.E. Paynter, N. Pearce, D. Stevenson, J.E. Trosko, H. Vainio, G. Williams, J. Woods, and S.H. Zahm. "Carcinogenic Effects of Pesticides," in: *The Effects of Pesticides on Human Health,* S.R. Baker and C.F. Wilkinson, Eds. pp. 201-260, Princeton Scientific Publishing Co., Princeton, NJ, 1990.

5. American Medical Association Council on Drugs. "Registry on blood dyscrasias: Report to the AMA Council," *JAMA* 148-150, 1962.

6. Agency for Toxic Substances and Disease Registry. "Toxicological profile for alpha-, beta-, gamma- and delta- hexachloro-cyclohexane (update)," U.S. Department of Health and Human Services, Pub. No. TP-93/09:43, May 1994.

7. D. Parent-Massin, D. Thouvenot, B. Rio, and C. Riche. "Lindane hemotoxicity confirmed by *in vitro* tests on human and rat progenitors," *Human Exp. Toxicol.* 13:103-106, 1994.

8. International Agency for Research on Cancer. "Hexachlorocyclohexanes," *Monographs on the Evaluation of Carcinogenic Risks to Humans: Overall Evaluations of Carcinogenicity* Supplement 7:220-222, 1987.

9. *Agency for Toxic Substances and Disease Registry* p. 142-149.

10. United Nations. "Consolidated list of products whose consumption and/or sale have been banned, withdrawn, severely restricted or not approved by governments," 4th Edition, p. 238-240, New York, 1991.

11. Food and Drug Administration. "Gamma Benzene Hexachloride (Kwell and Other Products) Alert " *FDA Drug Bulletin* 28, June-July 1976.

12. M. Wheeler. "Gamma Benzene Hexachloride (Kwell) Poisoning in a Child," *Western J. Med.* 127:518-521, 1977.

13. L.M. Solomon, D.P West, and J.F. Fitzloff. "Lindane" letter, *Arch. Dermtol.* 126:248, 1990.

14. *Agency for Toxic Substances and Disease Registry* p.51, 1994.

15. Food and Drug Administration, 1976.

Citizen Petition Seeking Labeling of Nitrite-Preserved Hot Dogs for Childhood Cancer Risk

April 25, 1995

David A. Kessler, M.D.
Commissioner
Food and Drug Administration, Room 1-23
12420 Parklawn Drive
Rockville, MD 20857

The undersigned submits on behalf of the Cancer Prevention Coalition, Inc. (CPC), Samuel S. Epstein, M.D., Chair, and on behalf of the Center for Constitutional Rights, Michael Deutsch, Esq., Legal Director. This citizen petition is based on accumulating scientific information on excess risks of childhood brain tumors and leukemia from the consumption of hot dogs containing nitrite preservatives.

The undersigned submits this petition under 21 U.S.C. 321 (n), 361, 362, and 371 (a); and 21 CFR 740.1, 740.2 of 21 CFR 10.30 of the Federal Food, Drug, and Cosmetic Act to request the Commissioner of the Food and Drug Administration (FDA) to label hot dogs that contain nitrites with a cancer risk warning.

A. Agency Action Requested

This petition requests that FDA take the following action:

1. Immediately require nitrite-containing hot dogs to be labeled with warnings such as "hot dogs containing nitrites have been shown to pose risks of childhood cancer."

2. Pursuant to 21 CFR 10.30 (h) (2), a hearing at which time we can present our scientific evidence.

B. Statement of Grounds

Nitrites are widely used as preservatives in hot dogs, besides other meat products. Nitrites combine with amines naturally present in meat to form carcinogenic N-nitroso compounds.[1-4] N-nitrosodimethylamine has been identified in nitrite-preserved meat products.[5,6] There is overwhelming evidence on the carcinogenicity of N-nitrosodimethylamine in animal experiments.[7] Furthermore, epidemiologic evidence has associated N-nitroso carcinogens with cancer of the oral cavity, urinary bladder, esophagus, stomach and brain.[8-10]

There is substantial evidence on the risks of childhood cancer from the consumption of meats containing nitrites.[11-13] In 1982, Preston-Martin, *et al.* found that "consumption during pregnancy of meats cured with sodium nitrite has been associated with development of brain tumors in the offspring."[14]

Recent case-control studies have confirmed the risks of cancer from consumption of hot dogs. Eating many hot dogs by children, as well as maternal hot dog consumption during pregnancy, has been shown to be associated with brain cancer and leukemia in children.[15-17]

Bunin, *et al.* studied children who were diagnosed with brain cancer before age six, between 1986 and 1989. Of 53 foods and beverages and three alcoholic beverages consumed by mothers during pregnancy, only hot dogs were associated with an excess risk of childhood brain tumors.[18]

Sarusua and Savitz studied 234 childhood cancer cases in Denver and found a strong association between the consumption of hot dogs and brain cancer. Children born to mothers who consumed hot dogs one or more times per week during pregnancy had approximately double the risk of developing brain tumors. Children who ate hot dogs one or more times per week were also at higher risk of brain cancer. In addition, children who ate hot dogs and took no vitamins, which retard the formation of N-nitroso carcinogens, were more strongly associated with both acute lymphocytic leukemia (ALL) and brain cancer.[19] Sarusua and Savitz concluded:

The results linking hot dogs and brain tumors (replicating an earlier study) and the apparent synergism between no vitamins and meat consumption suggest a possible adverse effect of dietary nitrites and nitrosamines.[20]

Peters, *et al.* studied the relationship between the intake of certain foods and the risk of leukemia in children from birth to age 10 in Los Angeles County between 1980 and 1987. The researchers found that children who ate 12 or more hot dogs per month had approximately seven times the normal risk for developing childhood leukemia. A strong risk for childhood leukemia also existed for those children whose fathers' intake of hot dogs was 12 or more per month.[21] Peters, *et al.* concluded:

> Our results provide evidence for an association between consumption of hot dogs and risk of childhood leukemia. Adjustments for all factors thought to be potential confounders did not affect these associations. Independent risks were associated with both children's and fathers' consumption. . . . The findings, if correct, suggest that reduced consumption of hot dogs could reduce leukemia risks, especially in those consuming the most. [22]

These findings are of particular significance considering a 38 percent increase in the incidence of brain and nervous system cancers in children from 1973 to 1991.[23] Brain tumors account for about one in five childhood cancers.[24]

C. Claim for Categorical Exclusion

A claim for categorical exclusion is asserted pursuant to 21 CFR 25.24 (a) (11).

D. Certification

The undersigned certifies, that, to the best knowledge and belief of the undersigned, this petition includes all information and views on which the petition relies, and that it includes representative data and information known to the petitioner which are unfavorable to the petition.

This petition is submitted by:

Samuel S. Epstein, M.D.
Cancer Prevention Coalition
520 North Michigan Avenue, Suite 410
Chicago, Illinois 60611
Phone: 312-467-0600
Fax: 312-467-0599

Council to the Cancer Prevention Coalition:
Michael E. Deutsch, Esq.
Legal Director
Center for Constitutional Rights
666 Broadway
New York, NY 10012
212-614-6427

References
1. W. Lijinsky and S. Epstein. "Nitrosamines as Environmental Carcinogens," *Nature* 225(5227):21-12, 1970.
2. Anonymous. "Nitrates and Nitrites in Food," *Medical Letter on Drugs & Therapeutics,* 16(18): 75-6, 1974.
3. P. Issenberg. "Nitrite, Nitrosamines, and Cancer," *Federation Proceedings* 35(6): 1322-1326, 1976.
4. IARC. "Monograph on the evaluation of the carcinogenic risk of chemicals to humans: some N-nitroso compounds," 17:36-38, 136-144, 1978.
5. Ibid.
6. P. Issenberg. "Nitrite, Nitrosamines, and Cancer," *Federation Proceedings* 35(6): 1322-1326, 1976.
7. IARC. "Monograph on the evaluation of the carcinogenic risk of chemicals to humans: some N-nitroso compounds."
8. P. Fraser *et al.* "Nitrate and Human Cancer: A Review of the Evidence," *Int. J.*

Epidemiol. 9:3-11, 1980.

9. P. Reed. "The Role of Nitrosamines in Cancer Formation," *Blblthca. Ntur. Dieta* 37:130-8, 1986.

10. V.M. Craddock. "Nitrosamines, Food and Cancer: Assessment in Lyon," *Fd. Chem. Toxic.* 28(1):63-65, 1990.

11. S. Preston-Martin *et al.* "N-nitroso compounds and childhood brain tumors: A case-control study," *Cancer Res.* 42:5240-5245, 1982.

12. G.R. Bunin *et al.* "Relation between maternal diet and subsequent primitive neuroectodermal brain tumors in young children," *N. Engl. J. Med.* 329:53641, 1993.

13. G.R. Bunin *et al.* "Maternal diet and risk of astrocytic glioma in children: a report from the children's cancer group (United States and Canada)," *Cancer Causes & Control* 5:177-87, 1994.

14. S. Preston-Martin *et al.* "*N*-nitroso compounds and childhood brain tumors: A case control study."

15. G.R. Bunin *et al.* "Maternal Diet and Risk of Astrocytic Glioma in Children."

16. S. Sarasua and D. Savitz. "Cured and broiled meat consumption in relation to childhood cancer: Denver, Colorado (United States)," *Cancer Causes & Control* 5:141-8, 1994.

17. J. Peters *et al.* "Processed Meats and Risk of Childhood Leukemia (California, USA)," *Cancer Causes & Control* 5:195-202, 1994.

18. G.R. Bunin *et al.* "Maternal Diet and Risk of Astrocytic Glioma in Children."

19. S. Sarasua and D. Savitz. "Cured and broiled meat consumption in relation to childhood cancer."

20. Ibid.

21. J. Peters, S. Preston-Martin, and S. London *et al.* "Processed Meats and Risk of Childhood Leukemia (California, USA)."

22. Ibid.

23. J. Reis *et al,* Eds. *SEER Cancer Statistics Review, 1973-1991: Tables and Graphs,* National Cancer Institute. NIH Pub. No. 94, 2789:428, Bethesda, MD, 1994.

24. G.R. Bunin *et al.* "Maternal Diet and Risk of Astrocytic Glioma in Children," 177:87.

Citizen Petition Seeking Cancer Warning on Cosmetics Containing DEA

October 22, 1996

David A. Kessler, M.D.
Commissioner
Food and Drug Administration
Room #14-71
Rockville, MD 20857

The undersigned submits on behalf of the Cancer Prevention Coalition, Inc., and its Chairman, Dr. Samuel S. Epstein, M.D., and on behalf of the Center for Constitutional Rights, Michael Deutsch, Esquire. This petition is based on scientific evidence of increased cancer risks from exposure to nitrosamines in cosmetics.

The undersigned submits this petition under 21 U.S.C. 321 (n), 361, 362, and 371 (a); and 21 CFR 740.1, 740.2 of 21 CFR 10.30 of the Federal Food, Drug, and Cosmetic Act to the Commissioner of Food and Drugs requiring that all cosmetic products containing diethanolamine (DEA) bear labels with a warning: "Caution — This product may contain N-nitrosodiethanolamine, a known cancer-causing agent."

A. Agency Action Requested

This petition requests that FDA take the following action:

1. Issue a regulation under the Federal Food, Drug and Cosmetic Act, Section 601 (a), stating that "All cosmetics containing diethanolamine (DEA), a constituent of diethanolamide soaps that may react with nitrosating agents to form N-nitrosodiethanolamine (NDEA), bear a label as an adulterated product containing poisonous and deleterious substances which may render it injurious to users under the conditions of use prescribed in the labeling thereof, or under such conditions of use as are custom-

ary or usual: That which contains DEA also bears the following legend conspicuously displayed thereon: 'Caution — This product may contain N-nitrosodiethanolamine, a known cancer-causing agent.' "

2. For purposes of enforcement of this act, the Secretary should conduct examinations and investigations of products which may be contaminated with NDEA through regular and routine analytical testing by officers and employees of the Department or through any health, food, or drug officer or employee of any State, Territory or political subdivision thereof, duly commissioned by the Secretary of the Department. Such examinations should result in removal of products from the shelves if products do not comply with labeling regulations.

3. Pursuant to 21 CFR 10.30 (h)(2), a hearing at which time we can present our scientific evidence.

B. Statement of Grounds

Widespread Contamination of Cosmetics with DEA and NDEA

Diethanolamine (DEA) is a high production chemical used in a wide range of cosmetic products, including shampoos, lotions and creams. In the presence of long-chain fatty acids DEA reacts to form neutral ethanolamide soaps, which are used as wetting agents in cosmetics. These soaps contain unreacted DEA. Triethanolamine (TEA), also used widely in cosmetics, may also be contaminated with DEA.[1]

According to the Cosmetics, Toiletries, and Fragrance Association,

Cocamide DEA, Lauramide DEA, Linoleamide DEA and Oleamide DEA are fatty acid diethanolamides which may contain 4 to 33 percent diethanolamine. These ingredients are used in cosmetics at concentrations of < 0. 1 percent to 50 percent, with

most products containing 1 percent to 25 percent diethanolamide.[2]

As of 1980, FDA reported that approximately 42 percent of all cosmetic products were contaminated with NDEA at the following concentrations: facial cosmetics from .042 to 49 mg/kg, lotions from less than .010 to .140 mg/kg, shampoos from less than 10 to 160 mg/kg.[3] In two surveys of cosmetics, 27 out of 29 American products contained up to 48 mg/kg NDEA.[4] A more recent FDA analysis (1991-1992) found that NDEA is present in some products at mg/kg concentrations.[5]

DEA is a Precursor of NDEA

N-nitrosodiethanolamine (NDEA), is readily formed in cosmetics by nitrosation of DEA. Even small amounts of DEA in cosmetics can react with nitrosating agents to form nitrosamines. According to the Cosmetics, Toiletries and Fragrance Association,

Nitrosamine contamination of diethanolamine and fatty acid diethanolamides, and nitrosamine formation in formulations are potential problems in using these diethanolamides. The diethanolamides used in cosmetic products should be free of nitrosamines, and the finished product should not contain nitrosating agents as ingredients.[6]

Nitrosating agents are added to cosmetics in one of three ways:

(1) Nitrites are added directly as anti-corrosive agents;
(2) Nitrites are released by the degradation of 2-nitro-1,3-propanediol (BNDP); and
(3) Nitrites are contaminants in the raw materials or resulting from the exposure of cosmetics to air. Secondary amines, such as DEA, are rapidly nitrosated by nitrogen oxides. Nitrosamine formation from nitrite and amines is accelerated under specific conditions by formaldehyde, paraformaldehyde, thiocyanate, nitrophenols

and certain metal salts ZnI_2, $CuCl$, $AgNO_3$, $SnCl_2$. [7-11]

Cosmetics remain on store shelves and in cabinets of consumers for long periods of time, allowing nitrosamines to form. If DEA is present, nitrosamines can continue to form throughout storage, especially at elevated temperatures. [12]

Acidic pH is an optimal reaction condition for nitrosamine formation. Although cosmetics generally have neutral pH, [13] N-nitrosamines can be formed at neutral or alkaline pH by the reaction of a nitrosating agent with an amine in the presence of carbonyl compounds such as formaldehyde. [14,15] Formaldehyde is present in cosmetics either from *in situ* formaldehyde-releasing agents, such as BNDP, or from its use as a preservative. [16]

Dermal Absorption of NDEA

There is substantial evidence of the dermal absorption of NDEA in both rodents and humans. "[NDEA] is a known carcinogen in laboratory animals; it is absorbed through the skin. The absorption rate is a function of the nature of the cosmetic; absorption is fastest in nonpolar vehicles." [17] Dermal absorption of NDEA was demonstrated by Lijinsky *et al.* in 1981. [18] As a fat-soluble chemical NDEA can be absorbed dermally in rats and humans. [19,20]

NDEA Increases Cancer Risk

There is substantial evidence of potent carcinogenicity of NDEA in a wide range of animal species. [21-29] According to the International Agency for Research on Cancer (IARC),

> There is sufficient evidence of a carcinogenic effect of N-nitrosodiethanolamine. . . . In view of the widespread exposure to appreciable concentrations of N-nitrosodiethanolamine, efforts should be made to obtain epidemiological information. [30]

The National Toxicology Program similarly concluded: "There is sufficient evidence for the carcinogenicity of N-nitrosodiethanol-amine in experimental animals." [31] Of over 44 different species in which N-nitroso compounds have been tested, all have been susceptible. [32] Humans are most unlikely to be the only exception to this trend.

In 1978, the IARC concluded that "although no epidemiological data were available, nitrosodiethanolamine should be regarded for practical purposes as if it were carcinogenic to humans." [33] In 1987 the IARC further confirmed the carcinogenicity of NDEA.

Based on early evidence of the carcinogenicity of NDEA and evidence of cutting fluid contamination, 20 years ago NIOSH recommended that action be taken to protect workers including elimination of nitrosamines from the fluids. [34] More recently, NIOSH published a hazard review of cutting fluids used in metal working that contain NDEA among other nitrosamines. This hazard review indicates that, based on epidemiological evidence in human beings, "increased cancer risk has been generally attributed to worker exposure to nitrosamine or PAH (polyaromatic hydrocarbon) contaminants in metal working fluids." [35]

The Failure of the FDA to take Appropriate Regulatory Action

In the *Federal Register* of April 10, 1979, the FDA called for industry "to take immediate measures to eliminate to the extent possible [NDEA] and any other N-nitrosamines from cosmetic products," and further insisted that "cosmetic products may be analyzed by FDA for nitrosamine contamination and that individual products could be subject to enforcement action."

FDA has taken no subsequent enforcement actions despite the limited compliance with this *Federal Register* order. According to the FDA officials Don Havery and Hardy Chou in 1994,

> In the United States . . . the personal care industry has invested resources in understanding both the mechanisms of N-nitrosamine formation in cosmetic systems and

the means of inhibiting N-nitrosamine formation. However, there is still room for improvement. New products containing nitrosatable amines with formaldehyde and nitrite-releasing preservatives are still appearing on the U.S. market. Manufacturers have a responsibility to be aware of the potential for N-nitrosamine formation and to take steps necessary to keep N-nitrosamine levels as low as possible as part of their good manufacturing practices.[36]

The goal of good manufacturing practices is to reduce "human exposure to N-nitrosamines to the lowest level technologically feasible by reducing levels in all personal care products. With the information and technology currently available to cosmetic manufacturers, N-nitrosamine levels can and should be further reduced in consumer products."[37]

The FDA has failed to act on the *Federal Register* recommendation made in 1979. More recently, the FDA has not fully recognized the consumer hazards of this carcinogen. Measurements have not been made to determine total daily exposure to nitrosamines and it is inappropriate to quantify exposures without such data.

Cosmetic Industry Response to FDA Action

In response to the FDA *Federal Register* order, the Nitrosamine Task Force of the Cosmetics, Toiletries and Fragrance Association failed to eliminate the use of DEA, but rather, they investigated ways to inhibit the formation of NDEA.[38]

There are no known nitrosation inhibitors that eliminate nitrosamine contamination. Inhibitors have failed for the following reasons:

• The compound a-tocopherol has been used as an inhibitor but this compound is useful only when the nitrosating agent is nitrite itself. It is not effective against nitrogen oxide, a gas found in polluted air. It has also been shown to be ineffective in some cosmetic systems.[39]

• Many cosmetics make inhibition of nitrosamine formation more difficult. If they are two-phase emulsion systems the inhibitor must be soluble in both hydrophilic and hydrophobic media to be effective as an inhibitor.[40, 41]

• Ascorbic acid, sodium bisulfite, butylated hydroxyanisole (BHA), butylated hydroxytoluene (BHT), sodium ascorbate, ascorbyl palmitate and a-tocopherol have all been used in attempts to inhibit nitrosamine formation. None of these inhibitors has been adequate against all possible nitrosation agents to which a shelved cosmetic is exposed.[42]

Industry has had no success in reducing NDEA below 1984 levels.[43] As a result, in 1996 the Cosmetics, Toiletries, and Fragrance Association stated: "These chemicals [Cocamide DEA, Lauramide DEA, Linoleamide DEA, and Oleamide DEA] should not be used as ingredients in cosmetic products containing nitrosating agents."[44] Nevertheless DEA is still widely used by major cosmetic manufacturers.

In contrast, some other manufacturers such as Aubrey Organics® have ceased to use diethanolamide soaps entirely. According to Aubrey Hampton of Aubrey Organics,® "None of our products performs less effectively because they do not contain DEA. There are many alternative soap bases available without DEA that can be used by cosmetic manufacturers. In short, the removal of DEA does not pose a manufacturing problem to the cosmetic industry."[45] There is no reason for high levels of NDEA to be found in cosmetic products. With safe alternatives available, the elimination of DEA should not be an economic burden for the cosmetics industry.

Response of National Institutes for Occupational Safety and Health

In striking contrast to the FDA's position on NDEA. National Institutes for Occupational Health and Safety (NIOSH) has issued two reports, one as early as 1976, stating that protective measures should be taken when workers are exposed to levels of NDEA similar to those found in cosmetics.[46, 47]

Response of German Industry and European Union

The German Federal Health Office issued a request to eliminate all secondary amines from cosmetics in 1987 and in response, the German manufacturers' association has voluntarily complied and sharply reduced the use of secondary amines in cosmetics and toiletries.[48] Included in the specifications of the German Federal Health Office were that fatty acid diethanolamides contain as low as achievable contamination by unreacted diethanolamine. Eisenbrand *et al.* explained:

> Commercially available products from the German market analyzed six to 18 months after the recommendation had been issued showed that only 15 percent were contaminated with [NDEA] or NDHPA . . . The overall results of this study demonstrate, however, a strong downward trend in both levels and frequency of contamination. They prove that nitrosamine contamination of cosmetics can be minimized by simple preventive measures."[49]

The European Union has stated specific maximum allowable concentrations of inadvertently formed N-nitrosodialkanolamine. In legislation that was most recently amended in 1993, the European Union asserted that monoalkanolamines and trialkanolamines must be stored in nitrite free containers, cannot be used in nitrosating systems, must have purity of at least 99% and can contain no more than .5% secondary alkanolamine. With regard to N-nitrosodialkanolamine specifically, the maximum content that the EU allows is 50 micrograms per kilogram[50] (50 ppb). In comparison, U.S. cosmetic levels for NDEA as high as 2,960 parts per billion were re-

ported in 1992.[51]

Conclusion

There is strong evidence proving: the widespread use of DEA in cosmetics, nitrosation of DEA to form NDEA, contamination of cosmetics with NDEA, the potent carcinogenicity of NDEA, and the availability of alternatives to DEA. The FDA should take prompt action to require labels on all products containing DEA that reads: "Caution — This product may contain N-nitrosodiethanolamine, a known cancer-causing agent."

C. Claim for Categorical Exclusion

A claim for categorical exclusion is asserted pursuant to 21 CFR 25.24 (a)(11).

D. Certification

The undersigned certifies, that, to the best knowledge and belief of the undersigned, this petition includes all information and views on which the petition relies, and that it includes representative data and information known to the petitioner which are unfavorable to the petition.

This petition is submitted by:

Samuel S. Epstein, M.D.
Cancer Prevention Coalition
520 North Michigan Avenue, Suite 410
Chicago, Illinois 60611
312-467-0600 - phone
312-467-0599 - fax

Council to the Cancer Prevention Coalition:
Michael Deutsch, Legal Director
666 Broadway
New York, NY 10012
212-614-6427

References

1. Donald C. Havery and Hardy J. Chou. "N-

Nitrosamines in Cosmetic Products," *Cosmetics & Toiletries* 109(5):53, May 1994.

2. Cosmetics, Toiletries, and Fragrance Association. "1996 CIR Compendium," *Cosmetic Ingredient Review,* Washington, D.C., 1996.

3. NTP. *Seventh Annual Report on Carcinogens,* U.S. Department of Health and Human Services, Public Health Service, National Toxicology Program, National Institute of Environmental Health Sciences, and Technical Resources Inc., Rockville, MD, 1994.

4. G. Eisenbrand, M. Blankar, H. Sommer, and B. Weber. "N-Nitrosoalkanolamines in Cosmetics," in: *Relevance to Human Cancer of N-Nitroso Compounds, Tobacco Smoke and Mycotoxins,* Ed. I. K. O'Neill, J. Chen and H. Bartsch, International Agency for Research on Cancer, Lyon, 1991.

5. Donald C. Havery and Hardy J. Chou. "Nitrosamines in Sunscreens and Cosmetic Products," Nitrosamines and Related N-Nitroso Compounds, *ACS Monograph,* No. 553. Richard N. Loeppky and Christopher J. Michejda, Eds. American Chemical Society, Washington, D.C., 1994.

6. Cosmetics, Toiletries, and Fragrance Association. "1996 CIR Compendium," *Cosmetic Ingredient Review*, Washington, D.C., 1996.

7. L.K. Keefer and P.P. Roller. "N-nitrosation by nitrite ion in neutral and basic medium," *Science* 181:1245-1246, 1973.

8. M.C. Archer and J.D. Okum. "Kinetics of nitrosamine formation in the presence of micelle-forming surfactants," *Journal of the National Cancer Institute* 58:409, 1977. (Cited In: National Institutes for Occupational Safety and Health. "Draft Criteria for Recommended Standards: Occupational Exposures to Metal Working Fluids," U.S. Department of Health and Human Services, February 19, 1996.)

9. R. Davies and D.J. McWeeny. "Catalytic effect of nitrosophenols on N-nitrosamine formation," *Nature* 266:657-658, 1977. (Cited In: National Institutes for Occupational Safety and Health. "Draft Criteria for Recommended Standards: Occupational

Exposures to Metal Working Fluids," U.S. Department of Health and Human Services, February 19, 1996.)

10. B.D. Challis, A. Edward, R.R. Hunma, S.A. Kyrtopoulos, and J.R. Outram. "Rapid formation of N-nitrosamines from nitrogen oxides under neutral and alkaline conditions," *IARC Scientific Publication* Lyon, France, 19:127, 1978. (Cited In: National Institutes for Occupational Safety and Health. "Draft Criteria for Recommended Standards: Occupational Exposures to Metal Working Fluids," U.S. Department of Health and Human Services, February 19, 1996.

11. R.N. Loeppky, T.J. Hansen, and L.K. Keefer. "Reducing nitrosamine contamination in cutting fluids," *Fd. Cosmet. Toxicol.* 21(5):607-613, 1983. (Cited In: National Institutes for Occupational Safety and Health. "Draft Criteria for Recommended Standards: Occupational Exposures to Metal Working Fluids," U.S. Department of Health and Human Services, February 19, 1996.)

12. Donald C. Havery and Hardy J. Chou. "Nitrosamines in Sunscreens and Cosmetic Products," Nitrosamines and Related N-Nitroso Compounds, *ACS Monograph,* No. 553. Richard N. Loeppky and Christopher J. Michejda, Eds. American Chemical Society, Washington, D.C., 1994.

13. Donald C. Havery and Hardy J. Chou. "N-Nitrosamines in Cosmetic Products," *Cosmetics & Toiletries* 109(5):53, May 1994.

14. Ibid.

15. L.K. Keefer and P.P. Roller. "N-Nitrosation by Nitrite Ion in Neutral and Basic Medium," *Science* 181:1245-46, 1973.

16. Donald C. Havery and Hardy J. Chou. "N-Nitrosamines in Cosmetic Products," *Cosmetics Toiletries* 109(5):53, May 1994.

17. Donald C. Havery and Hardy J. Chou. "Nitrosamines in Sunscreens and Cosmetic Products," Nitrosamines and Related N-Nitroso Compounds, *ACS Monograph,* No. 553. Richard N. Loeppky and Christopher J. Michejda, Eds. American Chemical Society, Washington, D.C., 1994.

18. W. Lijinsky, A.M. Losikoff, and E.B.

Sansone. *Journal of the National Cancer Institute* 66:125-127, 1981.

19. G. S. Edwards, M. Peng, D. J. Fine, B. Spiegelhalder, and J. Kann. "Detection of N-nitrosodiethanolamine in human urine following application of contaminated cosmetics," *Toxicol. Lett.* 4:217-222, 1979. (Cited In: National Institutes for Occupational Safety and Health. "Draft Criteria Recommended Standards: Occupational Exposures to Metal Working Fluids," U.S. Department of Health and Human Services, February 19, 1996.)

20. R. Preussman, "Occurrence and Exposure to N-Nitroso Compounds and Precursors," in: *N-Nitroso Compounds: Occurrence, Biological Effects and Relevance to Human Cancer,* I.K. O'Neill, R. C. Von Borstel, C.T. Miller, J. Long and H. Bartsch, Eds., IARC Scientific Publications No. 57, IARC, Lyon, 1984.

21. H. R. Preussman Druckrey, S. Ivankovic, and D. Schmahl. "Organotrope carcinogene Wirkungen Bei 65 verschiedenen N-Nitroso-verbindugen an BD-ratten," *Z. Krebsforsch.* 69:103-201, 1967. (Cited In: National Institutes for Occupational Safety and Health. "Draft Criteria for Recommended Standards: Occupational Exposures to Metal Working Fluids," U.S. Department of Health and Human Services, February 19, 1996.)

22. J. Hilfrich, I. Schmeltz, and D. Hoffmann. "Effects of N-nitrosodiethanolamine and 1, 1-diethanolhydrazine in Syrian Golden Hamsters." *Cancer Letters* 4:55-60, 1978. (Cited In: National Institutes for Occupational Safety and Health, "Draft Criteria for Recommended Standards: Occupational Exposures to Metal Working Fluids," U.S. Department of Health and Human Services. February 19, 1996.)

23. International Agency for Research on Cancer. "Monograph on the Evaluation of the Carcinogenic Risk of Chemicals to Humans: Some N-Nitroso Compounds," 17:77-82, 1978.

24. W. Lijinsky, M.D. Reuber, and W.B. Manning. "Potent Carcinogenicity of Nitrosodiethanolamine in Rats," *Nature* 288:589-590, 1980.

25. P. Pour and L. Wallcave. "The carcinogenicity of N-Nitrosodiethanolamine, an Environmental Pollutant, in Syrian Hamsters," *Cancer Letters* 14:23-27, 1981.

26. R. Preussman, M. Habs, H. Habs, and D. Schmahl. "Carcinogenicity of N-Nitrosodiethanolamine in Rats at Five Different Dose Levels," *Cancer Research* 42:5167-5171, 1982.

27. W. Lijinsky and M.D. Reuber. "Dose-response Study with N-nitrosodiethanolamine in F344 rats," *Fd. Cosmet. Toxicol.* 22(1):23-26, 1984.

28. W. Lijinsky and R.M. Kovatch. "Induction of liver tumors in rats by nitrosodiethanolamine at low doses," *Carcinogenesis* 6(12):1679-1681, 1985.

29. NTP. "Seventh Annual Report on Carcinogens," U.S. Department of Health and Human Services. Public Health Service, National Toxicology Program, National Institute of Environmental Health Sciences, Technical Resources Inc., Rockville, MD, 1994.

30. International Agency for Research on Cancer. "Monograph on the Evaluation of the Carcinogenic Risk of Chemicals to Humans: Some N-Nitroso Compounds," 17:77-82, 1978.

31. NTP. "Seventh Annual Report on Carcinogens," U.S. Department of Health and Human Services, Public Health Service, National Toxicology Program, National Institute of Environmental Health Sciences, Technical Resources Inc., Rockville, MD, 1994.

32. William Lijinsky. *Chemistry and Biology of N-Nitroso Compounds,* Cambridge University Press, New York, 1992.

33. International Agency for Research on Cancer. "Monograph on the Evaluation of the Carcinogenic Risk of Chemicals to Humans: Some N-Nitroso Compounds," 17:77-82, 1978.

34. NIOSH. "Nitrosamines in Cutting Fluids," *Current Intelligence Bulletin* October 6, 1976.

35. NIOSH. "Draft Criteria for Recommended Standards: Occupational Exposures to Metal Working Fluids," U.S. Department of Health and Human Services. Public

Health Service, Center for Disease Control and Prevention, National Institute for Occupational Safety and Health, Division of Standards Development and Technology Transfer, February 19, 1996.

36. Donald C. Havery and Hardy J. Chou. "N-Nitrosamines in Cosmetic Products," *Cosmetics & Toiletries* 109(5):53, May 1994.

37. Ibid.

38. B.L. Kabacoff, R.J. Lechnir, S.F. Vielhuber, and M.L. Douglass. "Formation and Inhibition of N-Nitrosodiethanolamine in Anionic Oil-Water Emulsion," *ACS Monograph*, American Chemical Society, 1981.

39. Donald C. Havery and Hardy J. Chou. "N-Nitrosamines in Cosmetic Products" *Cosmetics & Toiletries* 109(5):53, May 1994.

40. B.L. Kabacoff, R. J. Lechnir, S. F. Vielhuber, and M. L. Douglass. "Formation and Inhibition of N-Nitrosodiethanolamine in Anionic Oil-Water Emulsion," *ACS Monograph*, American Chemical Society, 1981.

41. Donald C. Havery and Hardy J. Chou. "N-Nitrosamines in Cosmetic Products," *Cosmetics & Toiletries* 109(5):53, May 1994.

42. Ibid.

43. Donald C. Havery and Hardy J. Chou. "Nitrosamines in Sunscreens and Cosmetic Products," Nitrosamines and Related N-Nitroso Compounds, *ACS Monograph* No. 553. Richard N. Loeppky and Christopher J. Michejda, Eds. American Chemical Society, Washington, D.C., 1994.

44. Cosmetics, Toiletries, and Fragrance Association. "1996 CIR Compendium," *Cosmetic Ingredient Review* Washington, D.C., 1996.

45. Aubrey Hampton. *Personal Communication,* May 30, 1996.

46. NIOSH. "Nitrosamines in Cutting Fluids," *Current Intelligence Bulletin*, October 6, 1976.

47. NIOSH. "Draft Criteria for Recommended Standards: Occupational Exposures to Metal Working Fluids," U.S. Department of Health and Human Services, Public Health Service, Center for Disease Control and Prevention, National Institute for Occupational Safety and Health, Division of Standards Development and Technology Transfer, February 19, 1996.

48. G. Eisenbrand, M. Blankar, H. Sommer, and B. Weber. "N-Nitrosoalkanolamines in Cosmetics," in: *Relevance to Human Cancer of N-Nitroso Compounds, Tobacco Smoke and Mycotoxins*, I.K. O'Neill, J. Chen, and H. Bartsch, Eds. International Agency for Research on Cancer, Lyon, 1991.

49. Ibid.

50. *Council Directive of 27 July 1976, on the approximation of the Laws of the Member States Relating to Cosmetic Products,* DIR. 76/768/EEC, DIR. Amendment 93/35/EC.

51. Donald C. Havery and Hardy J. Chou. "Nitrosamines in Sunscreens and Cosmetic Products," Nitrosamines and Related N-Nitroso Compounds, *ACS Monograph* No. 553. Richard N. Loeppky and Christopher J. Michejda, Eds. American Chemical Society, Washington, D.C., 1994.

Appendix XI

Cancer Risks of Hormonal Meat

As of 1990, more than 95 percent of American beef cattle were implanted with carcinogenic growth-promoting hormones. The European Economic Community banned hormone-treated meat in 1989, and does not allow U.S. or other producers to export their meat into the EEC. This ban was recently (February 1998) upheld by a World Trade Organization appellate body. The story behind hormonal meat is a scandal of regulatory irresponsibility, as documented below.

The Chemical Jungle: Today's Beef Industry

By Samuel S. Epstein, M.D.
From *International Journal of Health Services*, 1990*

In the absence of effective federal regulation, the meat industry uses hundreds of animal feed additives, including antibiotics, tranquilizers, pesticides, animal drugs, artificial flavors, industrial wastes, and growth-promoting hormones, with little or no concern about the carcinogenic and other toxic effects of dietary residues of these additives. Illustratively, after decades of misleading assurances of the safety of diethylstilbestrol (DES) and its use as a growth-promoting animal-feed additive, the United States finally banned its use in 1979, some 40 years after it was first shown to be carcinogenic. The meat industry then promptly switched to other carcinogenic additives, particularly the natural sex hormones estradiol, progesterone, and testosterone, which are implanted in the ears of more than 90 percent of commercially raised feedlot cattle. Unlike the synthetic DES, residues of which can be monitored and use of which was

* *International Journal of Health Services.* 20:277-280, 1990.

conditional on a seven-day pre-slaughter withdrawal period, residues of natural hormones are not detectable, since they cannot be practically differentiated from the same hormones produced by the body. The relationship between recently increasing cancer rates and the lifetime exposure of the U.S. population to dietary residues of these and other unlabeled carcinogenic feed additives is a matter of critical public health concern.

The United States is isolated among meat-exporting countries, such as Argentina and Australia, in having threatened retaliatory sanctions against the European Economic Community (EEC) and accusing it of unfair trade practices because of its January 1, 1989, ban on hormone-treated U.S. meat. The accusations ignore serious questions about the carcinogenic and other risks of hormonally contaminated meat that are of major concern to European consumers who, over two years ago, pressured the EEC into banning the use of all hormone additives.

Growth-promoting hormone additives, fed, implanted, or injected in more than 95 percent of U.S. cattle, are mostly synthetic nonsteroids such as Zeranol, natural sex steroids such as estrogens, or synthetic pituitary hormones such as bovine growth hormone.[1] Although the carcinogenicity of the synthetic diethylstilbestrol (DES) in test animals was known as early as 1938, its use as a feed additive was approved by the U.S. Department of Agriculture (USDA) and the Food and Drug Administration (FDA) in 1947. After repeated hearings on the hazards of DES in 1958, Congress passed the Delaney Amendment to the Federal Food, Drug, and Cosmetic Act, banning the deliberate addition of any level of carcinogens into food. This law reflected the overwhelming scientific consensus, which still prevails, that there is no way of setting safe levels or tolerances for carcinogens. Nevertheless, the USDA and the FDA allowed continued use of DES on the alleged grounds that this did not result in detectable and illegal residues in meat products and that the Delaney Amendment could not be applied retroactively. By 1971, DES was being used in 75 percent of U.S. cattle. In spite of infrequent federal sampling and insensitive monitoring, DES residues were found in cattle and sheep at levels in excess of those inducing cancer experimentally. At about the same time, vaginal cancers were reported in the daughters of women treated with DES during pregnancy. Based on these findings, DES-treated meat was subsequently banned in more than 20 foreign countries, mostly European. However, misleading assurances of safety and stonewalling by the FDA and USDA, including the deliberate suppression of residue data, managed to delay a U.S. ban on DES until 1979.

The meat industry then promptly switched to other carcinogenic additives, particularly natural sex hormones, which are implanted in the ears of commercially raised feedlot cattle. Unlike the synthetic DES, whose residues can be monitored and whose use was conditional on a seven-day pre-slaughter withdrawal period, residues of natural hormones are not routinely detectable because they cannot be differentiated from the same hormones produced by the body. Since 1983, the FDA has allowed virtually unregulated use of these natural additives right up to the time of slaughter, subject only to the nonenforceable requirement that residue levels in meat must be less than 1 percent of the daily hormonal production in children.

A dramatic warning of the dangers of growth-promoting additives was triggered by an epidemic of premature sexual development and ovarian cysts involving about 3,000 Puerto Rican infants and children from 1979 to 1981. These toxic effects were traced to hormonal contamination of fresh meat products and were usually reversed by simple dietary changes. Using highly specialized research techniques, independent testing found that samples of the meat products were contaminated with estrogen residues more than tenfold in excess of normal ranges. Additionally, elevated levels of estrogen and the synthetic Zeranol were found in the blood of afflicted children. Increased rates of uterine and ovarian cancers in adult women were also associated with this epidemic.

More than a decade ago, Roy Hertz,[2] then director of endocrinology of the National Cancer Institute and a world authority on hormonal cancer, warned of the carcinogenic risks of estrogenic feed additives, particularly for hormonally sensitive tissues such as breast tissue, because they could increase normal body hormonal levels and disturb delicately poised hormonal balances. Hertz pointed to evidence from innumerable animal tests and human clinical experience that such imbalance can be carcinogenic. Hertz also warned of the essentially uncontrolled and unregulated use of these extremely potent biological agents, no dietary levels of which can be regarded as safe. Even a dime-sized piece of meat contains billions or trillions of molecules of these carcinogens.

Virtually the entire U.S. population consumes, without any warning, labeling, or information, unknown and unpredictable amounts of hormonal residues in meat products over a lifetime. In 1986, as many as half of all cattle sampled in feedlots as large as

600 animals were found to have hormones illegally implanted in muscle rather than the ear skin, to induce further increased growth. This practice results in very high residues in meat, which even the FDA has admitted could produce "adverse effects." Left unanswered is whether such chronic and uncontrolled estrogen dosages are involved in increasing cancer rates (now striking one in three Americans), particularly the alarming 50 percent increase in the incidence of breast cancer since 1965. These questions are of further concern in the light of recent evidence confirming the association between breast cancer and oral contraceptives, whose estrogen dosage over a fraction of a lifetime is known and controlled, in contrast with that from residues of growth hormones in meat products.

Hormonal feed contamination in the United States is only part of a much larger problem caused by the use of thousands of feed additives. These include antibiotics, tranquilizers, pesticides, animal drugs, artificial flavors, and industrial wastes, many of which are carcinogenic in addition to their other harmful effects. The runaway technologies of the meat-product and pharmaceutical industries are supported by an eager cadre of academic consultants, contractees and apologists, tremendous lobbying pressures, and a revolving door between senior personnel in industry and regulatory agencies. This was personified by Reagan administration agriculture secretaries John Block, a former Illinois hog farmer, and Richard Lyng, a former head of the American Meat Institute.

As clearly evidenced in a series of General Accounting Office investigations and Congressional hearings, USDA inspection and FDA registration and residue-tolerance programs are in near total disarray, aggravated by brazen denials and cover-ups by these agencies. A January 1986 report, "Human Food Safety and the Regulation of Animal Drugs," unanimously approved by the House Committee on Government Operations, concluded that the "FDA has consistently disregarded its responsibility — has repeatedly put what it perceives are interests of veterinarians and the livestock industry ahead of its legal obligation to protect consumers — jeopardizing the health and safety of consumers of meat, milk, and poultry."[3] The great majority of feed additives are used in the absence of evidence of efficacy, practical and sensitive monitoring methods, and minimal if any safety test data, apart from the widespread use of illegal and unapproved drugs. The hazards of U.S. meat have retrogressed from the random fecal and bacterial contamination of Upton Sinclair's *The Jungle* to the brave new world of deliberate chemicalization.

Any possible trade basis for the EEC embargo, as alleged by the U.S. administration, is extremely unlikely, particularly in view of tough regulations and criminal sanctions against use of hormonal additives in European beef. Contrary to repeated assertions by the U.S. meat industry, the EEC's 1985 Scientific Risk Assessment Committee did not exculpate the use of hormonal additives, but recommended against the use of synthetics and emphasized the need to further evaluate the safety of natural hormones. Rather than finger-pointing at Europe, the embargo should prompt a high-level, independent investigation and drastic reform of meat industry practices and federal regulation to include the use of hormones in particular and feed additives in general. Immediate action, not further study, is well overdue. The U.S. position also reflects a disturbing double standard, since the administration banned imports of Australian beef in 1987 on the grounds of excess residues of the carcinogenic pesticide heptachlor.

All hormonal and other carcinogenic feed additives should be banned immediately, as should all other animal additives in the absence of conclusive evidence of their efficacy and safety. Any additive use should be subject to explicit labeling requirements of use and of residue levels in all meat products, including milk and eggs.

Until then, initiatives at the state level, such as State Agriculture Commissioner Jim Hightower's "Texas Plan" (proposed in February 1989 and implemented two months later) to establish a hormone-free certification program for shipments to Europe, should be applauded and vigorously extended to the domestic market. Meanwhile, consumers should avoid chemicalized meat products in favor of organic ones. Consumers should also insist on their absolute right to know which additives have been used in their meat products, their residue levels, and their known adverse effects. Finally, they should demand independent certification and verification for hormones and other feed additives, such as the California Nutri-Clean program for testing pesticide residues on fruits and vegetables that is now available in about 600 supermarkets nationwide.

References

1. S.S. Epstein, "Potential public health hazards of biosynthetic milk hormones," *Int. J. Health Serv.* 20(1):73-84, 1990.
2. R. Hertz. "The estrogen-cancer hypothesis with special emphasis on DES," in Origins of Human Cancer, H. H. Hiatt, J. D. Watson, and J. A. Winston, Eds, pp. 1665-1682, Vol. 4 of *Cold Spring Harbor Conference on Cell Proliferation*, Cold Spring Harbor Laboratory, 1977.
3. U.S. House of Representatives, Committee on Government Operations. *"Twenty-seventh Report: Human Food Safety and the Regulation of Animal Drugs,"* 99th Congress, Washington, D.C., December 31, 1985.

Testimony in Support of the EU Ban on Trade in Hormone Beef

By Samuel S. Epstein, M.D.
Submitted to the World Trade Organization
Geneva, Switzerland
February 5, 1997

I am Professor of Environmental and Occupational Medicine at the School of Public Health, University of Illinois Medical Center Chicago. I am also Chairman of the Cancer Prevention Coalition, a nationwide coalition of independent experts in cancer prevention and public health, together with representatives of a wide range of consumer, environmental, women's health and labor groups (a copy of my curriculum is attached).

Based on a review of the scientific literature, Food and Drug Administration (FDA) Freedom of Information Summaries, other U.S. Government reports, and FAO/WHO reports, I conclude that the use of natural and synthetic anabolics in meat production poses serious carcinogenic and other hazards to consumers, with particular reference to breast and other reproductive cancers. This conclusion is based on the following 8 considerations:

1. The Carcinogenicity of Natural Anabolics

a. Estradiol-17B. Based on an exhaustive review of the scientific literature, the International Agency for Research on Cancer (IARC) confirmed the carcinogenicity of estradiol in experimental animals, inducing mammary, testicular, other reproductive tumors, and tumors at other sites, and concluded that it was of comparable potency to diethylstilbestrol, an illegal synthetic anabolic.[1] IARC subsequently concluded that the evidence of estradiol's carcinogenicity to animals was "sufficient,"[2] and that it was "causally associated" with reproductive cancers in women.[3]

b. Testosterone. On the basis of a review of the scientific literature, testosterone was classified by IARC as a Group 2A carcinogen (4). IARC concluded that the evidence of its carcinogenicity in rodents was "sufficient," and that it "may be involved in the genesis of (prostatic) tumors in humans." These carcinogenic effects have also been recognized by FAO/WHO. Following administration of testosterone to rodents, "the incidence of prostatic tumors was higher than in control animals (and) the incidence of uterine tumors was surprisingly high."[5]

c. Progesterone. On the basis of a review of the scientific literature, IARC concluded that the evidence for its carcinogenicity, based on the induction of mammary, ovarian and uterine cancers in rodents, was "sufficient."[6]

d. Enhanced infant sensitivity. There is substantial literature on the enhanced carcinogenic sensitivity of neonatal rodents to natural anabolics, both individually and in combination,[7-10] and to synthetic anabolics, such as diethylstilbestrol.[11] Illustratively, "neonatal exposure of mice to progesterone plus estradiol-17B resulted in an increased incidence of mammary tumors.[12] Furthermore, there is a substantial literature on the increased susceptibility of infant and young rodents and humans to a wide range of carcinogens,[13, 14] including natural anabolics and diethylstilbestrol (DES).

2. The Carcinogenicity of Synthetic Anabolics

a. Trenbolone Acetate. There are no published data on the carcinogenicity of Trenbolone, a synthetic steroid resembling testosterone. However, unpublished and inadequately documented industry data have demonstrated its carcinogenicity to mice and rats.[15] These findings included: "Significant increases in hepatic proliferative lesions (neoplasia and hyperplasia) in male and female (mice) — and an increased incidence of pancreatic islet tumors" in rats. These carcinogenic effects have also been recognized by FAO/WHO (16). However, these conclusions were dismissed by FDA "on the basis of direct and ancillary evidence."[17]

b. Zeranol. There are no published data on the carcinogenicity of Zeranol, a non-steroidal synthetic estrogen. However, unpublished and inadequately documented indus-try data have demonstrated the "induction of anterior lobe pituitary adenomas" in male rats.[18] These carcinogenic effects have also been recognized by FAO/WHO.[19]

c. Melengesterol Acetate (MGA). There are no valid published data on the carcinogenicity of MGA, a synthetic progestin. A 1966 Food Additive Petition to the FDA, summarizing the toxicology of MGA and on the basis of which its use was approved, omitted any reference to carcinogenicity.[20] However, an internal industry report documented the induction of a statistically significant incidence of mammary tumors in female mice;[21] these results were subsequently published.[22]

3. Residues of Anabolics Following Legal Administration for Meat Production

The legal route for administration of natural anabolics and of synthetic anabolics, other than MGA, is by subcutaneous implantation of pellets in the ear. In October 1989, FDA approved the re-implantation of steers with estradiol benzoate and progesterone (Synovex-S) in the midpoint of their feeding period.[23] There has been no requirement for any pre-slaughter withdrawal period for over three decades.

Both USDA and FDA have assured the public that meat products are routinely monitored for residues of animal drugs and other industrial chemicals:[24]

Since 1987, USDA and FDA have been monitoring violative levels of residues of animal drugs, pesticides, and industrial chemicals in food animals.

The program has expanded greatly since its inception, and because the use of many pesticides has declined, a greater emphasis is now placed on testing for animal drugs.

The program is designed to ensure that the compounds most likely to be present in food animals are included in the nationwide monitoring residue plan. The program has the flexibility to keep up with current usage of animal drugs.

Samples of meat and poultry products are collected from healthy-appearing animals at domestic slaughter establishments using a statistically based, random sampling plan.

Surveillance programs are designed to distinguish those areas of the livestock and poultry populations in which residue problems exist, to measure the extent of the problems, and to evaluate the impact of actions initiated to reduce the occurrence of residues.

FSIS (Food Safety and Inspection Service of USDA) collects samples for testing when a problem with residues is suspected.

Most residue violations have been detected in kidney, liver, or fat, not in the muscle tissue. Tissue samples depend upon the compound/drug/residue involved.

The residue monitoring program has been supported by an education program targeted at food animal producers, and its success has assisted in the decline of residue violators.

In 1993, approximately one-fourth of one percent of animals tested showed positive for residue violation. In other words, almost 99.74 percent of animals tested showed no residue violations.[24]

However, in contrast to these highly misleading assurances, FSIS 1993 data indicate that none of approximately 130 million head of livestock slaughtered annually has been monitored for any residues of natural or synthetic anabolics.[25]

The only available residue data are provided in "New Animal Drug Application" (NADA) petitions to FDA by pharmaceutical companies manufacturing and formulating the anabolic drugs, as detailed in Freedom of Information Summaries obtained from the FDA. Residue levels were determined by specialized techniques, radioimmune assays, which are not practical for routine monitoring. Despite the requirement of Section 512 of the 1968 Animal Drug Amendments to the Federal Food Inspection Act, which stipulates that a manufacturer submitting a NADA must

provide "a description of practical methods" for analysis and monitoring of carcinogenic residues in food, no such methods were available in 1973;[26] over two decades later, none are still available. FDA, however, has circumvented this legislative mandate by claiming that "a regulatory method is not needed for the assurance of safety of the approved use of (anabolic) implants because the maximum increased exposure, even considering probable misuse of the drug, is demonstrated to be far below those concentrations considered unsafe."[27]

a. Estradiol. Following implantation of steers with Synovex-S (estradiol benzoate and progesterone), estradiol residues in liver, kidney, muscle and fat at 15 days were increased over normal background levels by 6, 9, 12 and 23-fold, respectively;[28] the average residue in fat of untreated controls was 1.8ppt (ng/kg). However, minimizing these data, FAO/WHO claimed that estradiol implants ". . . may produce two-fold to five-fold increases in residue levels and that these fall within the normal range found in untreated bovine animals . . . ,"[29] the comparability of which was, however, unspecified.

b. Testosterone. Following implantation of heifers with Synovex-H (estradiol benzoate and testosterone propionate), testosterone residues in kidney, liver, muscle and fat at 30 days were increased over normal background levels by 2, 3, 5 and 30-fold, respectively;[30] the average fat level in untreated animals was 26ppt (ng/kg). Similar increased residues have been reported by FAO/WHO.[31]

c. Trenbolone. Following implantation of heifers with Revalor (Trenbolone acetate and estradiol), the total average residues in beef liver were 50ppb (ug/kg) at 30 days, while "residues in muscle, kidney and fat were much lower."[32] In contrast to these data, FAO/WHO, however, claimed that the 50ppb liver residues were the "highest mean concentrations."[33]

d. Zeranol. Following implantation of Ralgro (Zeranol) in steers and heifers, total average residues in muscle, fat, kidney and liver at 15 days were 0.1, 0.3, 1.7, and 8.2ppb.[34] Similar residues have been reported by FAO/WHO.[35]

e. Melengesterol Acetate (MGA). Following feeding heifers with MGA, 139 of 174 fat samples contained residues below 10ppb, while the remainder had residues ranging from 10-19ppb at 12 to 24 hours after the last feeding;[36] the sensitivity level of this assay was only 10ppb. It should be noted that FAO/WHO has still failed to evaluate the use of MGA; this is in contrast to the requirement that it evaluate all veterinary drugs regulated in at least one country.[37]

4. Residues of Anabolics Following Illegal Administration

No data are available on the much higher local and distant residue levels anticipated following intramuscular implantation or injection. A 1986 USDA survey revealed that as many as half the cattle in 32 large feedlots had "misplaced implants."[38] FDA's response was limited in extreme: "part of the carcass containing pellets should continue to be condemned." Such action ignores the probability of high residues in distant organs and tissues due to the anticipated increased absorption of anabolics from highly vascular muscle in contrast to relatively avascular subcutaneous ear tissue. Furthermore, visual inspection and random monitoring could not reveal evidence of intramuscular injection, as opposed to implantation.

5. Public Health Hazards from Residues of Natural Anabolics in Meat Products

FDA has consistently dismissed concerns on hazards of natural anabolics in meat:

No harmful effects will occur in individuals chronically ingesting animal tissues that contain an incremental increase of endogenous steroid equal to 1% or less of the amount produced daily by the segment of

the population with the lowest daily production rate. In the case of Estradiol, prepubertal boys synthesize the least; in the case of testosterone, prepubertal girls synthesize the least. The calculated incremental increase permitted in beef muscle above the amount naturally present in untreated animals is 120ppt for Estradiol and 0.64ppb for Testosterone. Based upon relative consumption of other tissues versus muscle, safe incremental levels of 480ppt and 2.6ppb for Estradiol and Testosterone, respectively, are established for fat, 360ppt and 1.9ppb for kidney, and 240ppt and 1.3ppb for liver.

"When the sponsor can demonstrate with a suitable assay that under the proposed conditions of use the concentration of residue of the endogenous sex steroid in treated food-producing animals is such that the actual increase in exposure of people will not exceed the permitted increase, then the compound is shown to be safe."[39]

These assurances of safety are flawed for reasons including the following:

a. Consumption of meat products with incremental residues of a specific exogenous anabolic not only increases normal body hormonal levels, but also disturbs complex patterns of normal hormonal interaction and balances. Such imbalances pose carcinogenic hazards.[40]

b. The amount of endogenous steroids "produced by the segment of the population with the lowest daily production rate" are infants and young, rather than prepubertal children; daily estradiol production for prepubertal boys, 6.5 ug,[29] is 40-fold in excess of levels for children under 8, based on IARC data.[1 (p.42-46)] This is of particular significance in view of the enhanced sensitivity of infants to the carcinogenic effects of estrogens (Section 1d).

c. In the absence of routine monitoring,

there is no assurance that "the proposed conditions of use" of the anabolics corresponds to routine feedlot practice. There is in fact evidence to the contrary, resulting in unmonitored residue levels well in excess of those anticipated by FDA (Section 3).

d. FDA assurances are based on the alleged absence of "harmful effects" of individual anabolics. However, in practice, most implants contain two natural anabolics, or one natural and one synthetic anabolic, thus invalidating FDA's calculated assumptions. Furthermore, the probability of additive, let alone synergistic, hormonal effects has apparently not been considered by FDA (Section 1d). Of related concern is recent evidence that two xenobiotic pesticides induce synergistic estrogenic effects some 1000-fold greater than those resulting from individual exposures.[41]

e. FDA has failed to consider incremental, additive or synergistic, carcinogenic and estrogenic effects of anabolic steroids together with those of xenoestrogenic pesticides and other industrial chemical contaminants in meat products.

f. FDA has failed to recognize the longstanding evidence of the approximately 10,000-fold higher potency of estradiol than xenoestrogenic pesticides,[42-44] whose feminizing hazards are of increasing public health concern;[45, 46] such hazards may also include reduction in human male fertility.

6. Therapeutic Administration of Anabolics

The therapeutic uses of legal anabolics do not pose public health hazards. Such uses are extremely limited, compared to large-scale routine feedlot use, and are prescribed by qualified veterinarians, in contrast to feedlot operators. Furthermore, determination of therapeutic effectiveness necessitates pre-slaughter withdrawal.

7. Public Health Hazards from Residues of Synthetic Anabolics in Meat Products

The hazards of synthetic anabolics have been trivialized or dismissed by both FDA and FAO/WHO:

"Safe concentrations," or tolerances of ADI's (Acceptable Daily Intakes) have been established by FDA for residues of Trenbolone[47] in spite of explicit industry data on its carcinogenicity (see Section 2a); these tolerances range from 50-20ppb for different organs and tissues. Similarly, FAO/WHO has established "Maximum Residue Levels" (MRL) based on "Acceptable Daily Intakes" (ADI) for meat and dairy products.[48]

"Safe concentrations" for total Zeranol residues have also been established by FDA,[49] in spite of explicit industry carcinogenicity data, recognized by FAO/WHO. Similarly, FAO/WHO have established ADI-based "Acceptable Residue Levels."[50]

FDA has established a tolerance "in edible tissues" for MGA[51] in spite of explicit industry carcinogenicity data (Section 2c). FAO/WHO has failed to evaluate MGA in spite of its use in the U.S. for nearly three decades.

The public health hazards of synthetic anabolics are in general comparable to those of natural anabolics. Of particular concern, however, are the much higher residues of synthetic (in the ppb range) than the natural anabolics (in the ppt range). The concepts of tolerances, ADI and MRL, are inappropriate in the extreme for any carcinogen, let alone for high residues of carcinogens deliberately introduced into the food supply.

There is substantial evidence challenging the validity of classifying carcinogens as epigenetic, on the basis of bacterial gene mutation tests, for which thresholds or Acceptable Daily Intake (ADI) levels are claimed, as genotoxic. It should be emphasized that asbestos, benzene, arsenic and non-steroidal and steroidal estrogens, all IARC recognized potent Group I carcinogens, are inactive in bacterial tests and hence classified as epigenetic. However, they are all mutagenic and thus genotoxic in mammalian systems.[52] Apart from this, hormonal anabolics are mutagenic in mammalian test systems and are thus genotoxic (Tables XI.1 and XI.2). There is also substantial scientific evidence challenging the existence of thresholds for any carcinogen. This evidence is even more persuasive for exposures involving infants and young children, in view of their enhanced sensitivity to carcinogens, and for exposures involving unpredictable synergistic interactions. There is no scientific basis for FAO/WHO claims that ADI levels can be set for natural and synthetic anabolic carcinogens, or for claims that ADI levels can be based on "no-hormonal-effect levels" of synthetic anabolic carcinogens.[53]

8. Misleading Assurances of Safety by U.S. Regulatory Agencies and "Expert Committees"

The repeated misleading assurances by USDA and FDA since 1979 on the safety of natural and synthetic anabolics are consistent with a similar prior record with regard to DES, including suppression of residue data.[26, 54] Compounding these concerns is long-standing evidence of conflicts of interest in senior agency personnel and their consultants.[54]

As clearly evidenced in a series of General Accounting Office investigations and Congressional hearings, USDA inspection and FDA registration and residue-tolerance programs are in near total disarray. A 1986 report, "Human Food Safety and Regulation of Animal Drugs," unanimously approved by the House Committee on Government Operations, concluded that the "FDA has consistently disregarded its responsibility . . . has repeatedly

TABLE XI.1 Carcinogenicity and genotoxicity of hormonal anabolics*

Anabolic	Carcinogencity	Mammalian Genotoxicity
Estradiol-17B	+(1)	+
Testosterone	+(2)	+
Progesterone	+(3)	+
Trenbolone-17B	+(4)	+
Zeranol	+(5)	-(7)
Melengesterol	+(6)	ND (8)

* Citations in parens
1. Group 1 (IARC, 1987)
2. Group 2A WC, 1987)
3. Group 2B (IARC, 1987)
4. FDA, NADA No. 138-612, 1987; FAO/WHO, 32nd Rep. No. 763, 1988
5. FDA, NADA No. 38-233, 1989; FAO/WHO, 32nd Rep. No. 763, 1988; Coe *et al.*, 1992; Metzler, 1997
6. Lauderdale & Goyins, Upjohn Report, 1972; Lauderdale *et al*, 1977 (Note failure Codex to evaluate MGA)
7. Bacterial genotoxin
8. No data available

TABLE XI.2 Genotoxicity of hormonal anabolics

Anabolic	Genotoxic Test System*
Estradiol-17B	Aneuploidy, aberrant nucleotides and UDS rodent cells *in vitro* (1, 2) Micronuclei human cells *in vitro* (1) Transformation, and DNA adducts by metabolites (2) Chromosome aberrations by metabolites *in vitro* (3)
Testosterone	As for estradiol in view of in vivo aromatization (4) Transformation hamster cells *in vitro* (5)
Progesterone	Chromosome aberrations human cells *in vitro* (6) Chromosome aberrations dog and hamster meiotic cells *in vivo* (7)
Trenbolone-17B	Micronuclei and transformation hamster cells by metabolites *in vitro* (8)
Zeranol	Positive Rec-assay B. subtilis (9)

* Citation in parens
1. IARC, 1987; Tsutsui, 1987
2. Hayashi *et al.*, 1996; Liehr, 1996
3. Nutter *et al.*, 1994; Han & Liehr, 1994; Seegers *et al.*, 1989
4. IARC, 1979
5. Lasne *et al*, 1990; Tsutsui *et al.*, 1995
6. Seroya & Kerkis, 1974
7. Williams *et al.*, 1972
8. Schiffman *et al.*, 1988; Lasne *et al.*, 1990
9. Scheutwinkel *et al.*, 1986

put what it perceives are interests of veterinarians and the livestock industry ahead of its legal obligation to protect consumers . . . jeopardizing the health and safety of consumers of meat, milk, and poultry."[55] These criticisms appear equally appropriate today. Illustratively, in response to questions on hormonal meat raised in February 1996 by the European Commission Washington Delegation, the USDA responded with assurances that less than 0.25% of animals tested annually proved positive for "residue violations."[24] In fact, however, no cattle have been monitored for sex hormones.[25]

Similar concerns relate to exculpatory reports by Joint FAO/WHO Expert Committees on Food Additives. The membership of these committees reflects disproportionate representation of U.S. senior regulatory officials and of veterinary and food scientists, with minimal if any involvement of independent experts in preventive medicine, public health and carcinogenesis. The European Commission Scientific Conference of November 29-December 1, 1995 also reflects such imbalanced representation. While Conference participation of "scientists directly employed" by industry was "generally refused," no apparent attempt was made to identify or exclude industry consultants, contractees or grantees. Furthermore, the Conference based its findings and conclusions largely on unpublished industry data. As admitted by Steering Committee member Dr. F. W. Kenny, "all assessment data are provided by companies and this implies a regulatory gap," particularly in view of the confidentiality of these data;[56] industry is "capable of giving good results, but they will not necessarily always do so." Similar constraints in data generated and interpreted by industry and their consultants have been well documented.[e.g. 57]

9. Conclusions

Some two decades ago, Roy Hertz, then director of endocrinology of the National Cancer Institute and world authority on hormonal cancer, warned of the carcinogenic risks of estrogenic feed additives, particularly for hormonally sensitive tissues such as breast tissue, because they could increase normal body hormonal levels and disturb delicately poised hormonal balances.[54] Hertz pointed to evidence from innumerable animal tests and human clinical experience that such imbalance can be carcinogenic. Hertz also warned of the essentially uncontrolled and unregulated use of these extremely potent biological agents, no dietary levels of which can be regarded as safe. These warnings are even more apt today.

Lifelong exposure to hormonal anabolics poses significant carcinogenic risks, particularly for breast and other reproductive cancers, whose rates have sharply escalated over recent decades.[58, 59] Such exposures may also pose serious feminizing risks.

Concerns of European consumers about hormonal meat and the EU ban are well based on valid scientific data and considerations.

References

1. IARC. 21:131, 1979
2. IARC. Supp. 7:284, 1987
3. IARC. Supp. 7:280, 1987
4. IARC. Supp. 7:96-97, 1987
5. FAO/WHO Joint Expert Committee. Report No. 763:22, Geneva, 1988.
6. IARC. Supp. 7:296, 1987.
7. H.A. Bern *et al.* "Use of the Neonatal Mouse in Studying Long-term Effects of Early Exposure to Hormones and Other Agents," *J. Toxicol. Env. Hlth.* Supp 1:103-116, 1976.
8. T. Mori *et al.* "Long-term Effects of Neonatal Steroid Exposure on Mammary Gland Development and Tumorogenesis in Mice," *J. Nat. Cancer Inst.* 57:1057-1062, 1976.
9. L.A. Jones and H.A. Bern. "Long-term effects of neonatal treatment with progesterone alone, and in combination with estrogen, on the mammary gland and reproductive tract of female balb/cfC3H mice," *Cancer Res.* 37:67-75, 1977.
10. IARC. Supp. 7:272-308, 1987.
11. IARC, Supp. 7:275, 1987.
12. IARC. Supp. 7:303, 1987.
13. IARC. "Perinatal and Multigeneration Carcinogenesis," *IARC Scientific Pub.* No. 96, L. Tomatis and H. Yamasaki, Lyon, 1989.
14. "Intolerable Risk: Pesticides in Our Children's Food," Natural Resources Defense Council, February 27, 1989.
15. FDA. "Freedom of Information Summary for Finaplix (Trenbolone Acetate)," *NADA* No. 138,612:8-9, May 1987.
16. FAO/WHO Joint Expert Committee on Food Additives. "Thirty Second Report," *Technical Report* Series 763:24, WHO, Geneva, 1988.
17. FDA. "Freedom of Information Summary for Finaplix (Trenbolone Acetate)," *NADA* No. 138-612:9, May 1987.
18. FDA. "Freedom of Information Summary for Ralgro Brand of Zeranol Implants," *NADA* 38-233V:XI-14, January, 1989.
19. FAO/WHO Joint Expert Committee. Report No. 763:27, Geneva, 1988.
20. Upjohn Co. FDA Petition No. 67-1957, March 31, 1966.
21. J. W. Lauderdale and L. S. Goyins. *Upjohn Report* No. 610-9610-LSG-71-7, June 7, 1972.
22. J. W. Lauderdale *et al. J. Toxicol. & Environ. Hlth.* 3:5-33, 1977.
23. FDA. "Freedom of Information Summary,

Environmental Assessment, Synovex-S," *NADA* 9-576 Supplement, October 1989.

24. USDA. "Food Safety Inspection Service (FSIS), Residue Testing Program," Washington, D.C., February 8, 1996.

25. USDA. "FSIS, Domestic Residue Data Book, Science and Technology, National Residue Program," 1993.

26. S.S. Epstein. "Testimony on the federal food inspection act of 1973 and on deficiencies in current procedures for monitoring animal food for carcinogenic and toxic residues of animal drugs," hearing before the U.S. Senate Committee on Commerce, 93rd Congress, March 21, 1973.

27. FDA. "Freedom of Information Summary for Synovex-S," *NADA* No. 9-576, October 5, 1983.

28. FDA. "Freedom of Information Summary for Synovex-S," *NADA* No. 9-576:3, October 5, 1983.

29. FAO/WHO. "Thirty Second Joint Expert Committee Report on Food Additives (JECFA)," *WHO Tech. Rep.* Series No. 763:18-19, Geneva, 1988.

30. FDA. "Freedom of Information Summary for Synovex-H," *NADA* No. 11-427, undated.

31. FAO/WHO Joint Expert Committee. Report No. 763:22, Geneva, 1988.

32. FDA. "Freedom of Information Summary for Revalor," *NADA* No. 140-992, December 13, 1994.

33. FAO/WHO Joint Expert Committee. Report No. 763:24, Geneva, 1988.

34. FDA. "Freedom of Information Summary for Ralgro," *NADA* No. 38-233V, January 1989.

35. FDA. "Freedom of Information Summary for Ralgro," *NADA* No. 38-233V:XI-18, January 1989.

36. FDA. "Freedom of Information Summary for MGA," *NADA* Nos. 034-254 and 039-402, June 29, 1994.

37. FAO/WHO Joint Expert Committee. Report No. 763:11, Geneva, 1988.

38. "FDA Evaluating Health Hazards of Cattle Hormone Implants Misuse," *Food and Chemical News* July 28, 1986, pp. 37-38.

39. FDA. "Freedom of Information Summary for Heifer-oid (Estradiol benzoate and Testosterone propionate)," *NADA* No. 135-906, June 15, 1984.

40. R. Hertz. "The Estrogen-cancer Hypothesis With Special Emphasis on DES," in: *Origins of Human Cancer*, H. H. Hiatt, J. D. Watson, J. A. Winston, Eds., Vol. 4:1665-1682 of *Cold Spring Harbor Conference on Cancer Proliferation*, Cold Spring Harbor Laboratory, 1977.

41. S.F. Arnold *et al.* "Synergistic activation of estrogen receptor with combinations of environmental chemicals," *Science* 272:1489-1492, 1996.

42. H. Burlington *et al.* "Effect of DDT on testes and secondary sex characters of white leghorn cockerels," *Proc. Soc. Exptl. Biol. Med.* 74:48-51, 1950.

43. R.M. Wlech. "Estrogenic Action of DDT and Its Analogs," *Toxicol. Appl. Pharmacol.* 14:358-367, 1969.

44. W.H. Bulger and D. Kupfer. "Estrogenic activity of pesticides and other xenobiotics on the uterus and male reproductive tract," *Endocrine Toxicol.*, J.A. Thomas *et al*, Eds., Raven Press, New York, 1985, p.1-33.

45. T. Colborn *et al.* "Development effects of endocrine-disrupting chemicals in wildlife and humans," *Environ. Hlth. Perspec.* 101(5):378-284, 1993.

46. T. Colborn, J.P. Myers, and D. Dumanowski. *Our Stolen Future: Are We Threatening our Fertility, Intelligence and Survival*, Dalton Press, New York, 1996.

47. FDA. "Freedom of Information Summary for Revalor," *NADA* No. 140-992, December 13, 1994.

48. FAO/WHO Joint Expert Committee on Food Additives. "34th Report," *Technical Report* Series 788:42, WHO, Geneva, 1989.

49. FDA. "Freedom of Information Summary for Zeranol," *NADA* No. 38-233V:XI-22, January 1989.

50. FAO/WHO Joint Expert Committee on Food Additives (JECFA). "37th Report," *Technical Report* Series 763:28, WHO, Geneva, 1988.

51. FDA. "Freedom of Information Summary for MGA," *NADA* Nos. 034-254 and 039-402, June 29, 1994.

52. J.C. Barrett. *Environ. Hlth. Perspec.* 100:9-20, 1993.
53. FAO/WHO Thirty Second Joint Expert Committee Report on Food Additives (JECFA). *WHO Tech. Rep.* Series No. 763:18-19, Geneva, 1988.
54. S.S. Epstein. "The Chemical Jungle: Today's Beef Industry," *Int. J. Hlth. Services* 20:277-280, 1990.
55. U.S. House of Representatives Committee on Government Operations. "27th Report: Human Food Safety and the Regulation of Animal Drugs," 99th Congress, Washington, D.C., December 31, 1985.
56. European Consumer Organization. "Notes from E.U. Conference on Growth Promotion," BEUC/007/96, November 29-December 1, 1995.
57. S.S. Epstein. "Corporate Crime: Why We Cannot Trust Industry-derived Safety Studies," *Intl. J. Hlth. Services* 20(3):443-458, 1990.
58. S.S. Epstein *et al.* "Losing the War Against Cancer: A need for Public Policy Reforms," *Intl. J. Hlth. Services* 22(3): 455-469, 1992.
59. S.S. Epstein. "Environmental and Occupational Pollutants are Avoidable Causes of Breast Cancer," *Intl. J. Hlth. Services* 24:144-150, 1994.

None of Us Should Eat Extra Estrogen

By Samuel S. Epstein, M.D.
From *The Los Angeles Times*
March 24, 1997

When U.S. and Canadian beef cattle go to feedlots, hormone pellets are implanted under the ear skin, a process that is repeated at the midpoint of their 100-day fattening period. The hormones increase the weight of the cattle, adding to profits by about $80 per animal.

The most common hormone in current use is estradiol, a potent cancer-causing and gene-damaging estrogen. The FDA maintains that residues of estradiol and other hormones in meat are within "normal" levels, and has waived any requirements for monitoring and chemical testing.

Europe, however, has rightly eyed U.S. claims with great skepticism and since 1989 the European Union has forbidden the sale of beef from hormone-treated cattle. The opening of global markets has placed that ban under attack.

On Feb. 17, a panel of World Trade Organization judges began closed hearings on a U.S. and Canadian challenge charging that the European ban is merely protectionist and is costing North America $100 million a year in lost exports.

The FDA's claims of safety were endorsed by a 1987 report of two U.N. bodies, the Food and Agriculture Organization and the World Health Organization, an endorsement that is the main basis of the U.S. and Canadian action against Europe. The joint committee that prepared the report, however, has minimal expertise in public health and high representation of veterinary scientists and senior FDA and U.S. Department of Agriculture officials. Relying heavily on unpublished industry information and outdated scientific citations, the committee claimed that hormone residues in legally implanted cattle are so low that eating treated meat could not possibly induce any hormonal or carcinogenic effects.

However, confidential industry reports to the FDA, obtained under the Freedom of Information Act, reveal high hormone residues in meat products even under ideal test conditions. Following a single ear implant in steers of Synovex-S, a combination of estradiol and progesterone, estradiol levels in different meat products were up to 20-fold higher than normal. The amount of estradiol in two hamburgers eaten in one day by an 8-year-old boy could increase his total hormone levels by as much as 10%, based on conservative assumptions, because young children have very low natural hormone levels.

In real life, the situation may be much worse.

An unpublicized random USDA survey of 32 large feedlots found that as many as half the cattle had visible illegal "misplaced implants" in muscle, rather than under ear skin. This would result in very high local concentrations of hormones, and also elevated levels in muscle meat at distant sites. Such abuse is very hard to detect.

Responding to European concerns, the USDA recently claimed that, based on standard residue monitoring programs, drug levels in violation of regulations have not been detected in meat products. However, of 130 million livestock commercially slaughtered in 1993, not one was tested for estradiol or any related hormone.

The question we ought to be asking is not why Europe won't buy our hormone-treated meat, but why we allow beef from hormone-treated cattle to be sold to American and Canadian consumers. Untreated meat is currently hard to find and expensive; if it were widely produced and available, the price would come down. At the least, meat produced from hormone-treated animals should be explicitly labeled.

These hormones are linked ever more closely to the escalating incidence of reproductive cancers in the U.S. since 1950 — 55% for breast cancer, 120% for testicular cancer and 190% for prostate cancer. The endocrine-disruptive effects of estrogenic pesticides and other industrial food contaminants known as xenoestrogens are now under intensive investigation by federal regulatory and health agencies. But the contamination of meat with residues of the far-more-potent estradiol remains ignored.

The world trade judges ought to listen to one of the top FDA officials involved in meat safety, David Livingston. In Orville Schell's 1984 meat industry exposé, "Modern Meat," Livingston is quoted as saying, "Well, if you're going to have enough inexpensive meat for everyone, you're going to have to use some of these drugs. But personally, I'd rather eat meat that was raised without them." In other words, what's good enough for the rest of us is not something he wants to eat.

New Challenges on the Safety of U.S. Meat

By Samuel S. Epstein, M.D.
Press Release, Cancer Prevention Coalition
February 2, 1998

The World Trade Organization (WTO) ruled in favor of the 1989 European ban on the use of sex hormones for growth promotion of cattle in feedlots prior to slaughter. While subject to further assessment before it can be made permanent, this ruling is a major victory for European consumers. It is also a major defeat for the United States and Canada, which challenged the European ban claiming that it was "protectionist," costing over $100 million a year in lost exports, and that it reflected "consumerism versus science." The WTO ruling also raises serious concerns about the safety of U.S. meat, recently questioned on different grounds by Oprah Winfrey, based on the following considerations:

• Confidential industry reports to the FDA, obtained under the Freedom of Information Act, reveal high residues of natural and synthetic sex hormones in meat products even under ideal test conditions. This is contrary to repeated and explicit assurances by the FDA and USDA.

• Following legal implantation in the ear of steers of Synovex-S, a combination of estradiol and progesterone, estradiol levels in meat products ranged up to 20-fold in excess of the normal. Based on conservative estimates, the amount of estradiol in two hamburgers eaten by an 8-year-old boy could increase his hormone levels by 10%.

• Much higher hormone residues are found in meat products following illegal implantation in cattle muscle which is commonplace in U.S. feedlots. The WTO ruled that such abuse alone would justify the European ban.

• Contrary to repeated and explicit assurances by the FDA and USDA, none of the approximately 130 million U.S. livestock slaughtered annually are tested for residues of cancer-causing and gene-damaging estradiol or any related sex hormones. This misrepresentation has been confirmed by European Commission inspectors, in a November 1997 survey of U.S. control programs, who reported that there was no monitoring for residues of sex hormones nor for illegal animal drugs, including antibiotics, and that U.S. residue monitoring was totally inadequate to meet European standards.

• Repeated assurances on the safety of hormonal meat by two World Health Organization bodies, the Food and Agriculture Organization and the Codex Alimentarius Commission (FAO/CODEX), reflect minimal expertise in public health, high representation of senior FDA and USDA officials and industry consultants, reliance on unpublished industry and outdated scientific information, and conflicts of interest. Paradoxically, the same Codex Commission which approved hormonal meat, explicitly warned over a decade ago that baby meat foods "shall be free from residues or hormones."

• The endocrine-disruptive effects of estrogenic pesticides and other industrial food contaminants, known as xenoestrogens, are now under intensive investigation by U.S. regulatory and health agencies. But contamination of meat with residues of the thousands-fold more potent estradiol remains ignored.

• Lifelong exposure to high residues of natural and synthetic sex hormones in meat products poses serious risks of breast and other reproductive cancers, whose incidence in the U.S. has sharply escalated since 1950 — 55% for breast cancer, 120% for testicular cancer, and 230% for prostate cancer. Those residues have also been incriminated in increasing trends of precocious sexual development.

Commenting on these facts, Samuel S. Epstein, M.D., Professor of Environmental Medicine at the University of Illinois Chicago, School of Public Health, stated, "The European ban on hormonal meat should serve as a long-overdue wake-up call for U.S. consumers to demand an immediate ban on hormone use or, minimally, the explicit labeling of hormonal meat products. It should also lead to a congressional investigation of the FDA and USDA for gross regulatory abdication besides suppression of information vital to consumer health. The dangers of U.S. hormonal meat can no longer be ignored."

Cancer Risks of Hormonal Milk

Virtually the entire U.S. population is now consuming unlabeled milk from cows treated with synthetic bovine growth hormone (rBGH). Evidence of the hazards of rBGH milk is presented below.

A Needless New Risk of Breast Cancer

By Samuel S. Epstein, M.D.
From *The Los Angeles Times*
March 20, 1994

The Food and Drug Administration recently warned dairy producers, distributors and retailers against "hormone-free" labels on milk from cows that have not been given the biotech milk-production stimulant known as recombinant bovine growth hormone. The FDA states that such labeling could be "false or misleading" under federal law, as there is "no significant difference between milk from treated and untreated cows." Monsanto, maker of the hormone, is already suing one large Midwest milk producer for using the label.

The confusing FDA guidelines were, according to the consumer publication *Daily Citizen*, written by Deputy Commissioner Michael Taylor, a former counsel for Monsanto and a biotech umbrella organization. The guidelines are scientifically flawed and reckless and reflect flagrant disregard of consumers' right to know. Furthermore, the FDA ignores evidence linking milk from treated cows with increased risk of breast cancer. The concerns, based on published research:

• The biotech hormone induces a marked and sustained increase in levels of insulin-like growth factor-1, or IGF-1, in cow's milk.
• IGF-1 regulates cell growth, division and differentiation, particularly in infants. While human and normal bovine IGF-1 are identical, they are largely bound to protein and thus probably less biologically active than the unbound IGF-1 in treated milk.

• IGF-1 is not destroyed by pasteurization or digestion and is readily absorbed across the intestinal wall. In a 1990 FDA publication disclosing toxicity tests conducted by Monsanto, feeding the hormone (trade name Posilac) to mature rats for only two weeks resulted in statistically significant increases in body and liver weights and bone length. These effects were seen at a small fraction of injected doses given to control rats. But by gerrymandering these explicit data, the FDA alleged that IGF-1 "lacks oral toxicity."

Neither the FDA nor Monsanto has investigated the effects of long-term feeding of IGF-1 and treated milk on growth, or on more sensitive sub-cellular effects in infant rats or infants of any other species.

• Cows injected with the biotech hormone show heavy localization of IGF-1 in breast (udder) epithelial cells; this does not occur in untreated cows.
• IGF-1 induces rapid division and multiplication of normal human breast epithelial cells in tissue cultures.
• It is highly likely that IGF-1 promotes transformation of normal breast epithelium to breast cancer.
• IGF-1 maintains the malignancy of human breast-cancer cells, including their in-

vasiveness and ability to spread to distant organs.

• The breast tissues of female fetuses and infants are sensitive to hormonal influences. Imprinting by IGF-1 may increase future breast-cancer risks and sensitivity of the breast to subsequent unrelated risks such as mammography and the carcinogenic and estrogen-like effects of pesticide residues in food, particularly in premenopausal women.

These concerns are not new. In a 1989 letter to the FDA, I warned that the effects of IGF-1 "could include premature growth stimulation in infants, [breast enlargement] in young children and breast cancer in adult females." More recently, the Council on Scientific Affairs of the American Medical Association stated: "Further studies will be required to determine whether the ingestion of higher-than-normal concentrations of bovine insulin-like growth factor is safe for children, adolescents, and adults." The opposite of "further study" is uncontrolled, unlabeled sales of treated milk to unwitting consumers.

Apart from risks of breast cancer and other IGF-1 effects, the FDA and industry have down-played additional differences between hormonal and non-hormonal milk. The FDA-approved label insert for Posilac, a pamphlet that only dairy farmers see, admits that its "use is associated with increased frequency of use of medication in cows for mastitis and other health problems." Monsanto's own data further show up to an 80% incidence of mastitis, an udder infection, in hormone-treated cattle and resulting contamination of milk with statistically significant levels of pus; this will necessitate virtually routine use of antibiotics, with attendant risks of allergic reactions and antibiotic resistance.

Congress should insist that, at the very least, the FDA immediately revoke its restrictions on labeling of milk from untreated cows.

More prudently, it should ban the use of these hormones.

Unlabeled Milk from Cows Treated with Biosynthetic Growth Hormones: ### A Case of Regulatory Abdication

By Samuel S. Epstein, M.D.
From *International Journal of Health Services**
January, 1996

Levels of insulin-like growth factor-1 (IGF-1) are substantially elevated and more bioactive in the milk of cows hyperstimulated with the biosynthetic bovine growth hormones rBGH, and are further increased by pasteurization. IGF-1 is absorbed from the gastrointestinal tract, as evidenced by marked growth-promoting effects even in short-term tests in mature rats, and absorption is likely to be still higher in infants. Converging lines of evidence incriminate IGF-1 in rBGH milk as a potential risk factor for both breast and gastrointestinal cancers.

In 1985, the Food and Drug Administration (FDA) approved the commercial sale of unlabeled milk and meat from large-scale veterinary trials on cows treated with the synthetic bovine growth hormones (rBGH); these hormones are manufactured using recombinant DNA biotechnology by Monsanto, American Cyanamid, Dow Chemical, Upjohn, and Eli Lilly companies. FDA and industry claimed that rBGH had no adverse veterinary effects and that rBGH milk was indistinguishable from natural milk and safe for human consumption.

By 1990, evidence from published and unpublished industry sources had raised a wide range of concerns about the safety of rBGH milk.[1-3] These included: contamination of rBGH milk with pus from mastitis and with

* *International Journal of Health Services.* 26:173-185, 1996.

antibiotics used in its treatment; contamination of milk with rBGH that FDA admitted differed significantly in its molecular structure from the natural growth hormone; and contamination of milk with excess levels of insulin-like growth factor-1 (IGF-1). In spite of these unresolved veterinary and public health concerns, in November, 1993 FDA approved large-scale commercial use and sale of rBGH milk, and shortly after issued regulatory guidelines effectively banning the labeling of such milk[4, 5] This article presents an analysis of available information on potential risks of breast and gastrointestinal cancers from IGF-1 in rBGH milk.

Insulin-like growth factor-1 is a potent low molecular weight polypeptide growth factor that mediates the action of the pituitary growth hormone on somatic growth. IGF-1 induces profound metabolic effects through endocrine, paracrine, or autocrine mechanisms,[6-10] including regulation of transport processes, macromolecular synthesis, cell growth, replication and differentiation, and milk production. Although the gene encoding IGF-1 is expressed in many tissues, most circulating IGF-1 is produced by liver cells where transcription is regulated by a complex hypothalamic-pituitary-hepatic axis.[6, 7] IGF-1 is also synthesized at the local level by both normal and malignant cells.[7, 8] It should be further noted that the amino acid sequences of human and bovine IGF-1 are identical.[9, 10]

Elevated IGF-1 Levels in rBGH Milk

In an early report relating IGF-1 milk levels to natural BGH isolated from bovine pituitaries, administration of the hormone increased IGF-1 levels in goat's milk from a mean pretreatment level of 16 ng/ml to 25 ng/ml within four days.[11] Normal cow's milk collected just after parturition contained high IGF-1 levels, about 150 ng/ml, which rapidly fell to about 25 ng/ml within one week and then declined to only 1 to 5 ng/ml by 200 days, when levels of IGF-1 induced by rBGH

ranged from 6 to 20 ng/ml, up to a 20-fold increase.[12] In a subsequent short-term study on 35-47 weeks postpartum cows, a six-fold increase in IGF-1 milk levels was reported as early as 7 days following rBGH treatment.[13] Of particular interest was the finding that "a significant proportion [19 percent] of the total IGF-1 was present in the [protein] free unbound form,"[13] and was thus probably more bioactive or potent than the protein-bound form.[14] Furthermore, pasteurization increases milk IGF-1 levels by some 70 percent, presumably by disrupting protein binding.[15] The significance of these findings is emphasized by recent evidence that free IGF-1 levels in human serum are as low as 0.38 percent.[16] No data are available, however, on the ratios of free to unbound IGF-1 in the sera and milk of cows treated or untreated with rBGH, and in the sera of humans drinking milk from cows treated or untreated with rBGH.

In some six unpublished, confidential industry studies, disclosed by FDA in a highly abbreviated summary form, IGF-1 levels in rBGH milk were consistently increased;[15] these increases were statistically significant, ranging from 25 to 70 percent.[17] Illustratively, in a 1989 Monsanto trial, milk IGF-1 levels in cows increased from control levels of 3.5 ng/ml to 5.9 ng/ml and 6.1 ng/ml following intramuscular or subcutaneous rBGH injections, respectively; higher levels still, up to 25 ng/ml, were subsequently reported by Monsanto.[18] More recently, Lilly Industries, in its application for marketing authorization to the European Community Committee for Veterinary Medicinal Products, has admitted that rBGH milk may contain more than a 10-fold increase in IGF-1 concentrations.[19]

A summary report of the 1990 National Institutes of Health Technology Conference noted that IGF-1 levels in unspecified samples of rBGH milk were 3.5 to 13 ng/ml, approximately three to four times the levels in human milk, in contrast to 1.5 to 8 ng/ml in untreated cows.[20] This report also noted that IGF-1 levels in meat of rBGH animals were approximately twice as high as in untreated controls.

The results of virtually all these studies are, however, based on flawed analytic techniques that underestimated IGF-1 levels, as recognized by the technique developers and others.[17, 21, 22] Problems with these techniques included their inability to separate the IGF-1 molecule from a complex of associated large carrier proteins to which IGF-1 is usually bound. These problems were further extended by the finding that standard IGF-1 analytic techniques underestimate, by a factor of four, levels of a truncated form of IGF-1 (-3N:IGF-1) which is approximately 10 times more potent in stimulating protein and DNA synthesis than normal IGF-1, resulting in a potential 40-fold underestimate of levels in rBGH milk.[14, 23] The significance of these considerations was further emphasized: "The presence in colostrum of -3N:IGF-1 and of large amounts of free IGF-1 may be pointers to likely changes occurring in milk in response to bST [rBGH] treatment, since a strong parallel has been suggested between the increased milk secretion which occurs postpartum and that following bST treatment."[14]

Absorption of IGF-1 from the Gastrointestinal Tract

There is unequivocal evidence that a wide range of intact proteins are absorbed across the gut wall in a wide range of species including humans.[15, 24] In humans, this evidence is largely based on the detection of serum antibodies to food proteins.[25] The infant gut is more permeable to protein than the adult gut, particularly pre-term and prior to "closure" at about 3 months of age.[26-28] Infants and young children have higher serum levels of cow's milk protein antibodies than adults.[24, 29] These varying lines of evidence on absorption of intact proteins further confirm that smaller molecular weight polypeptides, such as IGF-1, can also be absorbed from the gut. Even more compelling is evidence of marked

systemic effects following short-term IGF-1 feeding tests in rats.[15]

FDA recently responded to this evidence with a wide range of tenuous and inconsistent claims.[30] These include: "There is no evidence that IGF-1 survives digestion in humans," in contrast to FDA's prior publication of Monsanto/Hazleton data on systemic effects of IGF-1 following short-term oral administration.[15] And "the IGF-1 content of milk is not altered by BST supplementation" on the basis of "more comprehensive [industry] studies,"[31] although these studies in fact conclude that "mean IGF-1 levels in the [rBGH] treated animals are always higher than those found in the controls." Excess IGF-1 milk levels were trivialized in comparison with endogenous levels in human saliva and blood by FDA's use of highly speculative and misleading calculations.[30]

More appropriate calculations should be based on the following considerations and data: Adult humans produce daily about 1.2 liters of saliva containing an IGF-1 level of about 3 ng/ml, equivalent to a daily recycling of some 3 μg of IGF-1;[32] corresponding intake levels in infants are substantially lower. This should be contrasted with an infant's daily consumption of 1 liter of rBGH cow's milk containing the maximum 25 μg level of IGF-1 admitted by Monsanto,[18] well over an order of magnitude of excess exogenous exposure. While exaggerating endogenous in relation to exogenous exposures from rBGH milk in infants, neither FDA nor industry has presented any data on salivary and blood levels of IGF-1 in infants. A 1990 letter from Monsanto to NIH claimed that plans to obtain the salivary data "will be forthcoming;"[33] however, no such data are yet available. FDA's quantitative comparison between IGF-1 levels in bovine milk and human blood is equally misleading.[30] Assuming an adult blood volume of 3.5 liters and adult IGF-1 levels of 100 ng/ml, adults have a total circulatory level of 350 μg of IGF-1, rather than the 600 μg calculated by FDA (30). Thus, assuming a neonate blood volume of 0.25 liters, based on a body weight of 3 kg and a volume of 80 ml/kg, this would correspond to a circulatory level of about 25 μg. This should be contrasted with a daily intake of up to 25 μg/l of IGF-1 in rBGH milk, which may be up to 40 times more potent or bioactive than blood IGF-1,[14] constituting a daily intake of 1000 μg blood equivalents.

Such calculations not only are based on a wide range of assumptions, but also reflect very substantial data gaps despite over a decade of industry experience with rBGH. What is clear, however, is that simplistic quantitative comparisons by FDA and industry that trivialize milk versus endogenous IGF-1 levels are not meaningful. Alternative calculations raise serious concerns on the potential hazards, particularly to infants, of excess IGF-1 levels in rBGH milk.

Oral Activity of IGF-1

There are no published studies, in the scientific literature or in FDA or industry reports, on the oral activity of IGF-1. FDA, however, in 1990 released a highly condensed summary of 1989 toxicity tests by the two major rBGH industries, Eli Lilly & Co. (Elanco) and Monsanto Agricultural Co.[15] The Elanco test was conducted at the company. The Monsanto test was contracted out to Hazleton Laboratories. Apart from a wide range of other flaws, the relevance of both these studies is questionable, as they were short- rather than long-term, were conducted on adult rather than infant rats, and were conducted on rIGF-1 rather than on IGF-1 — containing rBGH milk or IGF-1 isolated from rBGH milk.

The FDA report on the Elanco oral toxicity test was cryptic, even more so than that on the Monsanto/Hazleton study.[15] The Elanco test used groups of 10 male and female hypophysectomized adult rats, given oral doses of rIGF-1 for two weeks at 0.01, 0.1, or 1.0 mg/kg/day, with a subcutaneous infusion positive control at 1.0 mg/kg. Gross organ weights were increased in positive control rats but not test rats. No data were presented on epiphyseal width and tibia length. On the basis of these minimal parameters, rIGF-1 was alleged to be devoid of oral toxicity.

In the Monsanto/Hazleton test, groups of 20 male and female 36-day-old rats were dosed orally for two weeks with rIGF-1 at concentrations of 0.02, 0.2, or 2.0 mg/kg/day.[15] Two groups of rats served as positive controls. The first was infused subcutaneously with rIGF-1 doses of 0.05 or 0.2 mg/rat/day corresponding to about 1 to 4 mg/kg/day, and the second with porcine growth hormone (pGH) at doses of 4.0 mg/rat/day corresponding to about 80 mg/kg/day, assuming a 36-day-old rat weighs approximately 50 g. Statistically significant increases in body weight were seen with male test rats at 2.0 mg/kg, with a positive linear trend at all dose levels in test females. In addition, statistically significant increases in liver weight and tibia length and decreases in epiphyseal width were seen in test males at doses of 2.0 mg/kg, significant increases in tibia length of test males at 0.02 mg/kg, and significant decreases in epiphyseal width of test females at 2.0 mg/kg. The statistically significant lowest observed effect level (LOEL) of 0.02 mg/kg/day is thus approximately 1/4000 of the positive infusion control pGH dose and approximately 1/50 of the positive infusion control rIGF-1 LOEL.

In spite of the tabulated Monsanto data on the statistically significant sensitivity of rats to oral administration of rIGF-1, FDA asserted "that rIGF-1 is orally inactive at doses up to 2 mg/kg per day."[15] This conclusion conflicts with the cited data and was based on a series of tenuous claims that have been subject to detailed criticism.[14, 34] FDA claimed that there were no significant increases in body weight of orally dosed females in contrast to males, even though a similar difference in sensitivity was noted in female rIGF-1 controls injected at 0.05 mg/rat/day. FDA also claimed (a) that the increase in body weight of test males should be discounted as it only occurred in one "block" of half the control rIGF-1 rats, raising questions about the validity of the experimental design of the test on which FDA based its conclusion; (b) that there were no increases in serum IGF-1 of test rats, although no supportive data were cited; and (c) that decreases in epiphyseal width and increases in tibia lengths in test animals should be disregarded as "contradictory [and] sporadic," even though such effects in rIGF-1 control groups were also inconsistent and not even cited at the 0.05 mg/rat dose.

FDA's flawed analysis of their cited test data is compounded by a misleading presentation of the data. Notably, in Tables 4 and 5 of the Monsanto/Hazleton report, the dosages of test rats are presented in mg/kg, while those for the positive infused controls are presented in mg/rat, thus using incomparable dose units for test and control animals.[15] This resulted in a misleading reduction of oral dose levels in test rats compared with control rats by a factor of some 20, thus substantially underestimating their sensitivity to oral IGF-1.[34] Such data manipulation is consistent with the documented track record of Hazleton Laboratories.[35] Under the circumstances, it is not surprising that FDA and Monsanto refused to comply with a May 1994 Congressional request for an unabridged copy of the 1988 Hazleton report on which FDA bases its near-exclusive reliance for the alleged nontoxicity of IGF-1 in rBGH milk.[36]

The unpublished Monsanto/Hazleton oral toxicity test was conducted on rIGF-1, rather than more relevantly on IGF-1 in rBGH milk, which may differ from rIGF-1.[14] This study is also seriously flawed as it violated standard protocols on routine lifetime chronic toxicity and carcinogenicity tests based on two species. This study was only two weeks long and included groups of only 20 male and female adult rats. Maximally tolerated doses

(MTD) were not determined and test doses were not extended up to this range, nor was testing extended below 0.02 mg/kg in order to determine the no-observable-effect level (NOEL). No autopsy data were provided, except body and organ weight and epiphyseal width; and no histological data were reported. Moreover, no three-generation and transplacental tests were conducted, nor any tests involving neonatal rodents or neonatal and adult subhuman primates. Finally, no investigations were undertaken on sensitive subcellular effects, including IGF-1 binding and receptor levels in tests and controls.

Of further interest, a recent industry report noted a statistically significant increase in the body weight at weaning of calves from rBGH-treated cows compared with calves from untreated cows.[37] While this result suggests that increased IGF-1 milk levels induce growth factor effects, in the absence of paired feeding data it is not possible to exclude the effect of increased availability of milk.

Absence of Safety Margins for IGF-1 Following Consumption of rBGH Milk

As recently emphasized,[14] consumption of rBGH milk would expose infants and young children to IGF-1 levels substantially in excess of the safety margin based on the 0.02 mg/kg (20 µg/kg) LOEL identified in the Monsanto/Hazleton oral toxicity test.[15] Assuming a 10 kg child consumes 1 liter daily of rBGH milk with an IGF-1 concentration of 25 ng/ml (25 µg/l), this would then result in an intake of 2.5 µg/kg, one-eighth of the 20 µg/kg LOEL.[14] Safety margins for noncarcinogenic toxic effects are conventionally set on the basis of 1/100 of NOELs and 1/1000 of LOELs, which for IGF-1 would thus be 0.02 µg/kg. Thus, an intake of 2.5 µg/kg would actually be 125-fold in excess of the standard safety margin.

Such estimates are conservative for a range of reasons discussed above: pasteurization of rBGH milk increases IGF-1 levels by approximately 70 percent;[15] IGF-1 in rBGH milk is more bioactive than IGF-1 in untreated milk; standard analytic techniques underestimate IGF-1 levels by a factor of 4; and IGF-1 in rBGH milk may well be present, at least in part, in a truncated form that is some 10 times more potent than IGF-1 in untreated milk.[14]

IGF-1 in rBGH Milk as a Potential Risk Factor for Breast Cancer

FDA made its decision on the safety of rBGH milk in 1985 in the absence of data on a wide range of public health concerns, including information about excess IGF-1 levels in rBGH milk, and without consideration of the cellular proliferative effect of IGF-1. Over recent years, several converging lines of evidence have implicated IGF-1 in the initiation or promotion of breast cancer. This evidence raises serious concerns about the potential carcinogenic effects, particularly for female infants, of increased IGF-1 levels in rBGH milk and dairy products.

In the normal lactating bovine mammary gland, IGF-1 is almost exclusively located in intralobular stromal or connective tissue cells with minimal epithelial reactivity.[38] In contrast, there is a markedly prominent epithelial uptake of IGF-1 following increased serum levels induced by rBGH.[38] Furthermore, IGF-1 binds to specific surface receptors identified in cultured mammary epithelial cells of a wide range of species including pigs, cattle, and humans.[39-41] These receptors are proteins in the tyrosine kinase family, to which retrovirus oncogenes also belong.[42] IGF-1 receptors have also been identified in normal and malignant human breast tissue;[43, 44] levels in malignant tissue are some 10-fold elevated. Related growth factors, such as epidermal growth factor (EGF) and fibroblastic growth factor (FGF), also bind to receptors of breast cancer cells.[43] Of further interest, estradiol and progesterone regulate IGF-1 receptors in cultured normal and neoplastic human uterine endometrial cells.[45]

More direct evidence on the role of elevated levels of IGF-1 in rBGH milk as a potential risk factor for breast cancer is based on the following considerations: IGF-1 induces highly potent mitogenic effects in a variety of cell types,[46] including normal human breast cells maintained in long-term tissue culture.[39] IGF-1 is also a potent regulator of cultured human breast cancer cells[47, 48] and is more mitogenic than the potent estradiol.[49] While distinct from carcinogenesis, mitogenesis is likely to promote malignant transformation induced by estradiol in breast epithelium.[43] Furthermore, estrogens induce IGF-1 synthesis in both normal and malignant breast epithelia.[50, 51] Accordingly, it is now recognized that growth factors such as IGF-1 "are responsible at least in part for the evolution of normal breast epithelia to breast cancer."[52] IGF-1 and related growth factors are critically involved in the aberrant growth of human breast cancer cells, and maintain their invasive or metastatic phenotype.[43, 53] Of further interest is the fact that IGF-1 plasma concentrations are higher in breast cancer patients than healthy controls: "Even if there is no direct evidence that elevated plasma levels of IGF-1 reflect elevated levels of the growth factor at the tumor level, the possibility exists that increased levels of circulating IGF-1 may contribute to breast tumor growth."[44] Relevant in this connection is the suggestion that tamoxifen used in the chemotherapy of breast cancer acts by reducing blood IGF-1 levels.[49]

These unresolved concerns about the potential carcinogenicity of IGF-1 in rBGH milk are heightened by evidence that the undifferentiated prenatal and infant breasts are particularly susceptible to "imprinting" by hormonal influences.[54] This may implicate IGF-1 itself as a direct breast cancer risk factor. It may also act indirectly by sensitizing the breast to subsequent unrelated risk factors, such as carcinogenic and estrogenic pesticide contaminants in food, and radiation, particularly mammography in premeno-pausal women.[55, 56]

IGF-1 in rBGH Milk as a Potential Risk Factor for Gastrointestinal Cancer

IGF-1 stimulates proliferation of intestinal epithelial cells in culture.[57] Such mitogenic effects are induced at concentrations equivalent to those occurring in mature bovine milk. Furthermore, a related growth factor with similar biological effects on the human gut, epidermal growth factor, passes undigested through the stomach to the small intestine from where it is rapidly absorbed into the blood stream, suggesting the likelihood that IGF-1 is similarly absorbed.[57] Subsequent studies have demonstrated that IGF-1 is protected from digestion by casein, a protein in milk.[58] Reflecting these considerations, the 1990 NIH Technology Conference concluded: "Whether the additional amounts of IGF-1 in milk from [rBGH-treated] cows has a local effect in the esophagus, stomach or intestines is unknown." It was accordingly recommended: "Determine the acute and chronic action of IGF-1, if any, in the upper gastrointestinal tract."[20] However, no information is yet available on the local effects of IGF-1, particularly increased levels of the probably more bioactive IGF-1 in rBGH milk, on the gastrointestinal tract of infants and adults.

More recent studies have demonstrated that following consumption of rBGH milk, IGF-1 in the gastrointestinal lumen, unlike serum IGF-1, is not protein bound and thus more likely to "exert biological activity."[59] Intraluminal infusion of IGF-1 in rats at concentrations equivalent to those in bovine milk has been found to increase the cellularity of the intestinal mucosa.[60] In one study, rIGF-1 at concentrations of 100 ng/ml induced statistically highly significant mitogenic effects in crypt epithelial cells of cultured human duodenal explants.[61] The authors concluded: "The combination of IGF-1 in BST-milk and IGF-1 normally secreted into the human gastrointestinal lumen would augment intraluminal concentrations of this hormone, increasing the possibility of local mitogenic effects on gut tissues,"[61] and expressed concerns about local carcinogenic effects.[62] Research has also shown that human colorectal cancer cell lines are responsive to IGF-1,[63] and that IGF-1 is mitogenic to five of eight carcinoma cell lines and synergizes the effects of another growth factor, transforming growth factor (TGF). The authors concluded that their results illustrated the importance of IGF-1 as "stimulators of growth of colorectal carcinoma." There is also evidence that human gastric cancer cells have IGF-1 receptors.[64]

These results raise questions about IGF-1 residues in rBGH milk posing potential risks for the initiation or promotion of gastrointestinal cancer. An extensive recent review of rBGH milk further emphasized these concerns: "It could be considered an oversight for [the FDA] to suggest that ingested IGF-1 is inactive. . . . Many more potential effects of ingested IGF-1 on the gastrointestinal tract and the local immune system of the gut need to be explored."[65]

Discussion

Critical information on a wide range of potentially adverse health effects of IGF-1 is still unavailable.[e.g., 14, 17, 19, 63, 65, 66] This is particularly disturbing because FDA made its decision on the safety of rBGH milk in 1985, when there had been no consideration of the effect of IGF-1 on cell proliferation. Needed studies include (a) determination of free versus protein-bound IGF-1 in sera of cows treated with rBGH and of untreated cows; (b) study of the lifelong, three-generation, and subcellular effects in rodents and subhuman primates of rBGH milk and derived IGF-1; (c) chemical characterization of IGF-1 in rBGH milk; (d) radioactive label studies on gastrointestinal absorption of IGF-1 in rBGH milk; (e) pharmacological studies on binding to receptor sites; and (f) even more critically, extensive studies on humans who drink rBGH milk, with particular reference to absorption and characterization of serum IGF-1, determination of free versus bound forms, and subcellular binding. The significance of such data gaps is compounded by converging lines of evidence implicating IGF-1 in rBGH milk as a potential risk factor for breast and gastrointestinal cancers. Nevertheless, FDA has dismissed these concerns without investigation and on the basis of unpublished "confidential" short-term toxicity data, primarily from an industry consulting firm with a tainted track record. Furthermore, contrary to FDA and industry claims and in spite of misleading data, the results of this test revealed statistically significant growth-promoting effects.

In spite of these serious and still-unresolved public health concerns, in November 1993 FDA approved commercial sale of rBGH milk, some eight years after the agency approved the sale of unlabeled rBGH milk from large-scale veterinary trials. This was soon followed by regulatory guidelines effectively banning the labeling of such milk.[4, 5] The rationale for this continued denial of consumers' right to know was developed by Michael Taylor, then Deputy FDA Commissioner and formerly chief counsel for the International Food Biotechnology Council and Monsanto.[5] This ban has since been challenged by nationwide grassroots consumer groups and by two milk suppliers, both of whom have been sued by Monsanto.

In short, with the active complicity of the FDA, the entire nation is currently being subjected to an experiment involving large-scale adulteration of an age-old dietary staple by a poorly characterized and unlabeled biotechnology product. Disturbingly, this experiment benefits only a very small segment of the agrichemical industry while providing no matching benefits to consumers. Even more disturbingly, it poses major potential public health risks for the entire U.S. population.

Note added

The potential carcinogenicity of incremental IGF-1 in rBGH milk is confirmed by studies on acromegaly, in which levels of total and free serum IGF-1 are significantly elevated (Juul, A., *et al*. The ratio between serum levels of IGF-1 and the IGF binding proteins decreases with age in healthy patients and is increased in acromegalic patients. *Clin. Endocrinol.* 41:85-93, 1994). A recent review has reported increased rates of pre-malignant polyps and colon cancer and also of overall cancers in acromegalics (Tremble, J. M., and McGregor, A. M. Epidemiology, complications and mortality. In *Treating Acromegaly,* edited by J. A. H. Wass, pp. 5-12, Journal of Endocrinology Ltd, Bristol, England, 1994).

References

1. S.S. Epstein. "Potential Public Health Hazards of Biosynthetic Milk Hormones," letter and report to FDA Commissioner Frank Young, July 19, 1989.
2. S.S. Epstein. "Potential Public Health Hazards of Biosynthetic Milk Hormones," *Int. J. Health Serv.* 20: 73-84, 1990.
3. S.S. Epstein. "Questions and Answers on Synthetic Bovine Growth Hormones," *Int. J. Health Serv.* 20: 573-581, 1990.
4. Food and Drug Administration. "Interim guidance on the voluntary labelling of milk and milk products from cows that have not been treated with recombinant bovine somatotropin," *Federal Register* 59(28):6279-6280, 1994.
5. S.S. Epstein. "A Needless New Risk of Breast Cancer (commentary)," *Los Angeles Times* p. M5, March 20, 1994.
6. I.S. Matthews, G. Norstedt, and R.D. Palmiter. "Regulation of insulin-like growth factor I gene expression by growth hormone," *Proc. Natl. Acad. Sci. USA* 83:9343-9347, 1986.
7. A. Sekyi-Otu *et al.* "Metastatic behavior of the RIF-1 murine fibrosarcoma: Inhibited by hypophysectomy and partially restored

by growth hormone replacement," *J. Natl. Cancer Inst.* 86: 628-632, 1994.

8. J. Isgaard *et al.* "Pulsatile intravenous growth hormone (GH) infusion to hypophysectomized rats increases insulin-like growth factor I messenger ribonucleic acid in skeletal tissues more effectively than continuous GH infusion," *Endocrinology* 123:2605-2610, 1988.

9. A. Honegger and R.R. Humbel. "Insulin-like growth factors I and II in fetal and adult bovine serum," *J. Biol. Chem.* 261:569-575, 1986.

10. B.W. McBride, J.L. Burton, and J.H. Burton. "The influence of bovine growth hormone (somatotropin) on animals and their products," *Res. Dev. Agricult.* 5:1-21, 1988.

11. C.G. Prosser *et al.* "Changes in concentration of insulin-like growth factor I (IGF-1) in milk during bovine growth hormone treatment in the goat," *J. Endocrinol.* 112 (March Suppl.), Abstr. 65, 1987.

12. C.G. Prosser. "Bovine Somatotropin and Milk Composition," *Lancet* 1:1201, November 19, 1988.

13. C.G. Prosser, I.R. Fleet, and A.N. Corps. "Increased secretion of insulin-like growth factor I into milk of cows treated with recombinantly derived bovine growth hormone," *J. Dairy Res.* 56:17-26, 1989.

14. T.B. Mepham. "Public health implications of bovine somatotropin use in dairying: Discussion paper," *J. R. Soc. Med.* 85:736-739, 1992.

15. J.C. Juskevich and C.G. Geyer. "Bovine growth hormone: Human food safety evaluation," *Science* 249:875-884, 1990.

16. J. Frystyk *et al.* "Free insulin-like growth factors (IGF-1 and IGF-II) in human serum," *FEBS Lett.* 348:185-191, 1994.

17. M.K. Hansen. *Biotechnology and Milk: Benefit or Threat?*, p. 6, Consumer Policy Institute, New York, 1990.

18. D. Schams. "Secretion of somatotropin and IGF-1 into milk during BST administration," in *Sometribove: Mechanism of Action, Safety and Instructions for Use*, Monsanto, Basingstoke, 1991.

19. T.B. Mepham *et al.* "Safety of Milk from Cows Treated with Bovine Somatotropin," *Lancet* 2:197, 1994.

20. National Institutes of Health. "Technology Assessment Conference Statement on Bovine Somatotropin," *JAMA* 265:1423-1425, 1991.

21. W.H. Daughaday, M. Kapadia, and I. Mariz. "Serum somatomedin binding proteins: Physiologic significance and interference in radioligand assay," *J. Lab. Clin. Med.* 109:355-363, 1987.

22. S. Mesiano *et al.* "Failure of acid-ethanol treatment to prevent interference by binding proteins in radioligand assays for the insulin-like growth factors," *J. Endocrinol.* 119:453-460, 1988.

23. G.L. Francis *et al.* "Insulin-like growth factors I and 2 in bovine colostrum — Sequences and biological activities compared with those of a potent truncated form," *Biochem. J.* 251:95-103, 1988.

24. M.L. Gardner. "Gastrointestinal Absorption of Intact Proteins," *Annu. Rev. Nutr.* 8:329-350, 1988.

25. R.J. Levinsky. "Factors Influencing Uptake of Food Antigens," *Proc. Nutr. Soc.* 44:81-86, 1985.

26. D.M. Roberton *et al.* "Milk Antigen Absorption in the Preterm and Term Neonate," *Arch. Dis. Child.* 57:369-372, 1982.

27. M.C. Reinhardt. "Molecular Absorption of Food Antigens in Health and Disease," *Ann. Allergy* 53:597-601, 1984.

28. J.N. Udall. "Human digestion and absorption of milk and its components at different stages of development: Protein hormones and growth factors," in *NIH Technology Assessment Conference, Bovine Somatotropin*, pp. 91-97, Bethesda, MD, 1990.

29. E.J. Lee and C. Heiner. "Allergy to Cow's Milk-1984," *Pediatr. Rev.* 7:195-203, 1986.

30. R.H. Teske. Center for Veterinary Medicine FDA. Letter to S. Epstein, March 7, 1994, in response to Epstein's February 14, 1994 letter to FDA Commissioner Dr. Kessler.

31. FAO/WHO Expert Committee on Food Additives. "Evaluation of Certain Veterinary Drug Remedies in Food," *WHO Tech. Rep. Ser.* 832,4/5:113-142, 1992.

32. R.J. Collier. "Qualitative and quantitative changes in hormones and growth factors in milk as affected by the administration of

rBST to cattle," in *NIH Technology Assessment Conference,* pp.45-49, Bethesda, MD, 1994.

33. B. Hammond, Manager, Toxicology, Monsanto Agriculture Co. Letter to Jerry Elliott, Program Analyst, Office of Medical Applications of Research, NIH, December 19, 1990.

34. M.K. Hansen. Letter to FDA, May 24, 1993.

35. S.S. Epstein. "Polluted Data," *The Sciences* 18:16-21, 1978.

36. P. Carver, Staff Director to Rep. D. Obey, D-Wis., House Subcommittee on Labor, Health and Human Services. Personal communication, May 30, 1994.

37. J.D. Armstrong *et al.* (Hoffman-LaRoche/ Monsanto). Effects of sometribove or immunization against growth hormone releasing factor (GRFi) on milk yield and composition, calf gain, insulin and metabolites in multiparous beef cows," *J. Dairy Sci.* 77 (Suppl. 1): 182, 1994.

38. D.R. Glimm, V.E. Baracos, and J.J. Kennelly. "Effect of bovine somatotropin on the distribution of immunoreactive insulin-like growth factor-1 in lactating bovine mammary tissue," *J. Dairy Sci.* 71:2923-2935, 1988.

39. R.W. Furlanetto and J.N. DiCarlo. "Somatomedin-C receptors and growth effects in human breast cells maintained in long-term tissue culture," *Cancer Res.* 44:2122-2128, 1984.

40. P. Gregor and B.D. Burleigh. "Presence of high affinity somatomedin/insulin-like growth factor receptors in porcine mammary gland," *Endocrinology* 116 (Suppl. 1), Abstr. 223, 1985.

41. P.G. Campbell and C.R. Baumrucker. "Characterization of insulin-like growth factorI/somatomedin-C receptors in bovine mammary gland," *J. Dairy Sci.* 69 (Suppl. 1), Abstr. 163, 1986.

42. A. Ullrich and J. Schessinger. "Signal Transduction by Receptors with Tyrosine-kinase Activity," *Cell* 61:203-212, 1990.

43. M.E. Lippman. "The Development of Biological Therapies for Breast Cancer," *Science* 259:631-632, 1993.

44. V. Pappa *et al.* "Insulin-like growth factor-1 receptors are overexpressed and predict a

low risk in human breast cancer," *Cancer Res.* 53:3736-3740, 1993.

45. R.K. Reynolds *et al.* "Regulation of epidermal growth factor and insulin-like growth factor I receptors by estradiol and progesterone in normal and neoplastic endometrial cell cultures," *Gynecol. Oncol.* 38(3):396-406, 1990.

46. M.M. Rechler and S.P. Nissley. "The nature and regulation of the receptors for insulin-like growth factor," *Annu. Rev. Physiol.* 47:425-442, 1985.

47. C.K. Osborne, D.R. Clemmons, and C.L. Arteaga. "Regulation of Breast Cancer Growth by Insulin-like Growth Factors," *J. Steroid Biochem. Mol. Biol.* 37:805-809, 1990.

48. N. Rosen *et al.* "Insulin-like Growth Factors in Human Breast Cancer," *Breast Cancer Res. Treat.* 18 (Suppl.):555-562, 1991.

49. M.N. Pollak, H.T. Huynh, and P. Lefebvre. "Tamoxifen Reduces Insulin-like Growth Factor-1 (IGF-1)," *Breast Cancer Res. Treat.* 22:91-100, 1992.

50. R.C. Baxter *et al.* "High molecular weight somatomedin-C/IGF-1 from T47D human mammary carcinoma cells: Immunoreactivity and bioactivity," in *Insulin-like Growth Factors Somatomedins: Basic Chemistry, Biology, Clinical Importance,* E. M. Spencer, Ed. pp. 615-618, DeGruyter, New York, 1983.

51. K.K. Huff *et al.* "Secretion of an insulin-like growth factor-1-related protein by human breast cancer cells," *Cancer Res.* 46:4618-4619, 1986.

52. J.R. Harris *et al.* "Breast Cancer," *N. Engl. J. Med.* 7:473-480, 1992.

53. A. Lippman. "Growth Factors, Receptors and Breast Cancer," *J. Natl. Inst. Health Res.* 3:59-62, 1991.

54. M. Ekbom *et al.* "Evidence of Prenatal Influence on Breast Cancer Risk," *Lancet* October 24, 1992, pp. 1015-1018.

55. S.S. Epstein. "Environmental and Occupational Pollutants are Avoidable Causes of Breast Cancer," *Int. J. Health Serv.* 24:145-159, 1994.

56. J.M. Elwood, B. Cox, and A.K. Richardson. "The effectiveness of brest cancer screening by mammography in

younger women," *Online J. Current Clin. Trials* 193, No. 32, 1993.

57. A.N. Corps and K.D. Brown. "Stimulation of intestinal epithelial cell proliferation in culture by growth factors in human and ruminant mammary secretions," *J. Endocrinol.* 113:285-290, 1987.

58. R.J. Playford *et al.* "Effect of Luminal Growth Factor Preservation on Intestinal Growth," *Lancet* 2:843-848, 1993.

59. O.P. Chaurasia *et al.* "Insulin-like Growth factor-1 in Human Gastrointestinal Exocrine Secretions," *Regul. Pept.* 50:113-119, 1994.

60. H. Olanrewaju, L. Patel, and E.R Siedel. "Trophic action of local intraileal infusion of insulin-like growth factor-1: Polyamine dependence," *Am. J. Physiol.* 263:E282-E286, 1992.

61. D.N. Challacombe and E.E. Wheeler. "Safety of Milk from Cows Treated with Bovine Somatotropin," *Lancet* 344:815-816, 1994.

62. D. Coghlan. "Arguing Till the Cows Come Home," *New Scientist* October 26, 1994, pp. 11-12.

63. H. Lahm *et al.* "Growth regulation and co-stimulation of human colorectal cancer cell lines by insulin-like growth factor I, II and transforming growth factor alpha," *Br. J. Cancer* 65(3):341-346, 1992.

64. Y.S. Guo. "Insulin-like growth factor-binding protein modulates the growth response to insulin-like growth factor-1 by human gastric cancer cells," *Gastroenterology* 104(6):1595-1604, 1993.

65. J.L. Burton *et al.* "A Review of Bovine Growth Hormone," *Can. J. Animal Sci.* 74:167-201, 1994.

66. American Medical Association Council on Scientific Affairs. "Biotechnology and the American Agricultural Industry," *JAMA* 265:1429-1436, 1991.

Evidence of Monsanto's Coverup of the Hazards of rBGH Milk

Three terms are used interchangeably to refer to milk from cows treated with growth hormones: biosynthetic milk, rBGH milk, and hormonal milk. Although Monsanto — the ma-jor producer of genetically engineered bovine growth hormone — continues to insist that the hormone treatment poses few health risks, hard evidence to the contrary continues to mount inexorably, as witness the following two press releases from the Cancer Prevention Coalition.

Monsanto's Biosynthetic Milk Poses Risk of Prostate Cancer, Among Other Cancers

By Samuel S. Epstein, M.D.
Press Release
From Cancer Prevention Coalition
March 15, 1998

As reported in a January 23, 1998 article in *Science,* men with high blood levels of the naturally occurring hormone insulin-like growth factor (IGF-1) are over four times more likely to develop full-blown prostate cancer than are men with lower levels. The report emphasized that high IGF-1 blood levels are the strongest known risk factor for prostate cancer, only exceeding that of a family history, and that reducing IGF-1 levels is likely to prevent this cancer. It was further noted that IGF-1 markedly stimulates the division and proliferation of normal and cancerous prostate cells and that it blocks the programmed self-destruction of cancer cells thus enhancing the growth and invasiveness of latent prostate cancer. These findings are highly relevant to any efforts to prevent prostate cancer, whose rates have escalated by 180% since 1950, and which is now the commonest cancer in non-smoking men, with an estimated 185,000 new cases and 39,000 deaths in 1998.

While warning that increasing IGF-1 blood levels by treating the elderly with growth hormone (GH) to slow aging may increase risks of prostate cancer, the 1998 report appears unaware of the fact that the entire U.S. population is now exposed to high levels of IGF-1 in dairy products. In February 1995, the Food and Drug Administration approved the sale of unlabeled milk from cows injected with Monsanto's genetically engineered bovine growth hormone, rBGH, to increase milk production.

As detailed in a January 1996 report in the *International Journal of Health Services*, rBGH milk differs from natural milk chemically, nutritionally, pharmacologically, and immunologically besides being contaminated with pus and antibiotics resulting from mastitis induced by the biotech hormone. Most critically, rBGH milk is supercharged with high levels of abnormally potent IGF-1, up to 10 times the levels in natural milk and over 10 times more potent. IGF-1 resists pasteurization and digestion by stomach enzymes and is well absorbed across the intestinal wall.

Still-unpublished Monsanto tests, disclosed by FDA in summary form in 1990, showed that statistically significant growth-stimulating effects were induced in organs of adult rats by feeding IGF-1 at the lowest dose levels for only two weeks. Drinking rBGH milk would thus be expected to increase blood IGF-1 levels and to increase risks of developing prostate cancer and promoting its invasiveness. Apart from prostate cancer, multiple lines of evidence have also incriminated the role of IGF-1 as risk factors for breast, colon, and childhood cancers.

Faced with such evidence, FDA should immediately withdraw its approval of rBGH milk, whose sale benefits only Monsanto while posing major public health risks for the entire U.S. population. Failing early FDA action, consumers should demand explicit labeling and only buy rBGH-free milk.

Monsanto's Hormonal Milk Poses Serious Risks of Breast Cancer, Besides Other Cancers

By Samuel S. Epstein, M.D.
Press Release
From Cancer Prevention Coalition
June 21, 1998

As reported in a May 9, 1998 article in *The Lancet,* women with a relatively small increase in blood levels of the naturally occurring growth hormone insulin-like Growth Factor-1 (IGF-1) are up to seven times more likely to develop premenopausal breast cancer than women with lower levels. Based on those results, the report concluded that the risks of elevated IGF-1 blood levels are among the leading known risk factors for breast cancer, and are exceeded only by a strong family history or unusual mammographic abnormalities. Apart from breast cancer, an accompanying editorial warned that elevated IGF-1 levels are also associated with greater than any known risk factors for other major cancers, particularly colon and prostate.

This latest evidence is not unexpected. Higher rates of breast, besides colon, cancer have been reported in patients with gigantism (acromagely) who have high IGF-1 blood levels. Other studies have also shown that administration of IGF-1 to elderly female primates causes marked breast enlargement and proliferation of breast tissue, that IGF-1 is a potent stimulator of human breast cells in tissue culture, that it blocks the programmed self-destruction of breast cancer cells, and enhances their growth and invasiveness.

These various reports, however, appear surprisingly unaware of the fact that the entire U.S. population is now exposed to high levels of IGF-1 in dairy products. In February 1995, the Food and Drug Administration approved the sale of unlabeled milk from cows injected with Monsanto's genetically engineered bovine growth hormone, rBGH, to increase milk production. As detailed in a January 1996 report in the prestigious *International Journal of Health Services,* rBGH milk differs from natural milk chemically, nutritionally, pharmacologically and immunologically, besides being contaminated with pus and antibiotics resulting from mastitis induced by the biotech hormone. More critically, rBGH milk is supercharged with high levels of abnormally potent IGF-1, up 10 times the levels in natural milk and over 10 times more potent. IGF-1 resists pasteurization and digestion by stomach enzymes, and is well absorbed across the intestinal wall. Still-unpublished 1987 Monsanto tests, disclosed by FDA in summary form in 1990, revealed that statistically significant growth stimulating effects were induced in organs of adult rats by feeding IGF-1 at low dose levels for only two weeks. Drinking rBGH milk would thus be expected to significantly increase IGF-1 blood levels and consequently to increase risks of developing breast cancer and promoting its invasiveness.

Faced with escalating rates of breast, besides colon, prostate and other avoidable cancers, FDA should withdraw its approval of rBGH milk, whose sale benefits only Monsanto while posing major public health risks for the entire U.S. population. A Congressional investigation of FDA's abdication of responsibility is well overdue.

Monsanto apparently has a lot to lose in the event that the American people learn the whole truth about the hazards of hormonal milk. The article below, by Sheldon Rampton and John Stauber, was published in **PR Watch** *(www.prwatch.org) in the summer of 1998. The story shows how Monsanto uses its considerable financial, legal, and political clout to control and contain the dissemination of information about rBGH milk.*

Monsanto and Fox: Partners in Censorship

By all accounts, Jane Akre and Steve Wilson are tough, bulldog reporters — the sort of journalists you'd expect to make some enemies along the way.

That, according to Florida TV station WTVT, was why it hired the husband-and-wife team with much fanfare in November 1996 to head the station's "news investigative unit." Now, in the wake of their firing barely a year later, the Fox network affiliate is accusing them of theft for daring to independently publish the script of the story that they were never allowed to air.

"This is really not about a couple of disgruntled former reporters whining that their editors wouldn't let them do a story they thought was important," Wilson said in announcing that he and Akre are suing WTVT for breach of contract. "Jane and I have each spent more than 20 years in the news business. . . . It doesn't take that long for every reporter to learn that every now and then — usually when the special interest of your news organization or one of its friends is more important than the public interest — stories get killed. That's bad enough, but that's *not* what happened here. . . . Fox 13 didn't want to *kill* the story revealing synthetic hormones in Florida's milk supply. Instead, as we explain in great detail in our legal complaint, we were repeatedly ordered to go forward and broadcast demonstrably inaccurate and dishonest versions of the story. We were given those instructions after some very high-level corporate lobbying by Monsanto (the powerful drug company that makes the hormone) and also, we believe, by members of Florida's dairy and grocery industries."

The hormone in question is genetically-engineered recombinant bovine growth hormone (rBGH), the flagship product in Monsanto's campaign to take command of the ultra-high-stakes biotechnology industry. Injections of rBGH (sold under the brand name Posilac®) induce higher milk production in dairy cows, but critics warn of potential health risks to both cows and humans.

The Florida dispute offers a rare look inside the newsroom at the way stories get spun and censored. It also cracks the facade that Monsanto has erected through a highly effective, multi-million-dollar PR offensive aimed at preventing the news media from reporting the views of rBGH critics.

The Dairy Coalition

Coordinated by the DC-based PR/lobby firm of Capitoline/MS&L, the pro-rBGH campaign brings together drug and dairy industry groups in an ad hoc network called the Dairy Coalition, whose participants include university researchers funded by Monsanto, as well as carefully selected "third party" experts; the International Food Information Council, an industry funded coalition that attacks health and safety concerns about food as unwarranted and unscientific; the National Association of State Departments of Agriculture, representing the top executive of every department of agriculture in all fifty states; the American Farm Bureau Federation, the powerful right-wing lobby behind the movement to pass food disparagement laws like the one under which Oprah Winfrey was sued in Texas; the American Dietetic Association, the national association of registered dietitians which hauls in large sums of money advocating for the food industry; the Grocery Manufacturers of America; the Food Marketing Institute; and other dairy and food associations at the state and regional levels.

Immediately after FDA approval of rBGH, attorneys for Monsanto sued or threatened to sue stores and dairy companies that sold milk and dairy products advertised as being free of rBGH, to make sure that any dissenters within the well-organized food industry would be frightened into toeing the industry line.

Extensive media monitoring and aggressive intervention and punishment of offending journalists has been critical to the media management campaign. As early as 1989 the PR firm of Carma International was hired to conduct a computer analysis of every story filed on rBGH, ranking reporters as friends or enemies. This information was used to reward friendly reporters while complaining to editors about those who filed reports that were deemed unfriendly.

Leaked internal documents from the Dairy Coalition reveal how journalists who do not toe the line are handled. In January of 1996 dairy officials wrote Mary Jane Wilkinson, assistant managing editor of the *Boston Globe*, to complain about an upcoming food column by *Globe* writer Linda Weltner. "On February 23rd, [Dr.] Samuel Epstein . . . made unsupported allegations linking milk and cancer. We're concerned that Ms. Weltner will give Epstein a forum in the *Boston Globe* to disseminate theories that have no basis in science." The letter invoked carefully cultivated contacts to smear Epstein as a scaremonger with "no standing among his peers in the scientific community and no credibility with the leading health organizations in this country." It noted that "others in the news media who attended Epstein's press conference or reviewed his study — such as *The Wall Street Journal, The New York Times* and the *Washington Post* — chose not to run this 'story.' . . . *USA Today* was the only newspaper to print these allegations and we recently held a heated meeting with them."

Another internal dairy industry document bragged about the handling of *USA Today* health reporter Anita Manning, whose balanced article on the subject offended the rBGH lobbyists. "On Wednesday representatives of the Dairy Coalition met with reporter Anita Manning and her editor at *USA Today.* When Manning said that Epstein was a credible source, the Dairy Coalition's Dr. Wayne Callaway pointed out that Epstein has no standing among the scientific community. . . . When Manning insisted it was her responsibility to tell both sides of the story, Callaway said that was just a cop-out for not doing her homework. She was told that if she had attended the press conference, instead of writing the story from a press release, she would have learned that her peers from the *Washington Post, The New York Times, The Wall Street Journal,* and the Associated Press chose not to do the story because of the source. At this point Manning left the meeting and her editor assured the Dairy Coalition that any future stories dealing with [rBGH] and health would be closely scrutinized."

A February 1996 internal document of the Dairy Coalition notes that "The Coalition is convinced its work in educating reporters and editors at *The New York Times, The Wall Street Journal,* the *Washington Post,* and the Associated Press led to those organizations' dismissal of Samuel Epstein's pronouncements that milk from [rBGH] supplemented cows causes breast and colon cancer. They did not run the story."

The same document brags of knocking prominent *New York Times* food reporter Marian Burros off the beat entirely: "As you may recall, the Dairy Coalition worked hard with *The New York Times* last year to keep Marian Burros, a very anti-industry reporter, from 'breaking' Samuel Epstein's claim that milk from . . . supplemented cows causes breast and colon cancer. She did not do the story and now *The New York Times* health reporters are the ones on the [rBGH] beat. They do not believe Epstein. Marian Burros is not happy about the situation."

Given this climate of systematic intimidation and capitulation by news media management, the remarkable fact about the case in Florida is not that the story was killed. What makes this case unique is the dogged persistence that Akre and Wilson have shown in standing by their story.

The Deal That Soured

Steve Wilson is an Emmy award-winning former top investigative reporter for the TV news program "Inside Edition." His past work has produced stories that forced two recalls of faulty door latches in Chrysler minivans and exposed ABC news anchor Sam Donaldson's moves to accept farming subsidies while criticizing them on the air. *Washington Post*

media critic Howard Kurtz calls Wilson "a dogged and careful investigator" with a "high-decibel level of journalism." Jane Akre has been a reporter and news anchor for 20 years and has won a prestigious Associated Press award for investigative reporting.

The couple's contract with the station stipulated that Akre would be paid $149,500 over two years to file short investigative pieces every few days and anchor the station's weekend morning newscasts. Wilson's contract offered $85,500 for 10 hours of work per week on larger stories that would be timed for the all-important "sweeps" rating periods.

At the time of their hiring, it seemed like a good deal for all concerned. Akre had recently given birth to the couple's first child, and Wilson hoped signing up with a local station would give him the chance to spend more time at home and less on the road. "Jane and Steve, quite frankly, were only interested in a package deal . . . which suited me. They're both talented individuals who happen to be married," explained news director Daniel Webster.

A few months after their hiring, however, Webster was shown the door as part of a management shake-up following a $2.5 billion package deal in which WTVT and nine other stations were sold to the Fox network. By then, Webster had already given Wilson and Akre the editorial go-ahead for their first big investigative piece — an exposé about possible health risks of rBGH-treated milk, which also provided solid documentation of numerous disturbing facts about Monsanto and its product:

- Posilac® was never properly tested before FDA allowed it on the market. A standard cancer test of a new human drug requires two years of testing with several hundred rats. But rBGH was tested for only 90 days on 30 rats. Worse, the study has never been published, and the U.S. Food and Drug Administration has refused to allow open scientific peer review of the study's raw data.

• Some Florida dairy herds grew sick shortly after starting rBGH treatment. One farmer, Charles Knight — who lost 75% of his herd — says that Monsanto and Monsanto-funded researchers at University of Florida withheld from him the information that other dairy herds were suffering similar problems.

• Interviewed on camera, Florida dairy officials and scientists refuted Monsanto's claim that every truckload of milk from rBGH-treated cows is tested for excessive antibiotics.

• Also on camera, Canadian government officials described what they called an attempt at bribery by Monsanto, which offered $1 to $2 million to gain rBGH approval in Canada.

• A visit by Akre to seven randomly-selected Florida dairy farms found that all seven were injecting their cows with the hormone. Wilson and Akre also visited area supermarket chains, which two years previously had promised to ask their milk suppliers not to use rBGH in response to consumer concerns. In reality, store representatives admitted that they have taken no steps to assure compliance with this request.

• Finally, the story dwelt heavily on concerns raised by scientists such as Epstein and Consumers Union researcher Michael Hansen about potential cancer risks associated with "insulin-like growth factor-1" (IGF-1). Treatments of rBGH lead to significantly increased levels of IGF-1 in milk, and recent studies suggest IGF-1 is a powerful tumor growth promoter.

Sudden Death

The resulting story, a four-part series, was cleared by management and scheduled to be-

gin airing on Monday, February 24, 1997. As part of the buildup to network ratings sweeps, the story was already being heavily promoted in radio ads when an ominous letter arrived at the office of Fox News chairman Roger Ailes, the former Republican political operative who now heads Rupert Murdoch's Fox network news. The letter came from John J. Walsh, a powerful New York attorney with the firm of Cadwalader, Wickersham & Taft, who accused the reporters of bias and urged the network to delay the story in order to ensure "a more level playing field" for Monsanto's side of the story. "There is a lot at stake in what is going on in Florida, not only for Monsanto but also for Fox News and its owner," Walsh wrote.

"Monsanto hired one of the most renowned lawyers in America to use his power and influence," Wilson says. "Even though our stories had been scheduled to run, even though Fox had bought expensive radio ads to alert viewers to the story, it was abruptly cancelled on the eve of the broadcasts within hours of receiving the letter from Monsanto's lawyer."

Initially, the story was postponed for a week, during which station editors and lawyers fine-combed the story but could find no inaccuracies. Akre and Wilson also offered to do a further interview with Monsanto and supplied a list of topics to be discussed. In response, Walsh fired back an even more threatening letter: "It simply defies credulity that an experienced journalist would expect a representative of any company to go on camera and respond to the vague, undetailed — and for the most part accusatory — points listed by Ms. Akre. Indeed, some of the points clearly contain the elements of defamatory statements which, if repeated in a broadcast, could lead to serious damage to Monsanto and dire consequences for Fox News."

What followed next, according to Wilson and Akre, was a grueling nightmare of perpetual delays and station-mandated rewrites — 73 in all, none of which proved satisfactory to station management. "No fewer than six airdates were set and cancelled," Wilson recalls. "In all my years as a print and radio and local and national television reporter, I've never seen anything like it."

At one point, their lawsuit claims, WTVT general manager David Boylan told them he "wasn't interested" in looking at the story himself and pressured them to follow the company lawyer's directions, adding, "Are you sure this is a hill you're willing to die on?" On another occasion, Boylan allegedly told them, "We paid $3 billion for these television stations. We will decide what the news is. The news is what we tell you it is." Boylan then notified them they would be fired for insubordination within 48 hours and another reporter would make the requested changes.

"When we said we'd file a formal complaint with the FCC if that happened," notes Wilson, "we were not fired but were each offered very large cash settlements to go away and keep quiet about the story and how it was handled." The reporters refused the settlement, which amounted to nearly $200,000, and ultimately were fired in December 1997.

The Perfect Case

Notwithstanding the dramatic issues and allegations at stake for reporters everywhere, the lawsuit has generated almost no national media attention and only a few stories in the Florida press — most of which are couched in timid "he said, she said" language that is sure to please Monsanto. One editorialist could not resist putting quotation marks around the word "facts" in discussing the case: "The 'facts' at issue were as slippery as a just-milked cow. . . . And the lines between advocacy, truth, integrity, and insubordination thin to pencil width when an expensive lawsuit's in the offing."

"Is this an example of local TV's growing reluctance to air hard-hitting investigative news pieces?" asked Eric Deggans of the *St. Petersburg Times* before concluding that "The truth, as always, lies somewhere in the middle." After examining "the personality conflicts and lack of definitive scientific evidence" about rBGH, Deggans concludes that "Wilson's and Akre's case may not be the perfect example to illustrate the trend of increasingly irrelevant reporting in TV news."

Actually, the case *is* a perfect example to illustrate that trend. In fact, Deggan's response to the case shows how corporate interests have succeeded in dramatically shifting the terms of acceptability in journalistic discourse.

Good journalism — in particular, good *investigative* journalism — is almost always controversial and accompanied by "personality conflicts." In dealing with technologically novel products like genetically-engineered hormones, "lack of definitive scientific evidence" is part of what makes the story controversial.

"Is there smoking-gun, ironclad evidence available today that drinking milk from hormone-treated cows will lead to cancer in you or your children?" asks Wilson. "No. Many scientists will tell you because this is a drug injected into animals and not directly into humans the testing of its effects on milk-drinkers has never been thorough enough to know for sure. But ask yourselves this: how long did it take us all to learn about the effects of tobacco while the special interests insisted there was no evidence of any harm? Was it wrong to raise those issues before the link was indisputable? Or how about Agent Orange, dioxin, PCBs — all Monsanto products, by the way, all approved by the government, sworn by Monsanto to be safe. Was it wrong to raise those issues before we knew for certain?"

In reality, journalistic reluctance to discuss hypothetical, as-yet unproven health risks is driven more by fear of corporate lawsuits than by a desire to be "responsible." One such lawsuit by the Food Lion grocery store chain resulted in a $5.5 million judgment against

ABC-TV in January 1997 — just one month prior to Monsanto's threatening letter aimed at killing the Akre-Wilson story. It was a verdict that Monsanto's attorney made sure to mention in his letter to Roger Ailes. "What has Monsanto concerned . . . is the assault on their integrity . . . blatantly carried on by Ms. Akre and Mr. Wilson," Walsh wrote. "In the aftermath of the Food Lion verdict, such behavior would alone be cause for concern."

"A lot of people now are more fearful of doing investigative journalism since Food Lion . . . which is why we have so many lawyers involved," admits Phil Metlin, who took over as WTVT's news director in July 1997. "We have to be careful . . . and prudent."

The result, of course, has been that attorneys rather than reporters are empowered to make journalistic decisions.

For its part, WTVT insists that this system of institutional self-censorship must be defended in order to avoid "chilling the give-and-take essential in any newsroom in getting the news on the air in a timely and responsible manner." In legal court filings, the station insists that its "editorial discretion and judgment should not and cannot be the subject of second-guessing by a judge or jury, consistent with the First Amendment."

WTVT also objects to the fact that Akre and Wilson "conducted two press conferences the day they filed their suit" and "have also created a web site to publicize their issues, where they have posted the complaint and exhibits and where they are soliciting public comments." Worse yet, the web site includes two complete scripts of their controversial rBGH report — one version showing how they wanted to write the story, and the other showing how the network wanted it edited. Neither version has ever aired. In fact, its filings in court claim that by posting the scripts on their web site, Akre and Wilson "have misappropriated . . . property. . . . This misconduct by Plaintiffs is in itself a material and serious breach of the employment agreements

[and] amounts to theft."

Theft it may be, in some strange legal sense, but Akre and Wilson don't care at this point. "I am risking my career by doing this, and I will probably never work in television again," Wilson said, "But we wanted to get this story out."

"As a mother, I know this is important information about a basic food I've been giving my child every day," Akre said. "As a journalist, I know it is a story that millions of Floridians have a right to know. The television station we worked for promised the story would be told. Instead, we spent nearly a year struggling to tell it honestly and accurately, and four months after we were fired for standing up for the truth, the station has done nothing but continue to keep this important news secret. It is not right for the station to withhold this important health information, and solely as a matter of conscience we will not aid and abet their effort to cover this up any longer. Every parent and every consumer has the right to know what they're pouring on their children's morning cereal."

In May 1998, a month after Wilson and Akre filed suit, the station aired an rBGH story by the investigative reporter who was hired to replace them. His story, predictably, omitted many of their criticisms of Monsanto.

A version of this article appeared in the June 1998 issue of The Progressive *magazine. Further information about the Akre-Wilson lawsuit is available on their web site at <http://www.foxBGHsuit.com>.*

Summary of Scientific Evidence on the Hazards of rBGH Milk 1985-1998

A. Adverse Veterinary Effects

Eppard *et al*, **Unpublished "Confidential" Monsanto Report, January 13, 1987**

"Small, multifocal adhesions were scattered in 16 of 33 cows administered (CP11-5099-F (rBGH), while none were observed in the six control cows. The adhesions were associated with chronic pleuritis, chronic pericarditis, hyperplasia of pericardial membranes, epicardial fibrosis and/or villus hyperplasia of visceral pleura." Leakage of this report prompted Cong. J. Conyers (D. Michigan), Chairman of The House Committee on Government Operations, to charge Monsanto and FDA with "abdication of regulatory responsibility (as they) have chosen to suppress and manipulate animal health data, in efforts to approve commercial use of rBGH."

Monsanto, 1993

The Package Insert for Posilac (rBGH) lists over 20 toxic effects. These include mastitis, injection site reactions, bloat and other digestive disorders, retained placenta and other uterine disorders, enlarged hocks, foot disorders, and the need for medication for such toxic effects.

FDA Freedom of Information Summary for POSILAC, 1994

"The relative risk of a treated animal showing signs of clinical mastitis during the treatment period was about 1.79 times that of a control animal."

Kronfeld, J. Am. Vet. Med. Ass. 204,116-130,1994

In the Monsanto toxicity study (Eppard *et al*, 1987), "the frequency of renal, pulmonary, mammary gland and joint lesions is related linearly to rBGH use up to 5 times the approved dose."

Willeburg, J. Am. Vet. Med. Ass. 204, 538-541, 1994

"The result of introducing rBGH will be an increase in incidence of mastitis in the dairy cattle population, the health of dairy cows will be at risk, and doubts about the welfare aspect have caused the European Commission to delay its decision."

B. Misrepresentation of Adverse Veterinary Effects by Industry and Indentured Scientists

1. Animal Welfare

Monsanto's rBGH-drug, Posilac, has over 20 toxic effects listed on its label. At least nine are painful and disabling diseases. Use of this drug is thus inhumane. (Willeburg, Livestock Production Science 36:55, 1993; Willeburg, J. Am. Vet. Assn., 205:538-541, 1994).

FDA's approval of Posilac was based partly on the assumption that Posilac-induced mastitis is manageable. However, no experimental basis for this hypothesis has ever been reported. Moreover, a peer-reviewed scientific publication concluded that current preventive medical methods would probably be ineffective (Kronfeld, J. Am. Vet. Med. Assn., 204:116-130, 1994). Statistical analysis of the FDA's mastitis data has further confirmed this conclusion (Kronfeld, Am. Coll. Vet. Int. Med., Forum 12:632-684, 1994).

2. Scientific Misrepresentation

Documents released in 1994 (Posilac Labeling: FDA Freedom of Information summary; White *et al.*, J. Dairy Science, 77:2249-2260, 1994) disclosed previous false denials of adverse health effects of rBGH. Illustrative was a large-scale outbreak of mastitis in rBGH-treated cows at Cornell University. Four of 42 control cows, in contrast with 14 of 42 rBGH-treated cows, developed mastitis. This statistically significant observation was at first trivialized: "Health variables were not affected by treatment" (Bauman *et al.* J. Dairy Sci. 71:205, 1988), and then clearly misrepresented: "No adverse health effects were observed . . . animals were in good health throughout the study" (Bauman *et al.* J. Dairy Sci. 72:642-651, 1989). These false denials of rBGH-induced mastitis have been repeated elsewhere.

3. Distortion of Public Policy

Dale E. Bauman is an endowed professor at Cornell University, and consultant to Monsanto Company and the U.S. Congress Office of Technology Assessment (OTA). He authored the biologic basis for the OTA's economic predictions for rBGH(1991) as follows: "Catastrophic effects such as . . . mastitis have been postulated to occur. However, no such effects have been observed in any scientifically valid public health studies" (OTA, Special Report, F-470, 1991).

This industry consultant also had substantial input into a USDA economic study in 1987. Claiming no adverse effects, the study recommended approval of rBGH to help American farmers be competitive in a global market. Also, Bauman's allegation that there are no adverse effects of rBGH on animal welfare was accepted by the White House (1994).

Thus, U.S. public policy on rBGH has been misled by the indentured scientific literature. This mischaracterization or suppression of evidence on serious adverse health effects has misled Federal agencies, such as the USDA and OTA, and heavily pressured the FDA to approve rBGH.

C. Major Differences Between rBGH and Natural Milk (apart from IGF-1)

Bauman et al, J. Dairy Sci. 68:1352-1362, 1985

Monsanto's rBGH stimulated twice the increase in milk yield than an equal dose of BGH.

USAN & the USP Dictionary of Drug Names, page 510, 1988

Sometribove is "methionyl growth hormone (ox)." This alternative name revealed that Monsanto's rBGH does not have a natural amino acid sequence, but instead, has an extra methionine at the 191-position, which reflects manufacture by genetically altered bacteria rather than by the cow.

Baer et al, J. Dairy Sci. 72:1424-1434, 1989

In milk from untreated and rBGH treated cows, "serum protein (.65, 71 %) and lactose (4.7, 4.80%) were higher, and casein as a percent of true protein (80.2, 78.8%) was lower, with the somatotropin treatment. Proportions of short-chain (11.6, 10.5%) and medium-chain fatty acids (58.6, 56.0%) were reduced and long-chain fatty acids increased (26.9, 30.4%) for control and somatotropin milks, respectively."

Capuco, et al, J. Endocrinol. 121:205-211, 1989

Mammary activity of an enzyme, thyroxine-5'-monodeiodinase, which converts the hormone thyroxine to a more active form tri-iodothyronine, is doubled by rBGH treatment. Both hormones are present in normal milk, and the increased enzyme activity suggests that more tri-iodothyronine will be present in rBGH milk. The effects of tri-iodothyronine in rBGH milk on the thyroid status of human consumers needs serious investigation.

Food and Drug Administration, G. B. Guest Director for Veterinary Medicine, Letter to Senator W. P. Winkle, State Capitol, Madison, Wisc., May 9, 1989.

FDA admitted that rBGH is "about 0.5 to 3 percent different in molecular structure" from the natural hormone.

Epstein, International Journal Health Services, 20:73-84, 1990

. . . "it is clear that the hormones induce a wide range of measurable changes in milk composition. Increased fat yields and concentrations have been noted. Additionally, there is a statistically significant increase in long-chain fatty acids and decrease in short-chain fatty acids; this is associated with reduction in casein, in relation to both total and true protein, which is likely to decrease cheese yields."

Kronfeld, J. Am. Med. Assn. 265:1389, 1991

"Significant dose-response relationships

indicate that the concentration of methionyl-rBST in milk of cows treated with methionyl-rBST is raised progressively above the zero concentration of methionyl-rbST in milk of untreated cows."

Kronfeld, Science, 251:256,1991

Cited a 1987 Monsanto toxicology report to the FDA which listed 9 drugs used as therapy for illness and infertility in rBGH-treated cows that are not approved by the FDA for lactating cows. The use of unapproved drugs is likely to escape detection in routine screening of milk for drug residues, ". . . thus adverse effects of rBGH on the cow's health and fertility could indirectly affect human health through secondary drugs entering milk." This proposal of indirect human health risks posed by the increased use of medication, especially unapproved antibiotics to control extra illness induced by rBGH in cows, was subsequently endorsed by the U.S. General Accounting Office (1992), which regards the milk monitoring system as ineffective, but it was rejected by the FDA (1993), which regards the milk monitoring system as effective and which expects farmers to use all drugs legally.

Eppard *et al*, (Monsanto), J. Endocrinol. 132:47-59, 1992

rBGH is more potent than BGH in increasing milk yields of lactating cows.

Mepham, J. Royal Soc. Med. 85:736-739,1992

"Milk fat concentrations increase and those of protein decline. . . . there are reports of increases up to 27% in the concentration of long-chain fatty acids. . . . mean values seem likely to change in directions detrimental to the nutritional quality of milk . . . health risks to individual consumers . . . would thus depend on how much of the milk consumed was from cows treated with BST."

Harbour *et al*, Techniques in Protein Chemistry 111:487-495, 1992

This study demonstrated further deviations of rBGH from natural amino acid sequences, namely the presence of N-epsilon-acetyl groups attached to lysine at various positions. Monsanto's rBGH is 191-methionyl-144-N-epsilon-acetyl-BGH (Violand *et al*. Protein Science 3:1089-4 097, 1994); it is chemically different from any of the natural variants of BGH.

Toutain *et al*, J. Animal Sci. 71:1219-1225, 1993

Several dose-dependent pharmacokinetic parameters differ significantly between bacteria-made rBGH and cow-made BGH. rBGH thus differs pharmacologically from BGH.

Monsanto, 1993, Posilac Package Insert

The packing insert for Posilac (rBGH) states: "The use of Posilac is associated with increased frequency of use of medication in cows for mastitis and other health problems."

Erhard *et al*, J. Immunoassay 15:1-19,1994

This study demonstrated that methionyl-rBGH is immunologically different from natural BGH; however a specific assay for rBGH has not yet been required by the FDA. This finding also raises the possibility of immune interactions between human growth hormone and rBGH.

Kessler Federal Register 59(28):6279-6280, 1994

The FDA stated that there is "no significant difference" between the milks of rBGH treated and untreated cows. However, numerous statistically significant differences have been reported in the composition of rBGH milk compared to controls.

Millstone *et al*, Nature 371-647-648, 1994

Milk from rBGH treated cows contains significantly more somatic cells (dispersed pus cells), which reflect the bacteria present in the mammary gland. High somatic cell counts are regarded as unwholesome, and both American and European authorities are striving to lower somatic cell counts in milk to make it more wholesome and to protect public health.

Conclusion

rBGH milk thus differs from natural milk nutritionally, pharmacologically, immunologically and hormonally. It is also contaminated by rBGH, which differs chemically from BGH levels, by a thyroid hormone enzyme, and often by pus and antibiotics, besides by increased levels of IGF-1.

D. Increased IGF-1 LEVELS in rBGH Milk
Prosser, Lancet 1:1201, 1988

IGF-1 levels in rBGH milk are increased up to 20 fold.

Juskevich & Geyer, (FDA), Science 249: 875-884, 1990

Based on six unpublished industry studies, FDA admitted that IGF-1 levels in rBGH milk were consistently increased and that these increases were statistically significant. These levels were still further increased following pasteurization.

National Institutes of Health, Technology Assessment Conference Statement on Bovine Somatotropin, JAMA 265: 1423-1425, 1991

IGF-1 levels in rBGH milk are increased up to 8.5 fold; levels are also increased in meat.

Joint FAO/WHO Expert Committee on Food Additives, Fortieth Report, Geneva. June 9-18, 1992

Cited six unpublished industries studies confirming increased IGF-1 levels in rBGH milk. These included one by Monsanto (Schams *et al*, 1988) reporting a four-fold increase, and another (Miller *et al*. 1989) reporting a further 50% increase following pasteurization.

Mepham, Journal Royal Soc. Med. 85:736-739, 1992

Increased levels of IGF-1 in rBGH milk are probably underestimated because of flawed and analytical techniques. Also, the IGF-1 may be more potent than normal as it is not bound to milk proteins. Furthermore, some IGF-1 is likely to exist in modified (truncated) form; this is underestimated by four-fold in standard measurements and is ten times more potent than normal IGF-1. (This may result in a forty-fold underestimate of IGF-1 levels in rBGH milk.)

Mepham *et al*, The Lancet 2:197,1994

In their 1993 European marketing application, Lilly admitted that IGF-1 levels in rBGH milk could be increased by more than ten-fold.

Mepham & Schofield, International Dairy Federation Nutrition Week, Paris, June 1995

"There seems to be no doubt that the concentration of IGF-1 in milk is increased by rBGH treatment although the extent of increase appears variable."

Epstein, International Journal of Health Services 261:173-185, 1996

Details evidence of major increases of IGF-1 levels, besides its increased potency, in rBGH milk.

E. Public Health Hazards from Increased IGF-1 Levels in rBGH Milk (apart from cancer)

Prosser *et al*, J. Endocrinol. 112:65, 1987

"The implications of IGF-1 in milk for the human infant cannot be determined until we know more about the activity and function of milk IGF-1 in the newborn."

McBride *et al*, Res. Dev. Agricult. 5:1-21,1988

"Investigation of IGF-1 requires attention, particularly where animal health and food residues are concerned since they possess many biological activities and are immunologically and biologically similar among species . . . Some concerns arise as to the possibility of abnormal levels of IGF-1 in the milk of BGH-treated cows and, with it, consumer health."

Epstein, Int. J. Health Serv. 20:73-84, 1990

Adverse effects of increased IGF-1 levels in rBGH milk "could include premature growth stimulation in infants."

Juskevich & Geyer, (FDA), Science 249:375-83,1990

FDA reported summaries of still unpublished (1983 Monsanto toxicity tests) on IGF-1. Oral administration of IGF-1 to mature rats for only two weeks induced statistically significant evidence of growth-promoting (mitogenic) effects even at the lowest doses tested. Nevertheless, FDA relies on these tests in its claim that IGF-1 is "orally inactive."

American Medical Association, Council on Scientific Affairs, Biotechnology and the American Agriculture Industry, JAMA 265:1429-1436, 1991

"Further studies will be required to determine whether the ingestion of higher than normal concentrations of bovine insulin-like growth factor is safe for children, adolescents and adults."

National Institutes of Health, Technology Assessment Conference on Bovine Somatotropin, JAMA 265:1423-1425, 1991

"Milk from rBST-treated cows contains higher concentrations of IGF-1. The importance of the increased amounts of IGF-1 in milk from rBST-treated cows is uncertain."

Mepham, Journal Royal. Soc. Med. 85:736-739, 1992

"It would be imprudent to assume that the increased concentration of IGF-1 in milk rBST-treated cows presents no risks to human health." Based on conservative assumptions, infants drinking rBGH milk would be exposed to levels of IGF-1 substantially in excess of recommended safety margins de-

rived from 1988 Monsanto oral toxicity tests published in summary form by FDA (Juskevich & Geyer) in 1990.

Lasmezas *et al*, Biochem, Biophys. Res. Comm., 196:1163-1169, 1993

IGF-1 induced a dose-dependent increased expression of the protein prion gene (PrP) in cultured rat neuroblastoma (PC12) cells. PrP is "a housekeeping gene which is responsible for susceptibility to transmissible spongiform encephalopathies." This study raises unresolved questions on the possible effects of increased IGF-1 levels on susceptibility to bovine (BSE) and human prion disease (CJD).

Mepham *et al*, The Lancet 2:197, 1994

"We believe that the safety of rBST-milk has not been established with adequate scientific rigor because of possibly adverse effects of substantially increased concentrations of Insulin-like Growth Factor-1 (IGF-1) in the milk of rBST treated cows.

Graefe zu Baringdorf, Friederich-Wilhelm, Letter to FDA Commissioner David Kessler, December 7, 1994

"We feel fairly confident in being able to demonstrate that the safety of European citizens who consume rBST products cannot be guaranteed. More and more scientific evidence, such as the recent pieces in the British medical journal *The Lancet*, is accumulating to support this position."

Geier *et al*, Cancer Invest.13:480-486, 1995

The authors reported that IGF-1 specifically inhibited the lethal effects of different anti-cancer drugs on cultured human breast cancer cells. This suggests that IGF-1 is involved in the development of drug resistance "a major obstacle to the ultimate success of cancer therapy."

Resnicoff *et al*, Cancer Res. 55:2463-2469, 1995

The authors reported that IGF-1, interacting with its receptor, is highly protective against programmed cell death (apoptosis) of human and cancer cells in biodiffusion chambers in vivo. The practical implication of these findings was stressed. "The rate of cell death is an important determinant of tumor growth, and the extent of apoptosis could have a profound effect on the aggressiveness of a tumor." Anti-apoptotic effects could thus stimulate the growth and invasiveness of latent cancers.

Mepham & Schofield, International Dairy Federation Nutrition Week, Paris. June 1995

"It is recommended that the safety of milk and milk products from cows treated with BST be reexamined in the light of recent reports which suggest that insulin-like growth factor-1 (IGF-1) in such milk is both bioactive in intestinal tissues and protected from degradation by casein in milk. . . . It is a matter of concern that were BST use to result in widespread milk avoidance, there might be significant adverse effects on public health."

Xian *et al*, J. Endocrinol., 146:215-225, 1995

Casein, the major milk protein, is highly effective in protecting IGF-1 from intestinal digestion, and preserving receptor binding activity in stomach and duodenal fluid in the presence of casein. (In striking contrast, salivary IGF-1 could be rapidly digested).

Epstein, International Journal Health Services. 26:173-185, 1996

Based on conservative estimates, an infant consuming rBGH milk would be exposed to IGF-1 levels over 100-fold in excess of standard safety margins, which would double its normal blood level over the course of one day. Furthermore, the extra IGF-1 could be up to 40 times more potent.

Schofield & Mepham, International Dairy Federation Conference, Johannesburg, South Africa, October 23,1996

"It is now clear that the main action of the IGFs in transformation is through the inhibition of apoptosis induced by primary oncogenic mutations. . . ."

Hansen *et al*, Consumers Union Report to the FAO/WHO Joint Expert Committee on Food Additives, September 1987.

Summarizes evidence on public health hazards of excess IGF-1 levels in rBGH milk with regard to: excess antibiotic levels in milk and antibiotic resistance; colon, breast, pediatric and other cancers; and potentially increased risk of human prion disease (CJD).

F. rBGH Milk is a Breast Cancer Risk Factor

Furlanetto & DiCarlo, Cancer Res. 44:2122-2128,1984

IGF-1 induces highly potent stimulatory (mitogenic) effects in cultured human breast cells. Furthermore, IGF-1 binds to specific surface receptors of these cells.

Pines *et al*, Gastroenterol., 80:266-269, 1985

An "enhanced risk" of breast cancer (SIR=3.5), besides a statistically significant increase in gastrointestinal cancers, was reported among a small group of acromegalics.

Glimm *et al*, J. Dairy Sci. 71:2923-2935, 1988

Administration of rBGH to cows results in increased blood levels of IGF-1, and its uptake and heavy concentration in mammary epithelial cells.

Reynolds *et al*, Gynecol. Oncol. 38:396-406, 1990

IGF-1 plasma concentrations are higher in breast cancer patients than in healthy controls. "Even if there is no direct evidence that elevated plasma levels of IGF-1 reflect elevated levels of growth factor at the tumor level, the possibility exists that increased levels of circulating IGF-1 may contribute to breast tumor growth."

Lipman, J., National, Inst. Health Res. 3:59-62, 1991

IGF-1 and related growth factors are critically involved in the development of breast cancer and maintaining its invasiveness.

Rosen *et al*, Breast Cancer Res. Treat. 18(Suppl.):555-562, 1991

IGF-1 is a potent regulator of cultured human breast cancer cells.

Harris *et al*, New Engl. J. Med., 7:473-480,1992

"It now appears highly likely that a series of growth factors are responsible, at least in part, for the evolution of normal breast epithelia to breast cancer, and that breast cancer cells maintain their malignant phenotype as a result of the effects of these growth factors. These factors include the insulin-like growth factor."

Pollak *et al*, Breast Cancer Res. Treat 22:91-100, 1992

IGF-1 is more mitogenic to breast cells than the highly potent and carcinogenic estradiol. (While distinct from carcinogenesis, mitogenesis is likely to promote malignant transformation induced by estradiol.)

Lippman, Science 259:631-632,1993

"A number of proteins have been shown to participate in aberrant growth of breast cancer cells. These proteins include several families of cell surface growth factor receptors (including) the IGF-1 family."

Pappa *et al*, Cancer Res. 53:3736-3740, 1993

". . . plasma IGF-1 concentrations are higher in primary breast cancer patients . . . the possibility exists that increased levels of circulating IGF-1 may contribute to breast tumor growth." Furthermore, levels of IGF-1 breast cell receptors are some ten-fold higher in cancer than normal cells.

LeRoith, D., Ann. Int. Med. 122:54-59,1995

In a summary of information presented at a 2/23/94 NIH Conference on IGF-1, it was concluded: "IGF's are important mitogens in many types of malignancies. IGFs are likely to be involved in breast cancer at the level of tumor growth and perhaps at the level of initial development and later metastases."

Epstein, International Journal of Health Services 26l:173-185, 1996

Documents a wide range of converging lines of evidence strongly incriminating excess IGF-1 levels in rBGH milk as a risk factor for breast cancer.

Orme *et al*, J. Endocrinol. Suppl. No., OC22, June 1996

Based on a retrospective study of some 1400 acromegalics in 15 British centers, a statistically significant excess of breast cancer mortality, and also of colon and overall cancer mortality, was reported.

Schofield & Mepham, International Dairy Federation Conference, Johannesburg, South Africa, October 23, 1996

"High levels of circulating IGF seem to be predisposing for the generation of breast cancer, but it is unclear whether this reflects a direct effect." However, contrary to explicit evidence on the systemic effects following oral administration of IGF-1 to adult rats (Juskevich & Geyer, 1990), the authors stated that "quantitative considerations based on the uptake of IGF-1 from the gut into the circulation also indicate minimal risk." Furthermore, the authors appear surprisingly unaware of epidemiological evidence on the increased incidence of breast cancer in acromegalics.

NG *et al*, Nature Medicine 3:1141-1144, 1997

Dosing aged monkeys with IGF-1, over a broad range of concentrations extending down to the physiological, induced a highly significant increase in breast size and potent mitogenic effects an mammary epithelia. The authors warned of risks of breast cancer from treating postmenopausal women with IGF-1 or growth hormone, which acts by increasing IGF-1 levels, to delay the effects of aging.

Hankinson *et al,* The Lancet 351:1393-1396, 1998

In a prospective study of 300 healthy nurses, those with elevated IGF-1 blood levels, about 10% in excess of controls, were shown to be strongly associated with up to a 7-fold subsequent risk of premenopausal breast cancer. This risk factor appears greater than most others with the exception of a strong family history.

G. rBGH Milk Is a Colon Cancer Risk Factor

Pines *et al,* Gastroenterol. 80:266-269, 1985

A statistically significant increased incidence of gastrointestinal cancers was reported among a group of 48 acromegalics. Additionally, an "enhanced risk" of breast cancer was observed (SIR=3.5).

National Institutes of Health. Technology Assessment Conference Statement on Bovine Somatotropin. JAMA 265:1423-1425, 1991

"Whether the additional amount of IGF-1 from (rBGH) cows has a local effect in the esophagus, stomach or intestines is unknown."

Olanrewaju *et al,* Am. J. Physiol. 263: E282-E286, 1992

Infusion of IGF-1 into the intestine of rats at concentrations equivalent to those found in rBGH milk markedly increased the cellularity of mucosal cells.

Lamm, *et al,* Brit. J. Cancer 65:41-42, 1992

IGF-1 was shown to have potent mitogenic effects on 5 of 8 human colon cancer cell lines.

Sleisenger & Fordtran, eds. Gastrointestinal Disease, p. 1412, W. B. Saunders, Philadelphia, 1993

"Patients with acromegaly seem to have an increased tendency to develop colon cancers and adenomas. Although these studies inherently involve few subjects, consistently high prevalence rates of 6.3 to 25 percent for colon cancer and 14 to 35 percent for adenomatous polyps were observed in acromegalics."

Burton *et al,* Can. J. Animal Sci. 74:167-201, 1994

Based on evidence including the presence of specific IGF-1 receptors in intestinal epithelial cells and the stimulation of enzymes of these cells by IGF-1 at levels 1/1000 below those claimed inactive by the FDA, the authors concluded: "It could be considered an oversight (for the FDA) to suggest, that ingested IGF-1 is inactive. . . . Many more potential effects of ingested IGF-1 on the gastrointestinal tract and the local immune system of the gut need to be explored."

Challacombe & Wheeler, The Lancet 344:815-816, 1994

"The combination of IGF-1 in BST milk and IGF-1 normally excreted into the human gastrointestinal lumen would augment . . . concentrations of this hormone, increasing the possibility of local mitogenic effects on gut tissues."

Chaurasia *et al,* Regul. Pept. 50:113-119, 1994

"Since the growth factor is not protein-bound, its concentration in gut lumen may be high enough to exert biological activity."

Donovan & Odle, Annual Review Nutrition 14:147-167, 1994

"Studies suggest that orally administered IGF-1 at least partially survives digestion, binds to the GI tract . . . and may stimulate cell proliferation. In addition, IGF-1 can be absorbed into the blood, where it may effect the secretion of other hormones."

Juul *et al,* Clin. Endocrinol. 41:85-93, 1994

Blood levels of IGF-1 are significantly elevated in patients with gigantism (acromegaly) due to anterior pituitary tumors or hyperplasia.

Tremble & McGregor, In Treating Acromegaly, ed. Wass, pp. 5-12, Journal of Endocrinology Ltd., Bristol, England, 1994.

Increased rates of pre-cancerous polyps and colon cancer have been reported in acromegalics in whom levels of IGF-1 are significantly elevated.

Epstein, S. S., International Journal Health Services 26l:173-185, 1996

Documents a wide range of converging lines of evidence strongly incriminating excess IGF-1 levels in rBGH milk as a risk factor for colon cancer.

Orme *et al*, Endocrinol. Supp. No., OC22, June 1996

Based on a retrospective study of some 1400 acromegalics in 15 British centers, a statistically significant excess incidence and mortality of colon cancer, and also of overall and breast cancer mortality, was reported.

Wheeler & Challacombe, Gut. In Press 1996

IGF-1, and to a lesser extent Human Growth Hormone (HGH) and insulin, "alone or in combination," are involved in the regulation of crypt cell proliferation in the human intestine in vitro and possibly also in vivo.

Schofield & Mepham, International Dairy Federation Conference, Johannesburg, South Africa, October 23, 1996

"The effects of IGF-1 on gut proliferation and the acute sensitivity of the gut to IGF suggest that we should be most concerned about the generation of hyperplastic states in the gut, polyps, or ultimately, adenocarcinoma."

Hansen *et al*, Consumers Union Report to the FAO/WHO Joint Expert Committee On Food Additives, September 1997

Confirms and extends evidence detailed by Epstein, 1996 that excess IGF-1 levels in rBGH milk are a risk factor for colon cancer.

H. rBGH Milk Is a Prostate Cancer Risk Factor

Epstein, S. S., P. R. Newswire, March 16, 1998

As reported in a January 23, 1998 article in *Science,* men with high blood levels of IGF-1 (>270 ng/ml), are over four times more likely to develop full-blown prostate cancer than men with lower levels (<250 ng/ml). The report emphasized that high IGF-1 levels are the strongest known risk factor for prostate cancer, exceeding that of a family history, and that reducing IGF-1 levels is likely to prevent prostate cancer. It was further noted that IGF-1 stimulates the growth of normal and cancerous prostate cells, and that it blocks apoptosis of cancer cells thus stimulating the growth and invasiveness of prostate cancer.

Wolk *et al*, J. Nat. Cancer Inst. 90:911-915, 1998

A study on 210 men under the age of 70 with newly diagnosed prostate cancer revealed statistically significant excess blood levels of IGF-1 compared to matched controls. The authors concluded that: "IGF-1 likely plays an important role in the etiology of the disease."

Appendix XIII

The "Research Cures Cancer" Campaign

"Research Cures Cancer" Campaign Misleads Public and Congress

Press Advisory
From the Cancer Prevention Coalition
January 25, 1995

Introduction

A statement by national organizations representing over 5 million Americans warned of misleading efforts by treatment groups and the cancer drug industry to allocate more tax dollars towards funding cancer research.

The statement responded to a Washington, D.C. kickoff of the National Coalition for Cancer Research's industry-sponsored "Research Cures Cancer" campaign, which is lobbying Congress to increase support for the National Cancer Institute's (NCI) programs.

The statement sent a message to policymakers that further funding is not going to cure cancer. It stressed that NCI's priorities are fixated on research, on treatment, and molecular biology, while issues of environmental and workplace-induced cancers are trivialized. The reason for the failed war against cancer is not a shortage of funds but their gross misallocation. NCI has devoted minimal funding to cancer prevention. Furthermore, NCI has failed to inform Congress and the public of a wide range of avoidable causes of environmental and occupational cancers.

The organizations concluded by calling

for an appointment of a new director at NCI who is more responsive to growing national concerns on prevention of the cancer epidemic.

The Statement

On January 25, 1995 in Washington, D.C., the National Coalition for Cancer Research will launch an industry-funded "Research Cures Cancer" campaign which misleads Congress and the public into the groundless belief that further research is the answer to the cancer epidemic. The Coalition, sponsored by the American Cancer Society and the cancer drug industry, is lobbying Congress and taxpayers to provide the National Cancer Institute (NCI) with more research funding.

Twenty-five years since President Nixon and Congress inaugurated the National Cancer Act, the war against cancer has failed. In spite of over $25 billion of taxpayers funding, cancer rates have escalated to epidemic proportions while our ability to treat and cure most cancers remains largely unchanged.

For decades, NCI policy and priorities have remained narrowly fixated on research, on treatment, and basic molecular biology. Despite its questionable relevance, molecular biology receives over 50% of NCI's $2 billion annual budget. Nevertheless, molecular biologist and current director of the National Institutes of Health, Dr. Harold Varmus, is encouraging still more emphasis on basic molecular biology research in the NCI.

The reason for the failed war against cancer is not a shortage of funds but their gross misallocation. NCI has directed a minimal priority to cancer prevention. Furthermore, NCI has failed to inform Congress and the public of a wide range of avoidable carcinogens in the air, water, food, consumer products and the workplace. Research on such exposures receives a minuscule 5% of NCI's annual budget. Reduction of exposures to carcinogens in the workplace and the environment are likely to reverse the current epidemic.

With the NCI directorship being vacated next month, it is time to see the NCI face up to escalating cancer rates and its imbalanced preoccupation with research on treatment and molecular biology. As organizations representing 5 million Americans, we demand that President Clinton appoint a leading scientist with strong credentials and clear commitment to cancer prevention as director of the NCI.

The Cancer Prevention Coalition and the co-signing organizations also demand:

• NCI must be held accountable for its failed policies and the $25 billion in taxpayer support in the war against cancer.

• NCI must undergo radical reforms in its programs, priorities, and leadership.

• Cancer prevention must receive greater emphasis in NCI policies.

• The NCI budget must be held hostage to such reforms under the terms of the Government Performance and Results Act of 1993.

The Signatories

Breast Cancer Action
San Francisco, CA

Cancer Prevention Coalition
Chicago, IL

Center for Constitutional Rights
New York, NY

Center for Media & Democracy
Madison, WI

Citizen Action
Washington, DC

Environmental Research Foundation
Annapolis, MD

Food and Water, Inc.
Marshfield, VT

Greenpeace USA
Chicago, IL

Mother Jones **magazine**
San Francisco, CA

Pesticide Action Network
San Francisco, CA

Project Impact
Oakland, CA

Pure Food Campaign
Washington, DC

Radiation and Public Health Project
New York, NY

Women's Community Cancer Project
Boston, MA

Women's Environment & Development Organization
New York, NY

Shopper Beware:
Cancer Risks from Consumer Products

This Appendix is based on extracts from The Safe Shopper's Bible, *co-authored with David Steinman, and with a foreword by Ralph Nader. The book identifies a wide range of undisclosed carcinogenic, besides other toxic, ingredients and contaminants in a wide range of consumer products, and also provides information on safe alternatives. Unwitting exposure of the entire U.S. population to these avoidable carcinogens continues to play an important causal role in escalating cancer rates. However, the cancer establishment has remained silent about these exposures, which are well documented in the scientific literature, and has failed to testify before Congress or advise the regulatory agencies concerned. The ACS has actually gone still further, in trivializing these risks and opposing their regulation.* *

Consumers today want to make intelligent, informed shopping decisions. Until now, however, most have been shopping in the dark. They receive little guidance from food producers and product manufacturers, whose advertising and labeling are too often misleading and not objective sources of information.

Nor are consumers provided such information from the responsible regulatory agencies: the Food and Drug Administration, for food and cosmetics; the Environmental Protection Agency for pesticides; and the Consumer Product Safety Commission for household products. (For further details, see *The Safe Shopper's Bible.*)

Industry

Quite apart from government, industry perhaps plays the most key role in ensuring the safety of foods and consumer products. Indeed, making foods and consumer products safer will be difficult, if not impossible, without the cooperation and leadership of responsible industry.

Our goal is to encourage industry to provide consumers more information and to produce safer foods and products by reducing reliance on toxic chemicals. In fact, many major corporations are now moving toward responsible production of foods and consumer products. Some 15 percent of all new products marketed in 1992 were advertised as being environmentally friendly. Furthermore, to ensure the integrity of such claims, many leading retailers, including Home Depot, are now requiring that such claims be scientifically screened by certification groups such as Green Seal or Scientific Certification Systems. Meanwhile the largest organic farmer in the United

---

* Reprinted with permission from *The Safe Shopper's Bible*, S.S. Epstein and D. Steinman, Macmillan, USA, 1995.

States is now Gallo Wine Company. The firm that fought the United Farm Workers in the 1960s now has six thousand acres of vineyards under organic cultivation. Major fashion manufacturers such as Esprit are producing clothing made with organic cotton and environmentally friendly zippers and snaps. And JC Penney is now offering a wholly natural line of nonpetrochemical cosmetics and personal care products known as Earth Preserv. These changes are only the beginning. They signify the changing attitudes of industry toward the environment and consumer safety. After all, consumer confidence and taking care of the environment make good business sense.

Consumers' Right to Know

Consumers have an inalienable right to know what ingredients are in products they use daily, and to be certain that chemicals posing chronic health risks will be phased out when alternatives are available. These are rights, regardless of one's perception of the risk of the ingredient. Yet walk down the aisle of any supermarket and you will quickly see how minimal regulation has led to grossly inadequate labeling.

1. Foods and Beverages

With regard to foods and beverages, when was the last time your supermarket or seafood shop told you which fish or other food item has chemicals that cause cancer or birth defects? For women who are pregnant or intend to have children and for parents who wish to minimize their children's exposure to such toxins, this information is essential. It is also important to know about other food hazards. For example, children who eat hot dogs containing nitrite preservatives (which are precursors of carcinogenic nitrosamines) about a dozen times a month have up to 4-fold excess risk of brain cancer and a 7-fold excess risk of leukemia (page 575).

Foods and beverages may be contaminated with a variety of chemicals that have been intentionally or unintentionally added during their production, handling, storage, and processing. Fruits, vegetables, nuts, seeds, and grains are contaminated primarily with pesticides and sometimes molds. Dairy, meat, seafood, and processed foods are also contaminated with industrial chemicals, additives, hormones, growth stimulants, antibiotics, and other animal drugs as well as occasionally molds and bacteria. Many of these chemicals have carcinogenic, neurotoxic, reproductive, or immunotoxic effects. In addition to threatening the health of workers involved in growing and processing agricultural crops and livestock, they are a threat to your health and your children's health.

Of primary concern to consumers is the wide range of animal drug, industrial, chemical, and pesticide residues that show up in the foods that are placed on the dining tables of families across America each day. In 1993, two important studies provided overwhelming evidence that the pesticides used in food production are a public health menace, especially to the nation's children. *Pesticides in the Diets of Infants and Children,* issued by the National Academy of Sciences, and *Pesticides in Children's Food,* prepared by the Environmental Working Group, a Washington-based nonprofit research organization, both concluded that infants and children are at high risk for future cancers because of their exposure to carcinogenic pesticides, quite apart from neurotoxic, teratogenic, and other toxic effects. These reports are merely the latest in a long line of such findings, dating from the 1960s and earlier, detailing the health hazards of our nation's farmers' reliance on pesticides. The tragedy is that these reports, like those produced earlier, have been largely ignored by U.S. policymakers. In fact, pesticide use on American farms has increased 125 percent over the past twenty-five years.

The push for change is coming, not from

Washington, but from citizens who have decided to boycott foods and beverages contaminated with carcinogens that pose health risks. But it is going to take a lot more consumer outrage and anger, and the willingness of shoppers to vote with their consumer dollars.

"We've got a lot of pesticides out there and we ought to be doing something to reduce them," said former FDA Commissioner Dr. David A. Kessler in 1993. However, Dr. Kessler's agency has not yet taken any action requiring labeling of foods for carcinogenic pesticides and other contaminants. Meanwhile, although Congress has passed consumer disclosure legislation forcing the food industry to list fat, cholesterol, and additional nutritional information on labels, consumers have no legal right to know of the carcinogenic and other toxic chemicals whose residues are found in the food supply. The bottom line is that consumers have a legal right to know about cholesterol and fat in the food supply; but when it comes to pesticides in the food supply, consumers have no such right.

Recent reports have focused on the risk to children posed by chemicals in the food supply. But adults are also at risk, from both their childhood and current exposures to chemical contaminants. A 1993 study found that women with the highest blood levels of DDT had four times the breast cancer risk of women with the least exposure. This study is only one of many since the 1970s — all largely unpublicized — to associate DDT and other related pesticides and industrial chemicals with breast cancer risk. In fact, there is growing evidence that the nation's present breast cancer epidemic is related to exposure to a wide range of environmental contaminants, including DDT, other carcinogenic pesticides, and estrogenic stimulants.

Many other cancers related to toxic exposures, including brain cancer, non-Hodgkin's lymphoma, bladder cancer, prostate cancer, testicular cancer, and leukemia, have also shown major (age-adjusted) increases in inci-dence since 1950. Consumers, anxious about the presence of carcinogenic residues in the food supply, have been told that there is no cause for concern and that these amounts are trivial. But when one in three Americans is now stricken with cancer, up from one in four in 1950, reducing exposure to carcinogenic substances is prudent.

The regulatory system in place today can trace its origin to the enactment of the Federal Insecticide, Fungicide, and Rodenticide Act (FIFRA) in 1947. Congress intended FIFRA to "balance" the alleged economic benefits from pesticides with their established environmental and human health harm. In other words, rather than prevent cancer by preventing exposure to carcinogens in the food supply, the government attempts only to "manage" cancer, knowing that some people will be stricken and others will not.

The term used by scientists and government regulators to describe this system of cancer roulette is "quantitative cancer risk assessment (QCRA)." The scientific validity of QCRA has been seriously challenged, despite the government's reliance on the system to ensure your health and freedom from cancer (Appendix VII). These are "rubber" numbers that can vary by a factor of up to ten million. Furthermore, most independent and informed scientists agree that there is simply no such thing as a "safe" level of exposure to a carcinogen.

Carcinogens in Fruit

Artificial colors: Citrus Red No. 2 is used to dye the skins of Florida oranges to conceal color variations in the fruit so that they can compete with California oranges, which are not dyed. Citrus Red No. 2 is carcinogenic.

Pesticides: Fruits are contaminated with a wide range of carcinogenic pesticides. While you can always find safer fruits at any supermarket by using the accompanying shopping charts, your best bet is to buy organically grown produce whenever possible.

Table XIV.1 Carcinogenic contaminants commonly found in foods and beverages

1.	Acephate	17.	Dimethoate
2.	Azinphos-methyl	18.	Dioxin
3.	Benomyl	19.	Endrin
4.	Benzene hexachloride (BHC)	20.	Ethylenethiourea (ETU)
5.	Captafol	21.	Folpet
6.	Captan	22.	Heptachlor
7.	Chlordane	23.	Hexachlorobenzene (HCB)
8.	Chlorobenzilate	24.	Hormone additives
9.	Chlorothalonil	25.	Imidan/Phosmet
10.	Dacthal (DCPA)	26.	Mancozeb/Maneb (ethylene
11.	DDT, DDE, DDD		bisdithiocarbamate)
12.	Dicofol/Kelthane	27.	Permethrin
13.	Dieldrin	28.	Polychlorinated biphenyls
14.	o-Phenylphenol and Na salt		(PCB's)
15.	Oxadiazon	29.	Radioactive contaminants
16.	Pentachlorophenol ("Penta")	30.	Toxaphene

Radiation: Apple juice made from concentrate sometimes contains radioactive contaminants because of the Chernobyl nuclear explosion in 1986, reports the FDA's Radionuclides in Foods program. Most consumers do not know that some U.S. suppliers of apple juice made from concentrate import their raw materials from Austria, Germany, Hungary, and Yugoslavia. Government records indicate that cesium-137 isotopes, traced to the Chernobyl disaster, have been found in samples of apple juice concentrate from these nations. In the years since Chernobyl, levels have diminished dramatically, but Chernobyl-related contamination still is occasionally present. Since the concentration of radiation falls within what U.S. guidelines term *acceptable exposures,* such apple juice products are allowed to be sold legally.

Waxes: Waxes contain fungicides such as benomyl and sodium orthophenyl phenate; both are carcinogenic. Fruits most likely to be waxed include apples, avocados, cantaloupes, grapefruits, lemons, limes, melons, oranges, passion fruit, peaches, and pineapples.

Carcinogens in Vegetables

Pickling Vegetables: Traditional pickled vegetables from Asia have shown evidence of posing a cancer risk, based on epidemiological studies that have found a high rate of stomach and nasopharyngeal cancer among people consuming them.

Pesticides: As with fruits, vegetables are contaminated with a wide range of carcinogenic pesticides. It is always best to buy organically grown vegetables whenever possible.

Radiation: Some wild European mushrooms still have excess radiation because of the 1986 Chernobyl nuclear disaster. These include boletos and chanterelles, which are often found in gourmet shops and sections of stores.

Waxing: Waxes on vegetables may contain carcinogenic fungicides. Vegetables most likely to be waxed include cucumbers, eggplants, parsnips, peppers, pumpkins, rutabagas, squashes, and sweet potatoes.

Carcinogens in Grains

Conventionally grown grain products are

generally free from residues of carcinogenic pesticides (except for products from India); yet carcinogenic pesticides are used extensively in the production of grain products, and they pose a threat to the health of farmers and farm workers. Researchers have noted high rates of non-Hodgkin's lymphoma among farmers. The probable explanation is agricultural exposure to herbicides. Researchers from Sweden and the United States have found a five- to six-fold increase in the risk of non-Hodgkin's lymphoma and also excesses of brain cancer, multiple myeloma, and leukemia among persons frequently exposed to herbicides. You can do a lot for the health of farmers and farm workers by insisting on buying only organically grown grains.

Colors: Cereals should be avoided if they contain the following colors that have been shown to be carcinogenic or to contain carcinogenic impurities:

- FD&C Blue 1
- FD&C Green 3
- FD&C Red 4
- FD&C Red 40
- FD&C Yellow 5
- FD&C Yellow 6

Meat and Poultry

Meat and poultry contain a wide range of carcinogens, including pesticides, animal drugs, hormones, and radiation.

Pesticides: Pesticides remaining as residues in animal feed crops may be ingested by livestock and concentrate in their tissues. Pesticides may be applied directly on feed crops or come from general environmental contaminants in the soil, barns, or elsewhere. These include past use of chlordane, DDT, and dieldrin, which are among the potent pesticides commonly found in the food supply. A study by Dr. Mary S. Wolff, associate professor of community medicine at the Mount Sinai School of Medicine in New York City, found that women with blood levels of DDT in the top 10 percent had four times the breast cancer risk as women in the bottom 10 percent. In addition, several other pesticide contaminants found in meat and poultry have been implicated as causing breast cancer. Yet quite apart from those substances that induce breast cancer, many other carcinogens are found in meat and poultry products.

Animal drugs: Animal drugs are widely used nationwide. Drugs administered to livestock, which include antibiotics such as sulfas, are often misused, leaving illegal residues in animal tissues and subsequently in meat and poultry. Forty of the animal drugs and pesticides known to occur as residues in meat and poultry are carcinogens. Furthermore, another eighteen cause birth defects. There is virtually no monitoring of these substances — even though at least 143 pesticides and drugs are known to leave chemical residues in meat and poultry. Only 46 of the 143 drugs and pesticides found in edible animal tissues are monitored by the USDA, and they are poorly and rarely monitored. A 1985 congressional subcommittee concluded that FDA officials believe that as many as 90 percent or more of the twenty thousand to thirty thousand new animal drugs estimated to be on the market have not been approved by FDA as safe and effective and, therefore, are being marketed in violation of the Food, Drug, and Cosmetic Act. The committee went on to estimate that as many as four thousand of these new animal drugs could have potentially significant adverse health effects on animals or humans.

Simply choosing poultry instead of beef will not protect you from exposure to animal drugs. Unless raised organically, poultry is also contaminated. Says one former poultry industry executive who worked for one of the nation's major producers, "At Perdue we allocated three-quarters of a square foot for each animal. They are very crowded, and walking and pecking in their own excrement. That is why disease passes so rapidly through a flock of chickens. You go into a chicken house every week and do a post mortem and if there is a sick bird you treat the whole flock uniformly. They are medicated in the feed or in the water. Or you go into a [chicken] house with something that looks like a leaf blower and spray an atomized mixture of antibiotics in solution. It is like a fog."

One group of animal drugs that pose serious health risks is sulfa drugs. Sulfamethazine and other sulfa drugs have been used since the 1940s to prevent respiratory disease among market hogs and veal calves. Sulfamethazine is carcinogenic. Although in the past sulfamethazine residues have been found frequently in market pork as well as milk-fed veal, the USDA claims that the incidence is presently minimal. Certainly, there has been improvement among ranchers; however, the continued use of sulfamethazine remains a significant food safety issue, primarily because ranchers have replaced sulfamethazine, not necessarily with better animal husbandry and improved conditions, but with other structurally similar sulfa drugs. A report from the federal General Accounting Office (GAO) recognizes that if a structural feature in one compound is found to cause cancer, the presence of that same structural feature in other compounds greatly increases the probability that they too can cause cancer.

Growth stimulating hormones: Sex hormones, both natural and synthetic, which are given to up to 95 percent or more of the cattle raised for slaughter in the United States, also leave residues in edible portions of meats (Appendix XI). Industry experts claim there is no danger to humans from these hormones when they are used properly. But, like antibiotics, growth hormones are sold to ranchers over the counter without a veterinary prescription, and the federal system of inspection for hormone levels in meat and poultry is notoriously inadequate — despite the fact that hormones are listed as known human carcinogens by the International Agency for Research on Cancer. Only 1 in 8,000 livestock and 1 in 700,000 poultry are tested in USDA laboratories for chemical residue content and rarely ever for hormones. That means that a consumer who carefully checks the meat and poultry she buys to determine that it has a USDA-inspected stamp on it is merely getting a product that has been inspected for cleanliness and general health — but in no way does that imply that there has been any testing to determine whether or not it has high residues of carcinogenic hormones. Most meat and poultry products containing illegal levels of chemical residues are sold to the public. Most of this meat bears the USDA inspection stamp.

While the body produces hormones and hormones are naturally present in foods, the use of natural and synthetic hormones should be banned. Federal regulators and the beef industry claim that the hormones implanted in cattle are not harmful. The facts tell a different story. Although the government banned the synthetic hormone DES (diethylstilbestrol) in 1979, its illegal use by American meat producers continued until at least 1983, when nearly fifteen hundred veal calves from five different farms in upstate New York were found to be contaminated with residues of this illegal growth stimulator. Furthermore, rather than finding safe alternatives following the DES ban, the meat industry promptly switched to other carcinogenic additives, particularly forms of the natural sex hormones estradiol, progesterone, and testosterone, which are legally implanted in the ears of commercially raised feedlot cattle. These substances are carcinogenic. And unlike the synthetic DES, whose residues can be monitored and whose use was conditional on a seven-day pre-slaughter withdrawal period, residues of natural hormones are not detectable, and they cannot be practically differentiated from the same hormones produced by the body, except by their higher levels. Since 1983, however, the FDA has allowed virtually unregulated use of these additives up to the time of slaughter, subject only to the theoretical and nonenforceable requirement that residue levels in meat must be less than 1 percent of the daily hormonal production of young children. The result is that virtually the entire U.S. population consumes, without any warning, labeling, or information, unknown and unpredictable amounts of hormonal residues in meat products over a lifetime.

In 1986, as many as half of all cattle sampled in feedlots as large as six hundred animals were found to have hormones illegally implanted in muscle, rather than the ear skin, to induce further increased growth. This practice results in very high residues in meat, which even the FDA has admitted could produce "adverse effects." Left unanswered is whether or not such chronic and uncontrolled estrogen dosages are involved in increasing cancer rates (now striking one in three Americans), particularly the alarming 50 percent increase in the incidence of breast cancer since 1965. These questions are of further concern in light of long-standing evidence confirming the association between breast cancer and oral contraceptives, whose estrogen dosage over a fraction of a lifetime is known and controlled, in contrast with that from residues of hormones in meat products.

More than a decade ago, Roy Hertz, then director of endocrinology of the NCI and a world authority on hormonal cancer, warned of the carcinogenic risks from lifelong exposure to estrogenic feed additives, particularly for hormonally sensitive tissues such as breast tissue, because they could increase normal body hormonal levels and disturb delicately poised hormonal balances. Hertz pointed to evidence from innumerable animal tests and human clinical experience that such imbalances can be carcinogenic. Hertz also warned of the essentially uncontrolled and unregulated use of these extremely potent biological agents, no dietary levels of which can be regarded as safe. Even a dime-sized piece of meat contains billions or trillions of molecules of these carcinogens. Such exposures are particularly critical for young children.

A dramatic warning of the dangers of growth-promoting additives was triggered by an epidemic of premature sexual development and ovarian cysts involving about three thousand Puerto Rican infants and children from 1979 to 1981. These toxic effects were traced to hormonal contamination of fresh meat products, and were usually reversed by simple dietary changes. The meat products were found to be contaminated with estrogen residues more than ten times above the normal ranges. The epidemic also was associated with increased rates of uterine and ovarian cancers in adult women.

Nitrites: Cured meats such as bacon, ham, beef jerky, salami, and luncheon meats contain nitrites. These substances inhibit the growth of dangerous botulism-causing bacteria, and maintain the meat's red color. Although nitrite itself is not carcinogenic, it combines with naturally-occurring chemicals called secondary or tertiary amines to form carcinogenic nitrosamines. This reaction will occur in the food itself while it is sitting on the shelf or in the refrigerator or when being fried, but it also occurs within the stomach once the food is ingested. Nitrite-contaminated food is thought to be a cause of stomach cancer in the United States, Japan, and other nations. Recently, researchers reported that children who eat hot dogs cured with nitrite a dozen or more times monthly have a risk of leukemia seven times higher than normal (page 575). Furthermore, children born to mothers who consume hot dogs once or more weekly during their pregnancy are twice as likely to have childhood brain tumors.

Charcoal broiling, grilling, oven cooking, and pan frying: In the 1700s, soot containing polycyclic aromatic hydrocarbons (PAHs) was linked to scrotal cancer in chimney sweeps. Today, grilled meat is the major source of PAHs in food. Heavy charring of meat produces high concentrations of carcinogenic PAHs such as benzopyrene.

Some eighteen different PAHs have thus far been found in food. Although the data are not entirely conclusive, researchers believe that at least five and perhaps as many as twelve of these eighteen PAHs cause cancer. PAHs form when fat from grilled meats falls down on flames or hot coals. The PAHs that are formed in this reaction rise with the smoke and permeate the meat.

Although the formation of PAHs appears limited primarily to barbecuing and grilling, you must be careful when broiling and pan frying meats to prevent formation of another group of cancer-causing chemicals known as heterocyclic amines (HAs), which are created when amino acids and other substances in meats are burned. The National Cancer Institute estimates that HAs may increase the number of human cancers in the United States by about two thousand cases annually. (It is of interest to note that NCI has made no such estimates for excess cancers related to exposure to pesticides, hormones, and industrial contaminants in meats.)

Occasionally eating grilled meat or meats cooked at high temperatures, as in broiling or frying, is not a problem. But if you like to grill your meats regularly, then you learn a few cooking techniques that can help make consuming grilled foods safer and healthier.

Radiation: Some meat products are contaminated by environmental radiation from nuclear accidents such as Chernobyl. Radiation is carcinogenic. The meat products of four countries that export significant amounts to the United States have been shown to have trace levels of radioactivity because of the 1986 Chernobyl explosion. Such products include canned ham from Poland, Hungary, Yugoslavia, and Brazil (which processes European meats), as well as other meat and poultry products from Finland and Switzerland. Countries whose meat products were least affected include France, Germany, Italy, and the Netherlands.

Carcinogens in Fish

Antibiotics: The raising of farm-raised fish is quite similar to the factory farmyard methods used for cattle. As with cattle, fish are given a wide range of antibiotics and other drugs.

This massive new industry is virtually unregulated. As a result farm-raised fish are likely to contain residues of a wide variety of animal drugs, some of which are carcinogenic. Prefer wild deep-water ocean fish whenever possible.

Industrial chemicals and pesticides: Seafood can be one of the most dangerously contaminated food sources in the diet today when uninformed shopping choices are made. In fact, the National Academy of Sciences estimated in 1991 that the risk of cancer to the average consumer who eats seafood can be some seventy-five times greater than normally acceptable guidelines. Some seafood items such as bluefish, farm-raised catfish, lake trout, Maine lobster, and striped bass are contaminated with concentrations of industrial chemicals and pesticides hundreds to thousands of times greater than other food groups. Yet when consumers make choices based on adequate information, seafood can be one of the safest, most nutritious foods.

Carcinogenic industrial chemicals and pesticides commonly found in contaminated seafood include benzene hexachloride, chlordane, DDT, dieldrin, dioxin, heptachlor, hexachlorobenzene, lindane, and polychlorinated biphenyls.

No fish from waters near agricultural and industrial areas or from the nation's major inland waterways or harbors are safe to consume due to industrial chemical and pesticide contamination.

Carcinogens in Dairy Products

Pesticides: Many carcinogenic pesticides — including BHC, chlordane, DDT, dieldrin, heptachlor, HCB, and lindane — accumulate in the most fatty dairy products (e.g., butter, ice cream, whole milk, high-fat cheeses).

Animal drugs: The FDA is responsible for assuring the safety of the billions of gallons of milk produced in the United States each year. Concerned about media reports that independent surveys had found a wide range of animal drugs in the milk supply, the FDA conducted three surveys to determine the presence of selected antibiotic drug residues in milk between 1988 and 1990. Although the FDA insists that these surveys confirmed their belief that the nation's milk supply is safe, we cannot support such statements because of flaws in the survey methods. For one thing, the number of samples tested was small; for another, the testing methods were grossly inadequate for detecting the many drugs used by the dairy industry.

One major concern is the use of sulfa drugs in dairy cows. Sulfamethazine is carcinogenic, and its residues are often found in milk. *FDA's own 1990 screening tests indicate that 46 percent of all milk samples tested contained more than one sulfa drug residue.* According to the GAO, other sulfa drugs exhibit toxic effects like those produced by sulfamethazine. In setting alleged safety levels, however, the FDA has allowed residues of up to ten parts per billion (ppb) for each sulfa drug, while ignoring their aggregate or synergistic effect.

The problem is compounded further because sulfamethazine metabolites (i.e., breakdown products) may also be present in milk. They also present carcinogenic risks; however, metabolites of sulfamethazine cannot be detected by the analytic methods FDA has used in past milk surveys.

Quite apart from sulfamethazine, other highly dangerous drugs such as chloramphenicol, which can cause the often fatal blood disease aplastic anemia, have also been found in the milk supply.

Dioxin: The Health Protection Branch of Canada has reported dioxin levels in the parts per trillion range in several samples of milk and cream packaged in bleached milk cartons manufactured in the United States. Dioxin, which is a by-product of the process used to bleach paper products at pulp and paper mills,

had migrated from the cartons to the milk. Very likely U.S. milk products are similarly contaminated with dioxin. Dioxin's carcinogenicity is up to 500,000 times more potent than that of DDT.

The use of rBGH raises fundamental ethical, social, and economic considerations, including the continued viability of the small family dairy farm and adverse veterinary effects. The past and expanding use of rBGH poses potential public health hazards that so far have not been investigated (Appendix XII).

The biotech industry claims that the hormones are natural, increase milk yields up to 25 percent, do not harm cows, do not alter milk quality, and are safe for humans. (The FDA also agrees that bovine growth hormones are safe and even allowed the sale of unlabeled milk and meat from rBGH cows for about five years before formal approval was required. Some twenty thousand cows were treated in the past with rBGH/BST in experimental trials, and their milk was allowed to be sold with the general milk supply. The figure now exceeds 5 percent of all cows and is rapidly increasing.) These claims, which are based on industry-contracted research at more than twenty U.S. university dairy science departments, are misleading.

Apart from the national surplus of milk and anticipated loss of thousands of small dairy farms if milk production is increased and milk prices are reduced, the effectiveness of rBGH is exaggerated. Furthermore, the nutritional quality of milk and cheese is altered; fat is increased as much as 27 percent, and casein (milk protein) is decreased. Stress effects have been noted in cows hyperstimulated by rBGH. These include increased susceptibility to infection, infertility, loss of fat, heat intolerance, and "burnout" or lactational failure. Severe stress diseases, including gastric ulcers, arthritis, and kidney and heart abnormalities, have also been induced in pigs. Additionally, rBGH may be misused as a growth promoter in calves, pigs, and sheep, particularly as there are no practical methods for detecting the hormone in meat.

Apart from economic and veterinary concerns, rBGH poses grave potential consumer health risks that have not yet been investigated by the industry or the FDA:

- Increased levels of cell-stimulating insulin-like Growth Factor-1 (IGF-1), apparently identical to those in humans, have been reported in rBGH milk. These could induce premature growth in infants and possibly promote colon cancer and breast cancer in women.

- Increased bacterial infections in rBGH cows will require treatment with antibiotics that will pass into milk. This is likely to result in antibiotic-resistant infections in the general population. Also, the stress effects of rBGH in cows could suppress immunity and activate latent viruses, such as bovine leukemia (leukosis) and bovine immunodeficiency viruses, which are related to cancer and the AIDS complex and may be infectious to humans.

- Steroids and adrenaline-type stressor chemicals induced in cows by these hormones are likely to contaminate milk and may be harmful, particularly to infants and young children.

- The fat and milk of cows are already contaminated with a wide range of carcinogenic contaminants, including dioxins and pesticides. rBGH reduces body fat and is likely to mobilize these carcinogens into milk, with cancer risks to consumers.

Radiation: Milk is a prime route by which consumers are exposed to radioactive contaminants released by nuclear plants. Milk is especially dangerous because it is quickly marketed, and short-lived radioactive isotopes are still present when it is consumed. Milk is associated with increased risk for breast cancer, and the combination of pesticides and radiation have been proposed as one possible explanation. If your dairy is near a nuclear plant, don't use their products.

Carcinogens in Preserved Foods:

Additives: Some additives such as coal tar food colors, potassium bromate, and BHA are carcinogenic or have shown suggestive evidence of carcinogenicity. Products with such ingredients should not be eaten.

Preserved foods: Especially in processed foods containing cured meats such as pepperoni pizza, sausages, and luncheon meats, the presence of nitrite preservatives deserves caution. Nitrites interact with other secondary or tertiary amines in the food, especially following cooking, or in the stomach, to form carcinogenic nitrosamines. While the preservative effect of nitrites is clearly important, safer alternatives are available. Avoid processed or preserved foods, meats, or fish containing nitrites.

Pesticides: In general, carcinogenic pesticides concentrate in processed foods. Brands using organic ingredients are preferable; so are nonfat and low-fat brands.

Carcinogens in Desserts and Snacks

Pesticides: Milk chocolate is highly contaminated with residues of BHC and lindane.

Peanut butter is highly contaminated with carcinogenic pesticides, including DDT, dieldrin, and toxaphene. Peanut butter can also be contaminated with the fungus aflatoxin which is carcinogenic as well.

Pumpkin pie is contaminated with dieldrin. Pumpkin pie made with organically grown pumpkins is a better choice.

Carcinogens in Vegetable Oil

Pesticides: Although most oils tend to be fairly free from carcinogenic pesticide residues, soybean oil is contaminated with residues of dieldrin. Safflower oil is contaminated with lindane, which is carcinogenic.

Rancidity: Oils that are improperly stored can become oxidized, leading to formation of oxygen-free radicals that are associated with carcinogenic processes.

Carcinogens in Sweeteners

Aspartame: Aspartame is used in Equal and NutraSweet, as well as in many brands of low-calorie diet foods, desserts, and soft drinks. In 1980, the FDA convened a public board of inquiry (PBOI) to review concerns over aspartame's potential ability to induce brain tumors. Although the PBOI concluded that ingestion of aspartame would not cause brain damage, scientists who had been asked to review scientific findings expressed doubts. The PBOI concluded that experimental data "do not rule out an oncogenic effect of aspartame, and that, to the contrary, they appear to suggest the possibility that aspartame, at least when administered in the 'huge' quantities employed in the studies, may contribute to the development of brain tumors." Until these controversial findings on brain cancer in experimental animals have been resolved, use this product sparingly, if at all.

Cyclamates: Used as a sweetener in Canada, cyclamates have shown limited evidence of carcinogenicity.

Saccharin: Used as a sweetener in the United States in soft drinks and table sweeteners such as Sweet 'n Low, saccharin is carcinogenic.

Carcinogens in Baby Foods

Pesticides: The embryo, fetus, infant, and young child are much more sensitive and susceptible to carcinogenic pesticide residues than the adult for the following reasons: (1) because of their smaller size, pound for pound babies receive a greater dose; (2) the baby's liver often lacks certain enzymes required for breaking down pesticides; (3) babies' and toddlers' immune systems are not as strong as those of adults; (4) the baby's cells undergo rapid growth and may be more susceptible to carcinogens than cells that are more static. In spite of these concerns the EPA's tolerance-setting procedures have always been calculated for adults.

One recent report notes that "millions of children in the United States receive up to 35 percent of their entire lifetime dose of some carcinogenic pesticides by age 5. . . . By the average child's first birthday, the combined cancer risk from just eight pesticides on 20 foods exceeds the EPA's estimated lifetime level of 'acceptable risk' of one-in-one-million additional cancers throughout the U.S. population." These exposures can result in a high incidence of childhood and subsequent adult cancers.

Carcinogens in Drinking Water

Arsenic: A major cancer risk, arsenic contaminates the drinking water of millions of Americans. One report notes that some 350,000 Americans drink water containing levels of arsenic in excess of lenient federal standards, and that 2.5 million people drink water containing more than twenty-five parts per billion (ppb) arsenic, about half the federal standard of fifty ppb. Even very low levels of arsenic in drinking water present a major cancer threat. A California study found that the EPA standard of fifty ppb presents a cancer risk of one cancer in every one hundred people, one thousand to ten thousand times greater than the government's so-called negligible risk guidelines.

Chlorination and trihalomethanes (THMs): The public water supplies of some two hundred million Americans are chlorinated to reduce bacterial levels. Chlorination is a major disinfecting method that successfully prevents bacterially related illnesses. However, chlorination of water already contaminated with organic compounds and other carcinogenic pollutants produces additional carcinogenic compounds called trihalomethanes. Most major municipal water supplies deliver water that has gone through activated carbon filtration, which sharply reduces the levels of THMs; still, the levels can be elevated to the point of posing clear cancer risks. In the case of small municipalities there may be insufficient water treatment, and levels may be elevated as well.

More than one hundred million Americans consume water contaminated with significant levels of THMs. There is growing evidence that chlorinated drinking water causes bladder cancer and rectal cancer. THMs are responsible for 10,700 or more rectal and bladder cancers annually. More people die each year from THMs than from fires and handguns. Because of widespread pollution of drinking water with organic contaminants, many water supplies that are chlorinated probably contain some amount of THM. If above about ten ppb, they should not be used for human consumption, cooking, showering, or other household chores unless they have gone through an effective home filtration system. THMs are highly volatile and exposure in the home results from all possible avenues, including inhalation and skin absorption.

Fluoride: There is limited evidence that fluoride is carcinogenic.

Industrial pollutants: Many public water supplies are contaminated with carcinogenic industrial chemicals such as perchloroethylene and trichloroethylene.

Lead: Lead is carcinogenic. Older cities may still be using lead pipes in public water systems built before the 1930s. Any city with soft (i.e., corrosive) water — particularly in northeastern states such as Massachusetts and Pennsylvania where acid rain is a problem — could be delivering lead-tainted water. The government will test water only up to the point of delivery to your home. Once water flows through your home's plumbing, you are on your own. *And most lead exposure results from home plumbing.* For example, in April 1994, the EPA reported that brass fittings on submersible well pumps are capable of leach-

ing high levels of lead into well water; the latest study showed that commonly used well pumps can contaminate drinking water with lead levels some five hundred times greater than federal regulations allow.

Pesticides: In rural agricultural areas, water drawn from a private well may be contaminated with a variety of chemicals ranging from carcinogenic, neurotoxic, teratogenic, and immunotoxic pesticides such as alachlor, aldicarb, atrazine, dibromochloropropane (DBCP), and ethylene dibromide (EDB). A recent study by the U.S. Geological Survey found that more than one-quarter of samples of water from the Mississippi River Basin contained atrazine at levels exceeding the EPA's maximum contaminant level. Atrazine, as with several other pesticides found in drinking water such as DBCP and EDB, causes breast cancer. Atrazine also causes human ovarian cancer. Although many people think of pesticide contamination as a problem associated with private wells, some one out of ten public water supply wells contain pesticides, and nearly ten thousand community drinking water wells contain pesticides. A body of evidence incriminates pesticides in drinking water as a cause of human cancer.

Radiation: More than forty-nine million Americans consume water with significant radioactive contamination, because of radon, radium, and alpha particle emitters, and most ominously because of beta particle emitters from man-made fission products such as strontium-90, which damage the immune cells of the bone marrow and are carcinogenic. There is suggestive evidence that radiation-contaminated water supplies are in part responsible for escalating breast cancer mortality in some areas of the country. Recent evidence suggests that increased breast cancer incidence in the Long Island counties of Suffolk and Nassau, as well as Westchester County north of New York City, are related to radiation-contaminated drinking water. This is due to radioactive contamination of the Croton River watershed reservoirs; the watershed is located only about five miles downwind to the northeast from the Indian Point nuclear plant that has released radioactive fission products since the early 1960s. As for Suffolk and Nassau counties, their drinking water supplies are derived largely from deep aquifer wells that have become contaminated slowly by nuclear fallout contaminated with radioactive strontium-90.

There are also natural sources of radiation contamination of drinking water. For example, areas with granite rock outcroppings often have elevated levels of radium, a breakdown product of uranium, in their drinking water, especially if their supply is derived from groundwater.

Radon, the breakdown product of radium, is also found in drinking water, especially in the northeastern states such as Maine, New Hampshire, Massachusetts, New Jersey, Pennsylvania, and Vermont.

Carcinogens in Alcoholic Beverages

Pure alcohol is not carcinogenic. However, there is substantial evidence that alcoholic beverages do contain carcinogens. Alcoholic beverages have long been associated with cancers of the mouth, esophagus, and liver. More recent evidence, from a wide range of sources, associates excessive consumption with increased risk for breast cancer, which may be due to alcohol's ability to stimulate women's bodies to produce toxic metabolites of estrogenic hormones. Furthermore, consumption of any kind of alcohol in excess may cause cirrhosis of the liver, which in turn can lead to liver cancer. The problem is compounded by the presence of other unwelcome contaminants, including the following:

Asbestos: Asbestos fibers have been found in a wide range of alcoholic beverages worldwide, probably because of the filters used in clarifying beverages, from water used during production processes, and from asbestos-cement water pipes. Asbestos is a known human carcinogen.

Lead: Many fine wines are contaminated with lead from the foil around their corks.

Pesticides: A wide range of pesticides is used in vineyards. Most commonly detected carcinogenic pesticides in U.S. and European wines include dimethoate and procyrmiclone. Other carcinogenic pesticide residues that may be found in wine include arsenic compounds, metalaxyl, carbendazim, vinclozolin, iprodione, trichlorfon and its metabolite dichlorvos, and ethylenethiourea (ETU), which is a degradation product of the family of ethylene bisdithiocarbamate fungicides zineb, maneb, mancozeb, and nabam. Dichlorvos causes breast cancer in rodents.

Urethane: Urethane is present in many kinds of alcoholic beverages. Urethane has caused breast cancers in 100 percent of experimental animals in one study and has caused them to appear almost twice as early. Urethane promotes the effects of X rays in causing these tumors. Urethane has caused cancers in single doses. Although urethane is a known contaminant of alcoholic beverages and has been known to cause mammary tumors in experimental animal studies since 1962, not a single epidemiological study has been performed. Its widespread presence in alcoholic beverages is troubling, especially considering its cancer-promoting and synergistic effects. The alcohol industry has taken no steps to remove this contaminant. Federal regulators allowed the liquor industry to continue to produce beverages with urethane. The urethane problem will persist for years to come.

Carcinogens in Food Packaging

Cling film: Cling film contains carcinogens such as di-2-ethylhexyl phthalate (DEHP) and di-2-ethylhexyl adipate (DEHA), which will migrate into foods, especially fatty foods. Such films are used for wrapping cheese and packaging fruit, vegetables, meat, and fish.

Microwave packaging: The FDA has recognized that chemical components of adhesives, polymers, paper, and paperboard products used in microwave packaging migrate into food but has developed virtually no regulations.

Microwaving some packaging may cause it to disintegrate, allowing carcinogens and other uncharacterized chemicals contained in the packaging to enter food. Heat susceptor packages, which help elevate temperatures during microwaving for browning foods, have been shown to contain chemicals that can migrate into foods. These chemicals have been poorly studied, and nobody really knows how much of a hazard they present to the consumer. But what is known is that one such chemical, contained in microwave packaging, that can migrate into foods — dimethylterephthalate — has shown suggestive evidence of carcinogenicity. Heat susceptor packaging, in particular, is used for microwaving products such as popcorn, pizza, french fries, fish sticks, and Belgian waffles.

"Dual ovenables" are containers that can be used in either conventional or microwave ovens. Some prepared foods packaged in disposable trays, for use in either conventional or microwave ovens, may be contaminated with packaging chemicals at far higher rates when used in a conventional oven. Again, how much these chemicals pose hazards is difficult to determine.

PET bottling and packaging: Polyethylene terephthalate (PET) is used extensively in soft drink containers. PET bottles can release small amounts of dimethylterephthalate into foods and beverages. Although the National Cancer Institute claims that dimethylterephthalate is noncarcinogenic, these results have been questioned. Some experts believe this compound to be carcinogenic.

Plastic wrap: Plastic wrap contains residual vinylidene chloride, which is carcinogenic.

Carcinogens in Irradiated Foods

Irradiation is the process of exposing foods to high-level radiation to kill bacteria, insects, and molds. Massive doses of ionizing radiation (100,000 rads, roughly equivalent to ten million medical X rays) are used.

Food irradiation was the brainchild of the Atomic Energy Commission's efforts during the Eisenhower administration to find practical uses for the flood of radioactive wastes from nuclear weapons.

Atomic Energy of Canada (Nordion Ltd.), with its virtual monopoly on cobalt-60 and with strong backing from the International Atomic Energy Agency, hopes to operate a chain of U.S. plants with U.S. irradiation companies.

Industry and the FDA insist that irradiated food has been thoroughly tested and is absolutely safe. Foods approved for treatment include fruits and vegetables, dry and dehydrated herbs, spices, teas, pork, poultry, white potatoes, wheat, and wheat flour. However, New York, New Jersey, and Maine have prohibited the sale and distribution of irradiated food, as have foreign governments, including Germany, Denmark, Sweden, Australia, and New Zealand.

Claims of safety are unproven at best. High-energy irradiation produces complex chemical changes in food with the formation of poorly characterized radiolytic products, including benzene. Radiolytic products kill bacteria, molds, and larvae, and thus prevent spoilage, a major attraction to the purveyors of produce and poultry contaminated with salmonella and E. coli. However, concentrated extracts of irradiated food products have never been tested for cancer and other delayed adverse effects. The need for such studies is overdue, especially in light of numerous reports of chronic toxic effects in studies on test animals that were fed unextracted, whole irradiated food. The studies found reproductive damage in rodents and chromosomal damage in rodents, monkeys, and children.

An Indian study discovered chromosomal abnormalities in malnourished children fed freshly irradiated wheat.

Irradiation also reduces levels of essential nutrients in food, especially vitamins A, C, E, and the B complex. Cooking irradiated food reduces these levels further. A Japanese study found vitamin C content of potatoes reduced nearly 50 percent. The industry admits to this but suggests that the problem could be taken care of by vitamin supplements. But the decrease in these vitamins suggests that other related nutrients and beneficial plant substances, not available through supplements, may also have been decreased.

Another area of possible carcinogenicity deals with workers who will be exposed to cobalt-60 or cesium-137 and communities where such radioactive materials are transported and stored. In 1988, at a Decatur, Georgia, plant that irradiated medical supplies, some steel rods corroded, exposing employees to radiation and contaminating twenty-five thousand gallons of water with radioactive isotopes.

Despite this evidence, the FDA approved food irradiation in 1986. The FDA based its decision on five questionable or allegedly negative tests and on theoretical estimates on cancer risk, which were claimed to be insignificant and "acceptable." This position is consistent with the FDA's revocation of the Delaney law, which banned the deliberate contamination of food with any amount of carcinogenic chemicals, and its substitution by flexible "rubber number" standards based on "acceptable" cancer risk. Furthermore, the now-approved use of irradiation to solve the bacteria contamination problem associated with poultry is ill-advised; such problems would be better solved through the use of more government inspection and tighter and higher standards for animal care and processing.

2. Household Products

How bad is the situation? Some leading household products do not disclose to the consumer that they contain carcinogens, such as crystalline silica and trisodium nitrilotriacetate; neurotoxins, such as formaldehyde; or other hazardous substances. Household products have changed radically since the post–World War II "petrochemical" revolution when industry discovered that a wide range of new chemicals could be synthesized from petroleum. Production rates for synthetic petrochemicals have burgeoned from 1 billion pounds per year in 1940 to over 400 billion pounds per year in the 1980s. Since 1965 more than four million distinct chemical compounds have been reported in the scientific literature — some six thousand per week. Of these, about seventy thousand are now in commercial production; many accumulate in the human body and cause cancer and other diseases, yet have been inadequately tested or remain completely untested for their safety, raising concern for their hazards. However, only about six hundred of these chemicals are known to cause cancer, making the task of labeling their presence in products much easier.

Furthermore, many chemicals used in household products are volatile. That means they become gaseous at room temperature or are sprayed from an aerosol can or hand pump and thus take the form of microscopic particles that are easily inhaled. In either case, they can cause damage to the lungs or other organs as they are taken into the bloodstream. Because indoor pollutants are not as easily dispersed or diluted as outdoor pollutants, concentrations of toxic chemicals may be much greater indoors than outdoors. Peak concentrations of twenty toxic compounds — some linked with cancer and birth defects — were two hundred to five hundred times higher inside some homes than outdoors, according to a five-year EPA study that surveyed six hundred individuals in six cities to find out what their exposure was to common air pollutants. Not surprisingly, EPA experts say that indoor air pollution is one of the nation's most pressing personal health concerns. "If we measured outdoors what we are measuring indoors," says EPA indoor air specialist Lance Wallace, "there would be a tremendous hue and cry to clean up outdoor air."

In the last few years consumers have discovered that some of the chemicals in household products whose safety was taken for granted are hazardous. For instance, methylene chloride (also known as dichloromethane), the propellant used in many aerosol products, is carcinogenic. Although some products containing methylene chloride have been pulled from the market, thanks to belated government regulations, this carcinogen continues to be found in many consumer products such as spray paint and stripper.

More recently, a limited number of shoppers learned that indoor latex paints used widely for decades contained highly neurotoxic mercury-based fungicides. But it was not until 1990 that manufacturers finally removed most of these potent neurotoxins.

3. Cosmetics and Toiletries

As for cosmetics, while consumers are told what ingredients have been intentionally added to products, they are not provided with information that would alert them, for example, to carcinogenic contaminants or preservatives that release formaldehyde; nor are they told about ingredients in hair color products likely to be associated with cancer, or substances in fragrances that are potentially neurotoxic or teratogenic. Not a single cosmetic company warns consumers of the presence of carcinogens in its products, despite the fact that several common cosmetic ingredients or their contaminants are carcinogenic themselves or are carcinogenic precursors (Chapter 17).

A recent government investigation of the cosmetics industry provides strong evidence of how poorly regulated it is:

- FDA officials have found that many cosmetic manufacturers lack adequate data on safety tests and have generally refused to disclose the results of these tests.

- The FDA estimates that only a tiny percentage — 3 percent — of the 4,000 to 5,000 cosmetic distributors have filed reports with the government of injuries to consumers.

- The FDA believes that less than 40 percent of the nation's 2,000 to 2,500 cosmetic manufacturers are even registered.

- Despite the cosmetic industry's reliance on its voluntary program of self-regulation, industry participation has actually declined slightly in the last decade.

- The National Institute of Occupational Safety and Health found that 884 of the chemicals available for use in cosmetics have been reported to the government as toxic substances. A General Accounting Office report notes that the FDA has committed no resources for assessing the safety problems of those chemicals that have been found to cause genetic damage, biological mutations, and cancer.

A wide range of undisclosed carcinogenic ingredients and contaminants are presently in mainstream brands of cosmetics and toiletries. These fall into the following main classes:

Formaldehyde-Releasing Preservatives

Cosmetics and personal care products require preservatives or they will become contaminated with bacteria, and it would be irresponsible for companies not to use preservatives. The choice of preservatives is especially important because this family of ingredients is, like fragrances, one of the leading causes of contact dermatitis.

Some of the most allergenic and irritating preservatives release small amounts of formaldehyde, which is an irritant and sensitizer as well as a carcinogen and neurotoxin. Many cosmetic companies do not use such ingredients because they can make the eyes sting and irritate the skin. But many companies do, and you should be able to identify these ingredients so you can avoid products containing them.

The *following ingredients contain formaldehyde,* may release formaldehyde, or may break down into formaldehyde:

- 2-bromo-2-nitropropane-1, 3-diol
- Diazolidinyl urea
- DMDM hydantoin
- Imidazolidinyl urea
- Quaternium 15

DEA, TEA, Bronopol, and Padimate-O

Many cosmetics, both natural and from mainstream companies, contain either diethanolamine or triethanolamine (used as wetting agents), abbreviated on labels as DEA and TEA, and generally shown bound to fatty acid compounds as in cocamide DEA or TEA sodium lauryl sulfate.

If products contain nitrites (used as a preservative or present as contaminants and not disclosed on cosmetics labels), their presence (especially DEAs) in cosmetics can cause a chemical reaction during formulation or even as products sit on store shelves. This reaction leads to the formation of *nitrosamines.* Most nitrosamines, including those formed from DEA or TEA, are carcinogenic (pages 579, 577).

Not all products containing DEA or TEA contain nitrosamines. Some may; others will not. Yet because of the failure of the FDA to request Congress to enact adequate label disclosure legislation, the consumer has no way of knowing which products are contaminated with nitrosamines. That leaves the consumer to play cancer roulette and hurts the entire cosmetic industry, making all products suspect.

The FDA accepts that the presence of DEA and TEA in cosmetics can pose a significant consumer health threat. In the 1970s it published a notice In the *Federal Register* in which it urged the industry to remove these products from cosmetics. The industry has made some progress by using higher quality control standards in its selection of raw materials. But an FDA report from the late 1980s noted that some 37 percent of the products tested contained carcinogenic nitrosamine impurities. It is unfortunate that low-level to high-level nitrosamine contamination is so prevalent, because this is a problem that could be easily eliminated.

German cosmetics, for example, are unlikely to contain nitrosamines. This is because of official recommendations by the German Federal Health Office in 1987 that discouraged manufacturers from using DEA and TEA. Thus, German cosmetics would make a good choice for concerned consumers.

Your best self-protection is to boycott any products containing DEA or TEA. That will send a clear message to the cosmetic industry.

Two more chemicals pose similar hazards for nitrosamine formation. The chemical 2-bromo-2-nitropropane (also known as *Bronopol*) may break down in products into *formaldehyde* and *also* cause the formation of carcinogenic *nitrosamines* under certain conditions. One of the most expensive lines of cosmetics today, Chanel, often uses this chemical. So do many leading brands of baby products. And the Body Shop, whose product sales are built on a reputation of containing natural ingredients, also offers products containing this chemical. There are many safer yet equally effective products available.

Padimate-O (also known as octyl dimethyl PABA) is found in cosmetics, especially sunscreens. It can also cause formation of nitrosamines. At present it is not known whether the particular nitrosamine formed in this product is carcinogenic. Some experts have recommended that consumers continue to use sunscreens with padimate-O. The jury, however, is still out on the nitrosamine formed from padimate-O, and nobody knows for sure whether it will prove carcinogenic. So the most prudent consumer will prefer sunscreens without padimate-O, until the industry proves that the nitrosamine by-product that may be formed is not carcinogenic.

Although many products contain DEA, TEA, 2-bromo-2-nitropropane-1, 3-diol, or padimate-O, some manufacturers have added ingredients such as antioxidants that may slow or retard, but do not prevent, formation of nitrosamines. It is always better to avoid buying products with potential nitrosamine-forming ingredients. Quite apart from the risks of DEA as a precursor of nitrosomines, DEA itself has also recently been shown to be carcinogenic (page 479).

Ethoxylated Alcohols and 1,4-Dioxane

Cosmetics containing ethoxylated wetting agents (e.g., detergents, foaming agents, emulsifiers, and solvents) may be contaminated with 1,4-dioxane, which is carcinogenic. Studies show that dioxane readily penetrates human skin. It can be removed from cosmetics through vacuum stripping during processing without an unreasonable increase in raw material cost. This process is not mandatory, but should be. At present, there is not enough information shown on product labels to enable you to determine whether products are contaminated. The best way to protect yourself is to recognize ingredients most likely to be contaminated with 1,4-dioxane. These include ingredients with the prefix, word, or syllable PEG, *Polyethylene, polyethylene Glycol, Polyoxyethylene, eth* (as in sodium laur*eth* sulfate), or oxynol. Both polysorbate 60 and polysorbate 80 may also be contaminated with 1,4-dioxane.

We provide this information as a general caution. It is impossible to determine which products are contaminated and which have gone through vacuum stripping, so some products we recommend may contain ingredients that possibly are contaminated with 1,4-dioxane.

Talc

Cosmetic talc is carcinogenic (page 569). Powdered products containing talc and used around the face must be assumed to expose the consumer or professional cosmetologist via inhalation. Inhaling talc and using it in the genital area, where its use is associated with increased risk of ovarian cancer, are the primary ways this substance poses a carcinogenic hazard. In most cases, we have designated a "minimal risk" rating to products containing talc. However, products containing talc that are used in the genital region are given the "caution" rating because of clear evidence that talc causes ovarian cancer. Although some recommended products contain talc, these are generally liquid formulations and pose minimal, if any, carcinogenic risk.

Silica

Some silica used in cosmetics, especially amorphous hydrated silica, may be contaminated with small amounts of crystalline quartz. Crystalline silica is carcinogenic. We simply cannot tell whether the silica used in specific cosmetics and personal care products contains small amounts of crystalline quartz, or none. Furthermore, exposure via inhalation is assumed to be limited to special use situations: for example, people who use facial makeup, especially powders, may inhale the silica. The situation is obviously more perilous for beauty care professionals, as they may end up inhaling contaminants continuously. There are inadequate data to determine that amorphous silica is not carcinogenic: therefore we have assigned products containing silica the minimal risk rating. The hazard of silica is primarily via inhalation. As with talc, although some recommended products contain silica, they are still better than their competitors.

Artificial Colors

Some artificial colors, such as Blue 1 and Green 3, are carcinogenic. Impurities found in commercial batches of other cosmetic colors such as D&C Red 33, FD&C Yellow 5, and FD&C Yellow 6 have been shown to cause cancer not only when ingested, but also when applied to the skin. Some artificial coal tar colors contain heavy metal impurities, including arsenic and lead, which are carcinogenic. Nevertheless, the FDA maintains that these color additives, impurities notwithstanding, do not pose a hazard when used in cosmetics and personal care products. We have recommended against many products containing artificial colors when clear evidence of their carcinogenic hazard is available. In some cases, products with artificial colors have been recommended in the absence of such information. Many consumers may simply want to avoid products containing artificial colors. Most alternative brands, sold in health food stores, do not contain them.

Lanolin

Lanolin itself is perfectly safe, and its presence in cosmetics is generally beneficial to your skin, especially when it is sore and cracked (although some people develop allergic reactions to this ingredient). But cosmetic-grade lanolin can be contaminated with carcinogenic pesticides such as DDT, dieldrin, and lindane, in addition to other neurotoxic pesticides. Some sixteen pesticides were identified in lanolin sampled in 1988 (including the neurotoxic organophosphate pesticide diazinon, which was found in twenty-one out of twenty-five samples and readily penetrates the skin).

These chemicals are likely to migrate through the skin into the bloodstream. The National Academy of Sciences has expressed concern over the frequency of contamination of cosmetics containing lanolin with pesticides. The FDA recognizes that the contamination of lanolin is a problem, especially in the case of skin products used by nursing mothers directly on their nipples, because their infants may end up ingesting these carcinogenic impurities. Furthermore, lanolin is often applied to children's and babies' skin with the potential for significant absorption of pesticides.

The FDA has done nothing to improve the quality of cosmetic lanolin, though the industry has voluntarily reduced, but not removed, the contamination of these carcinogens. The fact that labels need not disclose this information leaves the consumer unsure of which products are pure and which are contaminated with carcinogenic pesticides. Again, the lack of full label disclosure causes the entire industry to be suspect, rather than limiting the problem to those companies that are not purifying their lanolin-based ingredients.

Although the FDA believes the risk to consumers is small, interestingly, Dr. Stan Milstein, special assistant to the director of the FDA Office of Cosmetics and Colors, adds this caution: "Given all the carcinogens in the environment that the consumer is bombarded with, do we really need to be increasing our exposure even incrementally?"

Hair Dyes

The use of permanent or semipermanent hair color products, particularly black and dark brown colors, is associated with increased incidence of human cancer. These contain a wide range of carcinogenic ingredients, contaminants, and precursors Table XIV.2). As stated earlier, the use of these products places women at increased risk of non-Hodgkin's lymphoma, multiple myeloma, and Hodgkin's disease. In fact, there is growing evidence that the use of hair-coloring prod-

Table XIV.2 Hazardous ingredients in permanent and semi-permanent dark hair dye.

Ingredient	Hazard
Dyes	
C1 disperses Blue 1	Carcinogenic
D&C Red 33	Carcinogenic
Diaminoanisole	Carcinogenic
Diaminotoluene	Carcinogenic
HC Blue No. 1	Carcinogenic
Para-phenylenediamine	Carcinogenic when oxidized
Detergents/Solvents	
Diethanoloamine/ Triethanolamine	Combine with nitrite to form carcinogenic nitrosamines
Ceteareths and Laureths	Contaminated with the carcinogen 1,4-dioxane
Dyes	
Polyethylene glycol	Contaminated with 1,4-dioxane; degrades into the carcinogen formaldehyde
Preservatives	
DMDM-hydantoin, Imidazolidinyl urea, Quaternium 15	All release formaldehyde

ucts accounts for 20 percent of all non-Hodg-kin's lymphoma cases in all U.S. women. These products should be banned. Until that happens, they should be clearly labeled for their cancer hazard (Chapter 17).

Synthetic Fragrances

Fragrances are made up of hundreds of chemicals. Some, such as methylene chloride, are carcinogenic. Because manufacturers are not required to disclose hazardous chemicals used in manufacturing fragrances, consumers have no way of knowing whether their brands' fragrances contain carcinogens. The wise consumer will make the assumption that all synthetic fragrances contain carcinogens. However, in the absence of such information we are unable to evaluate fragrances for their presence. Although some brands containing synthetic fragrances are recommended in the absence of available information, some consumers may simply wish to avoid such products.

Activist and Resource Groups,
U.S. and Great Britain

In the United States

AFL-CIO
Occupational Safety & Health Dept.
815- 16th St., N.W.
Washington, D.C. 20006
(202) 637-5366

American Federation of State County and
Municipal Employees
Health and Safety Dept.
525 L St., N. W.
Washington, D. C. 20036
(202) 429-1232

Breast Cancer Action
55 New Montgomery Street, Suite 323
San Francisco, CA 94105
(415) 243-0301

Breast Cancer Fund
282 Second St.
San Francisco, CA 94105
(415) 543-2979

Cancer Control Society
2043 North Berendon Street
Los Angeles, CA 90027
(213) 663-7801

Center for Medical Consumers
237 Thompson Street
New York, NY 10012
(212) 674-7105

Center to Protect Workers' Rights
111 Massachusetts Avenue,
N.W. Washington, D.C. 20001
(202) 962-8490

Center for Science in the Public Interest
1875 Connecticut Avenue
N.W. Washington, D.C. 20009
(202) 332-9110

Center for the Study of Responsive Law
1530 P Street, N. W.
Washington, D.C. 20005
(202) 387-8034

Citizens Clearing House for
Hazardous Wastes
P.O. Box 6806
Falls Church, VA 22040
(703) 237-CCHW

Committee for Nuclear Responsibility
P.O. Box 421993
San Francisco, CA 94142
(415) 776-8299

Communication Workers
Safety & Health Dept.
501 Third St., N.W.
Washington, D. C. 20001
(202) 434-1160

Community Nutrition Institute
2001 South Street, N.W.
Washington, D.C. 20009
(202) 462-4700

DES Action
1615 Broadway
Oakland, CA 94612
(510) 465-4011

Environmental Health Coalition
1717 Kettner Blvd.
San Diego, CA 92101
(619) 235-0281

Environmental Defense Fund
257 Park Avenue
New York, NY 10010
(900) Call EDF

Environmental Research Foundation
P.O. Box 5036
Annapolis, MD 21403
(410) 263-1585

Environmental Working Group
1718 Connecticut Avenue
Washington, D.C. 20009
(202) 667-6982

Food & Commercial Workers Union
Safety & Health Dept.
1775 K. St., N.W.
Washington, D. C. 20006
(202) 223-3111

Food and Water Inc.
RR 1, Box 68D
Walden, VT 05873
(800) EAT-SAFE

Greenpeace
1436 U Street, N.W.
Washington, D.C. 20009
(202) 319-2472

Health Research Group
2000 P Street, N.W.
Washington, D.C. 20036
(202) 588-7735

Inform, Inc.
120 Wall Street
New York, NY 10005
(212) 361-2400

International Association of Machinists
Safety & Health Dept.
9000 Machinist Place
Upper Marlboro, MD 20772
(301) 967-4704

International Chemical Workers Union
Council (ICWUC)
Health & Safety Dept.
1655 W. Market St.
Akron, Ohio 44313
(330) 867-2444

Jacobs Institute of Women's Health
409 12th Street, S.W.
Washington, D.C.
(202) 863-4990

Massachusetts Breast Cancer Coalition
Pioneer Valley P.O. Box 536
Leeds, MA 01053
(413) 585-1222

Mothers and Others for a Livable Planet
40 West 20th Street
New York, NY 10011
(212) 727-4474

Mothers for Natural Law
P.O. Box 1177
Fairfield, Iowa 10011
(515) 472-2809

National Coalition Against Misuse of
Pesticides
701 East Street, S.E., Suite 200
Washington, D.C. 20003
(202) 543-5450

National Silicone Implant Foundation
4416 Willow Lane
Dallas, TX 75244
(972) 490-0800

National Women's Health Network
1325 G Street, N.W.
Washington, D.C. 20005
(202) 347-1140

Natural Resources Defense Council
71 Stevenson Street, Suite 1825
San Francisco, CA 94105
(413) 777-0220

New York Committee on Occupational Safety
and Health
275 - 7th Avenue
New York, NY 10001
(212) 627-3900

Northwest Coalition for Alternatives to
Pesticides
P.O. Box 1393
Eugene, OR 97440
(503) 344-5044

Office of Technical Assistance for Toxics use
Reduction
100 Cambridge Street
Boston, MA 02202
(617) 727-3260

Oil, Chemical, and Atomic Workers International Union
  Health & Safety Dept.
  255 Union Blvd.
  Lakewood, CO 80288
  (303) 987-2229

People Against Cancer
  P.O. Box 10
  Otho, Iowa 50569
  (515) 972-4444

Pesticide Action Network
  North America Regional Center
  116 New Montgomery, Suite 810
  San Francisco, CA 94105
  (415) 541-9140
  (202) 588- 1000

Physicians for Social Responsibility
  1000, 16th Street, N.W.
  Washington, D.C. 20036
  (202) 785-3777

Public Citizen
  1600 20th Street, N.W.
  Washington, D.C. 20009
  (202) 588-1000

Public Interest Research Group
  218 D Street, S.E.
  Washington, D.C. 20003
  (202) 546-9707

Pure Food Campaign
  1130 17th Street, N.W., Suite 300
  Washington, D.C. 20036
  (202) 775-1132

Service Employees International Union
  1313 L St., N.W.
  Washington, D. C. 20005
  (202) 898-3200

Sierra Club
  85 Second Street
  San Francisco, CA 94104
  (415) 977-5500

Toxics Use Reduction Institute
  University of Massachusetts Lowell
  One University Avenue
  Lowell, MA 01854
  (508) 936-3275

Triad Silicone Network
  P.O. Box 7631
  Greensboro, NC 27417
  (910) 854-5338

Union of Concerned Scientists
  1616 P Street, N.W., Suite 310
  Washington, D.C. 20036
  (202) 332-0900

Union of Needle Trades, Industrial and Textile Employees
  Occupational Safety & Health Dept.
  275- 7th Ave.
  New York, NY 10001
  (212) 691-1691

United Auto Workers
  Health & Safety Dept.
  8000 E. Jefferson Ave.
  Detroit, MI 48214
  (313) 926-5000

United Brothers of Carpenters & Joiners of America
  Safety & Health Dept.
  101 Constitution Avenue, N.W.
  Washington, D. C. 20001
  (202) 546-6206

United Mine Workers of America
  Dept. Health and Safety
  900-15th Street, N.W.
  Washington, D. C. 20005
  (202) 842-7200

United Steelworkers of America
  Department Health & Safety
  Five Gateway Center
  Pittsburgh, PA 15222
  (412) 562-2400

Women's Cancer Resource Center
1815 East 41st Street, Suite C
Minneapolis, MN 55407
(800) 908-8544

Women's Community Cancer Project
46 Pleasant Street
Cambridge, MA 02139
(617) 354-9888

Women's Environment & Development
Organization
845 Third Avenue, 15th Floor
New York, NY 10022
(212) 759-7982

In Great Britain

Communities Against Toxins
31 Station Road
Little Sutton
South Wirral L66- I NU
(0151) 339-5473

DES Action Group
52-54 Featherstone Street
London EC1Y -8RT
(0171) 251-6580

Environmental Law Foundation
Lincoln's Inn House
42 Kingsway
London WC2E-6EX
(0171) 404-1030

Food Additive Campaign Team
Science Policy Research Unit
Mantell Building
Sussex University
Brighton BNI- 9RF
(0273) 686758

Friends of the Earth
26-28 Underwood Street
London N1-7JQ
(0171) 490-1555

Genetics Forum
258 Pentonville Road
London N I -9JY
(0171) 278-6578

Green Network
9 Clairemont Road
Lexden, Colchester
Essex C03-5BE
(01206) 546-902

Green Audit
38 Queen Street
Aberkstwyth
Dyfed, SA23- I PU
(01597) 824-771

Greenpeace Environmental Trust
30 Islington Green
London N1-2PN
(0171) 354-5100

Greenpeace Nuclear Campaigns
30 Islington Green
London N1-2PN
(0171) 359-7396

Greenpeace U. K.
Canonbury Villas
30 Islington Green
London N1-2PN
(0171) 865-8212

Newham Occupational Health Project
81-91 Commerce Road
London E1-1RD
(0171) 655-6600

Parents for Safe Food
5-11 Worship Street
London EC2A-2BH
(0171) 628-2442

Sustainable Agriculture, Food and
Environment Alliance
21 Tower Street
London WC2H-9NS
(0171) 240-1811

The Food Commission
5-11 Worship Street
London EC2A-2BH
(0171) 628-7774

The Pesticides Trust
23 Beehive Place
London SW9-7QR
(0171) 274-8895

Trades Union Congress
    (Contact Owen Tudor)
    Great Russell Street
    London WCIB-3LS
    (0171) 636-4030

What Doctors Don't Tell You
    4 Wallace Road
    London N1-2PG
    (0171) 3544592

Women's Environmental Network
    87 Worship Street
    London EC2A-2BE
    (0171) 247-3327

Women's Health
    52 Featherstone Street
    London EC1Y-8RT
    (0171) 251-6580

Women's National Cancer Control
Campaign
    Suna House
    128-130 Curtain Road
    London EC2A-3AR
    (0171) 729-1735

VDU Workers Rights Campaign
    City Centre
    32-35 Featherstone Street
    London EC1
    (0171) 608-1338

Women's Nationwide Cancer Control
Campaign
    Suna House
    128-130 Curtain Road
    London EC2A-3AR
    (0171) 729-2229

The Cancer Prevention Coalition

*"Cancer prevention through reduction of carcinogens
in air, water, food, consumer products, and the workplace"*

Cancer Prevention Coalition
School of Public Health
University of Illinois
Medical Center, Chicago
2121 West Taylor
Chicago, Illinois 60612
312-996-2297
www.preventcancer.com

Statement of Purpose

The Cancer Prevention Coalition, Inc. (CPC), which opened its national office in Chicago in July 1994, is a unique nationwide coalition of leading independent experts in cancer prevention and public health, together with citizen activists and representatives of organized labor, public interest, environmental and women's health groups. Our goal is to reduce cancer rates through a comprehensive strategy of outreach, public education, advocacy and public policy initiatives to establish prevention as the nation's foremost cancer policy.

An overemphasis on the diagnosis and treatment of cancer and relative neglect of its prevention, coupled with ineffective regulation of carcinogens in air, water, food, consumer products, and the workplace, have contributed to escalating cancer rates and an annual death toll of over 500,000. The National Cancer Institute (NCI) and American Cancer Society (ACS) — which should be the chief advocates of cancer prevention — instead mislead the public and policymakers into believing that we are winning the war against cancer, and trivialize the role of avoidable exposures to industrial carcinogens.

The Coalition's activities are dual and complementary. The first is directed to cancer prevention on the personal level by informing consumers of their avoidable risks from undisclosed carcinogenic ingredients and contaminants in a wide range of foods and consumer products, such as cosmetics and home and garden pesticides. With this information, consumers will be empowered to demand safer alternatives and explicit food and product labeling. A major objective of our educational programs is to generate a critical mass of support for establishing prevention as a top priority in cancer and public health policies.

Our second activity is directed to advocating reform of national cancer policies, and the priorities of the NCI and ACS, to produce major emphasis on cancer prevention, particularly the elimination of avoidable exposures to environmental and occupational carcinogens. To this end, CPC advocates phasing out the manufacture, use, and disposal of industrial carcinogens and their replacement with noncarcinogenic alternatives. In this regard we will seek out and work with socially responsible industries.

The ultimate and longer-term objective of CPC is to truly advance the war against cancer by reducing modern epidemic cancer rates to their relatively low pre-1940 levels. The Coalition has developed a wide range of outreach programs in efforts to attain this objective. The following are illustrative:

Cancer Prevention Alerts

1. Talc: Questions and Answers
2. Lindane: Questions and Answers
3. Facts You Need to Know About Cancer
4. Facts on Carcinogens at Home
5. IGF-1 and Milk: Questions and Answers
6. Hot Dogs: Questions and Answers
7. Household Products: Questions and Answers
8. Hazardous Ingredients in Household Products
9. Cosmetics and Personal Care Products: Questions and Answers
10. Foods and Beverages: Questions and Answers
11. Industry Funds Breast Cancer Campaign
12. Produce and Pesticides: A Safe Shopping List
13. Diethanolamine (DEA): What Is It?
14. Hormones in Meat: Questions and Answers
15. Ritalin: Stimulant for Cancer
16. Indoor Air Pollution: Cleaning up Cleaning Habits
17. Home and Garden Pesticides: What You Should Know
18. Scourge (Resmethrin): Questions and Answers
19. The "Dirty Dozen" Consumer Products

Citizen Petitions To The FDA

1. Petition Seeking Carcinogenic Labelling on all Cosmetic Talc Products, 4/17/94
2. Petition Seeking to Ban the Use of Lindane as Treatment for Lice and Scabies, 1/17/95
3. Petition Seeking Labelling of Nitrite-preserved Hot Dogs for Childhood Cancer Risk, 4/25/95
4. Petition Seeking a Medical Alert for All Women with Silicone Gel and Polyurethane Breast Implants, 5/12/95
5. Petition Seeking Cancer Warning on Cosmetics Containing DEA, 10/22/96

Press Releases

1. "Environmental Pollutants as Unrecognized Causes of Breast Cancer," American Association for the Advancement of Sciences, San Francisco, CA, 2/22/94.
2. "CPC Calls for the Replacement of the Director of the National Cancer Institute. Letter to President Clinton," 6/9/94.
3. "Breast Cancer Deaths Linked to Nuclear Emissions" 9/8/94.
4. "$4.25 Billion Implant Settlement Ignores Risk of Breast Cancer," 9/13/94.
5. "Breast Cancer Unawareness Month," 10/14/94.
6. "National Mammoscam Day," 10/18/94.
7. "Dusting With Cancer: Coalition Urges Chicago Drugstores to Label Talc," 11/17/94.
8. "Lice Won't Kill You but Its Treatment Can: Experts Call for Ban on Lindane Shampoos," 1/17/95.
9. "Research Cures Cancer Campaign Misleads Public and Congress," 1/25/95.
10. "Cancer Expert Calls Dow Breast Implant Ads Deceptive," 5/11/95.
11. "National Mammography Day," 10/18/95.
12. "New Study Warns Implants Pose Risk of Breast Cancer," 11/8/95.
13. "Cancer War is Threatened by Environmental Protection Agency, Proposals." (CPC Critique By 25

Leading Scientists, and 50 Environmental and Public Interest Groups Representing a Constituency of Some 10 Million Citizens), 8/16/96.

14. "Cancer War Is Threatened by Recommendations of Presidential Commision," 8/30/96.

15. "Europe's Ban on Hormone-Raised Beef Is Based on Sound Science," 10/8/96.

16. "They Make You Smell, Feel, and Look Good — But Can Cosmetics Increase Your Risk of Cancer: CPC Calls for Tough Cosmetics Standards," 10/22/96.

17. "Public Health and Veterinary Risks of rBST Dairy Products," Co-sponsored by the Green Network, Great Britain, Presentation to the House of Commons, British Parliament, 12/11/96.

18. "We Are Losing the Winnable War Against Cancer," 12/18/96.

19. "New Challenges on the Safety of U.S. Meat: Oprah Is Right for Other Reasons," PR Newswire, 2/2/98.

20. "New Drug (Evista) Poses Risks of Ovarian Cancer," PR Newswire, 2/4/98.

21. "Major Cosmetics and Toiletry Ingredient Poses Avoidable Risks of Cancer," PR Newswire, 2/22/98.

22. "Monsanto's Biosynthetic Milk Poses Risks of Prostate Cancer, Besides Other Cancer," PR Newswire, 3/15/98.

23. "Cancer Report Card Gets a Failing Grade," PR Newswire, 4/1/98.

24. "Monsanto's Hormonal Milk Poses Serious Risks of Breast Cancer, Besides Other Cancers," PR Newswire, 6/21/98.

25. "FDA Urged to Reject Approval of Zeneca's Application of Tamoxifen for Preventing Breast Cancer in Healthy Women, as the Drug is Ineffective and Dangerous," PR Newswire, 9/1/98.

26. "The Cancer Drug Industry 'March' Seriously Misleads the Nation," PR Newswire, 9/24/98.

Press Conferences And Briefings

1. "Distinguished Experts Call on President to Redirect War on Cancer," National Press Club, Washington, D.C., 6/24/93.

2. "How the Clinton Administration Pesticide Proposal Addresses the Recommendations of the National Academy of Sciences Report Concerning Pesticide and Infants and Children," Co-sponsored by Citizen Action, Washington, D.C., 9/8/93.

3. "rBGH-Milk and Breast Cancer," Co-sponsored by the National Farm Coalition, U.S. Capitol, Washington, D.C., 3/14/94.

4. "Cancer Group and Ralph Nader Release First Annual 'Dirty Dozen' Consumer Product List," National Press Club, Washington, D.C., 9/21/95.

5. "Advocacy Groups Escalate Efforts Against rBGH: Study on Cancer Risks Released," Co-sponsored by Food & Water, National Press Club, Washington, D.C., 1/23/96.

6. "The Scientific Basis for the EU Ban on Hormonal Meat," International Press Conference, European Parliament, Brussels, Belgium, 5/21/97.

References

PART I
The Politics of Cancer, 1979

CHAPTER 1
The Impact of Cancer

1. Testimony before Subcommittee on Health, House Commerce Committee, March 21, 1977. See also B. J. Culliton, "Fight Over Proposed Saccharin Ban Will Not Be Settled for Months," *Science* 196 (1977), pp. 276-78.
2. S. S. Epstein, "Environmental Determinants of Cancer," *Cancer Research* 34 (1974), pp. 2425-35; "1978 Cancer Facts and Figures" (New York: American Cancer Society, 1977), p. 3.
3. J. L. Young, S. S. Devesa, and S. J. Cutler, "Incidence of Cancer in United States Blacks," *Cancer Res.* 35 (1975), pp. 3523-33.
4. Ibid., p. 3525.
5. Epstein, "Environmental Determinants of Cancer"; S. S. Epstein, "Cancer and the Environment," *Bulletin of the Atomic Scientists (of Chicago)* 26 (1977), pp. 22-30.
6. A. C. Upton, "The National Cancer Institute and its Redefined Mission," *Grants Magazine, 1* (1978), pp. 113-28.
7. D. Greenberg, "Cancer: Now the bad news," *Washington Post,* January 19, 1975; D. Greenberg, Science and Government Report, Washington, D.C., April 1, 1975; SEER Program, "Cancer Patient Survival," SEER Program Report no. 5 DHEW Publication (NIH) 77-992 (Washington, D.C., 1976). It should be noted that survival data are difficult to collect, and debates rage concerning their accuracy. See, for example, J. E. Enstrom and D. F. Austin, "Interpreting Cancer Survival Rates," *Science* 195 (1977), pp. 847-51.
8. "Cancer Patient Survival," SEER Program Report; M. H. Myers (NCI), Personal Communication, May, 1979.
9. S. S. Devesa, and M. A. Schneiderman, "Increase in the Number of Cancer Deaths in the United States," *American Journal of Epidemiology* 106 (1977), pp. 1-5.
10. M. S. Zdeb, "The Probability of Developing Cancer," *Am. J. Epidemiology* 106 (1977), pp. 6-16.
11. American Industrial Health Council, "AIHC Recommended Alternatives to OSHA's Generic Carcinogen Policy" (Scarsdale, N.Y., January 9, 1978).
12. R. Doll, "Prevention of Cancer: Pointers from epidemiology" (London: Nuffield Hospital Trust, 1967); J. Higginson, "Present Trends in Cancer Epidemiology," *Proceedings of the Canadian Cancer Conference* 8 (1969), pp. 40-75; J. Higginson, "The Role of Geographical Pathology in Environmental Carcinogenesis," in *Environment and Cancer* (Baltimore: Williams and Wilkins, 1972), pp. 69-89; Epstein, "Environmental Determinants of Cancer"; B. Armstrong and R. Doll, "Environmental Factors and Cancer Incidence and Mortality in Different Countries with Special Reference to Dietary Practices," *International Journal of Cancer* 15 (1975), pp. 617-31.
13. W. Haenszel, ed., *Epidemiological Study of Cancer and Other Chronic Diseases,* National Cancer Institute Monograph 19 (Bethesda, Md., 1966).
14. Doll, "Prevention of Cancer."
15. AIHC, "Alternatives to OSHA's Generic Carcinogen Policy"; E. L. Wynder and G. B. Gori, "Contribution of the Environment to Cancer Incidence," *Journal of the National Cancer Institute* 58 (1977), pp. 825- 32.
16. I. J. Selikoff, E. C. Hammond, and J. Churg, "Asbestos Exposure, Smoking, and Neoplasia," *Journal of the American*

Medical Association 204 (1968), pp. 106-12; R. Saracci, "Asbestos and Lung Cancer: An analysis of the epidemiological evidence on the asbestos-smoking interaction," *Intl. J. Cancer* 20 (1977), pp. 323-31.

17. T. J. Mason and F. W. McKay, "U.S. Cancer Mortality by County, 1950-1969," DHEW Publication (NIH) 74-615 (Washington, D.C., 1973); R. Hoover *et al.*, "Geographic Patterns of Cancer Mortality in the United States," in J. F. Fraumeni, Jr., ed., *Persons at High Risk of Cancer* (New York: Academic Press, 1975), pp. 343-60; W. J. Blot, "The Geography of Cancer," *The Sciences* 17 (1977), pp. 12-15.

18. H. M. Menck, J. T. Casagrande, and B. E. Henderson, "Industrial Air Pollution: Possible effect on lung cancer," *Science* 183 (1974), pp. 210-12.

19. C. Noller, *Chemistry of Organic Compounds* (Philadelphia: Saunders, 1957), p. 73; *Chemical and Engineering News,* Nov. 7, 1977, p. 16.

20. T. H. Maugh, "Chemicals: How many are there?" *Science* 199 (1978), p. 162.

CHAPTER 2
Cancer: The Human Experiment

1. A. M. Lilienfeld, *Foundations of Epidemiology* (Oxford University Press, 1976); B. MacMahon and T. F. Pugh, *Epidemiology: Principles and Methods* (Boston: Little, Brown, 1970); J. Mausner and A. K. Bahn, *Epidemiology* (Philadelphia: Saunders, 1973); R. Doll, "The Contribution of Epidemiology to Knowledge of Cancer," *Revue Epidemiologie et Sante Publique* 24 (1976), pp. 107-21.

2. U.S. Department of Health, Education, and Welfare, *Vital Statistics of the United States, 1970,* vol. 2, "Mortality," (Washington, D.C.: Department of Health, Education, and Welfare, Public Health Service, 1974).

3. See, for example, B. Christine, J. T. Flannery, and P. D. Sullivan, "Cancer in Connecticut, 1966-1968" (Hartford: Connecticut State Department of Health, 1971).

4. I. Adler, *Primary Malignant Growths of the Lung and Bronchi: A pathological and clinical study* (London: Longmans, Green and Co., 1912), p. 1.

5. F. H. Muller, "Tabakmissbrauch und Lungencarcinom," *Zeitschrift für Krebsforschung* 49 (1939), pp. 57-84.

6. "Smoking and Health: Report of the Advisory Committee to the Surgeon General of the Public Health Service" (Washington, D.C.: Department of Health, Education, and Welfare, Public Health Service, 1964). The classic "Surgeon General's Report" exhaustively summarizing the evidence that smoking causes cancer and many other health problems.

7. E. C. Hammond, "Smoking in Relation to Death Rates of One Million Men and Women," National Cancer Institute Monograph 19 (Washington, D.C., 1966), pp. 124-204.

8. E. C. Hammond *et al.*, " 'Tar' and Nicotine Content of Cigarette Smoke in Relation to Death Rates," *Environmental Research* 12 (1976), pp. 263- 74.

9. "The Health Consequences of Smoking — 1974" (Washington D.C.: Department of Health, Education, and Welfare, 1974); E. L. Wynder, and S. D. Stellman, "Comparative Epidemiology of Tobacco-Related Cancers," *Cancer Research* 37 (1977), pp. 4608-22; W. Haenszel, ed., *Epidemiological Study of Cancer and Other Chronic Diseases,* National Cancer Institute Monograph 19 (Bethesda, Md., 1966). A hard-to-find technical monograph containing much fundamental data on smoking and cancer. Also contains British-Norwegian migrant studies which form one of the cornerstones for belief in environmental rather than genetic causes of cancer.

10. D. Hoffmann and E. L. Wynder, "Environmental Respiratory Carcinogenesis," ch. 7 in C. E. Searle, ed., *Chemical Carcinogenesis,* American Chemical Society Monograph 173 (Washington, D.C., 1976); E. L. Wynder, M. Mushinski, and S. D. Stellman, "The Epidemiology of the Less Harmful Cigarette," *Proceedings of the Third World Conference on Smoking and Health* (1976), pp. 1-13.

11. "Smoking and Health: Report to the Surgeon General," p. 7.
12. See, for example, I. J. Selikoff, "Lung Cancer and Mesothelioma during Prospective Surveillance of 1,249 Asbestos Insulation Workers, 1963-1974," *Annals of the New York Academy of Sciences* 271 (1976), pp. 448-56.
13. A. J. Fox and P. F. Collier, "Low Mortality Rates in Industrial Cohort Studies Due to Selection for Work and Survival in the Industry," *British Journal of Preventive and Social Medicine* 30 (1976), pp. 225-30.
14. S. D. Walter, "Determination of Significant Relative Risks and Optimal Sampling Procedures in Prospective and Retrospective Comparative Studies of Various Sizes," *American Journal of Epidemiology* 105 (1977), pp. 387-97.
15. Testimony of J. Jandl at OSHA hearings on proposed benzene standard, 1977.
16. M. Segi and M. Kurihara, *Cancer Mortality for Selected Sites in 24 Countries,* Tohoku University School of Medicine, Department of Public Health Monograph 2 (Sendai, Japan, 1972).
17. Joint Iran-IARC Study Group, "Esophageal Cancer Studies in the Caspian Littoral of Iran: Results of population studies — a prodrome," *Journal of the National Cancer Institute* 59 (1977), pp.1127-77.
18. Segi and Kurihara, "Cancer Mortality for Selected Sites," p. 72.
19. D. J. Jussawalla and V. M. Deshpande, "Evaluation of Cancer Risk in Tobacco Chewers and Smokers: An epidemiological assessment," *Cancer* 28 (1971), pp. 244-52.
20. T. J. Mason *et al.*, *Atlas of Cancer Mortality for U.S. Counties: 1950-1969* (Washington, D.C.: Department of Health, Education, and Welfare, 1975).
21. T. J. Mason *et al.*, *Atlas of Cancer Mortality among U.S. Non-Whites: 1950-1969* (Washington, D.C.: Department of Health, Education, and Welfare, Public Health Service, 1976).
22. W. J. Blot *et al.*, "Cancer Mortality in U.S. Counties with Petroleum Industries," *Science* 198 (1977), pp. 51-53.

CHAPTER 3
Cancer: The Animal Experiment

1. S. S. Epstein, "Environmental Determinants of Cancer," *Cancer Research* 34 (1974), pp. 2425-35. Cites detailed references.
2. M. D. Kipling and H. A. Waldron, "Polycyclic Aromatic Hydrocarbons in Mineral Oil, Tar, and Pitch, Excluding Petroleum Pitch," *Preventive Medicine* 5 (1976), pp. 262-78. A semi-historical review.
3. K. Yamagiwa, and K. Ichikawa, "Uber die Kunstliche Erzeugnung von Papillom," *Verhandlungen der Japanischen pathologischen Geselschaft* 5 (1915), pp. 142-58.
4. J. A. Murray, "Experimental Tar Cancer in Mice," *British Medical Journal* 2 (1921), pp. 795-96.
5. E. L. Kennaway, "On Cancer-Producing Tars and Tar-Fractions," *Journal of Industrial Hygiene* 5 (1934), pp. 462-88.
6. See, for example, H. G. M. Fischer *et al.*, "Properties of High-Boiling Petroleum Products: Physical and chemical properties as related to carcinogenic activity," *Industrial Hygiene and Occupational Medicine* 33 (1951), pp. 315-24.
7. Kennaway, "Cancer-Producing Tars."
8. J. H. Cook, C. L. Hewitt, and I. Hieger, "Coal Tar Constituents and Cancer," *Nature* 130 (1932), pp. 926-27.
9. W. C. Hueper, *Occupational Tumors and Allied Diseases* (Springfield, Ill.: Charles C. Thomas, 1942).
10. W. C. Hueper, F. H. Wiley, and H. D. Wolfe, "Experimental Production of Bladder Tumors in Dogs by Administration of Beta-naphthylamine," *J. Ind. Hyg.* 20 (1938), pp. 46-84.
11. R. H. Glasser, *The Greatest Battle* (New York: Random House, 1977). A good general account of the cancer process.
12. National Academy of Sciences, National Research Council, Food and Nutrition Board, *Problems in the Evaluation of Carcinogenic Hazards from Food Additives,* Food Protection Committee Publica-

tion 749 (Washington, D.C.: National Academy of Sciences, 1960).

13. F. W. Sunderman, Jr., "A Review of the Carcinogenicities of Nickel, Chromium, and Arsenic Compounds in Men and Animals," *Prev. Med.* 5 (1976), pp. 279-94.

14. L. Tomatis, C. Partensky, and R. Montesano, "The Predictive Value of Mouse Liver Tumour Induction in Carcinogenic Testing: A literature survey," *International Journal of Cancer* 12 (1973), pp. 1-20; L. Tomatis, "Validity and Limitations of Long-Term Experimentation in Cancer Research," in U. Mohr, D. Schmahl, and L. Tomatis, eds., *Air Pollution and Cancer in Man,* International Agency for Research on Cancer Scientific Publication 16 (Lyon, France, 1977), pp. 299-307.

15. H. F. Kraybill, "The Toxicology and Epidemiology of Mycotoxins," *Tropical and Geographical Medicine* 21 (1969), pp. 1-18.

16. A. W. Horton, D. T. Denman, and R. P. Trosset, "Carcinogenesis of the Skin, 2: The accelerating properties of aliphatic and related hydrocarbons," *Cancer Res.* 17 (1957), pp. 758-66.

17. J. M. Sontag, N. P. Page, and U. Safiotti, "Guidelines for Carcinogenesis Bioassay in Small Rodents," NCI Carcinogenesis Technical Report Series, 1, February, 1976.

18. M. B. Shimkin, "Species and Strain Selection," in L. Golberg, ed., *Carcinogenesis Testing of Chemicals* (Cleveland, Ohio: CRC Press, 1973), pp. 15-16.

19. J. M. Sontag, N. P. Page, and U. Safiotti, "Carcinogenesis Bioassay in Small Rodents."

20. M. G. Hanna, Jr., P. Nettesheim, and J. R. Gilbert, eds., "Inhalation Carcinogenesis," U.S. Atomic Energy Commission Symposium Series, 18 (1970); Epstein, "Environmental Determinants of Cancer."

21. Epstein, "Environmental Determinants of Cancer."

22. Ibid.

23. D. B. Clayson and R. C. Garner, "Aromatic Amines and Related Chemicals," in C. S. Searle, ed., *Chemical Carcinogenesis* (Washington, D.C.: American Chemical Society, 1976).

24. Epstein, "Environmental Determinants of Cancer."

25. For a comprehensive review see R. Montesano, H. Bartsch, and L. Tomatis, eds., *Screening Tests in Chemical Carcinogenesis,* IARC Scientific Publication 12 (Lyon, France, 1976); U. Saffiotti and H. Autrup, eds., National Cancer Institute, *In Vitro Carcinogenesis: Guide to the literature, recent advances, and laboratory procedures,* Technical Report Series, 44 (Washington, D.C., 1978).

26. B. N. Ames, J. McCann, and E. Yamasaki, "Methods for Detecting Carcinogens and Mutagens with the Salmonella/ Mammalian Microsome Mutagenicity Test," *Mutation Research* 31 (1975), pp. 347-64.

27. S. J. Rinkus and M. S. Legator, "Mutagenicity Testing Under the Toxic Substances Control Act," *Cancer Res.* (in press); T. H. Maugh, "Chemical Carcinogens: The scientific basis for regulation," *Science* 201 (1978), pp. 1200-5. Also discusses emerging regulatory implications and problems of carcinogenicity testing.

28. C. A. H. Bigger, J. E. Tomaszewski, and A. Dipple, "Differences between Products of Binding of 7,12-dimethylbenz(a)anthracene to DNA in Mouse Skin and in a Rat Microsomal Liver System," *Biochemical and Biophysical Research Communications* 80 (1978), pp. 229-35.

29. U. Saffiotti and H. Autrup, "In Vitro Carcinogenesis."

30. Maugh, "Chemical Carcinogens: The scientific basis for regulation."

CHAPTER 5
The Workplace: Case Studies

1. U.S. Department of Labor, Bureau of Labor Statistics, "Occupational Outlook Handbook," 1974-75 ed., bull. 1785 (Washington, D.C.: 1974); N. A. Ashford, *Crisis in the Workplace* (Cambridge, Mass.: MIT Press, 1976).

2. National Institute for Occupational Safety and Health, "The Right to Know" (Washington, D.C.: NIOSH, July, 1977).

3. "Chemical Dangers in the Workplace,"

Thirty-Fourth Report by the Committee on Government Operations (Washington, D.C., September 27, 1976).

4. "The Medical/ Industrial Complex," *Lancet,* 2 (1973), pp. 1380-81.

5. U. Saffiotti and J. K. Wagoner, eds., *Occupational Carcinogenesis,* Annals of the New York Academy of Sciences, vol. 271 (New York, 1976). Proceedings of a conference on occupational carcinogenesis held March 24-27, 1975, at the New York Academy of Sciences. Many papers present up-to-date reviews and data on occupational cancer studies. This is one of the best modern scientific references on occupational carcinogenesis; B. M. Boland, ed., *Cancer and the Worker* (New York: New York Academy of Sciences, 1977), a lay version of *Occupational Carcinogenesis* written specially for workers from the perspective of NIOSH scientists; L. McGinty, "Controlling Cancer in the Workplace," *New Scientist* 76 (1977), pp. 758-61; N. A. Ashford *et al.*, "Mobilizing National Resources for the Control of Occupational Cancer," Report to the Office of Technology Assessment, U.S. Congress, April, 1979.

Asbestos

1. P. Brodeur, *Expendable Americans* (New York: Viking, 1974). A good history of the occupational hazards of asbestos and the politics of their discovery and control.

2. H. Berger and R. E. Oesper, "Asbestos with Plastic and Rubber" (New York: Chemical Rubber Co., 1966).

3. I. J. Selikoff, "Cancer Risks of Asbestos Exposure" in H. H. Hiat, J. D. Watson, and J. A. Winsten, eds., *Origins of Human Cancer,* vol. 4 (Cold Spring Harbor Laboratory, 1977), pp. 1765-84; R. J. Levine, ed., "Asbestos: An information resource" (Stanford Research Institute, Contract No-1-55176), Division of Cancer Control and Rehabilitation, NCI, DHEW Publication No. (NIH) 78-168, May, 1978.

4. *Occupational Exposure to Asbestos: Criteria for a recommended standard* (Washington, D.C.: National Institute for Occupational Safety and Health, 1972), ch. 3, p. 4.

5. Ibid., ch. 3.

6. R. Doll, "Mortality from Lung Cancer in Asbestos Workers," *British Journal of Industrial Medicine* 12 (1955), pp. 81-97.

7. I. J. Selikoff and E. C. Hammond, "Multiple Risk Factors in Environmental Cancer," in J. F. Fraumeni, Jr., ed., *Persons at High Risk of Cancer* (New York: Academic Press, 1975).

8. Brodeur, *Expendable Americans,* pt. 3.

9. D. Kotelchuck, "Asbestos Research: Winning the battle but losing the war," *Health/PAC Bulletin* 61 (November/ December, 1974), pp. 1-32. A good summary of the interconnection between scientists and the asbestos industry.

10. W. J. Nicholson, "Occupational and Environmental Standards for Asbestos and Their Relation to Human Disease," In Hiatt, Watson, and Winsten, eds., *Origins of Human Cancer, pp.* 1785-96. A concise historical summary of the failure of government to regulate asbestos.

11. Ibid.; *Federal Register,* October 9, 1975, pp. 47652-65.

12. Quoted in Brodeur, *Expendable Americans, p.* 130.

13. J. C. McDonald *et al.*, "Mortality in the Chrysotile Asbestos Mines and Mills of Quebec," *Archives of Environmental Health* 22 (1971), pp. 677- 86.

14. H. L. Seidman, American Cancer Society statistician, letter submitted to U.S. Department of Labor at 1972 asbestos hearings.

15. J. C. McDonald to David Kotelchuck, published in *Health/PAC* Bull. 71 (July/ August, 1976).

16. National Cancer Institute, "Current Cancer Research on Environmental and Occupational Factors in Human Cancer, and Related Studies on Major Inorganic Carcinogens," Document NCI/ICRDB/ SL-76/53 (Washington, D.C., November 4, 1977).

17. J. D. Gillam *et al.*, "Mortality Patterns among Hard Rock Gold Miners Exposed to an Asbestiform Mineral," in U. Saffiotti

and J. K. Wagoner, eds., *Occupational Carcinogenesis,* Annals of the New York Academy of Sciences, vol. 271 (New York, 1976), pp. 336-44.

18. P. Kotin and G. R. Chase, "Comments on 'Mortality Patterns Among Hard Rock Gold Miners Exposed to an Asbestiform Mineral' and 'Asbestos Fiber Exposures in a Hard Rock Gold Mine'," Johns-Manville Corp., Health and Safety Department (Denver, Colo., 1976).

19. J. K. Wagoner, *et al.*, "Comments on 'Critique of Mortality Patterns among Hard Rock Gold Miners Exposed to an Asbestiform Mineral' and 'Asbestos Fiber Exposures in a Hard Rock Gold Mine'" (Washington, D.C.: National Institute of Occupational Safety and Health, 1976).

20. J. F. Finklea to Assistant Secretary for Health, "Evaluation of Data on Health Effects of Asbestos Exposure and Revised Recommended Numerical Environmental Limits," December 15, 1976.

21. P. A. Greene, "OSHA Serves a Corporate Client, Ignoring Asbestos in Vanderbilt Industrial Talc" (Washington, D.C.: Public Citizen Health Research Group, 1976).

22. Ibid., p. 18.

23. Occupational Safety and Health Review Commission, Docket 10757 OSHD 20, 947, June 28, 1976.

24. International Agency for Research on Cancer, *Asbestos,* IARC Monographs on the Evaluation of Carcinogenic Risks of Chemicals to Man, vol. 14 (Lyon, France, 1977). This is the best available summary on the carcinogenicity of asbestos.

25. H. Weinstein, "Did Industry Suppress Asbestos Data? Dangers Apparently Long Known," *Los Angeles Times,* October 23, 1978.

26. Kotelchuk, "Asbestos Research."

27. A. Lanza, "Effects of Asbestos Dust on the Lungs," Public Health Reports 50 (1935), p. 1.

28. K. W. Smith, "Industrial Hygiene-Survey of Man in a Dusty Area," unpublished Johns-Manville Report, 1949.

29. The Louisville Trust Company, Administrator of the Estate of William Virgil Sampson *vs.* Johns-Manville Corporation, Jefferson Circuit Court, Common Pleas Branch, Seventh Division, Deposition of Kenneth W. Smith, April 21, 1976, pp. 63-64.

30. I. J. Selikoff, J. Churg, and E. C. Hammond, "Asbestos Exposure and Neoplasia," *Journal American Medical Association* 188 (1964), pp. 22-26; I. J. Selikoff, J. Churg, and E. C. Hammond, "The Occurrence of Asbestosis Among Insulation Workers in the United States," *Annals New York Academy of Sciences* 132 (1965), pp. 139-55.

31. Minutes Asbestos Textile Institute Meetings, June 6, 1963 (Air Hygiene Committee), and October 8, 1964 (Air Hygiene Committee).

32. Minutes General Meeting Asbestos Textile Institute, February 4, 1971.

33. Selikoff, Churg, and Hammond, "Asbestos Exposure and Neoplasia," and "Asbestosis in Insulation Workers."

34. J. C. Wagner, C. A. Sleggs, and P. Marehand, "Diffuse Pleural Mesothelioma and Asbestos Exposure in the North Western Cape Province," *Brit. J. Ind. Med.* 17 (1960), pp. 260-71.

35. W. Nicholson, Mt. Sinai School of Medicine, New York, quoted in Brodeur, *Expendable Americans, p.* 172.

36. R. Nader and R. Harris, "Don't Drink the Water, Don't Breathe the Air," *Environmental Action,* September 15, 1973; E. W. Lawless, *Technology and Social Shock* (New Brunswick, N.J.: Rutgers University Press, 1977), pp. 288-307.

37. T. Temple, "Protecting Lake Superior," *EPA Journal* 4 (1978), pp. 5-9. Contains a chronological summary of the Reserve Mining case.

38. Selikoff, "Cancer Risks of Asbestos Exposure"; Nicholson, "Occupational and Environmental Standards for Asbestos"; IARC, *Asbestos.*

39. Nicholson, "Occupational and Environmental Standards for Asbestos"; IARC, *Asbestos.*

40. D. L. Bayliss *et al.*, "Mortality Patterns among Fibrous Glass Production Workers,"

in Saffiotti and Wagoner, eds., *Occupational Carcinogenesis, pp.* 324-35.

41. P. Kotin, *New Times,* November 25, 1977.

42. B. Castleman (1733 Riggs Place, N.W., Washington, D.C. 20009), "The Export of Hazardous Factories to Developing Nations," *Congressional Record,* June 29, 1978.

Vinyl Chloride

1. I. J. Selikoff and E. C. Hammond, eds., *Toxicity of Vinyl Chloride-Polyvinyl Chloride,* Annals of the New York Academy of Sciences, vol. 246 (New York, 1975). Proceedings of a conference on vinyl chloride with papers by most of the world's VC researchers, and with a detailed bibliography.

2. Environmental Protection Agency, "Scientific and Technical Assessment Report (STAR) on Vinyl Chloride and Polyvinyl Chloride," EPA-600/6-75-004 (Washington, D.C., June, 1975).

3. Ibid.

4. Ibid.; H. R. Simonds, *Handbook of Plastics,* 2nd ed. (Princeton, N.J.: D. Van Nostrand, 1949); E. A. Boettner and B. Weiss, "An Analytic System for Identifying the Volatile Pyrolysis Products of Plastics," *American Industrial Hygiene Association Journal* 28 (1967), pp. 535-40; E. A. Boettner, EPA Report 670/2-73/049, July, 1973.

5. EPA, "Report on Vinyl Chloride and Polyvinyl Chloride."

6. P. L. Viola, "Cancerogenic Effect of Vinyl Chloride" (abstract), *Proceedings, X International Cancer Congress,* Houston, Texas, *1970.*

7. R. N. Wheeler, Jr., Union Carbide Memo "MCA Occupational Health Committee: Vinyl Chloride Conference," November 23, 1971.

8. C. W. Heath, H. Falk, and J. L. Creech, "Characteristics of Cases of Angiosarcoma of the Liver Among Vinyl Chloride Workers in the U.S." in Selikoff and Hammond, eds., *Toxicity of Vinyl Chloride-Polyvinyl Chloride, pp.* 231-36; D. Byren, and B. Holmberg, "Two Possible Cases of

Angiosarcoma of the Liver in a Group of Swedish Vinyl Chloride-Polyvinyl Chloride Workers" in Selikoff and Hammond eds., *Toxicity of Vinyl Chloride-Polyvinyl Chloride, pp.* 249-50.

9. C. Maltoni, and G. Lefemine, "Carcinogenicity Bioassays of Vinyl Chloride: Current results," Selikoff and Hammond, eds., *Toxicity of Vinyl Chloride-Polyvinyl Chloride, pp.* 195-218.

10. C. Maltoni, "Vinyl Chloride Carcinogenicity: An experimental model for carcinogenesis studies," in H. H. Hiatt, J. D. Watson, and J. A. Winsten, eds., *Origins of Human Cancer,* vol. 4 (Cold Spring Harbor Laboratory, 1977), pp. 119-46.

11. J. T. Edsall, "Report of the AAAS Committee on Scientific Freedom and Responsibility," *Science* 188 (1975), pp. 687-93; M. Turshen, "Disaster in Plastic," *Health/PAC Bulletin* 71 (July/August, 1976), pp. 1-6.

12. R. N. Wheeler, Jr., Confidential Union Carbide Memo "Vinyl Chloride Research: MCA report to NIOSH," July 19, 1973.

13. Edsall, "Report of the Committee on Scientific Freedom and Responsibility."

14. B. W. Duck, J. T. Carter, and E. J. Coombes, "Mortality Study of Workers in a Polyvinyl Chloride Production Plant," *Lancet* 2 (1975), p. 1197.

15. "Exposure to Vinyl Chloride," *Federal Register* 39 (October 4, 1974).

16. S. Rattner, "Did Industry Cry Wolf?: Polyvinyl chloride health rules can be met," *New York Times,* December 28, 1975; N. Ashford, "Vinyl Chloride Industrial: Abstract of case study," Center for Policy Alternatives, MIT, Cambridge, Mass., 1976; D. D. Doniger "Federal Regulation of Vinyl Chloride: A short course in the law and policy of toxic substances control," *Ecology Law Quarterly* 7 (1978), pp. 497-677; Library of Congress, Congressional Research Service (report to Cong. Andrew Maguire), "Vinyl Chloride," December 8, 1978.

17. E. Mastromatteo *et al.,* "Acute Inhalation Toxicity of Vinyl Chloride to Laboratory Animals," *Am. Ind. Hyg. Assoc. J.* 21 (1960), pp. 395-401; T. R. Torkelson, F.

Oyen, and V. K. Rowe, "The Toxicity of Vinyl Chloride as Determined by Repeated Exposure of Laboratory Animals," *Am. Ind. Hyg. Assoc. J.* 22 (1961), pp. 354-61.

18. S. L. Tribukh *et al.*, "Working Conditions and Measures for their Sanitation in the Protection and Utilization of Vinyl Chloride Plastics," *Gigiena: Sanitariya* 10 (1949), p. 38.

19. R. J. Waxweiler *et al.*, "Neoplastic Risk Among Workers Exposed to Vinyl Chloride," in Selikoff and Hammond, eds., *Toxicity of Vinyl Chloride-Polyvinyl Chloride, pp.* 40-48.

20. University of Louisville, Health Education Program, Vinyl Chloride Project, "VC Health Notes," vol. 5 (Louisville, Ky., 1977).

21. W. N. Sokol, Y. Aelony, and G. N. Beall, "Meat-Wrapper's Asthma: A new syndrome?" *Journal of the American Medical Association,* 226 (1973), pp. 639-41.

22. J. K. Wagoner and P. Infante. "Vinyl Chloride-Polyvinyl Chloride: A review of carcinogenic and other toxicologic effects." Occupational Safety and Health Administration, U.S. Dept. of Labor, Washington, D.C., Draft Report, November, 1978.

23. A. M. Kuzmack and R. E. McGaughy, "Quantitative Risk Assessment for Community Exposure to Vinyl Chloride" (Washington, D.C.: EPA, December 5, 1976).

24. Environmental Protection Agency, Office of Enforcement, "Survey of Vinyl Chloride Levels in the Vicinity of Keysor-Century, Saugus, California," EPA-330/2-77-017 (San Francisco: National Enforcement Investigation Center, Region IX, June, 1977).

25. P. F. Infante, "Oncogenic and Mutagenic Risks in Communities with PVC Production Facilities," in Saffiotti and Wagoner, eds., *Occupational Carcinogenesis, pp.* 49-57.

26. G. P. Theriault and L. Goulet (Department of Social and Preventive Medicine, Laval University, Quebec, Canada), "Birth Defects in a Community Located near a Vinyl Chloride Plant," unpublished report, 1977.

27. B. W. Gay *et al.*, "Measurements of Vinyl Chloride from Aerosol Sprays," in Selikoff and Hammond, eds., *Toxicity of Vinyl Chloride-Polyvinyl Chloride, pp.* 286-95.

28. R. E. Shapiro (FDA) to K. Bridbord (NIOSH) on "Vinyl Chloride Migration Data," December 18, 1974.

29. "Vinyl Chloride Emission Control," *Chemical Engineering Progress* 71 (1975), pp. 1-62.

30. W. A. Mack, "VCM Reduction and Control," *Chemical Engineering Process 71 (1975), pp. 41-44.*

Bischloromethylether

1. H. E. Christensen and C. Zenz, "Compounds Associated with Carcinogenesis," in C. Zenz, ed., *Occupational Medicine: Principles & Practical Applications* (Chicago: Yearbook Medical Publishers, *1975), p. 859.*

2. W. S. Randall and S. D. Solomon, *Building Six: The Tragedy at Bridesburg* (Boston: Little, Brown, 1977). Expanded from the authors' award-winning *Philadelphia Enquirer* article, "54 Who Died," a well-researched account of the Rohm & Haas Company and how it dealt with the growing evidence that many of its employees were dying of occupationally-induced lung cancer.

3. Ibid., pp. 96-103.

4. Ibid., pp. 246-52.

5. Ibid., pp. 57-58.

6. Ibid.

7. Ibid., pp. 79-80.

8. S. Laskin *et al.*, "The Inhalation Carcinogenicity of Alpha Halo-Ethers, 2: Chronic Inhalation Studies with Chloromethyl Methyl Ether," *Archives of Environmental Health* 30 (1975), pp. 70-72; N. Nelson, "The Chloroethers — Occupational Carcinogens: A summary of laboratory and epidemiology studies," in U. Saffiotti and J. K. Wagoner, eds., *Occupational Carcinogenesis, Annals of the New York Academy of Sciences,* vol. 271 (New York, 1976), pp. 81-90.

9. W. Weiss and K. R. Boucot, "Respiratory

Effects of Chloromethyl Methyl Ether," *Journal of the American Medical Association* 234 (1975), pp. 1139-42.

10. W. G. Figueroa, R. Raszkowski, and W. Weiss, "Lung Cancer in Chloromethyl Methyl Ether Workers," *New England Journal of Medicine* 288 (1973), pp. 1096-97.

11. R. A. Lemen *et al.*, "Cytologic Observations and Cancer Incidence Following Exposure to BCME," in Saffiotti and Wagoner, eds., *Occupational Carcinogenesis, pp.* 71-80.

12. A. M. Thiess, W. Hey, and H. Zeller, "Zur Toxicologie von Dichlorodimethyl-äther-Verdacht auf Kanzeroge Wirkung auch beim Menschen," *Zentralblatt für Arbeitsmedizin und Arbeitsschultz* 23 (1973), pp. 97-102.

13. L. S. Frankel, K. S. McCallum, and L. Collier, "Formation of Bischloromethyl Ether from Formaldehyde and Hydrogen Chloride," *Environmental Science and Technology* 8 (1974), pp. 356-59.

14. W. C. Bauman, November 30, 1948, cited by M. Kelyman, Safety Manager, Midland Division, Dow Chemical USA, at OSHA hearings on Standards on Occupational Carcinogens, July 9, 1973.

15. H. M. Donaldson, and P. J. Shuler, "Field Survey of Dow Chemical Company Chloromethyl Ether Facilities, Midland, Michigan" (National Institute for Occupational Safety and Health, September 8, 1972).

Benzene

1. U.S. Department of Labor, Occupational Safety and Health Act, "Occupational Exposure to Benzene," *Federal Register* 42 (May 3, 1977), pp. 22516-29. Contains a general review of experimental and human studies on benzene carcinogenesis, with many references to the primary scientific literature.

2. "High Hazards Found," *Chemical Week*, October 12, 1977, p. 19.

3. S. J. Mara and S. S. Lee, "Human Exposures to Atmospheric Benzene," Center for Resource and Environmental Systems Studies Report 30 (Stanford, Calif.: Stanford Research Institute, 1977).

4. Ibid., p. 54.

5. Ibid., pp. 129-52.

6. Ibid., p. 13

7. Ibid., p. 63.

8. Ibid., p. 65.

9. Ibid., p. 38.

10. Ibid., p. 51.

11. Ibid., p. 87

12. R. J. Young *et al.*, "Benzene in Consumer Products," *Science* 199 (1978), p. 248.

13. M. McCann (Art Hazards Project, Center for Occupational Hazards, New York) to S. J. Byington (Chairman, Consumer Products Safety Commission), June 30, 1977.

14. For a narration of the Galaxy case, including an interview with Capurro, see L. Agran, *The Cancer Connection* (Boston: Houghton Mifflin, 1977).

15. "Doctor Links Galaxy, Cancer," *Washington Post,* December 14, 1977; see also P. V. Capurro and J. E. Eldridge, "Solvent Exposure and Cancer," *Lancet* 1 (1978), p. 942.

16. B. D. Goldstein, "Benzene Health Effects Assessment" (Washington, D.C.: EPA Office of Research and Development, 1977). This EPA report summarizes information on the toxic effects of benzene on animals and humans, including a critical review of epidemiological literature indicting benzene as a leukemogenic agent.

17. M. Aksoy *et al.*, "Acute Leukemia Due to Chronic Exposure to Benzene," *American Journal of Medicine* 52 (1972), pp. 160-66.

18. A. Forni, and L. Moreo, "Cytogenetic Studies in a Case of Benzene Leukemia," *European Journal of Cancer* 3 (1967), pp. 252-55; idem, "Chromosome Studies in a Case of Benzene-Induced Erythroleukemia," *Europ. J. Cancer* 5 (1969), pp. 459-63.

19. K. Freage, J. Reitalu, and M. Berlin, "Chromosome Studies in Workers Exposed to Benzene," unpublished report, University of Lund, Sweden, 1977.

20. M. Aksoy, S. Erdem, and G. Dincol, "Leukemia in Shoe-workers Exposed Chronically to Benzene," *Blood* 44 (1974),

pp. 837-41.

21. OSHA, "Occupational Exposure to Benzene"; Goldstein, "Benzene Health Effects Assessment"; E. C. Vigliani, "Leukemia Associated with Benzene Exposure," in U. Saffiotti and J. K. Wagoner, eds., *Occupational Carcinogenesis,* Annals of the New York Academy of Sciences, vol. 271 (New York, 1976), pp. 143-51.

22. J. J. Thorpe, "Epidemiologic Survey of Leukemia in Persons Potentially Exposed to Benzene," *J. Occup. Med.* 16 (1974), pp. 375-82.

23. S. M. Brown, "Leukemia and Potential Benzene Exposure," *J. Occup. Med.* 17 (1976), pp. 5-6.

24. P. F. Infante *et al.*, "Leukemia in Benzene Workers," *Lancet* 2 (1977), pp. 76-78.

25. Goldstein, "Benzene Health Effects Assessment," p. 105.

26. Ibid., p. 124-29.

27. I. M. Tough *et al.*, "Chromosome Studies on Workers Exposed to Atmospheric Benzene," *Europ. J. Cancer* 6 (1970), pp. 49-55.

28. S. Horiguchi, H. Okada, and K. Horiguchi, "Effect of Benzene on the Leucocytic Function of Mice," *Osaka City Medical Journal* 18 (1972), pp. 1-8.

29. American Conference of Governmental Industrial Hygienists, "Threshold Limit Values for Substances in Workroom Air Adopted by ACGIH for 1963" (Cincinnati, Ohio, 1963).

30. Aksoy *et al.*, "Leukemia in Shoe-workers"; Vigliani, "Leukemia Associated with Benzene Exposure."

31. National Institute for Occupational Safety and Health, "Criteria for Recommended Standard: Occupational exposure to benzene" (Washington, D.C., 1974), pp. 74-75.

32. National Academy of Sciences, Committee on Toxicology, "Health Effects of Benzene: A review" (Washington, D.C., June,1976).

33. National Institute for Occupational Safety and Health, "Occupational Exposure to Benzene: Revised criteria for a recommended standard" (Washington, D.C., August, 1976).

34. Infante *et al.*, "Leukemia in Benzene Workers."

35. Arthur D. Little, Inc., "Economic Impact Statement for Benzene" (March, 1977); see also *Chemical and Engineering News,* August 1, 1977, p. 12.

36. OSHA, "Occupational Exposure to Benzene."

37. Ibid.

38. Reported by Sylvia Krekel in *OCAW Lifelines,* July, 1977.

39. D. Hunter, *The Diseases of Occupations,* 4th ed. (Boston: Little, Brown, 1969), pp. 506-21.

40. I. R. Tabershaw, and S. H. Lamm, "Benzene and Leukemia," *Lancet* 2 (1977), pp. 867-68.

41. P. F. Infante *et al.*, reply to Tabershaw and Lamm "Benzene and Leukemia," *Lancet* 2 (1977), p. 868.

42. R. E. Olson, testimony before OSHA, Docket H-059, Washington, D.C., 1977.

43. Goldstein, "Benzene Health Effects Assessment."

44. Mara and Lee, "Human Exposures to Atmospheric Benzene."

45. R. E. Albert, "Carcinogen Assessment Groups Preliminary Report on Population Risk to Ambient Benzene Exposures" (Washington, D.C.: EPA, 1977).

46. J. D. Kilian and R. L. Daniel, "Cytogenetic Study of Workers Exposed to Benzene in the Texas Division of Dow Chemical USA," and M. C. Benge *et al.*, "Cytogenic Study of 290 Workers Exposed to Benzene," unpublished reports, February 27, 1978; see also R. Scott, "Danger of Low-Level Benzene Reported: Dow withheld report on danger," *Washington Post,* June 11, 1978.

47. W. J. Blot *et al.*, "Cancer Mortality in U.S. Counties with Petroleum Industries," *Science* 198 (1977), pp. 51-53.

48. Health Research Group petition to the Consumer Product Safety Commission, submitted by S. M. Wolfe and P. A. Greene, May 5, 1977.

CHAPTER 6
Consumer Products: Case Studies

Tobacco

1. B. Ramazzini, *De Morbis Artificum Diatriba,* trans. W. C. Wright (New York: Hafner, 1964).
2. Clearinghouse for Smoking and Health, "Adult Use of Tobacco, 1975" (Atlanta, Ga.: U.S. Public Health Service, Center for Disease Control, 1975).
3. U.S. Department of Health, Education, and Welfare, "The Health Consequences of Smoking — 1974" (Washington, D.C., 1974), a summary of relevant data and conclusions on smoking and health; see also U.S. Department of Health, Education, and Welfare, "Smoking Digest: Progress report on a nation kicking the habit" (Washington, D.C., October, 1977); U.S. Surgeon General's Report, "Smoking and Health," January 11, 1979.
4. E. L. Wynder, L. S. Covey, and K. Mabuchi, "Lung Cancer in Women: Present and future trends," *Journal of the National Cancer Institute* 51 (1973), pp. 391-402; see also E. L. Wynder and S. D. Stellman, "The Comparative Epidemiology of Tobacco-Related Cancers," *Cancer Research* 37 (1977), pp. 4608-22.
5. E. L. Wynder and S. Hecht, ch. 6 in E. L. Wynder and S. Hecht, eds., *Lung Cancer* (Geneva: International Union Against Cancer, 1976). A multiauthor monograph on causes of lung cancer, including sections on epidemiology, pathology of lung cancer, immunological aspects, animal experiments, and chemistry of tobacco smoke; E. L. Wynder and D. Hoffman, "Tobacco and Health: A societal challenge," *New England Journal of Medicine* 300 (1979), pp. 894-903.
6. E. C. Hammond *et al.,* "Some Recent Findings Concerning Cigarette Smoking" in H. H. Hiatt, J. D. Watson, and J. A. Winsten, eds., *Origins of Human Cancer,* vol. 4 (Cold Spring Harbor Laboratory, 1977), pp. 101-12; for sources and original literature, see Wynder and Hecht, *Lung Cancer,* ch. 2, and Wynder and Stellman, "Comparative Epidemiology of Tobacco-Related Cancers."
7. E. L. Wynder and K. Mabuchi, "Lung Cancer Among Cigar and Pipe Smokers," *Preventive Medicine* 2 (1972), pp. 529-42.
8. Ibid.
9. Wynder and Stellman, "Comparative Epidemiology of Tobacco-Related Cancers," p. 4615.
10. E. C. Hammond, "Tobacco," in J. F. Fraumeni, Jr., ed., *Persons at High Risk of Cancer* (Bethesda, Md.: National Cancer Institute, 1975), pp. 131-38.
11. Wynder and Stellman, "Comparative Epidemiology of Tobacco-Related Cancers," p. 4613.
12. Ibid.
13. E. L. Wynder, M. Mushinski, and S. D. Stellman, "The Epidemiology of the Less Harmful Cigarette," in E. L. Wynder, D. Hoffman, and G. B. Gori, eds., *Smoking and Health,* Proceedings of the Third World Conference on Smoking and Health, 1975, pp. 1-13; E. C. Hammond *et al.,* " 'Tar' and Nicotine Content of Cigarette Smoke in Relation to Death Rates," *Environmental Research* 12 (1976), pp. 263-74. The latter contains the latest results of the American Cancer Society's million-person prospective study, showing that smokers switching to low-tar cigarettes had a lower death rate from lung cancer than smokers of high- tar cigarettes; Wynder and Hoffman, "Tobacco and Health: A societal challenge."
14. Wynder and Hecht, eds., *Lung Cancer,* ch. 2.
15. S. J. Cutler and J. L. Young, "Demographic Patterns of Cancer Incidence in the United States," in Fraumeni, ed., *Persons at High Risk of Cancer,* pp. 307-42.
16. J. Berkson, "Smoking and Lung Cancer: Some observations on two recent reports," *American Statistical Association Journal* 53 (1958), pp. 28-38.
17. I. Schmeltz, D. Hoffman, and E. L. Wynder, "The Influence of Tobacco Smoke on Indoor Atmospheres," *Preventive Medicine* 4 (1975), pp. 66- 82.
18. W. S. Aronow, "Carbon Monoxide and

Cardiovascular Disease," in Wynder, Hoffman, and Gori, eds., *Smoking and Health,* pp. 321-28.

19. J. M. Stellman, *Women's Work, Women's Health* (New York: Pantheon, 1977).

20. E. Eckholm, "The Unnatural History of Tobacco," *Natural History,* May, 1977, pp. 22-32; see also B. R. Luce and S. O. Schweitzer, "Smoking and Alcohol Abuse: A comparison of their economic consequences," *New England Journal of Medicine* 298 (1978), pp. 569-71.

21. G. Gori, "Low-Risk Cigarettes, a Prescription," *Science* 194 (1976), pp. 1243-46.

22. G. B. Gori and C. J. Lynch, "Towards Less Hazardous Cigarettes," *Journal American Medical Association* 240 (1978), pp. 1255-59.

23. *Medical World News,* September 4, 1978.

24. J. L. Marx, "Health Officials Fired Up Over 'Tolerable' Cigarettes," *Science* 201 (1978), pp. 795-98.

25. Congressional Record, S. 13306, August 15, 1978.

26. *Wall Street Journal,* August 18, 1978.

27. *Washington Star,* January 11, 1977, p. 1.

28. *New York Times,* January 13, 1978.

29. Ibid.

30. P. R. J. Burch, *The Biology of Cancer: A New Approach* (London: MTP Press, 1975). Burch is the leading British proponent of the claim that smoking is not the main cause of lung cancer. This book summarizes his arguments, most of which have been rejected by scientists.

31. A. L. Fritschler, *Smoking and Politics: Policymaking and the Federal Bureaucracy* (New York: Appleton-Century-Crofts, 1969).

32. DHEW, "The Health Consequences of Smoking — 1974."

33. Quoted in *The New Yorker,* June 27, 1977, p. 23.

34. Quoted in letter from M. Daniel and M. F. Jacobson (Center for Science in the Public Interest) to V. Weingarten (Chairman, National Commission on Smoking and Public Policy), July 15, 1977.

35. Quoted in *The New York Times,* November 30, 1964.

36. Quoted in *The New York Times,* January 27, 1968.

37. Green *v.* American Tobacco Co. (5 Cir. 1969) 409 F.2d 1166.

38. Shimp *v.* New Jersey Bell Telephone Co., New Jersey Superior Court, Chancery Division, Para. 21, 421, December 20, 1976.

39. Clearinghouse for Smoking and Health, "Adult Use of Tobacco, 1975."

40. K. Friedman, Public *Policy and the Smoking-Health Controversy* (Lexington, Mass.: Lexington Books, 1975); F. Greve, "The Low Tar Cigarette Is Burning Up the Market," *The Miami Herald,* December 20, 1977.

Red Dyes #2 and #40

1. B. T. Hunter, *Food Additives and Federal Policy: The Mirage of Safety* (New York: Scribner, 1975). A well-documented general account of food additives and governmental failure to regulate them.

2. M. F. Jacobson, "Food Colors" (Washington, D.C.: Center for Science in the Public Interest, 1972).

3. C. R. Noller, *Chemistry of Organic Compounds,* 2nd ed. (Philadelphia: W. B. Saunders, 1957), pp. 672-73.

4. D. B. Clayson, "Occupational Bladder Cancer," *Preventive Medicine* 5 (1976), pp. 228-44.

5. A. J. Johnson and S. Wolfe, "Hazards of Food Colors," Report of Public Citizen, Health Research Group to FDA, January 11, 1977.

6. National Academy of Sciences, Food Protection Committee, "Food Colors" (Washington, D.C., 1971).

7. Report of the Comptroller General of the United States to Senator Gaylord Nelson, "Need to Establish the Safety of the Color Additive FD&C Red No. 2," MWD-76-40 (Washington, D.C., 1975); P. M. Boffey, "Death of a Dye," *New York Times Magazine,* February 29, 1976.

8. M. M. Adrianova, "Carcinogenic Properties of the Red Food Dyes Amaranth, Ponceaux SX, and Ponceaux 4R," *Voprosÿ Pitaniya* 29, no. 5 (1970).

9. Boffey, "Death of a Dye," p. 49.
10. Report of the Comptroller General, "Safety of the Color Additive FD&C Red No. 2."
11. Boffey, "Death of a Dye."
12. G. Moreland, "Warning: Red Dye #40 may be hazardous to your health," *Nutrition Action,* February, 1977, pp. 4-6; P. M. Boffey, "Color Additives: Is successor to Red Dye No. 2 any safer?" *Science* 191 (1976), pp. 832-34.
13. FDA, "Summary of Toxicological Evaluation of FD&C Red No. 40," Feb. 7, 1972.
14. Quoted in Moreland, "Red Dye #40 May Be Hazardous to Your Health," p. 4.
15. Joint FAO/WHO Expert Committee on Food Additives, 18th Report, 1974.
16. Moreland, "Red Dye #40 May Be Hazardous to Your Health."
17. Ibid.
18. Ibid.
19. M. F. Jacobson and S. S. Epstein, "Statement to FDA's Working Group on Red No. 40 Dye," December 16, 1976.
20. Interim Report of the FDA Working Group on FD&C Red No. 40, January 19, 1977, p. 4.
21. Quoted in "Red Dye No. 40 Given Initial Clearance As Not Cancer-Causing; More Study is Set," *Wall Street Journal,* April 28, 1978.

Saccharin

1. R. W. Rhein and L. Marion, *The Saccharin Controversy: A Guide for Consumers* (New York: Monarch Press, 1977). A good guide to the history and politics of saccharin in the United States.
2. R. Q. Brewster and W. E. McEwen, *Organic Chemistry,* 3rd ed. (Englewood Cliffs, N.J.: Prentice-Hall, 1961), p. 528.
3. *Chemical Week,* March 23, 1977, p. 13.
4. Calorie Control Council, news release, June 24, 1977.
5. E. Kun and I. Horvath, "The Influence of Oral Saccharin on Blood Sugar," *Proceedings of the Society for Experimental Biology and Medicine* 66 (1947), pp. 175-77; M. M. Thompson and J. Mayer, "Hypoglycemic Effects of Saccharin in Experimental Animals," *American Journal of Clinical Nutrition* 7 (1959), pp. 80-85; E. S. Valenstein and M. L. Weber, "Potentiation of Insulin Coma by Saccharin," *Journal of Comparative and Physiological Psychology* 60 (1965), pp. 443-46.
6. R. Friedhoff, J. A. Simon, and A. J. Friedhoff, "Sucrose Solution *vs.* No-Calorie Sweetener *vs.* Water in Weight Gain," *Journal of the American Dietetic Association* 59 (1971), pp. 485-86.
7. M. B. McCann, M. F. Trulson, and S. C. Stulb, "Non-Caloric Sweeteners and Weight Reduction," *J. Am. Diet. Assn.* 32 (1956), pp. 327-30.
8. National Academy of Sciences, Institute of Medicine, Committee on Saccharin, "Sweeteners: Issues and uncertainties" (Washington, D.C., 1975), p. 165.
9. S. M. Wolfe and A. Johnson, Public Citizens Health Research Group, testimony before Subcommittee on Health, House Commerce Committee Hearings on Saccharin, March 21, 1977.
10. *Congressional Record,* September 14, 1977.
11. M. D. Reuber, "Preliminary Review of the Carcinogenicity Studies on Saccharin," unpublished Report, September 12, 1977. Summarized in Wolfe and Johnson testimony, pp. 1-6.
12. C. Noller, *The Chemistry of Organic Compounds,* 2nd ed. (Philadelphia: W. B. Saunders, 1957), p. 557.
13. C. J. Kokoski (Division of Toxicology, FDA) to R. Ronk (Director, Division of Food and Color Additives), May 3, 1977.
14. Quoted in J. E. Brody, "Scientist Says Animal Cancer Tests Must Consider Number of Causes," *New York Times,* April 6, 1977.
15. "Saccharin and Health Studies: A history of safety" (Atlanta, Georgia: Calorie Control Council, June, 1977).
16. Ibid., p. 6.
17. R. M. Hicks, J. J. Wakefield, and J. Chowaniec, "Co-Carcinogenic Action of Saccharin in the Chemical Induction of Bladder Cancer," *Nature* 243 (1973), pp. 347-49.
18. R. P. Batzinger, S-Y. L. Ou, and E. Bueding, "Saccharin and Other Sweeteners: Mu-

tagenic Properties," *Science* 198 (1977), pp. 944-46.

19. F. Burbank and J. F. Fraumeni, Jr., "Synthetic Sweetener Consumption and Bladder Cancer Trends in the U.S.," *Nature* 227 (1970), pp. 296-97.

20. E. L. Wynder and R. Goldsmith, "The Epidemiology of Bladder Cancer: A second look," *Cancer* 40 (1977), pp. 1246-68; I. I. Kessler, "Non- Nutritive Sweeteners and Human Bladder Cancer: Preliminary findings," *Journal of Urology* 115 (1976), pp. 143-46.

21. I. I. Kessler, "Cancer Mortality in Diabetics," *Journal of the National Cancer Institute* 44 (1970), pp. 673-86.

22. G. R. Howe *et al.*, "Artificial Sweeteners and Human Bladder Cancer," *Lancet* 2 (1977), pp. 578-81.

23. General Accounting Office, "Need to Resolve Safety Questions on Saccharin," Publication HRD-76-156, August 16, 1976.

24. Calorie Control Council, "Why is the Verdict Almost in on Saccharin When All the Evidence Isn't?" *New York Times,* May 12, 1977.

25. *New York Times,* April 6, 1977.

26. K. Isselbacher, testimony before the Subcommittee on Health and Environment, House Interstate and Foreign Commerce Committee, March 21-22, 1977.

27. Wolfe and Johnson, testimony before Subcommittee on Health.

28. *Chemical and Engineering News,* March 28, 1977, p. 22.

29. "Cancer Testing Technology and Saccharin" (Washington, D.C.: Office of Technology Assessment, U.S. Congress, June 7, 1977). A detailed analysis of the problem, with a good bibliography.

30. *Congressional Record,* September 14, 1977.

31. "Saccharin: Technical assessment of risks and benefits," Assembly of Life Sciences/ Institute of Medicine, National Research Council/ National Academy of Sciences, Washington, D.C., November, 1978; R. J. Smith, "NAS Saccharin Report Sweetens FDA position, But Not by Much," *Science* 202 (1978), pp. 852-53.

Acrylonitrile

1. "Pepsi Finds Polyester Bottles to Its Taste," *Chemical and Engineering News,* March 7, 1977, p. 5.

2. J. F. Quast *et al.*, "Toxicity of Drinking Water Containing Acrylonitrile (AN) in Rats: Results after 12 months," unpublished report, Toxicology Research Laboratory, Dow Chemical USA, Midland, Michigan, March 1977.

3. F. J. Murray *et al.*, "Teratologic Evaluation of Acrylonitrile Monomer Given to Rats by Gavage," unpublished report, Dow Chemical USA, November 3, 1976.

4. S. Venitt, C. T. Bushell, and M. A. Osborne, "Mutagenicity of Acrylonitrile in *E. Coli,*" unpublished and undated report submitted to G. Newell, NCI, by Manufacturing Chemists Association (together with other attachments) on April 11, 1977.

5. M. T. O'Berg (Du Pont de Nemours Co.), "Epidemiologic Study of Workers Exposed to Acrylonitrile," unpublished report, May 13, 1977; see also I. Schwartz, "Facing up to Acrylo Problems," *Chemical Week,* June 22, 1977, pp. 38-40.

6. *Chemical Week,* January 25, 1978, p. 14.

7. "Emergency Standard Set for Acrylonitrile," *Chemical and Engineering News,* January 23, 1978, p. 4.

8. Ibid.

9. G. Speth (Council on Environmental Quality), "Towards a Better Bull's Eye: Corporate responsibility and accountability." Speech to the American Bar Association — National Resources Section, November 28, 1978. An important statement contrasting industry demands for deregulation with regard to pollution and health and their demands for continued regulation to limit free competition.

Female Sex Hormones

1. G. Pincus, *The Control of Fertility* (New York: Academic Press, 1965), a comprehensive medical text on fertility, drugs, and endocrinology; K. W. McKerns, *Steroid Hormones and Metabolism,* (New York: Appleton-Century-Crofts, 1969), a mono-

graph on the biochemistry and metabolism of sex hormones.

2. Forrestal, "Estrogen Hurting, Corticoids Healthy," *Chemical Week,* November 23, 1977, p. 23.

3. Ibid.; J. Rock, C. M. Garcia, and G. Pincus, "Synthetic Progestins in the Normal Human Menstrual Cycle," *Recent Progress in Hormone Research* 13 (1957), pp. 323-39; E. W. Lawless, "Oral Contraceptive Safety Hearings," in *Technology and Social Shock* (New Brunswick, N.J.: Rutgers University Press, 1977), pp. 28-45.

4. Lawless, "Oral Contraceptive Safety Hearings," p. 30.

5. Ibid., p. 31.

6. "Estrogen Replacement Therapy: The dangerous road to Shangri-la," *Consumer Reports,* November, 1976.

7. P. Weideger, *Menstruation and Menopause* (New York: Knopf, 1976).

8. E. B. Astwood, "Estrogens and Progestins," ch. 69 in L. S. Goodman and A. Gilman, eds., *The Pharmacological Basis of Therapeutics,* 4th ed. (New York: Macmillan, 1970), p. 1546.

9. J. M. Stellman, *Women's Work, Women's Health* (New York: Pantheon, 1977).

10. P. Christy, "Diseases of the Endocrine System," in P. B. Beeson and W. McDermott, eds., *Cecil-Loeb Textbook of Medicine,* 13th ed. (Philadelphia: Saunders, 1971), p. 1722.

11. R. I. Pfeffer, "Estrogen Use in Postmenopausal Women," *American Journal of Epidemiology* 105 (1977), pp. 21-29.

12. Astwood, "Estrogens and Progestins," pp. 1546-48.

13. Lawless, "The Diethylstilbestrol Ban," in *Technology and Social Shock*, pp. 70-82.

14. This incident is discussed in N. Wade, "DES: A Case Study in Regulatory Abdication," *Science 177* (1977), pp. 335-37; see also, J. N. S. White, "The Stilbestrol Conspiracy," *Natural Food and Farming,* March, 1973, pp. 15-19.

15. Discussed and quoted in M. Mintz, "Kennedy Sets Hill Hearings on Continued Use of DES," *Washington Post,* July 14, 1972.

16. Ibid.

17. *Sex Hormones,* International Agency for Research on Cancer monograph on the Evaluation of Carcinogenic Chemicals to Man, vol. 6 (Lyon, France, *1974).* A compendium of experimental data on carcinogenicity of male and female sex hormones.

18. Ibid.

19. J. A. McLachlan and R. L. Dixon, "Transplacental Toxicity of Diethylstilbestrol: A special problem in safety evaluation," ch. 13 in M. A. Mehlman, R. E. Shapiro, and H. Blumenthal, eds., *Advances in Modern Toxicology,* vol. 1, pt. *2,* "New Concepts in Safety Evaluation" (Washington, D.C.: Hemisphere Publishing Corp., 1976), pp. 423-48.

20. *Sex Hormones,* IARC monograph.

21. H. K. Ziel and W. D. Finkel, "Increased Risk of Endometrial Carcinoma among Users of Conjugated Estrogens," *New England Journal of Medicine 293* (1975), pp. 1167-70.

22. "Estrogen Drugs," *Science 191* (1976), pp. 838-41.

23. R. Hoover *et al.,* "Geographic Patterns of Cancer Mortality," ch. *20* in J. F. Fraumeni, Jr., ed., *Persons at High Risk of Cancer* (New York: Academic Press, 1975), pp. 343-60.

24. R. I. Horwitz and A. R. Feinstein, "Alternative Analytic Methods for Case-Control Studies of Estrogens and Endometrial Cancer," *New England Journal of Medicine 299* (1978), pp. 1089-94.

25. G. B. Hutchinson and K. J. Rothman, "Correcting a Bias?," *New England Journal of Medicine 299* (1978), pp. 1129-30; see also C.M.F. Antunes *et al.,* "Endometrial Cancer and Estrogen Use: Report of a large case-control study," *New England Journal of Medicine 300* (1979), pp. 9-13. This is the largest study so far performed which confirms the relation between estrogen and uterine cancer and which refutes the Horowitz-Feinstein-Averst hypothesis.

26. R. Hoover, L. A. Gray, and J. F. Fraumeni, Jr., "Stilbestrol and the Risk of Ovarian

Cancer," *Lancet* 2 (1977), p. 533.

27. R. Hoover *et al.*, "Menopausal Estrogens and Breast Cancer," *New England Journal of Medicine* 295 (1976), pp. 401-5.

28. M. R. Melamed *et al.*, "Prevalence Rates of Uterine Cervical Carcinoma *in situ* for Women Using the Diaphragm or Contraceptive Oral Steroids," *British Medical Journal* 3 (1969), p. 195.

29. E. Peritz, S. Ramcharan, J. Frank, W. L. Brown, S. Huang, and R. Ray, "The Incidence of Cervical Cancer and Duration of Oral Contraceptive Use," *American Journal of Epidemiology* 106 (1977), pp. 642-49.

30. V. Beral, S. Ramcharan, and R. Faris, "Malignant Melanoma and Oral Contraceptive Use Among Women in California," *British Journal of Cancer* 36 (1977), pp. 804-9.

31. J. K. Baum, J. J. Bookstein, and F. Holtz, "Possible Association Between Benign Hepatomas and Oral Contraceptives," *Lancet 2 (1973), pp. 926- 29;* H. A. Edmonson, B. Henderson, and B. Denton, "Liver-Cell Adenomas Associated with Use of Oral Contraceptives," *New England Journal of Medicine* 294 (1976), pp. 470-72.

32. J. Vana, G. P. Murphy, B. L. Aronoff, and H. W. Baker, "Primary Liver Tumors and Oral Contraceptives: Results of a survey," *Journal American Medical Association* 238 (1977), pp. 2154-58.

33. A. L. Herbst and R. E. Scully, "Adenocarcinoma of the Vagina in Adolescence: A report of 7 cases including 6 clear-cell carcinomas (so-called mesonephromas)," *Cancer* 25 (1970), pp. 745-57; A. L. Herbst, H. Ulfelder, and D. C. Poskanzer, "Adenocarcinoma of the Vagina: Association of maternal stilbestrol therapy with tumor appearance in young women," *New England Journal of Medicine* 284 (1971), pp. 878- 81; K. L. Noller, *et al.*, "Clear-Cell Adenocarcinoma of the Cervix After Maternal Treatment with Synthetic Estrogens," *Mayo Clinic Proceedings* 47 (1972), pp. 629-30.

34. W. J. Dieckmann *et al.*, "Does the Adminis-tration of Diethylstilbestrol during Pregnancy Have Any Therapeutic Value," *American Journal of Obstetrics and Gynecology* 66 (1953), pp. 1062-81.

35. M. Bibbo, *et al.*, "Follow-up Study of Male and Female Offspring of DES-Exposed Mothers," *Journal of the American College of Obstetrics & Gynecology* 49 (1977), pp. 1-8.

36. S. Wolfe (Public Citizen Health Research Group) to HEW Secretary Joseph Califano, December 12, 1977.

37. "Mortality Associated with the Pill," *Lancet* 2 (1977), pp. 747-48; "Mortality and Oral Contraceptives," *British Medical Journal* 2 (1977), p. 918.

38. M. Mintz, *By Prescription Only* (Boston: Houghton-Mifflin, 1967). An early report to laymen on potential hazards of pill usage.

39. W. H. W. Inmann and M. P. Vessey, "Investigation of Deaths from Pulmonary, Coronary, and Cerebral Thrombosis and Embolism in Women of Childbearing Age," *British Medical Journal* 2 (1968), pp. 193-99; M. Mintz, *The Pill: An Alarming Report* (Boston: Beacon Press, 1970). An update of Mintz's earlier book on the problems of pill usage.

40. Mintz, *The Pill.*

41. Royal College of General Practitioners' Oral Contraception Study, "Mortality Among Oral Contraceptive Users," *Lancet* 2 (1977), p. 727; M. P. Vessey, K. McPherson, and B. Johnson, "Mortality Among Women Participating in the Oxford Family Planning Association Contraceptive Study," *Lancet* 2 (1977), p. 731.

42. "OSHA Fines Dawes Labs $34,100," *OCAW Lifelines,* July, 1977.

43. Ibid.

44. U.S. Public Health Service, Center for Disease Control, *Morbidity and Mortality Weekly Report,* April 1, 1977.

45. *Sex Hormones,* IARC monograph.

46. Mintz, "Kennedy Sets Hearings on DES."

47. Wade, "DES: A case study in regulatory abdication"; White, "The Stilbestrol Conspiracy"; B. Doerschuk, "The DES Controversy: Beyond the tip of the ice-

berg," *Nutrition Action,* April, 1976; see also H. Wellford, *Sowing the Wind* (New York: Grossman Publishers, 1972).

48. Ibid.

49. Wade, "DES: A case study in regulatory abdication"; White, "The Stilbestrol Conspiracy."

50. Doerschuk, "The DES Controversy"; Wellford, *Sowing the Wind.*

51. Wade, "DES: A case study in regulatory abdication," pp. 336-37.

52. S. S. Epstein, "Federal Food Inspection Act of 1973," testimony before the Senate Commerce Committee, Hearings of Toxic Substances Control Act of 1973, U.S. Senate, March 21, 1973.

53. Ibid., quotation, p. 261.

54. "Food Producing Animals: Criteria and procedures for evaluating assay for carcinogenic residues," *Federal Register,* February 22, 1977, pp. 10412-37.

55. Lawless, "Oral Contraceptive Safety Hearings."

56. Pharmaceutical Manufacturers Association *et al. v.* Food and Drug Administration *et al.*, Civil No. 77-291, U.S. District Court for the District of Delaware, 1977.

CHAPTER 7
The General Environment:
Case Studies

Pesticides

1. U.S. Department of Health, Education, and Welfare, *Report of the Secretary's Commission on Pesticides and Their Relationship to Environmental Health* (Washington, D.C.: December, 1969), ch. 1; J. E. Blodgett, "Pesticides: Regulation of an evolving technology," in S. S. Epstein and R. Grundy, eds., *Consumer Health and Product Hazards: Cosmetics and Drugs, Pesticides, Food Additives,* Legislation of Product Safety, vol. 2 (Cambridge, Mass.: MIT Press, 1974), pp. 198-287.

2. W. Olkowski *et al.*, "Ecosystem Management: A framework for urban pest control," *Bioscience* 26 (1976), pp. 384-89; H. Olkowski and W. Olkowski, "How to Control Garden Pests without Killing

Almost Everything Else" (Washington, D.C.: Rachel Carson Trust for the Living Environment, 1976); M. F. Jacobson, "Agriculture's New Hero: IPM," *Nutrition Action,* January, 1978, pp. 3-12; "Farmers and the Environment," *EPA Journal* March, 1978; R. van den Bosch, *The Pesticide Conspiracy* (New York: Doubleday, 1978).

3. Van den Bosch, *Pesticide Conspiracy;* H. Wellford, *Sowing the Wind* (New York: Grossman Publishers, 1972), ch. 9.

4. Van den Bosch, *Pesticide Conspiracy.*

5. R. Carson, *Silent Spring* (Boston: Houghton-Mifflin, 1962).

6. F. Graham, *Since Silent Spring* (Boston: Houghton-Mifflin 1970).

7. Ibid., p. 57.

8. Carson, *Silent Spring,* p. 12.

9. Blodgett, "Pesticides: Regulation of an evolving technology."

10. International Agency for Research on Cancer, "Some Organochlorine Pesticides," IARC Monographs on the Evaluation of Carcinogenic Risk of Chemicals to Man, vol. 5 (Lyon, France, 1974).

11. Van den Bosch, *Pesticide Conspiracy;* Wellford, *Sowing the Wind;* L. Tallian, *Politics and Pesticides* (Los Angeles: People's Lobby Press, 1975).

12. Van den Bosch, *Pesticide Conspiracy.*

13. D. Pimentel, "Ecological Effects of Pesticides on Non-Target Species" (Washington, D.C.: Office of Science and Technology, June, 1971); see also E. H. Smith and D. Pimentel, *Pest Control Strategies* (New York: Academic Press, 1978); and D. Pimentel *et al.*, "Environmental and Social Costs of Pesticide Use," draft report to the EPA Pesticide Policy Committee, May 16, 1978.

Aldrin/Dieldrin

1. C. F. Wurster, "Aldrin and Dieldrin," *Environment* 13 (1971), pp. 33-45; U.S. Environmental Protection Agency, Office of the General Counsel, Attorneys for Respondent, "Respondent's Brief, Proposed Findings and Conclusion on Suspension," in re Shell Chemical Company *et al.*, Consolidated Aldrin/Dieldrin Hearing,

FIFRA Dockets 145 *et al.*, Washington, D.C., September 16, 1974. The latter is a good and concise account of environmental contamination, carcinogenicity and other hazards, and lack of efficacy of aldrin/dieldrin.

2. EPA, "Respondent's Brief," pp. 146-64.

3. Wurster, "Aldrin and Dieldrin."

4. B. D. Ayers, "Killing of Contaminated Chickens Begins in Missis*sippi,*" *New York Times,* March 14,1974; V. K. McElheny, "Animal Feed Oils Tainted by Insecticide Recalled," *New York Times,* April 19, 1974.

5. EPA, "Respondent's Brief," pp. 188-215.

6. EPA, "Respondent's Brief."

7. U.S. Department of Health, Education, and Welfare, "Reports of the Secretary's Commission on Pesticides and Their Relationship to Environmental Health" (Washington, D.C., December, 1969), p. 470.

8. EPA, "Respondent's Brief," pp. 28-56; see also L. Gibney. "EPA Broadens Approach to Pesticide Decisions," *Chemical and Engineering News,* November 3, 1975, p. 15.

9. S. S. Epstein, "The Carcinogenicity of Dieldrin," *Science of the Total Environment* 4 (1975), pp. 1-52, 205-17; see also National Cancer Institute, "Bioassays of Aldrin and Dieldrin for Possible Carcinogenicity," Technical Report Series, 21 (1978); and idem, "Bioassay of Dieldrin for Possible Carcinogenicity," Technical Report Series, 22 (1978).

10. Ibid.

11. Ibid.

12. EPA, "Respondent's Brief," pp. 127-45; Epstein, "The Carcinogenicity of Dieldrin."

13. EPA, "Respondent's Brief," pp. 75-78.

14. Ibid., p. 131. See also EPA Suspension Hearings, 1974, testimony of P. Newberne, Shell Ex. S-9, p. 20.

15. Ibid., p. 95-98.

16. Ibid., p. 140.

17. K. W. Jager, *Aldrin, Dieldrin, Endrin, and Telodrin* (Amsterdam: Elsevier, 1970).

18. Epstein, "The Carcinogenicity of Dieldrin," pp. 15-16.

19. EPA, "Respondent's Brief," p. 113.

20. Epstein, "The Carcinogenicity of Dieldrin,"
pp. 15-16; EPA, "Respondent's Brief," pp. 109-13.

21. EPA, "Respondent's Brief," p. 109.

22. Ibid.

23. President's Science Advisory Committee, "Use of Pesticides" (Washington, D.C., April 15, 1963).

24. Epstein, "The Carcinogenicity of Dieldrin"; NCI, "Bioassays of Aldrin and Dieldrin"; idem, "Bioassay of Dieldrin."

25. U.S. Department of Health, Education, and Welfare, "Report of the Secretary's Commission on Pesticides."

26. National Academy of Sciences, National Research Council, "Advisory Committee Report on Aldrin/Dieldrin" (Washington, D.C., March, 1972).

27. Ayers, "Killing of Contaminated Chickens Begins"; McElheny, "Animal Feed Oils Recalled."

28. EPA, "Respondent's Brief."

29. H. L. Perlman (Chief Administrative Law Judge), "Recommended Decision, Aldrin/Dieldrin Suspension Hearings," FIFRA Dockets 145 *et al.*, September 20, 1974.

30. "Opinion of the Administrator, EPA, on the Suspension of Aldrin/Dieldrin," FIFRA Dockets 145 *et al.*, October 1, 1974.

31. Council for Agricultural Science and Technology (CAST), "The Environmental Protection Agency's Nine 'Principles' of Carcinogenicity," CAST Report 4 (Ames, Iowa: Iowa State University, Department of Agronomy, 1976); see also "Comments on Health Risk and Economic Impact Assessments of Suspected Carcinogens, Interim Procedures and Guidelines," CAST Report 73, December 30, 1977.

32. W. Appleby (Shell Chemical Company), "EPA-Dieldrin: Towards a sound cancer policy," in H. H. Hiatt, J. D. Watson, and J. A. Winston, eds., *Origins of Human Cancer,* vol. 4 (Cold Spring Harbor Laboratory, 1977), pp. 1709-13.

33. B. Gillespie, D. Eva, and R. Johnston, "A Tale of Two Pesticides," *New Scientist* 77 (1978), pp. 350-52.

Chlordane/Heptachlor

1. U.S. Environmental Protection Agency,

Office of the General Counsel, Attorneys for Respondent, "Respondent's Final Brief," in re Velsicol Chemical Corporation *et al.*, Chlordane and Heptachlor, FIFRA Docket 384, Washington, D.C., December 8, 1975. A good and concise account of environmental contamination, carcinogenicity and other hazards of chlordane/heptachlor.

2. Ibid., pp. 77-85.
3. Ibid., pp. 135-39.
4. Ibid., pp. 115-33.
5. Ibid., pp. 140-56.
6. S. S. Epstein, "The Carcinogenicity of Heptachlor and Chlordane," *Science of the Total Environment* 6 (1976), pp. 103-54.
7. U.S. Department of Health, Education, and Welfare, Report of the Secretary's Commission on Pesticides and Their Relationship to Environmental Health (Washington, D.C., December, 1969), p. 470.
8. National Cancer Institute, "Bioassay of Chlordane for Possible Carcinogenicity," Technical Report Series, 8 (Washington, D.C., 1977); idem, "Bioassay of Heptachlor for Possible Carcinogenicity," Technical Report Series, 9 (Washington, D.C., 1977).
9. Epstein, "Carcinogenicity of Heptachlor and Chlordane."
10. Ibid., pp. 116-17.
11. NCI, "Bioassay of Chlordane"; idem, "Bioassay of Heptachlor."
12. National Academy of Sciences, National Research Council, Advisory Center on Toxicology, Pesticide Information Review and Evaluation Committee, "An Evaluation of the Carcinogenicity of Chlordane and Heptachlor" (Washington, D.C., October, 1977).
13. EPA, "Respondent's Final Brief," p. 221.
14. Ibid., p. 222.
15. Ibid., pp. 230-40.
16. Ibid., p. 82-92.
17. P. F. Infante and S. S. Epstein, "Blood Dyscrasias and Childhood Tumors and Exposures to Chlorinated Hydrocarbon Pesticides," in *Proceedings of the June 17-19, 1976, Conference on Women and the Workplace* (Washington, D.C.: Society for Occupational and Environmental Health, 1977), pp. 51-74.
18. U.S. Environmental Protection Agency, Office of the General Counsel, Attorney for Respondent, "Respondent's First Pretrial Brief," in re Velsicol Chemical Corporation *et al.*, Consolidated Heptachlor/Chlordane Hearings, FIFRA Dockets 336 *et al.*, April 1, 1975.
19. Velsicol's first prehearing brief, FIFRA Dockets 336 *et al.*, May 1, 1975.
20. D. Zinman, B. Wyrick and D. Hevesi, "Scientist's Role is Questioned," *Newsday,* January 18, 1977; see also, "Rep. Obey Questions Contract on Cancer," *Washington Post,* June 12, 1977.
21. EPA, Respondent's Final Brief, pp. 331-41.
22. "NCI Carcinogenesis Draft Sparks Backlash," *Blue Sheet* 19, no. 4, January 28, 1976.
23. H. L. Perlman (Chief Administrative Law Judge), "Recommended Decision," in re Velsicol Chemical Corporation *et al.*, FIFRA Docket 384, December 12, 1975.
24. Ibid.
25. "Decision of the Administrator, EPA, on the Suspension of Heptachlor- Chlordane," in re Velsicol Chemical Corporation *et al.*, FIFRA Docket 3 84, December 24, 1975.
26. *Federal Register,* March 24, 1978, pp. 12372-75.
27. N. Sheppard, Jr., "Maker of Pesticides Indicted on Charges of Hiding Test Data," *New York Times,* December 13, 1977

Nitrosamines

1. W. Lijinsky and S. S. Epstein, "Nitrosamines as Environmental Carcinogens," *Nature* 225 (1970), pp. 21-23.
2. P. N. Magee, R. Montesano, and R. Preussmann, "N-Nitroso Compounds and Related Carcinogens," in C. E. Searle, ed., *Chemical Carcinogens* (Washington, D.C.: American Chemical Society, 1976), pp. 491-625; Lijinsky and Epstein, "Nitrosamines as Environmental Carcinogens."
3. J. Sander, "Formation of Carcinogenic Nitroso Compounds under Biological Conditions," in *Environment and Cancer* (Baltimore, Md.: Williams and Wilkins,

1972), pp. 109-17.

4. Magee, Montesano, and Preussmann, "N-Nitroso Compounds and Related Carcinogens"; Sander, "Formation of Carcinogenic Nitroso Compounds"; S. S. Mirvish, "Formation of N-Nitroso Compounds: Chemistry, kinetics and *in vivo* occurrence," *Toxicology and Applied Pharmacology* 31 (1975), pp. 325-51.

5. D. H. Fine *et al.*, "N-Nitroso Compounds: Detection in ambient air," *Science* 192 (1976), pp. 1328-30.

6. Magee, Montesano, and Preussmann, "N-Nitroso Compounds and Related Carcinogens."

7. International Agency for Research on Cancer, "Environmental N-Nitroso Compounds, Analysis and Formation," IARC Scientific Publication 14 (Lyon, France, 1976), an excellent collection of a wide range of multi- authored chapters; D. H. Fine *et al.*, "Human Exposure to N-Nitroso Compounds in the Environment," in H. H. Hiatt, J. D. Watson, and J. A. Winsten, eds., *Origins of Human Cancer* (Cold Spring Harbor Laboratory, 1977), pp. 293-307.

8. Fine *et al.*, "N-Nitroso Compounds: Detection in ambient air."

9. National Academy of Sciences, "Air Quality and Automobile Emission Control," vol. 2 (Washington, D.C., 1974), pp. 282-83.

10. IARC, "N-Nitroso Compounds, Analysis and Formation."

11. S. S. King, "Nitrate Reduction Ordered in Bacon," *New York Times,* May 16, 1978.

12. U.S. House of Representatives, Committee on Interstate and Foreign Commerce, Hearings before the Subcommittee on Oversight and Investigations, May 28 and September 20, 1976.

13. Ibid., pp. 302-21.

14. Ibid., p. 218.

15. Ibid., p. 281.

16. IARC, "N-Nitroso Compounds, Analysis and Formation."

17. Ibid.

18. "N-Nitrosamines Found in Sidestream Smoke," *Chemical and Engineering News,* June 13, 1977, p. 18.

19. Hearings before the Subcommittee on Oversight and Investigations, pp. 248-73.

20. Ibid.

21. Ibid., p. 71.

22. J. K. Wagoner *et al.* to Director, NIOSH, "NIOSH Investigation of Cancer Hazard at E.I. Du Pont de Nemour & Company, Belle Plant," February 2, 1977.

23. S. R. Tannenbaum, D. Fett, V. R. Young, P. D. Lang, and W. R. Bruce, "Nitrite and Nitrate are Formed by Endogenous Synthesis in the Human Intestine," *Science* 200 (1978), pp. 1487-89.

CHAPTER 8
How to Improve Industry Data

1. S. S. Epstein, "Cancer and the Environment," *Bulletin of the Atomic Scientists (of Chicago)* 26 (1977), pp. 22-30.

2. Ibid.

3. *Federal Register,* August 8, 1967.

4. U.S. Department of Health, Education, and Welfare, Report of the Secretary's Commission on Pesticides and Their Relationship to Environmental Health, Washington, D.C., December, 1969.

5. P. Boffey, "Color Additives: Is successor to Red Dye No. 2 any safer?" *Science* 191 (1976), pp. 832-34; see also G. Moreland, "Warning: Red Dye #40 may be hazardous to your health," *Nutrition Action,* February 4, 1977.

6. S. S. Epstein, "The Carcinogenicity of Dieldrin," *Science of the Total Environment* 4 (1975), pp. 1-52, 205-17; S. S. Epstein, "The Carcinogenicity of Heptachlor and Chlordane," *Science of the Total Environment* 6 (1976), pp. 103-54; see also idem, "The Carcinogenicity of Organochlorine Pesticides," in H. H. Hiatt, J. D. Watson, and J. A. Winsten, eds., *Origins of Human Cancer* (Cold Spring Harbor Laboratory, 1977), pp. 243-45.

7. Ibid.

8. M. D. Reuber, "Review of Toxicity Test Results Submitted in Support of Pesticide Tolerance Petitions," *Science of the Total Environment* 9 (1977), pp. 135-48.

9. Staff Report to the Subcommittee on Administrative Practice and Procedures of

the Committee on the Judiciary, U.S. Senate, "The Environmental Protection Agency and the Regulation of Pesticides," December, 1976.

10. S. S. Epstein, "The Delaney Amendment and Mechanisms for Reducing Constraints in the Regulatory Process in General, and as Applied to Food Additives in Particular," Hearings before the Select Committee on Nutrition and Human Needs, U.S. Senate, September 20, 1972.

11. A. M. Schmidt, Statement before the Subcommittee on Health of the Committee on Labor and Public Welfare, and the Subcommittee on Administrative Practice and Procedures of the Committee on the Judiciary, U.S. Senate, January 20, 1976.

12. S. S. Epstein, "Toxicological and Environmental Implications on the Use of Nitrilotriacetic Acid as a Detergent Builder," Staff Report to the Committee on Public Works, U.S. Senate, December, 1970; see also, S. S. Epstein, *International Journal Environmental Studies* 2 (1972), pp. 291-300; 3 (1972), pp. 13-21.

13. S. S. Epstein, "The Public Interest Overview," *Environmental Health Perspectives* 10 (1975), p. 173.

14. Epstein, "Cancer and the Environment."

15. Ibid.

16. J. R. M. Innes *et al.*, "Bioassay of Pesticides and Industrial Chemicals for Tumorigenicity in Mice: A preliminary note," *Journal of the National Cancer Institute* 43 (1969), pp. 1101-14.

17. U.S. Department of Labor, transcript, Occupational Safety and Health Advisory Committee, Proceedings Standards, Advisory Committee on Occupational Carcinogens, August, 1973.

18. B. A. Schwetz, G. L. Sparschu, and P. J. Gehring, "The Effect of 2,4-D and Esters of 2,4-D on Rat Embryonal, Foetal, and Neonatal Growth and Development," *Food Cosmetics Toxicology* 9 (1971), pp. 801-17.

19. S. S. Epstein, "Kepone: Hazard evaluation," *Science of the Total Environment* 9 (1978), pp. 1-62.

20. Epstein, "Carcinogenicity of Heptachlor and Chlordane"; idem, "Carcinogenicity of Organochlorine Pesticides."

21. "Hiding Danger of Pesticides," *New York Times,* December 18, 1977.

22. J. T. Edsall, "Report of the AAAS Committee on Scientific Freedom and Responsibility," *Science* 188 (1975), pp. 687-93.

23. See note 17 above.

24. "Lab Officials Admit Shredding Test Data," *Washington Post,* September 20, 1977; "Testing Lab Errors Hinder Army Food Project," *Chemical and Engineering News,* November 14, 1977; B. Richards, "Probers Say Pesticide Makers Knew of Faulty Lab Test Data," *Washington Post,* March 9, 1978.

25. Ibid.

26. Ibid.

27. "Filling in Toxicology Gaps," *Chemical Week,* November 17, 1976, pp. 36-37.

28. W. Reddig, "Industry's Preemptive Strike Against Cancer," *Fortune,* February 13, 1978.

29. S. S. Epstein, "The Delaney Amendment and Mechanisms for Reducing Constraints in the Regulatory Process in General, and as Applied to Food Additives, in Particular," testimony before the Select Committee on Nutrition and Human Needs, U.S. Senate, September 20, 1972.

30. M. L. Weidenbaum, "How Much Regulation is Too Much? A Call for Cost/Benefit Analysis," N. A. Ashford, "A Plea For A New Kind of Realism," *New York Times,* December 17, 1978, p. 16.

CHAPTER 9
Governmental Policies

1. Office of Science and Technology, Council on Environmental Quality Ad Hoc Committee, "Report on Environmental Health Research" (Washington, D.C., June, 1972).

2. S. P. Strickland, *Politics, Science, and Dread Disease: A Short History of United States Medical Research Policy* (Cambridge, Mass.: Harvard University Press, 1972). A historical analysis of the background and development of the National Cancer Institute and national policies on cancer research prior to 1971.

3. Public Law 92-218, 85 Stat. 778 (42 U.S.C.

218 *et seq.),* December 23, 1971.

4. L. Agran, *The Cancer Connection and What We Can Do about It* (Boston: Houghton Mifflin, 1977), pp. 171-86.

5. Ibid.

6. Examples of Hueper's 350 scientific publications on cancer include: *Occupational Tumors and Allied Diseases* (Springfield, Ill.: Charles C. Thomas, 1942); *Occupational and Environmental Cancers of the Respiratory System* (New York: Springer Verlag, 1966); *Occupational and Environmental Cancers of the Urinary System* (New Haven, Conn.: Yale University Press, 1969); "Medicolegal Considerations of Occupational and Nonoccupational Environmental Cancer," in C. J. Frankel and R. M. Patterson, eds., *Lawyers' Medical Cyclopedia,* vol. 5B, rev. (Indianapolis, Ind.: Allen Smith Company, 1972), pp. 293-568.

7. S. S. Epstein, "Presentation of the First Annual Award of the Society for Occupational and Environmental Health to Wilhelm C. Hueper," in U. Saffiotti and J. K. Wagoner, eds., *Occupational Carcinogenesis,* Annals of the New York Academy of Science, 271 (New York, 1976).

8. Agran, *The Cancer Connection, pp.* 171-86.

9. Strickland, *Politics, Science, and Dread Disease.*

10. R. A. Rettig, *Cancer Crusade: The Story of the National Cancer Act of 1971* (Princeton, N.J.: Princeton University Press, 1977). A blow-by-blow legislative history of the Act, describing the influences of the various pressure groups.

11. Rettig, *Cancer Crusade,* p. 79.

12. U.S. Senate, Report of the National Panel of Consultants on the Conquest of Cancer, S. Doc. 92-9, 92nd Cong. 1st Sess., 1971.

13. Rettig, *Cancer Crusade, pp.* 18-41.

14. H. L. Perlman (Chief Administrative Law Judge), "Recommended Decision," in re Velsicol Chemical Corporation *et al.,* FIFRA Docket 384, December 12, 1975.

15. D. Zinman, B. Wyrick, and D. Hevesi, "Scientist's Role is Questioned," *Newsday,* January 18, 1977.

16. Ibid.

17. Ibid.

18. Ibid.; see also K. Gage and S. S. Epstein, "The Federal Advisory Committee System," *Environmental Law Reporter* 7 (1977), pp. 50001- 12.

19. Zinman, Wyrick, and Hevesi, "Scientist's Role is Questioned."

20. "Rep. Obey Questions Contract on Cancer," *Washington Post,* June 12, 1977.

21. Report of the Comptroller General of the United States, "Need to Improve Administration of a Carcinogen Testing and Carcinogenesis Research Contract" (HRD-78-44), Washington, D.C., February 10, 1978.

22. L. Parrott, "Regent: HEW wants Eppley to repay," *Omaha World-Herald,* April 23, 1978; see also J. Shapiro, "Dr. Shubik and Eppley Institute: From hope to embarrassment," Sun newspapers of Omaha, special report, June 15, 1978; M. McGrath, "HEW Asks Eppley Institute for Refund," and "Eppley Inquiry Continues in Another Field," *Omaha World-Herald,* November 13, 1978; L. Parrott, "N. U. Inquiry into Eppley is Revealed," *Omaha World-Herald,* December 6, 1978.

23. D. Greenberg, "Cancer: Now the bad news," *Washington Post,* January 19, 1975; Greenberg, D., Science and Government Report, April 1, 1975; "Cancer Patient Survival," Surveillance, Epidemiology and End Results (SEER) Program, Report no. 5, Publication (NIH) 77-992 (Washington, D.C., 1976).

24. Report to the Congress by the Comptroller General of the United States, "Federal Efforts to Protect the Public From Cancer-Causing Chemicals Are Not Very Effective" (MWD-76-59), Washington, D.C., 1976.

25. U.S. House of Representatives, Cong. D. Obey, Hearings before the Subcommittee of the Committee on Appropriations, 94th Cong., National Cancer Institute, February 25, 1976, pp. 64-208.

26. U. Saffiotti to Director, NCI, April 23, 1976; see also, *Cancer Letter* 2 (1976), pp. 5-8; N. Wade, "Cancer Institute: Expert Charges Neglect of Carcinogenesis Studies," *Science* 192 (1976), pp. 529-31.

27. A. Upton, "On Cancer Cause and Preven-

tion Activities of NCI," testimony before the Subcommittee on Oversight and Investigation, House Committee on Interstate and Foreign Commerce, January 23, 1978.

28. Rettig, *Cancer Crusade,* p. 320.

29. Gage and Epstein, "Federal Advisory Committee System."

30. S. S. Epstein, "A Catch-all Toxicological Screen," *Experientia* 25 (1969), pp. 617-18.

31. National Institute of Occupational Safety and Health, Division of Criteria Documentation and Standards Development, "Summary of NIOSH Recommendations for Occupational Health Standards" (Washington, D.C., June, 1977).

32. "Occupational Carcinogenesis Program," DHEW (NIOSH) Publication 77-111 (Washington, D.C., September 30, 1976); see also Hearings before a Subcommittee of the Committee on Appropriations, House of Representatives, pt. 3, 1977, pp. 162-63.

33. *Chemical and Engineering News,* December 16, 1976.

34. U.S. Department of Health, Education, and Welfare, Center for Disease Control, National Institute for Occupational Safety and Health, *National Occupational Hazard Survey,* vol. 1, "Survey Manual," DHEW (NIOSH) Publication 74-127 (Rockville, Md., 1971); vol. 2, "Data Editing and Data Base Development," 77-213 (Cincinnati, Ohio, 1977); vol. 3, "Survey Analysis and Supplemental Tables," 78-114 (Cincinnati, Ohio, 1977).

35. U.S. Department of Health, Education, and Welfare, Center for Disease Control, National Institute for Occupational Safety and Health, "The Right to Know: Practical problems and policy issues arising from exposures to hazardous chemical and physical agents in the workplace" (Washington, D.C., July, 1977); see also, "Chemical Dangers in the Workplace," Thirty-Fourth Report of the Committee on Government Operations, House of Representatives, September 27, 1976.

36. NIOSH, "The Right to Know," p. 3.

37. Ibid., p. 33.

38. U.S. House of Representatives, C. Edwards testimony, Hearings before a Subcommittee on Agriculture and Related Agencies, House Appropriations Committee, April, 1971; see also *Food Chemical News,* April 26, 1971.

39. U.S. House of Representatives, FDA testimony Hearings before a Subcommittee on Agriculture and Related Agencies, House Appropriations Committee, pt. 5, 1975, pp. 141-42.

40. H. L. Stewart, "Report of the Director's *ad hoc* Committee on Testing for Environmental Chemical Carcinogens" (Washington, D.C.: NCI, August, 1973).

41. National Academy of Sciences, National Research Council, "The National Center for Toxicological Research: The evaluation of its program" (Washington, D.C., 1977).

42. "NCTR Conflict of Interest Allegation Referred to Justice Department," *Food Chemical News,* April 24, 1978, pp. 3-6.

43. Environmental Quality Improvement Act of 1970, Public Law 91-190, January 1, 1970.

44. E. Dolgin, *Federal Environmental Law* (St. Paul, Minn.: West Publishing, 1974); M. L. Karstadt, "Protecting the Public Health from Hazardous Substances: Federal regulation of environmental contaminants," *Environmental Law Reporter* 5 (1975), pp. 50165-78. A useful summary of scientific problems underlying regulation.

45. S. S. Epstein and R. Grundy, eds., *Consumer Health and Product Hazards,* vol. 1, "Chemicals, Electronic Products, Radiation"; vol. 2, "Cosmetics and Drugs, Pesticides, Food Additives," Legislation of Product Safety (Cambridge, Mass.: MIT Press, 1974).

46. Public Law 91-596, 91st Congress S. 2193, December 29, 1970; see also, Occupational Safety and Health Act of 1970 (Oversight and Proposed Amendments), Hearings before the Select Subcommittee on Labor, Committee on Education and Labor, House of Representatives, 92nd Cong., 1972, and 93rd Cong., 1974.

47. N. Ashford, *Crisis in the Workplace* (Cambridge, Mass.: MIT Press, 1976); N. A. Ashford *et al.,* "Mobilizing National Resources for the Control of Occupational

Cancer," Report to the office of Technology Assessment, U.S. Congress, April, 1978.

48. U.S. Department of Labor, Occupational Safety and Health Administration, "Identification, Classification and Regulation of Toxic Substances Posing a Potential Carcinogenic Risk," *Federal Regulation,* pt. 6, October 4, 1977.

49. L. Ember, "OSHA on the Move," *Environmental Science and Technology* 11 (1977), pp. 1142-47.

50. American Industrial Health Council, "AIHC Recommended Alternatives to OSHA's Generic Carcinogen Policy" (Scarsdale, N.Y., January 9, 1978).

51. "Chemical Dangers in the Workplace," p. 8.

52. U.S. Congress, *Clean Air Amendments of 1970,* Conference Report No. 91-1783, 91st Cong. 2nd Sess., 1970, U.S. *Congressional and Administration News* (1970), pp. 5378-79, 1970; see also W. H. Rodgers, *Handbook on Environmental Law* (St. Paul, Minn.: West Publishing Co., 1977).

53. U.S. Senate Committee on Public Workers, Federal Water Pollution Control Act Amendments of 1971, S. Rep. No. 1414, 92nd Cong. 1st Sess., 1971; See also Rodgers, *Handbook on Environmental Law,* p. 482.

54. J. E. Blodgett, "Pesticides: Regulation of an evolving technology," in Epstein and Grundy, eds., *Consumer Health and Product Hazards: Cosmetics and Drugs, Pesticides, Food Additives,* vol. 2, pp. 198-287; H. Wellford, *Sowing the Wind* (New York: Grossman, 1972), pp. 310-53.

55. Blodgett, "Pesticides: Regulation of an evolving technology."

56. Ibid.: Federal Environmental Pesticide Control Act, Public Law No. 92- 516, 1972.

57. *Federal Regulation* 40 (1975), p. 28241; see also "Pesticide Decision Making," report to the EPA from the Committee on Pesticide Decision Making, National Research Council, National Academy of Sciences (Washington, D.C., 1978).

58. Report to the Congress by the Comptroller General of the United States, "Federal Pesticide Registration Program: Is it protecting the public and the environment adequately from pesticide hazards?" (Washington, D.C., 1975); U.S. Senate, Committee on the Judiciary, Subcommittee on Administrative Practice and Procedure, "The Environmental Protection Agency and the Regulation of Pesticides" (Washington, D.C., December, 1976).

59. Comptroller General, "Federal Pesticide Regulation Program."

60. Ibid.

61. M. D. Reuber, "Review of Toxicity Test Results Submitted in Support of Pesticide Tolerance Petitions," *Science of the Total Environment* 9 (1977), pp. 135-48.

62. H. Eschwege (U.S. General Accounting Office), testimony before the Subcommittee on Oversight and Investigations, House Committee on Interstate and Foreign Commerce, February 14, 1978; See also "Cancer-Causing Chemicals in Food," Report of the Subcommittee on Oversight and Investigations of the House Committee on Interstate and Foreign Commerce, November, 1978.

63. Subcommittee on Administrative Practice and Procedure, "The Environmental Protection Agency and the Regulation of Pesticides," p. 4.

64. U.S. Environmental Protection Agency, Office of Water Supply Criteria and Standards Division, "Statement of Basis and Purpose for an Amendment to the National Interim Primary Drinking Water Regulations on Trihalomethanes" (Washington, D.C., January, 1978); U.S. Environmental Protection Agency, "Interim Primary Drinking Water Regulations: Control of organic chemical contaminants in drinking water," *Federal Regulation* pt. 2, February 9, 1978.

65. "AWWA Protests EPA Regulations," *Willing Water,* March, 1978, pp. 12-13; see also "State EPA Questions New Drinking Water Rules," *Illinois EPA News,* March 15, 1978.

66. Toxic Substances Control Act, Public Law 94-469, 90 Stat. 2003 (15 U.S.C. 2601-2629), October 11, 1976.

67. U.S. Environmental Protection Agency, "Toxic Substances Control: Inventory

reporting requirements," *Fed. Regulation,* pt. 6, December 23, 1977.

68. M. L. Miller, ed., "Toxic Substances Control," 11. Proceedings of the Second Annual Toxic Substances Control Conference, December 8-9, 1977 (Washington, D.C.: Government Institute, Inc., January, 1978).

69. A. E. Rawse, "The Consumer Agency Bill: Time for a Recall?" *Washington Post,* February 5, 1978.

70. J. Thomas, "Chairman of Consumer Panel Quits, Charging Political Harassment," *New York Times,* February 9, 1978.

71. J. Turner, "Principles of Food Additive Regulation," in Epstein and Grundy, eds., *Consumer Health and Product Hazards,* vol. 2, pp. 289- 321.

72. Ibid.

73. Public Law 85-929, September 6, 1958.

74. S. S. Epstein, "The Delaney Amendment," in "Delaney Clause Controversy," *Preventive Medicine* 2 (1973), pp. 140-49; see also "Cancer Prevention and the Delaney Clause," Public Citizens Health Research Group monograph (Washington, D.C.: 1973), revised 1977.

75. Comptroller General, "Federal Pesticide Registration Program," pp. 38-48.

76. Eschwege, testimony before the Subcommittee on Oversight and Investigations; G. J. Ahart, "Testimony on Federal Efforts to Regulate Toxic Residues in Raw Meat and Poultry," before the Subcommittee on Oversight and Investigations, House Committee on Interstate and Foreign Commerce, February 16, 1978; See also Subcommittee on Oversight Report, "Cancer-Causing Chemicals in Food," November, 1978.

77. W. Sinclair, "More than 100 Suspect Cosmetic Ingredients Unregulated, GAO Study Finds," *Washington Post,* February 3, 1978; M. Russell and T. R. Reid, "FDA Chief Asks Hill for More Power to Regulate Cosmetics," *Washington Post,* February 4, 1978.

78. R. G. Marks, "Pharmaceuticals," in Epstein and Grundy, eds., *Consumer Health and Product Hazard,* vol. 2, pp. 143-95.

79. Eschwege, testimony before the Subcom-

mittee on Oversight and Investigations; Ahart, "Efforts to Regulate Toxic Residues" See also Subcommittee on Oversight Report, "Cancer-Causing Chemicals in Food," November, 1978.

80. S. S. King, "Nitrate Reduction Ordered in Bacon," *New York Times,* May 16, 1978.

81. Freedom of Information Act, Hearings before a Subcommittee of the Committee on Government Operation, House of Representatives, 93rd Cong., May, 1973; see also S. J. Archibald, "Working: The revised F.O.I. law and how to use it," *Columbia Journalism Review,* July/August, 1977.

82. Gage and Epstein, "Federal Advisory Committee System."

83. P. Hausman, "As the Revolving Door Turns," *Nutrition Action,* August, 1976, pp. 3-12.

84. D. Kirsten, "The New War on Cancer: Carter team seeks causes not cures," *National Journal* 9 (1977), pp. 1220-25; see also, Ember, "OSHA on the Move."

85. G. Speth (Council on Environmental Quality), "Towards a Better Bull's Eye Corporate Responsibility and Accountability," Speech to the American Bar Association — National Resources Section, November 28, 1978.

86. R. B. Du Boff, "Environment and the G.N.P.," *New York Times,* July 10, 1978.

87. P. Blanc, "Corporate Causes of Cancer in California." Draft Report to the Campaign for Economic Democracy and the California Public Policy Center, August, 1978.

CHAPTER 10
Non-governmental Policies

1. Monsanto Co., "The Chemical Facts of Life" (St. Louis, Mo., n.d.), p. 1.

2. F. de Lorenzo *et al.*, "Mutagenicity of Diallate, Sulfallate, and Triallate and Relationship between Structure and Mutagenic Effects of Carbamates Used Widely in Agriculture," *Cancer Research* 38 (1978), pp. 13-15.

3. National Cancer Institute, "Bioassay of Sulfallate for Possible Carcinogenicity," DHEW Publication (NIH) 78-1370

(Washington, D.C., March 24,1978).

4. P. Kotin, Address to the American Occupational Medicine Association, Denver, Colo., October, 1977.

5. C. Mittman *et al.*, "Prediction and Potential Prevention of Industrial Bronchitis," *American Journal of Medicine* 57 (1974), pp. 192-99.

6. J. O. Morse *et al.*, "A Community Study of the Relation of Alpha-Antitrypsin Levels to Obstructive Lung Diseases," *New England Journal of Medicine* 292 (1975), pp. 278-81.

7. See, for example, "How They Shaped the Toxic Substances Law," *Chemical Week,* April 27,1977, p. 52.

8. American Industrial Health Council, "AIHC Recommended Alternatives to OSHA's Generic Carcinogen Proposal" (Scarsdale, N.Y., January 9, 1978).

9. B. Castleman (1738 Riggs Place, N.W., Washington, DC 20009), "The Export of Hazardous Factories to Developing Nations," *Congressional Record,* June 29, 1978.

10. R. Nader, M. Green, and J. Seligman, "Constitutionalizing the Corporation: The case for the federal chartering of giant corporations" (Washington, D.C.: Corporate Accountability Research Group, 1976); G. Speth (Council on Environmental Quality), "Towards a Better Bull's Eye: Corporate responsibility and accountability," speech to the American Bar Association National Resources Section, November 28, 1978.

11. "Federal Chartering of Giant Corporations," Commission for the Advancement of Public Interest Organizations, *Proceedings of a Conference held on 16 June 1976, Washington, D.C.,* p. iii.

12. M. Weidenbaum and K. Chilton, "All Hazards Are Not Equal," *The Sciences* 18 (1978), pp. 8-32; J. Palmer, "The Rising Risks of Regulation," *Time,* November 27, 1978, pp. 85-87.

13. R. B. Du Boff, "Environment and the G.N.P.," *New York Times,* July 10, 1978; C. S. Bell, "The Benefits of Regulation," *New York Times,* July 25, 1978.

14. G. Speth, "Towards a Better Bull's Eye."

15. University of Michigan, Survey Research Center, "Survey of Working Conditions: Final report on univariate and bivariate tables" (Ann Arbor, Mich., November, 1970).

16. L. Stein, *The Triangle Fire* (Philadelphia: Lippincott, 1962).

17. B. Hume, *Death and the Mines* (New York: Grossman, 1971).

18. B. Weisberg, *Our Lives are at Stake* (San Francisco: United Front Press, 1973).

19. *New York Times,* May 2, 1973.

20. J. M. Stellman and S. M. Daum, *Work Is Dangerous to Your Health* (New York: Pantheon, 1973), p. 22.

21. R. Nader, "Professional Responsibility Revisited," in *Proceedings of the Conference on Science Technology and the Public Interest,* October 8, 1973. Brookings Institutions, Washington, D.C. (Jeannette, Pa.: Monsour Medical Foundation, 1977).

22. L. I. Moss, "Pulling Together," *EPA Journal* 4 (1978), pp. 11-37.

23. Quoted in L. E. Demkovich, "Ralph Nader Takes on Congress as Well as Big Business," *National Journal* 10 (1978), p. 390.

24. G. Lanson, "Industry Doubted as Cancer Cause," [New Jersey] *Record,* March 9, 1978.

25. National Information Bureau, Inc. (N.Y.), "American Cancer Society," December 16, 1976; D. S. Greenberg and J. E. Randal, "Waging the Wrong War on Cancer," *Washington Post,* May 1, 1977; R. Rosenbaum, "Cancer Inc.," *New York Times,* November 25, 1977; P. B. Chowka, "The Cancer Charity Rip-off: Warning, The American Cancer Society may be hazardous to your health," *East/West Journal,* July, 1978; M. Daniel (Center for Science in the Public Interest), "Voluntary Health Organizations," in press, 1979.

26. F. Greve, "Cancer Society's Efforts Are Found Wanting," *Philadelphia Inquirer,* April 30, 1978.

27. American Cancer Society, "1979 Cancer Facts and Figures," New York, 1978.

CHAPTER 11
What You Can Do to Prevent Cancer

1. S. S. Epstein, "Information Requirements for Determining the Benefit–Risk Spectrum," in *Perspectives on Benefit–Risk Decision Making* (Washington, D.C.: National Academy of Engineering, Committee on Public Engineering Policy, 1972), pp. 50-55; see also "Uses and Limits of Benefit-Cost Analysis," in *Decision Making for Regulating Chemicals in the Environment* (Washington, D.C.: National Academy of Sciences, 1975).

2. R. Nader, "Sorry State of the Labor Press," *The Progressive,* October, 1977, pp. 29-31.

3. J. F. Fraumeni, Jr., ed., *Persons at High Risk of Cancer: An Approach to Cancer Etiology and Control* (New York: Academic Press, 1975). An excellent collection of multi-authored chapters, each with a full set of references, dealing with a wide range of factors including environmental (occupational, tobacco, alcohol, radiation, drugs) and geographic; also deals with recognition of individuals and groups at high cancer risk.

4. J. A. Turner, R. W. Sillett, and N. W. McNicol, "Effect of Cigar Smoking on Carboxyhemoglobin and Plasma Nicotine Concentrations in Primary Pipe and Cigar Smokers and Ex-Cigarette Smokers," *British Medical Journal* 2 (1977), pp. 1387-89.

5. K. J. Rothman, "Alcohol," in Fraumeni, *Persons at High Risk of Cancer,* pp. 139-50; see also E. L. Wynder and S. D. Stellman, "Comparative Epidemiology of Tobacco-Related Cancers," *Cancer Research* 37 (1977), pp. 4608-22.

6. A. J. Tuyns, "Cancer of the Esophagus: Further Evidence of the Relation to Drinking Habits in France," *International Journal of Cancer* 5 (1970), pp. 152-56.

7. A. Z. Keller, "Alcohol, Tobacco, and Age Factors in the Relative Frequency of Cancer among Males with and without Liver Cirrhosis," *American Journal of Epidemiology* 106 (1977), pp. 194-202.

8. E. M. Whelan and F. J. Stare, *Panic in the Pantry: Facts and Fallacies* (New York: Atheneum, 1975); see also Iowa State University Council for Agricultural Science and Technology (CAST) publications and reports such as "Comments on Health Risks and Economic Impact Assessments of Suspected Carcinogens: Interim Procedures and Guidelines," CAST Report 73 (Ames, Iowa, December 30, 1977). Examples of slanted and poorly-informed literature presenting the industry position that food additives and contaminants pose no dangers to health.

9. See, for example, *Nutrition Action,* an excellent monthly publication of the Center for Science in the Public Interest dealing with problems of nutrition, food additives, and contaminants; M. F. Jacobson, *Eaters Digest* (New York: Doubleday and Co., 1972); see also "Chemical Cuisine," a poster on food additives produced by the Center for Science in the Public Interest, 1978.

10. Good sources include: J. S. Turner, *The Chemical Feast* (New York: Grossman, 1970); J. Verett and J. Carper, *Eating May Be Dangerous to Your Health* (New York: Simon and Schuster, 1974); B. T. Hunter, *Food Additives and Federal Policy: The Mirage of Safety* (New York: Charles Scribner & Sons, 1975); M. Burros, *Pure and Simple: Delicious Recipes for Additive-Free Cooking* (New York: William Morrow, 1978).

11. Congressman B. Rosenthal and M. F. Jacobson, "Study Finds Nutrition Professors 'Feeding at the Company Trough'," press release, August 15, 1976; see also J. Mintz, "Boston's Agri-Biz Academics: Go Ahead and Eat It," *Real Paper* (Cambridge, Mass.), December 4, 1976.

12. J. Hess, "The Man Who Loves Additives," *Saturday Review,* September 2, 1978.

13. D. Reuben, *The Save-Your-Life Diet* (New York: Ballantine, 1975).

14. C. Fredericks, *High Fiber Way to Total Health* (New York: Pocket Books, 1976); see also C. Fredericks, *Breast Cancer: A Nutritional Approach* (New York: Grosset & Dunlap, 1977).

15. R. D. Smith, "Checking Out the Fiber Fad," *The Sciences,* March/April, 1976, pp. 25-29.

16. American Heart Association, *The Prudent Diet* (New York: McKay, 1973).

17. E. L. Wynder *et al.,* "Environmental Factors in Cancer of the Upper Alimentary Tract: A Swedish study with special reference to Plummer-Vinson's (Paterson-Kelly) Syndrome," *Cancer* 10 (1957), pp. 470-87.

18. M. Harris, "Eating Oil: From the kitchens of Amoco comes petroleum protein, the new 'natural' food," *Mother Jones,* August, 1977, pp. 19-33.

19. R. Harris and E. M. Brecher, "Is the Water Safe to Drink," *Consumer Reports* 39 (June-August, 1974), pp. 436-43, 538-42, 623-27 (subtitled, respectively, "The Problem," "How to Make It Safer," and "What You Can Do").

20. R. Hoover, and J. F. Fraumeni, Jr., "Drugs," in Fraumeni, ed., *Persons at High Risk of Cancer,* pp. 185-200.

21. S. Jablon, "Radiation," in Fraumeni, ed., *Persons at High Risk of Cancer,* pp. 151-65; see also P. Laws, *Medical and Dental X-Rays: A Consumer's Guide to Avoiding Unnecessary Radiation Exposure* (Washington, D.C.: Public/Citizens Health Research Group, 1974); I. Illich, *Medical Nemesis* (New York: Pantheon Books, 1976); L. R. Tancredi and J. A. Barondess, "The Problem of Defensive Medicine," *Science* 200 (1978), pp. 879-82.

22. J. C. Bailar III, "Screening for Early Breast Cancer: Pros and cons," *Cancer* 39 (1977), pp. 2783-95; D. S. Greenberg and J. C. Randal, "The Questionable Breast X-Ray Problem," *Washington Post, May 1,* 1977; O. H. Bears *et al.,* "Report of the Working Group to Review the NCI-ACS Breast Cancer Demonstration Projects," *Journal of the National Cancer Institute* 62 (1979), pp. 641-709.

23. *New York Times,* January 30, 1976.

24. *New York Times,* January 28, 1976.

25. B. E. Henderson, V. R. Gerkins, and M. C. Pike, "Sexual Factors in Pregnancy," in Fraumeni, ed., *Persons at High Risk of Cancer,* pp. 267-84.

26. S. J. Cutler and J. L. Young, Jr., "Demo-graphic Patterns of Cancer Incidence in the United States," in Fraumeni, ed., *Persons at High Risk of Cancer,* pp. 307-42.

27. T. J. Mason and F. W. McKay, "U.S. Cancer Mortality by County: 1950-69," DHEW Publication (NIH) 74-615 (Washington, D.C.: U.S. Government Printing Office, 1973).

28. R. P. Ouellette and J. A. King, *Chemical Week Pesticides Register* (New York: McGraw-Hill, 1977).

29. M. Blumer, W. Blumer, and W. Reich, "Polycyclic Aromatic Hydrocarbons in Soils of a Mountain Valley: Correlation with highway traffic and cancer incidence," *Environmental Science and Technology* 11 (1977), pp. 1082-84.

30. J. L. Young, S. S. Devesa, and S. J. Cutler, "Incidence of Cancer in United States Blacks," *Cancer Res.* 35 (1975), pp. 3523-36.

31. B. Doerschuk, "West Virginia Schools Ban Junk Foods," *Nutrition Action,* April, 1976, pp. 10-12.

32. B. S. Trenk, "Health Hazards in the Science Classroom," *American Lung Association Bulletin,* May, 1977, pp. 2-9.

33. D. P. Murphy and H. Abbey, *Cancer in Families* (Cambridge, Mass.: Harvard University Press, 1959).

34. Cooper and Company, Stanford, Conn., "Promptness of Payment in Workers Compensation," Report to the Interdepartmental Workers Compensation Task Force, Washington, D.C., August 31, 1976. A detailed critique of the inequitable state of the workman's compensation system; Thomas C. Brown (Office of the Assistant Secretary for Policy Evaluation and Research, Department of Labor), "Denial and Compromise of Workers' Compensation Claims for Occupational Diseases," Address to the American Public Health Association, Annual Meeting, Los Angeles, October 16, 1978; Howard Vincent (Office of the Assistant Secretary for Policy Evaluation and Research, Department of Labor), "Who Pays for the Compensation of Victims of Occupational Diseases?" Address to the Asbestos-Associated Diseases Meeting,

New York City, November 28, 1978. (These various reports are background material for a Department of Labor "Policy Study on Compensation for Occupational Diseases," due to be presented to Congress in September, 1979.)

PART II
The Politics of Cancer, 1998

CHAPTER TWELVE
1987: Report to Congress

1. Based on keynote presentations at the National Safety and Health Conference of the International Association of Machinists, Washington, DC., March 9, 1987, the Fifth National pesticide Forum of the National Coalition Against the Misuse of Pesticides, Washington, DC., March 21, 1987 and the Conference on Global Development and Environment Crisis, Friends of the earth (Sahabat Alam), Penang, Malaysia, April 8, 1987. Copyright, 1987, Samuel S. Epstein.

2. **Bibliography:** This bibliography is selective and designed to provide illustrative key references on cancer prevention and its politics.

B. Ames *et al.* "Ranking Possible Carcinogenic Hazards," *Science* 236:271-280, 1987.

N. A. Ashford *et al.* Center for Policy Alternatives of the MIT. "Benefits of Environmental Health and Safety Regulation," Report to the U.S. Senate Committee on Governmental Affairs, 96th Congress, March 25, 1980.

N. A. Ashford and C. C. Caldart. "The Right to Know: Toxic information transfer in the workplace," *Ann. Rev. Pub. Hlth.* 6:383-401, 1985.

O. Axelson. "The Health Effects of Phenoxy Acid Herbicides," *Recent Advances in Occupational Health,* J. M. Harrington, Ed. No. 2, Sec. 5:253-266, Churchill Livingston, New York, 1984. (See also O. Axelson. "Rebuttals of the Final Report on Cancer by the Royal Commission on the Use and Effects of Chemical Agents on Australian Personnel in Vietnam," Linkoping University, Sweden, January 21, 1986.)

J. C. Bailar and E. M. Smith. "Progress Against Cancer?" *New England J. Med.* 314:1226-1232, 1986. See also comments on this article by S. S. Epstein and J. Swartz, *New Eng. J. Med.* 316:753, 1987.

M. S. Baram. "Cost-Benefit Analysis: An inadequate basis for health, safety, and environmental regulatory decision making," *Ecology Law Quarterly* 8(3):473-531, 1980.

P. M. Boffey. "Cancer Survival Rate Progress Reported, But Skeptics Object," *New York Times,* November 27, 1984, pp. 21-22.

K. Bridbord *et al.* "Estimates of the Fraction of Cancer in the United States Related to Occupational Factors," *Califano Report,* National Cancer Institute, National Institute of Environmental Health Sciences, and National Institute for Occupational Safety and Health, Bethesda, Md. September 15, 1978.

Center for Science in the Public Interest. "Voodoo Science, Twisted Consumerism: The golden assurances of the American Council on Science and Health," CSPI, Washington, D.C., 1982.

Center for Science in the Public Interest *et al.* "Petition to the Environmental Protection Agency to Develop Testing Methods to Assess Neurotoxic and Neurobehavioral Effects of Pesticide Active and Inert Ingredients," Washington, D.C., February 1987.

M. B. Clinard and P. C. Yeager. *Corporate Crime,* Free Press, New York and London, 1980.

F. Cohen. "Workplace Hazards: Do we have a right to know?" *Hofstra Environmental Law Digest* 2:10-11, Spring 1985.

R. Crawford. "Cancer and Corporations," *Society* 18:20-27, 1981.

D. L. Davis *et al.* "Cancer Prevention: Assessing cancer, exposure, and recent trends in mortality for U.S. males, 1968-1978," *Teratogenesis, Carcinogenesis and Mutagenesis* 2:105-135, 1982.

L. N. Davis. *The Corporate Alchemists: Profit*

Takers and Problem Makers in Chemical Industry, W. Morrow & Co., New York, 1984.

S. Diamond. "Problem of Toxic (Air) Emissions," *New York Times,* May 20, 1985, p. 19.

R. Doll and R. Peto. "The Causes of Cancer: Quantitative estimates of available risks of cancer in the United States today," *J. Natl. Cancer Inst.* 66:1191-1308, 1981.

J. Elder *et al.* "Toxic Air Pollution in the Great Lakes Basin: A call for action," Great Lakes Basin Working Group, March 1987.

Environmental Protection Agency. "Health Assessment Document for Polychlorinated Dienzo-p-Dioxins," EPA, September 1985.

S. S. Epstein. "Polluted Data," *The Sciences* 18:16-21, 1978.

S. S. Epstein. *The Politics of Cancer,* Sierra Club Books, San Francisco, 1978. Revised and Expanded Edition, Anchor Press/Doubleday, New York, 1979.

S. S. Epstein and J. Swartz. "Fallacies of Lifestyle Cancer Theories," *Nature* 289:127-130, 1982.

S. S. Epstein. "Cost-Benefit Analysis: Inspired by rational economics or a protectionist philosophy," *The Amicus Journal* pp. 41-47, Spring 1982.

S. S. Epstein, L. L. Brown, and C. Pope. *Hazardous Waste in America,* Sierra Club Books, San Francisco, 1981.

S. S. Epstein and J. Swartz. "Rebuttal to Ames on Cancer and Diet," *Science* 224:660-668, 1984. (This letter was co-signed by some 20 nationally recognized authorities in the fields of public health, and environmental and occupational carcinogenesis.)

S. S. Epstein and J. Swartz. "Testimony in Support of a Zero Tolerance for EDB," Public Hearings on Final Regulations of EDB, Massachusetts, March 19, 1984.

N. Freudenberg. "Citizen Action for Environmental Health: Report on a survey of community organizations," *Am. J. Public Health* 74:444-448, 1984.

Friends of the Earth, Natural Resources Defense Council. "Indictment: The case against the Reagan environmental record," The Wilderness Society, Sierra Club, National Audubon Society, Environmental Defense Fund, Environmental Policy Center, Environmental Action, Defenders of Wildlife, and Solar Lobby, Washington, D.C., March 1982.

General Accounting Office. "Report on Progress in Cancer Treatment: Patterns of survival, 1950-1982," April 15, 1987.

J. Gould. *Quality of Life in American Neighborhoods: Levels of Affluence, Toxic Waste, and Cancer Mortality in Residential Zip Code Areas,* Council of Economic Priorities, Westview Press, Boulder & London, 1986.

M. Green, Ed. *The Big Business Reader,* Pilgrim Press, New York, 1983.

W. F. Hunt *et al.* "Office of Air and Radiation, Environmental Protection Agency, Estimated Cancer Incidence Rates for Selected Toxic Air Pollutants Using Ambient Air Pollution Data," EPA, April 23, 1985.

J. H. Ives, Ed. *The Export of Hazard: Transnational Corporations and Environmental Control Issues,* Routledge and Kegan Paul, Boston & London, 1985.

M. Karstadt and R. Bobal. "Availability of Epidemiological Data on Humans Exposed to Animal Carcinogens. II, Chemical Uses and Production Volume. Teratogenesis, Carcinogenesis and Mutagenesis 2:151-167, 1982.

J. King. *Troubled Water,* Rodale Press, Emmaus, Pennsylvania, 1985.

H. Kjuus *et al.* "A Case Report Study of Lung Cancer, Occupational Exposure, and Smoking: III Etiologic Fraction of Occupational Exposures," *Scan. J. Work Environ. Hlth.* 12:210-215, 1986.

M. S. Legator, B. L. Harper, and M. J. Scott. *The Health Detectives Handbook,* John Hopkins Press, Baltimore & London, 1985.

C. G. Moertel. "On Lymphokines, Cytokines, and Breakthroughs," *J. Am. Med. Assoc.* 256:3141, 1986.

Cong. G. V. Molinari. "Ill Winds: A look at relationships between respiratory cancer deaths and petrochemical industry locations affecting Staten Island, N.Y. and 155 counties across the nation," U.S. Congress H.R., Washington, D.C., June 15, 1985.

J. J. Morgester. "Results of Measurement and Characterization of Atmospheric Emissions from Petroleum Refineries," In, proceedings of Symposium on Atmospheric Emission from Petroleum Refineries, November 1979, Environmental Protection Agency, March 1980.

R. Nader, M. Green, and J. Seligman. "Constitutionalizing the Corporation: The case for the federal chartering of giant corporations," The Corporate Accountability Research Group, Washington, D.C., 1978.

National Cancer Institute, Division of Cancer Prevention and Control. "Cancer Control Objectives for the Nation, 1985-2000," Greenwald and Sondik, Eds., *NCI Monographs,* No. 2:1-101, 1986.

National Research Council. *Toxicity Testing: Strategies to Determine Needs and Priorities,* National Academy Press, Washington, D.C., 1984.

New York State Department of Environmental Conservation. "Final Environmental Impact Statement on Amendments to 6 NYCRR Part 326 Relating to the Restriction of the Pesticides Aldrin, Chlordane, Chlorpyrifos, Dieldrin, and Heptachlor," Albany, New York, December, 1986.

Occupational Safety and Health Administration (OSHA). "Identification, Classification, and Regulation of Potential Occupational Carcinogens," *Fed. Reg.* 45(15):5001-5296, Jan. 22, 1980.

OSHA/Environmental Watch. "Industry Corrupts WHO Agency (IARC)," Vol I, No. 5, September 1982.

Office of Science and Technology Policy. "Chemical Carcinogens: A review of the science and its associated principles," *Federal Register* 50:10372-10442, 1985.

V. I. Pye, R. Patrick, and J. Quarles. *Groundwater Contamination in the United States,* University of Pennsylvania Press, Philadelphia, 1983.

Registrar General's Decennial Supplement for England and Wales. "Occupational Mortality, 1970-72," *OPCS* Series DS No. 1, 1978.

U. Saffiotti and J. K. Wagoner, Eds. "Occupational Carcinogenesis," *Ann. New York Acad. Sci.* 271:1-516, 1976.

H. Seidman *et al.* "Probabilities of Eventually Developing or Dying of Cancer: United States, 1985," *CA-A Cancer Journal for Clinicians* 35:35-56, 1985.

UAW. "The Case of the Workplace Killers: A manual for cancer detectives on the job," International Union UAW, November 1980.

U.S. House of Representatives, Democratic Study Group, Special Report. "Reagan's Toxic Pollution Record: A public health hazard," Washington, D.C., July 31, 1984.

U.S. National Center for Health Statistics. "Age-adjusted Death Rates for 72 Selected Cancers by Color and Sex, 1979-1983."

W. C. Willett *et al.* "Dietary Fat and The Risk of Breast Cancer," *New Eng. J. Med.* 316:22-28, 1987.

CHAPTER THIRTEEN
1992-1993: Challenge to the Cancer Establishment

Evaluation of the National Cancer Program and Proposed Reforms

1. J. Conyers, Congressman. Are we really winning the war against cancer? *Congressional Rec.*, April 2, 1992, pp. E947-E949.

2. S.S. Epstein, *et al.* "Losing the 'War Against Cancer': A need for public policy reforms," *Int. J. Health Serv.* 22:455-469, 1992.

3. D. Obey, Congressman. Hearings before a House Subcommittee of the Committee on Appropriations: Part 3. National Institutes of Health, National Cancer Institute, March 16, 1992.

4. "The Cancer War and Its Critics," (editorial), *Washington Post*, February 16, 1992.

5. J. Lawrence. "Cancer Cause and Prevention," (letter from the president of the American Cancer Society), *Washington Post,* February 12, 1992.

6. S.S. Epstein. "The Cancer Establishment," (Taking Exception/Op-Ed), *Washington Post*, March 10, 1992.

7. D. Greenberg. "In Tumultuous Meeting at NIH, Severest Critic Gets a Hearing on the

War on Cancer," *Sci. Government Rep.* 22(9):1-4, 1992.

8. D. Greenberg. "Washington Perspective: The two-by-four factor in critics of cancer politics," *Lancet* 339:1343-1344, 1992.

9. National Cancer Institute. *Cancer Control Objectives for the Nation*: 1985-2000, Monograph No. 2, pp. 1-105, Bethesda, Maryland, 1986.

10. U.S. Department of Health and Human Services/NCL *Health Status Objectives, 16.1. Cancer*, pp. 416-440, Bethesda, Maryland, 1991.

11. National Cancer Institute. *Cancer Statistics Review 1973-1988*, NIH Publication No. 91-2789, Bethesda, Maryland, 1991.

12. J. Bailar. "Cancer Control," *Science* 236:1049-1050, 1987.

13. J.C. Bailar. "Progress Against Cancer?" *N. Engl. J. Med.* 314:1226-1232, 1986.

14. General Accounting Office. *Cancer Patient Survival: What Progress Has Been Made?* GAO/PEMD-87-13. Report to the Committee on Government Operations, Washington, D.C., March 1987.

15. V. DeVita, NCI response to article by Dr. Samuel S. Epstein published in the September 9, 1987 issue of the Congressional Record. Letter to Cong. H.A. Waxman, 1987.

16. R. Doll. "Health and the Environment in the 1990s," *Am. J. Public Health* 82:933-941, 1992.

17. P.L. Landrigan. "Commentary: Environmental disease: A preventable catastrophe," *Am. J. Public Health* 82:941-943, 1992.

18. D.L. Davis, *et al.* "International Trends in Cancer Mortality in France, West Germany, Italy, Japan, England and Wales, and the United States," *Lancet* 336:474-481, 1990.

19. A.D. Lopez. "Competing Causes of Death: A review of recent trends in mortality in industrialized countries with special reference to cancer," *Ann. N.Y. Acad. Sci.* 609:58-76, 1990.

20. D.G. Hoel, *et al.* "Trends in Cancer Mortality in 15 Industrialized Countries, 1969-1986," *J. Natl. Cancer Inst.* 84:313-320, 1992.

21. S.S. Epstein. "Losing the War Against Cancer: Who's to blame and what to do about it?" A position paper on the politics of cancer, *Congressional Rec.,* September 9, 1987, pp. E3449-E3454.

22. R. Rifkind in *Natural Obsessions: The search for the Oncogene*, by N. Angier, p. 15. Houghton Mifflin, Boston, 1988.

23. U. Abel. *Chemotherapy of Advanced Epithelial Cancer: A Critical Survey*. Hippokrates Verlag, Stuttgart, 1990.

24. B.A. Chabner and M.A. Friedman. "Progress Against Rare and Not-so-rare Cancers," *N. Engl. J. Med.* 326:563-565, 1992.

25. P.J. Landrigan. Testimony before NCAB, Publication participation Hearings, Philadelphia, April 19, 1988.

26. S. Broder. Testimony before the House Appropriations Subcommittee on Labor Health and Human Services and Related Agencies, March 16, 1992.

27. D. Baltimore in *Natural Obsessions: The search for oncogene*, by N. Angier, pp. 12 and 15, Houghton Mifflin, Boston, 1988.

28. M. Barbacid in *Natural Obsessions: The search for oncogene*, by N. Angier, pp. 12, Houghton Mifflin, Boston, 1988.

29. Varmus in *Natural Obsessions: The search for oncogene*, by N. Angier, pp. 13, Houghton Mifflin, Boston, 1988.

30. D. Obey, Congressman. *House Congressional Rec.*, November 6, 1991, pp. H9457- H9458.

31. H. Waxman, Congressman. To amend the Public Health Service Act to revise and extend the programs of the National Institutes of Health and for other purposes, and report to accompany H.R. 2507, pp. 95-96, June 28, 1991.

32. "President's budget vs. NCI's bypass: A tale of missed opportunities," *Cancer Lett.* 18(8):4-7, 1992.

33. R. Doll, and R. Peto. "The Causes of Cancer: Quantitative estimates of avoidable risks of cancer in the United States today," *J. Natl. Cancer Inst.* 66:1191-1308, 1981.

34. I. Hermann. "Oxford Medicine Gains a College," *New Scientist* p. 653, March 9, 1978.

35. J.E. Enstrom. "Rising Lung Cancer

Mortality Among Nonsmokers," *J. Natl. Cancer Inst.* 62:755-760, 1970.

36. D.L. Davis, K. Bridbord, and M. Schneiderman. "Cancer Prevention: Assessing causes, exposures, and recent trends in mortality for U.S. males 1968-1978," *Teratogenesis Carcinog. Mutagen.* 2:105-135, 1982.

37. U.S. Department of Health and Human Services, USDHS Report No. PHS 83-1232, Washington, D.C., December 1982.

38. M.A. Schneiderman, D.L. Davis, and D.K. Wagener, "Smokers: Black and white," *Science* 249:228-229, 1990.

39. International Agency for Research on Cancer. *Tobacco Smoking* 38:1-421, 1986.

40. J. Wagoner, P. Infante, and D. Bayliss. "Beryllium: An etiologic agent in the induction of lung cancer, non-neoplastic respiratory diseases, and heart disease among industrially exposed workers," *Environ. Res.* 21:15-34, 1980.

41. S.S. Epstein, and J. Swartz. "Cancer and Diet: A rebuttal to Ames, B.," *Science* 224:660-667, 1984.

42. F.F. Perera. Presentation to the President's Cancer Panel, April 5, 1990, pp. 82-96.

43. P. Stocks. "On the Relations Between Atmospheric Pollution in Urban and Rural Localities and Mortality from Cancer, Bronchitis, and Pneumonia: With particular reference to 3,4-benzopyrene, beryllium, molybdenum, vanadium, and arsenic," *Br. J. Cancer* 14:397-418, 1960.

44. National Panel of Consultants on the Conquest of Cancer, *National Program for the Conquest of Cancer,* report to the Senate Committee on Labor and Public Welfare, November 27, 1970.

45. National Academy of Sciences, *Biologic Effects of Atmospheric Pollutants: Particulate Polycyclic Organic Matter,* National Academy Press, Washington, D.C., 1972.

46. International Agency for Research on Cancer, *Air Pollution and Cancer in Man,* Scientific Publication No. 16, 1977.

47. National Academy of Sciences, *Potential Risk of Lung Cancer from Diesel Engine Emissions,* National Academy Press, Washington, D.C., 1981.

48. National Institute for Occupational Safety and Health, *Carcinogenic Effects of Exposure to Diesel Exhaust,* NIOSH Current Intelligence Bulletin 50, Bethesda, Maryland, August 1988.

49. M.S. Gottlieb, *et al.* "Lung Cancer in Louisiana: Death certificate analysis," *J. Natl. Cancer Inst.* 63:1131-1137, 1979.

50. Environmental Protection Agency, *Toxic Release Inventory,* Washington, D.C., 1990.

51. M.A. Schneiderman, D.L. Davis, and D.K. Wagener. "Lung Cancer That is Not Attributable to Smoking," *JAMA* 261:2635-2636, 1989.

52. I.J. Selikoff and E.C. Hammond. "Asbestos-associated Disease in U.S. Shipyards," *CA Cancer J. Clin.* 28:87-99, 1978.

53. P.F. Infante and G.K. Pohl. "Living in a Chemical World: Actions and reactions to industrial carcinogens," *Teratogenesis Carcinog. Mutagen.* 8:225-249, 1988.

54. C. Maltoni and I.J. Selikoff. "Living in a Chemical World: Occupational and environmental significance of industrial carcinogens," *Ann. N.Y. Acad. Sci.* 534:1-1045, 1988.

55. National Institute for Occupational Safety and Health, *NIOSH National Occupational Hazard Survey* (NOHS), Bethesda, Maryland, 1982.

56. R. Peto and M.A. Schneiderman. Afterward in *Quantification of Occupational Cancer,* Banbury Report 9, edited by R. Peto and M.A. Schneiderman, pp. 695-697, Cold Spring Harbor, New York, 1981.

57. P.J. Landrigan and S. Markowitz. "Current Magnitude of Occupational Disease in the U.S.: Estimates from New York State," *Ann. N.Y. Acad. Sci.* 572:27-45, 1989.

58. W.J. Nicholson, G. Perkel, and I.J. Selikoff. "Occupational Exposure to Asbestos: Populations at risk and projected mortality, 1980-2030," *Am. J. Ind. Med.* 3:259-311, 1982.

59. L.M. O'Leary, *et al.* "Parental Occupational Exposures and Risk of Childhood Cancer: A review," *Am. J. Ind. Med.* 20:17-35, 1991.

60. R. Peto. "Saturated Fat Avoidance," *Science* 235:1562, 1987.

61. G. Kolata. "Dietary Fat: Breast cancer link

question," *Science* 235:436, 1987.

62. W.C. Willett, *et al.* "Dietary Fat and the Risk of Breast Cancer," *N. Engl. J. Med.* 316:22-28, 1987.

63. B.E. Henderson, R.K. Ross, and M.C. Pike. "Toward the Primary Prevention of Cancer," *Science* 254:1131-1138, 1991.

64. E. Marshall. "Breast Cancer: Stalemate in the war on cancer," *Science* 254:1719-1720, 1991.

65. General Accounting Office, *Breast Cancer, 1971-1991: Prevention, Treatment, and Research*, GAO/PEMD-92-12, report to the Committee on Government Operations. Washington, D.C., December 1991.

66. S.S. Epstein. "Mammography Radiates Doubt," [OP/ED] *Los Angeles Times*, January 28, 1992.

67. A.I.T. Walker, *et al.* "The Toxicology and Pharmacodynamics of Dieldrin: Two-year oral exposure of cats and dogs," *Toxicol. Appl. Pharmacol.* 15:345-373, 1969.

68. National Cancer Institute, *Bioassay of Chlordane for Possible Carcinogenicity*, Carcinogenesis Technical Report Series No. 8, Bethesda, Maryland, 1977.

69. D. Rall. "Laboratory Animal Toxicity and Carcinogenesis Testing: Underlying concepts, advantages, and constraints," *Ann. N.Y. Acad. Sci.* 534:78-83, 1988.

70. J.D. Scribner and N.K. Mottet. "DDT Acceleration of Mammary Gland Tumors Induced in the Male Sprague-Dawley Rat by 2-acetamidophenanthrene," *Carcinogenesis* 2:1235-1239, 1981.

71. M. Wasserman *et al.* "Organochlorine Compounds in Neoplastic and Adjacent Apparently Normal Breast Tissue," *Bull. Environ. Contamin. Toxicol.* 15:478-484, 1976.

72. F. Falk *et al.* "Pesticides and PCB Residues in Human Breast Lipids and Their Relation to Breast Cancer," *Arch. Environ. Health* 47:143-146, 1992.

73. J. B. Westin and E. Richter. "The Israeli Breast Cancer Anomaly," *Ann. N.Y. Acad. Sci.* 609:269-279, 1990.

74. R. Hertz. "The Estrogen-Cancer Hypothesis with Special Emphasis on DES," in *Origins of Human Cancer, Book C. Human Risk Assessment*, edited by H. H. Hiatt *et al.*, pp. 1665-1682, Cold Spring Harbor Laboratory, Cold Spring Harbor, New York, 1977.

75. A. Segaloff and W. S. Maxfield. "The Synergism between Radiation and Estrogen in the Production of Mammary Cancer in the Rat," *Cancer Res.* 31:166-168, 1971.

76. C. J. Shellabarger, J. P. Stone, and S. Holtzman. "Rat Strain Differences in Mammary Tumor Induction with Estrogen and Neutron Radiation," *J. Natl. Cancer Inst.* 61:1505-1508, 1978.

77. T. Dao. "The Role of Ovarian Hormones in Initiating the Induction of Mammary Cancer in Rats by Polynuclear Hydrocarbons," *Cancer Res.* 22:973-984, 1962.

78. National Academy of Sciences. "The Effects on Populations of Exposure to Low Levels of Ionizing Radiation," report to the Advisory Committee on the Biological Effects of Ionizing Radiation (BEIR), National Research Council Washington, D.C., November 1972.

79. N. Berlin. Quoted in D. S. Greenberg. "X-ray Mammography: A background to decision," *Med. Public Aff.* 295:739-740, 1976 (1973).

80. J. C. Bailar. "Mammography: A contrary view," *Ann. Intern. Med.* 84:77-84, 1976.

81. F. L. Greene *et al.* "Mammography, Sonomammography, and Diaphanography (light scanning)," *Am. Surg.* 51:58-60, 1985.

82. R. LaFreniere, F. S. Ashkar, and A. S. Ketcham. "Infrared Light Scanning of the Breast," *Am. Surg.* 52:123-128, 1986.

83. J. C. Bailar. "Mammography Before Age 50 Years," *JAMA* 259:1548-1549, 1988.

84. "Breast Cancer Screening in Women Under 50," (editorial) *Lancet* 337:1575-1576, 1991.

85. K. Smigel. "Breast Cancer Prevention Trial Takes Off," *J. Natl. Cancer Inst.* 84:669-670, 1992.

86. S. S. Epstein and S. Rennie. "A Travesty at Women's Expense," (Op-Ed) *Los Angeles Times*, June 22, 1992.

87. A. Fugh-Berman and S. S. Epstein. "Tamoxifen: Disease prevention or disease substitution," (Viewpoint) *Lancet* 340:1143-1145, 1992.

88. X. Han and J. G. Liehr. "Induction of covalent DNA adults in rodents by tamoxifen," *Cancer Res.* 52:1360-1363, 1992.

89. ICI Pharmaceutical Group. "Data presented at the FDA Oncology Drugs Advisory Committee Meeting," Bethesda, Md., June 29, 1990.

90. S. G. Nayfield *et al.* "Potential role of tamoxifen in prevention of breast cancer," *J. Natl. Cancer Inst.* 83:1450-1459, 1991.

91. "Tamoxifen trial controversy," *Lancet* 339:735, 1992.

92. L. E. Rutqvist *et al.* "Contralateral primary tumors in breast cancer patients in randomized trial of adjuvant tamoxifen therapy," *J. Natl. Cancer Inst.* 83:1299-1306, 1991.

93. S. B. Gusberg. "Tamoxifen for Breast Cancer: Associated endometrial cancer," *Cancer* 65:1463-1464, 1990.

94. S. S. Epstein. *The Politics of Cancer,* Anchor Press/Doubleday, New York, 1979.

95. National Research Council. *Toxicity Testing: Strategies to Determine Needs and Priorities,* National Academy Press, Washington, D.C., 1984.

96. L. Tomatis. "The contribution of the IARC Monographs program to the identification of cancer risk factors," *Ann. N.Y. Acad. Sci.* 534:31-38, 1988.

97. National Academy of Sciences. *Regulating Pesticides in Food: The Delaney Paradox,* National Academy Press, Washington, D.C., 1987.

98. Natural Resources Defense Council. "Intolerable Risks: Pesticides in Our Children's Food," February 27, 1989.

99. S. S. Epstein and J. Feldman. "Opening the door for carcinogens: Assaults on nation's food safety laws multiply," (Op-Ed) *Los Angeles Times*, February 27, 1989.

100. S. S. Epstein and J. Feldman. " 'Negligible Risk' is still much too great," (Op-Ed) *Los Angeles Times*, November 16, 1989.

101. National Coalition Against the Misuse of Pesticides. "Testimony of NCAMP before the Senate Subcommittee on Toxic Substances, Environmental Oversight, Research and Development," Committee on Environment and Public Works, May 9, 1991.

102. A. Blair *et al.* "Cancer among farmers: A review," *Scand. J. Environ. Health* 11:397-407, 1985.

103. L. M. Brown *et al.* "Pesticide exposures and other agricultural risk factors for leukemia among men in Iowa and Minnesota," *Cancer Res.* 50:6585-6591, 1990.

104. H. M. Hayes *et al.* "Case control study of canine malignant lymphoma: Positive association with dog owners use of 2, 4-dichlorophenoxyaetic acid herbicides," *J. Natl. Cancer Inst.* 83:1226-1231, 1991.

105. L. Fisher. "Environmental Protection Agency. Communication to Senate Committee on Labor and Human Resources," March 30, 1992.

106. S. S. Epstein. "Carcinogenicity of heptachlor and chlordane," *Sci. Total Environ.* 6:103-154, 1976.

107. S. S. Epstein. "Testimony on H.R. 262," House Subcommittee on Health and the Environment, Committee on Energy and Commerce, June 24, 1987.

108. National Research Council. "Chlordane in Military Housing. Committee on Toxicology," National Academy of Sciences, Washington, D.C., 1979.

109. National Academy of Sciences. "An Assessment of the Health Risks of Seven Pesticides Used for Termite Control," National Academy Press, Washington, D.C., August 1982.

110. U.S. Air Force. "Review of NCI proposed protocol for epidemiological feasibility study," B. R. Chappell, memo to AFMSC/SGPA, February 6, 1984.

111. S. K. "Letter to the USAF Colonel Smead," September 19, 1983.

112. R. W. Moss. *The Cancer Industry: Unraveling the Politics,* Paragon House, New York, 1989.

113. S. S. Epstein. "Losing the war against cancer: Who's to blame and what to do about it?" *Int. J. Health Serv.* 20:53-71, 1990.

114. S. S. Epstein. "Letter to J. Hallum," NIH Office of Scientific Integrity, May 7, 1992.

115. S. S. Epstein, D. Steinman, and S. LeVert, *The Breast Cancer Prevention Program,* MacMillan, USA, 1997, pp. 303-305.

116. M. Eliot. "NCI Director, Samuel Broder, M.D., resigned: 'Broder to join exodus from NCI.'" *Science* 267:24, 1995.

117. F. S. Mahaney, Jr. "Dr. Frank Rauscher resigned in 1976: 'Dr. Frank J. Rauscher, Jr.: An appreciation,'" *Journal of the National Cancer Institute*, 85(3):174-175, 1993.

118. J. Bleifuss. "NCI allowed Bristol-Myers to sell Taxol at inflated price."

CHAPTER FOURTEEN
The Academic Apologists Rebutted

Doll and Peto:
The "Lifestyle" Theorists

Sir Richard Doll: Discredited Pillar of the British Cancer Establishment

1. M.R. Law, J.K. Morris, and N.J. Wald. "Environmental tobacco smoke exposure and ischaemic heart disease: an evaluation of the evidence," *BMJ* 315:73, 1997.
   A.K. Hackshaw, M.R. Law, and N.J. Wald. "The accumulated evidence on lung cancer and environmental tobacco smoke," *BMJ* 315:980-8, 1997.
   R.M. Davis. "Passive smoking; history repeats itself," (Editorial) *BMJ* 315:961-2, 1997.

2. "Farming Today," BBC Radio Four. October 17, 1997.

3. *Guardian,* October 18, 1997.

4. Hill A. Bradford and R. Doll. "1950 Smoking and carcinoma of the lung," *BMJ* ii:1271, 1950.

5. Medical Research Council, Annual Report 1948.

6. R. Doll. "Mortality from lung cancer in asbestos workers," *Br. J. Indust. Med.* 12:81-6, 1955.

7. *The Times,* June 8, 1967.

8. *Ibid.*

9. *Daily Express,* April 25, 1968.

10. *Guardian,* October 31 1977.

11. S.S. Epstein and J.B. Swartz. "Fallacies of lifestyle cancer theories," *The Ecologist* Vol. 11, No. 5.

12. *Daily Telegraph,* August 28, 1985.

13. "Cancer: a killer 'moving into retreat.,'" *Guardian,* September 27, 1990.

14. *The Times,* January 10, 1980.

15. Hill A. Bradford and R. Doll. "The mortality of doctors in relation to their smoking habits. A preliminary report," *BMJ* i:15, 1954.
    Hill A. Bradford and R. Doll. "Lung cancer and other causes of death in relation to smoking. A second report on the mortality of British doctors.," *BMJ* ii:1071, 1956 .

16. *Daily Mail,* June 29, 195 1.

17. See Epstein in this issue.

18. J.L. Roberts and P.A. Graveling (eds.). "The big kill: smoking epidemic in England and Wales. Published for the Health Education Council and the British Medical Association. 15-volume series. Manchester: North Western Regional Health Authority, 1985.

19. Typescript of interview by Andrew Baron with Sir Richard Doll, April 7, 1993.

20. "Smoking or health," Royal College of Physicians of London. London: RCP. 1983.

21. Typescript of interview by Andrew Baron with Simon Wolff, May 13 1993.

22. R. Doll and R. Peto. "The causes of cancer: quantitative estimates of avoidable risks of cancer in the United States today," *Guardian* November 27, 198 1. Oxford: OUP, 1981.

23. Imperial Cancer Research Fund. Scientific Report, 1981.

24. T. Margerison and M. Wallace and D. Hallenstein. *The Superpoison,* Macmillan, London, 1981.

25. O. Axelson and L. Hardell. "Herbicide exposure, mortality and tumour incidence: An epidemiological investigation on Swedish railroad workers," *Work Env. Hlth.* 11:21-28, 1974.
    O. Axelson. "Herbicide exposure and turnout mortality: an updated epidemiological investigation on Swedish railroad workers," *Scand. J. Work Environ. Health* 6:73-79, 1980.
    L. Hardell and A. Sanderskin. "Case control study: Soft tissue sarcomas and

exposure to phenoxy acids and chlorophenols," *Br. J. Cancer* 39:711-717, 1979.
L. Hardell. "Epidemiological studies on soft tissue sarcoma and malignant lymphoma and their relation to phenoxy acid or chlorophenol exposure." Umea University, Medical Dissertations. New Series No. 65. Umea 1981.

26. O. Axelson and L. Hardell. "Australian epidemonology (sic): On Royal misruling in the realm of epidemiology," Presented at the 5th International Symposium, Epidemiology in Occupational Health, 1986.

27. Letter from Richard Doll to Hon. Mr. Justice Phillip Evatt. December 4, 1985.

28. Cited in: J.M. Gould and B.A. Goldman. *Deadly Deceit; Low Level Radiation High Level Cover Up,* Four Walls Eight Windows, New York, 199 1.

29. Cited *ibid.*.

30. G. Jones. "From Cancer to Cholesterol," *New Scientist* November 21, 1992.

31. D. Forman, P. J. Cook-Mozaffari, S.C. Darby, and Doll R. *et al.* "Cancer near nuclear installations," *Nature* 329:499-505, December 8-14, 1987.

32. M.J. Gardner, A.J. Hall, S. Downes and J.D. Terrell. Follow up study of children born to mothers resident in Seascale, West Cumbria," (birth cohort) *BMJ* 295:822-7, 1987.
M.J. Gardner, A.J. Hall, S. Downes, and J.D. Terrell. "Follow up study of children born elsewhere but attending schools in Seascale, West Cumbria," (schools cohort) *BMJ* 295:819-22, 1987.

33. D. Black. "Investigation of the possible increased incidence of cancer in West Cumbria," *London: HMSO* 1984.

34. P. Cook-Mozaffari, S.C. Darby and R. Doll. "Cancer near sites of nuclear installations," *Lancet* 2:1145-7, November 11, 1989.

35. *Sunday Telegraph,* November 26, 1989 and later in *The Times,* March 13, 1992.

36. *The Times,* July 1, 1989.

37. *The Times,* March 13, 1992.

38. S.C. Darby, G.M. Kendall and R. Doll, *et al.* "A summary of mortality and incidence of cancer in men from the United Kingdom who participated in the United Kingdom's atmospheric nuclear tests and experimental programs," *BMJ* 296:332-8, January 30, 1988.
In *The Times* of January 29, 1988, Doll is reported as saying that the statistical difference was curious, Darby on the other hand was reported in the *Guardian* of the same date saying that they were puzzling.

39. S.C. Darby and R. Doll. "Radiation and exposure rate," *Nature* 344:824, 1990.

40. R. Doll. "Mortality from lung cancer in asbestos workers," *Br. J. Indust. Med.* 12:81-6, 1955.
Reprinted in the *Br. J. Indust. Med.* 50(6):485-90, June 1993.

41. R. Doll, R. Peto. "Effects on Health of Exposure to Asbestos," *HMSO* 1985.

42. Letter from SPAID to the *Sunday Times,* April 26, 1985.

43. W.J. Rea. *Chemical Sensitivity. Vol. 3.* Boca Raton. Fl: Lewis, 1995.

44. Paper on the health of anesthetists, *BMJ* April 1979.

45. *Daily Telegraph,* May 4, 1979.

46. "Health damaging effects of fluoride," *JAMA* October 1944.

47. Royal College of Physicians of London. "Fluoride, teeth and health," London: Pitman Medical, 1976.

48. *Daily Telegraph,* January 7, 1976.

49. D. Wilson. *The Lead Scandal,* Heinemann Educational Books, London, 1983.

50. *Lead and Health,* DHSS, 1980. The Lawther Working Party.

51. R. Lansdown, W. Yule, M. Urbanowicz, and I. Millar. "Relationship between blood-lead intelligence, attainment and behavior in school children: Overview of a pilot study," Paper presented at CLEAR Int. Symp. London, 1982. M. Rutter and R. Russell Jones (ed). *In Lead versus health.*

52. Smith D. Bryce and R. Stephens, "Lead or Health: A review of the Lawther Report," The Conservation Society, 1983.

53. Cited in: D. Wilson, *op. cit.* 48.

54. *Daily Telegraph,* February 7, 1983.

55. Medical Research Council Annual Report 1947.
In 1947 the Council established a Toxicology Research Unit. Under the direction of

Dr. J. M. Barnes, to assist in the solution of toxicological problems referred to them by other bodies, and to pursue research on fundamental questions which may emerge during routine work. The Unit has had accommodation at the Chemical Defence Experimental Station, Porton, by arrangement with the Ministry of supply.

56. 1956 MRC Annual Report.
57. M. Walker, *Dirty Medicine,* Slingshot Publications, BM 8314, London WCIN 3XX, 1993.
58. M. Walker. *Ibid.*
59. C. Busby. *Wings of Death: Nuclear Pollution and Human Health,* Green Audit., Wales, 1995.
60. *Waste Paper,* published by CORE (Cumbrians Opposed to a Radioactive Environment), August 1989.
61. Sir Richard Doll. Interview with Andrew Baron. April 7, 1993.
62. Letter from Richard Doll to Miss Jean McSorley of CORE. May 10, 1989.
63. S.S. Epstein. "Corporate crime: Why we cannot trust industry-derived safety studies," *Int. J. of Health Services* Vol 20, 443-458, November 3, 1990.
    S. Beder *Global Spin: The corporate assault on environmentalism,* Green Books, Dartington, 1997.
64. D. Fagin, M. Lavelle, and the Centre for Public Integrity. *Toxic Deception; How the chemical industry manipulates science, bends the law, and endangers your health,* Carol Publishing Group, New Jersey, 1996.
65. *Ibid.*
66. *Ibid.*
67. *Ibid.*
68. *Ibid.*
69. *Daily Telegraph,* February 7, 1983.
70. *Daily Mail,* June 3, 1992.
71. *Ibid.*
72. *Ibid.*
73. *Ibid.*
74. Glyn Jones. "From Cancer to Cholesterol," *New Scientist* November 21, 1992.

Destroying the Epidemiology of Cancer: The Need for a More Balanced Overview

1. J. Cornfield. *Science* 198:693, 1977.
2. N. Mantel and M. A. Schneidermann. *Cancer Research* 35:1379, 1975.
3. K. S. Crump *et al. Cancer Research* 36:2973, 1976.
4. W. A. Guess *et al. Cancer Research* 37:3475, 1977.
5. Office of Technology Assessment of the U.S. Congress. "Cancer Testing Technology and Saccharin," 1977.
6. E. C. Hammond *et al.,* in *Origins of Human Cancer,* Cold Spring Harbor, New York, 1977.
7. E. L. Wynder *et al.,* in U.S. government DHEW publication *NIH* 76:1221, 1976.
8. O. Auerbach *et al. N. Engl. J. Med.* 300:381, 1979.
9. K. K. Caroll. *Cancer Research* 35:3374, 1975.
10. B. K. Armstrong and R. Doll. *Int. J. Cancer* 15:617, 1975.
11. D. G. Jose. *Nutrition and Cancer* 1(3):58, 1979. (Many other papers in all the 1979 issues of this journal are of great general interest e.g. 1(3):35, 67 and 27. See also part 2 of November 1975 *Cancer Research* devoted wholly to mutation and cancer).
12. R. Doll. *Proc. Roy. Soc. Lond. (B)* 205:47, 1979.
13. W. J. Blot and J. F. Fraumeni. *Natl. Cancer Inst.* 61:1017, 1978.
14. F. J. C. Roe and M. J. Tucker. *Excerpta Medica* (Int. Congress Series) 311:171, 1974.
15. I. J. Selikoff, in *Origins of Human Cancer,* Cold Spring Harbor, New York, 1977.
16. A. Norman. *Nature* 280:623, 1979.
17. R. Doll. *Nature* 265:589, 1977.
18. R. Doll. *Nutrition and Cancer* 1(3):35, 1979.
19. IARC working group. *Cancer Research* 40:1, 1980.
20. D. L. Davis and B. H. Magee. *Science* 206:1356, 1979.

Fallacies of Lifestyle Theories

1. R. Peto. *Nature* 284:297-301, 1980.
2. S. S. Epstein. *Politics of Cancer,* Sierra Club Books, San Francisco, 1978. Revised and expanded in Anchor/Doubleday, New York, 1979; quotations refer to the 1979 edition.

3. "AIHC Recommended Alternatives to OSHA's Generic Carcinogen Proposal, Occupational Safety & Health Administration (OSHA) Docket No. H-090," American Industrial Health Council, February 24, 1978.

4. "Vital Statistics — Special Reports, U.S. DHEW," 43:163, 1956; "Vital Statistics of the U.S.," 2, 1970.

5. E. S. Pollack and J. W. Horm. *J. Natl. Cancer Inst.* 64:1091, 1980.

6. "Trends in Mortality, 1951-1975," U.K. Office of Population Censuses and Surveys, Series DH1, No. 3, 1978.

7. "Third National Cancer Survey, 1969-1971," NCI, Bethesda; "Cancer Surveillance Epidemiology and End Results (SEER) Program."

8. M. Schneiderman. "Occupational Safety & Health Administration OSHA Docket 090," April 4, 1978.

9. M. S. Zdeb. *Am. J. Epidemiol.* 106:6, 1977.

10. D. L. Davis and B. H. Magee. *Science* 206:1356, 1979; see also U.S. International Trade Commission Reports.

11. "Chemical Dangers in the Workplace," 34th Report of the Committee on Government Operations, House of Representatives, September 27, 1976.

12. J. E. Enstrom. *J. Natl. Cancer Inst.* 62:755, 1979.

13. T. D. Sterling. *Int. J. Hlth. Services* 8:437, 1978.

14. M. L. Newhouse and J. C. Wagner. *Br. J. Ind. Med.* 26:302, 1969.

15. E. L. Wynder and S. D. Stellman. *Cancer Res.* 37:4608, 1977.

16. J. K. Wagoner, P. F. Infante, and D. L. Bayliss. *Envir. Res.* 21:15, 1980.

17. T. F. Mancuso and T. D. Sterling. *J. Natn. Med. Ass.* 67:107, 1975.

18. V. E. Archer, J. D. Gillam, and J. K. Wagoner. *Ann. N.Y. Acad. Sci.* 271:280, 1976.

19. O. Axelson and L. Sundell. *Scand. J. Work Envir. Hlth.* 4:46, 1978.

20. A. Yamada. *Acta path. Jap.* 13:131, 1963.

21. S. S. Pinto. *Archs. Envir. Hlth.* 33:325, 1978.

22. W. Weiss and K. R. Boucot. *J. Am. Med. Ass.* 234:1139, 1975.

23. J. T. Mason and F. W. McKay. *Atlas of Cancer Mortality for U.S. Counties*: *1950-1969,* Dept H.E.W., Washington, D.C., 1975; *Atlas of Cancer Mortality for U.S. Counties Among U.S. Non-Whites,* Dept H.E.W., Washington, D.C., 1976.

24. W. J. Blot *et al. Science* 198:51, 1977.

25. B. Carnow. *Envir. Hlth. Perspect.* 22:17, 1978.

26. B. K. Armstrong and R. Doll. *Int. J. Cancer* 15:617, 1975.

27. P. Cole, R. R. Monson, H. Haning, and G. H. Friedell. *New Engl. J. Med.* 284:129, 1971.

28. E. L. Wynder, K. Mabuchi, N. Maruch, and J. G. Fortner. *Cancer* 31:641, 1973.

29. P. Cole and R. Goldman. *Persons at High Risk of Cancer: An Approach to Cancer Etiology and Control,* J. F. Fraumeni, Jr., Ed., 167-184, Academic, New York, 1975.

30. W. J. Blot and J. Fraumeni. *J. Natl. Cancer Inst.* 61:1017, 1978.

31. R. Hoover and J. Fraumeni. *Envir. Res.* 9:196, 1975.

32. J. Milham, in *Occupational Carcinogenesis,* J. Wagoner and U. Saffiotti, Eds., 243-249, New York Academy of Sciences, 1976.

33. J.W. Berg, in *Persons at High Risk of Cancer: An Approach to Cancer Etiology and Control,* J.F. Fraumeni, Jr., Ed., 201-224, Academic, New York, 1975.

34. R.L. Phillips. *Cancer Res.* 35:3513, 1975.

35. A.B. Miller *et al. Am. J. Epidemiol.* 107:499, 1978.

36. R. Doll. *Cancer Res.* 45:2475, 1980.

37. K.K. Carroll. *Cancer Res.* 35:3374, 1975.

38. J. Higginson and C.S. Muir. *J. Natl. Cancer Inst.* 63:1291, 1979.

39. E.L. Wynder and G.B. Gori. *Am. J. Publ. Hlth.* 66:359, 1977.

40. T.H. Maugh. *Science* 205:1363, 1979.

41. R. Doll. *Nature* 265:589, 1977.

42. I.J. Selikoff and C.E. Hammond. *J. Am. Med. Ass.* 242:458, 1979.

43. K. Bridbord *et al.* "Estimates of the Fraction of Cancer in the United States Related to Occupational Factors," National Cancer Institute, National Institute of Environmental Health Sciences, and

National Institute for Occupational Safety and Health, September 15, 1978.

44. J.M. Stellman and S.D. Stellman. "What Proportion of Cancer is Attributable to Occupation; Statistical and Social Consideration," American Society for Preventive Oncology, Chicago, March 6-7, 1980.

45. Report of an IARC Working Group. *Cancer Res.* 40:1, 1980.

46. "Toxic Chemicals and Public Protection," Report to the President of the Toxic Substances Strategy Committee of the Council on Environmental Quality, May, 1980.

47. R.A. Stallones and T. Downs. "A Critical Review of K. Bridbord *et al.,*" prepared for the American Industrial Health Council, 1979.

Peto's Misrepresentations

1. S.S. Epstein. *The Politics of Cancer,* Sierra Club Books, San Francisco, 1978, revised and expanded in Anchor/Doubleday, New York, 1979, to which quotations refer.

2. R. Peto. *Nature* 234:297-300, 1980.

3. "Cancer Testing Technology and Saccharin," U.S. Congress, Washington, D.C., June 7, 1977.

4. S.M. Wolfe and A. Johnson. "Public Citizens Health Research Group Testimony Before Subcommittee on Health. House Commerce Committee Hearing on Saccharin," March 21, 1977.

5. M.D. Robert, *Envir. Hlth. Perspect.* 25:193, 1978.

6. Report to the Surgeon General. USPHS. "Evolutions of Environmental Carcinogens," Ad Hoc Committee on the Evaluation of Low Levels of Environmental Chemical Carcinogens, April 22, 1970.

7. K. Bridford, *et al.* "Estimates of the Factors of Cancer in the United States Related to Occupational Factors," NCI, National Institute of Environmental Health Sciences, and National Institute of Occupational Safety and Health, September 15, 1970.

8. *Lancet* 11:1380, 1973.

9. S. J. Rinkus. "M.S. Cancer Res." *Legator* 39:3289, 1979.

10. "International Program for the Evolution of Short Term Tests for Carcinogenicity," National Toxicology Program, Dept. of Health and Human Services, April 1980.

Ames: The "Natural Carcinogen" Proponent

Rebuttal

1. R. Doll, R. Peto, and J. Nail. *Cancer Inst.* 66:1191, 1981.

2. *Trends in Mortality 1971-1975,* Series DHI, U.K. Office of Population, Censuses and Surveys. London, 1978, No. 3. E. Pollack, J. Horm, and J. Nail. *Cancer Inst.* 64:1091, 1980.

3. S.S. Epstein. *The Politics of Cancer,* Anchor, New York, 1979. S.S. Epstein and J.B. Swartz, *Nature* (London) 289:127, 1981.

4. D.L. Davis, K. Bridbord, and M. Schneiderman. *Teratogen. Carcinogen. Mutagen.* 2:105, 1982.

5. E. Sondik (National Institutes of Health). Personal communication to Congressman J. Conyers.

6. J. Enstrom and J. Nail. *Cancer Inst.* 62:755, 1979.

7. C. Harris. *Cancer Chemother. Rep.* 4:39, 1973. Part 3. E. Wynder and S. Stellman. *Cancer Res.* 37:4608, 1977. J. Wagoner, P. Infante, and D. Bayliss. *Environ. Res.* 21:15, 1980.

8. *Smoking and Health: A Report of the Surgeon General,* Government Printing Office, Washington, D.C., 1979. J.L. Harris. *Natl. Cancer Inst.* 71:73, 1983.

9. *Advance Data from Vital and Health Statistics of National Center for Health Statistics,* No. 52, Department of Health, Education, and Welfare, Washington, D.C., September 19, 1979. *Health United States,* No. [PHS] 83-1232. Department of Health and Human Services, Washington, D.C., December 1982.

10. J. Mason and F. McKay. *Atlas of Cancer Mortality for U.S. Counties: 1950-1969,* Department of Health, Education, and Welfare, Washington, D.C., 1975. *Atlas of Cancer Mortality for U.S. Counties among U.S. Non-Whites,* Department of Health, Education, and Welfare, Washington, D.C., 1976. W.I. Blott, L.A. Brinton, J.F. Fraumeni, Jr., and B.J. Stone. *Science*

198:51, 1977. B. Carnow. *Environ. Health Perspect.* 22:17, 1978. L.S. Robertson. *Ibid.* 36:197, 1980.

11. K. Bridbord *et al.* "Estimates of the fraction of cancer in the United States related to occupational factors," National Cancer Institute, National Institute of Environmental Health Sciences, and National Institute for Occupational Safety and Health. Washington,. D.C., 1978.

12. G.W. Kneale, T. E. Mancuso, A.M. Stewart, *Br. J. Ind. Med.* 38:156, 1981.

13. J. Stellman and S. Stellman. Paper presented at the annual meeting of the American Society for Preventive Oncology. Chicago, Ill., 6 and 7, March 1980.

14. U. Mohr, D. Schmähl, L. Tomatis, and IARC (Int. Agency Res. Cancer) *Sci. Publ.* 16, 1977.

15. C. Johnson. Paper presented at the AAAS Annual Meeting. Washington, D.C., 1982.

16. S.W. Lakagos, B.J. Wessen, and M. Zelen. Unpublished manuscript.

17. Office of the General Counsel, Environmental Protection Agency. Respondent's brief proposed findings, and conclusion on suspension in the Shell Chemical Company *et al.* consolidated Aldrin/Dieldrin Hearing. FIFRA Dockets 145 *et al.*, Washington, D.C., September 16, 1974. S. Epstein. *Sci. Total Environ.* 4:1, 1975.

18. Office of the General Counsel, Environmental Protection Agency. Respondent's final brier, in the Velsicol Chemical Corporation *et al.*, Chlordane and Heptachlor. FIFRA Docket 384, Washington, D.C., December 8, 1975. S. Epstein. *Sci. Total Environ.* 6:103, 1976.

19. *An Assessment* of *the Health Risks* of *Seven Pesticides Used for Termite Control,* National Academy Press, Washington, D.C., 1982.

20. *Ambient Water Quality Criteria for Chlordane,* Environmental Protection Agency, Washington, D.C., 1980.

21. "Ethylene dibromide: Position document 2/3," Environmental Protection Agency, Washington, D.C., 1980.

22. B. Ames. *Wall Street J.* p. 30, February 14, 1994.

23. *Diet, Nutrition, and Cancer*, National Academy Press, Washington, D.C., pp. 8-50, 1982.

24. B. Armstrong and R. Doll. *Int. J. Cancer* 15:617, 1975.

25. J. Berg, in *Persons at High Risk* of *Cancer: An Approach to Cancer Etiology and Control.* J. Fraumeni, Jr., Ed. Academic Press, New York, 1975. pp. 201-224. K. Carroll. *Cancer Res.* 35:3374, 1975.

26. R. Phillips. *Cancer Res.* 35:3513, 1975. A. B. Miller *et al. Am. J. Epidemiol.* 107:499, 1978.

27. J.M. Concon, D.S. Newburg, and T.W. Swerczek. *Nutr. Cancer* 1:22, 1979.

28. I. Weinstein, M. Wigler, and C. Pietropaolo, in *Origin of Human Cancer.* H. Hiatt, J. Watson, J. Winston, Eds. Cold Spring Harbor Laboratory, Cold Spring Harbor, N.Y., 1977, pp. 751-772. L. Weinstein, *et al.,* in *Carcinogens: Identification and Mechanisms of Action,* A. Griffin and C. Shaw, Eds., Raven, New York, 1979, pp. 399-418. H. Rubin, J. Nail, "Cancer Inst." 64:995, 1980. J. Cairns. *Nature,* London, 289:353, 1981. I.L . Sager. *Chromosome Mutation and Neoplasia,* Liss., New York, 1983. p. 333.

29. S.J. Rinkus and M.S. Legator. *Cancer Res.* 39:3289, 1979.

30. H. Glastt, M. Protie-Sabijie, and F. Oesch. *Science* 220:961, 1983.

31. R. Peto, R. Doll, J.D. Buckley, and M.B. Sporn. *Nature*, London, 290:201, 1981.

32. W.C. Willen *et al. N. Engl. J. Med.* 310:430, 1994.

33. A. Blum and B.N. Ames. *Science* 195:17, 1977. B.N. Ames. *Ibid.* 204:597, 1979.

Carcinogenic Risk Estimation

1. J. Swartz *et al. Teratog. Carcinog. Mutagen.* 2:179, 1982. L. Davies, P. Lee, and P. Rothwell. *Brit. J. Cancer* 30:146, 1974. E. Hulse, K. Mole, and D. Papworth. *Int. J. Rad. Biol.* 114:437, 1978.

2. W. Hooper *et al. Science* 203:602, 1979.

3. J. Marshall and P. Groer. *Rad. Res.* 71:149, 1977.

4. A. Tannenbaum. *Proc. Am. Ass. Cancer Res.* 1:56, 1953.

5. R. Innis *et al. J. Natl. Cancer Inst.* 42:1101, 1969.

6. I. Berenblum. *Carcinogenesis as a Biological Problem,* American Elsevier, New York, 1974, chapter 5.

7. N. Kuratsune *et al. Gann* 62:395, 1971. C. Griciute *et al.*, in *Modulators of Experimental Carcinogenesis*, V. Turosov and K. Montesano, Eds., Publication 51, International Agency for Research on Cancer, Lyon, France, 1982. N. Schwartz and A. Buchanan, in *Models, Mechanisms and Etiology of Tumor Promotion*. M. Borzonyi *et al.*, Eds., International Agency for Research on Cancer, Lyon, France, 1984.

8. W. Willett *et al. N. Engl. J. Med.* 316:1170, 1987. A. Schankin *et al. Ibid.* p. 1170. S. Graham. *Ibid.* p. 1211.

9. H.L. Newmark. *Can J. Physiol. Pharmacol.* 65:461, 1987.

10. D. Davis and B. McGee. *Science* 206:1356, 1979.

11. S.S. Epstein. *The Sciences* 18:16, 1978. S.S. Epstein. *The Politics of Cancer,* Anchor/Doubleday, New York, 1979. National Research Council, *Toxicity Testing: Strategies to Determine Needs and Priorities,* National Academy Press, Washington, D.C., 1984.

12. D. Davis. *Teratog. Carcinog. Mutagen.* 2:105, 1982.

13. R.A. Lowengart *et al. J. Natl. Cancer Inst.* 79:39, 1987.

14. W.J. Nicholson, G. Perkel, and I. J. Selikoff, *Am. J. Ind. Med.* 3:259, 1982.

15. National Research Council, *Regulating Pesticides in Food*: *The Delaney Paradox,* National Academy Press, Washington, D.C., 1987.

16. C.R. Cothern, W.A. Coniglio, and W.L. Marcus. *Environ. Sci. Technol.* 20:111, 1986.

17. S. Lagakos *et al. J. Am. Stat. Ass.* 81:580, 1986.

18. National Research Council, *Drinking Water and Health,* National Academy Press, Washington, D.C., 1980, vol. 3. K.P. Cantor. *Environ. Health Perspect.* 46:187, 1982. K.P. Cantor. *J. Natl. Cancer Inst.* 79:1269, 1987.

19. National Research Council, *Drinking Water and Health,* National Academy Press, Washington, D.C., 1977.

20. P. Stocks and J. Swartz. *Nature* London 289:127, 1981.

21. Committee on Biologic Effects of Atmospheric Pollutants, National Academy of Sciences, *Particulate Polycyclic Organic Matter,* National Academy Press, Washington, D.C., 1972.

22. N. Karch and M. Schneiderman. "Explaining the Urban Factor in Lung Cancer Mortality," report to the Natural Resources Defense Council, New York, 1981.

23. W. Hunt, R. Faoro, T. Curran, and J. Muntz. *Estimated Cancer Incidence Rates for Selected Toxic Air Pollutants Using Ambient Air Pollution Data,* Office of Air Quality Planning and Standards, Environmental Protection Agency, Washington, D.C., 1985. These estimates of excess cancer rates are supported by epidemiological studies on cancer clustering in highly urbanized and highly industrialized communities. For example: R. Hoover and J.F. Fraumeni. *Environ. Res.* 9:196, 1975. W.J. Blot *et al. Science* 198:51, 1977. M.S. Gottlieb *et al. J. Natl. Cancer Inst.* 63:113, 1979. J. Kaldor *et al. Environ. Health Perspect.* 54:319, 1984.

24. R. Doll and R. Peto. *J. Natl. Cancer Inst.* 66:1191, 1981.

25. H. Seidman *et al. Ca A Cancer J. Clin.* 35:36, 1985.

26. S.S. Devesa *et al. J. Natl. Cancer Inst.* 79:701, 1987. *National Cancer Statistical Review,* 1950-1985, National Cancer Institute, Bethesda, MD, 1988. J.L. Davis and J. Schwartz. *Lancet* i:633, 1988.

27. S.S. Epstein *et al. Science* 224:660, 1984. U. Pastorini *et al. Int. J. Cancer* 33:23, 1984. S.S. Epstein and J. Swartz. *N. Engl. J. Med.* 316:753, 1987. J.B. Scheonberg *et al. J. Natl. Cancer Inst.* 79:13, 1987.

28. E. Pollack and J. Horm. *J. Natl. Cancer Inst.* 64:1091, 1980. *Trends in Mortality 1951-1975,* U.K. Office of Population Censuses and Survey, London, England, 1978. *Third National Cancer Survey 1969-1971,* National Cancer Institute, Bethesda, MD, 1975. Cancer Surveillance Epidemiology and End Results (SEER) Program, *Age*

Adjusted Death Rates for 72 Selected Causes by Color and Sex, 1979-1983, National Center for Health Statistics, Hyattsville, MD, 1984.

29. P.H. Abelson. *Science* 237:473, 1987. Further illustrations of the relationship between Ames and the editors of *Science* is provided in B. Ames *ibid.* 226:1396, 1984.

30. In 1977, Blum and Ames warned that the synthetic carcinogenic pesticide ethylene dibromide (EDB) is a "potent carcinogen" whose structural similarity to the flame retardant tris is one of the reasons why the synthetic chemical tris "should not be used." They also pointed to "enormous possible [carcinogenic] risks" from using an untested chemical in [a fire retardant in] pajamas, predicted that a "steep increase in the human cancer rate from these suspect . . . chemicals may soon occur" "as the 20 to 30 year lag time of chemical carcinogenesis in humans is almost over." [A. Blum and B. Ames, *Science* 193:17, 1977]. Blum and B. Ames also emphasized the need for high-dose testing in an effort to compensate for the "inherent statistical limitation in animal cancer tests" and expressed concerns about "the effects of the large-scale human exposure to the halogenated carcinogens [including] vinyl chloride, Strobane-toxaphene, aldrin-dieldrin, DDT, trichloro-ethylene . . . [and] heptachlor-chlordane." In 1979, Ames and his colleagues demonstrated that carcinogenesis dose-response curves usually rise less steeply than linear curves and criticized the view that many carcinogens have activity only at very high doses [W. Hooper, R. Harris, and B. Ames, *ibid.* 203:602, 1979]. Ames also stressed the need to establish "priorities for trying to minimize human exposure to these [synthetic] chemicals. [B. Ames, *ibid.* 204:587, 1979]. Four years later, however, he reversed himself and concluded that cancer rates were not rising, that synthetic carcinogens posed only trivial risks, and that the real culprits were natural carcinogens and faulty lifestyles, tobacco, and high-fat diets, citing Doll and Peto (24), who "guesstimated" that diet, particularly fat, is incriminated in 35% of all cancer deaths, as the basis for this statement [B. Ames, *ibid.* 221:1256, 1983]. Now, the carcinogenic hazards of high-fat diets are virtually dismissed in a few parenthetic words "[a possible risk factor in colon cancer . . .]," presumably reflecting Peto's recent reversal on the role of fat [R. Peto, *ibid.* 235:1562, 1987], and in its place alcohol now emerges, alongside tobacco, as [one of the two] "largest identified cause of neoplastic death in the United States."

31. S.S. Epstein. *Congr. Rec.,* 133:E3449, 1987.

32. We thank M. Jacobson, T. Mancuso, M. Schneiderman, and A. Upton for their helpful comments.
September 4, 1987, revised November 30, 1987, accepted March 11, 1988.

CHAPTER FIFTEEN
The British Parallel

The Science and Politics of Cancer in Britain

Place of publication is London unless stated otherwise.

1. S. Sontag. *Illness as Metaphor,* New York, Vintage Books, 1979.

2. See Peto's discussion, Chapter 14.

3. For a summary of his position, see Chapter 14.

4. ASTMS *The Prevention of Occupational Cancer,* 1980. GMWU *A Preliminary Cancer Prevention Campaign* 1980. NGA *Occupational Cancer in the Printing Industry* 1980. For details of where to obtain these, see appendix 6.

5. The most significant recent example of these are reproduced in Chapter 14.

6. ASTMS *The Prevention of Occupational Cancer* 1980. CIA *Cancer in Modern Mortality* 1980. J. Keir Howard. *The Prevention of Occupational Cancer: A Review* CIA, 1980.

7. Report of an IARC Working Group, "Cancer Research," vol. 40, no. 1, 1980.

8. J. Robinson. "Cervical cancer: a feminist critique," *Times Health Supplement,* November 27, 1981. J. Robinson. "Cancer

of the cervix: occupational risks of husbands and wives and possible preventive strategies," Proceedings of the Ninth Study Group of the Royal College of Obstetricians and Gynecologists, RCOG, 1982.

9. D. Forman, "The Politics of Cancer," *Marxism Today,* August 1981.

The Cancer Problem in Britain

1. T. McKeown, R.G. Record and R.D. Turner, "An interpretation of the decline in mortality in England and Wales during the twentieth century" *Population Studies* 29:391-422, 1975.

2. *Mortality Statistics: Cause 1980,* series DH2 no. 7, OPCS, 1982.

3. For the American data, see S. Epstein. *THE POLITICS OF CANCER Revisited,* Chapter 1. For British data, see *Cancer Statistics: Survival 1971-73 Registrations,* series MBI, no. 3, OPCS, 1980. See also D. Gould. "Cancer — a conspiracy of silence," *New Scientist* December 2, 1976, pp. 522-23.

4. *Trends in Mortality 1951-75,* series DH1 no. 3, OPCS, 1978.

5. *Ibid.*

6. *Ibid.*

7. *Ibid.*

8. For a discussion of this evidence, see Epstein, *Politics of Cancer,* pp. 14-16.

9. The best source of evidence for these differences is *Occupational Mortality: The Registrar General's Decennial Supplement for England and Wales, 1970-72* series DS, no. 1, OPCS, 1978. This is the most recent in a series of reports provided at ten-year intervals.

10. The Standardized Mortality Ratio (SMR) is the percentage ratio of the number of deaths observed in a specific group studied to the number that would be expected from the age-specific death rates for the total population of England and Wales.

11. This refers to the five "social class" categories often used in the presentation of British official statistics. The categories are based on occupation, social class I being the "highest" (professional and manage-

rial) and social class V the "lowest" (unskilled).

12. There is a useful discussion of this in *Occupational Mortality.* See also, A.J. Fox and A. M. Adelstein. "Occupational mortality: work or way of life?," *Journal of Epidemiology and Community Health* 32:73-78, 1978.

13. For a more detailed discussion of this point and its relationship to health issues, see L. Doyal with I. Pennell. *The Political Economy of Health,* Pluto Press, 1979, Chapter 2.

14. For a detailed account of this evidence, see Chapter 13.

15. ASTMS, *The Prevention of Occupational Cancer* 1980, p. 55.

16. These figures are published annually by the Department of Health and Social Security.

17. See letters to the *New Statesman* by R. Peto, September 10, 1982, and D. Gee, October 1, 1982.

18. ASTMS, *Prevention of Occupational Cancer* p. 17.

19. J. Robinson. "Cervical cancer: a feminist critique," *Times Health Supplement,* November 27, 1981.

20. For a discussion of these trends see B. Jacobson. *The Ladykillers: Why Smoking is a Feminist Issue* Pluto Press, 1981 and S. Stellman and J. Stellman. "Women's occupations, smoking, cancer and other diseases," *Cancer Journal for Clinicians* 3:29-41, 1981.

21. Doyal with Pennell. *Political Economy of Health,* pp. 83-92. *"Food and Profit,"* Politics of Health Group, Pamphlet no. 1, 1979. C. Wardle. *Changing Food Habits in the U.K. — An Assessment of the Social, Technological, Economic and Political Factors which Influence Dietary Patterns,* Friends of the Earth, 1977.

22. For a summary of these developments see: *Our Bodies Ourselves: A Health Book by and for Women,* Boston Women's Health Book Collective, British edition by A. Phillips and J. Rakusen, Harmondsworth, Penguin, 1978.

23. P. Stocks. "On the relations between

atmospheric pollution in urban and rural localities," *British Journal of Cancer* 14:397-418, 1960.

24. S.S. Epstein, L.O. Brown, and C. Pope, *Hazardous Waste in America,* Sierra Club Books, San Francisco, 1982.

25. O.L. Lloyd. "Respiratory cancer clustering associated with localized industrial air pollution," *Lancet* 1:318-20, 1978.

26. M.J. Gardner, P.D. Winter, and E.D. Acheson. "Variations in cancer mortality among local authority areas in England and Wales: relations with environmental factors and search for causes," *British Medical Journal,* 284:794-87, 1982.

How Carcinogens Are Controlled

1. *Chemical and Engineering News,* June 9, 1980.

2. J. Walsh. "EPA and toxic substances law: dealing with uncertainty," *Science* 202:598-602, 1978. "Scheme for the Notification of Toxic Properties of Substances," *Health and Safety Executive* 1977.

3. See Appendix XV for a list of those organizations which do exist in fields related to the fight against cancer.

4. Office of Science and Technology, Council on Environmental Quality Ad Hoc Committee. "Report on Environmental Health Research," Washington, D.C., June 1972, quoted in S. Epstein, *The Politics of Cancer,* New York, Anchor Press, 1979, p. 321.

5. NIEHS, *Report to the Senate Appropriation Committee on Federal Support for Environmental Health Research,* 1977, quoted in Epstein, *Politics of Cancer,* p. 321.

6. *Fortune,* February 13, 1978, p. 116.

7. Medical Research Council, *Annual Report,* 1978-79.

8. Royal Society, *Long-term Hazards to Man from Man-made Chemicals in the Environment,* 1978, quoted in "Royal Society slams routine toxicity tests," *Nature* 274:413, 1978.

9. The first major legislation of this sort was the Factory Act of 1833. See K. Marx, *Capital,* vol. 1, pp. 389-416, Harmondsworth, Penguin, 1976.

10. The most recent moves in this campaign are discussed in G. Wilson *et al., Cancer at work: Dyes,* Cancer Prevention Society, 1980. See also new HSE Guidance Note, *Health and Safety Precautions for Benzidine-based Dyes,* EH/34 August 1982.

11. "Toxic Substances: A Precautionary Policy," *Health and Safety Executive* note EH18, 1977.

12. H.J. Dunster. "Carcinogens in the Workplace," Technical Report, *Health and Safety Executive* 1982.

13. Quoted in the *Guardian,* March 1, 1982.

14. *Chemistry and Industry,* p. 504, April 15, 1978.

15. "Chemical company suppresses dioxin report," *Nature* 284:2, 1980. ASTMS, *Report on Coalite Chemicals,* May 1980.

16. *Official Journal of the European Community* no. L 259/10, October 15, 1979.

17. *European Chemical News,* p. 19, January 8, 1979, and p. 17, July 2, 1979.

18. ASTMS, *The Prevention of Occupational Cancer* p. 52, 1980.

19. "Toxic Substances: A Precautionary Policy," *Health and Safety Executive.*

20. Health and Safety Commission, *Notification of New Substances,* consultative document, HMSO, 1981.

21. The Nightwear (Safety) Order, 1978, and the Balloon-making Compounds (Safety) Order 1979, respectively.

22. These relate to the emission of hydrochloric acid gas from alkali works, to sulphuric acid works and to muriatic acid works.

23. This list is taken from Department of Environment Central Unit on Environmental Pollution, *Pollution Control in Great Britain — How it Works,* Pollution Paper no. 9, pp. 86-89, HMSO, 1978.

24. See Health and Safety Executive, *Lists of Registrable Works and Noxious or Offensive Gases Specified in the Acts and Orders,* 1977.

25. Royal Commission on Environmental Pollution, Fifth Report, *Air Pollution Control: An Integrated Approach,* HMSO, p. 24, 1976.

26. Quoted in M. Frankel, *The Alkali Inspectorate,* Social Audit, p. 8, 1974.

27. H.M. Chief Inspector of Factories, *Annual*

Report 1972, HMSO, 1973.

28. Frankel. *The Alkai Inspectorate,* p. 27.

29. Royal Commission on Environmental Pollution, Fifth Report, *Air Pollution Control,* pp. 33-4.

Call for Accountability

1. T. Reynolds. "Proposed Reign on Charity Spending for Research Unleashed U.K. Debate," *J. Natl. Cancer Inst.,* 90:1030-1031, 1998.

2. J. G. McVie. Letter to *The London Times,* May 26, 1998.

CHAPTER SIXTEEN

American Cancer Society: The World's Richest "Nonprofit" Institution

1. J.T. Bennett. "Health research charities: Doing little in research but emphasizing politics." *Union Leader,* p. 10, Manchester, New Hampshire, September 20, 1990.

2. J.T. Bennett and T.J. DiLorenzo. *Unhealthy Charities: Hazardous to Your Health and Wealth,* Basic Books, New York, 1994.

3. H. Hall and G. Williams. "Professor vs. Cancer Society," *The Chronicle of Philanthropy,* p. 26, January 28, 1992.

4. T.J. DiLorenzo. "One charity's uneconomic war on cancer," *Wall Street Journal,* March 15, 1992, A10.

5. J.D. Salant. "Cancer society gives to governors," *A. P. Release,* March 30, 1998.

6. S.S. Epstein, D. Steinman, and S. LeVert. *The Breast Cancer Prevention Program,* p. 306-314, MacMillan, USA, 1997.

7. S.S. Epstein, "Losing the war against cancer: Who's to blame and what to do about it," *International Journal of Health Services* 20:53-71, 1990.

8. S.S. Epstein. "Evaluation of the National Cancer Program and proposed reforms," *International Journal of Health Services* 23(1):15-44, 1993.

9. *The Breast Cancer Prevention Program,* p. 145-15 1.

10. American Cancer Society. "Upcoming television special on pesticides in food." Memorandum from S. Dickinson, Vice-President, Public Relations and Health, to Clark W. Heath, Jr., M.D., Vice-President, Epidemiology and Statistics, March 22, 1993.

11. American Cancer Society, *Cancer Facts & Figures — 1998,* p. 1-32, 1998.

12. *The Breast Cancer Prevention Program,* Chapter 6.

13. *The Breast Cancer Prevention Program,* p. 311-314.

14. S. Kaplan. "PR Giant Makes Hay from Client 'Cross-pollination': Porter/Novelli plays all sides," *PR Watch,* First quarter, 11994:4.

15. S. Kaplan. "Porter-Novelli plays all sides," *Legal Times* 16(27):1, November 2 3, 1993.

16. R.W. Moss. *Questioning Chemotherapy,* Equinox Press, Brooklyn, New York, 1995.

17. U.S. Congress Office of Technology Assessment (OTA). "Unconventional cancer treatments," U.S. Government Printing Office, Washington, D.C., 1990.

18. R.W. Moss. *Cancer Therapy: The Independent Consumer's Guide To Non-toxic Treatment and Prevention,* Equinox Press, Brooklyn, New York, 1992. See also the Moss Reports on alternative and complementary cancer treatments. (Tel: 718-636-4433; Fax: 718-636-0186.)

19. L. Castellucci. "Practitioners Seek Common Ground in Unconventional Forum," *J. Natl. Cancer Inst.,* 90:1036-1037, 1998.

CHAPTER SEVENTEEN

1994-1998: Track Record of the NCI

1. S. S. Epstein. "Evaluation of the National Cancer Program and Proposed Reforms," Testimony submitted for the Record Hearing, House Subcommittee on Labor, Health and Human Services, and Education, Committee on Appropriations, March 20, 1998.

2. NCI. *SEER (Surveillance Epidemiology and End Results) Cancer Statistics Review* 1973-1994.

3. NCI press release. "20th Anniversary: the National Cancer Program," December 16,

1996.

4. J. C. Bailar. "Diagnostic Drift in the Reporting of Cancer Incidence," *J. Natl. Cancer Inst.* 901:563-864, 1998.

5. D. L. Davis and D. Hoel. "Trends in Cancer Mortality in Industrial Countries," *Ann. N.Y. Acad. Sci.* 60:1990.

6. D. L. Davis and D. Hoel. "Figuring out Cancer," *Int. J. Hlth. Services,* 22:447-453, 1992.

7. J. C. Bailar and H. L. Gornik. "Cancer Undefeated," *New Eng. J. Mod.* 336:1569-1574, 1997.

8. J. R. Smeltz. "Common Ground Found: Overall Cancer Mortality Rates are Failing," *J. Natl. Cancer Inst.* 12:1001, 1997.

9. U. Abel. *Chemotherapy of Advanced Epithelial Cancer: A Critical Survey*, Hippokrates Verlag, Stuttgart, Germany, 1990.

10. NCI press release. "New Report on Declining Cancer Incidence and Death Rates. Report Shows Progress in Controlling Cancer," March 12, 1998.

11. P. A. Wingo *et al.* "Cancer incidence and mortality 1973-1995: A Report Card for the U.S.," *Cancer* SZ:1197-2207, 1998.

12. S. G. Stolberg. "New Cancer Cases Decreasing in U.S., As Deaths Do, Too," *The New York Times* March 13, 1998, pp. A1 & A12.

13. E. Marshall. "Cancer Warriors Claim A Victory," *Science* 279:1842-1843, 1998.

14. NCI. "SEER, 1973-1990."

15. NCI. Unpublished Report, "SEER, 1973-1995."

16. L. A. Ries, co-editor. "SEER reports personal communication," March 23, 1998.

17. S. S. Epstein. " 'Cancer Report Card' Gets A Failing Grade," PR Newswire, April 1, 1998.

18. R. Doll and R. Peto. "The Causes of Cancer: Quantitative Estimates of Avoidable Risks of Cancer in the United States Today," *J. Natl. Cancer Inst.* 66:1191-1308, 1981.

19. S. S. Epstein. "Evaluation of the National Cancer Program and Proposed Reforms," *Am. J. Ind. Mod.* 24:109-133, 1993.

20. S. S. Epstein, D. Steinman, and S. LeVert.

The Breast Cancer Prevention Program, second edition, Macmillan Books, New York, 1997. See also revised edition, 1998.

21. D. Steinman and S. S. Epstein. *The Safe Shopper's Bible: A consumer's guide to nontoxic household products, cosmetics and food*, Macmillan Books, New York, 1995. See also revised edition, 1998.

22. T. J. Moore. *Prescription for Disaster*, Simon & Schuster, 1998.

23. IMS America. "Leading 50 Drugs in 1995 By Total R_XRetail Market," 1995.

24. T. Moore. Personal Communication, April 16, 1998.

25. B. Seaman. *The Doctor's Case Against the Pill*, updated edition, Hunter House, Alameda, CA, 1995.

26. T. S. Davis and A. Monro. "Marketed Human Pharmaceuticals Reported to be Tumorigenic in Rodents," *J. Am. College Toxicol.* 14:90-107, 1995.

27. National Toxicology Program. "Carcinogenesis Studies on Methylphenidate Hydrochloride (Ritalin)," National Institute of Environmental Health Sciences, July 1995.

28. Environmental Health Letter. "National Toxicology Program Weighs Changes in Determining Cancer Risks," September 4, 1992, p. 173.

29. L. Ford. "Letter to J. W. Stratton, California Environmental Protection Agency," NCI, June 23, 1995.

30. NCI. "Research Dollars By Various Cancers," Budget Statement, February 1997.

31. NCI. "Cancer Control Objectives for the Nation, 1985-2000," *Monograph* No 2: 1-105, 1986.

32. National Cancer Advisory Board. "Cancer at a Cross Roads: A report to Congress for the nation," NCI, September 1994.

33. "Cancer Review Panel Recommends A Major Overhaul Of Prevention Research," *J. Natl. Cancer Inst.* 82:1187-1198, 1997.

34. "NCI Selects First Director's Consumer Liaison Group," *J. Natl. Cancer Inst.* 89:1755, 1997.

35. NCI director Klausner's response to a request for budgetary information on cancer prevention from the House Committee on Government Reform and Oversight,

July 3, 1998.

36. J. Nelson. "Anti-estrogens Come of Age: As pioneer looks back," *J. Natl. Cancer Inst.* 90:646-647, 1998.

37. K. Smigel. "Breast Cancer Prevention Trial Show Some Benefit, Some Risk," *J. Natl. Cancer Inst.* 20:647-648, 1998.

38. Editorial, "Breast Cancer Breakthrough." *The New York Times,* April 8, 1998: A22.

39. AP. "British Scientists Criticized U.S. for Ending Trial of Cancer Drug," *The New York Times* April 8, 1998, p. A14.

40. S. S. Epstein and S. Rennie. "A Travesty at Women's Expense," *Los Angeles Times* editorial, June 22, 1992.

41. A. Fugh-Berman and S. S. Epstein. "Tamoxifen for Breast Cancer Prevention: A cautionary review," *Reviews on Endocrine-related Cancer* 43:43-53, 1993.

42. News Roundup, "Tamoxifen's Use for Some Women Being Questioned," *The Wall Street Journal,* July 10, 1998: B7

43. K. I. Pritchard. "Is Tamoxifen Effective in Breast Cancer Prevention?" *The Lancet* 352(9122):80-81, 1998.

44. K. C. Fendi and S. J. Zimniski. *Cancer Res.* 52:235-237, 1992.

45. L. Ford. NCI "Letter to J. W. Stratton," California Environmental Protection Agency, Sacramento, California, June 23, 1995.

46. A. Fugh-Berman and S.S. Epstein. *The Lancet* 340:1143-1145, 1992.

47. A. Fugh-Berman and S. S. Epstein. *Reviews on Endocrine-related Cancer* 43:43-53, 1993.

48. X. Han and J. G. Liehr. *Cancer Res.* 52:1360-1363, 1992.

49. C. J. Jolles, et al. *J. Reprod. Med.* 35:299-300, 1990.

50. B. Kramer, Deputy Director NCI. *The Wall Street Journal,* July 10, 1998, p. 10.

51. S. G. Nayfield. *J. Natl. Cancer Inst.* 83:1450-1459, 1991.

52. NCI Unpublished report and press release, April 6, 1998.

53. T. Powles, et al. *The Lancet* 352:98-101, 1998.

54. K. I. Pritchard. *The Lancet* 352:80-81, 1998.

55. D. V. Spicer, et al. *The Lancet,* 337:1414,

56. J. Topham. Testimony before the FDA Oncologic Drugs Advisory Committee, June 29, 1990.

57. U. Veronesi, et al. *The Lancet* 352:93-97, 1998.

58. A.S. Whittemore. *Am, J. Epidemiol.* 136:1184-1203, 1992.

59. L. K. Altman. "Studies Show Another Drug Can Prevent Breast Cancer," *The New York Times* April 21, 1998, p. A16.

60. R. E. Harris *et al.* "Nonsteroidal Anti-inflammatory Drugs and Breast Cancer," *Epidemiology* 2:203-205, 1996.

61. E. Pennisi. "Building a Better Aspirin: Does aspirin ward off cancer and Alzheimer's?" *Science* 280:1191-1191, 1998.

62. M. Mezzetti *et al.* "Population Attributable Risks for Breast Cancer: Diet, nutrition and physical exercise," *J. Natl. Cancer Inst.* 20:389-394, 1998.

63. R. W. Moss. *Questioning Chemotherapy,* Equinox Press, New York, 1995.

64. M. Walker. *Dirty Medicine,* Slingshot Publications, London, England, 1994.

65. R. Pear. "Report Says Clinical Tests Put Patients' Rights At Risk," *The New York Times* May 30, 1998, p. A8.

66. S. Dickman. "Antibodies Stage a Comeback in Cancer Treatment," *Science* 280:1196-1197, 1998.

67. N. Wade. "Researchers Block Cancer from Developing Defenses," *The New York Times* November 17, 1997, p. A15.

68. N. J. Nelson. "Inhibitors of Angiogenesis Enter Phase III Testing." *J. Natl. Cancer Inst.* 90:960-962, 1998

69. F. Barringer. "Reporters, Book Deals, and Conflicts: As a new cancer therapy emerged, so did a question," *The New York Times* May 8, 1998, p. A15.

70. M. Dowie. "What's Wrong with *The New York Times's* Science Reporting," *The Nation* July 6, 1998, pp. 13-19.

71. "Special Hearings on Alternative Medicine," Subcommittee of the House Committee on Appropriations, June 24, 1993, p. 69.

72. I. W. Lane and L. Comac. *Sharks Don't Get Cancer,* Avery Publishing Group, Garden City Park, New York, 1992.

73. R. Weiss. "Cancer Research Gains Seen in Terms of Treatments, Not Cure," *Washington Post*, May 24, 1998, p. A3.

74. M. Eliott. "Broder to Join Exodus from the NCI," *Science* 267:24, 1995.

75. E. S. Mahoney, Jr. "Dr. Frank Rauscher Jr.: An appreciation," *J. Natl. Cancer Inst.* 85:174-175 1993.

76. J. Bleifuss. "Cancer Politics, In These Times," May 1, 1995.

77. L. Fellers. "Taxol Is One of the Best Cancer Drugs Ever Discovered by the Federal Government: Why Is It Beyond Some Patients' Reach?" *The Washington Post Magazine,* May 31, 1998.

78. J. P. Love. "Comments on the Need for Better Federal Government Oversight of Taxpayer-supported Research and Development," Center for Study of Responsive Law, Washington, D.C. Testimony before the Subcommittee on Business Opportunities, and Technology of the Committee on Small Business, U.S. House of Representatives, July 11, 1994.

79. L. D. Davis and H. P. Freeman. "An Ounce of Prevention," *Scientific American,* September 1994, p. 11.

80. A. Blair and S. H. Zahm. "Cancer Among Farmers," *Occupational Medicine* 6:335-354, 1991.

81. P. Cantor *et al.* "Pesticides and Other Agricultural Risk Factors for Non-Hodgkin's Lymphoma Among Men in Iowa and Minnesota," *Cancer Research* 52:2447-2455, 1992.

82. S. H. Zahm. "Use of Hair Coloring Products and the Risks of Lymphoma, Multiple Myeloma and Chronic Lymphocytic Leukemia," *Am. J. Public Health* 82:990-997, 1992.

CHAPTER EIGHTEEN

How to Win the Losing "War Against Cancer"

1. D. Steinman and S. S. Epstein. *The Safe Shopper's Bible: A Consumer's Guide To Non-toxic Household Products, Cosmetics, and Food,* Macmillan, USA, 1995.

2. D. Steinman and S. S. Epstein. *The Safe Shopper's Bible: A Consumer's Guide To Non-toxic Household Products, Cosmetics and Food,* updated edition, Macmillan, USA, 1998.

3. J. Harte, C. Holden, R. Schneider, and C. Shirley. *Toxic A to Z: A Guide to Everyday Pollution Hazards,* University of California Press, Berkeley, California, 1991.

4. M. K. Levenstein. *Everyday Cancer Risks and How to Avoid Them,* Avery Publishing Group Inc., Garden City Park, New York, 1992.

5. J. Hollender. *How to Make the World A Better Place,* W. W. Norton, New York, London, 1995.

6. T. J. Moore. *Prescription for Disaster,* Simon & Schuster, 1998.

7. J.H. Cushman, "Bill Would Give Water Consumers Pollution Notice," *The New York Times,* 6/23/98.

8. Environmental Health Letter. "EDF Creates Easy-to-Use Web site with Information on Local Toxics," May 1998.

9. Prevent Cancer Web site. "WWW.Prevent Cancer.Com," Health World on Line.

10. Cancer Prevention Coalition Web site. "WWW.Healthy.Net/CPC," Health World on Line.

11. Toxics Use Reduction Institute. *The Massachusetts Toxic Use Reduction Program,* University of Massachusetts, Lowell, 1997.

12. M. Becker and K. Geiser. "Evaluating Progress: A report on the findings of the Massachusetts Toxic Use Reduction Program Evaluation," Toxic Use Reduction Institute, University of Massachusetts, Lowell, March 1997.

13. "Government Performance and Results Act: Technical Amendments of 1998."

14. Institute of Medicine, National Academy of Sciences, "Scientific Opportunities and Public Needs," National Academy Press, Washington, D.C., July, 1998.

15. P. J. Greenberg. "More Science, Less Spice," *Washington Post,* July 15, 1998: A17.

16. S. S. Epstein, D. Steinman, and S. LeVert. *The Breast Cancer Prevention Program,* updated edition, Macmillan, USA, 1998.

Abbreviations

Agencies

ABPI	Association of the British Pharmaceutical Industry
ACGIH	American Conference of Government Industrial Hygienists
ACP	Advisory Committee on Pesticides (Great Britain)
ACR	American College of Radiology
ACS	American Cancer Society
ACS	American Chemical Society
ACTS	Advisory Committee on Toxic Substances (Great Britain)
AFL-CIO	American Federation of Labor-Congress of Industrial Organizations
AI	Alkali and Clean Air Inspectorate (Great Britain)
AIHC	American Industrial Health Council
AIM	Accuracy in Media
AMA	American Medical Association
API	American Petroleum Institute
ASTMS	Association of Scientific, Technical and Managerial Staffs (Great Britain)
BNFL	British Nuclear Fuels
CAST	Council for Agricultural Science and Technology
CCOP	Community Clinical Oncology Program
CCR	Committee on Cancer Research (Great Britain)
CDC	Center for Disease Control
CEQ	Council on Environmental Quality
CIA	Chemical Industries Association (Great Britain)
CODEX	Codex Alimentarius Commission
CORE	Cumbrians Opposed to a Radioactive Environment
COSH	Committees on Occupational Safety and Health
COWPS	Council on Wage and Price Stability
CPC	Cancer Prevention Coalition
CPI	Center for Public Integrity
CPRP	Cancer Prevention Research Program
CPSC	Consumer Product Safety Commission
CRC	Cancer Research Campaign
CRM	Committee on the Review of Medicines (Great Britain)
CSM	Committee on the Safety of Medicines (Great Britain)
CU	Consumers Union
DCE	Division of Cancer Etiology
DCPC	Division of Cancer Prevention and Control
DES	Department of Education and Science (Great Britain)
DHHS	Department of Health and Human Services
DHSS	Department of Health and Social Security (Great Britain)
DOE	Department of the Environment (Great Britain)
DOI	Department of Industry (Great Britain)
DOT	Department of Trade (Great Britain)
EPA	Environmental Protection Agency
ERDA	Engery Research and Development Administration
FACC	Food Additives and Contaminants Committee (Great Britain)
FAO	Food and Agriculture Organization
FCC	Federal Communications Commission

FDA	Food and Drug Administration
FSIS	Food Safety and Inspection Service
FTC	Federal Trade Commission
GAO	General Accounting Office
GMAG	Genetic Manipulation Advisory Group
GMWU	General and Municipal Workers' Union (Great Britain; became General Municipal, Boilermakers' and Allied Trades' Union)
HEW	Health, Education and Welfare
HRG	Health Research Group
HSC	Health and Safety Commission (Great Britain)
HSE	Health and Safety Executive (Great Britain)
IARC	International Agency for Research on Cancer
ICRF	Imperial Cancer Research Fund (Great Britain)
ICWUC	International Chemical Workers Union Council
IOCU	International Organization of Consumers Union
MAFF	Ministry of Agriculture Fisheries and Food (Great Britain)
MRC	Medical Research Council
MSHA	Mine Safety and Health Administration
NCAB	National Cancer Advisory Board
NCAP	National Cancer Advisory Panel
NCI	National Cancer Institute
NCTR	National Center for Toxicological Research
NEDO	National Economic Development Organization
NGA	National Graphical Association (Great Britain)
NIEHS	National Institute of Environmental Health Sciences
NIGMS	National Institute of General Medical Sciences
NIH	National Institutes of Health
NIOSH	National Institute for Occupational Safety and Health
NRPB	National Radiological Protection Board (Great Britain)
NUAAW	National Union of Agricultural and Allied Workers (Great Britain; became Transport and General Workers' Union, Agricultural and Allied Workers' National Trade Group)
OAM	Office of Alternative Medicine
OCAW	Oil, Chemical and Atomic Workers' Union
OSHA	Occupational Safety and Health Administration (in Department of Labor)
OTA	Office of Technology Assessment
PAC	People Against Chlordane
PBOI	Public Board of Inquiry
PCP	President's Cancer Panel
PHS	Public Health Service
QAMA	Quebec Asbestos Mining Association
RCEP	Royal Commission on Environmental Pollution (Great Britain)
SPAID	Society for the Prevention of Asbestosis and Industrial Diseases
TUC	Trades Union Congress (Great Britain)
UKAEA	United Kingdom Atomic Energy Authority
USDA	United States Department of Agriculture
WHO	World Health Organization
WTO	World Trade Organization

Chemicals

A/D	Aldrin/dieldrin
AF2	Furylfuramide
AN	Acrylonitrile
BCME	Bischloromethylether
BHA	Butylated hydroxyanisole
BHC	Benzene hexachloride
BHT	Butylated hydroxytoluene
BNDP	2-nitro-1,3-propanediol
C/H	Chlordane/heptachlor

CMME	Chloromethylmethylether			acetic acid
COX-2	Cyclooxygenase-2		2,4,5-T	2,4,5-Trichlorophenoxyacetic
DBCP	Dibromochloropropane			acid
DCPA	Dacthal		TEA	Triethanolamine
DDT	Dichlorodiphenyl-		TDI	Toluene diisocyanate
	trichloroethane		THMs	Trihalomethanes
DEA	Diethanolamine		VC	Vinyl chloride

CMME Chloromethylmethylether
COX-2 Cyclooxygenase-2
DBCP Dibromochloropropane
DCPA Dacthal
DDT Dichlorodiphenyl-
trichloroethane
DEA Diethanolamine
DEHA Di-2-ethylhexyl adipate
DEHP Di-2-ethylhexyl phthalate
DES Diethylstilbestrol
DMBA 7,12-dimethylbenzanthracene
DMN Dimethylnitrosamine
DNA Deoxyribonucleic acid
DP Depo-Provera
EDB Ethylene dibromide
EGF Epidermal growth factor
ETU Ethylenethiourea
FGF Fibroblastic growth factor
GH Growth Hormone
HAs Heterocyclic amines
HCB Hexachlorobenzene
HGH Human Growth Hormone
IGF-1 Insulin-like Growth Factor-1
MGA Melengesterol acetate
MOCA 4,4'-Methylene bis(2-chloro-aniline)

NDEA N-nitrosodiethanolamine
NMOR Nitrosomorpholine
NNN Nitrosonornicotine
NO$_x$ nitrogen oxides
NTA Nitrilotriacetic acid
OP organophosphate
OPP Orthophenylphenol
OTS Ortho-toluenesulfonamide
PABA Padimate-O
PAHs Polycyclic aromatic hydrocar-bons
PCBs Polychlorinated biphenyls
PET Polyethylene terephthalate
pGH Porcine growth hormone
PVC Polyvinyl chloride
rBGH Recombinant Bovine Growth Hormone
TCDD 2,3,7,8-Tetrachlordibenzo-p-dioxin
2,4-D Sodium 2,4-Dichlorophenoxy-

acetic acid
2,4,5-T 2,4,5-Trichlorophenoxyacetic acid
TEA Triethanolamine
TDI Toluene diisocyanate
THMs Trihalomethanes
VC Vinyl chloride

Units

g Gram (1/1000 kilogram)
kg Kilogram (2.2 pounds)
LOEL Lowest Observed Effective Level
µg Microgram (1/1000 milligram)
mg Milligram (1/1000 gram)
MRL Maximum Residue Levels
ppb Parts per billion (1 ppb = one ten-millionth of one percent)
ppm Parts per million (1 ppm = one ten-thousandth of one percent)
ppt Parts per trillion (1 ppt = one thousandth of a ppb)

Other

ADI Acceptable Daily Intakes
AIDS Acquired Immunodeficiency Syndrome
AIM Accuracy in Media
BASIS British Agrochemicals Supply Industry Scheme
BCDDP Breast Cancer Detection and Demonstration Program
BCPT Breast Cancer Prevention Trial
CAM Complementary Alternative Medicine
CAT Computerized Axial Tomography
CBS Columbia Broadcasting System
CCSP Cancer Control Science Program
CLI Consumer Labeling Initiative
CPCP Chemical and Physical Carcino-genesis Program
CPSA Consumer Product Safety Act
DNA Deoxyribonucleic acid
EDCOP Early Detection and Community Oncology Program

EDF	Environmental Defense Fund	NDA	New Drug Application
EEC	European Economic Community	NHL	Non-Hodgkin's Lymphoma
EHDs	Environmental Health Departments (Great Britain)	NSAIDS	Nonsteroidal Anti-inflammatory Drugs
EU	European Union	NTP	National Toxicology Program (USA)
FD&C	Food, Drug, and Cosmetic		
FEPCA	Federal Environmental Pesticide Control Act	OCEDPF	Ovarian Cancer Early Detection and Prevention Foundation
FIFRA	Federal Insecticide, Fungicide, and Rodenticide Act	PBS	Public Broadcasting Service
		PDR	Physicians' Desk Reference
GNP	Gross National Product	POMES	Practice Outcomes Monitoring and Evaluation Systems
GRAS	Generally Recognized as Safe		
HERP	Human Exposure Dose/Rodent Potency Dose	PSPS	Pesticides Safety Precautions Scheme
HRT	Hormone Replacement Therapy	PTA	Parent-Teacher Association
ICI	Imperial Chemical Industries (Great Britain)	QCRA	Quantitative Cancer Risk Assessment
JAMA	Journal of the American Medical Association	RPAR	Rebuttable Presumption Against Registration
MCS	Multiple Chemical Sensitivities	SEER	Surveillance, Epidemiology, and End Results
MRI	Magnetic Resonance Imaging		
MRL	Maximum Residue Levels	SERMs	Selective Estrogen Receptor Modulators
MSKCC	Memorial Sloan-Kettering Comprehensive Cancer Center	SMR	Standard Mortality Ratio
		TLV	Threshold Limit Value
MTD	Maximally Tolerated Doses	TOSCA	Toxic Substances Control Act (USA)
NADA	New Animal Drug Application		
NBCAM	National Breast Cancer Awareness Month	VAT	Validation Assistance Team

Index

Books

1. *The Mutagenicity of Pesticides,* S. S. Epstein and M. Legator, eds. Cambridge, Mass., and London, 1971: M.I.T. Press.
2. *Drugs of Abuse: Genetic and Other Chronic Non-Psychiatric Hazards,* S. S. Epstein, ed. Cambridge, Mass., and London, 1971: M.I.T. Press.
3. *The Legislation of Product Safety: Consumer Health and Product Hazards,* Vol. I: Chemicals, Electronic Products, Radiation. S. S. Epstein and D. Grundy, eds. Cambridge, Mass., and London, 1974: M.I.T. Press.
4. *The Legislation of Product Safety: Consumer Health and Product Hazards,* Vol. II: Cosmetics and Drugs, Pesticides, Food Additives. S. S. Epstein and D. Grundy, eds. Cambridge, Mass., and London, 1976: M.I.T. Press.
5. *The Politics of Cancer,* S. S. Epstein. San Francisco, 1978: Sierra Club Books; Revised and expanded edition, New York, 1979: Anchor/Doubleday Press.
6. *Hazardous Wastes in America,* S. S. Epstein, C. Pope, and L. Brown. San Francisco, 1982: Sierra Club Books.
7. *Cancer in Britain: The Politics of Prevention,* L. Doyal and S. S. Epstein. London, 1983: Pluto Press.
8. *The Safe Shopper's Bible,* D. Steinman and S. S. Epstein. New York, September, 1995: MacMillan Publishing Company.
9. *The Breast Cancer Prevention Program,* S. S. Epstein, D. Steinman, and S. LeVert. New York, 1997: MacMillan Publishing Company. 2nd edition, 1998.
10. *THE POLITICS OF CANCER Revisited,* S. S. Epstein. Fremont Center, New York, 1998: East Ridge Press.

Scientific Publications

1. Epstein, S. S., and Winston, P. Intubation granuloma. J. Laryngol. Otol., *71:*17-38, 1957.
2. Epstein, S. S., et al. The vocal cord polyp. J. Laryngol. Otol., *71:*673-688, 1957.
3. Epstein, S. S. and Shaw, H. J. Metastatic cancer of the larynx as a cause of carotid-sinus syndrome. Cancer, *10:*933-937, 1957.
4. Epstein, S. S. An intra-oral inoculation technique for the production of experimental pneumonia in mice. J. Hygiene, *56:*73-79, 1958.
5. Epstein, S. S. and Stratton, K. Further studies on the mouse intra-oral inoculation technique. J. Hygiene, *56:*81-83, 1958.
6. Epstein, S. S. and Shaw, H. J. Multiple malignant neoplasms in the air and upper food passages. Cancer, *11:*326-333, 1958.
7. Winston, P. and Epstein, S. S. Papilloma of the larynx: A clinico-pathological study. J. Laryngol. Otol., *72:*452-464, 1958.
8. Epstein, S. S. and Friedmann, I. *Klebsiella* serotypes in infections of the ear and upper respiratory tract. J. Clin. Path., *2:*359-362, 1958.
9. Epstein, S. S. A "stripping" technique for the examination of the total epithelial surface of the larynx. J. Path. Bact., *75:*472-473, 1958.
10. Freeman, T., Wakefield, G. S., and Epstein, S. S. Platelet-agglutinating factor in glandular fever complicated

by jaundice and thrombocytopenia. Lancet, 383-385, Oct. 25, 1958.

11. Epstein, S. S. and Bradbeer, T. L. A case of primary diptheritic otitis media. J. Laryngol. Otol., *72:*1001-1003, 1958.

12. Epstein, S. S. Experimental *Klebsiella* pneumonia in mice with particular reference to periarterial changes. J. Path. Bact., *78:*389-396, 1959.

13. Epstein, S. S. The biochemistry and antibiotic sensitivity of the *Klebsiellae.* J. Clin. Path., *12:*52-58, 1959.

14. Epstein, S. S. and Payne, P. M. The effect of some variables on experimental *Klebsiella* infections in mice. J. Hygiene, *57:*68-80, 1959.

15. Shaw, H. J. and Epstein, S. S. Cancer of the epiglottis. Cancer, *12:*246-256, 1959.

16. Epstein, S. S. and Weiss, J. B. The extraction of pigments from *Euglena gracilis.* Biochem. J., *75:*247-250, 1959.

17. Timmis, G. M. and Epstein, S. S. New antimetabolites of Vitamin B12. Nature, *184:*1383-1384, 1959.

18. Epstein, S. S., et al. Multiple primary malignant neoplasms in the air and upper food passages. Cancer, *13:*461-463, 1960.

19. Epstein, S. S. and Weiss, J. B. Measuring the size of isolated cells. Nature, *187:*461-463, 1960.

20. Epstein, S. S. Effects of some benzimidazoles on a Vitamin B12-requiring alga. Nature, *188:*143-144, 1960.

21. Epstein, S. S., et al. Vitamin B12 and growth of *Euglena gracilis.* Fed. Proc., *20*(1):450, 1961.

22. Epstein, S. S. and Timmis, G. M. "Simple" Vitamin B12 antimetabolites. Proc. Amer. Assoc. Cancer Res., *3*(3):223, 1961.

23. Epstein, S. S. and Burroughs, M.

Some factors influencing the photodynamic response of *Paramecium caudatum* to 3,4-benzpyrene. Nature, *193:*337-338, 1962.

24. Epstein, S. S., et al. The photodynamic toxicity of polycyclic hydrocarbons. Proc. Amer. Assoc. Cancer Res., *3*(4):316, 1962.

25. Epstein, S. S., et al. Influence of Vitamin B12 on the size and growth of *Euglena gracilis.* J. Protozool., *9:*336-339, 1962.

26. Epstein, S. S. and Timmis, G. M. Effect of Vitamin B12 antagonists and other compounds on the C1300 tumor. Biochem. Pharmacol., *11:*743-746, 1962.

27. Epstein, S. S. and Timmis, G. M. Simple antimetabolites of Vitamin B12. J. Protozool., *10:*63-73, 1963.

28. Epstein, S. S., et al. The photodynamic effect of the carcinogen 3,4-benzpyrene on *Paramecium caudatum.* Cancer Res., *23:*35-44, 1963.

29. Epstein, S. S., et al. Photodynamic bioassay of benzo(a)pyrene using *Paramecium caudatum.* J. Nat. Cancer Inst., *31:*163-168, 1963.

30. Epstein, S. S., et al. A photodynamic bioassay of atmospheric pollutants. Proc. Amer. Assoc. Cancer Res., *4*(1):18, 1963.

31. Epstein, S. S. Photodynamic activity of polycyclic hydrocarbon carcinogens. Acta Unio Internat. Contra Cancrum, *19:*3/4, 599-601, 1963.

32. Epstein, S. S., et al. Photodynamic bioassay of polycyclic air pollutants. A.M.A. Arch. Env. Health, *7:*531-537, 1963.

33. Small, M., Jones, H., and Epstein, S. S. Photodynamic activity of polycyclic compounds. Fed. Proc., *22:*316, 1963.

34. Epstein, S. S., et al. On the association between photodynamic and carcino-

genic activities in polycyclic compounds. Cancer Res., *24:*855-862, 1964.

35. Foley, G. E. and Epstein, S. S. Cell culture and cancer chemotherapy. In "Advances in Chemotherapy," *1:*1964, Academic Press, New York.

36. Epstein, S. S., et al. Charge-transfer complex formation, carcinogenicity and photodynamic activity in polycyclic compounds. Nature, *204:*750-754, 1964.

37. Epstein, S. S., et al. Charge-transfer complex formation, carcinogenicity and photodynamic activity in polycyclic compounds. Fed. Proc., *232:*287, 1964.

38. Epstein, S. S. Photoactivation of polynuclear hydrocarbons. A.M.A. Arch. Env. Health, *10:*233-239, 1965.

39. Epstein, S. S., et al. Photodynamic bioassay of polycyclic atmospheric pollutants. J. Air Poll. Control Assoc., *15:*174-176, 1965.

40. Epstein, S. S. A simple photodynamic assay for polycyclic atmospheric pollutants. World Health Organization Report, WHO/EBL/51, 1965.

41. Epstein, S. S., et al. A simple bioassay for antioxidants based on protection of *Tetrahymena pyriformis* from the photodynamic toxicity of benzo(a)-pyrene. Nature, *208:*655-658, 1965.

42. Small, M., Brickman, E., and Epstein, S. S. Uptake of polycyclic compounds by phagotropic protozoan. Fed. Proc., *24:*684, 1965.

43. Epstein, S. S., et al. A simple bioassay for antioxidants. Fed. Proc., *24:*623, 1965.

44. Epstein, S. S. Bioassay for polycyclic atmospheric pollutants and for antioxidants based on photodynamic response of protozoa. Abstract from Second International Conference on Protozoology, London. Reprinted from Excerpta Medica International Congress, Series 91, August, 1965.

45. Epstein, S. S. The lung as a transplant site for malignant tumors in rodents. Cancer, *19:*454-457, 1966.

46. Epstein, S. S. and Joshi, S. R. Obstructive renal failure in random-bred Swiss mice. Fed. Proc., *25:*237, 1966.

47. Epstein, S. S., et al. Interactions between antioxidant and photosensitizer in the photodynamic bioassay for antioxidants. Life Sciences, *5:*783-793, 1966.

48. Epstein, S. S., et al. An exploratory investigation on the inhibition of selected photosensitizers by agents of varying antioxidant activity. Rad. Res., *28:*322-335, 1966.

49. Epstein, S. S. and Tabor, F. B. Photosensitizing compounds in extracts of USA drinking water. Science, *154*(3746):261-263, 1966.

50. Epstein, S. S. Two sensitive tests for carcinogens in the air. J. Air Poll. Control Assoc., *16*(10):545-546, 1966.

51. Epstein, S. S., et al. Carcinogenicity of organic particulate pollutants in urban air after administration of trace quantities to neonatal mice. Nature, *212:*1305-1307, 1966.

52. Small, A., Mantel, N., and Epstein, S. S. The role of cell-uptake of polycyclic compounds in photodynamic injury of *Tetrahymena pyriformis.* Exp. Cell Res., *45:*206-217, 1967.

53. Epstein, S. S., et al. The null effect of antioxidants on the carcinogenicity of 3,4,9,10-dibenzpyrene to mice. Life Sci., *6:*225-233, 1967.

54. Epstein, S. S. and Niskanen, E. E. Effects of Tween 60 on benzo(a)-pyrene uptake by *Tetrahymena pyriformis.* Exp. Cell Res., *46:*211-234, 1967.

55. Epstein, S. S., et al. The synergistic toxicity and carcinogenicity of Freons and piperonyl butoxide. Nature, *214:*526-528, 1967.

56. Epstein, S. S., et al. Cytotoxicity of antioxidants to *Tetrahymena pyriformis.* J. Protozool., *14:*238-244, 1967.

57. Nagata, C., Fujii, K., and Epstein, S. S. Photodynamic activity of 4-nitroquin-oline-1-oxide and related compounds. Nature, *215:*972-973, 1967.

58. Epstein, S. S., et al. Hepatocarcin-ogenicity of griseofulvin following parenteral administration to infant mice. Cancer Res., *27:*1900-1906, 1967.

59. Epstein, S. S., et al. Carcinogenicity of the herbicide maleic hydrazide. Nature, *215:*1388-1390, 1967.

60. Epstein, S. S. Carcinogenicity of organic extracts of atmospheric pollutants. J. Air Poll. Control Assoc., *17:*728-729, 1967.

61. Epstein, S. S., et al. Enhancement by piperonyl butoxide of acute toxicity due to Freons, benzo(a)pyrene, and griseofulvin in infant mice. Toxicol. Appl. Pharmacol., *11:*442-448, 1967.

62. McCarthy, R. E. and Epstein, S. S. Cytochemical and cytogenetic effects of maleic hydrazide on cultured mammalian cells. Life Sci., *7:*1-6, 1968.

63. Epstein, S. S., et al. Photodynamic assay of neutral sub-fractions of organic extracts of particulate atmospheric pollutants. Env. Sci. Tech., *2:*132-141, 1968.

64. Epstein, S. S. and Mantel, N. Hepatocarcinogenicity of maleic hydrazide following parenteral administration to infant Swiss mice. Internat. J. Cancer, *3:*325-335, 1968.

65. Rondia, D. and Epstein, S. S. The effect of antioxidants on photodecom-position of benzo(a)pyrene. Life Sci., *7:*513-518, 1968.

66. Epstein, S. S. Carcinogenicity of tetraethyl lead. Experientia, *24:*580, 1968.

67. Epstein, S. S. and Shafner, H. Use of mammals in a practical screening test for chemical mutagens in the human environment. Nature, *219:*385-387, 1968.

68. Jaffe, J., Fujii, K., Sengupta, M., Guerin, H., and Epstein, S. S. *In vivo* inhibition of mouse liver microsomal hydroxylating systems by methylene-dioxyphenyl insecticidal synergists and related compounds. Life Sci., *7:*1051-1062, 1963.

69. Epstein, S. S. Irradiated Foods. Science, *161:*739, 1968.

70. Fujii, K., Jaffe, H., and Epstein, S. S. Factors influencing the hexobarbital sleeping time and zoxazolamine paralysis time in mice. Toxicol. Appl. Pharmacol., *13:*431-438, 1968.

71. Epstein, S. S. and Saporoschetz, I. B. On the association between lysogeny and carcinogenicity in nitroquinolines. Experientia, *24:*1245-58, 1968.

72. Jaffe, H., Fujii, K., Sengupta, M., Guerin, H., and Epstein, S. S. The bi-modal effect of piperonyl butoxide on o- and p-hydorxylation of biphenyl by mouse liver microsomes. Biochem. Pharmacol., *18:*1045-1051, 1969.

73. Pagnatto, L. D. and Epstein, S. S. The effects of antioxidants on ozone toxicity in mice. Experientia, *25:*703-704, 1969.

74. Epstein, S. S. A *catch-all* toxicologi-cal screen. Experientia, *25:*617-618, 1969.

75. Epstein, S. S. and St. Pierre, J. S. Mutagenicity in yeast of nitro-quinolines and related compounds. Toxicol. Appl. Pharmacol., *15:*451-460, 1969.

76. Epstein, S. S. Introduction to symposia on toxicologic and epidemiologic bases for air quality criteria. J. Air Pollution Control Assoc., *19:*629-630, 1969.

77. Epstein, S. S. Chemical hazards in the human environment. Ca-A Cancer Journal for Clinicians, *19:*277-281, 1969.

78. Epstein, S. S. Biological approaches to estimation of environment hazards. Drug Information Bulletin, *3:*150-152, 1969.

79. Epstein, S. S., et al. Cyclamate ban. Science, *166:*1575, 1969.

80. Lijinsky, W. and Epstein, S. S. Nitrosamines as environmental carcinogens. Nature, *225:*21-23, 1970.

81. Epstein, S. S., et al. Carcinogenicity testing of food additives and antioxidants by parenteral administration to infant Swiss mice. Toxicol. Appl. Pharmacol., *16:*321-334, 1970.

82. Fujii, K., Jaffe, H., Bishop, Y., Arnold, E., Mackintosh, D., and Epstein, S. S. Structure-activity relations for methylenedioxyphenyl and related compounds and hepatic microsomal enzyme functions, as measured by prolongation of hexobarbital narcosis and zoxazolamine paralysis in mice. Toxicol. Appl. Pharmacol., *16:*482-494, 1970.

83. Epstein, S. S., et al. Abnormal zygote development in mice after paternal exposure to a chemical mutagen. Nature, *225:*1260-1261, 1970.

84. Epstein, S. S. and Lederberg, J. Chronic non-psychiatric hazards of drugs of abuse. Science, *168:*507-509, 1970.

85. Epstein, S. S., et al. The mutagenicity of trimethyl phosphate in mice. Science, *168:*584-586, 1970.

86. Mailing, H. V., Wassom, J. S. and Epstein, S. S. Mercury in our environment. Environmental Mutagen Society Newsletter, *3:*7-9, 1970.

87. Epstein, S. S., et al. Mutagenic and antifertility effects of TEPA and METEPA in mice. Toxicol. Appl. Pharmacol., *17:*23-40, 1970.

88. Epstein, S. S., et al. The failure of caffeine to induce mutagenic effects or to synergize the effects of known mutagens in mice. Fd. Cosmet. Toxicol., *8:*381-401, 1970.

89. Epstein, S. S. A family likeness: 2,4,5-T and 2,4-D. Environment, *12:*16-25, 1970.

90. Epstein, S. S. Mutagenitatsprufung in der Toxikologie. Unschau, *15:*475-476, 1970.

91. Epstein, S. S., et al. Effects of methylenedioxyphenyl insecticidal synergists *in vitro* on hydroxylations of biphenyl by mouse liver microsomes. Biochem. Pharmacol., *19:*2605-2607, 1970.

92. Joshi, S. R., Page, E. C., Arnold, E., Bishop, Y., and Epstein, S. S. Fertilization and early embryonic development subsequent to mating with TEPA-treated male mice. Genetics, *65:*483-494, 1970.

93. Epstein, S. S. and Fujii, K. Synergism in carcinogenesis with particular reference to synergistic effects of piperonyl butoxide and related insecticidal synergists. Chapter, pp. 21-42. In, Chemical Tumor Problems. Nakahara, W., ed. Pub. Japanese Society for the Promotion of Science, Tokyo, Japan, 1970.

94. Epstein, S. S. I. Adverse biological effects due to chemical pollutants: General Principles. II. Potential carcinogenicity, mutagenicity and teratogenicity due to community air pollutants. Appendix M. pp. 1-54. Project Clean Air. Task Force Assessments. Vol. 2. Project Clean Air,

Regents of the Univ. of California, Sept. 1, 1970.

95. Epstein, S. S. The failure of caffeine to induce mutagenic effects or to synergize the effects of known mutagens in mice. Chapter 25, pp. 404-419. In, Chemical Mutagens, ed. Vogel, F., and Rohrborn, G., Publ. Springer-Verlag, Berlin, Heidelberg, New York, 1970.

96. Friedman, M. and Epstein, S. S. Stability of piperonyl butoxide. Toxicol. Appl. Pharmacol., *17:*810-812, 1970.

97. Epstein, S. S. NTA. Environment, *12:*2-11, 1970.

98. Epstein, S. S. Control of chemical pollutants. Nature, *228:*816-819, 1970.

99. Bateman, A. and Epstein, S. S. Dominant lethal mutations in mammals. Chapter in, Environmental Chemical Mutagens. Hollaender, A., ed., Plenum Publishing Co., New York, 1971.

100. Alam, B. S., Saporoschetz, I. B., and Epstein, S. S. Formation of N-nitrosopiperidine and sodium nitrite in the stomach and the isolated intestinal loop of the rat. Nature, *232:*116-118, 1971.

101. Epstein, S. S., et al. Sterility and semi-sterility in male progeny of male mice treated with the chemical mutagen TEPA. Toxicol. Appl. Pharmacol., *19:*134-146, 1971.

102. Epstein, S. S., et al. Bioassay for antioxidants based on protection of isolated rat liver mitochondria against the photodynamic toxicity of benzo(a)pyrene. Fd. Cosmet. Toxicol., *9:*367-377, 1971.

103. Epstein, S. S., et al. On the association between photodynamic and enzyme-inducing activities in polycyclic compounds. Cancer Res., *13:*1087-1094, 1971.

104. Alam, B. S., Saporoschetz, I. B., and Epstein, S. S. The synthesis of nitrosopiperidine from nitrate and piperidine in the stomach and small intestine and in isolated gastric contents of the rat. Nature, *232:*199-200, 1971.

105. Epstein, S. S. and Rohrborn, G. Recommended procedures for testing genetic hazards due to chemicals, based on the induction of dominant lethal mutations in mammals. Nature, *230:*459-460, 1971.

106. Epstein, S. S., et al. Eye on our Defenses. Environment, *13:*43-47, 1971.

107. Friedman, M. A., Millar, G., McEvoy, A., and Epstein, S. S. Rapid and simplified method for liquid scintillation counting of radioactive proteins utilizing aquasol. Anal. Chem., *43:*780, 1971.

108. Bishop, Y., Fujii, K., Arnold, E., and Epstein, S. S. Censored distribution technique in analysis of toxicological data. Experientia, *27:*1056-1059, 1971.

109. Asahina, S., Friedman, M., Arnold, E., Millar, G., Mishkin, M., and Epstein, S. S. Acute synergistic toxicity and hepatic necrosis following oral administration of sodium nitrite and secondary amines to mice. Cancer Res., *31:*1201-1205, 1971.

110. Friedman, M. A., Sengupta, M., Arnold, E., Bishop, Y., and Epstein, S. S. Additive and synergistic inhibition of mammalian microsomal enzyme functions by piperonyl butoxide, safrole and other methylenedioxyphenyl derivatives. Experientia, *27:*1052-1054, 1971.

111. Adler, I. D., Ramarao, G., and Epstein, S. S. *In vivo* cytogenetic effects of trimethylphosphate and of TEPA

on bone marrow cells of male rats. Mutation Res., *13:*263-273, 1971.

112. Epstein, S. S. Environmental pathology: A review. Am. J. Path., *66:*352-374, 1972.

113. Friedman, M. A., Sengupta, M., and Epstein, S. S. Paradoxical effects of piperonyl butoxide on the kinetics of mouse liver microsomal enzyme activity. Toxicol. Appl. Pharmacol., *21:*419-427, 1972.

114. Epstein, S. S. Information requirements for determining the benefit-risk spectrum. In, Perspectives on Benefit-risk Decision Making, pp. 50-62. Committee on Public Engineering Policy, National Academy of Engineering, Washington, D. C., 1972.

115. Epstein, S. S. Identification of hazards in the environment: Introductory remarks. In, Environment and Cancer, pp. 56-68. Williams and Wilkins Pub. Co., Baltimore, 1972.

116. Friedman, M. A., Millar, G., Sengupta, M., and Epstein, S. S. Inhibition of mouse liver protein and nuclear RNA synthesis following combined oral treatment with sodium nitrite and dimethylamine or methylamine or methylbenzylamine. Experientia, *28:*2-22, 1972.

117. Epstein, S. S. Toxicological and environmental implications on the use of nitrilotriacetic acid as a detergent builder – I. Int. J. Environ. Studies, *2:*291-300, 1972.

118. Toxicological and environmental implications on the use of nitrilotriacetic as a detergent builder – II. Int. J. Environ. Studies, *3:*13-21, 1972.

119. Friedman, M. A., Green, E. J., and Epstein, S. S. Rapid gastric absorption of sodium nitrite in mice. J. Pharm. Sci., *61:*1492-1494, 1972.

120. Epstein, S. S., et al. Detection of chemical mutagens by the dominant lethal assay in the mouse. Toxicol. Appl. Pharmacol., *23:*288-325, 1972.

121. Asahina, S., Andrea, J., Carmel, A., Arnold, E., Bishop, Y., Joshi, S., Coffin, D., and Epstein, S. S. Carcinogenicity of organic fractions of particulate atmospheric pollutants in New York City following parenteral administration to infant mice. Cancer research, *32:*2263-2268, 1972.

122. Epstein, S. S. Teratological hazards due to Phenoxy Herbicides and Dioxin Contaminants. Chap. 12, pp. 708-729. In, Pollution: Engineering and Scientific Solutions. Barrekette, E. S., ed., Pub. Plenum Publ. Co., New York, 1972.

123. Epstein, S. S. *In vivo* studies on interactions between secondary amines and nitrites or nitrates, pp. 109-115. In, N-Nitroso Compounds. Analysis and Formation. International Agency for Research on Cancer, Lyon, France. Scientific Publication No. 3, 1972.

124. Friedman, M. A., Millar, G. N., and Epstein, S. S. Acute dose-dependent inhibition of liver nuclear RNA synthesis and methylation of guanine following oral administration of sodium nitrite and dimethylamine to mice. Int. J. Environ. Studies, *4:*219-222, 1973.

125. Lavappa, K. S., Fu, M. M., Sing, M., Beyer, R. D., and Epstein, S. S. Banding patterns of chromosomes in bone marrow cells of the Chinese hamster as revealed by acetic-saline-Giemsa, urea and trypsin techniques. Lab. Animal Sci., *23:*546-550, 1973.

126. Lavappa, K. S., Yerganian, G., and Epstein, S. S. Autosomal heteromorphism in the Armenian hamster. Genetics, *74:*S151, 1973.

127. Epstein, S. S. The Delaney Amend-

ment. Ecologist, *3:*420-431, 1973.

128. Epstein, S. S. The Delaney Amendment. Preventive Med., *2:*140-149, 1973.

129. Epstein, S. S. Environment and Teratogenesis. Chapter 8, pp. 105-113. In, Pathobiology of Development. Perrin, E. V. and Finegold, M. J., eds., Pub. Williams and Wilkins Co., Baltimore, 1973.

130. Joshi, S. R., Bishop, Y., and Epstein, S. S. Reduced fertility in mice following treatment with Niridazole. Experientia, *29:*1253-1255, 1973.

131. Epstein, S. S. Use of the dominant lethal test to detect genetic activity of environmental chemicals. Environ. Health Perspec., *6:*23-26, 1973.

132. Fine, D. H., Rufeh, F., Lieb, D., and Epstein, S. S. A possible nitrogen oxide-nitrosamine cancer link. Bull. Environ. Contam. Toxicol., *11:*18-19, 1974.

133. Epstein, S. S. Definition of risk: Priority for safety, pp. 241-248. In, Environmental Quality and Food Supply. White, P. L., ed., Futura Publ. Co., Inc., 1974.

134. Epstein, S. S. Chronic biological hazards due to chemicals. In, Birth Defects and Fetal Development. Chapter 9, pp. 136-166. Moghissi, H., ed., C. C. Thomas Publ., Springfield, IL, 1974.

135. Alarif, A. and Epstein, S. S. Chemical synthesis of methyl C14 and H3 labeled N-methylnitrosourethane. J. Labeled Comp., *10:*161-164, 1974.

136. Epstein, S. S. Introductory Remarks to Sessions on "Mutagens in the Biosphere." First International Conference on Environmental Mutagens. Asilomar, Calif., 1973. Mutation Res., *26:*219-223, 1974.

137. Epstein, S. S. The carcinogenicity of Dieldrin. Testimonies at Hearings on Aldrin/Dieldrin, Environmental Protection Agency and Environmental Defense Fund *vs.* Shell. Cancellation Hearings, March, 1974: Suspension Hearings, Sept., 1974.

138. Epstein, S. S. Environmental determinants of human cancer. Cancer Res., *34:*2425-2435, 1974.

139. Epstein, S. S. Multiple factors in carcinogenesis. Environ. Health Perspec., *9:*319-324, 1974.

140. Amacher, D. D., Alarif, A., and Epstein, S. S. The effects of ingested chrysotile on DNA synthesis in the gastrointestinal tract and liver of the rat. Environ. Health Perspec., *9:*319-324, 1974.

141. Alarif, A. and Epstein, S. S. The uptake and metabolism of 14C-labeled nitrosomethyl urethane and methyinitrosourea in guinea pigs and their *in vitro* metabolism in the guinea pig and human pancreas. International Agency for Research of Cancer. Lyon, France, 215-219, 1974.

142. Billmaier, D., Yee, T., Allen, N., Craft, R., Williams, N., Fontaine, R., and Epstein, S. S. Peripheral neuropathy in a coated fabrics plant. J. Occupational Medicine, *16:*655-671, 1974.

143. Epstein, S. S. and Hattis, D. Regulatory aspects of occupational carcinogens. Proceedings XI International Cancer Congress. Florence, October 20-26, 1974. In, Vol. 3, Cancer Epidemiology, Environmental Factors, 1974.

144. Epstein, S. S. Carcinogens in industry: needed studies. In, the New Multinational Health Hazards, pp. 172-188, Proceedings of the ICF International Occupational Health Conference, Geneva, October 20-30, 1974.

145. Legator, M. S. and Epstein, S. S. Testing for chemically-induced

mutations. Chapter 9, Environmental Problems on Medicine, Ed., McKee, W. Published by C. C. Thomas, Springfield, IL, 1974.

146. Epstein, S. S. and Hattis, D. Adverse health effects and chemical pollutants of the environment. Chapter 8. In Environment: Resources, Pollution and Society, 2nd edition. Ed., Murdoch, W. N., Publisher, Sinauer Associates, 1975.

147. Epstein, S. S. Impact of mobile emissions control. The public interest overview. Conference on Health Consequences of Environmental Controls. Environmental Health Perspectives, *10:*173-179, 1975.

148. Hasumi, K., Iqbal, Z. M., Alarif, A., and Epstein, S. S. DNA repair synthesis following exposure of guinea pig pancreatic slices to methyl-N-nitrosourethane *in vitro.* Experientia, *31:*467, 1975.

149. Epstein, S. S. The carcinogenicity of Dieldrin. I. The Science of the Total Environment, *4:*1-52, 1975.

150. Epstein, S. S. The carcinogenicity of Dieldrin. II. The Science of the Total Environment, *4:*205-217, 1975.

151. Fine, D. H., Rounbehler, D. P., Huffman, F., and Epstein, S. S. Analysis of volatile N-nitroso compounds in drinking water at the part per trillion level. Bull. Environ. Contam. Toxicol., *14:*404-408, 1975.

152. Hasumi, K., Wilber, J. H., Berkowitz, J., Wilber, R. G., and Epstein, S. S. Pre- and post-natal toxicity induced in guinea pigs by N-nitrosomethyl urea. Teratology, *12:*105-110, 1975.

153. Fine, D. H., Rounbehler, D. P., Belcher, N. M., and Epstein, S. S. N-Nitroso Compounds in the Environment. International Conference on Environmental Sensing and Assessment. Las Vegas, September 14-19, 1975.

154. Amacher, D. E., Alarif, A., and Epstein, S. S. The dose-dependent effect of ingested chrysotile on DNA synthesis in the gastrointestinal tract, liver and pancreas of the rat. Environ. Res., *10:*208-216, 1975.

155. Lavappa, K. S., Fu, M. M., and Epstein, S. S. Cytogenetic studies on chrysotile asbestos. Environ. Res., *10:*165-173, 1975.

156. Page, T., Harris, R. H., and Epstein, S. S. Drinking water and cancer mortality in Louisiana. Science, *193:*55-57, 1976.

157. Hasumi, K., Iqbal, Z. M., and Epstein, S. S. DNA repair synthesis in guinea pig slices following *in vitro* exposure to nitrosomethylurethane. Chem.-Biol. Interactions, *13:*279-286, 1976.

158. Epstein, S. S. and Varnes, M. The short-term effects of ingested chrysotile asbestos on DNA synthesis in the pancreas and other organs of a primate. Experientia, *32:*602-604, 1976.

159. Fine, D. H., Rounbehler, D. P., Belcher, N. M., and Epstein, S. S. N-nitroso compounds: Detection in ambient air. Science, *192:*1328-1330, 1976.

160. Epstein, S. S. Potential Carcinogenic Hazards Due to Contaminated Drinking Water. Proceedings of the International Conference on Biological Control of Water Pollution, pp. 73-84, Eds., Tourbier, J. and Pierson, R. W., University of Pennsylvania Press, 1976.

161. Iqbal, Z. M., Majdan, M., and Epstein, S. S. Evidence of repair of DNA damage induced by 4-hydroxyaminoquinoline-1-oxide in guinea pig pancreatic slices *in vitro.* Cancer Res., *36:*1108-1113, 1976.

162. Epstein, S. S. Aldrin and dieldrin: Suspension based on environmental

evidence and evaluation of societal needs. Conference on Occupational Carcinogenesis, March 24, 1976. New York Academy of Sciences, *271:*187-195, 1976.

163. Epstein, S. S. The political and economic basis of cancer. Technology Review, *79:*34-43, 1976.

164. Iqbal, Z. M. and Epstein, S. S. Effects of N-methyl-N-nitrosourethane on DNA synthesis in the guinea pig pancreas. Chem. Biol. Interactions, *15:*131-137, 1976.

165. Epstein, S. S. The carcinogenicity of heptachlor and chlordane. The Science of the Total Environment, *6:*103-104, 1976.

166. Iqbal, Z. M. and Epstein, S. S. Kinetics of DNA repair synthesis in guinea pig pancreatic slices following *in vitro* exposure to N-methyl-N-nitrosourethane. Experientia, *32:*1055-1056, 1976.

167. Iqbal, Z. M. and Epstein, S. S. DNA repair synthesis in guinea pig pancreas following exposure to nitrosomethylurethane. International Agency for Cancer Research, WHO, Publication No. 141, pp. 411-424, Lyon, France, 1976.

168. Epstein, S. S. et al. Pre-natal and post-natal toxicity induced in guinea pigs by nitrosomethylurea. International Agency for Cancer Research, WHO, Publication No. 14, pp. 435-442, Lyon, France, 1976.

169. Fine, D. H., Rounbehler, D. P., Belcher, N. M., and Epstein, S. S. N-nitroso compounds in air and water. International Agency for Cancer Research, WHO, Publication No. 14, pp. 401-408, Lyon, France, 1976.

170. Epstein, S. S. Developing Health Policies and Standards; Responsibility of the scientist in developing and interpreting "Public Interest" view-points. LASL Third Life Sciences Symposium, Los Alamos, New Mexico, October 15-17, 1975, pp. 42-50. In "Impact of Energy Production in Human Health," eds. E. C. Anderson and E. M. Sullivan, Energy Res. and Development Adm., 1976.

171. Gage, K. and Epstein, S. S. The federal advisory committee system. Environmental Law Reporter, *7:*50001-50002, 1977.

172. Epstein, S. S. Cancer and the environment. Bull. Atomic Scientists, *33*(3):22-30, 1977.

173. Iqbal, Z. M., Varnes, M. E., Yoshida, A., and Epstein, S. S. Metabolism of benzo(a)pyrene by guinea pig pancreatic microsomes. Cancer Res., *37:*1011-1015, 1977.

174. Fine, D. H., Rounbehler, D. P., Ross, R., Song, L., Silvergleid, A., Iqbal, Z. M., and Epstein, S. S. Quantitation of dimethylnitrosamine in the whole mouse following biosynthesis from trace levels of precursors. Science, *197:*917-918, 1977.

175. Epstein, S. S. The case for a Consumer Protection Agency. Bull. Atomic Scientist, *33*(7):6-7, 1977.

176. Epstein, S. S. et al. Protection by antioxidants against the toxicity of ozone to microbial systems. Environmental Res., *14:*187-193, 1977.

177. Yoshida, Q., Iqbal, Z. M., and Epstein, S. S. Hepatocarcinogenic effects of N-methyl-N-nitrosourea in guinea pigs. Cancer Res., *37:*4043-4048, 1977.

178. Epstein, S. S. The carcinogenicity of organochlorine pesticides, pp. 243-265. In "Origins of Human Cancer," eds. H. H. Hiatt, J. D. Watson, and J. A. Winsten, Cold Spring Harbor Laboratory, 1977.

179. Epstein, S. S. Kepone: hazard evaluation. The Science of the Total Envi-

ronment, *9:*1-62, 1978.

180. Iqbal, Z. M. and Epstein, S. S. Evidence of DNA repair in the guinea pig pancreas *in vivo* and *in vitro,* following exposure to N-methyl-N-Nitrosourethane. Chem.-Biol. Interactions, *20:*77-87, 1978.

181. Epstein, S. S. Polluted Data. The Sciences, *18:*16-21, 1978.

182. Infante, P. F., Newton, W. A., and Epstein, S. S. Blood dyscrasias and childhood tumors following exposure to chlorinated hydrocarbon pesticides. Scand. J. Work Environment, *4:*137-150, 1978.

183. Epstein, S. S. Carcinogenicity of a composite organic extract of urban particulate atmospheric pollutants following subcutaneous injection in infant mice. Environmental Res., *19:*163-176, 1979.

184. Fujii, S. and Epstein, S. S. Effects of piperonyl butoxide on the toxicity and hepatocarcinogenicity of 2-acetyl-aminofluorene and 4-acetylamino-biphenyl, and their N-hydroxylated derivatives, following administration to newborn mice. Oncology, *36:*105-112, 1979.

185. Iqbal, Z. M., Yoshida, A., and Epstein, S. S. Uptake and excretion of benzo(a)pyrene and its metabolites by the rat pancreas. Drug Metabolism and Disposition, *7:*44-48, 1979.

186. Yoshida, A., Iqbal, Z. M., and Epstein, S. S. Spontaneous pancreatic islet cell tumors in guinea pigs. J. Comp. Pathol., *89:*471-480, 1979.

187. Epstein, S. S. Cancer and inflation. The Ecologist, *9:*236-246, 1979.

188. Epstein, S. S. Polluted data. The Ecologist, *9:*264-268, 1979.

189. Epstein, S. S. The Polluters hit back. The Ecologist, *9:*269-272, 1979.

190. Epstein, S. S. Information, requirements of the public. American Industrial Health Association Journal, pp. 48-54, December, 1979.

191. Epstein, S. S. Cancer, inflation and the failure to regulate. Technology Review, *82:*42-53, 1979.

192. Epstein, S. S., et al. Geographic Distribution of Cancer in Illinois. Illinois Institute of Natural Resources, Document No. 79/40, December, 1979.

193. Iqbal, Z. M., Dahl, K., and Epstein, S. S. Role of nitrogen dioxide in the biosynthesis of nitrosamines in mice. Science, *207:*1475-1477, 1980.

194. Whalley, C. E., Iqbal, Z. M., and Epstein, S. S. The separation of N-nitroso-di-n-propylamine and its B-oxidized carcinogenic metabolites by high pressure liquid chromatography. J. Liquid Chromat., *3:*693-703, 1980.

195. Epstein, S. S. and Swartz, J. Fallacies of lifestyle cancer theories. Nature, *289:*127-130, 1981.

196. Whalley, C. E., Iqbal, Z. M., and Epstein, S. S. *In vivo* and microsomal metabolism of the pancreatic carcinogen N-Nitrosobis(2-oxopropyl)amine by the Syrian golden hamster. Cancer Res., *41:*482-486, 1981.

197. Iqbal, Z. M. and Epstein, S. S., et al. Kinetics of nitrosamine formation in mice following oral administration of trace-level precursors. International Agency for Research on Cancer (IARC), Proceeding of VIth International Symposium on N-Nitroso Compounds, Budapest, October 16-20, 1979, pp. 195-206, IARC Scientific Publication No. 31, Lyon, France, 1980.

198. Epstein, S. S., et al. *In Vivo* Nitrosation of Morpholine in Mice by Inhaled NO2. International Agency for Research on Cancer (IARC), Proceeding of VIth International

Symposium of N-Nitroso Compounds, Budapest, October 16-20, 1979, pp. 195-206, IARC Scientific Publication No. 31, Lyon, France, 1980.

199. Epstein, S. S. "The Price We Pay for Progress: The Hazards of the Halogenated Hydrocarbons." Proceedings International Conference, "Chemistry-Man-Environment: Halogenated Hydrocarbons," Gottlieb Duttweiler Institute, Zurich, Switzerland, October 13-15, 1980.

200. Epstein, S. S. "The Politics of Cancer: The Costs of Failure to Regulate." Proceedings of the Warner-Lambert Science and Public Policy Colloquium, The University of Michigan, Collegiate Institute for Values and Science, November 1-2, 1980.

201. Epstein, S. S. The role of the scientist in toxic tort case preparation. Trial, *17:*38-78, 1981.

202. Epstein, S. S. Focus on Food Safety: Evaluating Risk Measurements. Proceedings Fourth National Food Policy Conference. Community Nutrition Institute and Food Marketing Institute, pp. 48-57, Washington, D. C., April 7, 1981.

203. Iqbal, Z. M., Dahl, K., and Epstein, S. S. Biosynthesis of dimethylnitrosamine in dimethylamine-treated mice after exposure to nitrogen dioxide. J. Nat. Cancer Inst., *67:*137-141, 1981.

204. Epstein, S. S. Surviving in the petrochemical age: Social and economic pressures needed to improve toxic waste disposal. Journal of Alternative Human Services, *7*(5):18-24, 1981.

205. Epstein, S. S. It costs us all more not to regulate. In These Times, pp. 16-77, August 12-25, 1981.

206. Iqbal, Z. M. and Epstein, S. S. *In vivo* nitrosation of amines by inhaled nitrogen dioxide and inhalation biosynthesis of nitrosamines. International Agency for Research in Cancer (IARC), Scientific Publication, Proceedings of VIIth International Symposium on N-Nitroso Compounds, Tokyo, Japan. September 28 - October 1, 1981.

207. Swartz, J. B. and Epstein, S. S. Problems in assessing risks from occupational and environmental exposure to carcinogens, pp. 559-575. Banbury Report 9: Qualification of Occupational Cancer, Cold Spring Harbor Laboratory, 1981.

208. Epstein, S. S. Cost-benefit analysis: Inspired by rational economics or a protectionist philosophy. The Amicus Journal, *3*(4):41-47, 1982.

209. Epstein, S. S. Public Health Concerns on the Proposed Alaska Petrochemical Complex. Proceedings of the VIIth Alaska Health Conference on Energy, Health and the Environment: The Health Impact of Petrochemical Development, Anchorage, Alaska, May 6-8, 1982.

210. Swartz, J. B., Riddiough, C. R., and Epstein, S. S. Analysis of carcinogenesis dose response data: Implications for carcinogenic risk assessment. Teratogenesis, Carcinogenesis and Mutagenesis, 2(2):179-204, 1982.

211. Epstein, S. S. The ideal solution: Options for hazardous wastes. The Amicus Journal, pp. 6-7, Spring, 1983.

212. Epstein, S. S. Agent Orange diseases: Problems of causality, burdens of proof and restitution. Trial, *19:*91-99, 1983.

213. Epstein, S. S. Hazardous Waste Management. Hazardous Materials and Waste Management Magazine, Kutztown, PA, pp. 17-23, May/June, 1983.

214. Epstein, S. S. and Gofman, J. Irradiation of foods. Science, *223:*1354, 1984.

215. Epstein, S. S. and Swartz, J. B. Cancer and diet: A rebuttal to B. Ames (Science, *221:*1256-1264, 1983) Science, *224:*660-667, 1984. (Endorsed by 16 co-signatories)

216. Dwyer, J. H. and Epstein, S. S. Cancer and Clinical Epidemiology: An Overview. Chapter 6, pp. 123-129. In, Herbicides in War, The Long-Term Ecological and Human Consequences, ed. A. H. Westing, Stockholm International Peace Research Institute, Stockholm, Sweden, 1984.

217. Epstein, S. S. The Toll of Chemical Warfare at Home: The Politics of Cancer, pp. 85-90. In, Issues '84, Dear Mr. President-Elect, eds. Green, M. and Siegal, J., The Democracy Project, New York, September 1984.

218. Epstein, S. S. Billions for cures, barely a cent to prevent. Environmental Action, pp. 10-11, November/December 1984.

219. Epstein, S. S. Environmental Issues in Medicine: A Dissenting View. In, Dissent in Medicine, ed. R. Mendelsohn, Contemporary Books, Chicago, Illinois, 1985.

220. Epstein, S. S. The environmental question: Beyond lifestyle change. Health and Medicine, *3:*19-21, 1985.

221. Epstein, S. S. U.S. Veterans and Agent Orange. International symposium on the Long-term Ecological and Human Consequences of Chemical Warfare in Vietnam. Jan. 14, 1983, published in "Herbicides in War." Ed. A. H. Westing, Stockholm International Peace Research Institute, Taylor & Francis, London/Philadelphia, 1984.

222. Epstein, S. S. Natural products and cancer: A rebuttal to P. Abelson. In, Readers Forum, Remote Sensing of the Planet: Impact of Science on Society, UNESCO, France, September 1985.

223. Epstein, S. S. and Briggs, S. Silent spring in retrospect. Environmental Law Reporter, *17:*10180-10184, 1987.

224. Epstein, S. S. Losing the war against cancer. The Ecologist, *17:*91-101, 1987.

225. Epstein, S. S. Are we losing the war against cancer? Congressional Record, *133:*E3449-E3454, 1987.

226. Epstein, S. S. and Ozonoff, D. Leukaemias and blood dyscrasias following exposure to chlordane and heptachlor. Carcinogenesis, Mutagenesis and Teratogenesis, *7:*527-540, 1987.

227. Epstein, S. S. The politics of cancer. Multinational Monitor, *9*(3):6-13, 1988.

228. Epstein, S. S. and Swartz, J. B. Carcinogenic risk estimation. Rebuttal to B. Ames (Science, *236:*271, 1987) Science, *240:*1043-1047, 1988. (Endorsed by 15 co-signatories)

229. Epstein, S. S. Carcinogenic Pesticides in Food and the Delaney Amendment. National Coalition Against Misuse of Pesticides, Annual Meeting. Washington, D. C., Keynote Address, March 18, 1989.

230. Epstein, S. S. The Externalized Public Health and Environmental Costs of Gasoline. National Conference on Octane and Oxygenated Fuels, San Francisco, March 22, 1989.

231. Epstein, S. S. Corporate crime: Can we trust industry-derived safety studies? The Ecologist, *19:*23-30, 1989.

232. Epstein, S. S. The real cost of petrol. The Ecologist, *19:*137-138, 1989.

233. Epstein, S. S. The chemical jungle: Today's beef industry. Multinational Monitor, *10*(5):8-9, 1989.

234. Epstein, S. S. Potential health hazards of biosynthetic milk hormones. Report

to the Food and Drug Administration, July 19, 1989.

235. Epstein, S. S. BST: The public health hazards. The Ecologist, *19:*191-195, 1989.

236. Epstein, S. S. Losing the war against cancer: Who's to blame and what to do about it. International Journal of Health Services, *20:*53-71, 1990.

237. Epstein, S. S. Potential public health hazards of biosynthetic milk hormones. International Journal of Health Services, *20:*73-84, 1990.

238. Epstein, S. S. The chemical jungle: Today's beef industry. International Journal of Health Services, *20*(2):277-280, 1990.

239. Epstein, S. S. Editorial misconduct in *Science.* International Journal of Health Services, *20*(2):349-352, 1990.

240. Epstein, S. S. Corporate crime: Why we cannot trust industry-derived safety studies. International Journal of Health Services, *20*(3):443-458, 1990.

241. Lashner, B. and Epstein, S. S. Industrial risk factors for colorectal cancer. International Journal of Health Services, *20*(3):459-483, 1990.

242. Clapp, R. W., Commoner, B., Constable, J. D., Epstein, S. S., et al. Human Health Effects Associated with Exposure to Herbicides and/or Their Associated Contaminants, Chlorinated Dioxins. Report to the American Legion and Vietnam Veterans of American, April 1990.

243. Epstein, S. S. Questions and answers on synthetic bovine growth hormones. International Journal of Health Services, *20*(4):573-582, 1990.

244. Lashner, B. and Epstein, S. S. Industrially related colorectal cancer: Eminently preventable. Chicago Medicine, *93*(18):30-31, 1990.

245. Epstein, S. S. Summary public health perspectives on rBGH. National Institutes of Health, Technology Assessment Conference on Bovine Somatotropin. National Institutes of Health, December 5-7, 1990.

246. Epstein, S. S., et al. Losing the war against cancer: A need for public policy reforms. Int. J. Health Services, *22*(3):455-469, 1992.

247. Epstein, S. S. The cancer war and its critics. Int. J. Health Services, *22*(4):747-749, 1992.

248. Epstein, S. S. Profiting from cancer. The Ecologist, *22:*233-240, 1992.

249. Fugh-Berman, A. and Epstein, S. S. Tamoxifen: Disease prevention or disease substitution? The Lancet, *340:*1143-1145, 1992.

250. Fugh-Berman, A. and Epstein, S. S. Should healthy women take tamoxifen? New Eng. J. Med., *327:*1596, 1992.

251. Epstein, S. S. Evaluation of the national cancer program and proposed reforms. Int. J. Health Services, *23*(1):15-44, 1993.

252. Epstein, S. S. Evaluation of the national cancer program and proposed reforms. American J. Ind. Med., *24:*109-133, 1993.

253. Fugh-Berman, A. and Epstein, S. S. Tamoxifen for breast cancer prevention. A cautionary review. Reviews on Endocrine-Related Cancer, *43:*1-11, 1993.

254. Epstein, S. S. Breast Cancer and The Environment. The Ecologist, *23*(5):192-193, 1993.

255. Epstein, S. S. Environmental pollutants as unrecognized causes of breast cancer. Int. J. Health Services, *24*(1):145-150, 1994.

256. Swartz, J. B. and Epstein, S. S. What is responsible for the rise in lung cancer mortality? New Solutions pp. 62-70, Spring 1995.

257. Epstein, S. S. Response to criticisms

of the September 1994, Los Angeles Times Guest Commentary on cancer risk of breast implants. Medical-Legal aspects of breast implants, Medical Monitor, Leader Publications, *3*(2):7-8, 1995.

258. Epstein, S. S. Implants pose poorly recognized risks of breast cancer. Int. J. Occup. Med. Toxicol., *4*(3):315-342, 1995.

259. Epstein, S. S. Unlabeled milk from cows treated with biosynthetic growth hormones: A case of regulatory abdication. Int. J. Health Services, *26*(1):173-185, 1996.

260. Epstein, S. S. Avoidable toxins in condos: how to go green. Condo Lifestyles, *1*(3):6-10, 1997.

261. Black, D. L., Fugate, M. E., and Epstein, S. S. Poly(ester) urethane foam covered Breast Implants: biodegradation and release of toluene diamines. Clinical Chemistry, In press, 1998.